Handbook of Infant
Mental Health
Second Edition

Handbook of Infant Mental Health

Second Edition

Edited by

Charles H. Zeanah, Jr.

The Guilford Press
NEW YORK   LONDON

KH

© 2000 The Guilford Press
A Division of Guilford Publications, Inc.
72 Spring Street, New York, NY 10012
www.guilford.com

Paperback edition 2005

Printed in the United States of America

This book is printed on acid-free paper.

Last digit is print number: 9 8 7 6

Library of Congress Cataloging-in-Publication Data

Handbook of infant mental health / Charles H. Zeanah, Jr., editor.—2nd ed.
    p. ; cm.
    Includes bibliographical references and indexes.
    ISBN 1-57230-515-0 (hardcover : alk. paper)   ISBN 1-59385-171-5 (pbk.)
    1. Infant psychiatry—Handbooks, manuals, etc.   2. Infants—Mental health—Handbooks, manuals, etc.   I. Zeanah, Charles H.
    [DNLM: 1. Mental Health—Infant.   2. Developmental Disabilities.   3. Mental Disorders—Infant. WS 350.6 H2375 2000]
    RJ502.5.H36 2000
    618.92'89—dc21

                                        99-051343

3/17/08

*With love and appreciation to my father, Charles H. Zeanah,
and my mother, Sarah Martin Zeanah*

About the Editor

❖

Charles H. Zeanah, Jr., MD, is Professor of Psychiatry and Pediatrics, Vice-Chairman of Psychiatry, and Director of Child and Adolescent Psychiatry at the Tulane University School of Medicine. He also directs an intensive intervention program for maltreated infants and toddlers in the New Orleans area. During the past two decades, his clinical and research interests have concerned development and psychopathology in the early years. A member of the MacArthur/McDonnell Research Network on Early Experience and Brain Development, he has been on the editorial board of the *Infant Mental Health Journal* since 1988 and for the past eight years has edited *The Signal,* a newsletter of the World Association for Infant Mental Health.

Contributors

❖

J. Lawrence Aber, PhD, National Center for Children in Poverty, Columbia University, New York, New York

Thomas Anders, MD, Department of Psychiatry, University of California, Davis, Davis, California

Marianne L. Barton, PhD, Department of Psychology, University of Connecticut, Storrs, Connecticut

Leila Beckwith, PhD, Department of Pediatrics, University of California, Los Angeles, Los Angeles, California

Anne Leland Benham, MD, Department of Psychiatry and Behavioral Science, Stanford University School of Medicine, Palo Alto, California

Diane Benoit, MD, Department of Psychiatry, Hospital for Sick Children, and University of Toronto, Toronto, Ontario, Canada

Karyn Kaufman Blane, PsyD, E. P. Bradley Hospital, Brown University School of Medicine, East Providence, Rhode Island

Neil W. Boris, MD, Department of Community Health Sciences, Tulane University School of Public Health and Tropical Medicine, and Department of Psychiatry, Tulane University School of Medicine, New Orleans, Louisiana

Michelle Bosquet, PhD, Institute of Child Development, University of Minnesota, Minneapolis, Minnesota

C. F. Zachariah Boukydis, PhD, Department of Psychiatry and Human Behavior, Brown University School of Medicine, Infant Development Center, Women and Infants' Hospital, Providence, Rhode Island

Susan J. Bradley, MD, Child Psychiatry Program, Child and Adolescent Gender Identity Clinic, Centre for Addiction and Mental Health, Clarke Division, University of Toronto School of Medicine, Toronto, Ontario, Canada

Celia A. Brownell, PhD, Department of Psychology, University of Pittsburgh, Pittsburgh, Pennsylvania

Susan B. Campbell, PhD, Department of Psychology, University of Pittsburgh, Pittsburgh, Pennsylvania

Doreen A. Cavanaugh, PhD, Heller Graduate School, Brandeis University, Waltham, Massachusetts

Jennifer Cohen, MA, Department of Psychology, Clinical Psychology Doctoral Program, City University of New York, New York, New York

Lisa J. Cohen, PhD, Department of Psychiatry, Beth Israel Medical Center, New York, New York

Susan Crockenberg, PhD, Department of Psychology, University of Vermont, Burlington, Vermont

Susan Dickstein, PhD, Division of Child and Adolescent Psychiatry, E. P. Bradley Hospital, Department of Psychiatry and Human Behavior, Brown University School of Medicine, East Providence, Rhode Island

Tiffany Field, PhD, Touch Research Institutes, Nova Southeastern University, Fort Lauderdale, Florida, and University of Miami School of Medicine, Miami, Florida

Barbara H. Fiese, PhD, Department of Psychology, Syracuse University, Syracuse, New York

Theodore J. Gaensbauer, MD, Department of Psychiatry, University of Colorado Health Sciences Center, Denver, Colorado

Linda Gilkerson, PhD, Erikson Institute, Chicago, Illinois

Walter S. Gilliam, PhD, Yale Child Study Center, Yale University School of Medicine, New Haven, Connecticut

Miles Gilliom, MS, Department of Psychology, University of Pittsburgh, Pittsburgh, Pennsylvania

Joyce Giovannelli, MS, Department of Psychology, University of Pittsburgh, Pittsburgh, Pennsylvania

Beth Goodlin-Jones, PhD, Department of Psychiatry, University of California, Davis, Davis, California

Sydney L. Hans, PhD, Department of Psychiatry, University of Chicago, Chicago, Illinois

Sherryl Scott Heller, PhD, Department of Psychiatry and Neurology, Tulane University School of Medicine, New Orleans, Louisiana

Christopher Henrich, MA, Department of Psychology, Yale University, New Haven, Connecticut

Anne Hungerford, MS, Department of Psychology, University of Pittsburgh, Pittsburgh, Pennsylvania

Stephanie Jones, BA, Department of Psychology, Yale University, New Haven, Connecticut

Michael D. Kaplan, MD, Yale Child Study Center, Yale University School of Medicine, New Haven, Connecticut

Joan Kaufman, PhD, Department of Psychiatry, Yale University, New Haven, Connecticut

Ami Klin, PhD, Yale Child Study Center, Yale University School of Medicine, New Haven, Connecticut

Kathleen Koenig, MSN, Yale Child Study Center, Yale University School of Medicine, New Haven, Connecticut

Julie A. Larrieu, PhD, Department of Psychiatry and Neurology, Tulane University School of Medicine, New Orleans, Louisiana

Esther Leerkes, MA, Department of Psychology, University of Vermont, Burlington, Vermont

Barry M. Lester, PhD, Department of Psychiatry and Human Behavior, Department of Pediatrics, Brown University School of Medicine, Infant Development Center, Women and Infants' Hospital, Providence, Rhode Island

Marva L. Lewis, PhD, School of Social Work, Tulane University, New Orleans, Louisiana

Alicia F. Lieberman, PhD, Child Trauma Research Program, University of California, San Francisco, San Francisco, California

John A. Lippitt, MMHS, MS, Heller Graduate School, Brandeis University, Waltham, Massachusetts

Joan L. Luby, MD, Department of Psychiatry (Child), Washington University School of Medicine, St. Louis, Missouri

Linda C. Mayes, MD, Yale Child Study Center, Yale University School of Medicine, New Haven, Connecticut

Susan C. McDonough, PhD, MSW, School of Social Work and Center for Human Growth and Development, University of Michigan, Ann Arbor, Michigan

Klaus Minde, MD, Department of Psychiatry, McGill University, Montreal Children's Hospital, Montreal, Quebec, Canada

David A. Mrazek, MD, Department of Psychiatry and Behavioral Sciences, The George Washington University Medical Center, Washington, DC

Charles A. Nelson, PhD, Institute of Child Development and Department of Pediatrics, University of Minnesota, Minneapolis, Minnesota

Jeree H. Pawl, PhD, Infant–Parent Program, University of California, San Francisco, San Francisco, California

Barry M. Prizant, PhD, Childhood Communication Services, Cranston, Rhode Island, and Center for the Study of Human Development, Brown University, Providence, Rhode Island

Kyle D. Pruett, MD, Yale Child Study Center, Yale University School of Medicine, New Haven, Connecticut

Joanne E. Roberts, PhD, Frank Porter Graham Child Development Center, University of North Carolina, Chapel Hill, Chapel Hill, North Carolina

Diana Robins, MA, Department of Psychology, University of Connecticut, Storrs, Connecticut

Emily Rubin, MA, Yale Child Study Center, Yale University School of Medicine, New Haven, Connecticut

Avi Sadeh, PhD, Department of Psychology, Tel Aviv University, Tel Aviv, Israel

Arnold J. Sameroff, PhD, Center for Human Growth and Development, University of Michigan, Ann Arbor, Michigan

Michael S. Scheeringa, MD, Department of Psychiatry and Neurology, Tulane University School of Medicine, New Orleans, Louisiana

Ronald Seifer, PhD, Division of Child and Adolescent Psychiatry, E. P. Bradley Hospital, Department of Psychiatry and Human Behavior, Brown University School of Medicine, East Providence, Rhode Island

Stephen Seligman, DMH, Infant–Parent Program, San Francisco General Hospital, Department of Psychiatry, University of California, San Francisco, San Francisco, California

Daniel S. Shaw, PhD, Department of Psychology, University of Pittsburgh, Pittsburgh, Pennsylvania

Jack P. Shonkoff, MD, Heller Graduate School, Brandeis University, Waltham, Massachusetts

Robin Silverman, PhD, Child Trauma Research Program, University of California, San Francisco, San Francisco, California

Arietta Slade, PhD, Department of Psychology, City University of New York, New York, New York

Frances Stott, PhD, Erikson Institute, Chicago, Illinois

Jean E. Twomey, PhD, Infant Development Center, Women and Infants' Hospital, Providence, Rhode Island, and E. P. Bradley Hospital, East Providence, Rhode Island

Jean Valliere, MSW, BCSW, Department of Psychiatry, Louisiana State University School of Medicine, New Orleans, Louisiana

Fred R. Volkmar, MD, Yale Child Study Center, Yale University School of Medicine, New Haven, Connecticut

Lauren S. Wakschlag, PhD, Department of Psychiatry, University of Chicago, Chicago, Illinois

Anne S. Walters, PhD, E. P. Bradley Hospital, Brown University School of Medicine, East Providence, Rhode Island

Amy M. Wetherby, PhD, Department of Communication Disorders, Florida State University, Tallahassee, Florida

Charles H. Zeanah, Jr., MD, Department of Psychiatry and Neurology, Tulane University School of Medicine, New Orleans, Louisiana

Paula Doyle Zeanah, PhD, Department of Psychiatry and Neurology, Tulane University School of Medicine, New Orleans, Louisiana

Kenneth J. Zucker, PhD, Child Psychiatry Program, Child and Adolescent Gender Identity Clinic, Centre for Addiction and Mental Health, Clarke Division, University of Toronto School of Medicine, Toronto, Ontario, Canada

Preface

❖

The response to the first edition of the *Handbook of Infant Mental Health* was, for me, overwhelming. Then, I expressed optimism that the field was coming of age. Now, only seven years later, it seems clear that the infant mental health field is well established. The idea that mental health is a legitimate area of concern for the youngest members of our society is accepted with less surprise and irony than ever before.

Part of the evidence of the emergence of the infant mental health field is the increasing number of questions about its identity. I have heard many discussions among senior-level luminaries in the field about whether or not "infant mental health" is a term that is appropriate for what we do, how we think, and what we are about. It is not surprising that a field that has been multidisciplinary from its beginnings would struggle with these issues, and some of the tension inherent in our blending of professional cultures is apparent in this volume.

Whatever term we decide to apply to this field of study, we must still insist that every infant has a right to mental health. I am always impressed by how much we tend to idealize babies, but I fear that, at times, this leads us to minimize or dismiss real and serious problems that young children may have because it is too uncomfortable for us to acknowledge them. And yet, there are important differences between the problems of infants and toddlers and the problems of older children. This dilemma illustrates the first major theme of this book—that infants are both like and unlike older children and adolescents. Thus, one purpose of this volume is to examine these similarities and differences and their implications.

A cartoon one of my former fellows drew for me a few years ago illustrates two other major themes of this book. The drawing depicts a psychiatrist (who bears a distinct resemblance to Freud) sitting in a comfortably furnished and well-credentialed office and listening intently to a patient. The patient on the couch is a baby. I had the drawing made into a slide that I use occasionally to begin a talk, saying something like, "Here is the answer to the question 'What does an infant psychiatrist do?'"

The drawing is clearly preposterous, mainly because of the developmental inappropriateness of a preverbal, cognitively limited infant lying on a therapist's couch where older patients verbally describe symptoms, feelings, memories, and fantasies. This represents a second major theme of this book—namely, that infants must be understood within a developmental context. Infants *are* developmentally limited, but they also are changing rapidly, constantly reinventing themselves with new capacities. Any consideration of infant mental health must incorporate a dynamic developmental perspective.

Another reason the drawing is preposterous is that the infant is alone with an intervener, without the presence of a primary caregiver. Implicitly, this introduces the third major theme of this volume—that the caregiving context of infancy is essential. There can be no assessment, no treatment, no predictions about development without a central focus on the infant as embedded within a variety of dynamically interacting contexts. This second edition emphasizes the infant's endogenous characteristics transacting continually with the primary caregiving relationship as the most "experience-near" contexts of infant development, recognizing that these contexts develop within myriad other contexts.

As in the first edition, this second edition has been a team effort. The most obvious team members are the contributors. It is a great pleasure to be able to include chapters from such a distinguished group; I am a great supporter of their work, and I appreciate their efforts.

Other vital team members are the staff at The Guilford Press. Seymour Weingarten, Editor-in-Chief, deserves tremendous credit for sensing the need for the first edition. He has my thanks for that and for supporting the idea of this second edition. Kitty Moore and Carolyn Graham have been consistently helpful and supportive over the years and especially about this new edition, and Anna Nelson skillfully oversaw the production of this volume with both care and alacrity.

Closer to home, Sherry Juul worked tirelessly and cheerfully for many hours on this edition, editing, organizing, communicating, etc., etc. In my office, she was the "go-to guy" for this book, and I could not have done it without her help. Nona Whitman had the thankless job of reminding me repeatedly that there was a bit more to my job than just completing this book. I appreciate her keeping the roller coaster mostly on the track. The entire Infant Team at Tulane University has been consistently supportive and incredibly patient with me over the years. I appreciate their help, insights, and innumerable contributions to my education about infant mental health.

Paula Doyle Zeanah, who indirectly contributed a tremendous amount to the first edition of this book, has contributed even more to this edition, including writing a chapter. I am forever indebted to her for her efforts to edit not only my writing but the rest of my life as well. I know she joins me in thanking our favorite teachers of development: Emily, Katy, and Mel. It is ever exhilarating, fascinating, and humbling to be their parents. We appreciate their support more than they know.

CHARLES H. ZEANAH, JR.

Contents

❖

Handbook of Infant
Mental Health
Second Edition

I

CONTEXT OF INFANT MENTAL HEALTH

❖

Anyone involved with the mental health of infants must be concerned fundamentally with the context in which they are developing. As the chapters in this section illustrate, contexts exist at multiple levels, ranging from the molecular and cellular to the cultural and societal. These levels do not merely coexist, they interact in complex ways. Because infants are developing at a pace that is unprecedented in the human lifespan, the interaction of multiple contexts continues over time, spurred on by infants' newly emerging capacities.

Because of the crucial importance of the primary caregiving relationship for infant mental health, a relational view dominates contemporary thinking about risk, psychopathology, assessment, and intervention. Still, the primary caregiving relationship itself exists within and depends on other multiple contexts.

Contexts provide the framework within which an infant develops. Models of development describe the process by which development proceeds, including the influences of genetic and biological dispositions and environmental influences. These models of development are not mere academic constructs. They are directly related to social policy and deployment of resources. This was brought home to me powerfully during a visit I made recently to institutions for "irrecuperable" children in another part of the world. Children in these institutions were housed in unspeakably horrific conditions because they were believed to be beyond hope of recovery. Many of the children I saw had treatable medical problems (e.g., congenital anomalies, Tourette's disorder, or hemophilia) that seemed to have led to their diagnosis as "irrecuperable." Nevertheless, once diagnosed and placed in these institutions, their development had become a grimly self-fulfilling prophecy. Remarkable recoveries in at least some of the children adopted out of these institutions indicates how a different model of development may have enormous implications for vast numbers of unfortunate children.

For the last 25 years, Sameroff's transactional model has dominated thinking about the process of development. In Chapter 1, he and Fiese use principles of systems theory to describe individual–environment transactions over time. In considering multiple contexts of infant development and their transactions over time, they emphasize that the individuals' states and potentialities constrain their experience of the shaping forces of development. Much of the rest of this volume examines in detail various components of the model they outline in the first chapter.

In Chapter 2, Cohen and Slade review the psychological experience of pregnancy, which represents the genesis of the infant–parent relationship. Importantly, they document that this relationship begins to form even before there is a baby. Focusing on the pregnant woman's internal self-reorganization and transformation, these authors are careful to include in their description the external and internal contextual forces that contribute to the woman's experience of pregnancy and of the developing baby.

Nelson and Bosquet, in Chapter 3, focus on the intrinsic aspect of prenatal development in their discussion of the context of neurobiology. In their careful, selective review, they provide an overview of what we know and do not know about brain development in the early years. In the current atmosphere of hyperbole about how experiences shape and sculpt the brain, they point to how little is actually understood about human central nervous system development. They emphasize the enormous need to close the gap between the approaches of neuroscience to understanding brain functioning and the pressing questions we would like to answer about the importance of early experiences.

In Chapter 4, Crockenberg and Leerkes describe infant social and emotional development as they unfold in the context of the primary caregiving relationship with mother and with father. In this chapter, they focus on the most clinically salient aspects of infant development and emphasize the inseparability of infants and their caregiving contexts. They conclude that although we have learned a great deal about the importance of dyadic interaction on the developing infant, we have a long way to go before we can approach the complexities inherent in triadic and even more complex family relationships.

In the final chapter (Chapter 5), Lewis describes the overarching context of culture and considers its implications for infant development. She draws our attention to important parallels between the study of culture and infant mental health, especially the transdisciplinary nature of each. She describes culture as the developmental niche of the infant–caregiver relationship and illustrates its importance in defining norms by which we evaluate behavior. She reminds us that risk is itself a cultural construction, and that any consideration of infant mental health must address the crucial contexts of race, ethnicity, culture, and minority status.

1

Models of Development and Developmental Risk

❖

ARNOLD J. SAMEROFF
BARBARA H. FIESE

A handbook of infant mental health must begin with both a positive and a negative definition. It must lay out what we can expect to gain from an understanding of infant social and emotional development and what we cannot. At one extreme are those who believe that a child's future is determined by early behavior. As a consequence, making sure that the infant has positive mental health is important for everything that follows. At the other extreme are those who believe that infancy is a passing period that will have little relation to what follows (Lewis, 1997; Kagan, 1998). According to this view, the foundation of later mental health is found in later stages of development, with each period's good and bad experiences determining concurrent mental health. In the first view, infancy is the most crucial period of development, and according to the second, it is only of transient interest. A third view takes elements from both perspectives and sees each developmental stage as laying a foundation for the next. If the foundation is one of competence, the following stage will proceed more easily than if the foundation is problematic, but the outcome of each following stage will be a product not of what the child brings to the situation alone or what is experienced alone but of the interplay between these two domains (Sameroff & Chandler, 1975). To be sure, proponents of all views support the notion that infants should be happy, but they differ as to whether this happiness has consequences for later mental health.

When we examine the circumstances that produce early mental health, we are immediately mired in the nature–nurture debate, in which the literature is filled with advocates for characteristics of either the infant or the caregivers as primary determinants. From the academic perspective there is no debate, for most scientists recognize the inextricability of one from the other (Ford & Lerner, 1992; Sameroff, 1995). Moreover, there is a dynamic transactional relation between nature and nurture in which both are constantly being changed by their experience with each other. However, on the clinical side, frequently there is a need to separate nature from nurture. Although some interventions with infants are directed at the interaction between parent and child (e.g., McDonough, 1995 and Chapter 31, this volume), many others are aimed at either changing the child or changing aspects of the caregiving environment. As one moves toward more distal influences, such as neighborhood characteristics or socioeconomic status, interventions deal with aspects of the environment on a level at which the child is not a participant. In this vein, a transactional model of intervention is reviewed where interventions can be targeted at different aspects of the developmental system: the infant alone, the parent alone, or their interaction (Sameroff & Fiese,

1999). However, the main focus here is on the social environment as the primary source of positive or negative development, leaving to others to describe the infant characteristics that place the child at risk.

INFANT RESOURCES

The birth of an infant is a physical separation that appears to produce an independent individual who will mature into a psychological adult. This material independence from other family members gives rise to the idea that there is a psychological independence so that whatever levels of achievement and health the child attains can be attributed to internal resources. Dramatic advances in molecular biology, which permit the identification of individual genes, have fostered a view that these genes play deterministic roles in the growth process. Such a perception leads to a maturational view of development in which there is an unfolding of intrinsic characteristics. From this perspective, individual differences in intelligence or personality or more categorical differences, such as retardation or mental disorder, can be explained by differences in initial circumstances, the genetic endowment of the individual. However, equally dramatic biological advances have demonstrated the intimate interplay between genes and context.

Biologists concerned with early development were divided into geneticists and embryologists (Waddington, 1962). The early geneticists focused on searching for single genes that produced specific structural outcomes, with little attention to developmental processes, whereas embryologists studied the interplay of cells and tissues as they interacted to produce the organs of the body, with little attention to gene contributions. After the Piagetian revolution, most developmental psychologists affiliated more with embryological models, which fit the organic cognitive processes they were studying. Developmental models, preferred by behavioral geneticists, tended to be linear, with the path from genes to behavior conceived as an unfolding process, much like photographic development where there is nothing in the resulting picture that was not contained in the negative. In this view, the study of infant behavior is merely to document the expression of what was in the hereditary material.

As the complexity of early biological processes is uncovered, this early dichotomy in biology is being replaced with a new synthesis in molecular biology in which genes and dynamic developmental processes are being integrated. Plomin and Rutter (1998) described the implications of complex multifactorial genetic processes for understanding behavior. These include the ideas that (1) most developmental risks arise from normal gene variants, not mutations; (2) genetic effects are indirect, producing risk factors rather than disorder; (3) genes affect dimensions of behavior that are not pathological in themselves; (4) for complex processes many genes act in combination; and, most important for our discussion, (5) genetic effects on behavior are probabilistic. These effects are manifest only if other conditions are also met. Contemporary genetic research fits squarely in the developmental camp because of concerns with the emergence over time of complex behaviors that have multiple causal influences.

Progress within neuroscience has also shown the necessity of studying complex systems in embryology if the goal is to understand the processes of development. The path from fertilized egg to the newborn infant has been described as one of the most complex phenomenon in biology. Nelson and Bloom (1998) contrasted earlier misconceptions that perinatal brain development reflects rigidly deterministic genetic programs with current knowledge that experience has a critical role in the development of the infant's brain and that neural plasticity can be found even in human adults (see Nelson & Bosquet, Chapter 3, this volume). Positive or negative life experiences can alter both the structure and the function of the brain. This intimate relation between the developing organism and experience is extended into the behavioral domain, where the transactional model is used to understand cognitive and socioemotional functioning during infancy. For example, Fox, Calkins, and Bell (1994) contrasted an insult model, where early brain deviations lead to later problems, and an environmental model, where the brain is seen as completely plastic, with the transactional model, where genetically coded programs for developmental processes interact with environmental modifiers of the code. In their review of research on behavioral development during the first 2 years of life, they found much evidence for brain plasticity in response to new experiences but constraints imposed by the developmental status of the nervous system. This, of course, is what the transactional model would lead us to expect.

TRANSACTIONAL RESEARCH

Research based on the transactional model is difficult because it requires assessment of the infant and the environment over time to determine if they are affecting each other. Behavioral researchers have developed powerful methodologies for the measurement of child behavior even during infancy but have been far less successful in the assessment of environments and even less so in the assessment of experience. More complicated designs are necessary to separate the effects of contemporary environmental effects from the continuity and accumulation of risk conditions. Many studies have examined the stability of child characteristics over time, but few have examined continuities of contextual risk. In one such effort Duncan, Brooks-Gunn, and Klebanov (1994) found the best predictor of competence during early childhood was not the current economic circumstance of the family but the number of previous years the family had spent in poverty.

Despite the interest of developmentalists in the effects of the environment, the analysis and assessment of context has fallen more in the domain of sociology than in the domain of developmental psychology (Elder, 1984; Mayer & Jencks, 1989). The magnitude of a social ecological analysis involving multiple settings and multiple systems has daunted researchers primarily trained to focus on individual behavioral processes. A further daunting factor has been the increasing necessity to use multicausal models to explain developmental phenomena (Sameroff, 1983).

Depending on disciplinary background, different variables have been proposed to explain the sources of emotional problems. Economists have focused on poverty and deprivation as the roots of social maladjustment, sociologists have implicated problems in the community and family structure as the variables that promote deviancy, educators blame the school system, and psychologists have focused on processes within the family and its members as the environmental influences that most profoundly affect successful development. But rather than viewing them as competing, these variables can be seen as making additive contributions to a positive or negative trajectory through life. It will not be any one of these factors that is damaging or facilitating for infants but their accumulation in the life of any one child. Children reared in families with a large number of negative influences will do worse than children in families with few risk factors. In regard to clinical concerns, such a view militates against any simplistic proposal that by changing one thing, we will change the fate of our infants. Competence is the result of a complex interplay between infants with a range of personalities, the variations in their families, and their economic, social, and community resources. Only by attending to such complexity will the development of mental health be understood and perhaps altered for the better.

REGULATIONS

The description of the contexts of development is a necessary prologue to the understanding of developmental problems and to the eventual design of intervention programs. Once an overview of the complexity of systems is obtained, we can turn to the search for nodal points at which intervention strategies can be directed. These points are found in the interfaces among the child, the family, and the cultural systems, especially where regulations are occurring.

Despite a tendency to see infants as objects existing in a material world where their talents unfold in some maturational sequence, the reality is that, from conception, the infant is embedded in relationships with others who provide the nutrition for both physical and psychological growth. In Figure 1.1, the developmental changes in this relationship between individual and context is represented as an expanding cone. The balance between other-regulation and self-regulation shifts as the child is able to take on more and more responsibility for his or her own well-being. At birth the infant could not survive without the environment's providing nutrition and warmth. Later the child is able to put on a jacket and find the refrigerator although someone else still has to buy the clothing and food for the family. But eventually the child reaches adulthood and can become part of the other-regulation of a new infant, beginning the next generation. All the ingredients of the regulation by others will be the subject of our analysis of the environment.

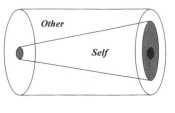

FIGURE 1.1. Changing balance between other-regulation and self-regulation as child develops into adult.

ENVIRONMENTAL ANALYSIS

The Rochester Longitudinal Study (RLS), was an effort to examine the effects of environmental factors over time on the development of several hundred children from birth (Sameroff, Seifer, & Zax, 1982) through adolescence (Sameroff, Seifer, Baldwin, & Baldwin, 1993; Baldwin et al., 1993). We assessed environmental factors as well as the cognitive and mental health of the children at four points in time, when the children were 1, 4, 13, and 18 years of age. At each age we assessed a set of 10 environmental variables ranging from proximal variables that were directly experienced by the child, such as interactions with parents, to distal ones that could only have indirect effects, such as the occupational status of the head of household. We then tested whether cognitive competence and mental health were related to the number of environmental risk factors (Sameroff, Seifer, Barocas, Zax, & Greenspan, 1987; Sameroff, Seifer, Zax, & Barocas, 1987). The 10 variables were (1) a history of maternal mental illness, (2) high maternal anxiety, (3) a parental perspectives score derived from a combination of measures that reflected rigidity in the attitudes, beliefs, and values that mothers had in regard to their child's development, (4) few positive maternal interactions with the child observed during infancy, (5) head of household in unskilled occupations, (6) minimal maternal education, (7) disadvantaged minority status, (8) reduced family support, (9) stressful life events, and (10) large family size. Each of these proposed risk factors has a large literature documenting its potential for deleterious developmental effects (Cichetti & Cohen, 1995; Damon & Eisenberg, 1998; Sameroff, Lewis, & Miller, 2000).

When we compared the risk groups for each variable separately, the cognitive and mental health outcomes for the low-risk group were better than those for the high-risk group at each age. Although studying the effects of individual risk factors is important for an analysis of each variable's contribution to infant mental health, a different approach is needed if the desire is to get a comprehensive view of environmental advantage or adversity. Such an overall perspective can be obtained by examining the accumulation of risk factors.

Rutter (1979) argued that it was not any particular risk factor but the number of risk factors in a child's background that led to psychiatric disorder. Psychiatric risk for a sample of 10-year-olds he studied rose from 2% in families with zero or one risk factor, to 20% in families with four or more. Similarly, Williams, Anderson, McGee, and Silva (1990) related behavioral disorders in 11-year-olds to a cumulative disadvantage score based on number of residence and school changes, single parenthood, low socioeconomic status, marital separation, young motherhood, low maternal cognitive ability, poor family relations, seeking marriage guidance, and maternal mental health symptoms. For the children with less than two disadvantages, only 7% had behavioral problems, whereas for the children with eight or more disadvantages, the rate was 40%. Fergusson, Horwood, and Lynsky (1994), in a study of the effects of 39 measures of family problems on the adolescent mental health of a sample of New Zealand children, used even more risk factors. Again, the result was the more risk factors, the more behavioral problems.

Although there were statistically significant effects for the single risk factors in the RLS at the population level, most children with only a single risk factor did not have a major developmental problem. However, when we created a multiple risk score that was the total number of risks for each individual family, found major differences on mental health and intelligence measures between those children with few risks and those with many at each of our assessment ages. At 4 years, children with no environmental risks scored more than 30 points higher on the intelligence test than children with eight or nine risk factors. On average, each risk factor reduced the child's IQ score by 4 points. No preschoolers in the zero-risk group had IQs below 85, whereas 26% of those in the high-risk (five or more risk factors) group did. Four-year-

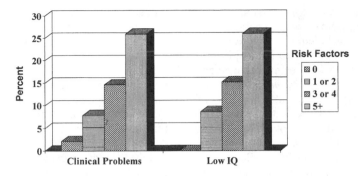

FIGURE 1.2. Percentage of children with Rochester Adaptive Behavior Inventory global rating scores in the clinical range and children with Wechsler Preschool and Primary Scale of Intelligence Verbal IQ scores below 85 in different multiple-risk groups.

olds in the high-risk group were 12.3 times as likely as low-risk children to be rated as having clinical mental health symptoms (see Figure 1.2).

The multiple pressures of environmental context in terms of amount of stress from the environment, the family's resources for coping with that stress, the number of children that must share those resources, and the parents' flexibility in understanding and dealing with their children all play a role in the contemporary development of child intelligence test performance and mental health.

COMMUNITY STUDIES OF RISK

To establish a normative base for the prevalence of risk factors and their association with mental health outcomes, a study requires a large representative sample and a clearly conceptualized model of risk. Unfortunately, as yet, there has not been a large epidemiological study of children's mental health, much less one for infants. Moreover, most studies of the effects of risk on development have not applied an ecological perspective in their conceptualization. As a consequence, ecological analyses usually are post hoc rather than a priori.

An example of such a study is an analysis of the progress of several thousand young children from kindergarten to third grade, using community samples from 30 sites (Peck, Sameroff, Ramey, & Ramey, 1999). From the data collected, investigators chose 14 risk factors that tapped ecological levels from parent behavior to neighborhood characteristics. They summed the number of risk factors and found a linear re-

lation between the multiple environmental risk score and school outcomes of academic achievement and social competence, supporting the findings from the RLS. Although this study used a large sample in multiple sites, the children were not a representative sample of the community, and the risk factors were selected from available data rather than planned in advance.

A study of adolescents in a group of Philadelphia families provided another set of data on the effects of multiple environmental risks on child development (Furstenberg, Cook, Eccles, Elder, & Sameroff, 1999). Mothers, fathers, and offspring were interviewed in nearly 500 families that had a youth between the ages of 11 and 14. Although not a representative sample, the families varied widely in socioeconomic status, from middle class to families living in poverty; the racial composition included African Americans and non-Hispanic and Hispanic whites.

An advantage of the Philadelphia project was that it took a more conceptual approach (Bronfenbrenner, 1979) in the design of the project so that environmental measures were available at a number of ecological levels. For our analyses of environmental risk, we examined variables within systems that affected the child, from those microsystems in which the youth was an active participant to those systems more distal where any effect had to be mediated by more proximal variables. The risk factors were from five groupings reflecting different ecological relations to the adolescent. We selected 16 variables to serve as risk factors, with the intention of being able to have multiple factors in each of our five ecological levels.

Family Process was the first grouping and included risks that were directly experienced by the child. These included a negative family emotional climate, poor marital quality, lack of behavior control, and lack of encouragement. The second grouping was *Parent Characteristics*, which included the parent's poor mental health, low sense of efficacy, low resourcefulness, and less than a high school education. The third grouping was *Community Connectedness* and comprised risk variables that reflected low levels of community involvement, lack of social support, and a lack of social resources. The fourth grouping, *Peers*, included indicators of the extent to which a youth was not associated with prosocial peers and was associated with antisocial peers. *Neighborhood*, the fifth grouping, represented the social level most distal to the youth and the family. Risks were a census tract variable reflecting low average income and educational level of the neighborhood in which the family lived, a parental report of many problems in the neighborhood, and a poor educational climate in the adolescent's school.

The project considered three outcomes that characterize successful development from a number of perspectives: parent reports of adolescent psychological adjustment; youth reports of problem behavior with drugs, delinquency, or early sexual behavior; and academic performance as reflected in grades.

MULTIPLE-RISK SCORES

To examine the effects of the total environment, investigators calculated multiple environmental risk scores for each family. When the three developmental outcome scores were plotted against the number of risk factors, a large decline in each outcome was found with increasing risk. The cumulative risk score meaningfully increased predictive efficiency, as demonstrated by analyses of relative risk for bad outcomes in high- versus low-environmental-risk families. The 25% of children who were doing the most poorly in terms of mental health, problem behavior, or academic performance were considered to have a bad outcome.

The relative risk in the high-risk group for each of the bad outcomes was substantially higher than in the low-risk group. The strongest effects were for mental health and academic performance, where the relative risk for a bad outcome increased from 3% in the zero-risk group to 50% in the high-risk group, an odds ratio of 17 to 1. There was a smaller effect for problem behavior where the risk rose from 3 to 45%. These data illustrate how the accumulation of environmental risk factors seems to have powerful negative effects on the important cognitive and mental health outcomes of youth (see Figure 1.3).

From the scientific data, it seems that the multiplicity of environmental risks is determinant of adverse child outcomes. However, common perceptions are that some single factors have overwhelming importance. Two such risk factors that economists and sociologists have been concerned about are income level and marital status. We did not find such effects when these single variables were put into a broader ecological framework. Any differences in child competence attributable to income and marital status disappeared when we controlled

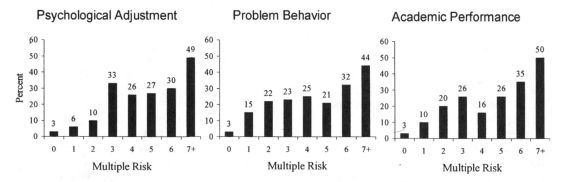

FIGURE 1.3. Percent of youth in lowest quartile for three youth outcomes in the Philadelphia study for each environmental risk group. Odds are calculated as the ratio between percentage of youth in the lowest quartile in the high-risk and low-risk groups.

for the number of other environmental risk factors in each family. Surprisingly, in each case there were no differences in the relation to child competence when we compared groups of children with the same number of risk factors raised in rich or poor families or families with one or two parents (Sameroff, Bartko, Baldwin, Baldwin, & Siefer, 1998).

Children from poorer and richer families had similar negative outcomes if there were many other risk factors and similar positive outcomes if there were no other risk factors. Children in two-parent families with many other risk factors had worse outcomes than did children in single-parent families who had few other risk factors. It is not single environmental factors that make a difference in children's lives but the accumulation of risks in each family's life. The reason that income and marital status seem to make major differences in child development is not because they are overarching variables in themselves but because they are associated with a combination of other risk factors. For example, whereas 60% of poorer children lived in high-risk families with more than six risk factors, only 25% of wealthier children did, and whereas only 17% of poorer youth had two or less risk factors, 46% of wealthier children did. Income or marital status taken alone may have statistically significant effects on adolescent behavior, but these differences are small in comparison with the effects of the accumulation of multiple negative influences that characterize our high-risk groups. One way that poverty compounds risk is through the depression it causes in single parents who cannot pay their bills and the worsening of parenting behavior as a consequence of the depression (McLoyd, 1998). Rather than one risk there are four: single parenthood, poverty, parental depression, and poor parenting. Many successful adults were raised in poverty or came from broken homes and many unsuccessful ones were raised in affluence or with two parents. But few successful adults came from multirisk families whether rich or poor.

PERSONAL FACTORS AND INFANT MENTAL HEALTH

It cannot be denied that personal characteristics are important ingredients in each infant's development. The nature of children (e.g., their temperament or intellect) may contribute to their development, but there is little evidence that it can explain their later success or failure when studied in context. Individual characteristics are only single ingredients in the dynamic system that characterizes human development (Sameroff & Chandler, 1975; Lewis, 1997), just as poverty and single parenthood are single characteristics. Therefore, we would not expect to see infant qualities be predictive of mental health unless they were examined in context. Unfortunately, few studies of infants have addressed the complexities of development directly from an ecological perspective, especially when the issue of personal resiliency is raised. Infancy is a starting point, and much of our concern is with the consequences of what happens during that period, requiring longitudinal designs wherein one can examine the relation of infant life to what follows.

To test the relative contribution of infant behavioral variables to the child's later performance in the RLS, we created an infant behavior score using 13 first-year variables that could be related to infant mental health. The score was based on a combination of measures of physical health, developmental status, and temperament, including subscores of the infant's perinatal physical condition from the Research Obstetrical Scale (Sameroff et al., 1982); and stress from the Brazelton Neonatal Behavioral Assessment Scales (Brazelton, 1973); the Mental Development Index at 4 and 12 months and the Psychomotor Development Index at 4 and 12 months from the Bayley Scales of Infant Development; and level of activity and crying at 4 and 12 months of age from home observations of infant behavior.

Based on the infant behavior score, we divided the sample into low and high competence groups of infants and examined as outcomes their 4-year IQ and mental health functioning scores (see Figure 1.4). There was no relation between infant competence scores and their 4-year IQ or mental health scores (Sameroff et al., 1998). High competent infants in high-risk environments did worse as 4-year-olds than did low competent infants in low-risk environments. Although we tend to see infants as having physical continuity over time and infer that there is mental continuity, there is little evidence for a strong longitudinal relationship. If one wants to predict the developmental course of infant psychological competence, attention to the accumulation of environmental risk factors appears to be a better strategy than concen-

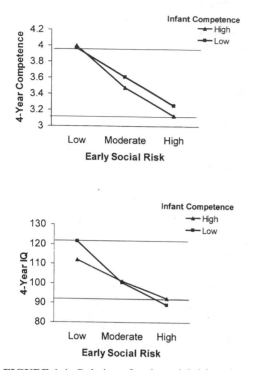

FIGURE 1.4. Relation of early social risk to 4-year intelligence and mental health for groups of children who were high and low on infant competence.

trating on individual characteristics. A focus on individual characteristics of individuals or families can only explain small proportions of variance in behavioral development. To truly appreciate the determinants of mental health fully requires attention to the broad constellation of ecological factors in which these individuals and families are embedded.

TRANSACTIONAL MODEL

In these ecological analyses, we have emphasized the role of the environment in affecting child development and argued that understanding the sources of mental health requires a sophisticated view of environmental action that includes attention to many social factors. However, this is not to say that individual differences in infant behavior have no role. Within a contextual emphasis we cannot lose sight of the important role child characteristics play in terms of what the child elicits from the environment and what the child is able to take from the environment

One such developmental model that appears to apply in a number of scientific domains is

the transactional model (Sameroff, 1983, 1993; Sameroff & Chandler, 1975). In this approach developmental outcomes are a function of neither the individual alone nor the experiential context alone. Outcomes are a product of the combination of an individual and his or her experience. To predict outcome, a singular focus on the characteristics of the individual, in this case the child, frequently will be misleading. An analysis and assessment of the experiences available to the child need to be added.

Within this transactional model, the development of the child is seen as a product of the continuous dynamic interactions of the child and the experience provided by his or her family and social context. What is innovative about the transactional model is the equal emphasis placed on the effects of the child and the environment, so that the experiences provided by the environment are not viewed as independent of the child. The child may have been a strong determinant of current experiences, but developmental outcomes cannot be systematically described without an analysis of the effects of the environment on the child. An emphasis on the eliciting power of child characteristics may be taken to an extreme, as when some behavioral geneticists argue that genes determine environments (Scarr & McCartney, 1983). In the niche-picking model, environments have powerful effects on development, but children choose environments that match their individual differences. Thus, genes produce both child and environment. This self-selection model would be all right if all children had a full array of environments from which to choose. Unfortunately, only certain environments are available to certain children, and more developmentally enhancing environments are more available to more affluent children (Jencks, 1979).

THE ENVIRONTYPE

The transactional model is an effort to provide a comprehensive view of how nature and nurture work together without degenerating to a discussion of what percentage of development is nature and what percentage is nurture. An elaboration of the model focuses on the developmental relations between biological organization, the genotype, the organization of the individual, the person or phenotype, and the organization of experience—the environtype (Sameroff, 1989). Just as the genotype regulates the physical outcome of each individual, the environtype is the organization of social influences or the ecological niche that regulates the way human beings develop in society. We have described many of the domains of environmental organization in the earlier discussion of risk factors in the family and community. The child's behavior at any time is a product of the transactions between the phenotype, the environtype, and the genotype (see Figure 1.5). The importance of identifying the sources of regulation of human development is obvious if one is interested in understanding changing that development, as in the case of prevention or intervention programs. It is beyond the scope of even the most ambitious clinical program to manipulate all the parameters that influence child development. The alternative is to understand determinants of development in sufficient degree to choose a level of complexity appropriate to the problem to be solved, the developmental stages of the child and family, and available resources.

Levels of environmental factors contained within the culture, the family, and the individual parent have been reviewed previously (Sameroff, 1993). Developmental regulations at each of these levels are carried within codes: the cultural code, the family code, and the individual code of the parent. These codes regulate cognitive development and mental health so that the child ultimately will be able to fill a role within the opportunity structure provided by society. They are hierarchically related in their evolution and in their current influence on the child. The experience of the developing child is partially determined by the beliefs, values, and personality of the parents, partially by the family's interaction patterns and transgenerational history and partially by the socialization beliefs, controls, and supports of the culture. There is a dis-

tinction that must be recognized between codes and behaviors, between environment and experience. The environtype is no more a description of what the child experiences than the genotype is a description of the biological phenotype. The genotype is just a list of available alleles. Whether any one of them will be expressed depends on the state and biochemical composition of the physical environment. There may be potential psychological experiences in the environtype, but depending on the infant's attentional focus, motivational level, intellectual competence, and social skills at a particular point in time, he or she will be more or less available to experience what is available.

Traditional research on child development has emphasized the child's use of biological capacities to gain experience and the role of experience in shaping child competencies, but there has been far less attention to how that experience is organized. Indeed, the organization of experience is explicit in the great amount of attention given to curriculum development and behavior modification plans, but far less attention is given to the implicit organization of experience found in the environtype to be described here. The discussion of ecological risk factors listed the variety of influences that need to be considered but in a cursory fashion. The analysis of risk factors is helpful for identifying infants highly likely to have mental health problems but offers little information on how one may change them. Next we take one aspect of the environtype, the family code, and detail many of the processes that need to considered. Discussions of the cultural code and individual code of parents that also influence the child can be found elsewhere (Sameroff & Fiese, 1999).

Family Code

The family code regulates child development through a combination of factors that extend across generations, include the coordinated efforts of more than two people, and provide a sense of belonging to a group. Traditional approaches to regulation in the family system have focused on the directly observable interaction patterns associated with individual adaptation, such as sensitive, intrusive, or neglectful behaviors directed toward the child (e.g., Clarke-Stewart, 1973). In these cases the repetitive patterns of neglect or intrusiveness are proposed to lead to maladaptive development. Recent extensions to family management and dyadic interac-

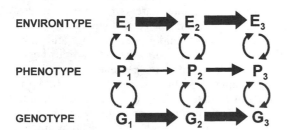

FIGURE 1.5. Regulation model of development with transactions among genotype, phenotype, and environtype.

tion have also been proposed (Grych & Fincham, 1990; Parke & Bhavnagri, 1989). Regulation in the family system has also been approached from the perspective that family beliefs directly affect behavior through working models that guide behavior and impart expectations to children. This approach is evident in the attachment literature as well as in generational influences on development (Main & Goldwyn, 1984; Zeanah, Boris, & Lieberman, 2000).

To appreciate the effects of family interactions and beliefs on child development, it is important to identify the central tasks of the family. Family life extends across a variety of domains and families are responsible for multiple aspects of their members' development. For example, Landesman, Jaccard, and Gunderson (1991) proposed six domains of family functioning: physical development and health, emotional development and well-being, social development, cognitive development, moral and spiritual development, and cultural and aesthetic development. Families organize their behavior around these goals, and adaptation is linked to whether they reach them successfully. Families also change over the lifespan with shifts in membership through marriage, divorce, birth, and death that are often accompanied by changes in roles and responsibilities that affect individual adaptation (McGoldrick, Heiman, & Carter, 1993). The family code regulates development so that the tasks of the family may be fulfilled.

The Represented and Practicing Family

Family influence may be better understood through the two ways in which families organize experiences: (1) through the beliefs that they hold, family representations, and (2) through the ways in which they interact with each other, family practices (Sameroff & Fiese, 1999). Reiss (1989) theorized that family regulatory processes can be detected and observed through the study of the represented and practicing family. The represented family highlights the internal representation of relationships and how working memories provide a sense of stability. Working models of relationships develop within the context of the family, are retained in memory, and guide the individual's behavior over time. To study the represented family, we must explore how families impart values and make sense of personal experiences. The practicing family, in contrast, stabilizes and regulates family members through observable interaction. The interaction patterns are repetitive and provide a sense of family coherence and identity. Not only does family life reside in the minds of individuals, but it is evident in the observed, coordinated practices of the group (Grych & Fincham,1990; Reiss, 1981).

The family code is a cause and a consequence of what families do on a regular basis and how family values and beliefs are directly imparted to children. One way to access the family code, while considering family ecology, is to examine family stories (Fiese, Hooker, Kotary, Schwagler, & Rimmer, 1995) as part of the represented family and family rituals (Fiese, Hooker, Kotary, & Schwagler, 1993) as part of the practicing family.

Family Stories

Family stories deal with how the family makes sense of its world, expresses rules of interaction, and creates beliefs about relationships. When family members are called on to recount an experience, they set an interpretive frame, reflecting how individuals grapple with understanding events, how the family works together, and how the ascription of meaning is linked to beliefs about relationships in the family and social world. The stories that families tell about their personal experiences aid in constructing a meaningful picture of the family's theory of how the world works and the familiy's expectations for family members' behavior (Bruner, 1990). Family stories may be examined by their thematic content, on the one hand, and by the process of storytelling itself, on the other.

Parents may use stories as a means to highlight expected developmental tasks of family members. During the early stages of parenting, both mothers and fathers told stories of an affiliative nature, focusing on the needs of others and being close. Consistent with the demands of raising an infant, parents recall experiences that incorporate themes of belonging. However, when the oldest child is preschool age and gaining a sense of autonomy, parents' stories begin to include themes of personal success and achievement, perhaps preparing the child for roles as a student and an achiever. In addition to the thematic content of family stories, the relative coherence of family narratives may impart to children that the world can be understood and mastered. The importance of family stories for clinical work is highlighted by the kinds of stories imparted by high-risk parents. In a study of psychiatrically ill parents Dickstein and colleagues found that depressed mothers told stories that provided a less coherent image of family life (Dickstein, St. Andre, Sameroff, Seifer, & Schiller, 1999). In this regard, the child in a depressed family may be at risk not only because of inconsistent interaction patterns but also because of the transmission of family messages that are inconsistent, poorly organized, and demonstrate a mismatch between affect and content. One only has to speculate what it is like for a child to be raised in an environment that is marked by difficulties in creating coherent images of personal experiences.

Family Rituals

Family rituals are powerful organizers of family life and are associated with both the practicing and represented aspect of the family code. Family rituals range from highly stylized religious observances (e.g., first communion) to less articulated daily interaction patterns (e.g., dinnertime) to problem-solving routines (e.g., anger management). Family rituals appear to affect family life by pairing meaning and affect with patterned interactions (Fiese, 1992, 1995). During the child-rearing years, creating and maintaining rituals on a daily basis are an integral part of family life (Bennett, Wolin, & McAvity, 1988). The organized experience of the family in its daily practices is sensitive to developmental changes in the family and may aid in the preservation of close relationships during periods of transition. In families with young children, investigators found that families of preschool-age children establish more dinnertime, weekend, and annual celebration rituals than do parents of infants. Furthermore, families of preschool-age children also report the occurrence of more family rituals, a greater attachment of affect and symbolic significance to family rituals, and more deliberate planning around ritual events, with a stated commitment to continue the family rituals into the future (Fiese et al., 1993). As children are able to take on a more active role in the family, daily activities appear to be reorganized to incorporate the child's participation (Goodnow & Delaney, 1989). Over time, these practices come to have meaning for the family and aid in the creation of a family identity.

Family stories and rituals are integrated into the developmental demands of raising young children and reflect transactional processes over time. Both the practicing and represented family code behavior across time and affect each other. Family practices take on meaning over time and become translated into the symbolic aspect of the represented family. The represented family, in turn, may affect how the family regulates and interprets their practices. As an example, consider the transactional consequences of negative affect expressed at the dinner table in the context of a parent with generational patterns of abuse and neglect (see Figure 1.6). The parent does not expect relationships to be rewarding and has created a representation of family as unfulfilling

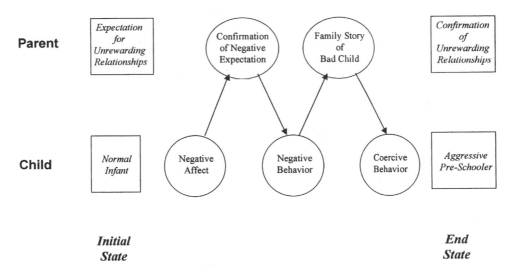

FIGURE 1.6. Transactional process leading from parent expectations of unrewarding relationships to child conduct problems.

and disappointing (Cicchetti & Toth, 1995). The infant's expression of negative affect confirms the parent's expectation for unrewarding family interactions and stimulates negative responses in the parent. Such direct exposure to negative affect may then lead to acting-out behaviors on the part of the child (Katz & Gottman, 1993). The acting-out behaviors may reinforce the parent in the belief that the parent cannot expect his or her offspring to behave in a positive manner, and a family story is created labeling the child as "bad" and uncontrollable with coercive consequences. This transactional process results in escalation of problem behavior and an entrenchment of beliefs that makes it more difficult to alter maladaptive patterns of interaction. The storied representation of family behavior becomes tainted with expectations for unfulfilling family relationships, confirmed in the directly observable interaction among family members (Fiese & Marjinsky, 1999).

As with other transactional systems, there is no direct causal link between parental expectations for unrewarding relationships and child coercive behavior. The relation is mediated by a chain of reciprocal events that could lead to many other outcomes with appropriate interventions. Changing parental behavior at dinnertime, negative expectations of the child, or family stories may significantly alter the outcome for the child. A transactional understanding of such processes helps in identifying both problematic developmental processes and potential interventions.

In summary, the operation of the family code is characterized by a series of regulated transactions. Parents may hold particular concepts of development that influence their caretaking practices. As children are exposed to different role expectations and listen to the family stories, they make their own contribution by their particular styles. The child's acting out of roles within the family is incorporated into family stories, rituals, and myths. By becoming an active transactor in the family code, the child ultimately may affect the child-rearing practices of the parents and even influence the code to be passed down to the next generation.

TRANSACTIONAL MODEL OF INTERVENTION

So far, we have been emphasizing the utility of such ecological and systems approaches as the

transactional model for understanding infant development as part of an academic agenda. However, the transactional model also has implications for a clinical agenda—the desire to improve the lives of infants. The utility of the model is especially evident in the prescription of intervention programs for young children, particularly for identifying therapeutic targets and strategies of intervention. The premise that the relation between infant mental health and later adaptive functioning is a property of the child-rearing system (i.e., the environtype) provides a rationale for an expanded focus of intervention efforts. Changes in behavior are the result of a series of regulatory interchanges between individuals within a shared social ecology. By examining the strengths and weaknesses of the regulatory system, targets can be identified that minimize the necessary scope of the intervention while maximizing cost efficiency. In some cases, small alterations in child behavior may be all that is necessary to reestablish a well-regulated developmental system. In other cases, changes in the parents' perception of the child may be the most strategic intervention. A third category comprises cases that require improvements in the parents' ability to take care of the child. These categories have been labeled remediation, redefinition, and reeducation, respectively, or the "three R's" of intervention (Sameroff, 1987).

Figure 1.7 depicts an abstraction of the regulatory model that focuses only on the three R's of early intervention. Remediation changes the way the child behaves toward the parent. For example, when children present with known organic disorders, intervention may be directed primarily toward remediating biological dysregulations. By improving the child's physical status, the child will be better able to elicit caregiving from the parents. Redefinition

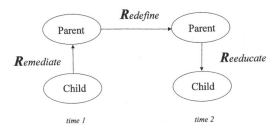

FIGURE 1.7. The three R's of early intervention within a transactional model.

changes the way the parent interprets the child's behavior. Attributions to the child of difficulty or willfulness may deter a parent from positive interactions. By refocusing the parent on other, more acceptable attributes of the child, positive engagement may be facilitated. Reeducation changes the way the parent behaves toward the child. Providing training in sensitive parenting or positioning techniques for parents of handicapped children is an example of this form of intervention. The framework for designing early interventions based on a transactional model has been described for infants with failure to thrive (Sameroff & Fiese, 1990) and for low birthweight infants (Sameroff & Fiese, 1999).

Remediation

As represented in Figure 1.7, the strategy of remediation is the class of intervention techniques designed to change the child, with eventual changes occurring in the parent (upward arrow). Remediation is not aimed at changing the family or cultural codes. The intervention goal is to fit the child to preexisting caregiving competencies that could operate adequately given appropriate infant triggering responses. Remediation is typically implemented outside the family system by a professional whose goal is to change an identifiable condition in the child (e.g., improving the physical condition and behavior of the infant). Once the child's condition has been altered, intervention is complete.

Premature infants are born ill-equipped to deal with the sensory environment outside the womb (Als, 1992), but if they receive gentle tactile stimulation and passive limb movements, stress associated with being in a neonatal intensive care unit can be reduced, resulting in greater weight gain and wakefulness and more mature habituation and orientation (Field et al., 1986). This example of remediation is an intervention aimed at changing the child, with the expectation that the child will become a more responsive interaction partner. In this regard, remediation allows the child to more fully participate in the practicing family.

Redefinition

Redefinition strategies are directed primarily toward the facilitation of more optimal parenting interactions through an alteration in parent beliefs and expectations. Redefinition is represented by the horizontal arrow between the parents at time 1 and time 2 in Figure 1.7. Difficulties in caregiving may arise from a variety of sources, including a failure of parents to adapt to a disabling condition in the child, failure of the parents to distinguish between their emotional reactions to the child and the child's actual behavior, and maladaptive patterns of care that extend across generations.

Low birthweight infants are often sent home in a biologically vulnerable state. Parents may be called on to continue massage techniques provided in the neonatal intensive care unit, monitor the child's sleep patterns, and adjust feeding practices to meet the needs of a small infant. Whereas parents may feel competent to care for a healthy infant, they may feel overwhelmed by the demands of caring for a vulnerable low birthweight infant. In this instance, the parents define caregiving as an extraordinary experience that they are unable to manage. Redefinition interventions may be aimed at normalizing the rearing of the infant and decreasing the emphasis on "special care." Highlighting the normal developmental tasks of sleeping, eating, and play would redefine the parents' role as one that is familiar and consistent with the parents' image of caregiving. Once the parents consider the normative aspect of raising a low birthweight infant, they may then be able to proceed with their intuitive parenting (Barnard, Morissett, & Spieker, 1993; Papousek & Papousek, 1987).

Redefinition interventions are aimed at altering parental beliefs and expectations about the child. If beliefs that the child is deviant are changed, normative caregiving can begin or resume. The parents are freed to use the skills that are already in their repertoire. There are cases, however, in which the parents do not have requisite skills or knowledge base for effective parenting, and the strategy of reeducation is indicated.

Reeducation

Reeducation is directed toward parents who do not have the knowledge base to use a cultural code to regulate their child's development. Public health initiatives have been used on occasion to reeducate large segments of society to change their caregiving behaviors. For example, Keys to Caregiving (Spietz, Johnson-Crowley, Sumner, & Barnard, 1990) is a program aimed at instructing parents about what to expect from infants at different ages in terms of their behaviors, cues, state modulation, and feeding interactions.

The majority of reeducation efforts are directed toward the family or individual parent and provide information about specific caregiving skills. In the Infant Health and Development Project (IHDP, 1990), families received home visits that provided parents with information on child development, instruction in the use of age-appropriate games, and family support for identified problems. Intervention effects improved cognitive development and reduced reports of child behavioral problems 2 and 3 years after the intervention (Brooks-Gunn, Klebanov, Liaw, & Spiker, 1993).

Reeducation interventions are typically aimed at the practicing aspect of the family code. These interventions focus on the immediate and momentary exchanges between parent and child that are associated with optimal development. It is assumed that once parents have the requisite knowledge about their child's behavior, that caregiving will proceed to facilitate development in accord with the cultural code.

Specificity of Interventions

Remediation, redefinition, and reeducation have been described as distinct forms of interventions aimed at targeting specific aspects of the transactional process. However, development is part of a system that is organized to include influence from multiple aspects of the cultural, family, and individual code. An examination of instances in which interventions do not work or have differential effectiveness may point to choosing a form of intervention aligned with resources and characteristics of individual families and children (Spiker, Ferguson, & Brooks-Gunn, 1993).

When faced with limited resources for early intervention programs, it is beneficial to consider the most cost-effective form of intervention that would affect multiple domains of adaptation. If education efforts aimed at parents also influence how they interact with their children and the beliefs they hold about development, then focused education programs may be offered to large groups of parents. However, if the parent is unable to make use of the educa-

tional efforts because of a past history of poor caregiving or lack of social support, more intensive redefinition programs would be warranted. It is possible to frame the three forms of intervention in the form of a transactional diagnosis process.

Transactional Diagnosis and Environtype Codes

Intervention efforts may be more effective when the focus is on identifying which environtype code is maintaining the problem. Such a strategy would lead not only to better program design but to better evaluation models and research designs as well. In remediation, the child is the identified target; in redefinition the parents' representations of the infant are the target; in reeducation, the parent's practices become the focus.

When taking a systems perspective, it is tempting to consider intervention always occurring at the level of the family. However, the transactional model of diagnosis and intervention proposed here pinpoints how intervention at the level of the child or parent alone may affect other aspects of the caregiving system. The three types of intervention correspond to different aspects of the environtype. Whereas singular interventions may be more closely aligned with specific aspects of the cultural, family, or parental codes, it should be evident that interventions in one area may influence other parts of the developmental agenda. Remediation aimed at the individual child may effect the family code by facilitating parent–infant interaction, at the same time stimulating redefinition of the child.

The complex model that characterizes our modern understanding of the regulation of development seems an appropriate one for analyzing the etiology of developmental disorders. It permits the understanding of intervention at a level necessary to identify targets of intervention. It helps us to understand why initial conditions do not determine outcomes, either positively or negatively. The model also helps us to understand why early intervention efforts may not determine later outcomes. There are many points in development at which regulations can facilitate or retard the child's progress. The hopeful part of this model is that these many points in time represent opportunities for changing the course of development.

SUMMARY

The preceding discussion has been aimed at understanding the impact of contextual influences on development. However, the shaping force is constrained by the state and potentialities of the individual (Sameroff, 1983). The transactional model incorporates both aspects in a coherent picture of development. In our progress toward understanding infant development, we have reached a key theoretical breakthrough. The problems of children are no longer seen as restricted to children. Social experience is now recognized as a critical component of all behavioral developments, both normal and abnormal.

Counter to the view of an unfolding of behavior is an environmental perspective in which the child grows as a consequence of interactions with the environment. However, the form of these interactions permits a variety of interpretations of how experience affects development. The understanding of psychological growth leading to and from infant mental health can be simplified by the use of analogies such as models of physical growth based on nutrition. Maturation models based on simple understandings of biological processes treat experience as a constant and leave all the dynamism to the individual. The most simple version is a nutritional one in which the budding mind requires sustenance for growth, but the pattern of that growth has already been laid down. A more complicated version is that the nature of the nutrition will change the direction of growth such that experience can always change the direction of development. Another set of models emphasizes the dialectic or transactional nature of development with a more complicated view of environmental action. Here, the nature of experience is changed by the activity of the child. A simple form of this model is the niche-picking view that children select their environments and, therefore, the kinds of experience they receive. The more complicated version here is that the nature of the child transforms experiences that are socially available. Although analogies are useful for understanding complex phenomena by appeals to simpler models, at some point the complexity of the target processes force the analogies to break down, and one must directly confront the functions of interest. To understand infant mental health and the possibilities for improvement requires an understanding of a dynamic individual and a dynamic family and social environment, a complicated but necessary task.

REFERENCES

Als, H. (1992). Individualized, family-focused developmental care for the very low birthweight preterm infant in the NICU. In S. L. Friedman & M. D. Sigman (Eds.), *The psychological development of low birthweight children* (pp. 341–388). Norwood, NJ: Ablex.

Baldwin, A. L., Baldwin, C. P., Kasser, T., Zax, M., Sameroff, A., & Seifer, R. (1993). Contextual risk and resiliency during late adolescence. *Development and Psychopathology, 5*, 741–761.

Barnard, K. E., Morisset, C. E., & Spieker, S. (1993). Preventive interventions: Enhancing parent–infant relationships. In C. H. Zeanah, Jr. (Ed.), *Handbook of infant mental health* (pp. 386–401). New York: Guilford Press.

Bennett, L. A., Wolin, S. J., & McAvity, K. J. (1988). Family identity, ritual, and myth: A cultural perspective on life cycle transitions. In C. J. Falicov (Ed.), *Family transitions* (pp. 211–234). New York: Guilford Press

Brazelton, T. B. (1973). *Neonatal Behavioral Assessment Scale*. London: Heinemann.

Bronfenbrenner, U. (1979). *The ecology of human development*. Cambridge, MA: Harvard University Press.

Brooks-Gunn, J., Klebanov, P. K., Liaw, F., & Spiker, D. (1993). Enhancing the development of low-birthweight premature infants: Changes in cognition and behavior over the first three years. *Child Development, 64*, 736–753.

Bruner, J. (1990). *Acts of meaning*. Cambridge, MA: Harvard University Press.

Cicchetti, D., & Cohen, D. (Eds.). (1995). *Developmental psychopathology: Vol. 2. Risk, disorder, and adaptation*. New York: Wiley.

Cicchetti, D., & Toth, S. L. (1995). Developmental psychopathology and disorders of affect. In D. Cicchetti & D. J. Cohen (Eds.), *Developmental psychopathology* (Vol. 2, pp. 369–420). New York: Wiley.

Clarke-Stewart, A. (1973). Interactions between mothers and their young children: Characteristics and consequences. *Monographs of the Society for Research in Child Development, 38*(5–6, Serial No. 153).

Damon, W., & Eisenberg, N. (Eds.). (1998). *Handbook of child psychology* (5th ed.): *Vol. 3. Social, emotional, and personality development*. New York: Wiley.

Dickstein, S., St. Andre, M., Sameroff, A. J., Seifer, R., & Schiller, M. M. (1999). Maternal depression, family functioning, and child outcomes: A narrative assessment. In B. H. Fiese, A. J. Sameroff, H. D. Grotevant, F. S. Wamboldt, S. Dickstein, & D. L. Fravel (Eds.), The stories that families tell: Narrative coherence, narrative interaction and relationship beliefs. *Monographs of the Society for Research in Child Development 64*(2, Serial No. 257), 84–104.

Duncan, G., Brooks-Gunn, J., & Klebanov, P. (1994). Economic deprivation and early childhood development. *Child Development, 65*, 296–318.

Elder, G. H., Jr. (1984). Families, kin and the life course: A sociological perspective. In R. D. Parke (Ed.), *Review of child development research: The family* (Vol. 7, pp. 80–136). Chicago: University of Chicago Press.

Fergusson, D. M., Horwood, L. J., & Lynsky, M. T. (1994). The childhoods of multiple problem adolescents: A 15-year longitudinal study. *Journal of Child Psychology and Psychiatry, 35,* 1123–1140.

Field, T. M., Schanberg, S. M., Scafidi, F., Bauer, C. R., Vega-Lahr, N., Garcia, R., Nystrom, J., & Kuhn, C. M. (1986). Tactile/kinesthetic stimulation effects on preterm neonates. *Pediatrics, 77,* 654–658.

Fiese, B. H. (1992). Dimensions of family rituals across two generations: Relation to adolescent identity. *Family Process, 31,* 151–162.

Fiese, B. H. (1995). Family rituals. In D. Levinson (Ed.), *Encyclopedia of marriage and the family* (pp. 275–278). New York: Macmillan.

Fiese, B. H., Hooker, K. A., Kotary, L., & Schwagler, J. (1993). Family rituals in the early stages of parenthood. *Journal of Marriage and the Family, 55,* 633–642.

Fiese, B. H., Hooker, K. A., Kotary, L., Schwagler, J., & Rimmer, M. (1995). Family stories in the early stages of parenthood. *Journal of Marriage and the Family, 57,* 763–770.

Fiese, B. H., & Marjinsky, K. A. T. (1999). Dinnertime stories: Connecting family practices with relationship beliefs and child adjustment. In B. H. Fiese, A. J. Sameroff, H. D. Grotevant, F. S. Wamboldt, S. Dickstein, & D. L. Fravel (Eds.), The stories that families tell: Narrative coherence, narrative interaction and relationship beliefs. *Monographs of the Society for Research in Child Development 64*(2, Serial No. 257), 52–68.

Ford, D. H., & Lerner, R. M. (1992). *Developmental systems theory: An integrative approach.* Newbury Park, CA: Sage.

Fox, N. A., Calkins, S. D., & Bell, M. A. (1994). Neural plasticity and development in the first two years of life: Evidence from cognitive and socioemotional domains of research. *Development and Psychopathology, 6,* 677–696.

Furstenberg, F. F., Jr., Cook, T. D., Eccles, J., Elder, G. H., Jr., & Sameroff, A. (1999). *Managing to make it: Urban families and adolescent success.* Chicago: University of Chicago Press.

Goodnow, J. J., & Delaney, S. (1989). Children's household work: Task differences, styles of assignment, and links to family relationships. *Journal of Applied Developmental Psychology, 10,* 209–226.

Grych, J. H., & Fincham, F. D. (1990). Marital conflict and children's adjustment: A cognitive-contextual framework. *Psychological Bulletin, 108,* 267–290.

Infant Health and Development Program (IHDP). (1990). Enhancing the outcomes of low-birthweight, premature infants. *Journal of the American Medical Association, 263*(22), 3035–3042.

Jencks, C. (1979). *Who gets ahead? The determinants of economic success in America.* New York: Basic Books.

Kagan, J. (1998). *Three seductive ideas.* Cambridge, MA: Harvard University Press.

Katz, L. F., & Gottman, J. M. (1993). Patterns of marital conflict predict children's internalizing and external-

izing behaviors. *Developmental Psychology, 29,* 940–950.

Landesman, S., Jaccard, J., & Gunderson, V. (1991). The family environment: The combined influence of family behavior, goals, strategies, resources, and individual experiences. In M. Lewis & S. Feinman (Eds.), *Social influences and socialization in infancy* (pp. 63–96). New York: Plenum.

Lewis, M. (1997). *Altering fate: Why the past does not predict the future.* New York: Guilford Press.

Main, M., & Goldwyn, R. (1984). Predicting rejection of their infant from mother's representation of her own experience: Implications for the abused and abusing intergenerational cycle. *Child Abuse and Neglect, 8,* 203–217.

Mayer, S. E., & Jencks, C. (1989). Growing up in poor neighborhoods: How much does it matter? *Science, 243,* 1441–1445.

McDonough, S. C. (1995). Promoting positive early parent–infant relationships through interaction guidance. *Child and Adolescent Clinics of North America, 4*(3), 661–672.

McGoldrick, M., Heiman, M., & Carter, B. (1993). The changing family life cycle: A perspective on normalcy. In F. Walsh (Ed.), *Normal family processes* (2nd ed., pp. 405–443). New York: Guilford Press.

McLoyd, V. (1998). Socioeconomic disadvantage and child development. *American Psychologist, 53,* 185–204.

Nelson, C. A., & Bloom, F. E. (1998). Child development and neuroscience. *Child Development, 68,* 970–987.

Papousek, H., & Papousek, M. (1987). Intuitive parenting: A dialectic counterpart to the infant's integrative competence. In J. D. Osofsky (Ed.), *Handbook of infant development* (2nd ed., pp. 669–720). New York: Wiley.

Parke, R. D., & Bhavnagri, N. P. (1989). Parents as managers of children's peer relationships. In D. Belle (Ed.), *Children's social networks and social supports* (pp. 241–259). New York: Wiley.

Peck, S., Sameroff, A., Ramey, S., & Ramey, C. (1999, April). *Transition into school: Ecological risks for adaptation and achievement in a national sample.* Paper presented at the Biennial Meeting of the Society for Research and Development, Albuquerque, NM.

Plomin, R., & Rutter, M. (1998). Child development, molecular genetics, and what to do with genes once they are found. *Child Development, 69,* 1223–1242.

Reiss, D. (1981). *The family's construction of reality.* Cambridge, MA: Harvard University Press.

Reiss, D. (1989). The represented and practicing family: Contrasting visions of family continuity. In A. J. Sameroff & R. N. Emde (Eds.), *Relationship disturbances in early childhood: A developmental approach* (pp. 191–220). New York: Basic Books.

Rutter, M. (1979). Protective factors in children's responses to stress and disadvantage. In M. W. Kent & J. E. Rolf (Eds.), *Primary prevention of psychopathology, Vol. 3. Social competence in children* (pp. 49–74). Hanover, NH: University Press of New England.

Sameroff, A. J. (1983). Developmental systems: Contexts and evolution. In W. Kessen (Ed.), *Handbook of child psychology: Vol. 1. History, theories, and methods* (pp. 238–294). New York: Wiley.

Sameroff, A. J. (1987). The social context of development. In N. Eisenberg (Ed.), *Contemporary topics in developmental psychology* (pp. 273–291). New York: Wiley.

Sameroff, A. J. (1989). Models of developmental regulations: The environtype. In D. Cicchetti (Ed.), *Development and psychopathology* (pp. 41–68). Hillsdale, NJ: Erlbaum.

Sameroff, A. J. (1993). Models of development and developmental risk. In C. H. Zeanah, Jr. (Ed.), *Handbook of infant mental health* (pp. 3–13). New York: Guilford Press.

Sameroff, A. J. (1995). General systems theories and developmental psychopathology. In D. Cicchetti & D. Cohen (Eds.), *Manual of developmental psychopathology* (Vol. 1, pp. 659–695). New York: Wiley.

Sameroff, A. J., Bartko, W. T., Baldwin, A., Baldwin, C., & Seifer, R. (1998). Family and social influences on the development of child competence. In M. Lewis & C. Feiring (Eds.), *Families, risk, and competence* (pp. 161–185). Mahwah, NJ: Erlbaum.

Sameroff, A. J., & Chandler, M. J. (1975). Reproductive risk and the continuum of caretaking casualty. In F. D. Horowitz, M. Hetherington, S. Scarr-Salapatek, & G. Siegel (Eds.), *Review of child development research* (Vol. 4, pp. 187–244). Chicago: University of Chicago Press.

Sameroff, A. J., & Fiese, B. H. (1990). Transactional regulation and early intervention. In S. J. Meisels & J. P. Shonkoff (Eds.), *Handbook of early childhood intervention* (pp. 119–149). New York: Cambridge University Press.

Sameroff, A. J., & Fiese, B. H. (1999). Transactional regulation: The developmental ecology of early intervention. In S. J. Meisels & J. P. Shonkoff (Eds.), *Early intervention: A handbook of theory, practice, and analysis*. New York: Cambridge University Press.

Sameroff, A., Lewis, M., & Miller, S. (Eds.). (2000). *Handbook of developmental psychopathology*. New York: Plenum.

Sameroff, A. J., Seifer, R., Baldwin, A., & Baldwin, C. (1993). Stability of intelligence from preschool to adolescence: The influence of social and family risk factors. *Child Development, 64,* 80–97.

Sameroff, A. J., Seifer, R., Barocas, R., Zax, M., & Greenspan, S. (1987). Intelligence quotient scores of 4-year-old children: Social environmental risk factors. *Pediatrics, 79,* 343–350.

Sameroff, A. J., Seifer, R., & Zax, M. (1982). Early development of children at risk for emotional disorder. *Monographs of the Society for Research in Child Development, 47*(Serial No. 199).

Sameroff, A. J., Seifer, R., Zax, M., & Barocas, R. (1987). Early indicators of developmental risk: The Rochester Longitudinal Study. *Schizophrenia Bulletin, 13,* 383–393.

Scarr, S., & McCartney, K. (1983). How people make their own environments: A theory of genotype-environment effects. *Child Development, 54,* 424–435.

Spietz, A., Johnson-Crowley, N., Sumner, G., & Barnard, K. E. (1990). *Keys to Caregiving: Study guide.* Seattle: NCAST, University of Washington School of Nursing.

Spiker, D., Ferguson, J., & Brooks-Gunn, J. (1993). Enhancing maternal interactive behavior and child social competence in low birthweight premature infants. *Child Development, 64,* 754–768.

Waddington, C. H. (1962). *New patterns in genetics and development.* New York: Columbia University Press.

Williams, S., Anderson, J., McGee, R., & Silva, P. A. (1990). Risk factors for behavioral and emotional disorder in preadolescent children. *Journal of the American Academy of Child and Adolescent Psychiatry, 29,* 413–419.

Zeanah, C. H., Boris, N. W., & Lieberman, A. F. (2000). Attachment disorders in infancy. In A. J. Sameroff, M. Lewis, & S. Miller (Eds.), *Handbook of developmental psychopathology.* New York: Plenum.

2

The Psychology and Psychopathology of Pregnancy: Reorganization and Transformation

❖

*LISA J. COHEN
ARIETTA SLADE*

There are probably few experiences in a woman's life more transforming than the experience of pregnancy and, ultimately, motherhood. As Therese Benedek (1959) and Grete Bibring (1959) noted long ago, the requirement for redefinition of self and other that is intrinsic to pregnancy is perhaps approximated only by the onset of menarche and menopause. Each of these changes heralds the beginning of a dramatic reorganization across a number of spheres in a woman's life and transforms her relationship to her body, her significant others, her culture, and her self.

Unlike menarche and menopause, however, pregnancy is not a stage that simply and inevitably occurs naturally over the course of development. Whereas the developments that necessarily precede pregnancy—namely, the biological, cognitive, and psychological antecedents to sexual maturity—are inevitable, the creation of a baby is not. Pregnancy is the result of a sexual act, and as such can be planned, avoided, and even terminated. It can of course also be accidental and nonvolitional. The continuation of a pregnancy involves a choice to embark on the transition to motherhood as well as to remain in some kind of actual or psychological relationship to a sexual partner. Pregnancy leads to the creation of a

life, one that will change a woman's place in her own world forever. These realities make pregnancy different from the biologically driven transitions of menarche and menopause; indeed, they underlie much of what is so emotionally compelling and yet difficult about becoming a parent.

Pregnancy involves tremendous physical transformation. There is disruption of basic physiological processes such as sleep, digestion, and appetite, and hormonal surges regularly affect mood and cognition. Over the course of the 40-week gestational period, a woman gains a significant percentage of her body mass in extra weight and her body completely changes shape. The psychological implications of these changes, in body size and shape and of loss of physical control, are considerable in and of themselves. Moreover, her body temporarily contains two people; there is literally another person inside her. This physical reality prepares the mother-to-be, particularly if she is pregnant for the first time, for profound changes in psychological reality; in effect, for the transition into the role of mother and for the extraordinary responsibility associated with it. As a mother, she will devote enormous time and energy to the care of a child who will be dependent on her for years, and whose lifelong well-being will be significantly affected by her ability to provide such care. To this end, she must also transform her identity, expanding her sense of self to incorporate her child, all the while recognizing her child's separateness (Trad, 1991). Hence, the psychological challenges of pregnancy provide significant opportunities for growth and integration (Benedek, 1959; Bibring, 1959; Deutsch, 1945). Under less felicitous conditions, however, pregnancy constitutes a high-risk period for the development of psychopathology, which can, in turn, have far-reaching effects on the later mother–child relationship.

As described in the sections that follow, the dramatic and complex reorganization that is inherent to pregnancy takes place at all levels—physical, biological, cognitive, and emotional. From the level of the body to the level of intimate relationships, family relationships and societal relationships to the level of self-definition and identity formation, the woman's sense of herself and her relationships changes dramatically by the time she gives birth. In a real sense, the process of adaptation during the 10 months of gestation prepares the mother for motherhood and creates a mother for the child. As she begins to "hold the baby in mind" (Fonagy & Target, 1996), she begins to imagine herself as a mother. Optimally, these processes mark the first steps in her developing flexible and pleasurable representations of her baby and of herself as mother, and together these beginnings make it possible for her to create an emotionally secure and safe environment for her baby.

A number of factors determine the success of this complex adaptation. On the one hand, a number of what we consider "external," or contextual, factors contribute to adaptation, such as the resilience of the marital relationship, a woman's age, socioeconomic status, and the degree of social support she can expect from her spouse, her family, and her society at large. These factors play an enormous role in determining whether the woman is able to hold and manage the complexity of pregnancy. Equally important are "internal," psychological factors such as her psychological openness to becoming a mother, her capacity to tolerate negative affect and ambivalence, her readiness to form secure and balanced representations of her baby, and the degree to which she has herself developed mature object relations and achieved a degree of security, flexibility, and autonomy from her own parents.

This chapter begins by presenting a developmental overview of pregnancy. We then consider relevant theory and research concerning the impact of external and largely relational and social factors upon the pregnancy. Finally, we consider the impact of internal, psychological processes on successful adaptation to the transition to motherhood.

DEVELOPMENTAL OVERVIEW OF PREGNANCY

Becoming Pregnant

Central to the experience of pregnancy is a woman's experience of choice in deciding whether or not to have a child. For those who feel ready to have a child, for those for whom the decision to have a child is conscious and intentional, the discovery of pregnancy can often bring great joy and excitement. Women speak of pregnancy as representing a natural unfolding of their marriage and as providing an intense connection to the primordial rhythms of life (Callister, 1995; Leifer, 1977; Slade & Cohen, 1996). Making a baby is often viewed as inevitably deepening the richness, intensity, and complexity of the parental relationship. It must be said, however, that the reality of what is before them also leaves women (and men) daunted, anxious, and ambivalent; however, when pregnancies are planned and wanted, these feelings do not usually disrupt feelings of contentment and happiness in any substantial way (Cowan & Cowan, 1992; Leifer, 1977). They are part and parcel of the "working through" of pregnancy.

Of course, many women feel unprepared to have a child, perhaps because they lack adequate financial resources or social support, or because they are young and less psychologically mature. For these women, discovery of the pregnancy can well be a negatively toned experience (Leifer, 1977; Lydon, Dunkel-Schetter, Cohan, & Pierce, 1996); the joy that is necessary to modulate the anxiety and ambivalence of pregnancy is diminished, and negative affects dominate the response to pregnancy from the start. Also, women who become pregnant—by design or accident—despite unresolved and marked ambivalence about motherhood, feel intensely emotionally unprepared for pregnancy. Often, such ambivalence is reflective of long-standing maladaptation and marks the beginning of an emotionally stressful and difficult pregnancy (Leifer, 1977; Trad, 1991). In extreme cases, women can exhibit psychotic denial of the pregnancy, lasting even to the point of birth (Kaplan & Grotowski, 1996; Spielvogel & Hohener, 1995). There are, of course, instances in which such negative beginnings can be reversed or at least attenuated over the course of pregnancy; as with all major developmental transition periods, change of all sorts is possible. Nonetheless, even for those who do not want the baby, the emotional intensity of the mother–fetal bond remains profoundly compelling, as is evident in the distress, guilt, and ambivalence many women (and men) feel after abortions (Major et al., 1990; Lydon et al., 1996).

Some couples want to have a baby but cannot, and they turn to fertility treatments to help them conceive. The emotional implications of beginning and sustaining a pregnancy following infertility treatments are enormous. The fact of prior infertility and its attendant grief and anxiety sets the stage for pregnancy in a particular way. Problems with fertility are not a new problem; modern technology, however, has introduced numerous techniques of improving fertility. Couples undergoing such treatments may endure months, even years, of arduous and expensive medical procedures; many of the medications used to treat infertility cause mood disturbances, and the failure of such treatments can be profoundly disappointing (Newton, Hearn, & Yuzpe, 1990). Thus, the emotional turmoil of infertility is exacerbated by the treatments themselves. When they are successful, the pregnancy is a hard-won accomplishment, replete, however, with its own set of anxieties and conflicts. Despite their joy and relief at finally conceiving, many parents may feel conflicted at having conceived in an "unnatural" way. They may feel averse to disclosing such information to family, to friends, and even to the child when he or she is old enough to undertand (Nielsen, Pedersen, & Lauritsen, 1995). In part because the technology used to treat infertility has emerged at such a rapid pace, the psychological and physical complications endemic to such treatments are rarely addressed by treating physicians (McKinney, Downey, & Timor-Tritsch, 1995; McKinney, Tuber, & Downey, 1996; Nielsen et al., 1995). The

achievement of fertility becomes the driving goal of the intervention. It is important to note here that fertility treatments are, for the most part, available only to middle- and upper-middle-class couples living in technologically sophisticated countries. Thus, women with limited means, or who live in cultures that do not support or provide such interventions, are usually left with no options other than to adopt or remain childless.

The Sequence of Trimesters

Women's experience of pregnancy is intimately tied to the biological sequence of development (Benedek, 1970). The greatest amount of fetal development takes place in the first trimester of pregnancy, in which undifferentiated cells are transformed into articulated tissues and organs. It is at this time that the baby is most vulnerable to toxic influences. Thus, mothers are now advised to stop smoking cigarettes and drinking coffee and alcohol. For those who have been actively trying to conceive, they will have been advised to do this long before. At this time the body is awash with hormones (Fleming, Ruble, Kreiger, & Wong, 1997); morning sickness is most severe as are irritability and mood changes. Cognitive changes, such as decreased attention and memory, also have been reported (Brindle, Brown, Griffith, & Turner, 1991). Paradoxically, pregnancy is a time when women in most cultures are expected to feel blissful and serene (Leifer, 1977).

A woman may not realize she is pregnant until she misses her period, but numerous women feel some changes in their body within the first few weeks of pregnancy. Despite weight gain in the mother-to-be's abdomen and breasts, the baby is still largely an abstraction to her. Her body may feel different, but she does not look notably different. Thus, during the first trimester, pregnancy involves life changes and physiological discomfort but does not feel as real or permanent as it will in later trimesters (Leifer, 1977; Phipps, 1985). In fact, as almost 25% of pregnancies result in first-trimester miscarriages (Kohn & Moffitt, 1992), many couples do not disclose their pregnancy until after the first trimester.

In the second trimester, fetal growth is more observable and the baby begins to feel more real to many women. Morning sickness and irritability generally are less severe than in the preceding trimester. For these reasons, many women eagerly anticipate their second trimester. At this point the abdomen has expanded enough for the pregnancy to "show," and women start wearing clothes that signal their impending motherhood. For some, this is a time of enormous conflict about bodily changes. For some mothers, the sense of loss of bodily control is terrifying; others fear they will never lose the weight. Although some mothers enjoy the motherly voluptuousness of their bodily changes, others feel fat and unattractive, holding to current standards which equate beauty with thinness (Huganir, 1990; Jenkin & Tiggeman, 1997; Leifer, 1977).

Mothers begin to feel movement at 4–5 months, although undetected motion has been occurring since 7–8 weeks (Klaus & Klaus, 1985). Quickening is the woman's moment of direct contact with the fetus as a living, volitional being, and as such it is perhaps one of the most significant moments in her pregnancy. Although the now irrefutable fact of the baby's presence can often be joyful and exciting, it will of course often be a further trigger to ambivalence and anxiety for those women unresolved about their pregnancy. Today, most women can now see their baby using ultrasonographic techniques, usually beginning at about 15 weeks, although vaginal ultrasonography can allow a view of the fetus as early as 10 weeks. This relatively new technological development allows the parents to view their infant before it is born, which was impossible until only a few decades ago (Klaus & Klaus, 1985). This is often experienced as intensely exciting—certainly making the baby feel more real—and often deepening attachment to the child (McKinney et al., 1996; Jordan, 1990).

As described more fully later, many psychoanalytic theorists have noted that as the mother's body grows, and as the baby becomes easier to imagine, to be felt through kicks and seen in the ultrasound, her psychological orientation turns inward. The mother's emotional investment is drawn away from the outside world and refocused inward toward her baby and the transformations taking place inside her (Bibring, 1959; Bibring, Dwyer, Huntington, & Valenstein, 1961; Leifer, 1977; Phipps, 1985). At this point, the psychological transition accelerates; not only is she becoming a mother physically, she is now evolving into one psychologically.

In the third trimester, the baby is largely formed, and it is time for the fetus to reach its full neonatal size. The woman gains the most weight at this point, generally up to 35 pounds. The large size of her stomach may make it difficult to sleep, especially if the baby rests on her bladder. The woman's mobility is considerably restricted now and her sheer body mass can lead to notable discomfort, especially in the final month. Certain pregnancy complications become more common at this point, such as gestational diabetes and placenta previa, and mothers may be assigned to bed rest. Psychologically, the woman is now preparing for childbirth and for the arrival of the baby into the world; Winnicott (1956) termed this the beginning of the period of "primary maternal preoccupation." Women leave work and begin "nesting" in a variety of ways; internally and externally, they are more and more turned to the baby's arrival and to the enormous changes this will bring (Leifer, 1977; Lester & Notman, 1986; Pines, 1972).

The culmination of pregnancy is, of course, childbirth. Women anticipate labor and childbirth with intense and ambivalent emotions. It heralds the long-awaited arrival of their child and the cessation of their now quite cumbersome pregnancy. Yet, it is also likely to be among the most physically painful experiences of a woman's life. In labor, a woman is inescapably confronted with the limits of her bodily control and, ultimately, with her own mortality. Unsurprisingly, women's fantasies about labor and childbirth can vary tremendously; some women insist on "mind over matter," that labor pain is only for the weak and physically unfit, while others maximize their anxiety, ruminating about labor for months prior to the birth. Many studies confirm the commonsense notion that women who feel informed about and in some control of the childbirth process will be less distressed and emotionally resilient during and after birth (Green, Coupland, & Kitzinger, 1990; Heaman, Beaton, Gupton, & Sloan, 1992; Niven & Gijsbers, 1996).

In most cultures, the rituals of childbirth are well articulated and highly affect-laden (Callister, 1995). In modern Western society, such rituals incorporate a range of choices, such as the use of Lamaze classes, the presence of the husband in the birthing room, the use of midwives versus obstetricians, and natural births versus assisted births, in which the mother is given medication to block her pain. All these choices can help the woman feel more positively toward the childbirth process by giving her a greater sense of control. After labor is over, common folklore suggests that many women develop a convenient amnesia for the pain of labor. One study suggested that women actually retain detailed memories of labor but forget the emotional quality of the pain (Niven & Brodie, 1996).

SOCIAL CONTEXT

Pregnant women do not live in a vacuum but in a complex network of family and culture. In fact, because of the increased physiological and emotional demands of pregnancy, women grow more dependent on others. They need more support from the people in their world—husband, family, friends, and those whose job it is to help them bring the pregnancy to a healthy end. Extended families often grow more cohesive around childbirth and even strangers are more likely to engage with pregnant women, sometimes putting their hands on women's stomachs or giving unsolicited advice about childcare. Pregnancy dramatically changes the dynamics of the nuclear family, the parental marriage in particular, and the availability of support—from husbands and other extended social networks—has been found intrinsic to a healthy adaptation to pregnancy (Condon & Corklindale, 1997; Leifer, 1977). The woman's experience of pregnancy is strongly affected by her social context, by the relationship with her partner, her children, and her own family of origin, and by the culture in which she lives.

Fathers' Experience of Pregnancy

Although there is remarkably little literature on the subject, fathers' psychological experience of pregnancy is naturally quite powerful, and they too are confronted with a series of major transitions in becoming a father. Although not as physically involved as the mother, the father is certainly affected by the process. The first-time father, in particular, must also undergo a tremendous transformation in role and in identity (Jordan, 1990). The man also must renegotiate his representation of his father and mother as he becomes a father and his sexual partner becomes a mother (Benedek, 1959; Jordan, 1990). In addition, as with mothers, the father must assume the tremendous responsibility of caring for a dependent child.

Over the last several decades in modern Western society, changes in sex roles have changed cultural notions of fathers' roles in childcare. Although women still do the majority of child care, fathers are expected in many cases to assume more child-care responsibilities than their own fathers may have (Jordan, 1990; Jones & Heerman, 1992). Hence, there is considerable confusion as to what role fathers should play. A number of studies speak to fathers' lack of clarity with regard to their role as fathers: their feelings of confusion regarding their relevance to the whole process (Jordan, 1990), their difficulty appreciating the degree of stress their partner is undergoing (Chapman, Hobfoll, & Ritter, 1997), and their often unrealistic attitudes about parenting techniques (Tiller, 1995). Thus many men are faced with the challenge of developing an identity as a father while trying to disidentify with the more remote role endorsed by their own fathers.

For many fathers, incipient fatherhood is an exciting, compelling, and profoundly moving experience. Nonetheless, a new father may feel intimidated by the responsibilities of parenthood and anxiously doubt his capacity to handle such responsibility. Interestingly, men often experience their anxiety about the baby's dependency in financial terms and are intensely concerned with their capacity to provide concrete support for their growing family. Such anxieties about being able to fill the shoes of fatherhood may reflect unresolved childhood idealizations of their own father and of masculinity in general (e.g., in order to be a good father, one must be Superman).

A father also may feel intense and ambivalent feelings about the changes his wife or partner is undergoing. The father may enjoy the woman's bodily changes, feeling excited and awed by the life growing inside of her. Conversely, he may have some difficulty seeing his sexual partner's body in so clearly a maternal form. Some men feel intense anxiety about their wife and child's physical health ("That big head is supposed to come out of where?"). Moreover, a man may feel abandoned by his wife, who is now devoting enormous energy and attention to her pregnancy. Many men also feel excluded from a central role in the parenting process, relegated by both friends and family to the ancillary role of breadwinner and helpmate, as if pregnancy is an exclusive club to which only women can belong (Jordan, 1990). Such a focus on fathers' emotional experience illuminates a largely neglected dynamic of women's experience of pregnancy—that although women's need for social support is heightened during pregnancy, many women may be reluctant to share the power and emotional significance of parenthood with their mates. However, for men to become more active fathers, women have to sacrifice the hegemony in child rearing they have traditionally enjoyed (Jones & Heerman, 1992).

In sum, both partners in the marriage undergo considerable transformation during pregnancy, especially in a primiparous pregnancy. Inevitably, the marriage is transformed as well (Hackle & Ruble, 1992). The dyad becomes a triad and it will be almost two decades before any decision can be made without considering the needs of their child. Pregnancy marks a profound commitment to the marriage and demands that father and mother remain inextricably connected to each other the rest of their lives. In conceiving a child, the man and woman join their physical bodies and family histories to create a life, which, while undeniably separate, is nonetheless a part of each of them. As one expectant father stated, "She is carrying a part of me inside her body." Thus pregnancy profoundly deepens the intimate bond of marriage. Not surprisingly, pregnancy also brings numerous stresses to the marriage. Many women are concerned that their husbands will not be fully involved in the pregnancy and feel frustrated and insufficiently supported. Many men are stunned and bewildered by their wives' irritability, confusing demands, and emotional lability. Moreover, couples may have different views on pregnancy and parenthood. Couples must find ways of both coordinating their needs and roles as parents and also of maintaining their own relationship independent of the new baby. As in most transitions, the ability to fully talk about both the positive and negative feelings and to anticipate problem areas and problem solve in advance can buffer the couple from inordinate stress. A study of couples' adjustment after the birth of a firstborn showed that those whose expectations most clearly matched the postnatal reality had the least difficult adjustment (Hackle & Ruble, 1992).

An area that has been relatively unstudied, but whose importance clinicians have recognized for decades, is the need to prepare older siblings for the birth of a child. For older siblings, their mother's pregnancy heralds the arrival of equally profound changes in their lives. For firstborn children, in particular, the arrival of a second child can be a distressing intrusion. Effectively dethroned, they cease to be the sole recipient of their parents' attention. Anecdotes abound of children's responses to the birth of a sibling; upon the arrival of his new brother, a 3-year-old suggested to his mother that she put him in the toaster-broiler until he was "toasty and crispy." For siblings who have already experienced the birth of a new baby, the new pregnancy is not as cataclysmic, although it can certainly be quite difficult. Jonah had an older sister 3 years his senior and was 3 when his new baby brother arrived. He was very well behaved when Simon came home from the hospital. After a few days, however, his patience flagged, and he asked his father: "When's Simon going to go to his new house?" Thus, the birth of a new baby is always significant for an older sibling, bringing both greater competition for parental attention and a brother or sister with whom the older child will have his or her own powerful relationship.

Depending on the age of the older sibling, the child may or may not be capable of understanding the implications of pregnancy—that in the future a new baby will come to stay. Nonetheless, eventually even a very small child can notice the change in the mother's body and may sense a change in her physical and emotional responsivity. Furthermore, a study on the effect of preparing older siblings for the arrival of a new baby showed that those who received such preparation adjusted better than those who did not (Fortier, Benna Carson, Will, & Shubkagel, 1991). The latter findings highlight what clinicians have known since Freud's time (and that sages have recognized since the time of the Greeks): Young children must be helped to work through their anxieties and jealousies both prior to and after their sibling's birth. For the mother and father, already stressed and anxious in their own right, this can seem a difficult task. However, resolving such issues are intrinsic to a healthy beginning for children, their parents, and the new baby.

Age, Socioeconomic Status, and Culture

A number of sociodemographic variables also have great impact on a woman's experience of pregnancy, including age, socioeconomic status (SES), and culture. Women are physically capable of bearing children for much of their adult lives, from early in their second into their fifth decade of life. In many cases, physical maturity precedes emotional maturity. In fact, most girls are capable of bearing children before they are legally able to drive a car or even hold a job. However, younger women have less life experience and less mature coping skills; they are often still children themselves, not at all ready for the tasks and demands of motherhood. Unsurprisingly, many studies show young age to be a risk factor for increased anxiety and depression during pregnancy and postpartum, for decreased prenatal care, and for worsened pregnancy outcome (Barnet, Joffe, Duggan, Wilson, & Repke, 1996; Bhalerao, Desai, Dastur, & Daftary, 1990; Bluestein & Rutledge, 1992; Fraser, Brockert, & Ward, 1995). However, most of these effects are confounded by various psychosocial variables, such as socioeconomic status and social support (Barnet et al., 1996; Fraser et al., 1995; Gazmararian, Adams, & Pamuk, 1996). In many countries young women have children to no ill effect, largely due to extensive family support networks and established traditions which guide parenting.

A host of literature looks at the phenomenon of teenage pregnancies, primarily in inner-city, low-SES women. Teenage mothers are at risk for a variety of difficulties, including increased psychopathology during pregnancy and postpartum, decreased birthweight, less prenatal care, and unrealistic expectations of pregnancy and parenting (Abel, 1996; Bluestein & Rutledge, 1992; Gazmararian et al., 1996). In this context, the combined effects of low SES, lack of education, ethnicity (minority status), and lack of social support appear to have a specifically pernicious effect, one that is more powerful than any single factor alone (Abel, 1996; Bluestein & Rutledge, 1992; McGrady, Sung, Rowley, & Hogue, 1992). Thus, in order for the mother to provide the necessary support for the baby, she needs to be "held" herself, by her own family, her culture, and society.

Youth is not the only age-related risk factor affecting women's experience of pregnancy. A study of first-time mothers over the age of 35 found that these women suffered from their own set of problems and stressors and had higher scores of perceived stress than did several samples of younger cohorts. Older women generally have more established lifestyles and, thus, experience pregnancy and parenthood as more disruptive to their life in general and,

specifically, to their occupational roles than do younger women (Reece, 1995).

A woman's experience of pregnancy is also affected by the broader social culture in which she lives (see Lewis, Chapter 5, this volume). She is not only influenced by demographic variables, such as socioeconomic status and related social advantages or disadvantages, but also by the values and beliefs about pregnancy and a woman's role as childbearer which permeate every culture (Callister, 1995). Studies of Asian and non-Asian women living in East London (Woollett et al., 1995) and Arab women living in Jordan (Khalaf & Callister, 1997) illustrate how different cultures vary as to beliefs about health care, diet, body image, childbirth practices, women's roles, and the religious implications of pregnancy. Nonetheless, members of one culture who have immigrated to another are also influenced by the mores surrounding pregnancy in their host culture (Woollett et al., 1995). In cultures in which the extended family is the predominant family organization, many women have had considerable exposure to pregnancy and child rearing prior to their own first pregnancy. In these cases, we can posit the psychological transformation in role and identity may not be as abrupt and dramatic as in Western cultures. Nonetheless, we can also posit that, to some extent, the profound physical, physiological, and psychological changes that women undergo during pregnancy are universal. Rooted in our biological history, they both precede and transcend culture.

PSYCHOLOGICAL PROCESSES IN PREGNANCY

Affective Upheaval in Pregnancy

Unsurprisingly, given the external and internal demands of impending parenthood, emotional upheaval is the sine qua non of pregnancy. Faced with some of the most daunting developmental transitions in her life, the pregnant woman is awash in feelings, many of them positive, many of them negative, many of them overwhelming. Fears and anxiety abound, in many variations: Will the fetus be viable? Will the baby be healthy? Will I survive labor? And of course, most centrally: Will I love my baby? Will I be a good mother? Will I still be myself? Ambivalence, too, arises in a variety of forms (Trad, 1990a). In most cultures, women are expected to be blissful when pregnant (Leifer, 1980); however, when childbearing brings with it enormous changes in every aspect of a woman's internal and external reality, this is rarely the case. One man, whose pregnant wife had tossed his clothes out their window in a rage after finding them on the floor, lamented: "But I'm giving her everything she wants . . . a baby, a new house, and she's miserable!" This woman was not fragile or depressed, nor was she especially ambivalent or highly anxious. In fact, she was a mature, stable woman in a happy marriage, thrilled at the birth of their first child. She was just pregnant. And her husband was blindsided by her lability and unhappiness. Although certainly he knew that pregnant women have their quirks, he was not prepared for the storm that was before him.

Over the last four decades, a number of psychoanalytic writers have described the affective lability of pregnant women (Bibring, 1959; Bibring et al., 1961; Leifer, 1977, 1980; Trad, 1990a, 1990b, 1991). Bibring specifically noted that were their mental state evaluated outside the context of pregnancy, these women would seem very disturbed and unstable. This instability can be seen as part and parcel of the tremendous consolidations inherent in the adaptation to motherhood. These destabilizations can be seen as a form of "decalage" (Piaget, 1954), the uncoupling of structures in the face of a new and higher level organization. Every aspect of a woman's sense of herself is being reworked: her relationship to her body, her mind, her private spaces and inner life. Even more dramatically, she is shifting her sense of herself to encompass the notion of becoming a mother, whose primary, biologically driven job is to care for her dependent infant. From a unitary sense of self, she now expands her identity to encompass her child. So much of what has defined her is being reorganized. Instability and reintegration are intrinsic to the formation of new structures.

This process, with its concomitant regressions and lability, necessarily awakens unresolved identifications, conflicts, aggression, anxiety, which become a live and intense part of the present (Deutsch, 1945; Pines, 1972). The slow process of resolving and integrating these internal experiences is the emotional work of pregnancy, and it is central to a woman's preparing herself both for motherhood and for her relationship with her child (Ballou, 1978). When successful, it offers a significant

opportunity for repair and resolution (Benedek, 1959).

Naturally, the degree to which these emotions and concomitant regressions come to dominate the pregnancy or serve as a springboard for integration and organization vary from woman to woman (Frank, Tuber, Slade, & Garrod, 1994; Leifer, 1977). There is ample evidence, for instance, that premorbid psychiatric disturbance (depression, anxiety, or major psychiatric disorder) is a major risk factor for pregnant women, one that will vastly affect their capacity to prepare for motherhood (Condon & Corklindale, 1997; Leifer, 1977, 1980; Trad, 1990a, 1990b, 1991). Similarly, pregnant teenagers are typically quite unprepared for pregnancy and motherhood, due to the fact that they have not yet completed the tasks of psychological separation from their own parents, nor have they accomplished the adaptations intrinsic to the redefinition of self that occurs in adolescence. Thus, they are ill prepared for the complex reintegration central to becoming a mother (Pines, 1988). Thus, any prior instability, either developmental or internal, has the potential to overwhelm an already destabilizing and difficult process.

Tasks of Pregnancy

Over the course of her pregnancy, a woman must come to see herself as a caregiver, someone who can nurture and comfort her child (Solomon & George, 1996). In Bowlby's (1988) terms, she must come to see herself as able to provide a secure base for her child. She must begin to see herself as a mother. To do so, she invariably returns to her experiences with her own mother. This is often a difficult and fraught process, as conflicts and ambivalence are a natural part of such remembering (Deutsch, 1945; Pines, 1972). As the pregnancy proceeds, however, a woman's experience of herself as a child in relation to her mother will hopefully begin to give way to an identification with her mother and a sense of herself as a mother, like her mother. Often this reworking allows women to see their mothers in a more positive light. Even more important, women create—from a reintegration of their own experience of themselves as a child—a vision of themselves as a mother. They are now mothers together, rather than a child dependent on or in conflict with her mother.

As is amply documented in the clinical literature on pregnancy, there are many women for whom the anxiety, ambivalence, and conflict evoked by pregnancy are so powerful that such reworking is difficult, if not impossible (Ballou, 1978; Deutsch, 1945; Leifer, 1977, 1980; Lester & Notman, 1986, 1988; Pines, 1972, 1988; Trad, 1990a). For some, the reorganization of maternal identifications is compromised by deep rifts in a woman's relationship to her own mother, brought on by maternal unavailability, rejection, disparagement, or trauma. One woman in an investigation we conducted, for instance (see Slade & Cohen, 1996), described her own mother as unrelentingly critical and emotionally abusive. She had a shattered quality to her, of someone angrily waiting for the next barb, the next blow. She had waited a long time to have a child, hoping to find some internal peace before she took on the task of mothering. Her pregnancy, however, was a torment to her. She was dreadfully anxious throughout, but even more important, she was enraged at her fetus. She wanted it out and separate from her, and at the same time, she wanted it under her control. But she had no desire to nurture it. Faced with the painful memories of having been mothered, Susan still felt the victimized, needy, angry, and unloved child. How could she become a mother when all she knew of motherhood was rejection and resentment? How could she care for a child when she could not even imagine a child who could be comforted nor a mother who could provide it? For women who cannot find the good mother in their memories of their mothers, who cannot in any sense identify with their mothers, and who cannot expunge a concomitant sense of their own badness, becoming a mother is a terrifying process.

Intertwined with the task of reworking earlier attachment relationships is the task of becoming attached to the child while at the same time acknowledging its separateness (Ballou, 1978; Condon & Corklindale, 1997; Pines, 1972). (We note here that although attachment theorists reserve the term "attachment" to describe the baby's relationship with someone "stronger and wiser" [Bowlby, 1988], we are using it here in a more colloquial way to describe the mother's enduring feelings of deep emotional connection to the baby, as well as her sense of herself as able to care for and nurture her baby.) For some mothers, the fetus is experienced as a baby from early on, whereas for others, it is experienced as a foreign object,

"which can be dispensed with as easily as an inflamed appendix" (Pines, 1972, p. 335).

For some women, "motherhood does not imply motherliness," in which the mother is responsible to care for the child. In such instances, the urge to have a baby "represents the narcissistic wish for an object to repair earlier hurts and losses" (Lester & Notman, 1988, p. 198). The baby thus becomes an attachment object of a very different sort. In effect, the baby is seen as a new chance to receive mothering but not to give it.

Nonetheless, complexity and contradiction are inherent in the mother's developing attachment to the child. On the one hand—particularly during the latter stages of pregnancy and the early postnatal period—the woman must in some very real sense abandon herself to her child. Winnicott (1956) has called this "primary maternal preoccupation," referring to the mother's becoming utterly preoccupied and identified with her baby, with his needs, his rhythms, his very being. She and the baby are—profoundly—together as one. At the same time, however, the baby's separateness, separate within her own body, must remain real to her. She must imagine and hold in mind his or her autonomy, distinct from her fantasies, her desires, her projections, and her attributions. She must also feel secure in her own ability to retain an autonomous identity, even while surrendering her sense of self to her baby. For those with significant experiences of intrusion and coercion, this relinquishment of autonomy can be a terrifying experience. Achievement of appropriately flexible boundaries, at once loose enough to encompass the baby and firm enough to allow the mother to mentalize both the baby's and her own separateness (Fonagy & Target, 1996), is intrinsic to the mother's ability to see the baby as both part of her and apart from her, and will pave the way toward a relationship after birth that is at once reciprocal and intimate (Leon, 1986; Lester & Notman, 1988). By example, Lily, another mother from a study we conducted, could describe her fetus as "us," and at the same time as willful, with desires of his own. He was both in her and separate at the same time. A mother unable to relax her boundaries while still remaining separate from the baby will be unable to feel the sense of love and connection that is intrinsic to healthy attachment. She may experience her baby as an alien creature invading her body, one whose relentless needs threaten to overpower her own identity. The message she will then convey to her child will be that his or her needs are bad and devouring, thus continuing the cycle of attachment and identity disturbances into the next generation.

Representation and Reflection

Out of the gamut of these experiences, the mother begins to develop a representation of her child and of herself as mother. Even in pregnancy she imagines a "busy" baby, a "demanding" baby, a baby who "won't stop bothering her," a baby who "makes her sick all the time," a baby who "will make her feel good about life." And she will be a "good" mother, a "scared" mother, a mother who "won't be changed" by her baby, a mother with "too much to handle." In pregnancy, there is no known baby and mother, there is only an imagined baby and mother. Thus, these representations are truly creations, based not on reality but on an amalgam of the mother's projections, hopes, dreams, attributions (Lieberman, 1997), and unconscious fantasies. This representation is intrinsically tied to the mother's sense of herself in relationship to her parents and carries embedded within it the core conflicts and difficulties of earlier attachment relationships (Slade & Cohen, 1996). As such, the mother's representation of the child is inevitably imbued with layers of subjective meaning, rooted in an array of the mother's experiences of self and other. More important, however, both the content and structure of such representations speak volumes about the success of the woman's adaptation to the tasks of pregnancy: To what degree can she imagine her baby, both as part of and apart from her? To what degree can she imagine herself as a mother?

In talking to pregnant women toward the end of their third trimesters, it is striking to see how vastly they differ from one another in their capacity to imagine the baby and to imagine themselves as mothers. For some mothers, their unborn child is a mystery; these women are detached from the emotional turmoil of pregnancy, even from the act of imagining the child to come. They have no nicknames for the baby, no sense of affection or attachment. They "try not to think" about the complexities of life after the baby is born, and in a variety of ways, they deny the baby's profound dependency as well as their own neediness. Often, they are compulsively self-reliant (Reeves, 1990), describing themselves as needing little help during pregnancy. Representations of themselves as mothers are shallow and superficial. These women appear to have avoided the regressions that pave the way to allowing themselves to feel like a mother, presumably because such destabilization threatens vital, but rigid, defenses.

For others, the representation is a torment, a constant reminder of the chaos, depletion, and ambivalence they anticipate ahead. These women are overwhelmed with anxiety, with fears for the baby and for themselves. They may see the baby as eating them up, robbing them of their lives, or as simply diffuse and frightening. And their visions of themselves as mothers revolve around the effort to maintain a sense of control and an intact sense of self in the face of the baby's overwhelming dependency and neediness; such representations may also be diffuse and fragmented, reflecting women's internal chaos and ambivalence. Although so highly threatened by the demands made on them and by the self-surrender inherent in the transformation into motherhood, such women themselves are often intensely needy and demanding of those around them and, yet, find little true comfort in their relationships to their husband or family (Reeves, 1990). For women who are either detached from or tormented by the experience of pregnancy, there is little joy in anticipation of the baby and little capacity to integrate and manage the vast emotional complexity of the transition to parenthood.

And, finally, there are those whose representations of the child and of the self-as-mother encompass a wide range of affects and fantasies; there is joy in anticipation, fear of the unknown, pleasure in imagined intimacy, and the act of giving care and providing succor. What is intrinsic to these latter representations is their flexibility and coherence. And these representations are often infused with positive affect. A whole, real, baby—both like and unlike her parents, changeable, unpredictable—can be imagined, and the complex and multifaceted emotions that will accompany this relationship, as well as the woman's relationship to her body and to her family, can be described in a coherent way.

Given that pregnancy is a time of such profound destabilization, no woman will be flexible and coherent all the time. And women who are highly defended and detached from the experience of pregnancy will sometimes be overwhelmed and frightened, whereas women who are consumed with negative fantasies and expectations will shut down and try to maintain a distance between themselves and their anxieties. Nevertheless, by the third trimester, relatively stable patterns of representation of self and baby can be discerned. Unsurprisingly, the quality of such maternal representations will have a profound impact on the mother–child relationship (Aber, Belsky, Slade, & Crnic, in press; Slade, Belsky, Aber, & Phelps, 1999) and will likely play a significant role in ultimately determining the security and safety inherent in the child's experience of his mother (George & Solomon, 1996; Zeanah, Benoit, Hirshberg, Barton, & Regan, 1995).

The quality of a mother's representation of her unborn child and, indeed, her capacity to synthesize and integrate the vast and complex psychological demands of pregnancy must be seen as a function of a number of factors: the quality of her internalized object relations (Lester & Notman, 1986, 1988; Pines, 1972, 1988), her capacity to synthesize and organize primary process regressions intrinsic to pregnancy (Frank et al., 1994), the degree of prior psychiatric disturbance or symptomatology (Condon & Corklindale, 1997; Deutsch, 1945; Leifer, 1977; Trad, 1990b), and the severity of unresolved conflicts and ambivalence (Deutsch, 1945; Lester & Notman, 1986).

They are also linked in a number of ways to the quality of a mother's representation of her own early attachment relationships. Women secure in their representations of their own parents (Main, 1995) are far more likely than their insecure counterparts to be able to maintain flexible, coherent, and motherly representations of themselves and their baby throughout their pregnancy (Frank et al., 1994; Grunebaum, 1990; Huganir, 1990; Slade & Cohen, 1996; Slade et al., 1995). Security, of course, does not imply the absence of difficulty, trauma, or loss. It implies that such difficulties have—to a large extent—been resolved and integrated. For women who have suffered in relationship to their own mothers, the work of pregnancy may be complex and painful, but a "secure state of mind in relation to attachment" (Main, 1995) will in most instances make it possible to develop healthy representations of the self and of the child.

Intrinsic to healthy adaptation across these many spheres is the capacity for reflective functioning (Fonagy et al., 1995; Fonagy & Target, 1996). Reflective functioning refers to the ca-

pacity to reflect on one's own or another's mental states and to use such reflectiveness as a means to make emotions and behavior meaningful. The reflective capacity emerges out of the context of a secure relationship between mother and child, out of the mother's capacity to imagine her baby as an intentional, desiring, believing being with a mind of his own. It is through being experienced as distinct within his mother's mind that the child gains a sense both of security and separateness, of a mind separate but known. High reflective functioning is protective in both children and adults. In children, it protects them from the effects of abuse and trauma, and in adults, it protects them from feeling unknown, dysregulated, and uncontained. They can hold and reflect upon their own experience. Reflective functioning plays a particular and important role in pregnancy, because the mother is necessarily holding two minds in her mind: her own changing sense of self alongside her fluctuating and intense affects and the reality of her baby, both part of and apart from her. Reflective functioning allows her to retain a sense of herself as coherent and knowable in the face of the turmoil of pregnancy and of her child as coherent and knowable, both in her imagination and after he is born.

Pregnancy Loss

From the moment she discovers she is to have a baby, the pregnant woman embarks on a complex journey of redefinition, reorganization, and reintegration. In the case of miscarriage or other forms of pregnancy loss, this process—of identifying with one's own mother, and of becoming a mother to one's own increasingly known and imagined baby—is interrupted, with devastating emotional consequences to the mother. Women experience much greater grief following pregnancy loss than is commonly recognized (Dermer, 1995; Janssen, Cuisinier, Hoogduin, & de Grauw, 1996; Janssen, Cuisinier, de Grauw, & Hoogduin, 1997; Hunfeld, Wladmiroff, & Passchier 1997; Leon, 1986; Zeanah, 1989). Miscarriage halts transformation in its tracks, making resolution difficult and painful. It is a loss that cannot be anticipated or prepared for. Women are often sad, preoccupied, depressed, angry, guilty, and anxious following a miscarriage, and in some instances, pregnancy loss can revive prior psychiatric disturbance and lead to a variety of forms of disordered mourning (Janssen et al., 1996;

Hunfeld, Wladimiroff, et al., 1997; Hunfeld, Taselar-Kloos, Agterberg, Wladimiroff, & Passchier, 1997; Zeanah, 1989). Miscarriage may also reevoke earlier losses and, in particular, reawaken unresolved mourning (Dermer, 1995). Although the acute distress of a pregnancy loss may persist for some time (Janssen et al., 1996; Hunfeld, Wladimiroff, et al., 1997), such feelings will usually diminish eventually, although Zeanah (1989) reports that 20 to 30% of women who experience perinatal loss experience significant psychiatric morbidity during the first year after the loss. For some, pathological or disordered mourning may continue for years. Anecdoctal clinical evidence has long supported the notion that the shadows of such losses can persist for generations.

The intensity of such feelings, and their resonance throughout a woman's life after the miscarriage, must be understood as a function of what she has lost. She has lost a part of herself, the part identified in a profound way with her baby. And she has received a "traumatizing blow" to revived identifications with her mother and with herself as a baby (Leon, 1986, p. 315), and the adaptational "crisis" of pregnancy cannot be resolved. Indeed, it has been suggested that grief following pregnancy loss has unique characteristics that distinguish it from other types of grief and, in fact, render it similar to forms of pathological mourning. Pathological grief is characterized, in part, by lowered self-esteem because the bereaved feels the loss as a injury to the self (Horowitz, Wilner, Marmar, & Kurpnick, 1980). The mother's sense of herself—across an array of domains—is profoundly affected by such loss (Dermer, 1995). In losing the baby, the woman is losing a part of herself. Disordered mourning of pregnancy loss may take many forms: pathological and unremitting grief, denial of grief, fantasies of replacement, and feelings of intense guilt (Zeanah, 1989).

The natural ambivalence of pregnancy may suddenly be experienced as causal following pregnancy loss: I made my baby die because of my feelings. Because she has increasingly come to feel like a mother to this baby, the woman's guilt is so much the greater. Many women who have lost a baby also feel intense rage and envy toward other mothers and mothers-to-be. In addition, they often struggle terribly with relinquishing their wishes and hopes for the baby, as these fantasies, rooted in childhood strivings, hold tremendous power (Leon, 1986). Unsurprisingly, women who do not have other children, or who lose their babies late in the pregnancy, are most affected by pregnancy loss and are more vulnerable to disordered mourning. Prepregnancy psychopathology also predisposes women to severe and pathological grief reactions.

The impulse to have another child is often strong following pregnancy loss. Despite the strength of such feelings, it is necessary to grieve the loss before embarking on another pregnancy (Leon, 1986; Zeanah, 1989). Given the complexity of the task of mourning a lost baby and a lost pregnancy, conception too soon after the loss threatens to truncate the mourning process and even to affect the capacity to become attached to later children (Lewis, 1979; Cain & Cain, 1964). This is probably most true when miscarriage happens late in the pregnancy. However, conception once the issues of loss and grief are diminished or following a miscarriage that occurs very early in the pregnancy may actually help in resolution and recovery (Cuisinier, Janssen, de Graauw, Bakker, & Hoogduin, 1996; Hunfeld, Wladimiroff, et al., 1997; Leon, 1986; Zeanah, 1989). At the same time, great individual differences remain in the time each woman and couples require to fully heal from their loss (Zeanah, 1989).

Abortion

Abortion is, of course, a different type of pregnancy loss. Some women elect to terminate a pregnancy because they do not feel ready to mother the child they are carrying. Other women terminate pregnancy for medical reasons, such as the presence of genetic defects or of multiple fetuses. Elective and medical abortions are very different emotional events. Abortion in a viable pregnancy is rarely carried out without conflict and most women feel some distress after their decision. Nonetheless, how a woman feels about her abortion is highly related to the way she processes and integrates her choices. If a woman clearly admits her options and alternatives and fully acknowledges her ambivalence about the decision, she is less likely to have significant regrets. Her adjustment to the abortion is also influenced by her capacity to fully acknowledge the power and implications of her decision; that she is choosing to terminate the incipient life of her unborn child and to relinquish the chance to become a mother to her own baby. In an effort to avoid facing such difficult truths, many women actively struggle against the process of acknowledging the fetus as a potential child and of recognizing themselves as potential mothers-to-be. That is, they try hard not to allow themselves to be psychologically pregnant. Other women entertain unrealistic, idealized fantasies of the baby-that-could-have-been and of the magically reparative effect completion of the pregnancy would have had on their lives. For women who likewise do not admit their ambivalence, or who do not experience the decision to abort as one they fully made for themselves, unresolved guilt, regret, or resentment may haunt them for years.

One young woman, who became pregnant at 17, immediately began imagining married life with her long-term boyfriend, who was quite a bit older than she, and whom she perceived as vulnerable and needing her care. At the same time, she planned to attend college in another state. Her parents desperately wanted her to end the pregnancy; her own mother had given birth to a child at 18 and had given the child up for adoption. She continued to struggle with this decision 25 years later. Both parents very much wanted their daughter to have a life that they themselves had not been able to have. And they actively disliked her boyfriend, who was uneducated and quite limited emotionally. Bowing to the inevitable, the young woman set aside her fantasies of raising the baby, agreed to an abortion, and went off to college. She knew it was the right thing to do. Nevertheless, her decision haunted her, and she clung to the belief that she could have raised the baby with her boyfriend and lived a happy life. She maintained her relationship with the baby's father throughout college and maintained the fantasy that someday they could try again. She never made peace with her loss, and its echoes profoundly shaped her capacity to move ahead in her life, increasingly separate both from her parents and from immature and compromised choices. She remained wedded to both, and at some level she remained wedded to the fantasy of reviving and keeping in the family her mother's lost child. Clearly, had her decision to seek an abortion been less ambivalently held, she would have resolved the loss and its attendant conflicts far more easily.

The young woman had begun to imagine her baby and her self as a mother against the backdrop of adolescent immaturity, grandiosity, and limited reflectiveness. Had she been older and more mature and had more developed object re-

lations, more flexible defenses, and a more comfortable and stable attachment to her mother, the abortion would certainly have left a different kind of residue (Cozzarelli, Sumer, & Major, 1998; Major, Richards, Cooper, Cozzarelli, & Zubeck, 1998). Abortions are invariably experienced, just as is pregnancy, within the context of a woman's individual psychic life and history.

Medical abortions pose a far different challenge to women's sense of psychological well-being. In such instances, both the baby(ies) and the self-as-mother have been acknowledged; nevertheless, the mother ultimately agrees to terminate her pregnancy. This invariably complicates the intense conflict inherent in any abortion. Grief following abortions for fetal anomalies has been shown to be as intense as grief following spontaneous perinatal losses (Zeanah, Dailey, Rosenblatt, & Saller, 1993). In a study of multifetal abortions, women reported powerful feelings of guilt, anxiety, and sadness, despite the fact that selective terminations can increase the chances of carrying at least one fetus to full term, reduce risk to the mother, or reduce the often overwhelming burden of caring for multiple infants (McKinney et al., 1996). A number of women reported dreams of the lost fetus. Interestingly, the majority of these women appeared to recover from the acute distress following the abortions, apparently because of the relief of finally giving birth to one or two healthy infants. The situation facing women who elect to abort fetuses whose ultimate survival would be profoundly compromised by genetic defect is somewhat different, because such children are expected to survive the pregnancy and birth. It is life that will be difficult for them and for their parents. Women often feel both guilt and grief at such decisions; guilt at not raising the child despite his or her damages and grief at the loss of the fantasy of a perfect baby. For the medical profession, multifetal abortions and medical abortions are necessary and sensible; for mothers and fathers, however, such procedures bring with them intense and complex feelings. These, too, must be addressed before the couple moves on in creating their family.

CONCLUSIONS

Pregnancy is a time of tremendous physiological and psychological transition, wherein a woman is preparing to take on the enormous responsibility of caring for a dependent infant. In this transition, she must reorganize her representation of her self in relation to her own body, her marriage, and her culture and in regard to her past as the child of her own mother. She must expand her identity to encompass her developing child, for whose physical and psychological survival she will—for a time—have to surrender much of her own autonomy. She must come to recognize the child as both part of and apart from her, as a being to whom she is profoundly attached and yet separate from. Finally, she must begin to develop a representation of her unborn child that is flexible and multifaceted; that integrates negative affect but is overridingly loving and joyous. This process is inherently destabilizing and emotionally tumultuous. In addition to the direct impact of physiological upheaval on her emotional stability, the pregnant mother must integrate a wide range of intense and conflicting emotions over the course of her parity. When development proceeds felicitously, pregnancy provides enormous opportunities for growth and resolution of past conflicts.

The success of a woman's adaptation to the tasks of pregnancy is critical to the development of a healthy, flexible, and reciprocal mother–infant relationship. The capacity to manage ambivalence, regulate negative affect, and develop a flexible yet coherent identity as a mother is at the heart of a woman's ability to provide a secure and safe base for her baby. It is only through such extraordinary transformation that a woman can become a "good enough" mother (Winnicott, 1965). All the work of pregnancy has a purpose: to ensure the development of a healthy, secure, and loved child. A woman who is unable to manage the many adaptive tasks of pregnancy will find mothering more than difficult, and her child's development will inevitably suffer in myriad ways.

As Bibring (1959) noted long ago, pregnancy is a time ripe for intervention. The nature of the developmental crisis of pregnancy makes a woman particularly open to change, to reorganization, and transformation. However, it is also a time when rigid and distorted perceptions of the self and of the baby can be set in motion, setting the stage for a troubled pregnancy and a disturbed mother–child relationship. Thus, signs of trouble in a woman's adaptation to pregnancy should be taken seriously by obstetricians, nurse midwives, and mental health professionals. When rage, ambivalence, depression, unrelenting anxiety, excessive somatization, or emotional disengagement define the woman's emotional experience during this period, intervention can be critical. In such cases, psychotherapy should be initiated as soon as possible to set the mother's development back on course, to protect the mother's developing relationship with her unborn child, and, ultimately, to strengthen the foundation of the child's future development.

ACKNOWLEDGMENTS

We would like to thank the staff of the Pregnancy Project at the City University of New York for their many contributions to our longitudinal study of pregnancy and mothering; this project was supported by National Institutes of Health Grant No. HD24676.

REFERENCES

Abel, M. H. (1996). Maternal characteristics and inadequate prenatal care. *Psychological Reports*, *79*(3 Pt. 1), 903–912.

Aber, J. L., Belsky, J., Slade, A., & Crnic, K. (in press). Stability and change in maternal representations of their relationship with their toddlers. *Developmental Psychology*.

Ballou, J. (1978). The significance of reconciliative themes in the psychology of pregnancy. *Bulletin of the Menninger Clinic*, *42*, 383–413.

Barnet, B., Joffe, A., Duggan, A. K., Wilson, M. D., & Repke, J. T. (1996). Depressive symptoms, stress, and social support in pregnant and postpartum adolescents. *Archives of Pediatric and Adolescent Medicine*, *150*(1), 64–69.

Benedek, T. (1959). Parenthood as a developmental phase. A contribution to the libido theory. *Journal of the American Psychoanalytic Association*, *7*, 379–417.

Benedek, T. (1970). The psychobiology of pregnancy. In E. J. Anthony & T. Benedek, (Eds.), *Parenthood: Its psychology and psychopathology* (pp. 137–151). New York: Little, Brown.

Bhalerao, A. R., Desai, S. V., Dastur, N. A., & Daftary, S. N. (1990). Outcome of teenage pregnancy. *Journal of Postgraduate Medicine*, *36*(3), 136–139.

Bibring, G. (1959). Some considerations of the psychological processes in pregnancy. *Psychoanalytic Study of the Child*, *14*, 113–121.

Bibring, G., Dwyer, T. F., Huntington, D. C., & Valenstein, A. F. (1961). A study of the psychological processes in pregnancy and the earliest mother–child relationship. *Psychoanalytic Study of the Child*, *16*, 9–44.

Bluestein, D., & Rutledge, C. M. (1992). Determinants of delayed pregnancy testing among adolescents. *Journal of Family Practice, 35*(4), 406–410.

Bowlby, J. (1988*). A Secure base: Parent–child attachment and healthy human development.* New York: Basic Books.

Brindle, P. M., Brown, M. W., Griffith, H. B., & Turner, G. M. (1991). Objective and subjective memory impairment in pregnancy. *Psychological Medicine, 21*(3), 647–653.

Cain, A., & Cain, B. (1964). On replacing a child. *Journal of the American Academy of Child Psychiatry, 3,* 443–455.

Callister, L. C. (1995). Cultural meanings of childbirth. *Journal of Obstetrical and Gynecological Neonatal Nursing, 24*(4), 327–331.

Chapman, H. A., Hobfoll, S. E., & Ritter, C. (1997). Partners' stress underestimations lead to women's distress: A study of pregnant inner-city women. *Journal of Personality and Social Psychology, 73,* 418–425.

Condon, J. T., & Corklindale, C. (1997). The correlates of antenatal attachment in pregnant women. *British Journal of Medical Psychology, 70,* 359–372.

Cowan, C. P., & Cowan, P. A. (1992). *When partners become parents: The big life change for couples.* New York: Basic Books.

Cozzarelli, C., Sumer, N., & Major, B. (1988). Mental models of attachment and coping with abortion. *Journal of Personality and Social Psychology, 74*(2), 453–467.

Cuisinier, M., Janssen, H., de Graauw, C., Bakker, S., & Hoogduin, C. (1996). Pregnancy following miscarriage or perinatal loss: Course of grief and some determining factors. *Journal of Psychosomatics, Obstetrics and Gynaecology, 17* (3), 168–174.

Dermer, M. (1995). *Pregnancy following pregnancy miscarriage: A study of attachment and unresolved grief.* Unpublished dissertation, City University of New York.

Deutsch, H. (1945). *The psychology of women.* New York: Grune & Stratton.

Fleming, A. S., Ruble, D., Krieger, H., & Wong, P. Y. (1997). Hormonal and experiential correlates of maternal responsiveness during pregancy and the puerperium in human mothers. *Hormones and Behavior, 31*(20), 145–158.

Fonagy, P., Steele, M., Steele, H., Leigh, T., Kennedy, R., Mattoon, G., & Target, M. (1995). Attachment, the reflective self, and borderline states: The predictive specificity of the Adult Attachment Interview and pathological emotional development. In S. Goldberg, R. Muir, & J. Kerr (Eds.), *Attachment theory: Social, developmental, and clinical perspectives* (pp. 233–279). Hillsdale, NJ: Analytic Press.

Fonagy, P., & Target, M. (1996). Playing with reality. I: Theory of mind and the normal development of psychic reality. *International Journal of Psychoanalysis, 77,* 217–233.

Fortier, J. C., Benna Carson, V., Will, S., & Shubkagel, B. L. (1991). Adjustment to a newborn: Sibling preparation makes a difference. *Journal of Obstetrical and Gynecological Neonatal Nursing, 20,* 73–79.

Frank, M. A., Tuber, S., Slade, A., & Garrod, E. (1994).

Mother's fantasy representations and infant security of attachment: A Rorschach study of first pregnancy. *Psychoanalytic Psychology, 11,* 475–490.

Fraser, A. M., Brockert, J. E., & Ward, R. H. (1995). Association of young maternal age with adverse reproductive outcomes. *New England Journal of Medicine, 332* (17), 1113–1117.

Gazmararian, J. A., Adams, M. M., & Pamuk, E. R. (1996). Associations between measures of socioeconomic status and maternal health behavior. *American Journal of Preventive Medicine, 12,* 108–115.

George, C., & Solomon, J. (1996). Representational models of relationships: Links between caregiving and attachment. *Infant Mental Health Journal, 17,* 198–216.

Green, J. M., Coupland, V. A., & Kitzinger, J. V. (1990). Expectations, experiences, and psychological outcomes of childbirth: A prospective study of 825 women. *Birth, 17*(1), 15–24.

Grunebaum, L. (1990). *Adult attachment classification and its relationship to the psychological tasks of pregnancy.* Unpublished doctoral dissertation, City University of New York.

Hackle, L. S., & Ruble, D. N. (1992). Changes in the marital relationship after the first baby is born: Predicting the impact of expectancy disconfirmation. *Journal of Personality and Social Psychology, 62,* 944–957.

Heaman, M., Beaton, J., Gupton, A., & Sloan, J. (1992). A comparison of childbirth expectations in high-risk and low-risk pregnant women. *Clinical Nursing Research, 1*(3), 252–265.

Horowitz, M. J., Wilner, N., Marmar, C., & Kurpnick, J. (1980). Pathological grief and the activation of latent self images. *American Journal of Psychiatry, 137,* 1157–1162.

Huganir, L. S. (1990). *Body image in pregancy: An attachment perspective.* Unpublished dissertation, City University of New York.

Hunfeld, J. A. M., Taselar-Kloos, A. K., Agterberg, G., Wladimiroff, J. W., & Passchier, J. (1997). Trait anxiety, negative emotions, and the mothers' adaptation to an infant born subsequent to late pregnancy loss: A case-control study. *Prenatal Diagnosis, 17*(9), 843–851.

Hunfeld J. A. M., Wladimiroff, J. W., & Passchier, J. (1997). Prediction and course of grief four years after perinatal loss due to congenital anomalies: A follow-up study. *British Journal of Medical Psychology, 70,* 85–91.

Janssen, H. J. E. M., Cuisinier M. C. J., de Grauw, K. P. H. M., & Hoogduin, K. A. L. (1997). A prospective study of risk factors predicting grief intensity following pregnancy loss. *Archives of General Psychiatry, 54*(1), 36–61.

Janssen, H. J. E. M., Cuisinier M. C. J., Hoogduin, K. A. L., & de Grauw K. P. H. M. (1996). Controlled prospective study on the mental health of women following pregnancy loss. *American Journal of Psychiatry, 153,* 226–230.

Jenkin, W., & Tiggeman, M. (1997). Psychological effects of weight retained after pregnancy. *Women and Health, 25*(1), 89–98.

Jones, L. C., & Heerman, J. A. (1992). Parental division

of infant care: Contextual influences and infant characteristics. *Nursing Research, 41*(4), 228–234.

Jordan, P. L. (1990). Laboring for relevance: Expectant and new fatherhood. *Nursing Research, 39*(1), 11–16.

Kaplan, R., & Grotowski, T. (1996). Denied pregnancy. *Australian and New Zealand Journal of Psychiatry, 30*(6), 861–863.

Khalaf, I., & Callister, L. C. (1997). Cultural meaning of childbirth: Muslim women living in Jordan. *Journal of Holistic Nursing, 15*(4), 373–388.

Klaus, M. H., & Klaus, P. H. (1985). *The amazing newborn: Making the most of the first weeks of life*. Reading, MA: Addison-Wesley.

Kohn, I., & Moffitt, P. (1992) *A silent sorrow: Pregnancy loss*. New York: Dell.

Leifer, M. (1977). Psychological changes accompanying pregnancy and motherhood. *Genetic Psychology Monographs, 95*, 55–96.

Leifer, M. (1980). *Psychological effects of motherhood: A study of first pregnancy*. New York: Praeger.

Leon, I. G. (1986). Psychodynamics of perinatal loss. *Psychiatry, 49*, 312–324.

Lester, E., & Notman, M. T. (1986). Pregnancy, developmental crises and object relations: Psychoanalytic considerations. *International Journal of Psychoanalysis, 67*, 357–366.

Lester, E., & Notman, M. T. (1988). Pregnancy and object relations: Clinical considerations. *Psychoanalytic Inquiry, 8*, 196–221.

Lewis, E. (1979). Inhibition of mourning by pregnancy: Psychopathology and management. *Lancet, 2*, 28–29.

Lieberman, A. F. (1997). Toddlers' internalization of maternal attributions as a factor in quality of attachment. In L. Atkinson & K. J. Zucker (Eds.), *Attachment and psychopathology* (pp. 277–291). New York: Guilford Press.

Lydon, J., Dunkel-Schetter, C., Cohan, C. L., & Pierce, T. (1996). Pregnancy decision making as a significant life event: A commitment approach. *Journal of Personality and Social Psychology, 71*(1), 141–151.

Main, M. (1995). Recent studies in attachment: Overview, with selected implications for clinical work. In S. Goldberg, R. Muir, & J. Kerr (Eds.), *Attachment theory: Social, developmental, and clinical perspectives* (pp. 407–479). Hillsdale, NJ: Analytic Press.

Major, B., Cozzarelli, C., Sciacchitano, A. M., Cooper, M. L., Testa, M., & Mueller, P. M. (1990). Perceived social support, self-efficacy, and adjustment to abortion. *Journal of Personality and Social Psychology, 59*(3), 452–463.

Major, B., Richards, C., Cooper, M. L., Cozzarelli, C., & Zubeck, J. (1998). Personal resilience, cognitive appraisals, and coping: An integrative model of adjustment to abortion. *Journal of Personality and Social Psychology, 74*(3), 735–752.

McGrady, G. A., Sung, J. F., Rowley, D. L., & Hogue, C. J. (1992). Preterm delivery and low birth weight among first-born infants of black and white college graduates. *American Journal of Epidemiology, 136*(3), 266–276.

McKinney, M. K., Downey, J. I., & Timor-Tritsch, I. (1995). The psychological effects of selective fetal reduction. *Fertility and Sterility, 64*, 51–61.

McKinney, M. K., Tuber, S. B., & Downey, J. I. (1996, Winter). Multifetal pregnancy reduction: Psychodynamic implications. *Psychiatry, 59*, 393–407.

Newton, C. R., Hearn, M. T., & Yuzpe, A. A. (1990). Psychological assessment and follow-up after in vitro fertilization: Assessing the impact of failure. *Fertility and Sterility, 54*(5), 879–886.

Nielsen, A. F., Pedersen, B., & Lauritsen, J. G. (1995). Psychosocial aspects of donor insemination. Attitudes and opinions of Danish and Swedish donor inseminations patients to psychosocial information being supplied to offspring and relatives. *Acta Obstetricia Gynecologica Scandinavica, 74*(1), 45–50.

Niven, C. A., & Brodie, E. E. (1996). Memory for labor pain: Context and quality. *Pain, 64*(2), 387–392.

Niven, C. A., & Gijsbers, K. (1996). Coping with labor pain. *Journal of Pain Symptom Management, 24*(2), 116–125.

Phipps, S. (1985). The subsequent pregnancy after stillbirth: Anticipatory parenthood in the face of uncertainty. *International Journal of Psychiatry in Medicine, 15*, 243–264.

Piaget, J. (1954). *The construction of reality in the child*. New York: Basic Books.

Pines, D. (1972). Pregnancy and motherhood: Interaction between fantasy and reality. *British Journal of Medical Psychology, 45*, 333–343.

Pines, D. (1988). Adolescent pregnancy and motherhood: A psychoanalytic perspective. *Psychoanalytic Inquiry, 8*, 234–251.

Reece, S. M. (1995). Stress and maternal adaptation in first-time mothers more than 35 years old. *Applied Nursing Research, 8*(2), 61–66.

Reeves, M. E. (1990). *Self-reliance during pregnancy: A correlate with social support and adult attachment*. Unpublished dissertation, City University of New York.

Slade, A., Belsky, J., Aber, J. L., & Phelps, J. L. (1999). Mothers' representations of their relationship with their toddlers: Links to adult attachment and observed mothering. *Developmental Psychology, 35*, 611–619.

Slade, A., & Cohen, L. J. (1996). The process of parenting and the remembrance of things past. *Infant Mental Health Journal, 17*(3), 217–238.

Slade, A., Dermer, M., Gerber, J., Gibson, L., Graf, F., Siegel, N., & Tobias, K. (1995, March). *Prenatal representation, dyadic interaction and quality of attachment*. Paper presented at the biennial meetings of the Society for Research in Child Development, Indianapolis, IN.

Solomon, J., & George, C. (1996). Defining the caregiving system: Toward a theory of caregiving. *Infant Mental Health Journal, 17*, 183–197.

Spielvogel, A. M., & Hohener, H. C. (1995). Denial of pregnancy: A review and case reports. *Birth, 22* (4), 220–226.

Tiller, C. M. (1995). Fathers' parenting attitudes during a child's first year. *Journal of Obstetrical and Gynecological Neonatal Nursing, 24*(6), 508–514.

Trad, P. V. (1990a). Emergence and resolution of ambivalence in expectant mothers. *American Journal of Pscyhotherapy, 44*, 577–589.

Trad, P. V. (1990b). On becoming a mother: In the throes

of developmental transformation. *Psychoanalytic Psychology*, 7, 341–361.

Trad, P. V. (1991). Adaptation to developmental transformations during the various phases of motherhood. *Journal of the American Academy of Psychoanalysis*, *19*(3), 403–421.

Winnicott, D. W. (1956). Primary maternal preoccupation. In *Through pediatrics to psychoanalysis* (pp. 300–305). New York: Basic Books.

Winnicott, D. W. (1965). *Maternal processes and the facilitating environment*. New York: International Universities Press.

Woollett, A., Dosanjh N., Nicolson, P., Marshall, H., Djanbakhch, O., & Hadlow, J. (1995). The ideas and experiences of pregnancy and childbirth of Asian and non-Asian women in east London: Part 1. *British Journal of Medical Psychology*, *68,* 65–84.

Zeanah, C. H. (1989). Adaptation following perinatal loss: A critical review. *Journal of the American Academy of Child and Adolescent Psychiatry*, *28*(4), 467–480.

Zeanah, C. H., Benoit, D., Hirshberg, L., Barton, M., & Regan, C. (1995). Mothers' representations of their infants are concordant with infant attachment classifications. *Developmental Issues in Psychiatry and Psychology*, *1*, 1–14.

Zeanah, C. H., Dailey, J., Rosenblatt, M. J., & Saller, N. (1993). Do women grieve following termination of pregnancy for fetal anomalies? A controlled investigation. *Obstetrics and Gynecology*, *82*, 270–275.

3

Neurobiology of Fetal and Infant Development: Implications for Infant Mental Health

❖

CHARLES A. NELSON
MICHELLE BOSQUET

Earlier in this century, studies by Spitz (1945), among others, demonstrated that early deprivation could, under some circumstances, lead to horrific developmental outcomes. Indeed, the results of this work eventually contributed to the abolishment of institutionalized orphanages, a transformation that prevailed until fairly recently. Although subsequent studies revealed that the effects of institutionalization do not uniformly lead to disastrous consequences (e.g., see Skeels, 1966; Provence & Lipton, 1962; Tizard & Hodges, 1977; Tizard & Rees, 1975), the fact remains that many such children fair poorly. Unfortunately, in the past few years, unsettling reports of children reared in Romanian institutions and adopted by parents in the United States and Canada began to appear in the scientific literature (e.g., Benoit, Jocelyn, Moddemann, & Embree, 1996; Marcovitch et al., 1997), and the news was not good. A disproportionate number of these children showed deficits in cognitive, emotional, and linguistic functioning (e.g., Ames, 1997; Fisher, Ames, Chisholm, & Savoie, 1997; Marcovitch et al., 1997); they also suffered from growth retardation and a high morbidity rate due to a variety of infectious diseases (e.g., Albers et al., 1997; Hostetter, Iverson, Dole, & Johnson, 1989; Hostetter et al., 1991; Johnson et al., 1993; Johnson et al., 1996; Miller, Kiernan, Mathers,

& Klein-Gitelman, 1995). More recent studies have indicated that the severity of the handicap varies proportionally with how much time the child spends in the institution. In particular, children who are adopted before their first birthday appear to have better outcomes than do children adopted at a later age (Ames, 1997; Benoit et al., 1996).

Although the flow of Romanian adoptees into this country has now all but disappeared, current reports indicate that similarly deprived conditions exist on a large scale in sections of Russia and China. Indeed, recent information suggests that what we experienced with Romanian children will pale in comparison with what we will soon experience with children reared in Russia and China. (Adoptions of children from these countries into U.S. families have increased at an almost exponential rate over recent years: More than 7,000 such adoptions occurred in 1997 alone [Dana Johnson, personal communication, October, 1998].)

These early reports of poor outcomes of children reared under conditions of acute and tragic deprivation began to come to the attention of the news media in the mid-1990s. Recent articles in *Newsweek* and *Time* as well as various TV news shows began to report on these children in earnest, eventually raising two fundamental questions: First, what happened to the brains of these children as a result of early deprivation? And, more generally, how important *are* the first years of life in facilitating normal development? Seemingly overnight, and based on precious few data, it was concluded that the first 2 to 3 years of life are fundamental to fostering healthy development, and that this seemed to be true across all domains of functioning (e.g., sensory, linguistic, and emotional). A public debate then ensued, eventually leading to a conference sponsored by the White House in the spring of 1997. As a nation, what previously had been mere hypothesis suddenly became gospel: *The first 2 to 3 years of life are critical in fostering healthy brain development and, in turn, healthy behavioral development.*

For those who study the relation between brain and early behavioral development, this news was disconcerting. Certainly, there was irrefutable evidence that the first few years of life are critical in fostering normal development in the sensory, linguistic, and emotional domains. For example, it has been known for decades that visual deprivation or defects in the visual system (e.g., strabismus) can lead to visual impairments, such as the lack of stereoscopic depth perception (e.g., Blakemore, 1991; Hubel, Wiesel, & LeVay, 1977; LeVay & Stryker, 1979; LeVay, Wiesel, & Hubel, 1980). Similarly, children deprived of hearing spoken language, because of a hearing impairment, may not develop normal language (Curtis, 1977; Neville, 1991). Finally, infants or young children reared by abusive or neglectful caretakers may show atypical emotional development (e.g., Crittenden & DiLalla, 1988; Galenson, 1986; Schneider-Rosen & Cicchetti, 1984, 1991). Regardless, the reality is that we know little about brain development in the human and even less about the role of experience in sculpting the developing brain. Furthermore, there is strong evidence to suggest that although the most rapid period of brain development occurs toward the last third of gestation and during the first 2 postnatal years, the reality is that much of brain development begins long *before* the third trimester, and key aspects of brain development continue well *after* middle childhood. How, then, can we account for the disastrous outcomes of the children reared in Romanian orphanages and other institutions? More important, can we generalize from this and related work to normally developing children?

Overall, it is difficult to know exactly what is responsible for the poor outcomes of children who have experienced deprivation early in life. We know little about the brains of such children other than that they may be smaller (and even this is only surmised based on the circumference of the skull), nor do we know the mechanisms through which altered brain development comes to bear on behavioral and emotional development. The answers to these questions may lie in part in the fact that Romanian orphans and children reared under similarly horrific conditions were deprived of stimulation on a grand scale; they received little linguistic input, their movements were limited, they were not afforded much opportunity for human contact (including that with peers and caretakers), and they received few cognitive challenges (such as those that occur naturally by being read to, playing games, etc.). After spending a year or two in such conditions, these children were not only impaired emotionally—they also had smaller bodies and heads (and thus, brains), their motor and linguistic skills were impaired, and they suffered from various acute and chronic infections. In many respects, children reared under these drastic conditions are similar to children in our own society who suffer chronic physical and emotional neglect.

Although we have data from many quarters—notably from studies of deprivation—that clearly point to the importance of the first 2 to 3 years of life as playing a critical role in fostering healthy neural and psychological development, we have amazingly little information on exactly which aspects of experience are essential to development or how experience works itself into the structure of the developing brain. The reason for this paucity of knowledge is that there has been so little formal study, and efforts have been particularly scant in the area that focuses specifically on the relationship between brain and behavioral development.

A major goal of this chapter is to provide information about the importance of the first few years of life in influencing brain and behavioral development. We begin by providing an overview of what is known about the earliest stages of brain development, beginning with conception and ending at birth. We then describe brain development in both the immediate as well as the extended (i.e., through adolescence) postnatal period. What will be particularly apparent in this latter section is the important role experience plays in sculpting the developing brain. Thus, particular attention will be paid to the relation between experience and development, and what is commonly referred to as *neural plasticity.*

Once we provide this background, we turn our attention to some of the ways in which brain development has been studied in the human, with particular attention paid to the insight gained by studying both normally and atypically developing children. Because our goal is to focus on research that is grounded in the brain sciences and has implications for infant mental health, we restrict our discussion to work using physiological measures, such as measures of cortisol levels, and electrophysiological measures, such as the electroencephalogram. We conclude this chapter by offering suggestions for future research.

NEUROBIOLOGICAL DEVELOPMENT

In general, the development of the brain has an enormously long trajectory, beginning within a few weeks after conception and, at the cellular level, continuing through adolescence. The first stage of brain development (*neurulation*) involves the formation of the primitive neural tube. The tube itself is derived from the ectodermal (outer) layer of the embryo. As cells in this region of the embryo multiply, a groove forms along a longitudinal axis. As seen in the illustration in Figure 3.1, this groove gradually begins to fold over onto itself and forms a tube. The tube begins to close on the 18th day of gestation, and if all goes well is completely closed by the 24th day. Errors in neural tube closure (*neural tube defects*) include spina bifida and anencephaly.

Primitive neural cells (neuroblasts) trapped inside the tube go on to make up the central nervous system, whereas cells trapped between the outside of the tube and the ectodermal wall make up the autonomic nervous system (see Figure 3.1). Once the tube itself is closed, the neuroblasts continue their rapid proliferation and cell division. Between the time the neural tube closes and the sixth prenatal week, this proliferation results in the formation of first three and then five "vesicles" (see Figure 3.2). At the top of the tube the forebrain (*prosencephalon*) forms, which will eventually constitute the cerebral cortex and cerebral hemispheres (*telencephalon*), and the hypothalamus and thalamus (*diencephalon*). Below the forebrain lies the midbrain (*mesencephalon*), and

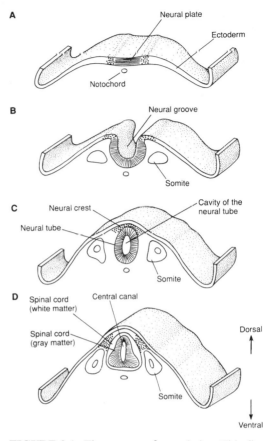

FIGURE 3.1. The process of neurulation. This figure illustrates the process whereby the primitive neural plate (derived from the outer layer of the ectodermal wall of the embryo) first thickens (due to cell proliferation) and then folds over onto itself (Panels A and B). Once this neural tube is formed, closure occurs at the top (rostral) and bottom (caudal) ends. Cells trapped inside the tube will give rise to the central nervous system, whereas those trapped between the outside of the tube and the ectodermal wall (see Panel C, "neural crest") will give rise to the autonomic nervous system. From Kandel, Schwartz, and Jessell (1991). Copyright 1991 by McGraw-Hill Cos. Reprinted by permission.

below the midbrain lies the hindbrain (*metecephalon*). The rest of the neural tube is the spinal cord. (For an excellent tutorial on cell proliferation, see McConnell, 1995.)

After neurulation and proliferation have run their course (generally by the sixth prenatal week), primitive neuroblasts and glioblasts (glial cell precursors) begin to migrate outward in a radial direction. In the cerebral cortex, neuroblasts are guided to their target destination by *radial glial cells,* which essentially act as long

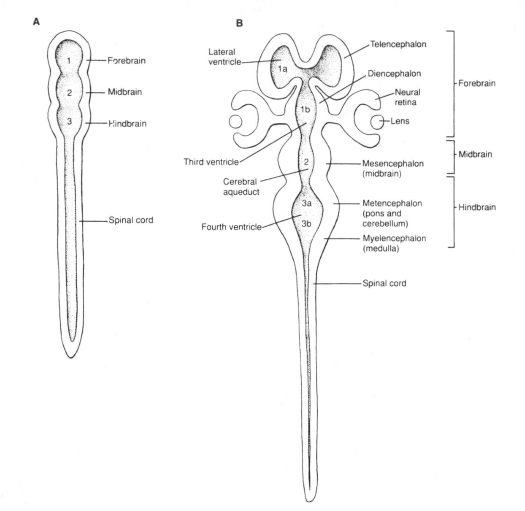

FIGURE 3.2. Once the primitive neural tube is formed and cells begin to differentiate, the central nervous system begins to form. This figure illustrates the early 3 (Panel A) and then 5 (Panel B) vesicle stage of development. Specifically, the three major structures (forebrain, midbrain, and hindbrain) gradually differentiate to give rise to more elaborated structures, including the telencephalon and diencephalon (forebrain), and the metencephalon and myelencephalon (hindbrain) (the midbrain changes little at this point in development). From Kandel, Schwartz, and Jessell (1991). Copyright 1991 by McGraw-Hill Cos. Reprinted by permission.

tentacles on which the migrating neuroblast attaches itself. (In the cerebellum, a different radial cell is used, so-called *Bergmann* cells. Moreover, in the cerebellum and cortex, different cells likely have different developmental trajectories; see Komuro & Rakic, 1998, for discussion.) The neuroblast is carried along the radial glial fiber until it reaches its target destination, at which point it detaches itself and takes up its final destination. As wave after wave of migrating neurons complete their cycles, eventually six layers (*laminae*) of the cortex are formed. Importantly, these layers are formed in an inside-out fashion, such that the deepest layers of the cortex are formed first, followed progressively by more superficial layers. Thus, the oldest part of the cortex is also the deepest part. Finally, because neuroblasts migrate in a radial direction, perpendicular to the cortical surface, columns of related cells also form. Many such columns are thought to subserve specific functions, such as the role of ocular dominance columns in vision.

As a rule, cell migration concludes by about the sixth prenatal month, after which these primitive cells begin their process of differentiation. Thus, these cells mature, begin to develop processes (axons and dendrites), and then make connections (synapses) among themselves. Moreover, in some parts of the brain the axons of neurons become coated with myelin, which increases the speed at which they conduct information from one neuron to another. These last two events—*synaptogenesis* and *myelination*—have variable courses of development, depending on what part of the brain is being discussed. With regard to myelination, we know that sensory and motor regions begin to myelinate before birth and, for the most part, are completely myelinated within the first months or possibly a year after birth. In contrast, the frontal lobe (particularly the prefrontal cortex) is probably not fully myelinated until close to adolescence (for discussion of myelination, see Jernigan & Tallal, 1990; Jernigan, Hesselink, Sowell, & Tallal, 1991; Yakovlev & LeCours, 1967). Similarly, in terms of synaptogenesis we know that (1) some regions of the brain form synapses before others,

and (2) all regions of the brain go through a phase of overproducing synapses, which is followed by a pruning back of these exuberant synapses until adult numbers are reached. For example, synapses in the visual areas of the brain reach their peak of overproduction by about the fourth postnatal month. This is followed by a gradual decline until about the end of the preschool period, when adult numbers of synapses are obtained. The auditory region of the brain follows a similar time course, although it is slightly displaced in time, so that the peak and pruning phases occur slightly later (see Huttenlocher & Dabhholkar, 1997). Finally, regions of the prefrontal cortex (e.g., middle frontal gyrus) do not reach their peak until closer to one year of age and then, show a much more gradual decline, so it is not until adolescence that adult numbers of synapses are obtained (for review of this literature, see Huttenlocher, 1994; see Figure 3.3 for an illustration of the differential time course of synaptogenesis).

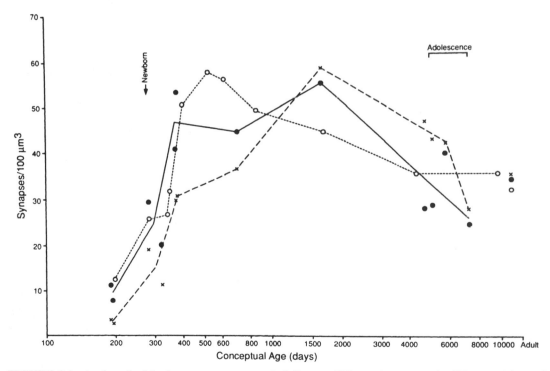

FIGURE 3.3. As described in the text, synaptogenesis follows a different time course in different regions of the human brain. For example, synapses in the visual cortex peak before those in the auditory cortex, which in turn peaks before those in the frontal cortex. Similarly, the retraction of synapses to adult numbers begins sooner and completes its course first in visual, then in auditory, and finally in the frontal cortex. From Huttenlocher and Dabhholkar (1997). Copyright 1997 by John Wiley and Sons. Reprinted by permission of Wiley-Liss, Inc., a division of John Wiley & Sons, Inc.

Summary

Overall, the *structural* development of the brain is completed largely before birth (at least in the case of the full-term birth; the neuroblasts of infants born at 25 weeks gestational age, for example, have not completed their migratory phase of development). However, the *functional* development of the brain is made possible by, in lay terms, the completion of the wiring diagram—the local and distal connections that are formed between and among areas by way of synapses and entire neural circuits, and by the efficacy with which the brain processes information. What is critical to note is that the formation and pruning of synapses depend, in many instances, largely on experience. Thus, it has been hypothesized that experience has a profound effect on the process of synapse elimination and, thus, the cultivation of synaptic circuits; that is, the development of these circuits is *activity dependent*. Note also that the role of the environment need not wait until postnatal life. We know, for example, that the fetus is powerfully affected by the extrauterine world, such as maternal nutritional status, drug abuse, exposure to acute or chronic stress (see subsequent sections), and so forth (for discussion, see Black, Jones, Nelson, & Greenough, 1998; Nelson, 2000).

To illustrate such effects, in the section that follows we turn our attention to how the structure of experience is incorporated into the structure of the brain. This phenomenon (neural plasticity) is critical to our thesis that brain development does not develop *in vacuo*; rather, brains need experience to grow.

MODELS OF NEURAL PLASTICITY

As described earlier in this chapter, *neural plasticity* is the process whereby the structure of experience is incorporated into the structure of the brain. Plasticity per se can be adaptive or maladaptive for the organism, depending on the experience and the brain's response to the experience. For example, recovery from brain injury and the sparing of function in the face of brain injury are both examples of positive adaptation. On the other hand, cell death due to exposure to teratogens, such as alcohol, is clearly maladaptive. In both cases, of course, the brain has been modified by some experience. It is important to ask how this occurs. We know that changes can occur at multiple levels, including physiological (e.g., the release of more neurotransmitters to compensate for cell death or damage), anatomic (e.g., the extension of existing axons into the space vacated by axons that have been deleted due to injury), and metabolic (e.g., the brain can "grow" new capillaries in response to the demand for oxygenated blood in an area being recruited for a new function, such as might occur with learning a new physical activity). All these changes can occur at virtually any point in the life cycle. However, in the context of development and the mission of this book, it would be useful to consider this problem at a more conceptual level. To do so brings us to describe models of plasticity offered by William Greenough and his colleagues (for general reviews, see Greenough & Black, 1992; Black et al., 1998).

Greenough has proposed two mechanisms whereby synapses are formed based on experience. *Experience-expectant* development refers to a process whereby synapses form after some minimal experience has been obtained. Greenough has proposed that the unpatterned, temporary overproduction of synapses dispersed within a relatively wide area of the brain during a sensitive period provides for the structural substrate of "expectation." Subsequent retraction of synapses that have not formed connections at all, or that have formed abnormal connections, then follows. The expected experience produces patterns of neural activity, targeting those synapses that will be selected for preservation. The assumption is that synaptic contacts are initially transient and require some type of confirmation for their continued survival. If such confirmation is not obtained, synapses will be retracted according to a developmental schedule or due to competition from confirmed synapses.

An example of an experience-expectant process is the development of ocular dominance columns in vision. It has been known for nearly three decades that stereoscopic vision (i.e., the ability of each eye to capture an image and then fuse this image so that it appears in depth) depends on regions of the visual cortex that receive separate inputs from each eye. These inputs (to layer IV of the visual cortex via the lateral geniculate) result in separate columns of cells that are distinct for the two eyes. Although these cells initially appear to form without benefit of experience, experience quickly becomes essential for the normal and complete elaboration of these columns (Crair, Gillespie, & Stryker, 1998). Thus, if the organism is deprived of vision in one eye or if the input a given eye receives is abnormal (such as might occur in an infant with strabismus), these ocular dominance columns fail to develop normally, and stereoscopic vision is compromised. Importantly, normal experience must occur at a certain time for these columns to develop normally; if this critical period is missed, the resulting deficit is permanent. This critical period coincides with the period of rapid overproduction of synapses in the visual cortex (see previous discussion; for a summary of the development of ocular dominance columns, see LeVay et al., 1980).

In contrast to experience-expectant development, *experience-dependent* development refers to those unique aspects of the environment that affect individuals. A classic example is learning. Each time we are exposed to new information, we modify our existing synapses and even make new ones. Unlike experience-expectant synaptogenesis, this process has no critical or sensitive period and can occur throughout the lifespan.

In summary, experience-expectant development is a time-limited function that depends on experience occurring during a sensitive or critical period of development. In contrast, experience-dependent development is not bound by time and can occur at any point in the life cycle. Experience-expectant development tends to apply particularly to sensory and perceptual functions (e.g., the development of vision or the ability to perceive speech), whereas experience-dependent development can apply to virtually all behaviors. Given the scope of this book, it would seem most fitting to focus on examples of experience-dependent development. We do so in the sections that follow; first, focusing on plasticity in the developing organism and then on plasticity in the so-called mature organism (for elaboration on some of these points, see Nelson, 2000; Nelson & Bloom, 1997).

Neural Plasticity in the Developing Organism: The Case of Early Stressful Experiences

Because of the difficulty in controlling for the many confounding variables that can contribute to the effects of stress on human brain develop-ment, researchers have made extensive use of animal models. Though animal brain development is, clearly, not identical to human brain development, parallels between animal and human brain systems have been found, and many researchers believe that animal data can be informative about human brain development. Animals are often used in place of humans as subjects when the use of human subjects would be impossible and/or unethical.

Research with rats suggests that maternal stress may affect fetal brain development via hyperactivity of the maternal hypothalamic–pituitary–adrenal (HPA) axis. Fameli, Kitraki, and Stylianopoulou (1994) administered adrenocorticotropic hormone (ACTH) to rats during the last third of their pregnancy to produce maternal adrenal hyperactivity. According to the authors, the results suggested that maternal HPA axis hyperactivity affected brain development in the offspring via corticosterone in a manner that led to malfunctioning of the offspring HPA axis. Data suggested that the adrenal glands of offspring animals hyperfunctioned under basal conditions, leading to adrenal exhaustion and to the animal's inability to react properly to stress. The authors noted that the effects of prenatal exposure to corticosterone affected all levels of the HPA axis, including monoamine levels. In particular, in the brains of the experimental offspring, serotonergic activity increased and dopaminergic activity decreased. The biological changes appeared to be permanent, as differences in monoamine levels were found in offspring brains when the rats were adults.

A number of other studies have found that prenatal stress is related to changes in levels of serotonin (5-HT) in the rat brain. Peters (1990) found that stress (crowding and saline injections) elevated maternal levels of tryptophan, which was associated with increased fetal and postnatal brain levels of 5-HT. Peters (1988) has suggested that the mechanism of change of the serotonergic system is a factor that is released during the stress response that interferes with the formation of and/or verification of synaptic contacts in the serotonergic system, resulting in permanent changes in the functioning of central serotonergic neurons. Peters (1982) hypothesized that stress may accelerate the onset of differentiation of nerve cells in regions containing 5-HT terminals.

Changes in the brain's serotonergic as well as catecholaminergic (dopamine and norepinephrine) activities are thought to be responsible for the abnormal behaviors documented in rats exposed to stress prenatally; such behaviors include altered emotional, reactive, sexual, and maternal behaviors. According to Peters (1986), alterations in the functional activity of 5-HT appears to affect virtually all behavioral and physiological processes, so 5-HT may have a modulatory role in the central nervous system. Fameli et al. (1994) suggested that changes in the monoamine levels of the offspring in response to prenatal exposure to stress may parallel underlying biological etiological factors in depression in humans because depression can be precipitated by stress in predisposed people, and elevated plasma glucocorticoids are commonly found in individuals suffering from depression; also, antidepressants act by modifying serotonergic and dopaminergic activities. Decreased activity of the serotonergic system has also been implicated in suicide and aggressive disorders, some personality disorders, Alzheimer's disease, and anxiety disorders in humans (Clarke et al., 1996). The serotonergic system also influences the differentiation of other neurons and is important in the regulation of brain development, especially in the early postnatal period (Trevarthen & Aitken, 1994). It may be related to calmness and sleep and feelings of well-being in the human infant (Trevarthen & Aitken, 1994).

Several studies have found that dopamine (DA) activity is affected in the brains of prenatally stressed rats. As mentioned previously, Fameli et al. (1994) found decreased levels of DA activity in the brains of prenatally stressed rats. Moyer, Herrenkohl, and Jacobowitz (1978) found that the female offspring of rats exposed to random heat, restraint, and bright light during pregnancy had less DA in the periventricular nucleus and more DA in the arcuate nucleus than did normal females. Fride and Weinstock (1988) found that prenatal stress created significant and long-lasting effects on dopamine activity and cerebral asymmetry. Prenatally stressed rats demonstrated increased rates of dopamine turnover in the right prefrontal cortex and a decrease in turnover in the left corpus striatum and right nucleus accumbens; these changes in rates led to a directional shift of the left–right differences in dopamine activity in all three areas. Prenatally stressed rats also showed increases in anxious behavior. The authors hypothesized that these findings may be related to the findings that anxiety in humans is related to relative activation of the

right frontal lobe (Fride & Weinstock, 1988). In the human infant, the dopaminergic system is hypothesized to be involved in the communication of emotion and in the active, exploratory, playful phases of infant development (Trevarthen & Aitken, 1994).

Research findings also suggest that levels of norepinephrine (NE) are affected by exposure to prenatal stress. Peters (1984) found that NE receptor binding was reduced by prenatal stress and suggested that there may be a delayed or impaired development of the postsynaptic elements of noradrenergic neurons in response to prenatal stress. However, Takahashi, Turner, and Kalin (1992) found that prenatal stress was linked to a significant increase in cerebral cortical NE concentrations in preweanling rats. According to Takahashi et al. (1992), animal and human studies indicate that NE neurons in the locus coeruleus may mediate attentional processes, stress responses, and affective and anxiety states. The increase in cerebral cortical NE concentrations in response to stress may account in part for the predisposition of prenatally stressed rats to exhibit, as adults, heightened stress-induced responses, such as freezing (Takahashi et al., 1992).

Prenatal stress is also thought to influence opiate levels in the brain. Insel, Kinsley, Mann, and Bridges (1990) found that the offspring of rats exposed to heat and restraint had a decreased number of brain opiate receptors. Opiates may have trophic roles during neural development, altering the elaboration of processes, the formation of synapses, and the normal rate of cell attrition (Insel et al., 1990). The opioid peptides have also been implicated in the perception of pleasure and pain and are thought to mediate positive emotions from social contact in humans. Furthermore, they are hypothesized to play a significant role in the formation of attachment relationships (Trevarthen & Aitken, 1994).

Rats are not the only animals that show deleterious responses to stress. Schneider has demonstrated that monkeys exposed to stress as fetuses (e.g., the mothers were exposed to unpredictable loud sounds) show symptoms of neurobehavioral dysregulation at birth and beyond; in fact, these symptoms appear to persist well into postnatal life (see Schneider, 1992). Furthermore, Schneider et al. (1998) have shown that exposing Rhesus monkeys to chronic, unpredictable stress as fetuses has long-lasting effects on noradrenergic and dopaminergic activity and behavior as long as 1.5 years after birth.

In the case of the human, some data suggest that stress experienced by the mother during pregnancy can adversely affect fetal brain development. Lou et al. (1994) compared the neonates of women who had experienced moderate to severe stressors during pregnancy to non-stressed women; group assignment was determined on the basis of ratings of stress according to the revised third edition of the *Diagnostic and Statistical Manual of Mental Disorders* (DSM-III-R; American Psychiatric Association, 1987). A multivariate logistic regression analysis of the data revealed that stress during pregnancy affected neonate head circumference, even when corrected for birthweight, indicating a specific effect of stress on brain growth (unfortunately, the authors did not test a competing hypothesis, which is the possibility that the effects were transmitted genetically). The authors noted that impaired head growth reflects cerebral maldevelopment and is a predictor of impaired neurological and cognitive development. Prenatal stress was related to neonatal neurological optimality as examined by the Prechtl neurological inventory between 4 and 14 days after birth. The authors hypothesized that the effects of maternal stress on fetal brain development may be mediated by glucocorticoids secreted by the adrenal cortex as a response to increased corticotropin release in stress. Research suggests that exposure to corticoids may be harmful because corticoids are involved in catabolic action and the inhibition of cell division in the brain (Lou et al., 1994). Also, we know that adults who have survived abuse as children show reduced hippocampal volume and, in some instances, impairments in memory as a result (Bremner et al., 1995, 1997; Stein, Koverola, Hanna, Torchia, & McClarty, 1997). It is thought that the mechanism for action is the neurotoxic effects of circulating glucocorticoids on the hippocampus, a structure rich in receptors for stress hormones and one that plays a key role in memory (see Nelson & Carver, 1998, for a review of the effects of stress on brain and memory development). Other areas of the brain, including the cingulate gyrus (which is thought to be involved in effortful attention, inhibitory control, and self-regulation of emotion and behavior), the amygdala (which has been implicated in fear and stress reactions), and frontal regions (which have been implicated in attentional

abilities) appear to have high levels of glucocorticoid receptors (Gunnar, 1997; Gunnar, 1998).

The effects of stress hormones on young children's development and the influence of the postnatal environment on the regulation of these hormones have been extensively studied by Gunnar and colleagues. In humans, cortisol is the glucocorticoid produced in response to stress (Gunnar, 1998). The HPA axis regulates the production of cortisol (Stansbury & Gunnar, 1994). Because the activity of the HPA axis is thought to be sensitive to emotion processes and because activity of the system can be measured noninvasively via levels of cortisol in samples of saliva, the HPA axis has been a popular area of investigation in the study of infant emotion processes and brain development (Stansbury & Gunnar, 1994).

According to Gunnar (1998), if elevated levels of glucocorticoids may deleteriously effect the development of the brain and, consequently, the development of competent cognitive and emotional functioning, evolution has likely built in mechanisms to keep these hormones at low levels during infancy. At birth, the neonate's HPA system is highly reactive and labile (Gunnar, Brodersen, Krueger, & Rigatuso, 1996). Between 2 and 6 months of age, the infant's stress systems are becoming organized via the transaction between the child and a sensitive caregiver, who buffers the reactivity of the HPA axis (Gunnar, 1997; Gunnar, Brodersen, & Rigatuso, 1993). Gunnar et al. (1993) found that infants who gave clear signals of their distress at 2 months and who had sensitive and responsive caregivers were likely to have an effective stress-regulatory system under maternal or dyadic regulation by 6 months of age. Stressful experiences that are not properly regulated by the caregiver before the infant is capable of self-regulation may not only influence the development of particular brain structures but also the reactivity of the HPA axis. According to Gunnar (1997), stressful experiences early in development may "program" the HPA system to be "hyper-" or "hypo-" reactive. Repeated or chronic activation of the HPA axis may promote the development of anxiety difficulties and/or more anxious temperaments (Gunnar, 1997).

The quality of the attachment relationship has been associated with the ability of the caregiver to buffer the activity of the HPA axis (Gunnar, 1997). Spangler and Grossmann

(1993) found that infants who demonstrate a secure attachment relationship demonstrate lower cortisol levels after the stressor of the Strange Situation than do insecurely attached infants. The variable mediating the relationship between attachment status and HPA axis activity may be the infant's sense of his or her ability to cope with stress. According to Gunnar (1993), it is not stressors but rather the child's appraisal of his or her ability to cope with stressors in the environment that influences the activity of the HPA axis. If adequate coping resources are available, including the child's own competencies and resources present in the environment, the child's HPA stress response may be reduced or prevented, even in the face of great stressors (Gunnar, 1994). Presumably, securely attached children have a history of responsive and sensitive caregiving, whereas insecurely attached children have a history of inconsistent and/or rejecting caregiving. Securely attached children can depend on their caregivers to respond appropriately as a buffer to stress, whereas the insecurely attached children cannot depend on their caregivers to respond appropriately. Therefore, securely attached children may be more likely than insecurely attached children to judge their coping resources to be adequate in the face of stressors and consequently show less of a physiological response to stress. Nachmias, Gunnar, Mangelsdorf, Parritz, and Buss (1996) found that infants who were both insecurely attached and temperamentally prone to approach new situations with caution were particularly at risk for elevated stress reactivity, as these infants are especially prone to experience novel events as possibly threatening and to expect their caregivers to be ineffective in buffering them from the effects of stress.

Collectively, it is clear that early deleterious experience can have significant negative effects on the developing brain that may be long term (for a tutorial on the role of stress and cognitive ability, see McEwen & Sapolsky, 1995). The likely explanation for these effects is that the brain is being affected at a critical point in its development. What is not known, unfortunately, are the effects of *positive* experiences on the developing *human* brain. We know such experiences have beneficial effects on the developing rat, and, as a society, we certainly hope such experiences have beneficial effects on the developing child. Although we know this is true at the behavioral level, the fact remains that there

have yet to be definitive studies examining the brain of the human child exposed to positive, enriching experiences.

It should be clear from the preceding section that the developing brain can be profoundly influenced by experience. It must be noted, however, that at least in some domains, experience can exert effects on the brain well beyond the first years of life.

Neural Plasticity in the Mature Organism: The Effects of Enrichment

Let us once again begin with a few examples from the rat. Greenough and colleagues have demonstrated that rats raised in complex, "enriched" environments (e.g., those filled with lots of toys and other rats) outperform rats reared in normal laboratory cages on a variety of cognitive tasks. Moreover, the "enriched" rats show a variety of changes in their brains, including improved synaptic contacts and a greater number of dendritic spines (suggesting more synapses; for review, see Greenough & Black, 1992; Black et al., 1998). It has also been observed that rats that receive extensive training in the use of one forelimb to reach through a tube to receive food show dendritic growth in the contralateral but not ipsilateral hemisphere. Finally, Black and Greenough have shown increased numbers of synapses per neuron within the cerebellum of rats that had been required to master several new complex motor coordination tasks; in contrast, animals exhibiting greater amounts of motor activity in running wheels or treadmills, where little information was learned, or yoked-control animals that made an equivalent amount of movement but in a simple straight alley, did *not* show significant alterations in synaptic connections in the cerebellum. Thus, learning, and not simply the repetitive use of the limb that may occur during dull physical exercise, led to synaptogenesis in the cerebellum. (For a select review of the literature on rearing rats in enriched environments, see Black et al., 1998.)

Reorganization of the brain based on selective experience is not limited to the rat. For example, in a study reported by Elbert, Pantev, Weinbruch, Rockstroh, and Taub (1995), magnetic encephalography (MEG) was used to map the somatosensory cortex of adults with and without experience playing a stringed instrument (e.g., guitar and violin). The authors observed that the area of the somatosensory cortex in musicians that represented the fingers of the left hand (the hand requiring greater fine motor learning, as it was used on the finger board) was larger than the area represented by the right hand (which was used to bow), and larger than the left-hand area in nonmusicians. This work suggests that the brain of the adult human can be reorganized based on positive experiences in the environment, in this case, musical training.

To complement this work, Paula Tallal has speculated that children with language learning impairments (LLI) have difficulty in parsing phonemes embedded in ongoing speech, which in turn results in difficulty discriminating speech sounds. Tallal and Merzenich (e.g., Merzenich et al., 1996; Tallal et al., 1996) recently reported significant improvements (e.g., a gain of 2 years) in both speech discrimination and language comprehension when children with LLI were given 4 weeks of intensive training in the processing of speech. Although the investigators did not examine changes in the brains of these children, it is not unreasonable to hypothesize that such changes were at the heart of the improved performance.

Summary

Overall, it is clear that the adult brain can be reorganized based on enriching experiences. This should come as no surprise, given that as a species we are capable of learning our entire lives. However, two points should be noted about this literature. First, a disproportionate number of examples of cortical reorganization come from the sensory and motor domains; we actually know little about reorganization at the level of social, emotional, or even cognitive development. Second, it is clear that there are still distinct limits on when reorganization can occur, at least in some domains of functioning. For example, early visual or auditory deprivation is likely to lead to lifelong disabilities in these domains. Thus, when talking about neural plasticity, we must be careful to specify (1) what domain of function is being discussed, (2) when this function emerges in development, and (3) the extent to which this function depends on experiences of a certain kind.

At least in some domains, the brain is capable of being modified by experience well after the infancy period. This has implications for the topic to which we next turn our attention: how one actually studies the relation between expe-

rience and brain development and the implications such study has for our understanding of infant mental health. We begin our discussion with some of the electrophysiological tools that have been used to look at the relation between brain and emotion—specifically, the electroencephalogram. We do so because this method has proved useful in examining the link between brain development and emotion, clearly an area that has implications for our understanding of infant mental health. We conclude the chapter with suggestions for future research.

FRONTAL LOBE DEVELOPMENT IN THE INFANT AND ITS ROLE IN EMOTION GENERATION AND REGULATION: EEG MEASURES

One method researchers have used to study infant brain development is the electroencephalogram (EEG). In particular, scientists have employed EEG methods to study regional brain activity that generates emotion and affective style (Davidson, 1994b). The EEG reflects the background electrical activity that exists in the brain at all times and ceases only with death. It reflects the summation of pools of neurons that conduct their electrical charges (brought about by synaptic activity) through extracelluar currents to the surface of the scalp. EEG recordings are taken by placing electrodes over several sites on the scalp, often by placing an electrode cap on the subject, which allows for accurate and quick placement of the electrodes on the head (Davidson, 1992). The electrical activity from each site is measured and analyzed compared to a baseline reference point. Analyses can also compare relative levels of activity at each of the sites.

Background to EEG and Emotion

Much of the research using EEG measures has explored the role of the frontal lobes in emotion generation and regulation. The frontal lobes have been the focus of research on emotion generation and regulation for several reasons. The experience and expression of emotions require several components, including subjective feelings, physiological changes, and facial and expressive signs (Fox & Bell, 1990). The regulation of emotions involves several additional components, including intentionality, planfulness, communication skills, motor control, and behavioral inhibition (Dawson, 1994a; Kopp, 1989). The frontal region is singularly capable of integrating all these elements. According to Nauta (1971), the frontal cortex has unique neural circuitry connecting it in reciprocal relationships to the parietal and temporal regions—which are involved in processing visual, auditory, and somatic sensory information—and to the telencephalic limbic system (and its subcortical components)—which is believed to receive information from the environment and to express itself in the form of affects and motivations. Because the frontal lobe has a reciprocal relationship with the limbic system, the former can monitor as well as modulate the latter (Nauta, 1971). According to Dawson (1994b), some theorists postulate that the amygdala of the limbic system is capable of quickly processing primitive emotional stimuli, while the frontal lobe is necessary for interpreting complex emotion stimuli and for modulating the affective and motivational states produced by the limbic system. The frontal lobe also plays a role in arousal and alerts the individual to respond to meaningful stimuli (Dawson, 1994a). There is evidence that each hemisphere may have its own cortical–limbic–reticular loop; this system would allow for different strategies in the hemispheres for emotion regulation and may express itself in EEG hemisphere asymmetries (Dawson, 1994a).

Researchers such as Davidson, Fox, and Dawson have hypothesized that the frontal lobes act in concert as an approach–withdrawal system, with the left hemisphere specialized for approach-related behaviors and emotions, such as joy, interest, and anger, and the right hemisphere specialized for withdrawal-related behaviors and emotions, such as distress, sadness, and disgust (Dawson, 1994a). Emotions associated with approach toward the environment have been found to activate the left frontal lobe, while emotions that prompt withdrawal have been found to activate the right frontal lobe (Dawson, 1994a). According to Davidson (1994a), the capacity of the left and right lobes to be differentiated as approach and withdrawal systems, respectively, is attained via two different circuits in the brain. Davidson (1994a) hypothesized that innervations from the basal ganglia, amygdala, sensory and association cortex, cingulate, and dorsolateral prefrontal cortex, particularly on the left side, are involved in the circuitry of the approach system. These brain regions are hypothesized to be involved in the memory and expression of a goal, motivation for action, and attention—all factors believed to be important for approach-related behavior. Davidson (1994a) hypothesized that the circuit for withdrawal emotions and behavior involves the amygdala, temporal polar regions, basal ganglia, and hypothalamus.

Activation and inhibition of the left and right frontal cortex are thought to serve different functions and lead to different results: Disinhibition of one side does not equal activation of the other side (Fox, 1994). Increased right frontal activation is thought to be related to anxiety, distress, and crying (Fox, 1994). For example, evidence suggests that social phobic adults exhibit increased right-anterior-hemisphere activation during periods of anticipatory anxiety compared to control subjects (Davidson, 1994a). Decreased right frontal activation is thought to result in indifference or impulsivity, and euphoria (Fox, 1994). Increased left frontal activation is hypothesized to be related to laughter and positive affect (Fox, 1994). Decreased left frontal activation is hypothesized to be linked to depression, inhibition, and negative thoughts and moods (Fox, 1994).

The frontal lobe is believed to be involved not only in the generation of emotions but in emotion regulation. The manner in which the left and right hemispheres interact to regulate emotional reactivity is not clear. One hypothesis is that the left hemisphere modulates the activity of the right hemisphere. One of the functions of positive affect is thought to be the inhibition of negative affect (Davidson, 1994a). Davidson (1994a) has speculated that negative emotion may be regulated via activation of the left frontal cortex. The left hemisphere is hypothesized to exert control over right-hemisphere arousal; therefore, with maturation and increased interhemispheric communication, the left hemisphere may regulate right-hemisphere negative affect (Fox, Bell, & Jones, 1992). Subjects with left prefrontal activation may differ from other subjects in the speed with which negative emotion is diminished once it is aroused, not in the frequency or initial amplitude of the negative emotion that is experienced. Individuals with right frontal activation may be deficient in their ability to terminate a negative affective response once it has been triggered (Wheeler, Davidson, & Tomarken, 1993). Alternatively, frontal asymmetry may reflect individuals' neural thresholds for experiencing particular emotions

(Tomarken, Davidson, Wheeler, & Doss, 1992). For example, individuals with right frontal asymmetry may experience a negative affective response to a low-intensity negative affect elicitor (Wheeler et al., 1993).

EEG and Emotion: Studies with Infants

Though the role of the frontal lobe in emotion expression and regulation has been recognized for decades, many researchers assumed that the frontal lobe is nonfunctional during infancy; therefore, the possibility that the frontal lobe may have an important role in infant affective development was largely ignored (Dawson, Grofer Klinger, Panagiotides, Spieker, & Frey, 1992; Dawson, Panagiotides, Grofer Klinger, & Hill, 1992). However, investigators have recently begun to explore the role of the frontal lobe in the infant's developing range of affective behaviors and in infant emotion regulation. There are now preliminary data to suggest that the frontal lobe is functional, albeit at a simplistic level, from birth (Fox & Davidson, 1986).

According to Fox (1991, 1994), the approach–withdrawal dichotomy is present at birth, and the neonate's initial responses to the environment are largely based on the approach versus withdrawal continuum rather than on discrete emotional responses. Infants expand their range of emotional states by adding and integrating new motor patterns associated with either approach or withdrawal so that by the end of the first year, the approach–withdrawal dichotomy has been differentiated to embody the "basic" emotions that most 1-year-olds experience, including joy, interest, anger, distress, disgust, and fear (Fox, 1991, 1994). Also, communication between the two cerebral hemispheres increases due to maturation of the corpus callosum (the bundle of fibers that connect the two hemispheres); consequently, emotional responses may become a combination of approach and withdrawal and become further differentiated and more complex (Fox et al., 1992). Fox et al. (1992) proposed that the combination of the level of arousal of each hemisphere and the communication between hemispheres interact to produce individual differences in response to specific emotional stimuli. According to Davidson (1994a), evidence suggests that these individual differences in emotional reactivity are influenced by trait-like individual differences in baseline asymmetry. Therefore, as the infant develops, the asymmetry patterns become more solidified, though still susceptible to short-term changes in response to contextual influences (such as exposure to strong affective elicitors). Studies have demonstrated that there is modest stability in asymmetry scores between individuals by the second half of the first year of life (Bell & Fox, 1994). For example, Fox et al. (1992) found modest stability in frontal asymmetry between 7 and 12 months of age. Infants who were more likely to cry at maternal separation across age demonstrated greater relative right frontal activation, whereas infants who were not likely to cry showed greater relative left frontal activation. Frontal asymmetry was modestly stable across the 6 months. Though they become "hard-wired," tendencies to approach or withdraw may be influenced by experiences that can "accentuate, attenuate, or even replace the approach or withdrawal patterns" (Davidson, Ekman, Saron, Senulis, & Friesen, 1990, p. 339). For example, fearful individuals may learn to approach rather than withdraw from the object they fear (Davidson et al., 1990). However, evidence suggests that although approach or withdrawal behavior patterns may change as the result of experience, the original frontal asymmetry patterns may remain (Fox, Calkins, & Bell, 1994).

Researchers have recently begun studying the development and differentiation of frontal lobe asymmetry patterns in neonates and infants. Fox and Davidson (1986) have presented evidence that patterns of asymmetric frontal lobe activation correlating with affective behavior are present in the neonate. When they analyzed newborns' electrocortical response to tasting solutions of water, sucrose, and citric acid, they found that administration of the water solution produced a disgusted response and activated the right hemisphere (frontal and parietal) whereas administration of the sucrose solution produced a significantly shorter disgust response and resulted in greater left-hemisphere activation than did the water solution.

Several studies indicate that asymmetric activation patterns become more specific to the frontal lobes throughout infancy. For example, Davidson and Fox (1982) showed 10-month-old infants a videotape of an actress displaying happy and sad facial expressions. They found that the infants demonstrated greater activity in the left frontal lobe during the happy epochs than during the sad epochs. Parietal recordings could not discriminate between the epochs. Fox and Davidson (1986) speculated that the newborns exhibited parietal asymmetries while the older infants did not because the newborn brain had yet to develop the functional specificity of the older infant brain. By 10 months of age, infants appear to display the same pattern of asymmetry that adults do. Dawson, Panagiotides, et al. (1992) replicated these patterns with a sample of 21-month-olds. These findings lend support to the proposition that the frontal lobe has a unique role in emotion generation/regulation.

In another study, Fox and Davidson (1988) found that when mothers approached their 10-month-old infants, the infants expressed joy with facial movement of two different muscles around the eyes, the zygomatic and orbicularis oculi. The infants responded to approaching strangers with smiles without orbicularis oculi movement. According to Fox and Davidson (1988), only smiles with orbicularis oculi movement are associated with happiness in adults; accordingly, only these smiles were correlated with relative left frontal activation. They speculated that the smiles toward strangers were "unfelt" smiles that signaled wariness and triggered the desire to withdraw; therefore, these types of smiles were correlated with relative right frontal activation. According to Fox and Davidson (1988), these results suggest that infants are able to regulate certain emotions and use subtle expressions, such as the "unfelt" smile, in certain situations by 10 months of age. These results also suggest that though behaviors may appear similar, the underlying motivations (approach or withdrawal) may differ.

Dawson and colleagues (e.g., Dawson, 1994b; Dawson, Panagiotides, et al., 1992) have suggested that it is necessary to study overall frontal activity level as well as electrocortical asymmetry to understand emotional reactivity and regulation. According to Dawson (1994b), emotions can be characterized along two domains: type and intensity. She has speculated that measures of asymmetry predict individual differences in types of emotions expressed, whereas measures of generalized frontal activity predict differences in emotional reactivity and intensity. The two measures are uncorrelated in individuals: Expressions of both happiness and sadness were associated with general increases in frontal lobe activity (Dawson, Panagiotides, et al., 1992). Therefore, individual differences in the intensity and types

of emotions experienced may vary independently (Dawson, 1994b). Dawson, Panagiotides, et al. (1992) hypothesized that the generalized increase in frontal lobe activity is a reflection of the pervasive influence of the subcortical structures on the cortex. Specifically, the subcortical structures activate the entire frontal lobe in order to alert the individual and prepare him or her to perceive and react to external stimuli.

The development of individual patterns of brain activation is believed to be the result of a continual transactional process between genetically coded programs for the formation of structures and the connections among structures and environmental influence (Fox et al., 1994). One manner in which genetic makeup is believed to exert its influence is via temperament.

Kagan and Snidman (1991) have defined temperament as the "variety of initial, inherited profiles that develop into different envelopes of psychological outcomes" (p. 856). According to Bell and Fox (1994) and Calkins, Fox, and Marshall (1996), a child's temperament may be represented by his or her pattern of frontal asymmetry via his or her threshold for positive and negative reactivity and the intensity of his or her reaction to stimuli. Wheeler et al. (1993) found that individual differences in the quality and intensity of adult subjects' responses to positive and negative film clips were related to baseline asymmetry measured 3 weeks prior to the viewing of the clips. Individuals with stable, increased left-sided and decreased right-sided frontal activation described more intense positive affect in response to positive films compared to the other subjects; subjects with increased right-sided frontal activation described more negative responses to the negative films compared to subjects with other patterns of baseline asymmetry. The authors concluded that frontal activation asymmetry acts as a diathesis that influences an individual's vulnerability to certain positive and negative emotions in response to affective elicitors.

Davidson and Fox (1989) found that 10-month-old infants' responses to emotional stressors could also be predicted from frontal activation asymmetry. Infants who demonstrated greater relative right-sided frontal activation at baseline were more likely to show more intense negative affect in response to the stressful event of maternal separation.

Studies measuring electrocortical activity

have begun to shed light on the possible underpinnings of the temperamental construct "behavioral inhibition." Calkins et al. (1996) have defined behavioral inhibition as the tendency to withdraw and display negative affect in response to new people, places, events, and objects. Behaviorally inhibited children tend to find unfamiliar or challenging events more stressful than do noninhibited children (Reznick et al., 1986). According to Kagan and colleagues, behavioral inhibition is a categorical construct, with 10% of healthy, Caucasian, American children displaying extreme behavioral inhibition; these children represent a qualitatively different group of individuals, both behaviorally and biologically, from the remaining 90% (Kagan & Snidman, 1991; Kagan, Reznick, & Gibbons, 1989; Reznick et al., 1986). There is support for the supposition that behaviorally inhibited children are physiologically different from their noninhibited counterparts. Research with inhibited children has found that extremely inhibited children demonstrate a pattern of frontal brain activity similar to that of depressed adult subjects. Compared to uninhibited and noninhibited children, inhibited children, like depressed adults, exhibit left frontal hypoactivation (Davidson, 1992, 1994a; Henriques & Davidson, 1990). Davidson (1994a) suggested that these findings indicate that inhibited children, who are wary to approach novel objects and people, may have an approach deficit (as opposed to an overactive withdrawal system).

Frontal asymmetry may also be related to vulnerability to experience certain psychopathologies. Davidson (1992) proposed that a small percentage of children with the physiological profile of the inhibited child may be vulnerable to psychopathology, such as an affective disorder, in the face of relatively extreme life stressors later in life. However, a larger percentage may be vulnerable to subclinical characteristics such as dysthymic mood, shyness, and decreased positive affect (Davidson, 1992).

Henriques and Davidson (1990) also found evidence in an adult sample that baseline asymmetry may reflect a vulnerability to experience certain emotions and, ultimately, certain psychopathologies. Compared to control subjects who had never been depressed, recovered depressed subjects exhibited decreased relative left-sided activation. Therefore, though they had not been experiencing depressive symptoms for at least 1 year, previously depressed subjects continued to show brain asymmetry patterns consistent with depression, suggesting that frontal asymmetry may reflect trait rather than state characteristics and a possible vulnerability to psychopathology.

The mechanisms by which the environment influences frontal lobe development are not clearly understood. Currently, the role of critical periods of sensitivity to environmental factors is not known (Davidson, 1994a). Many have speculated that the environment may exert its influence on brain asymmetry patterns via synapse formation and pruning (e.g., Dawson, Panagiotides, et al., 1992). According to Thatcher (1994), the frontal cortex has a dominant role in determining which synapses will survive and which will be pruned, exerting significant influence over the organization and reorganization of synapses in the posterior cortical regions. Neuronal groups of cells that are frequently and/or intensely stimulated through environmental stimulation are thought to be selectively amplified, forming cortical maps with defined functions (Dawson, Hessl, & Frey, 1994). Conversely, cells that do not form functional synapses are retracted (Huttenlocher, 1979, 1994; Huttenlocher & Dabbholkar, 1997).

Dawson and colleagues (e.g., Dawson, Grofer Klinger, Panagiotides, Hill, & Spieker, 1992; Dawson, Grofer Klinger, Panagiotides, Spieker, et al., 1992) have conducted a series of experiments to examine the relation between maternal depressive symptomatology and infant frontal lobe development, and they have found several differences in the EEG patterns between infants of nonsymptomatic and symptomatic mothers. For example, during a game of peek-a-boo with their mothers, 11- to 17-month-old infants of symptomatic mothers did not show differential frontal lobe activation, whereas infants of nonsymptomatic mothers demonstrated greater left than right frontal lobe activation. All the infants who scored one standard deviation below the mean for left frontal lobe activation during the play segment were infants of symptomatic mothers (Dawson, Grofer Klinger, Panagiotides, Hill, et al., 1992). Dawson, Frey, Panagiotides, Osterling, and Hessl (1997) also found, in a sample of 13- to 15-month-old infants, that infants of depressed mothers differed from infants of nondepressed mothers primarily in left frontal power. The patterns of brain activation appear to be trait rather than state characteristics: In both studies, the patterns of frontal lobe activation were not correlated with infant or maternal affective behavior. These results are consistent with the findings among adults that depression is associated with decreased left frontal lobe activation relative to right (Henriques & Davidson, 1990).

Field and colleagues (Field, Fox, Pickens, & Nawrocki, 1995) have found that infants as young as 3 months of age demonstrate brain activity patterns related to maternal depression status. Infants 3 to 6 months old who had mothers who endorsed a significantly high number of depressive symptoms were more likely to exhibit patterns of right frontal EEG asymmetry than were infants of nondepressed mothers. These findings are consistent with those of numerous observational studies that have found that infants of depressed mothers tend to demonstrate behaviors associated with right frontal hyperactivation as well as left frontal hypoactivation, including increased fussiness, withdrawal, frequent gaze aversion, tension, rapid deterioration under stress, lowered physical activity, and reduced positive affect (Cutrona & Troutman, 1986; Field et al., 1985; Gelfand & Teti, 1990; Hopkins, Campbell, & Marcus, 1987; Mayberry & Affonso, 1993; Ventura & Stevenson, 1986; Whiffen, 1988; Whiffen & Gotlib, 1989). Though the hypothesis that the negative affect and mood common among infants of depressed mothers may reflect an endogenous trait cannot be dismissed, several researchers have suggested that infants of depressed mothers demonstrate relative right frontal EEG asymmetry as the result of repeated exposure to a depressed mother. Dawson, Frey, et al. (1997) found that the number of postnatal months of maternal depression was significantly related to infant frontal EEG pattern, whereas the number of prenatal months of maternal depression was not. This finding suggests that exposure to the depressogenic environment may be necessary to produce the atypical EEG patterns seen in infants of depressed mothers.

The way in which maternal depression influences infant frontal lobe activity is not well understood. Researchers have speculated on how depression may influence brain development by considering what is known about depressed maternal behavior and what is thought to be critical for healthy emotional development in the infant. According to Field, Healy, Goldstein, and Guthertz (1990), in normal mother–infant interactions, the mother regulates her behavior to meet the needs of her infant so that the infant is appropriately stimulated. Optimally, the mother's and infant's attentive and affective behaviors become synchronized. In the depressed mother–infant dyad, the depressed mother is often emotionally unavailable or affectively unresponsive; consequently, the infant may experience behavioral disorganization, and the mother's and infant's attentive/affective behaviors would become desynchronized. Field et al. (1990) suggested that such desynchronization leads to failure of the infant to develop arousal modulation and organized attentive/affective behavior.

In a study of interactions between depressed and nondepressed mothers and their 3-month-old infants, Field et al. (1990) found that depressed mothers and their infants spent significantly less time in shared affective states and that their interactions tended to be less coherent than those of nondepressed mothers and their infants, suggesting that early interactions among depressed mothers and their infants may be less synchronous than those of nondepressed mothers and their infants. Also, infants of depressed mothers were more likely to share negative states with their mothers and less likely to share positive states than infants of nondepressed mothers. Field et al. (1990) suggested that the infants may be reflecting their mothers' predominant mood states. Several other studies have found that depressed mothers engage in less optimal interactional behavior with their infants than do nondepressed mothers. Livingood, Daen, and Smith (1983) found that compared to nondepressed mothers, depressed mothers gazed less at their infants and displayed less continuity of rocking and lower levels of unconditional positive regard toward their infants 2 days postpartum. According to Field et al. (1985), depressed mothers, in face-to-face interactions with their 4-month-old infants, looked more depressed or anxious and showed less contented facial expression (i.e., more flat or tense), less activity, fewer imitative behaviors, fewer contingent responses, and less game playing than did nondepressed mothers.

The lack of attentive/affective synchronization and the exposure to high levels of negative affectivity found among depressed mother–infant dyads may have a significant impact on the pruning of brain synapses and organization of neuronal groups, particularly during the first

2 years of life when the frontal lobe is undergoing rapid transformations. Exposure to increased levels of maternal negativity, including flat affect, withdrawal, and intrusiveness, may lead to amplification of neuronal groups associated with negative affectivity and withdrawal behavior (i.e., in the right frontal lobe), while lack of exposure to sufficient levels of positive affectivity may lead to pruning of synapses associated with positive, approach behavior (i.e., in the left frontal lobe). This pattern of amplification and pruning would be expected to be reflected in relative right frontal asymmetry, a pattern commonly found among infants of depressed mothers. Once established, the cortical maps become progressively less vulnerable to change (Dawson et al., 1994). These maps guide the infant in interpreting future experiences with the external environment (Dawson et al., 1994).

If such speculation is true, infants should demonstrate a particular sensitivity to long-term effects from exposure to maternal depression during the first few years of life. Although researchers have had difficulty separating the effects of chronicity and severity of maternal depression from that of timing, there is evidence to support the hypothesis that infants are particularly sensitive to the effects of maternal depression between 6 and 18 months of age (Alpern & Lyons-Ruth, 1993; Dawson, Frey, et al., 1997; Dawson et al., 1994). A number of studies have found that exposure to maternal depression during this period predicts emotional and cognitive difficulties during the preschool and early school years, regardless of mothers' depression status during these later years (Alpern & Lyons-Ruth, 1993; Coghill, Caplan, Alexandra, Robson, & Kumar, 1986; Wolkind, Zajicek-Coleman, & Ghodsian, 1980). Dawson et al. (1994) have noted that this vulnerability may be due to the state of the frontal lobe and the salient developmental tasks to be achieved during that period of development. During 6 to 18 months, there is a rapid growth of the frontal lobe as well as a period of synaptic excess in this region (Chugani & Phelps, 1986; Dawson et al., 1994; Huttenlocher, 1979). Because the frontal lobe plays a critical role in the development of self-regulatory behaviors during this time and because these self-regulatory behaviors are heavily influenced by parental behavior, the period of 6 to 18 months may be a time of particular vulnerability to the effects of maternal depression on frontal lobe development and the ability to regulate emotion (Dawson et al., 1994).

Dawson, Frey, et al. (1997) have evidence that may lend support to the hypothesis that exposure to maternal depression leads to hyperarousal of brain areas associated with experience and expression of negative emotion and/or hypoarousal of brain areas that moderate negative emotion. Among infants of depressed mothers, severity of maternal depression, as assessed by level of depressive symptomatology, was related to infant EEG asymmetry scores. Infants who were exposed to the most severe depressive symptoms exhibited the most extreme negative asymmetry EEG scores. Furthermore, Dawson, Panagiotides, Grofer Klinger, and Spieker (1997) found that compared to infants of nondepressed mothers, infants of depressed mothers showed increased frontal EEG activation during the display of negative emotions but not during the display of neutral expressions or positive emotions. They proposed that these findings may suggest that certain brain regions of the frontal lobe may be selectively activated early in life in infants of depressed mothers. They postulated that heightened activation of specific areas of the frontal lobes may be related to a greater likelihood of expressing certain emotions or to expressing certain emotions more intensely.

Evidence suggests that maternal depressive symptomatology interacts with other environmental factors to influence infant electrocortical activity. Dawson, Grofer Klinger, Panagiotides, Spieker, et al. (1992) reported an interaction between maternal depressive symptomatology, attachment status, and infant electrocortical activity. They found that during baseline and play with the mother, insecurely attached infants of symptomatic and nonsymptomatic mothers did not differ in frontal EEG asymmetry scores. Furthermore, among infants of symptomatic mothers, the insecurely attached demonstrated greater relative left frontal lobe activation than the securely attached during maternal separation (Dawson, Grofer Klinger, Panagiotides, Spieker, et al., 1992). The authors speculated that an insecure attachment may serve as a protective factor for infants of symptomatic mothers. All but one of the insecurely attached infants in their study were classified as avoidant; this suggests that the avoidant infants of symptomatic mothers may prevent the development of brain patterns found among securely attached infants of symptomatic mothers by reducing their exposure to their mothers (Dawson, Grofer Klinger, Panagiotides, Spieker, et al., 1992).

Summary

The frontal lobe plays a critical role in emotion generation and regulation from an early age. This region of the brain appears to be dichotomized into an approach–withdrawal system, with the approach system localized to the left frontal lobe and the withdrawal to the right frontal lobe. The relative activation and interaction of the left and right lobes are thought to be associated with individual patterns of emotional reactivity. Research also suggests that individual activation patterns are initially somewhat plastic and become more fixed over time. Individual patterns of activation appear to be influenced by environmental factors. Specifically, exposure to maternal depression during a critical period of frontal lobe development—most likely 6 to 18 months—has been linked to a specific pattern of frontal lobe activation found among depressed adults.

CONCLUSIONS

Our goal in writing this chapter was to provide a framework for considering how research in the brain sciences can facilitate our understanding of infant mental health. We began by providing an overview of brain development. Here we demonstrated that even as early as the first months after conception, the embryonic and fetal brain can be influenced by exogenous factors, such as maternal stress. We then proceeded to show that experiential effects on brain development continue postnatally. Indeed, outside sensory functions (e.g., the development of the visual system or the speech system onto which the language system scaffolds itself), and possibly some aspects of emotional development, we made it clear that experience can exert its influence on brain development well beyond the first years of life. It is likely that this is made possible by two events. The first is the relatively long trajectory of overproducing synapses and then the retraction of these exuberant connections based on experience. The second is the potential for synapses to be altered by experience at many points in the lifespan (e.g., increased dendritic arborization due to experience).

The potential for the brain to be modified by experience was richly illustrated by the next topic we discussed, the relation between brain and affect as measured by the EEG. Here it was made clear that infants of depressed mothers show altered patterns of EEG activity, suggesting that these patterns may have come about based on exposure to maternal depression. Unfortunately, receiving far less study are the effects of *positive* rearing experiences on infant brain development; for example, we do not know whether there are beneficial effects to being reared by highly competent, sensitive caretakers, and if there are, how these effects would be manifested by the EEG, and whether there is a critical or sensitive period for these effects to be realized. In a related fashion, we know nothing about protective factors, such as those that might transpire in a family with a depressed mother but with an infant of positive temperament and an otherwise high-functioning family. Finally, also unknown is the extent to which we can intervene in the life of the "at risk" (for depression or other internalizing disorders) infant, based on the principles of neuroscience. It is desirable to think that the trajectory of infants affected by negative experiences can be positively altered by intervening life events, such as by (1) successfully treating the mother's depression or (2) providing the infant with compensatory experiences.

It should be apparent that we have much work ahead of us. A particular need lies in the development of methods that are suitable for studying the relation between brain development and behavioral development (see Nelson & Bloom, 1997, for elaboration). A second area that needs investigation concerns conceptualizing what risk and protective factors mean in the context of neural plasticity. Despite the paucity of information on these topics, it is our belief that the time is right for research in the neurosciences to be filtered down to work in the behavioral sciences. It would be our hope that investigators in both camps join forces to present a unified front in improving our understanding of infant development and in developing intervention programs that are based on the sound principles of the brain sciences.

ACKNOWLEDGMENTS

Writing of this chapter was made possible, in part, by grants to Charles A. Nelson from the

National Institutes of Health (NS32976) and the John D. and Catherine T. MacArthur Foundation (through their research networks on *Psychopathology and Development* and *Early Experience and Brain Development*), and to Michelle Bosquet from a fellowship from the National Science Foundation.

REFERENCES

Albers, L., Johnson, D. E., Hostetter, M., Iverson, S., Georgieff, M., & Miller, L. (1997). Health of children adopted from the former Soviet Union and Eastern Europe: Comparison with pre-adoptive medical records. *Journal of the American Medical Association, 278,* 922–924.

Alpern, L., & Lyons-Ruth, K. (1993). Preschool children at social risk: Chronicity and timing of maternal depressive symptoms and child behavior at school and at home. *Development and Psychopathology, 5,* 371–387.

Ames, E. W. (1997). *The development of Romanian orphanage children adopted to Canada.* Final report to Human Resources Development, Canada.

Bell, M. A., & Fox, N. A. (1994). Brain development over the first year of life: Relations between electroencephalographic frequency and coherence and cognitive and affective behaviors. In G. Dawson & K. W. Fischer (Eds.), *Human behavior and the developing brain* (pp. 314–345). New York: Guilford Press.

Benoit, T. C., Jocelyn, L. J., Moddemann, D. M., & Embree, J. E. (1996). Romanian adoption: The Manitoba experience. *Archives of Pediatric and Adolescent Medicine, 150,* 1278–1282.

Black, J. E., Jones, T. A., Nelson, C. A., & Greenough, W. T. (1998). Neuronal plasticity and the developing brain. In N. E. Alessi, J. T. Coyle, S. I. Harrison, & S. Eth (Eds.), *Handbook of child and adolescent psychiatry: Vol. 6. Basic psychiatric science and treatment* (pp. 31–53). New York: Wiley.

Blakemore, C. (1991). Sensitive and vulnerable periods in the development of the visual system. In G. R. Bock & J. Whelan (Eds.), *The childhood environment and adult disease* (Ciba Symposium No. 156, pp. 129–154). Chichester, UK: Wiley.

Bremner, J. D., Randall, P., Scott, T. M., Bronen, R. A., Seibyl, J. P., Southwick, S. M., Delaney, R. C., McCarthy, G., Charney, D. S., & Innis, R. B. (1995). MRI-based measurement of hippocampal volume in patients with combat-related posttraumatic stress disorder. *American Journal of Psychiatry, 152,* 973–981.

Bremner, J. D., Randall, P., Vermetten, E., Staib, L., Bronen, R. A., Mazure, C., Capelli, S., McCarthy, G., Innis, R. B., & Charney, D. S. (1997). Magnetic resonance imaging-based measurement of hippocampal volume in posttraumatic stress disorder related to childhood physical and sexual abuse—a preliminary report. *Biological Psychiatry, 41,* 23–32.

Calkins, S. D., Fox, N. A., & Marshall, T. R. (1996). Behavioral and physiological antecedents of inhibited and uninhibited behavior. *Child Development, 67,* 523–540.

Chugani, H. T., & Phelps, M. E. (1986). Maturational changes in cerebral function in infants determined by 18FDG positron emission tomography. *Science, 231,* 840–843.

Clarke, A. S., Hedeker, D. R., Ebert, M. H., Schmidt, D. E., McKinney, W. T., & Kraemer, G. W. (1996). Rearing experience and biogenic amine activity in infant rhesus monkeys. *Biological Psychiatry, 40,* 338–352.

Coghill, S. R., Caplan, H. L., Alexandra, H., Robson, K., & Kumar, R. (1986). Impact of maternal postnatal depression on cognitive development of young children. *British Medical Journal, 292,* 1165–1167.

Crair, M. C., Gillespie, D. C., & Stryker, M. P. (1998). The role of visual experience in the development of columns in cat visual cortex. *Science, 279,* 566–570.

Crittenden, P., & DiLalla, D. (1988). Compulsive compliance: The development of an inhibitory coping strategy in infancy. *Journal of Abnormal Child Psychology, 16,* 585–599.

Curtis, S. (1977). *Genie: A psycholinguistic study of a modern-day "wild child."* London: Academic Press.

Cutrona, C. E., & Troutman, B. R. (1986). Social support, infant temperament, and parenting self-efficacy: A mediational model of postpartum depression. *Child Development, 57,* 1507–1518.

Davidson, R. J. (1992). Anterior cerebral asymmetry and the nature of emotion. *Brain and Cognition, 20,* 125–151.

Davidson, R. J. (1994a). Asymmetric brain function, affective style, and psychopathology: The role of early experience and plasticity. *Development and Psychopathology, 6,* 741–758.

Davidson, R. J. (1994b). Temperament, affective style, and frontal lobe asymmetry. In G. Dawson & K. W. Fischer (Eds.), *Human behavior and the developing brain* (pp. 518–536). New York: Guilford Press.

Davidson, R. J., Ekman, P., Saron, C. D., Senulis, J. A., & Friesen, W. V. (1990). Approach–withdrawal and cerebral asymmetry: Emotional expression and brain physiology: I. *Journal of Personality and Social Psychology, 58,* 330–341.

Davidson, R. J., & Fox, N. A. (1982). Asymmetrical brain activity discriminates between positive and negative affective stimuli in human infants. *Science, 218,* 1235–1237.

Davidson, R. J., & Fox, N. A. (1989). Frontal brain asymmetry predicts infants' response to maternal separation. *Journal of Abnormal Psychology, 98,* 127–131.

Dawson, G. (1994a). Development of emotional expression and emotion regulation in infancy: Contributions of the frontal lobe. In G. Dawson & K. W. Fischer (Eds.), *Human behavior and the developing brain* (pp. 346–379). New York: Guilford Press.

Dawson, G. (1994b). Frontal electroencephalographic correlates of individual differences in emotion expression in infants: A brain systems perspective on emotion. In N. A. Fox (Ed.), Emotion regulation: Behavioral and biological considerations. *Monographs of the Society for Research in Child Development, 59*(Serial No. 2–3), 135–151.

Dawson, G., Frey, K., Panagiotides, H., Osterling, J., & Hessl, D. (1997). Infants of depressed mothers exhibit atypical frontal brain activity: A replication and extension of previous findings. *Journal of Child Psychology and Psychiatry, 38,* 179–186.

Dawson, G., Grofer Klinger, L., Panagiotides, H., Hill, D., & Spieker, S. (1992). Frontal lobe activity and affective behavior in infants of mothers with depressive symptoms. *Child Development, 63,* 725–737.

Dawson, G., Grofer Klinger, L., Panagiotides, H., Spieker, S., & Frey, K. (1992). Infants of mothers with depressive symptoms: Electroencephalographic and behavioral findings related to attachment status. *Development and Psychopathology, 4,* 67–80.

Dawson, G., Hessl, D., & Frey, K. (1994). Social influences on early developing biological and behavioral systems related to risk for affective disorder. *Development and Psychopathology, 6,* 759–779.

Dawson, G., Panagiotides, H., Grofer Klinger, L., & Hill, D. (1992). The role of frontal lobe functioning in the development of infant self-regulatory behavior. *Brain and Cognition, 20,* 152–175.

Dawson, G., Panagiotides, H., Grofer Klinger, L., & Spieker S. (1997). Infants of depressed and nondepressed mothers exhibit differences in frontal brain electrical activity during the expression of negative emotions. *Developmental Psychology, 33,* 650–656.

Elbert, T., Pantev, C., Weinbruch, C., Rockstroh, B., & Taub, E. (1995). Increased cortical representation of the fingers of the left hand in string players. *Science, 270,* 305–307.

Fameli, M., Katraki, E., & Stylianopoulou, F. (1994). Effects of hyperactivity of the maternal hypothalamic–pituitary–adrenal (HPA) axis during pregnancy on the development of the HPA axis and brain monoamine of the offspring. *International Journal of Developmental Neuroscience, 12,* 651–659.

Field, T., Fox, N. A., Pickens, J., & Nawrocki, T. (1995). Relative right frontal EEG activation in three- to six-months-old infants of "depressed" mothers. *Developmental Psychology, 31,* 358–363.

Field, T., Healy, B., Goldstein, S., & Guthertz, M. (1990). Behavior–state matching and synchrony in mother–infant interactions of nondepressed versus depressed dyads. *Developmental Psychology, 26,* 7–14.

Field, T., Sandberg, D., Garcia, R., Vega-Lahr, N., Goldstein, S., & Guy, L. (1985). Pregnancy problems, postpartum depression, and early mother–infant interactions. *Developmental Psychology, 21,* 1152–1156.

Fisher, L., Ames, E. W., Chisholm, K., & Savoie, L. (1997). Problems reported by parents of Romanian orphans adopted to British Columbia. *International Journal of Behavioral Development, 20,* 67–82.

Fox, N. A. (1991). If it's not left, it's right: Electroencephalograph asymmetry and the development of emotion. *American Psychologist, 46,* 863–872.

Fox, N. A. (1994). Dynamic cerebral processes underlying emotion regulation. In N. A. Fox (Ed.), Emotion regulation: Behavioral and biological considerations. *Monographs of the Society for Research in Child Development, 59*(Serial No. 2–3), 152–166.

Fox, N. A., & Bell, M. A. (1990). Electrophysiological indices of frontal lobe development: Relations to cognitive and affective behavior in human infants over the first year of life. *Annals of the New York Academy of Sciences, 608,* 677–704.

Fox, N. A., Bell, M. A., & Jones, N. A. (1992). Individual differences in response to stress and cerebral asymmetry. *Developmental Neuropsychology, 8,* 161–184.

Fox, N. A., Calkins, S. D., & Bell, M. A. (1994). Neural plasticity and development in the first two years of life: Evidence from cognitive and socioemotional domains of research. *Development and Psychopathology, 6,* 677–696.

Fox, N. A., & Davidson, R. J. (1986). Taste-elicited changes in facial signs of emotion and the asymmetry of brain electrical activity in human newborns. *Neuropsychologia, 24,* 417–422.

Fox, N. A., & Davidson, R. J. (1988). Patterns of brain electrical activity during facial signs of emotion in 10-month-old infants. *Developmental Psychology, 24,* 230–236.

Fride, E., & Weinstock, M. (1988). Prenatal stress increases anxiety related behavior and alters cerebral lateralization of dopamine activity. *Life Sciences, 42,* 1059–1065.

Galenson, E. (1986). Some thoughts about infant psychopathology and aggressive development. *International Review of Psycho-Analysis, 13,* 349–354.

Gelfand, D. M., & Teti, D. M. (1990). The effects of maternal depression on children. *Clinical Psychology Review, 10,* 329–353.

Greenough, W. T., & Black, J. E. (1992). Induction of brain structure by experience: Substrates for cognitive development. In M. R Gunnar & C. A. Nelson (Eds.), *Minnesota Symposia on Child Psychology: Vol. 24. Developmental behavioral neuroscience* (pp. 155–200). Hillsdale, NJ: Erlbaum.

Gunnar, M. (1993, April). *Adrenocortical reactivity: Who is more stress vulnerable, the inhibited or bold child.* Paper presented at the symposium on the psychobiology of stress reactivity: Implications for emotional development at the biennial meeting of the Society for Research in Child Development, New Orleans.

Gunnar, M. (1994). Psychoendocrine study of temperament and stress in early childhood: Expanding current models. In J. Bates & T. D. Wachs (Eds.), *Temperament: Individual differences at the interface of biology and behavior* (pp. 175–198). New York: American Psychological Association Press.

Gunnar, M. R. (1997*). Links between stress physiology and environment in influencing the healthy development of children.* Paper prepared for the Workshop on "Research Ideas and Data Needs for Studying the Well-Being of Children and Families" sponsored by the Family and Child Well-Being Research Network and the National Institute of Child Health and Human Development.

Gunnar, M. R. (1998). Quality of early care and buffering of neuroendocrine stress reactions: Potential effects on the developing human brain. *Preventive Medicine, 27,* 208–211.

Gunnar, M. R., Brodersen, L., Krueger, K., & Rigatuso, J. (1996). Dampening of adrenocortical responses during infancy: Normative changes and individual differences. *Child Development, 67,* 877–889.

Gunnar, M., Brodersen, L., & Rigatuso, J. (1993). *Infant and parent contributions to the organization of adrenocortical stress reactivity.* Paper presented at the symposium on the development and organization of stress reactivity at the biennial meeting of the Society for Research in Child Development, New Orleans.

Henriques, J. B., & Davidson, R. J. (1990). Regional brain electrical asymmetries discriminate between previously depressed and healthy control subjects. *Journal of Abnormal Psychology, 99,* 22–31.

Hopkins, J., Campbell, S. B., & Marcus, M. (1987). Role of infant-related stressors in postpartum depression. *Journal of Abnormal Psychology, 96,* 237–241.

Hostetter, M. K., Iverson, S., Dole, K., & Johnson, D. E. (1989). Unsuspected infectious diseases and other medical diagnoses in the evaluation of internationally adopted children. *Pediatrics, 83,* 559–564.

Hostetter, M. K., Iverson, S., Thomas, W., McKenzie, D., Dole, K., & Johnson, D. E. (1991). Prospective medical evaluation of internationally adopted children. *New England Journal of Medicine, 325,* 479–485.

Hubel, D. H., Wiesel, T. N., & LeVay, S. (1977). Plasticity of ocular dominance columns in monkey striate cortex. *Philosophical Transactions of the Royal Society of London* [Biol], *278,* 377–409.

Huttenlocher, P. R. (1979). Synaptic density in human frontal cortex: Developmental changes and effects of aging. *Brain Research, 163,* 195–205.

Huttenlocher, P. R. (1994). Synaptogenesis, synapse elimination, and neural plasticity in human cerebral cortex. In C. A. Nelson (Ed.), *Minnesota Symposia on Child Psychology: Vol. 27. Threats to optimal development: Integrating biological, psychological, and social risk factors* (pp. 35–54). Hillsdale, NJ: Erlbaum.

Huttenlocher, P. R., & Dabhholkar, A. S. (1997). Regional differences in synaptogenesis in human cerebral cortex. *Journal of Comparative Neurology, 387,* 167–178.

Insel, T. R., Kinsley, C. H., Mann, P. E., & Bridges, R. S. (1990). Prenatal stress has long-term effects on brain opiate receptors. *Brain Research, 511,* 93–97.

Jernigan, T. L., Hesselink, J. R., Sowell, E., & Tallal, P. A. (1991). Cerebral structure on magnetic resonance imaging in language- and learning impaired children. *Archives of Neurology, 48,* 539–545.

Jernigan, T. L., & Tallal, P. (1990). Late childhood changes in brain morphology observable with MRI. *Developmental Medicine and Child Neurology, 32,* 379–385.

Johnson, D. E., Albers, L. H., Iverson, S., Mathers, M., Dole, K., Georgieff, M. K., Hostetter, M. K., & Miller, L. C. (1996). Health status of Eastern European orphans referred for adoption. *Pediatric Research, 39,* 134A.

Johnson, D. E., Miller, L. C., Iverson, S., Thomas, W., Franchino, B., Dole, K., Kiernan, M. B., Georgieff, M. K., & Hostetter, M. K. (1993). Post-placement catch-up growth in Romanian orphans with psychosocial short stature. *Pediatric Research, 33,* 89A.

Kagan, J., Reznick, J. S., & Gibbons, J. (1989). Inhibited and uninhibited types of children. *Child Development, 60,* 838–845.

Kagan, J., & Snidman, N. (1991). Temperamental factors in human development. *American Psychologist, 46,* 856–862.

Kandel, E. R., Schwartz, J. H., & Jessell, T. M. (Eds.). (1991). *Principles of neural science* (3rd ed.). New York: Elsevier Press.

Komuro, H., & Rakic, P. (1998). Distinct modes of neuronal migration in different domains of developing cerebellar cortex. *Journal of Neuroscience, 18,* 1478–1490.

Kopp, C. B. (1989). Regulation of distress and negative emotions: A developmental view. *Developmental Psychology, 25,* 343–354.

LeVay, S., & Stryker, M. P. (1979). The development of ocular dominance columns in the cat. In J. A. Ferrendelli (Ed.), *Society for Neuroscience Symposia: Vol. 4. Aspects of developmental neurobiology,* (pp. 83–98). Bethesda, MD: Society for Neuroscience.

LeVay, S., Wiesel, T. N., & Hubel, T. (1980). The development of ocular dominance columns in normal and visually deprived monkeys. *Journal of Comparative Neurology, 191,* 1–51.

Livingood, A. B., Daen, P., & Smith, B. D. (1983). The depressed mother as a source of stimulation for her infant. *Journal of Clinical Psychology, 39,* 369–375.

Lou, H. C., Hansen, D., Nordentoft, M., Pryds, O., Jensen, F., Nim, J., & Hemmingsen, R. (1994). Prenatal stressors of human life affect fetal brain development. *Developmental Medicine and Child Neurology, 36,* 826–832.

Marcovitch, S., Goldberg, S., Gold, A., Washington, L., Wasson, C., Krekewich, K. I., & Handley-Derry, M. (1997). Determinants of behavioural problems in Romanian children adopted in Ontario. *International Journal of Behavioral Development, 20,* 17–32.

Mayberry, L. J., & Affonso, D. D. (1993). Infant temperament and postpartum depression: A review. *Health Care for Women International, 14,* 201–211.

McConnell, S. K. (1995). Strategies for the generation of neuronal diversity in the developing central nervous system. *Journal of Neuroscience, 15,* 6987–6998.

McEwen, B. S., & Sapolsky, R. M. (1995). Stress and cognitive function. *Current Opinion in Neurobiology, 5,* 205–216.

Merzenich, M. M., Jenkins, W. M., Johnston, P., Schreiner, C., Miller, E., & Tallal, P. (1996). Temporal processing deficits of language-learning impaired children ameliorated by training. *Science, 271,* 77–81.

Miller, L. C., Kiernan, T., Mathers, M. I., & Klein-Gitelman, M. (1995). Developmental and nutritional status of internationally adopted children. *Archives of Pediatrics and Adolescent Medicine, 149,* 40–44.

Moyer, J. A., Herrenkohl, L. R., & Jacobowitz, D. M. (1978). Stress during pregnancy: Effect on catecholamines in discrete brain regions of offspring as adults. *Brain Research, 144,* 173–178.

Nachmias, M., Gunnar, M., Mangelsdorf, S., Parritz, R. H., & Buss, K. (1996). Behavioral inhibition and stress reactivity: The moderating role of attachment security. *Child Development, 67,* 508–522.

Nauta, W. J. H. (1971). The problem of the frontal lobe: A reinterpretation. *Journal of Psychiatric Research, 8,* 167–187.

Nelson, C. A. (2000). The neurobiological bases of early intervention. In J. P. Shonkoff & S. J. Meisels (Eds.), *Handbook of early childhood intervention* (2nd ed.). New York: Cambridge University Press.

Nelson, C. A., & Bloom, F. E. (1997). Child development and neuroscience. *Child Development, 68,* 970–987.

Nelson, C. A., & Carver, L. (1998). The effects of stress and trauma on brain and memory: A view from developmental cognitive neuroscience. *Development and Psychopathology, 10,* 793–809.

Neville, H. (1991). Neurobiology of cognitive and language processing: Effects of early experience. In K. R. Gibson & A. C. Petersen (Eds.), *Brain maturation and cognitive development: Comparative and cross-cultural perspectives* (pp. 355–380). Hawthorne, NY: Aldine de Gruyter Press.

Peters, D. A. V. (1982). Prenatal stress: Effects of brain biogenic amine and plasma corticosterone levels. *Pharamacology Biochemistry and Behavior, 17,* 721–725.

Peters, D. A. V. (1984). Prenatal stress: Effect on development of rat brain adrenergic receptors. *Pharmacology Biochemistry and Behavior, 21,* 417–422.

Peters, D. A. V. (1986). Prenatal stress: Effect on development of rat brain serotonergic neurons. *Pharmacology Biochemistry and Behavior, 24,* 1377–1382.

Peters, D. A. V. (1988). Effects of maternal stress during different gestational periods on the serotonergic system in adult rat offspring. *Pharmacology Biochemistry and Behavior, 31,* 839–843.

Peters, D. A. V. (1990). Maternal stress increases fetal brain and neonatal cerebral cortex 5-hydroxytryptamine synthesis in rats: A possible mechanism by which stress influences brain development. *Pharmacology Biochemistry and Behavior, 35,* 943–947.

Provence, S., & Lipton, R. C. (1962). *Infants in institutions: A comparison of their development with family reared infants during the first year of life.* New York: International Universities Press.

Reznick, J. S., Kagan, J., Snidman, N., Gersten, M., Baak, K., & Rosenberg, A. (1986). Inhibited and uninhibited children: A follow-up study. *Child Development, 57,* 660–680.

Schneider, M. L. (1992). The effect of mild stress during pregnancy on birthweight and neuromotor maturation in Rhesus monkey infants (Macaca mulatta). *Infant Behavior and Development, 15,* 389–403.

Schneider, M. L., Clarke, A. S., Kraemer, G. W., Roughton, E. C., Lubach, G. R., Rimm-Kaufman, S., Schmidt, D., & Ebert, M. (1998). Prenatal stress alters brain biogenic amine levels in primates. *Development and Psychopathology, 10,* 427–440.

Schneider-Rosen, K., & Cicchetti, D. (1984). The relationship between affect and cognition in maltreated infants: Quality of attachment and the development of visual self-recognition. *Child Development, 55,* 648–658.

Schneider-Rosen, K., & Cicchetti, D. (1991). Early self-knowledge and emotional development: Visual self-recogntion and affective reactions to mirror self-images in maltreated and non-maltreated toddlers. *Developmental Psychology, 27,* 471–478.

Skeels, H. M. (1966). Adult status of children with contrasting early life experiences. *Monographs of the Society for Research in Child Development, 31,* 1–65.

Spangler, G., & Grossmann, K. E. (1993). Biobehavioral organization in securely and insecurely attached infants. *Child Development, 64,* 1439–1450.

Spitz, R. (1945). Hospitalism: An inquiry into the genesis of psychiatric conditions in early childhood. In A. Freud, H. Hartmann, & E. Kris (Eds.), *The psychoanalytic study of the child* (pp. 53–74). New York: International Universities Press.

Stansbury, K., & Gunnar, M. R. (1994). Adrenocortical activity and emotion regulation. In N. A. Fox (Ed.), Emotion regulation: Behavioral and biological considerations. *Monographs of the Society for Research in Child Development, 59*(Serial No. 2–3), 108–134.

Stein, M. B., Koverola, C., Hanna, C., Torchia, M. G., & McClarty, B. (1997). Hippocampal volume in women victimized by childhood sexual abuse. *Psychological Medicine, 27,* 951–959.

Takahashi, L. K., Turner, J. G., & Kalin, N. H. (1992). Prenatal stress alters brain catecholaminergic activity and potentiates stress-induced behavior in adult rats. *Brain Research, 574,* 131–137.

Tallal, P., Miller, S. L., Bedi, G., Byma, G., Wang, X., Nagarajan, S. S., Schreiner, C., Jenkins, W. M., & Merzenich, M. M. (1996). Language comprehension in language-learning impaired children improved with acoustically modified speech. *Science, 271,* 81–84.

Thatcher, R. W. (1994). Psychopathology of early frontal lobe damage: Dependence on cycles of development. *Development and Psychopathology, 6,* 565–596.

Tizard, B., & Hodges, J. (1977). The effect of early institutional rearing on the development of eight-year-old children. *Journal of Child Psychology and Psychiatry, 18,* 99–118.

Tizard, B., & Rees, J. (1975). The effect of early institutional rearing on the behaviour problems and affectional relationships of four-year-old children. *Journal of Child Psychology and Psychiatry, 16,* 61–73.

Tomarken, A. J., Davidson, R. J., Wheeler, R. E., & Doss, R. C. (1992). Individual differences in anterior brain asymmetry and fundamental dimensions of emotion. *Journal of Personality and Social Psychology, 62,* 676–687.

Trevarthen, C., & Aitken, K. J. (1994). Brain development, infant communication, and empathy disorders: Intrinsic factors in child mental health. *Development and Psychopathology, 6,* 597–633.

Ventura, J. N., & Stevenson, M. B. (1986). Relations of mothers' and fathers' reports of infant temperament, parents' psychological functioning, and family characteristics. *Merrill–Palmer Quarterly, 32,* 275–289.

Wheeler, R. E., Davidson, R. J., & Tomarken, A. J. (1993). Frontal brain asymmetry and emotional reactivity: A biological substrate of affective style. *Psychophysiology, 30,* 82–89.

Whiffen, V. E. (1988). Vulnerability to postpartum depression: A prospective multivariate study. *Journal of Abnormal Psychology, 97,* 467–474.

Whiffen, V. E., & Gotlib, I. H. (1989). Infants of postpartum depressed mothers: Temperament and cognitive status. *Journal of Abnormal Psychology, 98,* 274–279.

Wolkind, S. N., Zajicek-Coleman, E., & Ghodsian, M. (1980). Continuities in maternal depression. *International Journal of Family Psychiatry, 1,* 167–182.

Yakovlev, P. I., & LeCours, A.-R. (1967). The myelogenetic cycles of regional maturation of the brain. In A. Minkowski (Ed.), *Regional development of the brain in early life* (pp. 3–70). Oxford: Blackwell Scientific.

4

Infant Social and Emotional Development in Family Context

❖

SUSAN CROCKENBERG
ESTHER LEERKES

With his provocative identification of the mother–infant relationship as the basis of all future love relationships, Freud (1905/1953) focused attention on the early family context in the search for greater understanding of the origins of emotional adjustment and psychopathology. In the last three decades the scope of that search has expanded significantly to include the web of family relationships in which infant social–emotional development occurs. Fathers, grandparents, and siblings have been studied as sources of influence on development in the first 3 years of life (see Crockenberg, Lyons-Ruth, & Dickstein, 1993, for a review).

The beneficial impact of family social support on maternal caregiving is well-documented, particularly support provided by the baby's father. Increasingly, the direct impact of fathers on infants has been recognized and investigated as well, due in part to the increase in the amount of time fathers in dual-earner families engage in child care. Recently, researchers have expanded their focus to consider the specific patterns of interactions that characterize fathers and infants, the links between these interactions and infant development, and the processes that explain them, as we discuss later.

Like fathers, grandmothers influence infant development indirectly, through their support of mothers, and directly, through their contact and interaction with infants themselves. They are often the major source of social support for adolescent mothers. Grandparents interact sim-

ilarly to parents with their grandchildren, and infants who see their grandmothers regularly treat them almost interchangeably with parents. Grandmothers serve also as primary caregivers of their infant grandchildren when parents are unable or unwilling to do so. As of 1990, there were 3.2 million children in the United States living with their grandparents or other kin, an increase of 40% in 10 years (as cited in Minkler & Roe, 1993). This practice has increased as male unemployment, drug addiction, and the number of "out of wedlock" births have increased, and the age of unmarried mothers decreased in low-income, minority communities (Burton & Dilworth-Anderson, 1991), but it is not limited to such families, as evidenced by the growth of grandparent support groups and publications oriented toward more affluent caregiving grandparents (Doucette-Dudman, 1996). Nor are grandparent effects limited to their current impact on children and grandchildren. As Fraiberg (1980) dramatized so effectively in her reference to "ghosts in the nursery," unbidden thoughts and feelings born in prior relationships influence parents' perceptions and reactions to their infants (van IJzendoorn, 1995).

Another significant shift in the study of infant social–emotional development is the recognition of the infant's role in the construction of caregiving relationships (Bell, 1971; Sameroff & Chandler, 1975). Since Thomas, Chess, and Birch's (1968) groundbreaking longitudinal study of infant temperamental differences, the possibility that infants contribute to their own development has become a near certainty (Rothbart & Bates, 1998), although the processes by which this effect occurs remain under active investigation. Infants' temperament or reactivity may elicit dysfunctional responses from caregivers, interact with caregiver behavior to influence development, and influence what regulatory strategies will be effective (Crockenberg, 1986).

In the review that follows, we present what is known about infant development in the context of multiple family relationships. Nevertheless, we focus on mothers and infants, given the reality that mothers, by birth or circumstance, remain the primary caregivers of infants under most circumstances. As a consequence, their dyadic relationship will likely have the greatest impact on infant social–emotional development and mental health.

From the first days of life, infants demonstrate awareness of their environment and evidence of learning (Stern, 1985), confirming that different family experiences likely affect infant development far earlier than once thought possible. At the same time, growing knowledge of basic processes involved in early developmental change provides a basis for understanding how early social interactions influence infant development. We integrate this knowledge below in an effort to more completely explain infant social–emotional development and to indicate why some interventions should be more effective than others in facilitating adaptive infant development at particular points in development.

DEVELOPMENTAL TRANSITIONS DURING INFANCY

The rapid shifts in physiological, motor, cognitive, social, and emotional development during the first 3 years of life, and evidence that experience and physiology act together to prompt these changes, identify infancy as a prime time for the emergence of developmental trajectories that increase or reduce the likelihood of later emotional and behavioral dysfunction. Three major periods of reorganization have been identified, 2 to 3 months, 7 to 9 months, and 18 to 20 months, with quantitative changes and smaller shifts occurring throughout the intervals between transition points.

2- to 3-Month Transition

At roughly 2 to 3 months of age infants become more focused, better organized, and more communicative and, hence, more efficient learners and more enjoyable social partners. Growth of synapses in the cortex, myelination of visual pathways, and other changes in the brain likely underlie infants' enhanced cognitive capacities, as reflected in classical and operant conditioning, habituation, and receptive and expressive communication, including social smiling. Infants remember longer, with less exposure, increasing the likelihood that repeated patterns of social interactions will be anticipated and alterations noted, with potentially disruptive effects on regulatory and interactive behavior. Patterns of vocal turn taking begin to appear, indicating infants' awareness of their caregivers' behavior and, hence, increasing its potential to have an impact on their development in a variety of areas (Tronick, Cohn, & Shea, 1986; Field, 1994). Specific emotions begin to emerge also, with joy differentiating from contentment, sadness, and, later, anger differentiating from general distress (Lewis, 1993).

7- to 9-Month Transition

Stern (1985) has termed the shift that occurs between seven and nine months "the discovery of intersubjectivity," based on behaviors indicating that infants now understand that their own thoughts and feelings can be shared and that they understand the thoughts and desires of others. Infants begin to detect different affective states in their social partners and use these to regulate their emotions and behavior (i.e., social referencing; Campos & Stenberg, 1981), and they exhibit means–end behavior in a range of contexts (e.g., using emotions and, later, gestures and words in pursuit of goals and directed toward specific others). These abilities underlie the development of emotional–behavioral strategies infants use to maintain contact with attachment figures, the basis for classifying relationships as secure, insecure, and disorganized (Ainsworth, Blehar, Walters, & Wall, 1978). Emde (1984) has termed the 7- to 9-month shift the "onset of focused attachment." Success in this arena likely contributes to an emerging sense of efficacy, the belief or expectation that they will be successful in attaining goals.

Infants also demonstrate object permanence,

the ability to retain a mental image of an object, which is thought to explain the development of stranger wariness and separation protest behaviors that mark the emergence of specific attachments. At the same time, the increased mobility associated with the onset of crawling and later walking increases infants' capacities to explore the world, providing additional opportunities for the development of feelings of efficacy. Extensive concurrent changes in brain development have been documented, including improved inhibitory control of higher centers and more sophisticated associations between neural pathways, which prompt behavioral advances and are stimulated by them.

18- to 20-Month Transition

A qualitative advance in symbolic representation characterizes the 18–20-month shift and is accompanied by an increase in localization and specialization of brain function associated with advances in language competence. Infants are better able to remember specific past events and sequences in the absence of those events, to form representations based on repeated events, and to use representations of past experience to inform future behavior, as in the "working models" of relationships infants are thought to develop through interactions with their primary caregivers. These representational abilities provide the basis also for an objective sense of self, apparent in toddlers' recognition of themselves in mirrors and photographs (Kagan, 1981; Lewis & Brooks-Gunn, 1979), in their use of personal pronouns as language expands rapidly during this period, and, subsequently, in their ability to label and evaluate themselves in relation to standards, as girls or boys, good or bad, and more or less effective in achieving goals.

The identification of personal goals and the ability to hold them in mind increases goal-directed behavior and also the possibility of conflict between infants and caregivers. At the same time, the emergence of self-conscious emotions, such as shame, guilt, and embarrassment, and of true empathy (Emde, Johson, & Easterbrooks, 1988; Lewis, Sullivan, Stanger, & Weiss, 1989), together with a greatly enhanced ability to comprehend and use language, allow toddlers to regulate their behavior in the service of social goals (i.e., to develop goal-corrected partnerships) and contribute to an emerging morality.

These accomplishments in social–emotional development during the first 3 years provide the organizational structure for this review. We begin by discussing emotion regulation, then attachment security, compliance and autonomy, and mastery/self-effectance. Although we organize these achievements chronologically and hierarchically, we believe that each of these developmental processes are ongoing throughout infancy and that they develop transactionally in relation to each other over time. Although economic circumstances and events external to families affect the nature of the relationships that evolve within them, impacting both parenting and infant development (Bronfenbrenner, 1979; see Aber, Jones, & Cohen, Chapter 6, this volume), we consider the broader social context below primarily in relation to designing appropriate and effective interventions for infants and families.

EMOTION REGULATION

Emotion regulation is the keystone of social–emotional development during infancy. The strategies infants develop to regulate emotion during the first year of life are theorized to underlie secure attachment relationships and to contribute to the achievement of autonomy and mastery in the second and third years of life, as well as the development of emotion-related behavior problems.

Parent–infant interaction is the primary context in which emotion regulation begins to emerge. A decade ago, Kopp (1989) articulated the view that infants first learn about modulating distress from their caregivers. Parents assist their infants in alleviating negative emotions, reinforce positive emotions, and structure the environments in which infants experience emotions (Thompson, 1994). Beyond this, parents influence how infants interpret situations as well as how and when infants regulate their emotions. Thus, we consider how parents, typically mothers, influence their infants' developing regulatory abilities and how infants contribute to this process.

Defining Emotional Reactivity and Emotion Regulation

Thompson (1994) defined emotion regulation as individuals' attempts to monitor, evaluate, and modify their emotional reactions, particularly in pursuit of a goal. These regulation attempts may involve internal or external processes, distinctions Eisenberg (1997) labeled emotion regulation and emotion-related behavior regulation. Emotion regulation involves the maintenance or modification of physiological arousal or internal feeling states. Emotion-related behavioral regulation refers to modulation of the overt expression of emotion (i.e., the frequency, intensity, or duration of the facial expressions, vocalizations, and actions that serve as external signals of internal states). These regulatory behaviors are typically goal-directed and, hence, may involve attempts to modify the context in which the emotion was elicited. As we discuss below, maintaining proximity to mother is a primary goal during the second half of the first year of life, and emotion-related behavioral regulation is undertaken in its service.

The centrality of intensity and duration of emotions in defining emotion regulation links it inextricably to emotional reactivity, that is, the onset, duration, and intensity of the infant's emotional arousal. Infant reactivity, or temperament, influences emotion regulation by determining the intensity range in which emotions are typically expressed and the signals to which parents react. Temperament also influences which regulatory strategies are effective and likely to be adopted by the infant (Cassidy, 1994). At least initially, a highly aroused infant is likely to express negative emotions strongly (e.g., by crying loudly). The intensity or duration of the infant's crying elicits emotional reactions and behaviors in the caregiver, inducing her to respond quickly or slowly, or in ways that are more or less effective in helping the infant to regulate. How a caregiver responds may interact also with the infant's reactivity to influence emotion regulation. Strategies that work with an infant who is not very reactive may be less effective with one who is highly reactive.

In the model outlined previously, reactivity is an internal characteristic of infants that together with exogenous factors contributes to differences in emotion regulation. In addition, constitutionally based differences in infants' capacity to regulate may both influence and be influenced by their reactive tendencies. An infant who becomes highly aroused in response to certain events may be unable to trigger internal mechanisms that lead to regulation (Fox & Calkins, 1993; Calkins, 1994), or, alternatively, an infant with a faulty regulatory system may

be easily aroused. Several types of data suggest that both reactivity and regulation are rooted in the infant's neurophysiology. In a 1982 study, Crockenberg and Smith reported that neonatal irritability in the first 2 weeks of life predicted time to calm during crying bouts at 3 months, independently of maternal responsiveness. Evidence that infants with colic differ from other infants in cry intensity/acoustic frequency, duration of crying bouts, as well as in observed and perceived consolability provides additional support for this thesis (Barr & Lehtonen, 1998; Gustafson & Green, 1998; St. James-Roberts, 1998; Stifter, 1998). In conjunction with caregiver behavior, these initial predispositions lay the groundwork for the development of temperament-linked emotion regulation strategies later in infancy. Mangelsdorf, Shapiro, and Marzolf's (1995) finding that wary 12-month-old infants used more self-soothing when they were exposed to novel stimuli, whereas bold infants used more self-distraction, is consistent with this thesis also, although longitudinal data are needed to elucidate the course of development during the infant's first year.

One implication of the intricate connections between infant emotional reactivity and regulation is that distinguishing the two constructs operationally is challenging. Studies must be carefully designed and findings interpreted cautiously to determine how patterns of emotional regulation develop in infants. Another is that it is essential to identify "effective" caregiver regulatory behaviors in relation to the infant's reactivity and capacity for regulation.

Caregiver Influence on Emotion Regulation

Explanations of the processes by which mother–infant interactions foster infant emotion regulation have focused on the ability of both mothers and infants to respond to and reinforce each other contingently. Tronick et al. (1986) refer to this process as mutual regulation; Field (1994) calls it attunement. Both propose that when mothers and infants are engaged in a contingent cycle of signals and responses, as indicated, for example, by matched affective states, the conditions needed to promote emotion regulation exist. The match indicates that the mother is aware of and is responding appropriately to her infant's affective cues, and vice versa, and that regulation either exists or is in the process of being reestablished. Lack of contingency, as indicated by mismatched affect, sets the stage for behavioral and physiological disorganization in the infant, although these mismatches serve also as opportunities for mothers to repair the interaction and, hence, contribute to the development of adaptive regulatory processes over time (Gianino & Tronick, 1988).

In the context of these early interactions with caregivers (typically mothers), infants learn to control their own emotion-linked behavior and the behavior of others in social interchanges. The quality of these exchanges depends in part on mothers' abilities to read and respond correctly to their infants' signals. Mothers must be able to interpret infant emotions accurately (Kropp & Haynes, 1987; Zeanah, 1998), that is, to recognize when an infant is afraid, angry, or interested, as different emotions call for different responses. To do so, mothers must be emotionally and physically available to their infants. Significantly, when their own working models of relationships as adults reflected ongoing insecurity, mothers perceived a narrower range of infant emotions and were less accurate in their identification of specific infant emotions than secure (autonomous) mothers (Blokland & Goldberg, 1998). Their emotional reactions to infant distress and failure to soothe differed also; in contrast to mothers with insecure (dismissive or preoccupied) models, secure mothers experienced more positive and less negative affect (Adam, Tanaka, Brodersen, & Gunnar, 1998).

According to attachment theorists, the primary goal of infancy is the maintenance of proximity to the primary attachment figure. Cassidy (1994) has argued that it is in the pursuit of this goal that infants first learn about emotion regulation. Essentially, infants tailor their behavior to fit their caregiving environment and optimize the likelihood that their attachment figure will remain close at hand. She identified three distinct patterns of emotion regulation that develop in response to differences in the caregiving environment. When mothers are sensitive to the entire range of infant emotions and respond consistently to their emotion signals, infants are expected to express and integrate the whole range of emotions freely because doing so facilitates proximity to mother. If mothers withdraw from and become emotionally unavailable when their infants are distressed, infants learn to minimize negative affect in an attempt to avoid rejection by the attachment figure. If mothers respond inconsis-

tently to negative emotions, infants learn to heighten or escalate their emotions to maximize the odds that their mothers will remain close or increase their proximity. As we discuss later, these patterns of emotion regulation are congruent with the three attachment classifications identified by Ainsworth et al. (1978).

Although the models described differ in specific ways, they are similar in their focus on contingent mother–infant interaction as the key context for the development of infant emotion regulation. In support of these models, there is increasing evidence that maternal sensitivity, the mother's ability to read her infant's cues and to respond appropriately, influences this process.

Maternal Sensitivity/Responsiveness and Emotion Regulation

Maternal sensitivity includes the timing of the mother's response and the match between her response and the infant's expressed affect. Sensitive responses include increasing contact or retreating briefly, depending on the infant's emotional signal and the context (e.g., backing off when the infant averts her gaze), and doing so promptly. Insensitive responses include a lack of response, poorly timed responses, or intrusive responses (e.g., continuing stimulation after the infant has responded negatively).

Researchers have used several methodologies to investigate the contribution of maternal sensitivity to infant emotion regulation. In the still-face procedure developed by Tronick, Als, Adamson, Wise, and Brazelton (1978), mothers are instructed to interact with their infants as they normally would for 2 minutes, then at a signal to display a face devoid of emotion, and, finally, to reengage their infants in normal interaction. Using this procedure, Tronick, Ricks, and Cohn (1982) found, as expected, that 6-month-old infants who attempted to elicit a maternal response during the still face had mothers who engaged in more elaboration and less over- or undercontrolling behavior during the initial interaction period. A number of investigators have replicated this finding and reported further that infants of intrusive or withdrawn mothers are more likely to display gaze aversion and other avoidant behaviors in the still-face paradigm and in other contexts as well (Belsky, Rovine, & Taylor, 1984; Braungart-Reiker, Garwood, Power, & Notaro, 1998; Cohn, Matias, Tronick, Connell, & Lyons-Ruth,

1986; Egeland & Farber, 1984; Isabella & Belsky, 1991; Isabella, Belsky, & von Eye, 1989; Lyons-Ruth, Connell, Zoll, & Stahl, 1987; Malatesta, Culver, Tesman, & Shepard, 1989).

More recently, researchers have examined infant and maternal behavior during the reengagement period that immediately follows the still face to identify possible carryover effects. Kogan and Carter (1996) found that during the reengagement period, 4-month-old infants of sensitive mothers looked at their mothers, vocalized, smiled, and reached to them. Infants of less sensitive mothers were either resistant (i.e., displayed high levels of negative affect or were unsoothable) or avoidant (i.e., averted their gaze and delayed responding to their bids). Both are indicative of limited or maladaptive regulatory behavior.

van den Boom (1994) confirmed the causal link between maternal sensitivity and infant regulatory behavior experimentally. She identified 100 irritable neonates and their mothers and assigned 50 to an intervention designed to foster maternal sensitivity and responsiveness by teaching mothers to identify their infants' signals, interpret them correctly, and select and implement appropriate responses. The other 50 were assigned to a control group. By the 9-month home observation, intervention mothers were significantly more responsive, stimulating, visually attentive, and appropriately controlling than control mothers. Their infants were more sociable, displayed more self-soothing and exploration, and cried less than infants of control mothers. A follow-up at 3½ years demonstrated the link between infant emotion regulation and children's subsequent ability to interact adaptively with their social and inanimate environments. Intervention mothers continued to show more age-appropriate sensitivity, and their children engaged in more positive social interactions and had fewer behavioral problems (van den Boom, 1995).

Taken together, these findings are congruent with the view that maternal sensitivity facilitates infants' emotion regulation and teaches them to use their caregivers to assist them in regulating emotions and emotion-related behavior. Although the underlying processes have not been fully explicated, it appears that mothers' ability to perceive their infants' emotions accurately is a key feature of maternal sensitivity. By 6 months, these regulatory patterns are well established. Moreover, there is evidence that infants who attempt to elicit maternal responses during the still-face procedure at 6 months are more likely to be securely attached at 12 months (Tronick et al., 1982; Cohn, Campbell, & Ross, 1991).

Paternal Behavior and Infant Emotion Regulation

Despite evidence that fathers have a unique opportunity to influence their infants' regulatory behaviors in the course of rough-and-tumble play, their contribution to infants' emotion regulation has been less well documented (see Parke & Tinsley, 1987, for a review). Fathers engage in more such play with infants than do mothers (Teti, Bond, & Gibbs, 1988), during which they may be instrumental in modulating their infants' emotional arousal. Initially, they may activate arousal and, subsequently, help their infants to reduce arousal before they become dysregulated. Fathers' lack of sensitivity to their infants' emotional signals in the course of physical play may contribute to problems with emotion regulation, particularly for males, with whom fathers are especially likely to play in rougher, more physically stimulating ways (Power & Parke, 1983).

Recently, investigators have documented links between fathers' sensitivity during play and infants' emotion regulation. Volling, Herrera, Notaro, and McElwain (1998) found that when fathers were more sensitive and less intrusive during free play, their 12-month-old infants were more emotionally competent in that context, as indicated by their expression of positive and negative affect, their use of gaze aversion to cope with intrusiveness, and their ability to reduce proximity seeking in the service of exploration and attention to objects. Only fathers' behavior during physical play was associated with male infants' emotional competence, confirming that fathers have a distinctive impact on boys' regulatory capacities through physical play. Diener, Mangelsdorf, McHale, and Frosch (1998) reported further that at 12 months, infants engaged in more proximity seeking toward fathers who had interacted with them more sensitively during structured play at 6 months, suggesting that fathers, like mothers, may influence their infants' regulatory strategies by the middle of the first year of life. Other investigators have failed to find comparable father effects, perhaps because they have not observed fathers in settings that elicit differences in fathers' regulatory behavior, such as physical play, or because fathers in different studies spent differing amounts of time with their infants, affecting their opportunity to influence development (Mangelsdorf, Frosch, & McHale, 1998).

Social Referencing and Emotion Regulation

Another way infants obtain regulatory assistance is through social referencing, that is, by looking to the caregiver for emotional guidance. In doing so, they are expected to be better able to resolve uncertainty, form appraisals of the situation, and regulate emotion and behavior (Campos & Stenberg, 1981). The information gleaned from social referencing alerts infants to the potential danger of a situation and prepares them to mount the behavioral strategies needed for emotion regulation.

Typically, social referencing is examined using Klinnert's (1984) procedure in which a novel stimuli is presented to the infant, and the parent is instructed to offer the infant specific facial and verbal cues. The infant's behavior prior to and following referencing of the parent is observed. Findings from studies of this type indicate that parental affect offers infants information that guides their behavioral and emotional responses. Positive parental affect during referencing is associated with approach behaviors (i.e., looking at, approaching, or touching a novel toy or person and displaying positive affect), whereas negative parental affect is associated with avoidant behaviors (i.e., looking away, distancing from a novel toy or person, and displaying negative affect [Klinnert, 1984; Walden & Ogan, 1988]). Infants reference mothers and fathers similarly (Dickstein & Parke, 1988; Hirshberg & Svejda, 1990), although they are more likely to reference mothers than fathers when no affective signals are offered (Hirshberg & Svejda, 1990).

These studies confirm both that infants reference parents in emotionally arousing contexts and that parents' affective cues likely influence infant behavior, possibly by stimulating or confirming their emotions and activating regulation strategies. Campos and Stenberg (1981) theorized that infants look to parents for an appraisal of an event only if the infant's own appraisal is inadequate. Others contend that by 1 year, infants continue to seek their parents' input even after they have formed their own appraisals (Hornik & Gunnar, 1988; Rosen,

Adamson, & Bakeman, 1992). Support for these divergent views is conflicting (Gunnar & Stone, 1984; Rosen et al., 1992), and other data indicate that parental negative affect, rather than the ambiguity of the situation, elicits social referencing. In Hornik, Risenhoover, and Gunnar's (1987) study, infants displayed fewer positive facial expressions and played less with toys when their mothers displayed negative affect, regardless of ambiguity. They continued to play less with the toys and to stay further away from them even after mothers shifted to neutral affect, indicating that appraisals constructed from mothers' displays of negative emotion continue to affect infants for at least a short time following exposure. Infants may need time to recover from the impact of mothers' negative affect before their negative emotion diminishes sufficiently to allow exploration.

Recently, researchers have identified behaviors other than facial expressions that serve as salient cues during social referencing. Vocalizations accompany mothers' facial expressions during referencing (Rosen et al., 1992) and mothers' fearful vocalizations are sufficient to elicit behavioral regulation in infants even when they are unaccompanied by matching facial expressions (Mumme, Fernald, & Herrera, 1996). Touch also conveys affective information. When depressed mothers touched their infants during the still-face procedure, infants displayed more positive affect than did comparable infants who were not touched (Pelaez-Nogueras, Field, Hossain, & Pickens, 1996). These affective behaviors serve as conduits for the transmission of negative emotions from mothers to infants and may interfere with regulatory processes. Alternatively, positive maternal affect may facilitate regulation in infants and therefore may be targeted in interventions with mother–infant dyads at risk for regulatory dysfunction (Field, 1998).

Infants employ regulatory behaviors other than social referencing, with the type of strategy differing in relation to mothers' availability and other features of the context. In an innovative extension of the social-referencing paradigm, Diener, Mangelsdorf, Fosnot, and Kienstra (1997) investigated how infants' regulatory strategies in response to potentially frightening or frustrating events differed as a function of mothers' availability. Ninety-four 18- and 24-month-old infants were exposed to each type of emotional event; first, with mothers present in the room but instructed to remain uninvolved with the infant and then with mothers directed to interact with their infants as they wished. During the fear episode, when mothers were uninvolved, toddlers engaged primarily in self-soothing, whereas when mothers were available, toddlers spent more time referencing and engaging them, engaging the stimulus, and problem solving. Unexpectedly, and in contrast to the results of a previous study (Grolnick, Bridges, & Connell, 1996), during frustration episodes toddlers engaged the stimulus more and fussed more toward mothers when they were uninvolved, whereas during the involved episode they used more self-soothing.

These divergent results may be due to the infants' assessment of the strategies most likely to be effective in each context, as Stein and Levine (1987) have proposed. Fear may activate withdrawal through self-soothing when mothers are not involved because that strategy is more effective than active engagement in reducing negative emotion when the situation does not lend itself to active infant control. In contrast, frustration may activate more engagement with the environment when mothers are not involved if infants believe they can attain the goal (i.e., get the cracker out of the zip-lock bag) and reduce negative emotion through their own efforts. When mothers were involved, the toddlers may have expected their mothers to assist them. When they failed to do so (i.e., mothers were directed not to open the bag), toddlers may have become more emotionally aroused and, as a consequence, unable to engage actively in the environment.

The gender of the parent available to provide affective information and support also may influence how infants regulate in emotionally arousing situations. Bridges and Grolnick (1998) found that 12-month-old infants employed different regulation strategies with mothers and fathers in a frustrating delay of gratification task, and that their strategies sometimes varied by gender. When the parent was present but not actively task oriented, infants played with the toys more if fathers rather than mothers were present. At 18 months, when the parent was available to interact, boys played with the toys more if the parent were the father rather than the mother. These differences in infant regulatory behavior may reflect differing expectations about the likely behavior of mothers and fathers in such situations. If fathers are less sensitive and more intrusive with their 12-month-old infants than are mothers, as Volling

et al. (1998) reported, infants may tailor their behavior accordingly.

In sum, infants use their parents as regulators through social referencing, and they use the information obtained to guide and monitor subsequent behavior. They respond to the same parental behaviors differently depending on the type of emotion experienced, the parent's gender, and possibly their own gender. The extent to which these early interactive processes contribute to the development of stable patterns of emotion regulation is less certain, though of considerable developmental importance.

Maternal Affect and Emotion Regulation

Researchers have attempted to assess the impact of persistent patterns of maternal affect on infant emotion regulation by comparing the affective behavior of depressed and nondepressed mothers and their infants. Consistently, infants of depressed mothers express more negative emotions and engage in more avoidant behavior during emotionally arousing mother–infant interactions than do infants of nondepressed mothers (Cohn et al., 1986; Field et al., 1988). However, depressed mothers may demonstrate either predominantly sad affect and withdrawn behavior or angry and intrusive behavior. Infant reactions vary as a function of these specific maternal styles. During a 3-minute face-to-face interaction in which no toys were available, infants of intrusive depressed mothers engaged in more gaze aversion, whereas infants of withdrawn depressed mothers used more distress and protest (Cohn et al., 1986). Although these findings confirm expected links between maternal depression, maternal behavior, and infant emotion regulation, they do not indicate the stability of these behaviors across contexts and over time. Withdrawn mothers may become angry and intrusive when their infants persist in attempts to elicit a response. As infants become more mobile and assertive, it may be difficult for withdrawn depressed mothers to ignore their behavior, and they may shift to a more intrusive pattern.

Tronick et al. (1982) used an experimental design to confirm that maternal affective behavior influences infants' emotion regulation, reducing the likelihood that this association is explained by infant characteristics. They observed 24 mothers and their 3-month-old infants under two conditions. In one, mothers were instructed to display sad or withdrawn affect and to speak more slowly than normal when interacting with their infants in a modified still-face procedure; in the second, they were instructed to interact as they normally would. Infants of mothers in the depressed interaction group spent more time fussing, glancing toward mothers with a sad face, and looking away. After normal interactions were resumed, they remained wary and difficult to reengage. Thus, emotion-linked infant behavior generated in one context carried over, introducing the possibility that it may elicit affective responses from others in new contexts.

Field et al. (1988) investigated this carryover effect further by observing 3- to 6-month-old infants interacting with their mothers and with a nondepressed stranger immediately afterwards. Consistent with the hypothesis that infants elicit depressive reactions from others, the nondepressed strangers behaved in a more depressed fashion when interacting with the infants of depressed mothers than with those of nondepressed mothers. Nonetheless, the timing of the stranger interaction leaves open the possibility that the carryover is only temporary, and the use of a stranger unfamiliar with the infant's regulation style and needs may have heightened this carryover effect (Field, 1995). When the order of mothers' and fathers' observations were counterbalanced, infants' interaction styles with depressed mothers did not generalize to interactions with their nondepressed fathers (Hossain et al.,1994). Similarly, infants of depressed mothers were less likely to display negative affect and low activity levels with a familiar nursery teacher than with their depressed mothers (Pelaez-Nogueras, Field, Cigales, Gonzalez, & Clasky, 1994). Thus, it appears that familiar caregivers may buffer infants from some of the adverse effects of maternal depression on emotion regulation.

In sum, there is considerable empirical support for the thesis that infants develop more or less adaptive affective communication and emotion regulation in the context of repeated interactions with mothers and that these patterns are apparent from the third month of life. When mothers successfully read and respond to their infants' emotional cues, infants are less fussy and engage in more exploration. Infants interpret their environments based in part on their parents' affective cues and appear to use parents to help regulate emotion-linked behavior. Importantly, relationships with other caregivers may serve as buffers against negative affective carryover by infants who experience withdrawn or angry interactions with their mothers.

Implications for Intervention

Although the processes linking caregiver behavior and infant emotion regulation are not entirely clear and intervention studies need to be replicated, the consistent empirical associations between maternal sensitivity, affective communication, and infant emotion regulation permit several preliminary recommendations. First, caregivers can be trained to respond to their infants' cues both sensitively and appropriately and, thereby, improve infants' emotion regulation, as van den Boom (1994) demonstrated in her intervention with mothers of irritable infants. Similarly, Malphurs et al. (1996) successfully altered the interactive behavior of both intrusive and withdrawn depressed mothers. Mothers became less intrusive with their infants when they were trained to imitate them and less withdrawn when they were taught to engage their infants' attention. Second, increasing parental awareness that infants look to them for affective signals and use them to regulate their behavior may allow parents to anticipate these opportunities and to provide clear and appropriate affective signals for their infants. If caregivers have difficulty offering affective facial signals, encouraging them to use appropriate vocalizations or touch may help infants regulate more effectively. Third, evidence that infants' relationships with fathers and other familiar caregivers buffer infants from the adverse effects of interacting with depressed mothers demonstrates the value of including them in interventions designed to enhance infant emotion regulation.

In the sections that follow, we consider how the early interactions that contribute to emotion regulation influence other aspects of social–emotional functioning and suggest how early preventive efforts may support adaptive development during the first 3 years of life.

ATTACHMENT AND INFANT MENTAL HEALTH

Bowlby (1969/1982, 1973) laid out a systems perspective of infant and caregiver attachment, emphasizing the development of a goal-corrected partnership between infant and caregiver. In the system, superficially dissimilar infant and caregiver behaviors are organized around the goal of maintaining the infant's proximity to the mother and sense of felt security. When the attachment system is activated by a potential threat to proximity, the infant attempts to increase or maintain proximity to the primary caregiver, retreating to her for a sense of safety and reduction of distress.

The concept of a goal-corrected attachment behavioral system provided the underpinnings for Ainsworth et al.'s (1978) identification of three patterned subtypes of the organization of infant–parent attachment behavior, secure, avoidant, and ambivalent, each characterized by a distinct strategy in relation to the achievement of proximity and apparent by the end of the first year. Main and Solomon (1990) later identified the disorganized/disoriented subtype.

In a secure attachment relationship, an infant may protest separation from the mother but greets her warmly when she returns, often seeks to be near or in direct physical contact with her, calms quickly if distressed, and returns relatively quickly to play and exploration. In contrast, when the attachment is avoidant, the infant typically does not protest a mother's departure in an unfamiliar setting but focuses instead on toys and other objects or persons in the room. Although this behavior appears quite independent and competent to a casual observer, the impression is misleading. The infant does not immediately acknowledge the mother's return, averting his or her gaze when she enters and possibly moving away from her if she approaches, suggesting a discrepancy between his or her overt behavior and underlying feelings. Ambivalent attachment is characterized by distress at the mother's absence and contact seeking at her return, mixed with direct or displaced anger and resistance, and a failure to be fully comforted.

The consistency and organization characterizing avoidant and ambivalent insecure attachment patterns distinguish them from the disorganized pattern. Although the particular combination of behaviors of infants in disorganized attachment relationships varies, they have in common behaviors that seem to lack a readily observable goal, intention, or explanation (Main & Solomon, 1990). These include unusual behaviors, such as prolonged freezing or stilling or slowed "underwater" movements. In addition, they may engage in both avoidant and resistant behaviors, and this lack of a consistent strategy for coping with threats to security may partially explain the link between disorganized attachment to mother and subsequent developmental problems (see Zeanah & Boris, Chapter 22, this volume).

Why infants develop distinct patterns of attachment with particular caregivers is a key question. Efforts to prevent and alter insecure attachments in the service of more adaptive future development depend on understanding the functions of attachment strategies and the conditions that give rise to their development. According to Bowlby (1969/1982, 1973), the attachment relationship serves two related functions: reducing distress and regulating emotion and promoting exploration. Both functions serve the broader goal of survival and are modulated through "felt security," or, more precisely, the emotions and cognitions that reflect infants' understanding of their position in the world. Although Bowlby argued that all human infants are biologically predisposed to maintain proximity to caregivers, he recognized that infants would differ in the ways they achieved this goal by virtue of their experiences with specific caregivers. Through their unique experiences, infants and children develop expectations, that is, "working models" or cognitive/emotional representations of their interactions with primary caregivers, which serve as guides for future relationships.

Origins of Infants' Working Models of Attachment

Sensitive Responsiveness

Bowlby (1969/1982) identified the primary caregiver's sensitive responsiveness to her infant's signals as one of the conditions influencing the development of a secure infant–caregiver attachment. According to this view, infants whose mothers respond quickly and appropriately to their cues (e.g., by attempting to soothe a crying baby) learn that they can count on their mothers to respond when they need assistance (i.e., feel secure) and begin to form an understanding or internal representation of themselves and others based on these experiences.

There is substantial empirical research linking mothers' sensitivity to their infants' signals to secure infant–mother attachments (Belsky et al., 1984; Egeland & Farber, 1984, and more recently, Gunnar, Brodersen, Nachmias, Buss, &

Rigatuso, 1996; Seifer, Schiller, Sameroff, Resnick, & Riordan, 1996). Infants from working- and middle-class two-parent families establish specific attachments to their fathers by the end of the first year, and similar associations have been reported between fathers' sensitive and engaged behavior and infant–father attachment security (Cox, Owen, Henderson, & Margand, 1992; Caldera, Huston, & O'Brien, 1995), although less consistently (e.g., Volling & Belsky, 1992). Nevertheless, in a recent meta-analysis of 21 studies, De Wolff and van IJzendoorn (1997) concluded that maternal sensitivity is not the only antecedent of attachment security, despite a moderately high combined effect size of .24 between observation-based ratings of maternal sensitivity and attachment security assessed in the Strange Situation. Other research reviewed next is consistent with this conclusion.

Main, Kaplan, and Cassidy (1985) elaborated further on the working-model thesis, proposing that infants tailor their behavior to a particular type of caregiving and that the manner in which they do so becomes a consistent, albeit not necessarily conscious, strategy. In the service of a strategy, the infant regulates feelings, behaviors, attention, memories, and cognitions (Cassidy, 1994). Thus, Main and Hesse (1990) interpreted the heightened distress and angry behavior shown by an infant with an ambivalent attachment as a strategy of exaggerating attachment behaviors to elicit a response from a less consistent caregiver. Although Main contends that the infant's strategy has an adaptive quality in that it helps ensure proximity to a particular caregiver, it may be less adaptive with respect to future relationships and development; hence, our concern with the patterns of insecure attachment that develop during infancy.

Like Main et al. (1985), Cassidy (1994) and Thompson (1994) focused on the impact of attachment relationships on emotion regulation, as one of Bowlby's two key attachment-related goals. They posited that children learn how to regulate emotion in the service of attaining their goals and that patterns of emotion regulation inherent in attachment patterns reflect what infants have learned about maintaining relationships with attachment figures. Infants who have not had their needs met consistently and appropriately by caregivers either minimize emotional displays (are avoidant) in an effort to reduce the risk of future disappointment or harm or they heighten their expression of negative emotions

(are ambivalent/resistant) in an effort to engage an inconsistently responsive caregiver. In each case, emotion regulation serves the function of maintaining proximity, and the selection of strategy reflects the infant's understanding of what works with a particular caregiver.

Empirical findings are consistent with these claims. As reviewed previously by Cassidy (1994) and Lyons-Ruth and Zeanah (1993), mothers of avoidant–insecure infants are more covertly rejecting of their infants, especially when the infants express negative affect (Escher-Graeub & Grossmann, 1983), and show a restricted range of emotional expressiveness in comparison to mothers of secure infants (Ainsworth et al., 1978; Main, Tomasini, & Tolan, 1979; Malatesta et al., 1989). Also consistent with conceptually based predictions, mothers of ambivalent–insecure infants are relatively unavailable in the home (Belsky et al., 1984; Grossmann, Fremmer-Bombik, Rudolf, & Grossmann, 1988; see Cassidy & Berlin, 1994, for a review).

With respect to disorganized infant–mother attachments, Main and Hesse (1990) proposed that such infants have been exposed to frightening experiences, or to frightened parents who themselves have experienced unresolved traumatic events. Because of these traumas, parents may behave in ways that are puzzling to the infant and, therefore, frightening. An infant frightened by a parent's behavior is less likely to seek comfort from that parent because the infant is simultaneously motivated to seek proximity (for comfort) and to avoid (because of fear) and, hence, is at risk for becoming disorganized. Lyons-Ruth, Bronfman, and Parsons (in press) expanded this conceptualization to include two types of disruptions in maternal affective communication. The first, "failure of repair," is characterized by unresponsiveness to the content or intention of the infant's communication and demonstrated by hostility, intrusiveness, withdrawal, or parent–infant role reversal. They reasoned that in the absence of a minimal level of appropriate parental responsiveness, infants are unable to employ either deactivation or heightened activation, leading to fear and a breakdown of behavioral strategies. The second type of disrupted communication, "competing strategies," refers to fear-based contradictory caregiving behaviors that both elicit and reject infant attachment behaviors and thereby undermine infants' ability to form coherent attachment strategies.

Support for these conceptualizations of disorganized attachment is growing (Lyons-Ruth & Jacobvitz, 1991). Scheungel, van IJzendoorn, Bakersmans-Kranenburg, and Bloom (1997) reported that a set of maternal disorganized, including frightening, behaviors predicted infant disorganized attachment behavior. Similarly, Lyons-Ruth et al. (in press) found that mothers of disorganized infants displayed more communication errors in the Strange Situation; they provided infants with contradictory messages and responded inappropriately or not at all to clear communications by the infant. In addition, mothers of disorganized–insecure infants engaged in more negative-intrusive behaviors and role confusions, as well as more frightening and other atypical behaviors, compared to mothers of both disorganized–secure infants and infants with organized attachment strategies. In contrast, mothers of disorganized–secure infants (i.e., those whose attachment relationships demonstrated both security and disorganization) engaged in elevated withdrawal and mild fearfulness that distinguished them from mothers of other infants. These findings are consistent with the thesis that disruptions of caregiving behavior that expose infants to inadequately modulated fear underlie the development of disorganized infant–mother attachments, which are associated, in turn, with children's later behavioral problems (Lyons-Ruth, Easterbrooks, & Cibelli, 1997).

Evidence that infants in high-risk families, characterized by maternal depression, maltreatment, and alcoholism, or by battering, are especially likely to be classified as disorganized also is consistent with the view that frightening and frightened parental behaviors are at the core of disorganized attachments (see Lyons-Ruth, Repacholi, McLeod, & Silva, 1991, for a review). More recently, Lyons-Ruth and Block (1996) reported that violence or abuse in the mother's childhood increased the tendency for insecure attachment to take disorganized rather than avoidant forms, with different types of childhood experience associated with different patterns of maternal caregiving. Violence or harsh punishment was associated with more hostile–intrusive maternal behavior, whereas abuse, including sexual abuse, was associated with maternal withdrawal. Thus, to be effective in altering maternal behavior related to disorganized infant–mother attachments, clinicians may need to address traumatic events in the mother's childhood in their treatment and interventions. We return to this point in discussing mothers' working models of attachment.

In sum, we can be reasonably confident that mothers' sensitive-responsiveness to their infants' negative emotions, as well as their own emotional expressiveness, contribute to the security of the infant–mother attachment, and that specific patterns of maternal caregiving affect the nature of the infant's attachment strategies. Fathers' behavior likely contributes to infant–father attachment security as well. It is important to keep in mind, however, that classification of an infant as insecurely attached does not necessarily implicate parental insensitivity as the primary causal factor in its development. There are multiple pathways to both types of insecure attachment, and parental sensitivity may be overridden by unfavorable experiences that occur concurrently or have occurred previously in the infant's life.

Separation and Trauma

Bowlby (1969/1982, 1973), citing Heinicke and Westheimer (1966), identified separation of infant from mother as a primary experience contributing to the development of an insecure infant–mother attachment. Recently, Sagi et al. (1994) provided support for the importance of separation from mother in the development of insecure attachments. Kibbutzim-raised infants who slept away from their mothers in communal houses were more likely than other kibbutz-raised infants to develop insecure attachments, despite evidence of sensitive maternal caregiving. Although these findings pertain to a specific type of separation and may be partially attributable to the variable responsiveness of the watchwomen who monitored the infants at night, they caution about focusing exclusively on maternal sensitivity as a contributor to attachment security.

Recognition that current caregiving is only one factor in the development of a secure infant attachment is especially important in serving the needs of adoptive and foster parents whose infants' attachment strategies may be shaped in part by experiences that occurred prior to their entry into their adoptive families. These could include neglect and abuse, painful health-related treatments, or even the separation from the previous caregiver. The older the infant at the time of placement, the greater the likelihood of having had such experiences and having devel-

oped the capacities that contribute to the formation of insecure models of attachment, which,
in turn, might undermine the security of the
new attachment relationship. Tyrrell and Dozier
(in press) found that foster parents reported
more attachment related difficulties with foster
infants placed after 6 months of age than
among infants placed earlier. Stovall and Dozier (in press) reported further that children
placed with foster parents after 12 months of
age were reported to show patterns of insecure
attachment behavior, even when placed with
foster parents whose own working models of
attachment were autonomous (secure). In view
of these infants' problematic caregiving histories, normal levels of parental sensitivity may
not be enough for secure attachments to develop in new relationships (Dozier, Stovall, & Albus 1999). Dozier and colleagues have proposed that foster parents need to be actively
therapeutic to promote a reorganization of the
infants' attachment strategies, and they have
developed an intervention to support therapeutic caregiving in foster parents.

In a recent review of programs designed to
prevent or ameliorate insecure infant–mother
attachments, van IJzendoorn, Juffer, and
Duyvesteyn (1995) reported that such attempts
had been more successful in changing maternal
behavior than in promoting secure infant–
mother attachment. This perplexing finding
makes sense if experiences and behaviors other
than maternal sensitivity contribute to the development of infant–mother attachment security. In addition to separation and trauma, the
caregiver's own working model of attachment
may affect the infant in ways not subsumed by
the specific maternal behaviors targeted for intervention.

Adult Working Models of Attachment and Infant Attachment Security

According to Cassidy (1994), parents have their
own working models of attachment, which they
strive unconsciously to maintain in their relationships with their children. Mothers who are
dismissing of attachment relationships convey
this orientation to their children, whereas mothers who are preoccupied with attachment convey their preoccupation. Children attempt to
regulate their emotions in specific ways in an
unconscious effort "to help the parent maintain
her own state of mind in relation to attachment"
(Cassidy, 1994, p. 248). They cooperate in

maintaining parental orientations by creating
their own psychological and emotional distance
(i.e., by behaving avoidantly) or by continuing
to engage parental caregivers in a tug-of-war
for their attention and involvement (i.e., by behaving ambivalently). Presumably, infants understand from repeated experiences with mothers (i.e., how they respond to negative emotions
in a variety of contexts and over time) that a
pattern exists in their interaction. These understandings are the core of infants' schema or
representations that function as "working models" of relationships.

Data linking mothers' adult attachment representations to specific patterns of infant–
mother attachment support the proposition that
parents' working models of attachment contribute to the type of attachment relationship
they develop with their infants (e.g., Ainsworth
& Eichberg, 1991; Crowell & Feldman, 1988;
Grossmann et al., 1988; Zeanah et al., 1993).
That adult models of attachment assessed prenatally predicted the security of infant–parent
relationships at 1 year lends additional cre-
dence to a parent-to-child effect (Fonagy,
Steele, & Steele, 1991; Ward & Carlson, 1995;
Benoit & Parker, 1994; see van IJzendoorn,
1995, for a meta-analysis), although genetic influences cannot be ruled out using a within-
family design. Ward and Carlson's (1995) finding that prenatal attachment models of
adolescent mothers predicted both their sensitivity to their infants and infants' attachment security extends the links between mothers' models of attachment, caregiving behavior, and
infants' attachment security to young, low-income, ethnic-minority mothers.

Evidence linking mothers' interpretations of
their infants' affective behaviors during the
still-face procedure with infants' attachment
classifications at 12 months is consistent also
with the view that mothers' representations of
relationships affect the attachment relationships
their infants develop (Ungerer & Sygall, 1998).
Consistent with Cassidy's (1994) predictions,
mothers of avoidant infants interpreted their infants' behavior at 4 months as rejecting of
them, whereas mothers of ambivalent infants
thought their infants felt rejected and were attempting to control them. These interpretations
may have led to different patterns of maternal
response to infants' emotional signals and,
hence, to differences in attachment security.
Differences in infant reactivity and regulation
during the still face may have contributed to

mothers' interpretations, as suggested earlier, perhaps in conjunction with mothers' working models of attachment.

There is evidence also linking unresolved parental trauma (i.e., experiences of intense fear, terror, or helplessness during childhood), as assessed by the Adult Attachment Interview (AAI) (Main & Goldwyn, in press), to classification of infants as disorganized (Main & Hesse, 1990). Other investigators have replicated and extended these findings by demonstrating that trauma characterized by physical and sexual abuse of the parent predicted disorganized infant attachment status (Ainsworth & Eichberg, 1991), and that unresolved loss predicted mothers' frightened or frightening behaviors toward their infants (Jacobvitz, Hazen, & Riggs, 1997; Scheungel et al., 1997), the same pattern of behavior linked previously to disorganized infant attachment relationships.

Acknowledgment of a parent-to-child influence in the development of working models of attachment does not imply that the infant plays only a passive role in his or her own development. The infant's gender, physical attributes, and temperament, or reactive style, may be important both in eliciting particular caregiving behaviors and in moderating the impact of those behaviors on the attachment relationship.

Infant Temperament and Infant Attachment Security

The infant's role in the development of a secure attachment relationship has been hotly debated. On one side of the debate, investigators have argued that the infant's temperament, in particular, the intensity and pervasiveness of her negative emotionality (i.e., irritability), is a primary determinant of attachment patterns (Goldsmith & Alansky, 1987). On the other, Ainsworth et al. (1978), Sroufe (1985), and Cassidy (1994) have emphasized the dominant role of maternal sensitivity in determining the course of the early infant-mother relationship. Each cites data to support his or her position (see Rothbart & Bates, 1998).

One approach to this divergence of opinion and data has been to craft conceptualizations in which both maternal behavior and infant temperament are recognized as contributors to attachment relationships. Early in the debate, Bell (1971) proposed that infant irritability or reactivity might elicit less sensitive and responsive maternal caregiving. If an infant cries intensely and frequently and is difficult to soothe, a mother must be extremely attentive, patient, and resourceful for the infant to develop the belief that his or her needs will be met, the core of a secure working model of attachment. To the extent that this pattern of infant behavior increases the likelihood that a mother may fail to read accurately or to respond to her infant's signals, it could be said that the infant's characteristics have elicited the lack of maternal sensitivity and contributed indirectly to the insecurity of the attachment relationship. Evidence in support of such a link is contradictory, and Crockenberg (1986) proposed that infant temperament may interact with other characteristics of the mother or her context to predict how she will behave with her infant. When mothers at risk for parenting problems by virtue of poverty or their own mental health have a temperamentally reactive baby, they may be at increased risk for responding less sensitively to their babies' cues.

Infant temperament/reactivity also may interact with maternal sensitivity to predict attachment security. According to this view, infants respond differently to the same maternal behavior by virtue of their own physiologically based reactivity. A mother's slowness to respond to her infant's cries may be experienced more often by a reactive infant, whose frequent crying serves as a potential elicitor of maternal behavior, and may have a greater negative impact on a reactive infant's regulatory competence than the same behavior experienced by a baby who reacts less intensely to stimulation. Thus, maternal insensitivity may act in concert with infant reactivity to influence the course of the infant-mother attachment relationship.

Empirical support for the interactive impact of infant temperament and maternal characteristics on the security of infant-mother attachment is growing. Manglesdorf, Gunnar, Kestenbaum, Lang, and Andreas (1990) reported that infants who were "prone to distress" were more likely than other infants to develop insecure attachments if their mothers had rigid personalities, replicating Crockenberg's (1981) finding that irritable infants with less responsive mothers were more resistant during reunion episodes of the Strange Situation. van den Boom (1994, 1995) experimentally confirmed that increasing mothers' sensitive responsiveness to their irritable infants' cues resulted in more secure infant-mother attachments.

Although van den Boom's (1994) research indicates the usefulness of teaching mothers of irritable infants to identify and respond to their infants' signals, it is important also to encourage mothers of reactive infants to seek help so they can maintain the high level of attentive care their babies require. The expectation that most mothers can continue to care for an irritable baby sensitively, over an extended period, ignores the stress and simple exhaustion that accompanies this task, especially when the needs of other family members or demands associated with pressing life circumstances require the caregiver's attention. Emotional and instrumental support that bolsters a mother's feelings of efficacy and reduces competing tasks help her to remain engaged and sensitively responsive and have been linked to development of secure attachments in irritable infants (see Crockenberg, 1988, for a review).

Implications for Intervention

An obvious implication of the theories and findings reviewed is that to promote the development of secure attachments and to alter insecure attachments in infants and young children, it is necessary to change the behavior of the primary caregiver, typically the mother. Nevertheless, improving maternal sensitivity may be insufficient to alter the infant's working model of attachment in some families. As Fraiberg (1980) proposed nearly 20 years ago, it may be necessary to provide therapeutic intervention oriented toward altering parents' working models of attachment, or, as Dozier et al. (1999) suggested, to help parents provide therapeutic caregiving to alter insecure infant–mother attachments once they have formed.

However, it is important to keep in mind Wakschlag, Chase-Lansdale, and Brooks-Gunn's (1996) caution about attributing intergenerational effects entirely to "ghosts in the nursery." Ongoing patterns of interaction between black adolescent mothers and their mothers in multigenerational families were associated with the young mothers' parenting independent of socioeconomic status and may partly explain associations between their working models of relationships and caregiving behavior. Others have reported that the family's socioeconomic context may increase infants' risk for exposure to traumatic events, as well as less sensitive parenting leading to insecure and disorganized attachments (Lyons-Ruth et al., in

press; McLoyd, 1990). Further, associations between maternal behavior and infant attachment are significantly weaker in studies with low-income samples (DeWolff & van IJzendoorn, 1997). Taken together, these findings suggest that present circumstances must be as much a target of prevention/intervention attempts as past experiences. It makes little sense to provide intensive, expensive psychotherapy for mothers without attempting to ameliorate ongoing life circumstances that undermine trust and self-esteem and adversely impact maternal sensitivity.

On the other hand, it is equally unrealistic to expect sustained improvement in attachment security simply by reducing poverty for mothers whose parenting problems are rooted in their own childhood experiences. It may be necessary both to reduce poverty and poverty-related stresses and to provide more intense, parenting-related interventions to alter or prevent the development of insecure and disorganized attachments (see Lieberman & Zeanah, 1999, for a review of dual-focused interventions). In the absence of multifaceted, continuous intervention, it may be difficult for mothers to maintain behaviors that support secure attachments, especially when living conditions are stressful.

An exclusive focus on maternal sensitivity as the goal of intervention may be unwarranted also. Other conditions known to affect attachment security (e.g., separations of infants from parents and exposure to traumatic events) must be addressed for interventions to have the broadest beneficial effect on infant attachment security. This might involve treatment for drug and alcohol abuse or marital therapy aimed at reducing the prevalence of family-based traumatic events and should include fathers as well as mothers. Not only are fathers implicated in traumatic family events, but recently Belsky (1996) found that father–infant attachments were more likely to be secure when fathers had more positive marriages and carried over positive emotions from their work to their family life.

Preventive intervention to protect infants and support secure attachments also must involve minimizing the amount of time infants spend in foster care and the frequency of caregiving disruptions, which further complicates the formation of secure attachment relationships when infants are placed permanently (Dozier et al., 1999). This may require faster removal of infants from families in which they are exposed to traumatic events when therapy is refused or ineffective (Barnett, 1997; Emery & Laumann-Billings, 1998).

Attachment as Risk Factor or Current Disorder

In the previous review, we discussed insecure attachment as a risk factor for subsequent disorder, depending on the occurrence of additional risk or protective factors. Zeanah (1996) has drawn attention to clinical work focusing on infants "who are not merely at risk for subsequent disorders, but are disordered already" (p. 42). According to his scheme, these clinically disordered infants are an extreme subgroup of insecurely attached infants. Thus, all disordered attachments are insecure, but not all insecure infants should be considered disordered. Drawing on the previous work of Zeanah, Mammen, and Lieberman (1993), Zeanah identified three criteria for identifying such disorders: (1) recognition that neither parental maltreatment nor lack of stable caregiving need be present for an attachment relationship to be disordered; (2) in defining an attachment as disordered, the focus must be on the infant's attachment–exploration balance, that is, the infant's ability to use the attachment figure as a source of comfort and a base for exploring the environment; and (3) given infants' capacity to construct differing relationships with different caregivers, an attachment relationship may be disordered even if it does not generalize to different relationships. He points out further that disordered attachments must be validated directly and distinguished from nondisordered insecure attachments, hence identifying directions for future clinical and developmental research efforts (see Zeanah & Boris, Chapter 22, this volume).

Insecure Infant–Mother Attachment and the Timing of Interventions

Identification of infancy as a prime time for the development of attachment relationships does not imply that later experiences are unimportant in the construction or modification of children's working models of attachment. Indeed, Bowlby (1969/1982, 1973) states explicitly that children develop expectations about relationships and future experiences over the course of infancy and childhood, even through the adolescent years. Nevertheless, he believed that ex-periences during the first 3 to 5 years of life are relatively more important than later experiences by virtue of both their primacy and other characteristics of infants and young children and their social contexts that support the formation of coherent working models of attachment. Typically, infants and children under the age of 5 have more extensive and dependent contact with primary caregivers than do older children. It follows that the opportunity for them to be influenced by their families and for professionals to help support change in families may be especially great during the first few years of life.

AUTONOMY AND COMPLIANCE IN THE SECOND YEAR OF LIFE

During the second year of life, infants direct their attention increasingly toward exploring the environment, typically increasing the distance they put between themselves and their primary caregivers. This shift is linked to changes in infants' motor behavior that occur during the second 6 months of the first year of life and accelerates with other changes that emerge around 18 months of age. As a consequence of these changes, toddlers are able to consider the impact of their behavior on others and also to keep their own goals in mind over longer sequences of activity, bringing them into conflict with others. This conflict in goals defines the so-called terrible twos. The way the conflict is resolved constitutes the model for the way 2-year-olds learn to "achieve one's own goals without violating the integrity of the goals of the other" (Bronson, 1974, p. 280). Although balancing one's own and others' goals is an issue throughout development, it has special significance during the toddler period because the way it is resolved then likely influences what occurs subsequently.

Developmental Origins of Differences in Exploration and Compliance

In his original conceptualization of the attachment process, Bowlby (1969/1982, 1973) identified exploration as a primary function of a secure mother–infant attachment, the consequence of a well-functioning goal-corrected partnership. Cassidy and Berlin (1994) elaborated on this thesis, arguing that when a mother is minimally or inconsistently responsive, infants increase their monitoring of her, resulting in extreme dependence which impedes exploration. If an infant needs to keep his mother in sight, he is less free to investigate the environment. Attention needs to remain focused on her to ensure that she remains available. Researchers have confirmed that insecure/ambivalent infants are more fearful about exploring new environments (Hazen & Durrett, 1982; Jacobson & Wille, 1986) and more fearful and withdrawn with peers (Renken, Egeland, Marvinney, Mangelsdorf, & Sroufe, 1989).

Cassidy (1994) posited further that ambivalent infants learn to heighten their expression of negative emotion in an effort to gain their mothers' attention. In doing so, an infant may both elicit more control attempts from the mother and engage in more angry and defiant and less compliant behavior in response to her control attempts. Londerville and Main's (1981) finding that infants who were insecurely attached at 12 months directed more anger, physical aggression, and noncompliance toward their mothers as toddlers than did securely attached infants is consistent with this conceptualization. In contrast, but consistent with what we would expect in a goal-corrected partnership, secure attachment is associated with more compliant toddler behavior (Londerville & Main, 1981; Kochanska, Aksan, & Koenig, 1995). As Cassidy, Kirsch, Scolton, and Parke (1996) have articulated, children may develop cognitive representations of themselves in relation to their mothers and strategies for maintaining contact with different types of mothers during the first 18 months of life, which they generalize to subsequent interactions with their mothers and to other relationships. According to this view, as conflicts arise during the second year of life, the way parents behave with their children is shaped both by their own predispositions and by characteristics their children have developed in the course of their earlier interactions. The same understandings that contribute to a mother's early sensitivity and, hence, a secure infant–mother attachment likely underlie her accommodation to her toddler's goals as she attempts to increase his acceptance of hers. Securely attached toddlers may be more inclined initially to comply with their mothers' bids because they expect her to be responsive to theirs (Parpal & Maccoby, 1985), and perhaps also because they are better able to empathize with her feelings, as discussed later.

Nevertheless, patterns of infant–mother at-

tachment change as life circumstances shift and children both develop greater cognitive competence and face new developmental challenges (Crittenden, 1994). Children who were securely attached earlier in infancy may shift to a more coercive style during the second and third years of life if parents are not attuned to their need for both limits and autonomy during this period of increasing assertiveness and exploration. Initially toddlers may "try out" coercive responses to restrictions of their autonomy and discover either that they are effective in threatening others into compliance or that they are not. According to this thesis, if parents capitulate in the face of a toddler's rage, in effect sacrificing their socialization goals to the child's will, the child learns that angry, coercive behavior is effective in obtaining important goals. If parents respond in kind, a pattern of coercive conflict may develop around autonomy issues.

A defining feature of such conflicts is the toddler's ability and willingness to say "no" to caregivers. Spitz (1957) described negation as an indicator of a new level of autonomy that accompanies the toddler's increasing awareness of the "other" and the "self" during the second year of life. He noted that with the child's assertion, the process of accommodation and negotiation begins. In response to the toddler's refusal, a mother may restate what she wants the child to do, establishing her concern for her own goal; she may escalate her demands in an attempt to force compliance and further restrict the child's autonomy, or she may respond in a way that allows both of them to achieve their goals. When her response is more balanced, the child complies more willingly because there is no significant cost and a likely benefit of doing so.

Following Erikson (1963), several researchers investigated specific aspects of maternal behavior during conflictual interactions as determinants of toddlers' autonomy and compliance (Crockenberg & Litman, 1990; Kuczynski, Kochanska, Radke-Yarrow, & Girnius-Brown, 1987; Parpal & Maccoby, 1985). As predicted, maternal behavior characterized by balancing of goals was associated with greater toddler compliance. Parpal and Maccoby (1985) found that children whose mothers were instructed to allow the child to control their interaction during a play period were subsequently more likely to comply when their mothers asked them to pick up the toys. Crockenberg and Litman (1990) reported similarly that 2-year-olds were significantly more likely to comply after first saying "no" when mothers combined control and guidance than when they used only control or only guidance in their attempts to influence child behavior. Control involves informing children of what you want them to do and, hence, clarifies adult goals. Guidance includes behaviors that provide opportunities for children to "choose" compliance (e.g., suggesting, compromising, and explaining) and, hence, to retain a sense of autonomy in relation to goal attainment. In contrast, 2-year-olds whose mothers escalated their attempts to control their toddlers' behavior following a refusal (i.e., used negative control characterized by threats, anger, and criticism) were more defiant than toddlers whose mothers used less coercive forms of control.

In addition to modeling aggressive methods of goal attainment, coercion may elicit negative emotional arousal from children, which they express as defiance when parents provide aggressive models. Calkins, Smith, Gill, and Johnson (1998) lend support to this thesis. When mothers used more negative control during goal-oriented tasks, toddlers showed poor physiological regulation (i.e., lower vagal suppression), less adaptive emotion regulation as indicated by lower use of distraction when their goals were frustrated, and more noncompliance. Maternal negative control was unrelated to baseline measures of physiological and emotional reactivity, supporting a maternal influence on toddler's regulatory capacities.

At the same time toddlers are constructing an understanding of parental standards, they begin to show empathy and guilt in response to the distress of others, which may affect their reactions to parental socialization efforts. Zahn-Waxler and colleagues identified concern, anxiety, remorse, and reparative behavior displayed by children between the ages of 18 months and 2 years when they caused or witnessed distress in others (Cummings, Zahn-Waxler, & Radke-Yarrow, 1981), and they linked differences in these behaviors to parents' use of explanations or love withdrawal (mild disapproval or physical withdrawal; Zahn-Waxler & Radke-Yarrow, 1990; Chapman & Zahn-Waxler, 1982). More extreme love withdrawal had less desirable effects, eliciting avoidant responses and attempts to make up with parents, interpreted as indicative of excessive guilt. However, these patterns may reflect children's reactions to parental emotions as much as to their behavior. When mothers were angry, rather than sad, toddlers were less empathic, perhaps focusing on self-protection and, thus, experiencing less concern for others (Crockenberg, 1985).

From these studies it appears that the way mothers engage with their children during the toddler period, specifically, their ability to share control during play and conflict, increases the likelihood that children will comply with mothers' socialization goals. There are several types of compliance, however, and not all have the same positive link with children's social–emotional development. If a child complies with a mother out of fear, as abused children sometimes do (Crittenden & DiLalla, 1988), compliance may be a form of avoidance and submission and serve as an antecedent of depression and suppressed hostility. On the other hand, if a toddler complies because she fully accepts her mother's goals, she may be demonstrating self-regulation and an early form of internalization (Kochanska et al., 1995). Kochanska and Aksan (1995) reported that committed compliance was accompanied by mutually positive maternal and child affect, which may reflect the quality of prior, as well as current, mother–infant interactions.

Fathers as Influences on Self-Regulation and Compliance

There are reasons to expect fathers to influence the development of compliance and self-regulation during toddlerhood. Fathers become more involved in the parenting process as their children get older (Belsky, Rovine, & Fish, 1989), and, like mothers, they experience their toddlers' growing assertiveness, the impetus for increasing parental control attempts. Power, McGrath, Hughes, and Manire (1994) have confirmed fathers' involvement in toddler socialization. By the time children were 2, fathers were more directive with them around compliance issues than were mothers, and 2-year-old boys, in particular, were more compliant to fathers than to mothers

The few investigators who have included fathers in studies of toddler self-regulation and compliance have provided empirical support for their impact on toddler development. Toddlers with less emotionally supportive fathers were more discontented (boys) and less task-oriented during problem solving (Belsky, Youngblade, Volling, & Rovine, 1989), and children with negative, intrusive fathers were more negative and disobedient at 3 years

(Goldberg & Easterbrooks, 1984). Belsky, Woodworth, and Crnic (1996) reported further that father variables reliably identified families that had trouble exercising appropriate control with their 15–21-month-old boys (i.e., made more control attempts and used less control with guidance, and whose toddlers were less compliant and more defiant). Men in more troubled families were less social, more negative, less considerate of others, and less satisfied with their social support than were men in less troubled families, and these associations were independent of correlated maternal behaviors.

Fathers may influence toddler development also through the "co-parenting" relationship, that is, the degree to which fathers and mothers support or undermine each others' parenting (Gable, Belsky, & Crnic, 1992). A father may back up a mother confronted by a coercive toddler, or he may contradict her, thus encouraging noncompliance; or he may simply withdraw from the fray, a pattern Patterson (1982) identified in families of clinically aggressive boys. In support of a co-parental effect, McHale and Rasmussen (1998) reported that a hostile–competitive co-parenting style during whole-family interactions when infants were 8 to 11 months old predicted higher aggressiveness at 3 years, especially for boys. Conflicts between fathers and mothers may affect toddler development in much the same way as direct parental behavior. When parents are physically or verbally aggressive with each other, they expose toddlers to aggressive models for behavior and also elicit negative emotional reactions (i.e., anger, sadness, and fear) that may prompt aggression or withdrawal. Some researchers have found stronger associations between marital quality and the father–infant than the mother–infant relationship (Lamb & Elster, 1985), although others have reported links for mothers as well (e.g., Dickstein & Parke, 1988; Howes & Markman, 1989).

In sum, it is likely that fathers have an impact on the development of toddlers' regulatory capacities, although the processes by which they exert their influence require further investigation. As we discuss later, recognition of father effects has important implications for intervention.

Temperament and Compliance

As proposed in relation to infant attachment, the type of parental socialization that promotes internalized, self-regulated toddler behavior is expected to vary as a function of the toddler's characteristics. Kochanska (1993) hypothesized that infant temperamental reactivity both elicits certain socialization practices and moderates the impact of those practices on developing self-regulation. Subsequently, she confirmed that maternal control styles interacted with infant fearfulness to predict internalization (Kochanska, 1995). Fearful toddlers engaged in more internalized behavior when mothers used gentle, non-power-oriented discipline; less fearful children were less affected by differences in maternal discipline strategies. It may be more important for the mother of an emotionally reactive toddler to avoid overcontrol because of its potentially greater disruptive impact on child behavior but also to employ firm control when necessary to limit the buildup of arousal and to support emotion regulation.

In a recent study, Spinard and Stifter (1998) reported that the interactive process apparent in toddlerhood originates during the infant's first year of life in the course of interactions with responsive mothers. Reactive infants with less responsive mothers at 5 months ignored mothers' bids for compliance more frequently at 18 months, and infants so identified at 10 months were more defiant at 18 months, in comparison to reactive infants with more responsive mothers. These data suggest that maternal responsiveness increases reactive infants' ability to self-regulate, or, alternatively, that unresponsiveness contributes to dysregulated behavior during the toddler period. They confirm an earlier finding that infants identified as slow to calm during crying bouts at 3 months were more angry and defiant during a toy cleanup task at 2 years when mothers used punitive, power-assertive strategies to control their behavior (Crockenberg, 1987).

Implications for Intervention

Although researchers have tended to choose either an attachment or a parenting model to direct their investigations of toddler development, the two perspectives are compatible. Attachment relationships establish the contexts in which parents' efforts to socialize toddlers takes place. Current parent–child interaction behaviors alone, although important, are unlikely to fully explain child behavior and adjustment (Goodnow & Collins, 1990), but neither are prior attachment relationships, as these may change in the course of subsequent interactions.

The interrelatedness of development in the first and second years of life has important implications for intervention. Although we have advocated preventive efforts during the first year, these may be insufficient to target all infants at risk for future mental health problems by virtue of maladaptive parental behavior. Changes in infant behavior during the second year of life create new challenges for mothers and may elicit less adaptive parental behavior in the absence of ongoing intervention. Continued intervention in some form through the second year of life may be useful also in solidifying changes begun earlier in infancy. The brevity of many interventions may explain in part why infant attachment security is less likely to change than maternal behavior in response to early interventions (van IJzendoorn et al., 1995). Once an attachment relationship is established, it may take consistent and sustained changes in maternal behavior to alter that pattern.

Although at this point the data are not definitive, it is reasonable to advise parents to adapt their socialization behaviors to their child's unique characteristics during the second and third years of life, keeping in mind the importance of balancing their own goals with those of the child. The growing evidence of fathers' influence on toddler development indicates the advisability and potential value of including fathers in interventions designed to foster emotion regulation and compliance and to reduce defiant toddler behavior. Interventions that focus exclusively on mothers will be less effective than hoped for because they disregard the impact of fathers, particularly on sons, and their potential to undermine mothers' socialization efforts.

THE DEVELOPING SENSE OF EFFECTANCE

Although the desire to effect change in the environment through self-initiated efforts may be intrinsic (White, 1959), an infant's belief in her ability to do so develops in the course of experiences in the social and physical world. Through their earliest contingent experiences with caregivers and the environments they create, infants begin to form a sense of themselves and of their ability to affect their environments

(Stern, 1985). As they develop new competencies in the second year, they become more aware of their separate selves and better able to explore the world independently and to direct their interactions with it. Infants who can express and regulate their emotions, have developed secure attachments, and have sufficient opportunity for autonomous behavior enter their third year believing in their capacity to effect change in the environment in pursuit of goals.

Investigators have coined different terms for this belief, "mastery motivation" (Frodi, Bridges, & Grolnick, 1985) or "a sense of effectance" (Tronick et al., 1986), distinguishing it from "competence," which they define as the successful achievement of some goal (Barrett, Morgan, & Maslin-Cole, 1993). To be competent, one must have both high hopes that one can be successful and the skills necessary to achieve success in a particular arena. Although the specific skills needed differ by whether the arena is social or object focused, a sense of effectance is relevant to both. Effectance is reflected in infant behaviors that create opportunities to develop skills and strategies necessary for goal attainment (i.e., attempts to directly control the environment and to persist in those attempts in the face of obstacles) and in the expression of a range of emotions in which interest, pleasure, and pride predominate. In this review, we consider the development of a sense of effectance throughout infancy and how this belief contributes to emotional and behavioral adjustment.

The Developmental Origins of a Sense of Effectance

Contingent Interaction

Infants' earliest opportunities for social mastery occur within the parent–infant relationship when caregivers respond contingently and appropriately to infants' emotional signals. According to Tronick et al. (1986), an important goal of early interaction is the attainment of mutual regulation, in which one partner tries to achieve his or her goals in coordination with those of the other through the interchange of emotional expressions. When infant and partner successfully read each other's signals and match their affect, the infant feels effective and conveys this sense of effectance through the expression of positive emotions. When repeated mismatches occur, feelings of effectance are undermined, and negative emotions result, although some degree of mismatch is adaptive because it provides infants with opportunities to try new responses (Gianano & Tronick, 1988).

With experience, infants express more pleasure at their accomplishments without maternal prompting and initiate more affective exchanges on their own. Mothers respond by expressing less pleasure at their infants' accomplishments and by initiating fewer affective exchanges, thus shifting greater control of their interactions to the infant (Grolnick, Cosgrove, & Bridges, 1996; Heckhausen, 1993). The gradual shift from initiator to responder represents mothers' sensitive adaptation to their infants' changing needs. It reflects infants' growing ability to regulate emotions and emotion-related behavior and is accompanied by an enhanced sense of effectance.

The results of several studies cited earlier are consistent with these claims. During still-face procedures in which mothers enacted depressed affect and did not respond to infants' emotional signals, infants displayed negative affect and looked away from their mothers when attempts to elicit responses from them failed (Tronick et al., 1982). Similarly, Termine and Izard (1988) reported that 9-month-old infants engaged in more gaze aversion and less play with toys following a face-to-face interaction in which mothers had displayed sadness in comparison to when they displayed joy. The infants' withdrawal, undertaken in the service of emotion regulation, deprives them of the opportunity to attain their goal of proximity or engagement and, hence, to develop feelings of effectance. Evidence that infants of depressed mothers were less persistent than other infants in their attempts to engage mothers during the still face and initiated fewer positive attempts to interact with adult strangers (Field et al., 1988) provides further support for this thesis. Through repeated experiences with affectively unresponsive mothers, infants' expectations that they will be successful in eliciting a response diminish, altering their subsequent engagement.

There is evidence also linking maternal affect and behavior to infants' persistence in relation to the inanimate environment. Redding, Harmon, and Morgan (1990) found that mothers with high levels of depressed affect had infants who displayed less task persistence in attempting to solve challenging tasks at both 1

and 2 years and less pleasure at 2 years than infants of nondepressed mothers across tasks of any difficulty level. Moreover, in another study, maternal responsivity, involvement, and provision of a high level of experiences (e.g., pretend play and problem solving) within a positive emotional context all correlated positively with task persistence at 24 months (Spangler, 1989).

In sum, contingent affective mother–infant interactions appear to elicit positive emotions in infants and behaviors indicative of a sense of effectance. Although in most studies the focus has been on effectance in social interactions, the expected links have been observed in relation to object mastery as well. This congruence across contexts may reflect the central role caregivers play in mediating infants' interactions with the physical environment. Much of the interaction between mothers and infants during the second half of the first year of life and thereafter occurs during play, and mothers' ability to stimulate interest in toys through her own affect and behavior, to assist in modulating negative emotion, and to shift control gradually to the infant are likely instrumental in the infant's continued engagement and pleasure, key features of a sense of effectance.

Attachment Security and Effectance

A secure attachment relationship is believed to contribute to the infant's sense of confident expectancy (Winnicott, 1971). As discussed previously, when mothers respond contingently and appropriately to their infants' emotional cues, infants come to believe that their needs will be met and construct a representation of themselves as able to get and deserving of what they need. As they become increasingly aware of their own self and their effects on others in the second year of life, they can identify themselves as the source of their accomplishments and, in doing so, develop a more enduring sense of effectance (Stern, 1985).

We believe this sense of effectance, in conjunction with the expectation that mother is available if needed and the associated reduction in negative emotions, accounts for the securely attached infant's ability to explore the environment freely and joyfully. Infants with ambivalent attachments engage in less exploratory behavior because they must remain focused on their mothers to ensure proximity, because the negative emotions they use to ensure her engagement interfere with their attentive engagement with the environment, and because they have less confidence than securely attached infants in their ability to attain goals independently. Infants with avoidant attachments, though less focused on mothers, make less effective use of the environment than do secure infants because their strategies for maintaining proximity involve suppression of emotions, including the positive emotions of interest and pleasure that reflect and promote active engagement, and because goal attainment may require active social engagement that infants with avoidant attachments eschew.

Consistent with these predictions, researchers have confirmed concurrent and predictive links between attachment security and mastery motivation (effectance), although the latter results have been less consistent. Frankel and Bates (1990) replicated Matas, Arend, and Sroufe's (1978) finding that infants who were securely attached at 13 months displayed more task persistence and less negativism during challenging tasks at 2 years. More recently, Riksen-Walraven, Meij, van Roozendaal, and Koks (1993) reported that attachment classification assessed at 12 months predicted mastery motivation (i.e., time spent exploring, eagerness/involvement, excitement, and self-reliance) at 30 months for tasks requiring exploration, but only for girls. In contrast, Frodi et al. (1985) found that, although infants who were either securely attached or avoidant displayed more task persistence than did ambivalent infants at both 12 and 20 months, and ambivalent infants displayed the most negative affect, attachment classification at 12 months did not predict persistence at 20 months. Similarly, Maslin-Cole, Bretherton, and Morgan (1993) found that attachment security was associated with concurrent task directedness at 18 months but did not predict task directedness at 25 months.

These conflicting results may be due to changes in attachment security over time or to other experiences that contribute to older infants' feelings of effectance and moderate the impact of attachment security on their effectance-related behavior. As they get older, infants interact increasingly with fathers and other caregivers who are likely to play important roles in their developing sense of effectance. Methodological issues such as the difficulty level of tasks used to assess mastery motivation may also explain the inconsistent results by impacting how engaging the task is for individual children and, hence, their pleasure and task persistence. Redding, Morgan, and Harmon (1988) have since developed a method to assess intraindividual task difficulty to eliminate this problem. In addition, parents' task-focused teaching strategies influence infants' feelings of effectance and mastery, as we discuss next.

Parental Scaffolding/Teaching and Effectance

Caregivers are the more knowledgeable partners in infant–parent interaction and, thus, have the ability to assist infants in learning skills just beyond their current abilities. This assistance occurs as scaffolding, providing infants with increasingly complex information about the task at hand that is appropriate for the infant's developmental level and contingent upon the infant's behavior. As such, we would expect scaffolding to promote both increasingly competent behavior and a sense of effectance that develops when infants believe they are responsible for their own goal attainment. Also, scaffolding provides infants with strategies to use in attempting to master particular aspects of the environment and may contribute in this way to their persistence in the face of initial failure.

By the middle of the first year of life, parental didactic interaction predicts several aspects of effectance in infants. Yarrow et al. (1984) found that both mothers' and fathers' sensory stimulation (e.g., stimulate with object and prompt motor act) was associated with infant persistence during problem solving at 6 months. By 12 months, the prediction held only for boys' persistence and, significantly, was accounted for by paternal behavior. Similarly, Hauser-Cram (1996) reported that maternal didactic interaction at 1 and 2 years (e.g., clarity of instructions, use of verbal description and modeling, and praising the infant) was positively associated with concurrent persistence, as well as competence, during several types of challenging tasks in a sample of infants with developmental disabilities.

Findings from a study conducted by Frodi et al. (1985) are consistent with the view that infants must experience a certain degree of autonomy of action if they are to attribute their accomplishments to their own efforts and feel effective. The authors found that at 12 and 20 months, infants of mothers who were controlling during play (i.e., changed the infant's activity) displayed less persistence and competence than did infants of mothers who supported their infants' autonomy. Intrusiveness, or overcontrol, may induce children to adopt a more passive stance in response to environmental challenges. Parents who provide infants with too much direction may promote efficient responding rather than a willingness to initiate and persist in mastery-directed behaviors (Busch-Rossnagel, Knauf-Jensen, & Des-Rosiers, 1995). Lawson, Parinello, and Ruff (1992) found that maternal responsiveness, involvement, and holding an object within reach during play all were associated positively with infants' focused exploration at 12 months, whereas maternal intrusiveness, restrictiveness, and manipulation of the objects were associated with more passive looking.

Similar to findings on the parental correlates of compliance reviewed earlier, scaffolding behaviors that direct infant behavior by encouraging attention and engagement with objects but allow autonomy to explore and experiment likely contribute to an infant's belief in his or her ability to alter the environment in pursuit of goals. However, in the absence of experimental studies, it is possible that infants elicit as well as respond to maternal behavior.

Temperament and Effectance

Temperamental characteristics may be alternate, direct pathways to behaviors that serve as markers for effectance, they may elicit caregiver behaviors that contribute to feelings of effectance, and they may interact with maternal behaviors to impact effectance (Vondra, 1995). To illustrate, behaviorally inhibited infants may engage in less exploration in the presence of strangers or novel toys because they are more highly aroused in those contexts and, thus, constitutionally predisposed to inhibit behavior in the service of regulation. Alternatively, highly active infants may engage or appear to engage in more exploration by virtue of their physical movement. Thus, differences in infant's exploratory behavior may be attributable to temperamental differences rather than to a lack of effectance, introducing "error" into tests of the association between maternal behavior and infant effectance and limiting its utility as an operational measure of the construct.

There have been few attempts to validate these propositions in relation to the temperamental constructs most often identified as likely contributors to exploratory behavior or persistence. In one such effort, Frankel and Bates (1990) found that infants who had difficulty adapting to new situations displayed dependency in joint problem-solving tasks by whining, proximity seeking, and seeking help from mothers, indicating that temperamental characteristics may affect infant behavior in challenging tasks in ways that mirror the impact of effectance on behavior. Spangler's (1989) findings that mothers were less responsive and involved during interactions with difficult infants, and that these maternal behaviors were, in turn, associated with lower task persistence, may reflect an indirect effect of infant characteristics on persistence through its impact on maternal behavior. Wachs (1987) reported also that infant characteristics and maternal behavior interacted to predict infant behavior; object naming prompted goal-directed behavior for less active infants, whereas it interfered with goal-directed behavior for highly active infants.

Implications for Intervention

Intervention to promote feelings of effectance may be warranted if we can identify links between those feelings and emotional–behavioral adjustment during infancy and beyond. Although empirical data are scant, a compelling argument can be made for the centrality of effectance in the infant's and young child's mental and emotional health. Belief in one's capacity to alter the environment in pursuit of goals is the basis of problem-focused coping, a behavioral response to stress characterized by active engagement with the environment to alter stressful events or moderate their impact on the self (Lazarus & Folkman, 1984). Without the belief that one might be successful, there would be no purpose for such behavior, no function it would serve. Moreover, in studies of older children, adolescents, and adults, problem-focused coping has been linked to lower levels of depression and fewer mental health problems of all kinds (Compas, Malcarne, & Fondacaro, 1988). Evidence that infants of depressed mothers engaged in fewer efforts to elicit a response during the still face and displayed depressed affect throughout their interaction offers a prototype for later findings (Cohn et al., 1986; Field et al., 1988; Tronick et al., 1982). In our view, this sense of effectance or confident expectancy is the essential ingredient of resilience, the individual's ability to overcome obstacles to achieve developmental goals across the lifespan.

As discussed previously, the infant's sense of effectance in the world develops from early infancy onward through the myriad encounters with caregivers, particularly mothers, who respond contingently, provide appropriate stimulation, and allow sufficient autonomy for infants to explore freely, experiment with behavior, and attribute their accomplishments to themselves. It follows that interventions, such as van den Boom's (1994, 1995), in which mothers are helped to provide contingent experiences for their infants in the service of emotional regulation and secure attachments, should support the development of effectance.

Attempts to encourage parents' scaffolding behavior during play in an effort to provide infants with well-timed stimulation that allows autonomy and encourages exploration and experimentation also should enhance infants' sense of effectance (Hauser-Cram & Shonkoff, 1995). Although play-based interventions may be introduced as early as the second half of the first year of life, infants' growing competencies and increasing desire for autonomy during the second and third years suggest that later interventions that include fathers as well as mothers may have an especially beneficial impact on infant effectance at that time.

CONCLUSION

There are several advances apparent in this review of research on the social–emotional bases of infant mental health, some clear implications for intervention, and promising directions for future research. The first is that both past and present interactive experiences of infants with mothers contribute transactionally to more or less adaptive patterns of development over time. Strategies infants develop to regulate negative emotions during the first year of life both influence and are influenced by attachment relationships and subsequent socialization practices. Changes in both family circumstances and infants' developmental competencies provide opportunities for the alteration of developmental trajectories. Crittenden (1994) has suggested that during periods of cognitive and social transitions, children may be especially receptive to changes in parental behavior, making interventions more effective at those times. The complexity of the developmental processes involved and the possibility of change during infancy are consistent with the concept of "multiple pathways," a term used in developmental psychopathology to indicate that different patterns of experience may produce equally adaptive or maladaptive outcomes. These features of early development are the basis for optimism in the potential effectiveness of interventions designed to foster infant mental health both early and later in infancy.

A second advance is the empirical confirmation that infant temperamental characteristics both elicit caregiving behavior and interact with it to influence emotion regulation and related aspects of infant emotional development. These findings underscore the infant's role in his or her own development and the interconnectedness of infant and context. They also emphasize the importance of developing interventions adapted to the needs of specific infants and caregivers.

A third advance is the documentation that mothers' working models of relationships, based in part on their own childhood experiences with parents, affect their perceptions of infant emotions and interpretations of their infants' behavior. It appears that grandparents influence infant development, even when they have little direct contact with their grandchildren, and that more intensive interventions focusing on mothers' developmental histories may be needed in some families to effect sustained improvement in infant social–emotional development.

Knowledge of fathers' contribution to individual differences in infant adaptation also has been advanced. There is empirical confirmation of earlier predictions that fathers play a role in fostering infant's emotion regulation, and that they exercise their influence partly in the course of rough-and-tumble play. In contrast to earlier findings, recent investigators have documented father effects and demonstrated that infants engage differently with mothers and fathers in emotionally arousing situations during the first year of life, perhaps because fathers are spending more time with their infants than in previous generations. They also have identified distinct patterns of father–son interaction as early as 12 months. Taken together, these findings warrant including fathers in early interventions designed to foster infant emotional development.

Although we have progressed in our understanding of infant development in the context of families during the last three decades, current knowledge does not yet reflect the complexity of the relationships that exist within families (Emde, 1991; McHale, Kuersten, & Lauretti, 1996). Such a perspective requires consideration of the multiple and transactional ways family members influence each other, rather than a simple, unilinear approach (Marvin & Stewart, 1990). Few investigators have considered triadic as well as dyadic influences and both interactive and main effects of mothers and fathers on infant development. Thus, the impact of the family context on the infant, and vice versa, may be even greater than is apparent from the extant research.

In future investigations, researchers need to combine consideration of complex family effects with efforts to understand the psychological processes involved in the development of maladaptive patterns of social–emotional development. In addition to longitudinal, correlational studies of multiple family members, we need qualitative data to expand knowledge of family systems and experimental designs to identify underlying processes and confirm causal links. We must evaluate the effectiveness of theoretically driven, empirically based interventions to determine whether they are having the desired effect and to assess how they could be improved.

REFERENCES

Adam, E. K., Tanaka, A., Brodersen, L., & Gunnar, M. R. (1998, April). *Adult attachment and maternal perceptions of toddler temperament and emotion.* Paper presented at the biennial International Conference on Infant Studies, Atlanta.

Ainsworth, M. D. S., Blehar, M., Waters, E., & Wall, S. (1978). *Patterns of attachment.* Hillsdale, NJ: Erlbaum.

Ainsworth, M. D. S., & Eichberg, C. G. (1991). Effects on infant–mother attachment of mother's unresolved loss of an attachment figure or other traumatic experience. In P. Marris, J. Stevenson-Hinde, & C. Parkes (Eds.), *Attachment across the life cycle* (pp. 160–186). New York: Routledge.

Barr, R. G., & Lehtonen, L. (1998, April). *Pathways to and from colic: Three complementary hypotheses.* Paper presented at the biennial International Conference on Infant Studies, Atlanta.

Barrett, K. C., Morgan, G. A., & Maslin-Cole, C. (1993). Three studies on the development of mastery motivation in infancy and toddlerhood. In D. J. Messer (Ed.), *Mastery motivation in early childhood: Development, measurement, and social processes* (pp. 83–108). New York: Routledge.

Barnett, D. (1997). The effects of early intervention on maltreating parents and their children. In M. J. Guralnick (Ed.), *The effectiveness of early intervention: Directions for second generation research.* Baltimore: Brookes.

Bell, R. Q. (1971). Stimulus control of parent or caretaker behavior by offspring. *Developmental Psychology, 4*(1), 63–72.

Belsky, J. (1996). Parent, infant, and social–contextual antecedents of father–son attachment security. *Developmental Psychology, 32*(5), 905–913.

Belsky, J., Rovine, M., & Fish, M. (1989). The developing family system. In M. Gunnar & E. Thelen (Eds.), *Minnesota Symposia on Child Psychology: Vol. 22. Systems and development* (pp. 119–166). Hillsdale, NJ: Erlbaum.

Belsky, J., Rovine, M., & Taylor, D. (1984). The Pennsylvania Infant and Family Development Project, III: The origins of individual differences in infant–mother attachment–maternal and infant contributions. *Child Development, 55,* 718–728.

Belsky, J., Woodworth, S., & Crnic, K. (1996). Trouble in the second year: Three questions about interaction. *Child Development, 67,* 556–578.

Belsky, J., Youngblade, L. M., Rovine, M., & Volling, B. L. (1989). *Patterns of marital change and parent–child interaction.* Paper presented at the biennial meeting of the Society for Research in Child Development, Kansas City, MO.

Benoit, D., & Parker, K. (1994). Stability and transmission of attachment across three generations. *Child Development, 65,* 1444–1456.

Blokland, K., & Goldberg, S. (1998, April). *Attachment and expectant mothers' responses to infant emotion.* Paper presented at the biennial International Conference on Infant Studies, Atlanta.

Bowlby, J. (1973). *Attachment and loss: Vol. 2. Separation: Anxiety and anger.* New York: Basic Books.

Bowlby, J. (1982). *Attachment and loss: Vol. 1. Attachment* (2nd ed.). New York: Basic Books. (Original work published in 1969)

Braungart-Reiker, J. M., Garwood, M. M., Powers, B. P., & Notaro, P. C. (1998, April). *Infant affect and affect regulation during still-face with mothers and fathers: The role of infant characteristics and parental sensitivity.* Paper presented at the biennial International Conference on Infant Studies, Atlanta.

Bridges, L. J., & Grolnick, W. S. (1998, April). *A longitudinal investigation of infant emotion regulation with mothers and fathers.* Paper presented at the biennial International Conference on Infant studies, Atlanta.

Bronfenbrenner, U. (1979). *The ecology of human development.* Cambridge, MA: Harvard University Press.

Bronson, W. (1974). Mother–toddler interaction: A perspective on studying the development of competence. *Merrill–Palmer Quarterly, 20,* 275–301.

Burton, L., & Dilworth-Anderson, P. (1991). The intergenerational family roles of aged Black Americans. *Marriage and Family Review, 16,* 311–330.

Busch-Rossnagel, N. A., Knauf-Jensen, D. E., & DesRosiers, F. S. (1995). Mothers and others: The role of the socializing environment in the development of mastery motivation. In I. E. Sigel (Series Ed.) & R. H. MacTurk & G. A. Morgan (Vol. Eds.), *Advances in applied developmental psychology: Vol. 12. Mastery motivation: Origins, conceptualizations, and applications* (pp. 117–145). Norwood, NJ: Ablex.

Caldera, Y., Huston, A., & O'Brian, M. (1995, April). *Antecedents of father–infant attachment: A longitudinal study.* Paper presented at the biennial meetings of the Society for Research in Child Development, Indianapolis, IN.

Calkins, S. (1994). Origins and outcomes of individual differences in emotion regulation. *Monographs for the Society for Research in Child Development, 59*(2–3, Serial No. 240) 53–72.

Calkins, S. D., Smith, C. L., Gill, K. L., & Johnson, M. C. (1998). Maternal interactive style across contexts: Relations to emotional, behavioral and physiological regulation during toddlerhood. *Social Development, 7*(3) 350–369.

Campos, J. J., & Stenberg, C. R. (1981). Perception, appraisal, and emotions: The onset of social referencing. In M. E. Lamb & L. R. Sherrod (Eds.), *Infant social cognition: Empirical and theoretical considerations* (pp. 273–314). Hillside, NJ: Erlbaum.

Cassidy, J. (1994). Emotion regulation: Influences of attachment relationships. *Monographs for the Society for Research in Child Development, 59*(2–3, Serial No. 240).

Cassidy, J., & Berlin L. J. (1994). The insecure/ambivalent pattern of attachment: Theory and research. *Child Development, 65,* 971–991.

Cassidy, J., Kirsh, S., Scolton, K., & Parke, R. (1996). Attachment and representations of peer relationships. *Developmental Psychology, 32,* 892–904

Chapman, M., & Zahn-Waxler, C. (1982). Young children's compliance and noncompliance to parental discipline in a natural setting. *International Journal of Behavior and Development, 5,* 81–94.

Cohn, J. F., Campbell, S. B., & Ross, S (1991). Infant response in the still-face paradigm at 6 months predicts avoidant and secure attachment at 12 months. *Development and Psychopathology, 3,* 367–376.

Cohn, J. F., Matias, R., Tronick, E. Z., Connell, D., & Lyons-Ruth, K. (1986). Face-to-face interactions of depressed mothers and their infants. In E. Z. Tronick & T. Field (Eds.), *New directions for child development: Vol. 34. Maternal depression and infant disturbances* (pp. 31–45). San Francisco: Jossey-Bass.

Compas, B. E., Malcarne, V. L., & Fondacaro, K. M. (1988). Coping with stressful events in older children and young adolescents. *Journal of Consulting and Clinical Psychology, 56,* 405–411.

Cox, M. J., Owen, M. T., Henderson, V. K., & Margand, N. A. (1992). Prediction of infant–father and infant–mother attachment. *Developmental Psychology, 28,* 474–483.

Crittenden, P. (1994). Peering into the black box: An exploratory treatise on the development of self in young children. In D. Cicchetti & S. Toth (Eds.), *Rochester Symposium on Developmental Psychopathology: Vol. 5. Disorders and dysfunctions of the self* (pp. 79–148). Rochester, NY: University of Rochester Press.

Crittenden, P. M., & DiLalla, D. L. (1988). Compulsive compliance: The development of an inhibitory coping strategy in infancy. *Journal of Abnormal Child Psychology, 16,* 585–599.

Crockenberg, S. (1981). Infant irritability, mother responsiveness, and social influences on the security of infant–mother attachment. *Child Development, 52,* 857–865.

Crockenberg, S. (1985). Toddler's reactions to maternal anger. *Merrill–Palmer Quarterly, 31* (4), 361–373.

Crockenberg, S. (1986). Are temperamental differences in babies associated with predictable differences in care giving? In J. V. Lerner & R. M. Lerner (Eds.), *New directions for child development: Vol. 31. Temperament and social interaction during infancy and childhood* (pp. 52–73). San Francisco: Jossey-Bass.

Crockenberg, S. (1987). Predictors and correlates of anger toward and punitive control of toddlers by adolescent mothers. *Child Development, 58,* 964–975.

Crockenberg, S. (1988). Social support and parenting. In H. Fitzgerald, B. Lester, & M. Yogman (Eds.), *Theory and research in behavioral pediatrics* (pp. 141–174). New York: Plenum.

Crockenberg, S., & Litman, C. (1990). Autonomy as competence in two-year-olds: Maternal correlates of child compliance, defiance, and self-assertion. *Developmental Psychology, 26,* 961–971.

Crockenberg, S., Lyons-Ruth, K., & Dickstein, S. (1993). The family context of infant mental health: II. Infant development in multiple family relationships. In C. II. Zeanah, Jr. (Ed.), *Handbook of infant mental health* (pp. 38–55). New York: Guilford Press.

Crockenberg, S., & Smith, P. (1982). Antecedents of mother–infant interaction and infant irritability in the first three months of life. *Infant Behavior and Development, 5,* 105–119.

Crowell, J. A., & Feldman, S. S. (1988). Mothers' internal models of relationships and children's behavioral and developmental status: A study of mother–child interaction. *Child Development, 59,* 1273–1285.

Cummings, E. M., Zahn-Waxler, C., & Radke-Yarrow, M. (1981). Young children's responses to expressions of anger and affection by others in the family. *Child Development, 52,* 1274–1282.

De Wolff, M. S., & van IJzendoorn, M. H. (1997). Sensitivity and attachment: A meta-analysis on parental antecedents of infant attachment. *Child Development, 68*(4), 571–591.

Dickstein, S., & Parke, R. D. (1988). Social referencing: A glance at fathers and marriage. *Child Development, 59,* 506–511.

Diener, M., Mangelsdorf, S., Fosnot, K., & Kienstra, M. (1997, April). *Effects of maternal involvement on toddlers' emotion regulation strategies.* Paper presented at the biennial meeting for the Society for Research in Child Development, Washington, DC.

Diener, M., Mangelsdorf, S. C., McHale, J. L., & Frosch, C. A. (1998, April). *Mother-father differences and paternal correlates of infant emotion regulation.* Paper presented at the biennial International Conference on Infant Studies, Atlanta.

Doucette-Dudman, D. (1996). *Raising our children's children.* Minneapolis, MN: Fairview Press.

Dozier, M., Stovall, K. C., & Albus, K. E. (1999). A transactional intervention for foster infants' caregivers. In D. Cicchetti & S. L. Toth (Eds.), *Rochester Symposium on Developmental Psychopathology: Vol. 9. Developmental approaches to prevention and intervention* (pp. 195–219). Rochester, NY: University of Rochester Press.

Egeland, B., & Farber, E. A. (1984). Infant-mother attachment: Factors related to its development and changes over time. *Child Development, 55*, 753–771.

Eisenberg, N. (1997, April). *Emotion-related regulation*. Paper presented at the biennial meeting for the Society for Research in Child Development, Washington, DC.

Emde, R. (1984). Infant psychiatry in a changing world: Optimism and paradox. In J. D. Call, E. Galenson, & R. L. Tyson (Eds.), *Frontiers of infant psychiatry, Vol. II*. New York: Basic Books.

Emde, R. N. (1991). The wonder of our complex enterprise: Steps enabled by attachment and the effects of relationships on relationships. *Infant Mental Health Journal, 12*, 164–173.

Emde, R., Johnson, W. F., & Easterbrooks, M. A. (1988). The do's and don'ts of early moral development: Psychoanalytic tradition and current research. In J. Kagan & S. Lamb (Eds.), *The emergence of morality* (pp. 245–277). Chicago: University of Chicago Press.

Emery, R. E., & Laumann-Billings, L. (1998). An overview of the nature, causes, and consequences of abusive family relationships: Toward differentiating maltreatment and violence. *American Psychologist, 53*(2), 121–135.

Erikson, E. H. (1963). *Childhood and society*. New York: Norton.

Escher-Graeub, D., & Grossmann, K. E. (1983). *Attachment security in the second year of life: The Regensburg cross-sectional study* [Research report]. Regensburg, Germany: University of Regensburg.

Field, T. (1994). The effects of mother's physical and emotional unavailability on emotion regulation. *Monographs for the Society for Research in Child Development, 59*(2–3, Serial No. 240), 208–227.

Field, T. (1995). Psychologically depressed parents. In M. H. Bornstein (Ed.), *Handbook of parenting: Vol. 4. Applied and practical parenting* (pp. 85–99). Mahwah, NJ: Erlbaum.

Field, T. M. (1998, April). *Touch and touch therapies*. Paper presented at the biennial International Conference on Infant Studies, Atlanta.

Field, T., Healy, B., Goldstein, S., Perry, S., Bendell, D., Schanberg, S., Zimmerman, E. A., & Kuhn, C. (1988). Infants of depressed mothers show "depressed" behavior even with nondepressed adults. *Child Development, 59*, 1569–1579.

Fonagy, P., Steele, H., & Steele, M. (1991). Maternal representations of attachment during pregnancy predict the organization of infant–mother attachment at one year of age. *Child Development, 62*, 891–905.

Fox, N. A., & Calkins, S. D. (1993). Multiple-measure approaches to the study of infant emotion. In M. Lewis & J. M. Haviland (Eds.), *Handbook of emotion* (pp. 167–184). New York: Guilford Press.

Fraiberg, S. (1980). *Clinical studies in infant mental health: The first year of life*. New York: Basic Books.

Frankel, K. A., & Bates, J. E. (1990). Mother–toddler problem solving: Antecedents in attachment, home

behavior, and temperament. *Child Development, 61*, 810–819.

Freud, S. (1953). Three essays on the theory of sexuality. In J. Strachey (Ed. and Trans.), *The standard edition of the complete psychological works of Sigmund Freud* (Vol. 7, pp. 123–245). London: Hogarth Press. (Original work published 1905)

Frodi, A., Bridges, L., & Grolnick, W. (1985). Correlates of mastery related behavior: A short term longitudinal study of infants in their second year. *Child Development, 56*, 1291–1298.

Gable, S., Belsky, J., & Crnic, K. (1995). Co-parenting in the child's second year. *Journal of Marriage and the Family, 57*, 609–616.

Gianino, A., & Tronick, E. Z. (1988). The mutual regulation model: The infant's self and interactive regulation, coping, and defense. In T. Field, P. McCabe, & N. Schneiderman (Eds.), *Stress and coping* (pp. 47–68). Hillsdale, NJ: Erlbaum.

Goldberg, W. A., & Easterbrooks, M. A. (1984). The role of marital quality in toddler development. *Child Development, 20*, 504–515.

Goldsmith, H. H., & Alansky, J. A. (1987). Maternal and infant predictors of attachment: A meta-analytic review. *Journal of Consulting and Clinical Psychology, 55*, 805–816.

Goodnow, J. J., & Collins, W. A. (1990). *Development according to parents: The nature, sources, and consequences of parents' ideas*. Hove, England: Erlbaum.

Grolnick, W. S., Bridges, L., & Connell, J. (1996). Emotion regulation in two-year-olds: Strategies and emotional expression in four contexts. *Child Development, 67*, 928–941.

Grolnick, W. S., Cosgrove, T. J., & Bridges, L. J. (1996). Age-graded changes in the initiation of positive affect. *Infant Behavior and Development, 19*, 153–157.

Grossmann, K., Fremmer-Bombik, E., Rudolph, J., & Grossmann, K. E. (1988). Maternal attachment representations as related to patterns of infant–mother attachment and maternal care during the first year. In R. A. Hinde & J. Stevenson-Hinde (Eds.), *Relationships within families: Mutual influences* (pp. 241–260). New York: Oxford University Press.

Gunnar, M. R., Broderson, L., Nachmias, M. C., Buss, K., & Rigatuso, J. (1996). Stress reactivity and attachment security. *Developmental Psychobiology, 29*(3), 191–204.

Gunnar, M. R., & Stone, C. (1984). The effect of positive maternal affect on infant responses to pleasant, ambiguous, and fear-provoking toys. *Child Development, 55*, 1231–1236.

Gustafson, G. E., & Green, J. A. (1998, April). *Perceiving the causes of infant crying*. Paper presented at the biennial International Conference on Infant Studies, Atlanta.

Hauser-Cram, P. (1996). Mastery motivation in toddlers with developmental disabilities. *Child Development, 67*, 236–248.

Hauser-Cram, P., & Shonkoff, J. P. (1995). Mastery motivation: Implication for intervention. In I. E. Sigel (Series Ed.) & R. H. MacTurk & G. A. Morgan (Vol. Eds.), *Advances in applied developmental psychology: Vol. 12. Mastery motivation: Origins, conceptual-*

izations, and applications (pp. 257–272). Norwood, NJ: Ablex.

Hazen, N., & Durrett, M. (1982). Relationship of security of attachment to exploration and cognitive mapping ability in two-year-olds. *Developmental Psychology, 18*, 751–759.

Heckhausen, J. (1993). The development of mastery and its perception within caretaker–child dyads. In D. J. Messer (Ed.), *Mastery motivation in early childhood: Development, measurement, and social processes* (pp. 55–79). New York: Routledge.

Heinecke, C. M., & Westheimer, I. J. (1966). *Brief separations*. New York: International Universities Press.

Hirshberg, L. M., & Svejda, M. (1990). When infants look to their parents: Infants' social referencing of mothers compared to fathers. *Child Development, 61*, 1175–1186.

Hornik, R., & Gunnar, M. R. (1988). A descriptive analysis of infant social referencing. *Child Development, 59*, 626–634.

Hornik, R., Risenhoover, N., & Gunnar, M. (1987). The effects of maternal positive, neutral, and negative affective communications on infant responses to new toys. *Child Development, 58*, 937–944.

Hossain, Z., Field, T. M., Gonzalez, J., Malphurs, J., Del Valle, C., & Pickens, J. (1994). Infants of "depressed" mothers interact better with their non-depressed fathers. *Infant Mental Health Journal, 15*(4), 348–357.

Howes, P. W., & Markman, H. J. (1989). Marital quality and child attachment: A longitudinal investigation. *Child Development, 60*, 1044–1051.

Isabella, R. A., & Belsky, J. (1991). Interactional synchrony and the origins of infant–mother attachment: A replication study. *Child Development, 62*, 373–384.

Isabella, R. A., Belsky, J., & von Eye, A. (1989). The origins of infant mother attachment: An examination of interactional synchrony during the infant's first year. *Developmental Psychology, 25*, 12–21.

Jacobson, J. L., & Wille, D. E. (1986). The influence of attachment pattern on developmental changes from the toddler to the preschool period. *Child Development, 57*(2), 338–347.

Jacobvitz, J. D., Hazen, N., & Riggs, S. (1997, April). *Disorganized mental processes in mothers, frightening/frightened caregiving, and disoriented/disorganized behavior in infancy.* Paper presented at the biennial meeting for the Society for Research in Child Development, Washington, DC.

Kagan, J. (1981). *The second year: The emergence of self-awareness*. Cambridge, MA: Harvard University Press.

Klinnert, M. D. (1984). The regulation of infant behavior by maternal facial expression. *Infant Behavior and Development, 7*, 447–465.

Kochanska, G. (1993). Toward a synthesis of parental socialization and child temperament in early development of conscience. *Child Development, 64*, 325–347.

Kochanska, G. (1995). Children's temperament, mothers' discipline, and security of attachment: Multiple pathways to emerging internalization. *Child Development, 66*, 597–615.

Kochanska, G., & Aksan, N. (1995). Mother–child mutually positive affect: The quality of child compliance to requests and prohibitions, and maternal control as correlates of early internalization. *Child Development, 66*, 236–254.

Kochanska, G., Aksan, N., & Koenig, A. (1995). A longitudinal study of the roots of preschoolers' conscience: Committed compliance and emerging internalization. *Child Development, 66*, 1752–1779.

Kogan, N., & Carter, A. S. (1996). Mother–infant reengagement following the still-face: The role of maternal emotional availability in infant affect regulation. *Infant Behavior and Development, 19*, 359–370.

Kopp, C. B. (1989). Regulation of distress and negative emotions: A developmental view. *Developmental Psychology, 25*(3), 343–354.

Kropp, J. P., & Haynes, O. M. (1987). Abusive and nonabusive mothers' ability to identify general and specific emotion signals of infants. *Child Development, 58*, 187–190.

Kuczynski, L., Kochanska, G., Radke-Yarrow, M., & Girnius-Brown, O. (1987). A developmental interpretation of young children's non-compliance. *Developmental Psychology, 23*, 799–806.

Lamb, M. E., & Elster, A. B. (1985). Adolescent mother–infant–father relationships. *Development Psychology, 21*, 768–773.

Lawson, K., Parinello, R., & Ruff, H. A. (1992). Maternal behavior and infant attention. *Infant Behavior and Development, 15*, 209–229.

Lazarus, R. S., & Folkman, S. (1984). *Stress, appraisal, and coping*. New York: Springer.

Lewis, M. (1993). The emergence of human emotions. In M. Lewis & J. M. Haviland (Eds.), *Handbook of emotions* (pp. 223–235). New York: Guilford Press.

Lewis, M., & Brooks-Gunn, J. (1979). *Social cognition and the aquisitional self* (pp. 223–226). New York: Plenum.

Lewis, M., Sullivan, M. W., Stanger, C., & Weiss, M. (1989). Self development and self-conscious emotions. *Child Development, 60*, 146–156.

Lieberman, A. F., & Zeanah, C. H. (1999). Contributions of attachment theory to infant–parent psychotherapy and other interventions with infants and young children. In J. Cassidy & P. Shaver (Eds.), *Handbook of attachment: Theory, research, and clinical applications* (pp. 555–574). New York: Guilford Press.

Londerville, S., & Main, M. (1981). Security of attachment, compliance, and maternal training methods in the second year of life. *Developmental Psychology, 17*(3), 289–299.

Lyons-Ruth, K., & Block, D. (1996). The disturbed caregiving system: Relations among childhood trauma, maternal caregiving, and infant affect and attachment. *Infant Mental Health Journal, 17*(3), 257–275.

Lyons-Ruth, K., Bronfman, E., & Parsons, E. (in press). Maternal disrupted affective communication, maternal frightened, frightening, or atypical behavior and disorganized infant attachment patterns. In J. Vondra & D. Barnett (Eds.), *Atypical patterns of attachment: Theory and current directions. Monographs of the Society for Research in Child Development.*

Lyons-Ruth, K., Connell, D. B., Zoll, D., & Stahl, J. (1987). Infants at social risk: Relations among infant maltreatment, maternal behavior, and infant attachment behavior. *Developmental Psychology*, *23*(2), 223–232.

Lyons-Ruth, K., Easterbrooks, M. A., & Cibelli, C. D. (1997). Infant attachment strategies, infant mental lag, and maternal depressive symptoms: Predictors of internalizing and externalizing problems at age 7. *Developmental Psychology*, *33*(4), 681–692.

Lyons-Ruth, K., & Jacobvitz, D. (1999). Attachment disorganization: Unresolved loss, relational violence, and lapses in behavioral and attentional strategies. In J. Cassidy & P. R. Shaver (Eds.), *Handbook of attachment: Theory, research, and clinical applications* (pp. 520–554). New York: Guilford Press.

Lyons-Ruth, K., Repacholi, B., McLeod, S., & Silva, E. (1991). Disorganized attachment behavior in infancy: Short-term stability, maternal and infant correlated and sick-related subtypes. *Development and Psychopathology*, *3*, 377–396.

Lyons-Ruth, K., & Zeanah, C. H., Jr. (1993). The family context of infant mental health: I. Affective development in the primary caregiving relationship. In C. H. Zeanah, Jr. (Ed.), *Handbook of infant mental health* (pp. 14–37). New York: Guilford Press.

Main, M., & Goldwyn, R. (in press). *Adult Attachment Classification System.* Unpublished manuscript, University of California, Berkeley.

Main, M., & Hesse, E. (1990). Parents' unresolved traumatic experiences are related to infant disorganized attachment status: Is frightened and/or frightening parental behavior the linking mechanism? In M. Greenberg, D. Cicchetti, & E. M. Cummings (Eds.), *Attachment in the preschool years: Theory, research and intervention* (pp. 161–184). Chicago: University of Chicago Press.

Main, M., Kaplan, N., & Cassidy, J. (1985). Security in infancy, childhood and adulthood: A move to the level of representation. *Monographs of the Society for Research in Child Development*, *50*(1–2, Serial No. 209), 66–104.

Main, M., & Solomon, J. (1990). Procedures for identifying infants as disorganized/disoriented during the Ainsworth Strange Situation. In M. Greenberg, D. Cicchetti, & E.M. Cummings (Eds.), *Attachment in the preschool years: Theory, research and intervention* (pp. 121–160). Chicago: University of Chicago Press.

Main, M., Tomasini, L., & Tolan, W. (1979). Differences among mothers of infants judged to differ in security of attachment. *Developmental Psychology*, *15*, 472–473.

Malatesta, C. Z., Culver, C., Tesman, J. R., & Shepard, B. (1989). The development of emotion expression during the first two years of life. *Monographs of the Society for Research in Child Development*, *54*(1–2, Serial No. 219), 1–104.

Malphurs, J. E., Field, T. M., Larraine, C., Pickens, J., Pelaez-Nogueras, M., Yando, R., & Bendell, D. (1996). Altering withdrawn and intrusive interaction behaviors of depressed mothers. *Infant Mental Health Journal*, *17*(2), 152–160.

Mangelsdorf, S. C., Frosch, C. A., & McHale, J. L. (1998, April). *Fathers' and mothers' parenting during the first three years: Predictors and correlates.* Paper presented at the biennial International Conference on Infant Studies, Atlanta.

Mangelsdorf, S., Gunnar, M., Kestenbaum, R., Lang, S., & Andreas, D. (1990). Infant proneness-to-distress temperament, maternal personality, and mother–infant attachment: Associations and goodness of fit. *Child Development*, *61*, 820–831.

Mangelsdorf, S. C., Shapiro, J. C., & Marzolf, D. (1995). Developmental and temperamental differences in emotion regulation. *Child Development*, *66*, 1817–1828.

Marvin, R. S., & Stewart, R. B. (1990). A family systems framework for the study of attachment. In M. T. Greenberg, D. Cicchetti, & E. M. Cummings (Eds.), *Attachment in the preschool years: Theory, research, and intervention* (pp. 51–86). Chicago: University of Chicago Press.

Maslin-Cole, C., Bretherton, I., & Morgan, G. A. (1993). Toddler mastery motivation and competence: Links with attachment security, maternal scaffolding, and family climate. In D. J. Messer (Ed.), *Mastery motivation in early childhood: Development, measurement, and social processes* (pp. 205–229). New York: Routledge.

Matas, L., Arend, R. A., & Sroufe, L. A. (1978). Continuity of adaptation in the second year: The relationship between quality of attachment and later competence. *Child Development*, *49*, 547–556.

McHale, J. P., Kuersten, R., & Lauretti, A. (1996). New directions in the study of family-level dynamics during infancy and early childhood. In J. P. McHale & P. A. Cowen (Eds.), *New directions for child development: Vol. 74. Understanding how family-level dynamics affect children's development. Studies of two-parent families.* San Francisco: Jossey-Bass.

McHale, J. P., & Rasmussen, J. L. (1998). Co-parental and family group-level dynamics during infancy: Early family precursors of child and family functioning during preschool. *Development and Psychopathology*, *10*, 39–59.

McLoyd, V. C. (1990). The impact of economic hardship on black families and children: Psychological distress, parenting, and socio-emotional development. *Child Development*, *61*, 311–346.

Minkler, R., & Roe, K. M. (1993). *Family caregiver application series, Vol. 2. Grandmothers as caregivers: Raising children of the crack cocaine epidemic.* Newbury Park, CA: Sage.

Mumme, D. L., Fernald, A., & Herrera, C. (1996). Infant's responses to facial and vocal emotional signals in a social referencing paradigm. *Child Development*, *67*, 3219–3237.

Parke, R. D., & Tinsley, B. J. (1987). Family interaction in infancy. In J. D. Osofsky (Ed.), *Handbook of infant development* (2nd ed., pp. 579–641). New York: Wiley.

Parpal, M., & Maccoby, E. E. (1985). Maternal responsiveness and subsequent child compliance. *Child Development*, *56*, 1326–1334.

Patterson, G. R. (1982). *Coercive family processes.* Eugene, OR: Castalia.

Pelaez-Nogueras, M., Field, T. M., Cigales, M., Gonzalez, A., & Clasky, S. (1994). Infants of depressed mothers show less "depressed" behavior with their nursery teachers. *Infant Mental Health Journal, 15* (4), 358–367.

Pelaez-Nogueras, M., Field, T. M., Hossain, Z., & Pickens, J. (1996). Depressed mothers' touching increases infants' positive affect and attention in still-face interactions. *Child Development, 67,* 1780–1792.

Power, T. G., Mcgrath, M. P., Hughes, S. O., & Manire, S. H. (1994). Compliance and self-assertion: Young children's responses to mothers versus fathers. *Developmental Psychology, 30*(6), 980–989.

Power, T. G., & Parke, R. D. (1983). Patterns of mother and father play with their 8 month old infant: A multiple analyses approach. *Infant Behavior and Development, 6,* 453–459.

Redding, R. E., Harmon, R. J., & Morgan, G. A. (1990). Relationships between maternal depression and infants' mastery behaviors. *Infant Behavior and Development, 13,* 391–395.

Redding, R. E., Morgan, G. A., & Harmon, R. J. (1988). Mastery motivation in infants and toddlers: Is it greatest when tasks are moderately challenging? *Infant Behavior and Development, 11,* 419–430.

Renken, B., Egeland, B., Marvinney, D., Mangelsdorf, S., & Sroufe, L. A. (1989). Early childhood antecedents of aggression and passive-withdrawal in early elementary school. *Journal of Personality, 57,* 257–282.

Riksen-Walraven, J. M., Meij, H. T., van Roozendaal, J., & Koks, J. (1993). Mastery motivation in toddlers as related to quality of attachment. In D. J. Messer (Ed.), *Mastery motivation in early childhood: Development, measurement, and social processes* (pp. 189–204). New York: Routledge.

Rosen, D., Adamson, L. B., & Bakeman, R. (1992). An experimental investigation of infant social referencing: Mother's messages and gender differences. *Developmental Psychology, 28*(6), 1172–1178.

Rothbart, M. K., & Bates, J. E. (1998). Temperament. In W. Damon (Series Ed.) & N. Eisenberg (Vol. Ed.), *Handbook of child psychology: Vol. 3. Social, emotional, and personality development* (pp. 105–176). New York: Wiley.

Sagi, A., van IJzendoorn, M. H., Scharf, M., Koren-Karie, N., Joels, T., & Mayseless, O. (1994). Stability and discriminant validity of the adult attachment interview: A psychometric study in young Israeli adults. *Developmental Psychology, 30,* 988–1000.

Sameroff, A. J., & Chandler, M. J. (1975). Reproductive risk and the continuum of caretaking casualty. In F. D. Horowitz (Ed.), *Review of child development research* (Vol. 4, pp. 187–244). Chicago: University of Chicago Press.

Scheungel, C., van IJzendoorn, M., Bakermans-Kranenburg, M., & Blom, M. (1997, April). *Frightening, frightened and/or dissociated behavior, unresolved loss and infant disorganization.* Paper presented at the biennial meeting for the Society of Research in Child Development, Washington, DC.

Seifer, R., Schiller, M., Sameroff, A. J., Resnick, S., & Riordan, K. (1996). Attachment, maternal sensitivity, and infant temperament during the first year of life. *Developmental Psychology, 32*(1), 12–25.

Spangler, G. (1989). Toddler's everyday experiences as related to preceding mental and emotional disposition and their relationships to subsequent mental and motivational development: A short-term longitudinal study. *International Journal of Behavioral Development, 12*(3), 285–303.

Spinard T. L., & Stifter, C. A. (1998, April). *Predicting individual differences in toddlers' behavioral control: Contributions of maternal responsivity and emotion regulation in infancy.* Paper presented at the biennial International Conference on Infant Studies, Atlanta.

Spitz, R. A. (1957). *No and yes: On the genesis of human communication.* Madison, CT: International Universities Press.

Sroufe, L. A. (1985). Attachment classification from the perspective of infant-caregiver relationships and infant temperament. *Child Development, 56,* 1–14.

St. James-Roberts, I. (1998, April). *What's distinct about infants' colic cries?* Paper presented at the biennial International Conference on Infant Studies, Atlanta, GA.

Stein, N. L., & Levine, L. (1987). Thinking about feelings: The development and organization of emotional knowledge. In R. Snow & M. Farr (Eds.), *Aptitude, learning and instruction* (Vol. 3, pp. 165–197). Hillsdale, NJ: Erlbaum.

Stern, D. (1985). *The interpersonal world of the infant.* New York: Basic Books.

Stifter, C. A. (1998). *The short and long-term consequences of infant excessive crying: A case for differentiating perceptions of "colic" from more objectively-based assessment.* Paper presented at the biennial International Conference on Infant Studies, Atlanta.

Stovall, K. C., & Dozier, M. (in press). The evolution of attachment in new relationships: Single subject analysis of ten foster infants. *Development and Psychopathology.*

Termine, N. T., & Izard, C. E. (1988). Infants' responses to their mothers' expressions of joy and sadness. *Developmental Psychology, 24*(2), 223–229.

Teti, D. M., Bond, L. A., & Gibbs, E. D. (1988). Mothers, fathers and siblings: A comparison of play styles and their influence upon infant cognitive level. *International Journal of Behavioral Development, 11,* 415–432.

Thomas, A., Chess, S., & Birch, H. G. (1968). *Temperament and behavior disorders in children.* New York: New York University Press.

Thompson, R. A. (1994). Emotion regulation: A theme in search of definition. *Monographs for the Society of Research in Child Development, 59* (2–3, Serial No. 240), 250–283.

Tronick, E. Z., Als, H., Adamson, L., Wise, S., & Brazelton, T. B. (1978). The infant's response to entrapment between contradictory messages in face-to-face interaction. *Journal of the American Academy of Child Psychiatry, 17,* 1–13.

Tronick, E. Z., Cohn, J., & Shea, E. (1986). The transfer of affect between mothers and infants. In T. B. Brazelton & M. W. Yogman (Eds.), *Affective development in infancy* (pp. 11–25). Norwood, NJ: Ablex.

Tronick, E. Z., Ricks, M., & Cohn, J. F. (1982). Maternal and infant affective exchange: Patterns of adaptation. In T. Field & A. Fogel (Eds.), *Emotion and early interaction* (pp. 83–100). Hillsdale, NJ: Erlbaum.

Tyrrell, C., & Dozier, M. (in press). Factors affecting foster parent sensitivity. *Adoption Quarterly*.

Ungerer, J. A., & Sygall, N. (1998, April). *A longitudinal study of maternal perceptions of emotions and the development of attachment relationships in the first year*. Paper presented at the biennial International Conference on Infant Studies, Atlanta.

van den Boom, D. C. (1994). The influence of temperament and mothering on attachment and exploration: An experimental manipulation of sensitive responsiveness among lower-class mothers with irritable infants. *Child Development, 65*, 1457–1477.

van den Boom, D. C. (1995). Do first-year intervention effects endure? Follow-up during toddlerhood of a sample of Dutch irritable infants. *Child Development, 66*, 1798–1816.

van IJzendoorn, M. H. (1995). Adult attachment representations, parental responsiveness, and infant attachment: A meta-analysis on the predictive validity of the adult attachment interview. *Psychological Bulletin, 117*(3), 387–403.

van IJzendoorn, M. H., Juffer, F., & Duyvesteyn, M. G. C. (1995). Breaking the intergenerational cycle of insecure attachment: A review of the effects of attachment-based interventions on maternal sensitivity and infant security. *Journal of Child Psychology and Psychiatry, 36*, 225–248.

Volling, B. L., & Belsky, J. (1992). Infant, father, and marital antecedents of infant father attachment security in dual earner and single earner families. *International Journal of Behavioral Development, 15*(1), 83–100.

Volling, B. L., Herrera, M. G., Notato, P. C., & McElwain, N. L. (1998, April). *Differences and similarities in maternal and paternal emotion socialization: Effects on infant affect and attention*. Paper presented at the biennial International Conference on Infant Studies, Atlanta.

Vondra, J. I. (1995). Contributions and confounds from biology and genetics. In I. E. Sigel (Series Ed.) & R. H. MacTurk & G. A. Morgan (Vol. Eds.), *Advances in applied developmental psychology: Vol. 12. Mastery motivation: Origins, conceptualizations, and applications* (pp. 165–199). Norwood, NJ: Ablex.

Wachs, T. D. (1987). Specificity of environmental action as manifest in environmental correlates of in-

fant's mastery motivation. *Developmental Psychology, 23*(6), 782–790.

Wakschlag, L. S., Chase-Lansdale, P. L., & Brooks-Gunn, J. (1996). Not just "ghosts in the nursery": Contemporaneous intergenerational relationships and parenting in young African-American families. *Child Development, 67*, 2131–2147.

Walden, T. A., & Ogan, T. A. (1988). The development of social referencing. *Child Development, 59*, 1230–1240.

Ward, M. J., & Carlson, E. A. (1995). Associations among adult attachment representations, maternal sensitivity, and infant–mother attachment in a sample of adolescent mothers. *Child Development, 66*, 69–79.

White, R. W. (1959). Motivation reconsidered: The concept of competence. *Psychological Review, 66*, 297–333.

Winnicott, D. W. (1971). *Playing and reality*. New York: Basic Books.

Yarrow, L. J., MacTurk, R. H., Vietze, P. M., McCarthy, M. E., Klein, R. P., & Mcquiston, S. (1984). Developmental course of parental stimulation and its relationship to mastery motivation during infancy. *Developmental Psychology, 20*(3), 492–503.

Zahn-Waxler, C., & Radke-Yarrow, M. (1990). The origins of concern. *Motivation and Emotion, 14*, 107–130.

Zeanah, C. H. (1996). Beyond insecurity: A reconceptualization of attachment disorders in infancy. *Journal of Clinical and Consulting Psychology, 64*(1), 42–52.

Zeanah, C. (1998, April). *Emotional development: Perspectives on the role of maternal perceptions of emotions and internal working models of attachment*. Discussant of symposium presented at the biennial International Conference on Infant Studies, Atlanta.

Zeanah, C. H., Benoit, D., Barton, M., Regan, C., Hirshberg, L. M., & Lipsitt, L. (1993). Representations of attachment in mothers and their one-year-old infants. *Journal of the American Academy of Child and Adolescent Psychiatry, 32*, 278–286.

Zeanah, C. H., Jr., Mammen, O. K., & Lieberman, A. F. (1993). Disorders of attachment. In C. H. Zeanah, Jr. (Ed.), *Handbook of infant mental health* (pp. 332–349). New York: Guilford Press.

5

The Cultural Context of Infant Mental Health: The Developmental Niche of Infant–Caregiver Relationships

❖

MARVA L. LEWIS

INTRODUCTION

There are well-documented, universal features of child development and parent–infant relationships across all ethnic and cultural groups. The areas of variability are equally important to understand (Nugent, 1994). Since the publication of the earliest volumes on culture, infancy, and psychological topics (e.g., Mead & MacGregor, 1951; Minturn & Lambert, 1964; Whiting & Child, 1953), there has been a growing number of articles, books, and studies on topics of cultural influences on infant development and parent behavior. The literature of the past decade goes beyond basic ethnographic descriptions of similarities and variations of child development in different cultural settings (Jessor, Colby, & Shweder, 1997; Tudge & Putnam, 1997) to topics important to infant mental health practitioners. Examples of these topics are cross-cultural studies of maternal responsiveness and a series of studies of family cosleeping practices, and clinical and educational approaches with linguistically and culturally different children (e.g., Gopaul-McNicol & Thomas-Presswood, 1998; LeVine, 1990; Weiss, McCarthy, Eastman, Caseate, & Suwanlert, 1997). The edited volume *Transcultural

Child Development: Psychological Assessment and Treatment (Johnson-Powell & Yamamoto, 1997) is devoted specifically to topics that address the interplay of cultural factors with psychological processes relevant to assessment and treatment of children and their families from diverse cultural groups. Each chapter focuses on how particular circumstances such as immigration, slave ancestry, or political migration may differentially contribute to psychological disorders in children in a variety of ethnic groups.

In addition, there are increasing numbers of studies conducted by scholars indigenous to the cultural group under consideration (e.g., Grossmann, Grossmann, Spangler, Suess, & Unzner, 1985; Jackson-Lowman, 1997; Lewis, Turnage, & Taylor, 1999; Miyake, Chen, & Campos, 1985; Nsamenang, 1992). The findings from these studies will help inform theories of child development and enable us to design more culturally valid interventions.

Garcia Coll and Meyer (1993) summarized several categories of theoretical models that help us understand the influence of culture and the broader ecological context on infant development and caregiver behavior. One category of theories provides a framework for understanding how the physical environment and historical circumstances are determinants of a societal maintenance system. The maintenance system includes the social structure, economy, and household type. In a second category of theories it is argued that group differences in child-rearing techniques are predicated on the cognitive, linguistic, motivational, and social competencies desired by the group. Further, there is a hierarchy of goals that begins with basic physical survival and proceeds to the inculcation of the child into the cultural groups' moral standards. Finally, ecological and transcultural theoretical frameworks highlight the complex contributions made at multiple levels of the infant and caregiving environment.

THE DEVELOPMENTAL NICHE

Super and Harkness (1986, 1997) provide a transcultural and ecologically derived approach to understanding how culture influences child development, which they call the developmental niche. This theoretical model describes the multiple levels of the caregiving environments of infant development. The developmental niche is composed of three primary areas: (1) the psychology of the caregivers, (2) the physical and social settings in which the child lives, and (3) the customs of child care and child rearing. These three levels of the niche interact synergistically and constitute the cultural context of parent–child relationships. Super and Harkness (1993) argue that because the developmental niche can be described for an individual child, it is a conceptualization that can be applied to the clinical analysis of developmental psychopathology.

In this chapter this conceptual model serves as an organizing framework to review recent literature and identify new areas for research related to the cultural context of infant mental health. At the first level of the developmental niche, the psychology of the caregiver, findings from cross-cultural and intracultural studies will be reviewed that highlight a key area of concern in infant mental health—caregiver sensitivity. In addition, a multidimensional definition of ethnicity of the caregiver will be presented as an important new area for research and practice. At the next level of the developmental niche, the physical and social settings, I propose that technology and innovations of the past decade are now a regulatory component of

the cultural context of infant development. Further, I argue that technology has established new cultural norms for parent behaviors and that infant mental health practitioners must embrace technology in order to effectively serve an increasingly diverse, multicultural, and global society. Finally, at the third level of the niche, which includes the customs of child care and child-rearing practices, I present a cultural practices approach (Miller & Goodnow, 1995) as an ideal entry point for intervention and research with families from diverse cultural groups.

GENERAL PRINCIPLES

Before reviewing the recent literature, there are several general principles to keep in mind when attempting to understand the cultural context of infancy.

Principle 1. To understand cultural influences we must first examine how we conceptualize culture. Each of us reflects a unique ethnobiography that provides the filter through which we make meaning of parent–child relationships. Ethnobiographies are our personal histories with the ethnic and cultural groups we were socialized into as children. Therefore, our first task in understanding the cultural context of the "other" is to become aware of our personal ethnotheories and beliefs about children, childhood, and the parental role.

Principle 2. A conceptual model of culture and development must provide a framework to separate the frequently confounded terms of culture, race, and ethnicity. As discussed more fully later, each of these constructs though closely related may have a different degree of influence on the caregiver, the child, and the caregiving environment. Whether we are conducting a clinical assessment in a hospital, educational, or physical therapy setting; designing a research study; or providing a psychiatric consultation, we should be able to distinguish clearly among these three ways to describe a population and understand aspects of their collective experience.

Principle 3. We must not let the intense emotions that often are associated with discussions of ethnicity or race serve as a reason to dismiss the assessment of culture and ethnicity as "a lower priority." In the face of flagrant psychopathology and pragmatic constraints of time and resources, it is sometimes too easy to dismiss culture as secondary or irrelevant. Because culture and ethnicity are basic building blocks for who we are and, therefore, basic to identity (Phinney, 1990), both our professional and personal explorations of culture and ethnicity are likely to be emotionally intense. Emotions may run high when an infant mental health practitioner's identity is Protestant while that of the client is Catholic and their mutual homeland is Ireland. Similarly, if the practitioner's identity is Arab and the client's Jewish and their homeland near the Gaza strip, or the practitioner's identity is White and the client is Black and their homeland is the United States, there may be intense emotions between each as members of their respective ethnic groups. The legacy of these group's relationships with each other may be the emotional "ghost in the nursery" of client–practitioner relationships.

Principle 4. It is not necessary to be an anthropologist to understand culture. Our best tools for understanding are simply to be open and willing to explore these new frontiers.

With these four principles in mind and using the developmental niche as a conceptual model, I review the selected literature from the past decade on the cultural context of infant development relevant for infant mental health practice and research.

What is presented next are the findings from recent cross-cultural and intracultural studies on caregiver sensitivity and the ethnicity of the caregiver at the first level of the developmental niche.

THE DEVELOPMENTAL NICHE: THE PSYCHOLOGY OF CAREGIVERS

This level of the developmental niche includes the values, goals, and beliefs of the parent.* Cultural topics that may be explored at this level include ethnotheories about feeding practices, sleeping, toilet training, values, and con-

cepts of independence and autonomy. Other topics include discipline standards and techniques; the quality and type of child's play; beliefs about spoiling, cuddling, or holding infants; and ethnotheories about what constitutes a responsive parent and optimal attachment behavior of developing children.

Cultural Influences on Internal Working Models

Bowlby's (1969) concept of internal working models of attachment relationships and Zeanah and Anders's (1987) concept of parents' working model of their relationship with their infant both emphasize the dominant role of cognitive and emotional processes in transmission of cultural practices and parenting beliefs.

Research on the cognitive and emotional processes in infant mental health has typically focused on the psychopathology of the caregiver (Doi, 1990; LeVine, 1990; Weiss et al., 1997). Recent studies focus on the cultural belief systems of parents on relevant topics such as the concept of interdependence (Doi, 1990), the underlying beliefs associated with sleeping arrangements in various cultures (Shweder, Jensen, & Goldstein, 1995), and perceptions of what constitutes the behavior of a securely attached child or child neglect by members of different cultural groups (Harwood, Miller, & Irizarry, 1995; Rose & Meezak, 1996).

Caregiver sensitivity is a core infant mental health construct. Cross-cultural studies on caregiver sensitivity and a new conceptualization of the construct of ethnicity illustrate the challenges and advances in our understanding of the role of culture at this psychological level of the developmental niche.

Caregiver Sensitivity

According to the Bowlby–Ainsworth theory of attachment, there are several primary parent and child behaviors that become organized into the child's attachment behavioral system. Maternal caregiving behaviors central to the formation of secure attachment have been studied under the constructs of parental acceptance/rejection, maternal sensitivity and, more recently, emotional availability (Ainsworth, Blehar, Waters, & Wall, 1978; Biringen & Robinson, 1991; Bowlby, 1988; Pederson, Gleason, Moran, & Bento, 1998; Rohner, 1986).

Maternal sensitivity and responsivity are de-

---

*Although caregivers of children include a wide variety of people across various cultural contexts, parents will be the primary focus of this discussion and used interchangeably with caregiver.

fined as the prompt, appropriate response by the caregiver to the infant's cues and include qualities of warmth and emotional availability (Ainsworth et al., 1978; Bornstein & Tamis-LeMonda, 1989; DeWolff & van IJzendoorn, 1997; Sorce & Emde, 1981). To react sensitively, the adult must be able to see things from the baby's point of view, interpret the infant's needs correctly, select an appropriate response and implement it effectively (Bretherton, 1987). Caregiver sensitivity also means the degree to which the mother's and infant's interactions are successfully coordinated (Raver & Leadbeater, 1992) and the appropriateness of dyadic emotional communication (Biringen & Robinson, 1991). A sensitive and warm response from an emotionally available caregiver begins a pattern for the quality of the interaction that evolves between the caregiver and the child. Caregiver sensitivity and attachment history have been identified as key factors for individual variation in the quality of security in mother–infant attachment relationships (Ainsworth et al., 1978; Main & Hess, 1990; Pianta, Sroufe, & Egeland, 1989; Spangler, Fremmer-Bombik & Grossmann, 1996).

Attachment researchers have neglected the identification of sociocultural antecedents to caregiver–child attachment relationships within minority populations in the United States and other countries (Harwood et al., 1995; Jackson, 1993; Rosser & Randolph, 1989; van IJzendoorn & Kroonenberg, 1988). Sociocultural factors include sociological factors such as racial group membership and socioeconomic status as well as cultural factors such as parental beliefs, culturally defined goals for socialization and emotional display rules, linguistic socialization, and the structure of the caregiving environment (Schiefflin, & Ochs, 1986; Super & Harkness, 1997; Valsiner, 1988, 1997; Valenzuela, 1997; Wang & Phinney, 1998; Whiting, 1994).

Several U.S. and cross-cultural researchers have argued that an improved conceptualization of the construct of maternal sensitivity is needed to gain a better understanding of the role of maternal behavior as an antecedent to attachment quality (Biringen, Robinson, & Emde, 1994; Bornstein, Tal, & Tamis-LeMonda, 1990; Grossmann, et al., 1985; Miyake et al., 1985; Sagi, 1990; Schaffer & Collis, 1986). The findings from the few empirical studies that examine the role of parental beliefs in parental sensitivity and responsive behaviors suggest significant variation in maternal sensitive and

contingent responsiveness to infants' cues based on the parent's beliefs related to children (Harwood et al., 1995; Skinner, 1985). In a sample of low- and middle-income two-parent U.S. families, significant correlations were found between child-rearing goals, the parent's child-rearing orientation, and maternal sensitive and contingent behaviors (Skinner, 1985). Similarly, Harwood (1992) concluded that Puerto Rican mothers' preference for infant behaviors that did not fit the traditional description of "secure" infant behavior were derived from cultural beliefs about children.

Three different constituents define maternal sensitivity at minimum: responding promptly; responding consistently; and responding appropriately. The global qualities of warmth and acceptance are the additional domains of this construct. Schaffer and Collis (1986) challenge the underlying assumption that these constituent elements belong together and make up one unitary entity. They suggest that the construct be reconceptualized and empirically separated. Further, the context in which the behavior occurs must also be assessed. There has been some support for this position from cross-cultural work on attachment.

Cross-Cultural Studies of Maternal Sensitivity

Conclusions from the findings from recent cross-cultural studies on the association of sensitivity to attachment security have been mixed (Bornstein et al., 1990; DeWolff & van IJzendoorn, 1997; Posada et al., 1995; Spangler et al., 1996). Nakagawa, Lamb, & Miyake (1989) found no significant associations between attachment classifications and maternal behavior (defined as accessibility, acceptance, cooperation, and sensitivity). In contrast, Vereijken, Riksen-Walraven, and Kondo-Ikemura (1997) reported that maternal sensitivity was a significant factor in the development of a secure attachment relationship in a longitudinal study they conducted with a Japanese sample of mothers. Grossmann et al. (1985), in their study of North German mothers, concluded that maternal sensitivity appeared to be driven by the cultural goals of the importance of independence and preference for a nonclingy child. Bornstein et al. (1990), in cross-cultural comparisons of contingent responsive behaviors of mothers from Japan and the United States, found areas of similarities and differences.

Tavecchhio and van IJzendoorn (1987) cite evidence for the existence of two independent dimensions of caregiver sensitivity: one for affective behaviors and one for instructional behaviors. In their study, both the mother's affective (e.g., smiling, distance from child, and encouragement) and cognitive (e.g., hints, feedback, and instruction) behaviors during joint problem-solving tasks were rated. Results indicated that these behaviors varied independently and formed two orthogonal factors in a factor analysis, suggesting that some mothers may provide adequate instruction and vice versa. Thus, despite structural similarities between two concepts (which suggests a global construct of sensitivity), in actuality, sensitive caregiving behavior may be specific to maternal teaching styles. The finding that individuals varied orthogonally along two dimensions of maternal sensitivity lend support to Schaffer and Collis's (1986) position that the construct of sensitivity must not be approached as a unitary entity.

These findings suggest that the conceptualizations of the behaviors that constitute a "sensitive mother" may vary cross-culturally and intraculturally. The findings from these studies highlight the need for a reconceptualization of the construct of maternal sensitivity from a more ecological and cultural perspective (Belsky & Isabella, 1988; Nicholls & Kirkland, 1996; Scheper-Hughes, 1990). Some of the antecedent factors suggested by these findings are parental beliefs. Few studies have explored the range of child-rearing attitudes and beliefs that comprise parental cognition of diverse cultures (Okagaki & Divecha, 1993). Korbin (1994) argues that to assess child maltreatment across cultures, an assessment must first be made of the parent's beliefs about children, childhood, and their parental role. Parental beliefs are a more fundamental construct in contrast to simple observations of parental style and may serve as a more robust mediator between parents' inner states and behaviors (Sigel, McGillicuddy-De Lisi, & Goodnow, 1992). Yet, there is a long-standing controversy surrounding the reliability of parental espoused beliefs as predictors of parenting behaviors. The other two levels of the developmental niche provide a culturally valid alternative choice point for deconstructing parental beliefs and contextualizing ethnotheories of children, childhood, and parenting roles.

Before moving to these other levels of the niche, there is yet another key factor that may contribute to variation in caregiver sensitivity. This factor, the ethnicity of the caregiver, may serve as the foundation for the parent's culturally driven belief systems. The ethnicity of the caregiver is the other new area for exploration to understand the role of culture and the psychology of the caregiver.

Ethnicity and the Psychology of Caregivers

In their discussion of the sociocultural context of infant development, Garcia Coll and Meyer (1993) highlighted the cultural variation of infant development within the borders of the United States. They noted that ethnic minority groups are disproportionately represented in a number of risk statuses that may contribute to psychopathology. There are also consistent family structural differences in that minority families tend to be characterized by a higher percentage of single mothers, younger mothers, and large extended families. They argue that these social status and sociological indices are important determinants to the family's world view and the infant's developmental experience. The concept of ethnicity then will be a salient concept in our discussions of intracultural variations.

The terms "race," "ethnicity," and "culture" are often used interchangeably to characterize individuals or groups. These same terms are often confounded in sampling strategies in research studies. As noted in Principle 2 outlined earlier, a clear distinction must be made among the terms "culture," "ethnicity," and "race." Briefly defined, culture is "the human-made part of the environment" (Lonner, 1994, p. 231) and includes the norms, values, attitudes, and behaviors of the group. Culture is transmitted primarily through language and the everyday social interactions of a caregiver and children (Harwood & Lewis, 1994; Schieffelin & Ochs, 1986). Ethnicity according to Helms (1990) is defined as "a social identity based on the culture of one's ancestors' national or tribal groups as modified by the demands of the [larger culture or society] in which one group currently reside" (p. 293). Thus, ethnic identity is "defined from the inside (of the person) out (to the world). And is self-defined and maintained because it 'feels good' rather than because it is necessarily imposed by powerful others" (Helms, 1990, pp. 293–294).

Finally, race has historically had a variety of meanings and been the basis for extensive debate as to its usefulness and validity as a means of distinguishing between groups of people. A racial group is biologically an isolated, inbreeding population with a distinctive genetic heritage (Healey, 1998). Socially, the term must be considered contextually and reflects patterns of inequality and power. The genotype (i.e., the genetic structure of foundation) and phenotype (the physical characteristics and appearance) approach has been the sociopolitical and historical basis for categorizing individuals into racial groups (such as Negroid, Caucasoid, or Mongoloid) and maintaining patterns of dominance and control (Schriver, 1998). Hence, individuals may also have a racial identity where they share a sense of identity and common experience. In this sense the construct of race can be a powerful tool, either for oppression or for group self-actualization. The aspect of ethnicity that is salient in the psychology of the caregiver at this level of the developmental niche is the ethnic identity of the caregiver.

The distinction between the constructs of ethnicity and race have fostered distinctive theoretical models of ethnic and racial identity formation. Several scholars have proposed that *ethnicity* is a complex, multidimensional construct (Camilleri & Malewska-Peyre, 1997; Phinney, 1990; Sellers, Smith, Shelton, Rowley & Chavous, 1998). Phinney (1990) argues that to understand how psychological outcomes are influenced by ethnicity, at least three dimensions must be explored: *culture*, *ethnic identity*, and *dominant or minority status*. These dimensions are not independent but overlapping and confounded.

Ethnic identity is the strength or degree of the individual's identification with the group and subjective sense of group membership. William Cross (1971) proposed one of the earliest models of racial identity formation of Black individuals. The Cross model emphasized that African Americans differ in their degree of identification with African American culture. Further, these individual differences are tied to stages of identity development. These stages are *preencounter*, characterized by idealization of the dominant culture of Whites and Europeans and denigration of Blacks and Black culture, and *encounter*, where the individual experiences significant events or situations such as housing discrimination because of skin color and then begin to search for

their Black identity. This transitional stage is also marked by rejection of White culture, confusion, and intense affect. The *immersion–emersion* stage of racial identity involves a transition to a new Black identity and immersion in "Blackness" and withdrawal from interactions with other ethnic groups. The final stage is *internalization,* where the person achieves an internally defined positive Black identity that transcends racism and acceptance of positive aspects of White culture. This conceptual model has been further developed and is the basis for a measure of White racial identity formation (Helms, 1990). Racial identity formation has also been conceptualized as a developmental process that individuals may recycle through the life span (Parham, 1989).

Dominant or minority group status includes the experiences associated with the status of the ethnic group within the larger society. Healey (1998) argues that the subsistence technology of the industrial revolution of European society profoundly affected the nature of dominant or minority group relationships. He states, "The new industrial technology changed the nature of work, altered the family institution, lowered birth and death rates, raised the average level of education, created new minority groups, and transformed other dominant–minority situations" (p. 191).

The psychological domains of dominant or minority group status experiences include feelings of powerlessness and in the extreme internalized racism and self-hatred based on their minority group membership (Abdullah, 1998; Fannon, 1968). For members of the dominant ethnic group of a society, these experiences may also include unexamined feelings of power, dominance, and privilege (Helms, 1990).

Ethnic minority parents must socialize their children from birth to be bicultural in order for them to be successful in the larger society as well as in their own minority ethnic group (Camilleri & Malewska-Peyre, 1997; Norton, 1993). The process of racial socialization has only recently received attention as a topic for research (Spencer & Markstrom-Adams, 1990; Thornton, 1997). Racial socialization may also develop important coping skills in children. In an ethnographic, longitudinal study of socialization practices of African American children in Sunday School, a number of themes were identified regarding the racial climate in which parents rear children. In this study, a number of proactive parental practices were identified, including warmth and positive acceptance of children and an emphasis on interdependence with adults and peers, and the use of biblical concepts to understand experiences in the child's life. These findings parallel findings from other cross-cultural studies that report faith and spirituality as characteristics of resilient children (Werner, 1990). The socioemotional domains of racial socialization and developmental outcomes for children are important areas for infant mental health practitioners.

This multidimensional conceptualization of ethnicity subsumes the less precise and politicized term "race." This conceptualization highlights the importance of assessment and exploration of the meaning of ethnicity for caregivers in order to understand ethnotheories of infants, childhood, and the parental role. Phinney (1990) also argues that the heterogeneity among members of ethnic groups is based on variability along each of the three dimensions of culture, ethnic identity, and dominant or minority group status.

Heterogeneity of Cultural and Ethnic Groups

The concept of the multilayered developmental niche also provides an opportunity to appreciate the heterogeneity among members of each cultural group. The areas of cultural, racial, and ethnic heterogeneity aid our understanding of individual differences in specific child-rearing practices. Other factors that may affect the degree of cultural allegiance and ethnic affiliation of the caregiver include immigration experience, language spoken at home, race and country of origin, neighborhood, education and socioeconomic status, social mobility, emotional processes in the family, and political and religious ties of the ethnic group.

Cultural practices may vary based on the individual's social class, language, level of assimilation, and acculturation and regional differences. A working-class, second-generation, highly assimilated, and monolingual, English speaking Japanese-American father living in the southern region of the United States will differ in substantive ways from his ethnic counterpart in the northeastern part of the United States. This father may be high income, with advanced degrees, but first generation, highly acculturated but not highly assimilated, and bilingual, still practicing many of the customs of his homeland in Japan. The common

Japanese ancestry of both fathers may be expressed in qualitatively different ways in the manner they rear their children. Issues of the influence of assimilation and acculturation on ethnotheories of child care and development are salient areas of assessment and research by infant mental health researchers and practitioners.

Theoretical advances for understanding intracultural variation also add to our ability to conceptualize research and enhance the validity of the results (Jackson, 1993; Rosser & Randolph, 1989; Vezeau, 1991). For example, Sinha (1981, 1988) has conducted a series of studies on the socialization and development of children in India. Doi (1990) has examined the concept of interdependence from a cultural perspective. The concept is important to infant mental health practitioners with its relationship focus. Similarly, Norton (1993) proposed that a "dual perspective" must be taken to conceptualize the experience of minority parents with their infants in the United States. A dual perspective outlines the dual cultural communities that ethnic minority parents and infants operate on a daily basis. Many studies have been conducted to describe the cultural discontinuities between home and school (for example, Colby, 1996). More work is needed to add to our understanding of the discontinuities between ethnic minority and other cultural groups' beliefs and practices regarding infants and those beliefs and practices of the dominant therapeutic community.

Paradoxically, research and practice with those low-income Black and Latina mothers whose racial status was synonymous with their "risk" status (e.g., Pascoe & Solomon, 1994; Sameroff, Seifer, & Zax, 1982) may provide future direction for practice of infant mental health in the dawning age of a global practice (Lewis, 1996).

Intracultural studies compare practices of individual members within one cultural group in a society who may differ on other key variables such as socioeconomic status. Intracultural studies may corroborate the universal nature of some parenting practices and customs of child care as well as highlight distinctive differences unique to a particular cultural group (Haight, 1998; Harwood, 1992; Kagitcibasi, 1996; Sanders-Phillips, 1998; Vezeau, 1991). An example of a finding from an intracultural sample that illustrates this point is from a study with a group of low-income, African American mothers (Burchinal, Follmer, & Bryant, 1996). In this study, women with larger support networks tended to be more responsive in interactions with their infants and provided more stimulating home environments than did mothers with smaller social networks. The authors concluded that supportive social networks may positively influence maternal caregiving. These findings reinforce the cross-cultural generalizability of the critical role of social support to optimal maternal caregiving behavior important to the formation of secure attachment (Crittenden & Bonvillian, 1984; Miller-Loncar, Erwin-Loeta, Landry, Smith, & Swank, 1998).

The next level of the developmental niche is the physical and social settings of the developing infant.

PHYSICAL AND SOCIAL SETTINGS OF THE DEVELOPMENTAL NICHE

This level of the developmental niche includes institutions such as schools, churches, and hospitals as well as urban or rural neighborhoods and communities. The social setting includes the people who frequent the settings as well as the social roles of the actors within the setting. The adaptation of the child and family to the different ecological and economic conditions of their environment is one concern in assessments by infant mental health practitioners (Norton, 1993). The physical settings of the developmental niche now include environmental toxins and waste sites in industrialized countries such as the United States. These toxins have been identified as life-threatening, prenatal teratogens. These toxins have also been linked to behavioral disorders in developing children (Sroufe, Cooper, DeHart, & Marshal, 1996).

Epidemic levels of community violence and chronic exposure to war-like conditions constitute new factors in the current physical settings of the cities, villages, neighborhoods, and homes of some children (Garbarino, 1995; Lewis, Osofsky, & Moore, 1997). We have only recently begun to understand the impact of these settings on the physical, social, emotional, and neurological development of children. Further, the behavioral changes and new cultural practices of parents rearing children in these conditions are another new area of study at this level of the developmental niche (Lewis, 1996; Osofsky, 1995).

There has long been recognition of the primacy of educational institutions in the socialization of children (Randolph, Koblinsky, & Roberts, 1998). Federally funded programs such as Head Start and private and public preschools all play a significant role in socializing children from a variety of cultural and linguistic backgrounds and inculcating them into the social roles of the dominant society (National Association for the Education of Young Children [NAEYC], 1996: Spencer, 1998). Though the family contextual influences on the educational outcomes of children also have been found to be a significant predictor, the specific directions of the paths of influence are still not clear (Luster & McAdoo, 1996). A recent observation by a middle-class, professional mother brings up a newly institutionalized method of education of the next generation of children.

The mother reported that her 36-month-old daughter had climbed onto her lap as she turned on her computer. The toddler matter-of-factly announced, "I have to check my e-mail." The ease with which she relayed these concepts that are technically beyond her cognitive capacity to understand reminds us to appreciate new ways young children are being culturally socialized in this era of technology. Technology has become a regulatory system at multiple layers of the developmental niche. The physical and social settings of children in industrialized countries now contain some form of technology that serves to regulate their development and relationship with their caregiver.

The Culture of Technology and Infancy

The concept of culture with its anthropological and sociological roots must be redefined in the new age of technological advancement, blurred national and local physical boundaries, and the global mobility of individuals and families. This level of the developmental niche as a cultural context for infant development and caregiver relationships is being transformed in ways we may not fully understand for decades. Using our broad definition of culture as the people-made part of the environment, computers, the Internet, and technology all have become part of our global culture (Stokols, 1999). The juxtaposition of technology and infant mental health, at first blush, appears to be an oxymoron. Technology connotes computers, machines, and cyberspace. Infancy connotes images of soft, round, cuddly babies. Culture, as noted before, conjures up images of far off, "exotic" people and villages. Yet, technology has already been an important determinant in both the normal expectable environments of infancy in developed cultures (LeVine, 1990) as well as in the practice and research for infant mental health.

Sameroff (1993) noted that advances in techniques of molecular genetics will provide the opportunity to better understand the etiology of mental disorders. A recent cover story in a news magazine detailed the advances made in scientific understanding and knowledge of which parts of the brain are involved in attention-deficit/hyperactivity disorder (ADHD) and which chemicals in the brain respond to Ritalin (methylphenidates), ("The age of Ritalin," 1998).

From conception through birth, medical advances have enhanced both the viability and the health of the developing fetus and premature neonate. Sameroff's (1993) transactional model of development is predicated on the assumption of a unity and coherence of developmental processes, both biological and behavioral. Given this premise, biological competence promoted by technological advances in the neonate will have a correlated impact on the caregiver's behavior and their evolving relationship.

The prolonged viability of heretofore premature infants as small as 2 pounds or born with a variety of congenital anomalies or disabilities brings up important ethical issues with which parents, mental health practitioners, and social policymakers will need to struggle. In fact, medical technology has become so advanced that choices about the gender of the fetus may now be accomplished through a controversial manipulation of the chromosomes. Though this procedure is new and available to only a small number of parents, given the speed that other technological advances have been made, this option should also become more widely available in the near future. The assessment of relationship dynamics among complex claimants of biological, legal, and surrogate parents with infants is an important new area to be addressed by infant mental health practitioners. The antecedents and correlated emotions of choices about when and how to conceive *in vitro* may accompany these decisions. These emotionally charged issues will be important components of the circumstances of the child's birth and areas for assessment and intervention by infant mental health practitioners and researchers (Lewis, 1998).

Technology and the Visualization Approach to Parent Education, Research, and Intervention

New parents have a vast amount of information readily available to them in their homes regarding infant development, parenting, and consumer advice on products via on-line chat rooms with other parents. Also available are the popular afternoon television talk shows dispensing sometimes controversial and often unbalanced advice on a wide range of parenting issues.

The advances in technology have made research on the subtle dynamics of parent–infant relationships in infant development more refined than ever. Developmental researchers have a vast array of highly complex audiovisual tools available to them for the study of parent–caregiver interaction and infant behavior. Miniaturized and highly affordable digital video recording systems and laptop computers permit not only microanalysis of behaviors but also highly accurate recordings in more naturalistic settings of the home.

Infant mental health practitioners have pioneered a visualization approach to interaction in troubled relationships and education for parents (Bakermans-Kranenburg, Juffer, & van IJzendoorn, 1998; McDonough, 1993; Carter, Osofsky, & Hann, 1991). The use of videotaped feedback with parents provides an opportunity for parents to visualize in a very concrete way the strengths and weaknesses of their relationship with their infant. In essence, the visualization approach operationalizes the concept of the observing ego in psychodynamic theory (Goldstein, 1995).

THE CUSTOMS OF CHILD CARE

Super and Harkness (1986) describe this final level of the developmental niche as "the behavioral strategies for dealing with children of particular ages in the context of particular environmental constraints" (p. 546). These social practices are regarded by the cultural group members as reasonable and the natural thing to do even though they are not given conscious thought. The customs of child care are also the methods of transmission of cultural values and traditions that serve to solidify the distinctive existence of the group (Super & Harkness, 1997; Valsiner, 1997).

Werner (1988) proposed that cultural characteristics of the caregiving environment include the contingent responsiveness of caregivers to infant cues; variations in the amount of tactile, social, and verbal stimulation to the infant; the routines of infant care; and deliberate teaching of skills valued in a given culture such as sitting, smiling, or vocalizing. How mothers interpret and respond to the infant's cry; the manner in which they provide such face-to-face stimulus as smiling, vocalizing, and looking at infants; and how they facilitate language learning are all influenced by cultural norms and cultural scripts (Minturn & Lambert, 1964; Schieffelin, & Ochs, 1986).

Parents have peer groups that teach them the group's expectations for socialization of children and ways a standard normal parent behaves (Bornstein et al., 1990). Considering the realities of cultural pluralism in the 21st century driven by global mobility and communicative access through technology of the Internet, "cultural group members" takes on a new, more expanded meaning.

Parent Peer Groups and Cultural Norms

In an age of mobility and frequent changes of residence, parents no longer have as much physical access to their parents and other extended family members to assist in the day-to-day rearing of children. These family members have traditionally served to reinforce family and community norms. In the past decades in the United States, child experts such as Dr. Benjamin Spock, the Child Guidance movement, and groups such as the Parent/Teacher Association were sources for setting norms for new parents. There is a new wave of "parent educators," either individuals or groups whose mission is to provide practical, hands-on information for new parents about the physical, emotional, and intellectual development of children. Groups such as "Birth to Three," first formed by parent educator Minalee Saks, in Eugene, Oregon in 1979, and Parents as Teachers (PAT), a project begun in 1981 by the Missouri Department of Education, are examples. The PAT program has exported its curriculum to 47 states in the United States and has trained more than 8,000 professional parent educators, who spend 1 hour a month in parents' homes (O'Donnell, 1997). These groups reflect specific beliefs about children, childhood, and values. Fueled by federal monies and the energy and enthusiasm of isolated parents, in part they define the cultural norms for what constitutes "a good parent."

Newsweek ("Television," 1997) conducted a poll of 506 parents of young children. The majority of the parents stated that they turn to a variety of sources, primarily their father/mother (87%), for advice and guidance about how to raise their child. Other sources of advice included books and magazines, friends, neighbors, television, babysitters, and religious leaders. It is important to note that these were the *conscious* sources of advice parents sought out. No one has examined the unconscious cultural influences on parents' behaviors.

The unconscious influences, such as media marketing and observations made of other parents sitting in a pediatrician's waiting room or the checkout line in the local grocery store, are the unexplored cultural influences. These unconscious influences are a powerful and unregulated component of this level of the niche, as is evidenced by the sweeping popularity of the newest toy product that both the parent and the child become convinced they must have. The recent program and accompanying toys of *Teletubbies,* a public television program imported from Great Britain, is an example. The creator of this show that has only been shown in the United States since April 1997 ("Television," 1997) stated that her goal was to create a fantasy world "that is technical but full of warmth." The four Teletubbies, Tinky-Winky, Dipsy, Laa-Laa, and Po, live in a high-tech world. At the center of their world, the warm sun merges with the round, laughing face of an infant. The Teletubbies talk to each other in baby talk that is perfectly understood by the enthralled preschool audience. The show has garnered support from linguists and child psychologists who argue that the format helps 2-year-olds learn the rudiments of language by repeating basic sounds.

Most parents of preschoolers can sing the songs from the popular toy dinosaur program *Barney* as well as those from *Sesame Street.* Visits to friends' homes and informal appraisals of children's clothing, bedroom furniture, and Winnie the Pooh decorations all serve as a kind of cultural peer pressure to conform to cultural standards of care.

Embracing the Culture of Technology

In the past 10 years the explosion of technological and scientific advances has created new and uncharted areas for the future practice of infant mental health. We can begin to speculate on and identify several areas that we can proactively explore from a prevention and intervention perspective. The increasing access to the Internet by parents in industrialized societies has the potential for globalization of dominant Western notions of mental health. It has been estimated that more than 47 million users in the United States will be on-line by the end of this year—19 million more than last year (Stokols, 1999). The demographic profiles of consumers or stakeholders in the area of infant mental health parallel the demographic profiles of some Internet users. They are typically better educated and have higher incomes. Chat rooms on the Internet, such as "Moms on Line," have bulletin boards for all manners of specialized interests, ranging from issues about being a stepparent to toilet training a toddler to coping with elderly parents.

A new cultural reality for infant mental health practitioners to grapple with may be the isolation that accompanies our high-tech reality. Technological innovations may inadvertently serve to disconnect individuals from each other. For example, the premature infant who spends his or her first days or even weeks of life in a sterile neonatal isolette is largely removed from human touch. The parent and child each positioned in front of colorful blinking computer monitors and fast-action video games may become isolated from one another. The researcher or practitioner positioned behind the camera may feel some disconnection as he or she videotapes a parent's interaction with her infant.

The antidote to the isolation created by technology may be a renewed interest in reconnection with the culture of one's family of origin and ethnic group. Infant mental health practitioners can be in the forefront by offering aid to individuals and families in reaffirming and resurrecting their ethnic identities and cultural heritages. Supporting alienated and isolated parents in the customs of child care that support the values and socialization goals of their ethnic group may become a new component that heals and facilitates healthy attachments between caregivers and their infants and communities. A conceptual window into identifying the customs of child care of various ethnic groups is the use of a cultural practices approach.

CULTURAL PRACTICES: A PRAGMATIC APPROACH

An important focus for infant mental health is cultural practices; in fact, these may represent a more effective focus for intervention than understanding parental beliefs and goals. Miller and Goodnow (1995) argue that cultural practices, that is, what people of a particular cultural group do, are an ideal focus for research and practice because they can be observed. The normative nature of these phenomena stem from the fact that they are engaged in by many members of the cultural group and carry with them normative expectations about how things should be done. Cultural practices are not neutral; they come packaged with values about what is natural, mature, morally right, or aesthetically pleasing. These, then, are actions that may easily become part of a group's identity. "As people learn the practice—its essential and optional features—they also develop values and a sense of belonging and identity within the community. At the same time, the shared quality of the practice means that it may be sustained, changed, or challenged by a variety of people" (p. 6). Miller and Goodnow (1995) propose a set of propositions about the efficacy of the cultural practices approach to understand the cultural context of development.

Proposition 1: Practices provide a way of describing development-in-context, without separating child and context and without separating development into a variety of separate domains.
Proposition 2: Practices reflect or instantiate a social and moral order.
Proposition 3: Practices provide the route by which children come to participate in a culture, allowing the culture to be "reproduced" and "transformed."
Proposition 4: Practices do not exist in isolation.
Proposition 5: The nature of participation has consequences. (pp. 8–13)

There are several recent examples of research using this approach, which illustrate the rich potential for infant mental health practitioners (Leslie, 1998; Miller, Wiley, Fung, & Liang, 1997). One example of the application of this model for understanding core values of a cultural group is the linguistic practice of the use of proverbs by parents. Proverbs represent the distillation of generations of wisdom that have been transmitted through the generations. These maxims provide guidelines, rules, and commentary about how individuals can make meaning of their world. Proverbs are readily psychically available to individuals and are easily articulated. Recent studies analyzing the use of proverbs and their reflection of parenting values support the value of proverbs as a viable method of study and intervention by infant mental health practitioners (McAdoo, 1991; Jackson-Lowman, 1997).

Another example of a new paradigm for research that uses a cultural practices approach was the use of the task of hair combing as a naturalistic context to study interaction between African American mothers and their daughters (Lewis, in press). With a multidimensional conceptualization of ethnicity, it is possible to examine how ethnicity influences African American mothers' parenting styles in the more culturally salient context of hair combing interaction as opposed to the more traditional context of a teaching task (Lewis, Turnage, Taylor, & Diaz, 1999).

The increasing need to tailor services to diverse ethnic and immigrant populations within the United States and around the world is the catalyst for reviewing lessons learned with ethnic minority populations and use of a cultural practices approach as a beginning point of study.

CONCLUSIONS

The cultural context of infant development provides a rich opportunity for infant mental health practitioners and researchers to further our understanding and support of infant–caregiver relationships. There are key conceptual and methodological parallels between the study of culture and human development and the field of infant mental health. For example, infant mental health focuses on understanding the emotional meaning of the relationship between the infant and caregiver (Bowlby, 1969; Zeanah & Anders, 1987), and the study of culture and human development focuses on the

cultural meaning underlying practices by caregivers (Bornstein et al., 1990; Super & Harkness, 1997). Both fields draw on observational techniques as one method to gain access to the subjective meaning of the relationship. The infant mental health practitioner observes and microanalyzes infant–caregiver interaction. Similarly, the cultural researcher may use participant observation and ethnographic or other qualitative methods to describe the customs of child care or caregiver behavior (Haight, 1998; Hewlett, Lamb, Shannon, Leyendecker, & Schoelmerich, 1998; Werner, 1988). Both fields draw from an interdisciplinary group of scholars and practitioners. Nurses, anthropologists, physicians, educators, social workers, psychiatrists, and psychologists have made important contributions in both fields. Finally, both fields have moved from a predominately intrapsychic focus toward inclusion of context in the design of studies and interventions (Cicchetti & Toth, 1997; Colby, 1996; Super & Harkness, 1997; Lutzker, Bigelow, Doctor, Gershater, & Greene, 1998; Sameroff, 1993; Valsiner, 1997; Whiting, 1994).

In this chapter I used the conceptual model of the developmental niche to look backward at the cultural roots of infant mental health and to look forward to directions for infant mental health in the next millennium. I proposed that technology is a new regulatory system in the customs of child care and that the ethnicity of the caregiver must be a part of any comprehensive evaluation of the parent–infant relationship. Using this model, I proposed that the field of infant mental health must move beyond an exclusive focus on the infant–mother dyad to focus on the customs of child care as an entry point into understanding the cultural contributions to parent–infant relationships. Further, cultural practice models offer important methodological directions for infant mental health in the areas of both intervention and research. The use of the hair-combing task as a cultural window into African American mother–child relationships is one example of the use of a cultural-practices model in research.

A strength of infant mental health is the interdisciplinary nature of both practitioners and researchers. Important work has come from early childhood educators, nursing, psychiatrists, social workers, and psychologists. This interdisciplinary history provides the setting for the type of collaborative work that awaits the future in order to understand the cultural meaning systems of the diverse cultural groups from an infant mental health perspective.

Almonte (1994) makes an important and underexplored observation about the growing practice of the use of indigenous members of cultural groups as paraprofessionals who provide infant mental health services to their own cultural group. She highlights the need for recognition of the cultural change and inherent issues surrounding professionalization of the indigenous worker.

We must remain vigilant to guard against the type of reductionistic tendency that has been the legacy of our positivist, cross-cultural mental health traditions (Whiting, 1994). Nugent (1994) reminds us, as he reviews the implications for infant mental health practitioners of the findings of cross-cultural research, that "risk" is a cultural construction. He states:

> These findings demonstrate that what constitutes risk in one setting may not in another. Definitions of risk are inevitably cultural constructions by virtue of the fact that they are derived from specific circumscribed empirical data sets that often have limited application across cultural setting. . . . Definitions of risk must be context-specific in order to provide appropriate guidelines for clinicians and policymakers who are trying to meet the needs of infants and families in at-risk settings. Thus, we must always examine the validity of the data bases on which many of our at-risk categories and diagnoses are based. (p. 6)

In this chapter I have also presented a new conceptualization of the concept of ethnicity that provides the framework to understand heterogeneity among members of the same cultural group. The impact of acculturation and assimilation on parent–infant relationships are important constructs for infant mental health professionals to explore in normative populations of specific ethnic groups. We are then in a more valid position to assess and intervene from a strengths perspective as we understand the dual contexts (Norton, 1993) in which ethnic minorities in the United States and diverse ethnic groups in countries around the world nurture and care for infants and toddlers.

These complex issues reinforce Garcia Coll and Meyer's (1993) argument that cultural competence in practice requires the substantial long-term commitment by researchers and practitioners to implement culturally competent service to infants and their caregivers.

ACKNOWLEDGMENT

I would like to express my appreciation to my colleagues Dr. Michael Cunningham and Dr. Dewana Thompson for their review and helpful comments of earlier versions of this chapter.

REFERENCES

Abdullah, A. (1998). Mammy-ism: A diagnosis of psychological misorientation for women of African descent. *Journal of Black Psychology, 24*, 196–210.

The age of Ritalin. (1998, September 7). *Newsweek*, pp. 52–60.

Ainsworth, M. D., Blehar, M. C., Waters, E., & Wall, S. (1978). *Patterns of attachment: A psychological study of the strange situation.* Hillsdale, NJ: Erlbaum.

Almonte, B. E. (1994, October/November). Professionalization as cultural change: Issues for infant/family community workers and their supervisors. *Zero to Three, 15*(2), 1–3.

Bakermans-Kranenburg, M. J., Juffer, F., & van IJzendoorn, M. H. (1998). Interventions with video feedback and attachment discussions: Does type of maternal insecurity make a difference? *Infant Mental Health Journal, 19*, 202–219.

Belsky, J., & Isabella, R. (1988). Maternal infant and social–contextual determinants of attachment security. In J. Belsky & T. Nezworski (Eds.), *Clinical implications of attachment* (pp. 41–94). Hillsdale, NJ: Erlbaum.

Biringen, Z., & Robinson, J. (1991). Emotional availability in mother–child interactions: A reconceptualization for research. *American Journal of Orthopsychiatry, 6*, 258–271.

Biringen, Z., Robinson, J. L., & Emde, R. N. (1994). Maternal sensitivity in the 2nd year: Gender-based relations in the dyadic balance of control. *American Journal of Orthopsychiatry, 64*, 78–90.

Bornstein, M. H., Tal, J., & Tamis-LeMonda, C. S. (1990). Parenting in cross-cultural perspective: The United States, France, and Japan. In M. H. Bornstein (Ed.), *Cultural approaches to parenting* (pp. 69–90). Hillsdale, NJ: Erlbaum.

Bornstein, M. H., & Tamis-LeMonda, C. S. (1989). Maternal responsiveness and cognitive development in children. In M. H. Bornstein (Ed.), *Maternal responsiveness: Characteristics and consequences, new directions for child development* (No. 43, pp. 49–61). San Francisco: Jossey-Bass.

Bowlby, J. (1969). *Attachment and loss: Vol. I. Attachment:* New York: Basic Books.

Bowlby, J. (1988). *A secure base.* New York: Basic Books.

Bretherton, I. (1987). New perspectives on attachment relations: Security, communication and internal working models. In J.D. Osofsky (Ed.), *Handbook of infant development* (pp. 1061–1100). New York: Wiley.

Burchinal, M. R., Follmer, A., & Bryant, D. M. (1996). The relationship of maternal social support and family structure with maternal responsiveness and child outcomes among African American families. *Developmental Psychology, 32,* 1073–1083.

Camilleri, C., & Malewska-Peyre, H. (1997). Socialization and identity strategies. In J. W. Berry, P. R. Dasen, & T. S. Saraswathi (Eds.), *Cross-cultural psychology: Vol. 2. Basic processes and human development* (pp. 41–68). Needham Heights, MA: Allyn & Bacon.

Carter, S., Osofsky, J., & Hann, D. M. (1991). Speaking for the baby: Therapeutic interventions with adolescent mothers and their infants. *Infant Mental Health Journal, 12,* 291–301.

Cicchetti, D., & Toth, S. L. (1997). Transactional ecological systems in developmental psychopathology. In S. S. Luthar, J. A. Burack, & D. Cicchetti (Eds.), *Developmental psychopathology: Perspectives on adjustment, risk, and disorder* (pp. 317–349). New York: Cambridge University Press.

Colby, A. (1996). The multiple contexts of human development. In R. Jessor, A. Colby, & R. A. Shweder (Eds.), *Ethnography and human development: Context and meaning in social inquiry* (pp. 327–338). Chicago: University of Chicago Press.

Crittenden, P. M., & Bonvillian, J. D. (1984). The relationship between maternal risk status and maternal sensitivity. *American Journal of Orthopsychiatry, 54,* 250–261.

Cross, W. E. (1971). Negro-to-Black conversion experience. *Black World, 20,* 13–27.

DeWolff, M., & van IJzendoorn, M. H. (1997). Sensitivity and attachment: A meta-analysis on parental antecedents of infant attachment. *Child Development, 68,* 571–591.

Doi, T. (1990). The cultural assumptions of psychoanalysis: A cross-cultural view. In J. W. Stigler, R. A., Shweder, & G. Herdt (Eds.), *Cultural psychology: Essays on comparative human development* (pp. 446–453). New York: Cambridge University Press.

Fannon, F. (1968). *The wretched of the earth.* New York: Grove Weidenfeld.

Garbarino, J. (1995). *Raising children in a socially toxic environment.* San Francisco: Jossey-Bass.

Garcia Coll, C. T., & Meyer, E. C. (1993). The sociocultural context of infant development. In C. H. Zeanah, Jr. (Ed.), *Handbook of infant mental health* (pp. 56–69). New York: Guilford Press.

Goldstein, E. G. (1995). *Ego psychology and social work practice.* New York: Free Press.

Gopaul-McNicol, S., & Thomas-Presswood, T. (1998). *Working with linguistically and culturally different children.* Needham Heights, MA: Allyn & Bacon.

Grossmann, K., Grossmann, K. E., Spangler, G., Suess, G., & Unzner, L. (1985). Maternal sensitivity and newborns' orientation responses as related to quality of attachment in northern Germany. In I. Bretherton & E. Waters (Eds.), Growing points in attachment theory and research. *Monographs of the Society for Research in Child Development, 50*(Serial No. 209), 233–256.

Haight, W. L. (1998). A gathering the spirit at First Baptist Church: Spirituality as a protective factor in the lives of African American Children. *Social Work, 43* (3), 213–221.

Harwood, R. L. (1992). The influence of culturally derived values on Anglo and Puerto Rican mother's perceptions of attachment behavior. *Child Development, 63,* 822–839.

Harwood, R. L., & Lewis, M. L. (1994). How parents construct culture in their everyday interactions with children. *Newsletter of the Louisiana Infant Mental Health Association, 2,* 1–3.

Harwood, R. L., Miller, J. G., & Irizarry, N. L. (1995). *Culture and attachment: Perceptions of the child in context.* New York: Guilford Press.

Healey, J. F. (1998). *Race, ethnicity, gender, and class: The sociology of group conflict and change* (2nd ed.). Thousand Oaks, CA: Pine Forge Press.

Helms, J. E. (1990). *Black and white racial identity: Theory, research, and practice.* Westport, CT: Greenwood.

Hewlett, B. S., Lamb, M. E., Shannon, D., Leyendecker, B., & Schoelmerich, A. (1998). Culture and early infancy among central African foragers and farmers. *Developmental Psychology, 34,* 653–661.

Jackson, J. F. (1993). Multiple caregivers among African Americans and infant attachment: The need for an emic approach. *Human Development, 36,* 87–102.

Jackson-Lowman, H. (1997). Using Afrikan proverbs to provide an Afrikan-centered narrative for contemporary Afrikan-American parental values. In J. K. Adjaye & A. R. Andrews (Eds.), *Language, rhythm, and sound: Black popular culture into the twenty-first century* (pp. 74–89). Pittsburgh: University of Pittsburgh Press.

Jessor, R., Colby, A., & Shweder, R. A. (Eds.). (1997). *Ethnography and human development: Context and meaning in social inquiry.* Chicago: University of Chicago Press.

Johnson-Powell, G., & Yamamoto, J. (Eds.). (1997). *Transcultural child development: Psychological assessment and treatment.* New York: Wiley.

Kagitcibasi, C. (1996). *Family and human development across cultures: A view from the other side.* Mahwah, NJ: Erlbaum.

Korbin, J. E. (1994). Sociocultural factors in child maltreatment. In G. B. Melton & F. D. Barry (Eds.), *Protecting children from abuse and neglect: Foundations for a new national strategy* (pp. 182–223). New York: Guilford Press.

Leslie, A. R. (1998). What African American mothers perceive they socialize their children to value when telling them Brer' Rabbit stories. *Journal of Comparative Family Studies, 29,* 173–185.

LeVine, R. A. (1990). Infant environments in psychoanalysis: A cross-cultural view. In J. W. Stigler, R. A. Shweder, & G. Herdt (Eds.), *Cultural psychology: Essays on comparative human development* (pp. 454–476). Cambridge, UK: Cambridge University Press.

Lewis, M. L. (1996, April 28–30). *Remembering mama: African-American mother–child relationships, a model for community parenting.* Plenary address, Michigan Association of Infant Mental Health, Ann Arbor, MI.

Lewis, M. L. (1998). *Assessment of families with infants*

and toddlers: A family systems and developmental approach. Unpublished manuscript, Tulane University, New Orleans.

Lewis, M. L. (in press). Hair combing task: A new paradigm for research with African American mothers and daughters. *American Journal of Orthopsychiatry.*

Lewis, M. L., Osofsky, J. D., & Moore, M. S. (1997). Violent cities, violent streets: Children draw their neighborhoods. In J. D. Osofsky (Ed.), *Children in a violent society* (pp. 277–299). New York: Guilford Press.

Lewis, M. L., Turnage, B., & Taylor, S. (1999, April). *The meaning of hair for African American mothers and daughters.* Poster session presented at the Society for Research in Child Development, Albuquerque, NM.

Lewis, M. L., Turnage, B., Taylor, S., & Diaz, L. (1999, April). *Ethnicity predicts parenting styles in African American mothers.* Poster session presented at the Society for Research in Child Development, Albuquerque, NM.

Lonner, W. J. (1994). Culture and human diversity. In E. J. Trickett & R. J. Watts (Eds.), *Human diversity: Perspectives on people in context* (pp. 230–243). San Francisco, CA: Jossey-Bass.

Luster, T., & McAdoo, H. P. (1996). Family and child influences on educational attainment: A secondary analysis of the High/Scope Perry preschool data. *Developmental Psychology, 32,* 26–39.

Lutzker, J. R., Bigelow, K. M., Doctor, R. M., Gershater, R. M., & Greene, B. F. (1998). An ecobehavioral model for the prevention and treatment of child abuse and neglect: History and applications. In J. R. Lutzker (Ed.), *Handbook of child abuse research and treatment* (pp. 239–266). New York: Plenum.

Main, M., & Hess, E. (1990). Parents' unresolved traumatic experiences are related to infant disorganized attachment status: Is frightened and/or frightening parental behavior the linking mechanism? In M. T. Greenberg, D. Cicchetti, & E. M. Cummings (Eds.), *Attachment in the pre-school years* (pp. 161–181). Chicago: University of Chicago Press.

McAdoo, H. P. (1991). Family values and outcomes for children. *Journal of Negro Education, 60,* 361–365.

McDonough, S.C. (1993). Interaction guidance: Understanding and treating early infant–caregiver relationship disturbances. In C. H. Zeanah, Jr. (Ed.), *Handbook of infant mental health* (pp. 414–426). New York: Guilford Press.

Mead, M., & MacGregor, F. C. (1951). *Growth and culture.* New York: Putnam.

Miller, P. J., & Goodnow, J. J. (1995). Cultural practices: Toward an integration of culture and development. In J. J. Goodnow, P. J. Miller, & F. Kessel (Eds.), *Cultural practices as contexts for development. New directions for child development* (pp. 5–16). San Francisco: Jossey-Bass.

Miller, P. J., Wiley, A. R., Fung, H., & Liang, C. (1997). Personal storytelling as a medium of socialization in Chinese and American families. *Child Development, 68,* 557–568.

Miller-Loncar, C. L., Erwin-Loeta, J., Landry, S. H., Smith, K. E., & Swank, P. R. (1998). Characteristics of social support networks of low socioeconomic status African American, Anglo American, and Mexican American mothers of full term and preterm infants. *Journal of Community Psychology, 26,* 131–143.

Minturn, L., & Lambert, H. (1964). *Mothers of six cultures: Antecedents to child rearing.* New York: Wiley.

Miyake, K., Chen, S. J., & Campos, J. (1985). Infant temperament, mother's mode of interaction, and attachment in Japan: An interim report. In I. Bretherton & E. Waters (Eds.), Growing points in attachment theory and research. *Monographs of the Society for Research in Child Development, 50*(Serial No. 209), 276–297.

Nakagawa, M., Lamb, M. E., & Miyake, K. (1989). Psychological experiences of Japanese infants in the Strange Situation. *Research and Clinical Center for Child Development Annual Report, 11*(1987–1988), 13–24.

National Association for the Education of Young Children (NAEYC). (1996, January). NAEYC position statement: Responding to linguistic and cultural diversity—recommendations for effective early childhood education, *Young Children,* 4–12.

Nicholls, A., & Kirkland, J. (1996). Maternal sensitivity: A review of attachment literature definitions. *Early Child Development and Care, 120,* 55–65.

Norton, D. (1993). Diversity, early socialization, and temporal development: The dual perspective revisited. *Social Work, 38,* 82–90.

Nsamenang, B. (1992). *Human development in cultural context.* Newbury Park, CA: Sage.

Nugent, J. K. (1994, October/November). Cross-cultural studies of child development: Implications for clinicians. *Zero to Three, 15*(2), 4–6.

O'Donnell, P. (1997, Spring/Summer). Will it be on the test?: Your child [Special issue]. *Newsweek,* pp. 15–17.

Okagaki, L., & Divecha, D. J. (1993). Development of parental beliefs. In T. Luster & L. Okagaki (Eds.), *Parenting: An ecological perspective* (pp. 35–67). Hillsdale, NJ: Erlbaum.

Osofsky, J. D. (1995). The effects of exposure to violence on young children. *American Psychologist, 50* (9), 782–788.

Parham, T. A. (1989). Cycles of psychological nigrescence. *The Counseling Psychologists, 17,* 187–226.

Pascoe, J. M., & Solomon, R. (1994). Prenatal correlates of indigent mothers' attitudes about spoiling their young infants: A longitudinal study. *Developmental and Behavioral Pediatrics, 15,* 367–369.

Pederson, D. R., Gleason, K. E., Moran, G., & Bento, S. (1998). Maternal attachment representations, maternal sensitivity, and the infant–mother attachment relationship. *Developmental Psychology, 34,* 925–933.

Phinney, J. S. (1990). Ethnic identity in adolescence and adulthood: A review and integration. *Psychological Bulletin, 108,* 499–514.

Pianta, R. C., Sroufe, L. A., & Egeland, B. (1989). Continuity and discontinuity in maternal sensitivity at 6, 24, and 42 months in a high-risk sample. *Child Development, 60,* 481–487.

Posada, G., Gao, Y., Wu, F., Posada, R., Tascon, M., Schoelmerich, A., Sagi, A., Kondo-Ikemura, K., Haaland, W., & Synevaag, B. (1995). The secure-base phenomenon across cultures: Children's behavior, mothers' preferences, and experts' concepts. In E. Waters, B. E. Vaughn, G. Posada, & K. Kondo-Ikemura (Eds.), Caregiving, cultural, and cognitive perspectives on secure-base behavior and working models: New growing points of attachment theory and research. *Monographs of the Society for Research in Child Development, 60*(2–3, Serial No. 244), 27–48.

Randolph, S. M., Koblinsky, S. A., & Roberts, D. D. (1998). Studying the role of family and school in the development of African American preschoolers in violent neighborhoods. *Journal of Negro Education, 65,* 282–294.

Raver, C. C., & Leadbeater, B. J. (1992). *Patterns of reciprocity in the play interactions of sensitive and controlling adolescent mothers and their 12-month-old infants.* Poster presented at the eighth annual International Conference on Infant Studies, Miami, FL.

Rohner, R. P. (1986). *The warmth dimension.* Newbury Park: CA: Sage.

Rose, S. J., & Meezak, W. (1996). Variations in perceptions of child neglect. *Child Welfare, 75,* 139–160.

Rosser, P. L., & Randolph, S. M. (1989). Black American infants: The Howard University normative study. In K. Nugent, B. Lester, & T. B. Brazelton (Eds.), *The cultural context of infancy* (pp. 133–165). Norwood, NJ: Ablex.

Sagi, A. (1990). Attachment theory and research from a cross-cultural perspective. *Human Development, 33,* 10–22.

Sameroff, A. J. (1993). Models of development and developmental risk. In C. H. Zeanah, Jr. (Ed.), *Handbook of infant mental health* (pp. 3–13). New York: Guilford Press.

Sameroff, A. J., Seifer, R., & Zax, M. (1982). Early development of children at risk for emotional disorder. *Monographs of the Society for Research in Child Development, 47* (7, Serial No. 199).

Sanders-Phillips, K. (1998). Infant feeding behavior and caretaker–infant relationships in Black families. *Journal of Comparative Family Studies, 29*(1), 161–171.

Schaffer, H. R., & Collis, G. M. (1986). Parental responsiveness and child behavior. In W. Sluckin & M. Herbert (Eds.), *Parental behavior* (pp. 283–315). New York: Basil Blackwell.

Scheper-Hughes, N. (1990). Mother love and child death in northeast Brazil. In J. W. Stigler, R. A. Shweder, & G. Herdt (Eds.), *Cultural psychology: Essays on comparative human development* (pp. 542–568). New York: Cambridge University Press.

Schieffelin, B. B., & Ochs, E. (Eds.). (1986). *Language socialization across cultures.* New York: Cambridge University Press.

Schriver, J. M. (1998). *Human behavior and the social environment.* Boston: Allyn & Bacon.

Sellers, R. M., Smith, M. A., Shelton, J. N., Rowley, S. A., & Chavous, T. M. (1998). Multidimensional model of racial identity: A reconceptualization of African American racial identity. *Personality and Social Psychology Review, 2,* 18–39.

Shweder, R. A., Jensen, L. A., & Goldstein, W. M. (1995). Who sleeps by whom revisited: A method for extracting the moral goods implicit in practice. In J. J. Goodnow, P. J. Miller, & F. Kessel (Eds.), *Cultural*

practices as contexts for development (pp. 41–86). San Francisco: Jossey-Bass.

Sigel, I. E., McGillicuddy-DeLisi, A. V., & Goodnow, J. J. (Eds.). (1992). *Parental belief systems: The psychological consequences for children* (2nd ed.). Hillsdale, NJ: Erlbaum.

Sinha, D. (Ed.). (1981). *Socialization of the Indian child.* New Delhi: Naurang Rai.

Sinha, D. (1988). The family scenario in a developing country and its implications for mental health: The case of India. In P. R. Dasen, J. W. Berry, & N. Sartorius (Eds.), *Health and cross cultural psychology: Toward applications* (pp. 48–70). Newbury Park, CA: Sage.

Skinner, E. A. (1985). Determinants of mother sensitive and contingent-responsive behavior: The role of child rearing beliefs and socioeconomic status. In I. E. Sigel (Ed.), *Parental beliefs systems: The psychological consequences for children* (pp. 25–41). Hillsdale, NJ: Erlbaum.

Sorce, J. F., & Emde, R. N. (1981). Mother's presence is not enough: The effect of emotional availability on infant exploration. *Developmental Psychology, 17,* 737–745.

Spangler, G., Fremmer-Bombik, E., & Grossmann, K. (1996). Social and individual determinants of infant attachment security and disorganization. *Infant Mental Health Journal, 17,* 127–139.

Spencer, M. B. (1998). Social and cultural influences on school adjustment: The application of an identity-focused cultural ecological perspective. *Educational Psychologist, 34*(1), 43–57.

Spencer, M. B., & Markstrom-Adams, C. M. (1990). Identity processes among racial and ethnic minority children in America. *Child Development, 61,* 433–441.

Sroufe, L. A., Cooper, R. G., DeHart, G., & Marshal, M. E. (1996). *Child development: Its nature and course* (3rd ed.). New York: McGraw-Hill.

Stokols, D. (1999). Human development in the age of the Internet: Conceptual and methdological horizons. In S. L. Friedman & T. D. Wachs (Eds.), *Measuring environment across the lifespan: Emerging methods and concepts* (pp. 327–335). Washington, DC: American Psychological Association.

Super, C., & Harkness, S. (1986). The developmental niche: A conceptualization at the interface of child and culture. *International Journal of Behavioral Development, 9,* 545–569.

Super, C., & Harkness, S. (1993). Temperament and the developmental niche. In W. B. Carey & S. A. McDevitt (Eds.), *Prevention and early intervention: Individual differences as risk factors for the mental health of children—a festschrift for Stella Chess and Alexander Thomas* (pp. 115–125). New York: Brunner/Mazel.

Super, C., & Harkness, S. (1997). The cultural structuring of child development. In J. W. Berry, P. R. Dasen, & T. S. Saraswathi (Eds.), *Cross-cultural psychology: Vol. 2. Basic processes and human development* (pp. 1–40). Needham Heights, MA: Allyn & Bacon.

Tavecchio, L. W., & van IJzendoorn, M. H. (1987). *Attachment in social networks: Contributions to the Bowlby-Ainsworth attachment theory.* Amsterdam, Netherlands: North-Holland.

Television: Sesame street it's not. (1997, October 13). *Newsweek*, pp. 89–90.

Thornton, M. C. (1997). Strategies of racial socialization among Black parents. In R. J. Taylor, J. S. Jackson, & L. M. Chatters (Eds.), *Family life in Black America* (pp. 201–215). Thousand Oaks, CA: Sage.

Tudge, J., & Putnam, S. E. (1997). The everyday experiences of North American preschoolers in two cultural communities: A cross-disciplinary and cross-level analysis. In J. Tudge, M. J. Shanahan, & J. Valsiner (Eds.), *Comparisons in human development: Understanding time and context* (pp. 252–284). New York: Cambridge University Press.

Valenzuela, M. (1997). Maternal sensitivity in a developing society: The context of urban poverty and infant chronic undernutrition. *Developmental Psychology, 33*, 845–855.

Valsiner, J. (Ed.). (1988). *Child development within culturally structured environments, parent cognition and adult-child interaction.* Norwood, NJ: Ablex.

Valsiner, J. (1997). *Culture and the development of children's action: A theory of human development.* New York: Wiley.

van IJzendoorn, M. H., & Kroonenberg, P. M. (1988). Cross-cultural patterns of attachment: A meta-analysis of the strange situation. *Child Development, 59*, 147–156.

Vereijken, C. M., Riksen-Walraven, J. M., & Kondo-Ikemura, K. (1997). Maternal sensitivity and infant attachment security in Japan: A longitudinal study. *International Journal of Behavioral Development, 21*, 35–49.

Vezeau, T. M. (1991). Investigating "greedy." *The American Journal of Maternal/Child Nursing, 16*, 337–338.

Wang, C. C., & Phinney, J. S. (1998). Differences in child rearing attitudes between immigrant Chinese mothers and Anglo-American mothers. *Early Development and Parenting, 7*, 181–189.

Weiss, J. R., McCarthy, C. A., Eastman, K. L., Caseate, W., & Suwanlert, S. (1997). Developmental psychopathology and culture: Ten lessons from Thailand. In S. S. Luthar, J. A. Burack, & D. Cicchetti (Eds.), *Developmental psychopathology: Perspectives on adjustment, risk, and disorder* (pp. 342–361). New York: Cambridge University Press.

Werner, E. E. (1988). A cross-cultural perspective on infancy: Research and social issues. *Journal of Cross-Cultural Psychology, 19*(1), 96–115.

Werner, E. E. (1990). Protective factors and individual resilience. In S. Meisels & J. Shonkoff (Eds.), *Handbook of early childhood intervention* (pp. 97–116). New York: Cambridge University Press.

Whiting, J. W. (1994). *A model for psychocultural research.* New York: Cambridge University Press.

Whiting J. W. M., & Child, I. L. (1953). *Child training and personality.* New Haven: Yale University Press.

Zeanah, C. H., & Anders, T. F. (1987). Subjectivity in parent–infant relationships: A discussion of internal working models. *Infant Mental Health Journal, 8*(3), 237–250.

II

RISK AND PROTECTIVE FACTORS

❖

An increasing amount of evidence suggests that risks and outcomes are not specifically linked in the early years. Equifinality describes similar outcomes deriving from a variety of different risk conditions, and plurafinality describes a variety of outcomes that derive from a single risk condition. In fact, in several studies, the number of risk factors is more predictive of maladaptive outcomes than is any particular combination of risk factors. All this raises the question of why a section on risk and protective factors should be organized by types of risk factors.

One answer to the question is that many interventions are organized around risk conditions. Many programs are organized to serve poor families or adolescent mothers or preterm infants, for example. For this reason, learning as much as possible about infants characterized by each of these categories has considerable merit. This leads to a second answer to the question; namely, the effects of risk conditions can be studied and comprehended more fully when considered in relative isolation. Still another answer to the question is that some specificity *is* known to exist; for example, adult attachment classifications are specifically predictive of infant attachment classifications (van IJzendoorn, 1995) and extremely low birthweight in infants may be specifically predictive of inattention/hyperactivity (Szatmari, Saigal, Rosenbaum, & Campbell, 1993). Clearly, we still have more to learn about specific and nonspecific relations of risks and outcomes.

From the clinical perspective, what is important to remember is that risk factors tend to cluster together and exert their effects synergistically. Having any one of the risk conditions described in the chapters in this section increases the risk of having any of the other risk conditions. Further, it is important to be as diligent about identifying protective factors as risk factors. Therefore, individual differences in adaptation within broad categories of risk are of great interest.

Poverty is perhaps the prototypical risk factor for infant mental health. Indeed, for a broad range of health and mental health outcomes, social class is the single best predictor of outcomes. In Chapter 6, Aber, Jones, and Cohen use Brofenbrenner's model to consider two major questions. First, they ask about the mechanisms by which poverty increases risk and affects the healthy development of very young children. Second, they review what is known about the impact of poverty on young children via these mechanisms. Throughout they consider potential protective factors that contribute to the diversity of outcomes.

In Chapter 7, Wakschlag and Hans review the important areas of early and unplanned parenthood. Concentrating on individual differences in young mothers, they describe the complex family relationships associated with early and unplanned parenthood and see this as a crucial variable related to outcome. They make an important distinction between adolescent parenting as an adaptive life choice versus adolescent parenting as a manifestation of a pattern of problematic behavior, and they describe crucial differences in domains of functioning that distinguish the two. They point to problems with interventions that have used a generic rather than an individualized approach. Finally, they suggest that the move to expand intervention efforts from a focus on mother alone to mother and infant have been promising, but they suggest that recent research supports a further expansion to grandmother, mother, and infant.

In Chapter 8, Seifer and Dickstein review what is known about parental mental illness and infant development. They review and critique the latest findings in this area, concentrating on children whose parents are diagnosed with schizophrenia and with depression. They point to a well-documented heterogeneity of outcomes in such infants, and they use a transactional model to explain these findings. Critically reviewing the literature, they point to a number of specific child risks associated with having parents with these disorders. Finally, they document new findings indicating that overall family functioning moderates intergenerational transmission of disorders.

A major policy debate in the United States in the past 20 years has concerned the proper responses to infants exposed prenatally to illicit substances. Some have favored criminalization of drug abuse, but others have suggested that from the standpoint of the infants, treatment is a better approach. Lester, Boukydis, and Twomey, in Chapter 9, review much of the literature on cocaine abuse to highlight the findings, controversies, and distortions associated with this policy debate. They emphasize that prenatal drug exposure occurs in psychological and social contexts that often are fairly enduring and may contribute risks that are often attributed to prenatal drug exposure. On the other hand, pregnancy and early infancy provide important opportunities for intervention. Throughout the chapter they document the advantages of conceptualizing drug abuse as a disease—not only for mothers but also for their young children—and they conclude by advocating for its inclusion as primarily a mental health rather than a criminal justice problem.

Minde, in Chapter 10, reviews the experiences of infants who are hospitalized for prematurity or other serious medical conditions. At first, this seems to provide an opportunity to consider the potential effects of biological adversity on infant development. Minde demonstrates, however, that prematurity, is associated with a variety of psychosocial risk factors that are inextricably linked to infants' low birthweights. After documenting the scope of the problem of prematurity and hospitalized infants, he reviews the challenges that they present as interactional partners. He also highlights some effective interventions designed to enhance the relationship between preterm and chronically ill infants and their parents. He concludes by advocating for efforts to make the hospital experience of these vulnerable infants more humane and to support their parents as primary caregivers.

Another increasing public health problem in this and other countries is the exposure of infants and young children to family and community violence. In Chapter 11, Kaufman and Henrich review effects of maltreatment and exposure to violence on infant development. They point out the complex effects of these experiences as they contribute to developmental and clinical deviance. Throughout, they note similarities and differences in the effects in the early years compared to other points in the life cycle, and they point to accumulating evidence that suggest that the first few years of life may be especially vulnerable. They challenge us to develop more comprehensive efforts to prevent exposure to and to minimize sequella of exposure to violence in young children.

REFERENCES

Szatmari, P., Saigal, S., Rosenbaum, P., & Campbell, D. (1993). Psychopathology and adaptive functioning among extremely low birthweight children at eight years of age. *Development and Psychopathology, 5,* 345–357.

van IJzendoorn, M. H. (1995). Adult attachment representations, parental responsiveness and infant attachment: A meta-analysis on the predictive validity of the Adult Attachment Interview. *Psychological Bulletin, 117,* 387–403.

6

The Impact of Poverty on the Mental Health and Development of Very Young Children

❖

J. LAWRENCE ABER
STEPHANIE JONES
JENNIFER COHEN

The basic facts are increasingly well-known. Young children (under 6 years of age) have the highest poverty rates of any age group in the United States (Shirk, Bennett, & Aber, 1999) and in most other major Western industrialized democracies (Rainwater & Smeeding, 1995). In addition, poverty experienced in early childhood, especially extreme poverty, is more detrimental to children's future development than poverty experienced later in life (Duncan, Brooks-Gunn, & Klebanov, 1994). And, although it is difficult to tease out the effects of family-level poverty compared to that of neighborhood-level poverty, when researchers do so, it appears that family-level poverty has the stronger influence on children's development, including their mental health (Aber, 1994; Brooks-Gunn, Duncan, & Aber, 1997).

Although these basic facts are well-known, a more refined scientific understanding of the effects of poverty on child health and development is still being constructed. Because poverty can be defined in many ways, and it so often occurs with other potent factors, studies must use complex measurement strategies to estimate the unique effects of poverty on development (Aber, 1997; Aber, Bennett, Conley, & Li, 1997). Further, because the healthy development of young children itself is quite complex

and unfolds dynamically over time, longitudinal studies of the precise mechanisms by which poverty affects the development of growing children have been undertaken. An increasing number of theoretically driven studies on the effects of poverty on early childhood development has been conducted since the last review on poverty and infant mental health (Halpern, 1993).

In this chapter, we review selectively the extant scientific literature, especially the literature of the last decade, to address two overarching questions:

1. What are the mechanisms by which poverty increases risk and affects the healthy development of very young children (newborn to 3 years of age)?
2. What is the impact of poverty on young children via those mechanisms?

These two questions help us cover the most important advances made in our scientific understanding over the last decade. They also help frame the issues in a manner in which the practice and policy implications of the research can be laid bare. For in understanding the causal mechanisms by which poverty affects infant development, including infant mental health, we find insights into targets for preventive interventions.

The next section defines poverty and describes its most important co-factors. It also briefly describes our conceptual framework for infant development, including infant mental health. We use this framework to organize the third section, which is a selective review of the extant literature. The next section highlights some of the most cutting-edge research and offers several recommendations for new research priorities. Finally, we suggest several implications of the research for the design and conduct of program interventions and social policies aimed at enhancing infant mental health and development.

CONCEPTUAL FRAMEWORK

Concepts of Poverty

The Random House Dictionary defines poverty as "the state or condition of having little or no money, goods or means of support" (p. 1127) and that simple definition begins to suggest the complexity of the concept. A family can be poor in money (income poverty), goods (material deprivation), or means of support (asset poverty). In the United States, poverty is most commonly conceived as "income poverty." Researchers distinguish among three measures of income poverty. *Absolute poverty* is measured by gross family income falling below an absolute threshold. In the United States, the current poverty threshold for a family of four is $16,400 a year. This absolute threshold in turn is based on (1) studies of the cost of a minimally adequate diet for four and (2) consumer expenditure studies of the percentage of a low-income family budget that goes to food. A recent report by the National Academy of Science has leveled serious criticism at the official poverty measure, but it remains in use today (Citro & Michael, 1995). The U.S. government uses the absolute measure as its official measure of poverty to define families' eligibility for programs and services. Consequently, it (or a variant of it, the income-to-needs ratio, defined as the ratio of families' gross income to the poverty threshold) is the most frequently used measure of poverty used by U.S. researchers.

Two alternative concepts and measures of income poverty are those of relative poverty and subjective poverty. *Relative poverty* is defined as a gross family income which falls below a certain percentage of a jurisdiction's median income (usually 40–50% of the national median income). Because the median family income in the United States is approximately $38,000 a year; relative poverty (at 50% of the national median) would be defined as a gross family income of $19,000 a year (a full $2,600 above the absolute poverty threshold). European governments and researchers use measures of relative poverty to facilitate cross-national comparisons. *Subjective poverty* is measured as the average answer to the following question, "What is the minimum income required for a family [of four] to just barely get by in your community?" Based on well-designed, highly representative surveys, the answer to this question averages $22,000 a year in the United States ($5,600 above the absolute poverty threshold), but it can increase to as high as $45,000 in high-cost states such as Connecticut. Clearly, the nature and extent of income poverty in a community, state or country depend on precisely how income poverty is conceptualized and measured.

It is useful to contrast income poverty to material deprivation and asset poverty. To illustrate, let us think of two families. Both families are headed by unemployed, single mothers who are (1) receiving cash assistance benefits from their state ($6,000), (2) working part time, part year at minimum wage ($ 4,000) and therefore receiving an earned income tax credit of approximately ($1,500). Their gross income of $11,500 falls below the poverty threshold of $13,500 for a family of three. Both families are poor by all three definitions of income poverty. But in the first family, the mother was recently divorced and lives in a modest house worth $65,000, owned by her ailing father, on which the mortgage is fully paid. In addition, this mother owns a 5-year-old car and has almost no outstanding credit card debt. In contrast, in the second family, the mother was recently evicted from public housing and pays a rent of $500 a month for a small two-bedroom apartment. This mother does not own a car and carries a credit card debt of several thousand dollars.

Both mothers are "income poor," but the first mother has considerably more assets than the second. Because fewer assets and greater debts translate into greater expenses in the second family, they also experience greater material deprivation on the same income (less nutritious meals, less heat in the winter, etc.). Of course, families that experience deeper income poverty for longer periods tend to be poorer in assets and more nutritionally deprived.

To understand the effects of poverty on infant mental health and development, it is important (1) to distinguish poverty conceptually from associated risk factors (referred to often as poverty co-factors) and (2) to tease apart the effects of poverty per se from the effects of co-factors on infant mental health and development. We recognize, of course, that there is a fine line between some poverty co-factors and the mechanisms by which poverty affects development.

Three demographic characteristics of parents are powerfully associated with whether their young children (less than 5 years of age) live in poverty: marital status, education, and employment status. In 1997, children under 6 living with single mothers were five times as likely to be poor as were those living with both parents (56–11%). Young children whose most educated parent did not finish high school were 4 times more likely to be poor than were children whose parents completed some college (63–15.2%) and 20 times more likely than were young children whose best educated parent finished college (63–3%). Not surprisingly, no matter the parents' education levels, if neither parent is employed, more than 70% of their young children live in poverty. Stated another way, among young children who live in two-parent families in which at least one parent has graduated high school and is working full time, the poverty rate is a mere 3.5%. But among children of single mothers who have not graduated high school and are not employed full time, the poverty rate reached an astounding 82%. In light of these figures, it is clearly necessary to consider these powerful poverty co-factors in any analysis of the effects of poverty on infant mental health and development.

In addition to these parent characteristics, family poverty is associated with a wide variety of risk factors, including poor neighborhoods, poor schools, poor basic services, and greater environmental health risks. Although some researchers also refer to these types of variables as poverty co-factors, we conceptualize most of them as "mediators" or the mechanisms by which poverty influences development. In any case, it is important to note that other parental factors and social conditions are associated with poverty and that a full scientific understanding of the effects of poverty on development requires clear thinking and analysis of their separate and combined influences.

Developmental–Contextual Approach

To organize the recent literature on the mechanisms by which poverty increases the risk and affects the health and development of very young children, we have adopted a developmental contextual approach. This theoretical approach, famously articulated by Bronfenbrenner (1979), has come to organize much of the field's thinking about both normal and abnormal development (Cicchetti & Aber, 1998; Ford & Lerner, 1992; Sameroff, 1983, Chapter 1, this volume). Developing persons are viewed as nested within micro-, meso-, and macro-level contexts. Development involves reciprocal transactions between persons and contexts, which both influence and are influenced by changes in the child's physical/biological, cognitive/linguistic, and social/emotional competencies. Working within this approach, we organize our review of the mechanisms by which poverty influences the health and development of young children by four levels: person, family, neighborhood, and other (including social policy).

By outlining some of the relationships among poverty and person (micro), family (meso), neighborhood (exo), and other contextual processes (macro), we hope to begin to sketch the large network of associations that characterize the multiple possible pathways from poverty to outcomes for very young children. There are several literature reviews that comprehensively describe the impact of poverty on families and their children (Aber et al., 1997; Huston, 1991; McLloyd, 1998). This review summarizes and provides examples of pertinent research focusing on very young children and their families, but by no means could describe all of the existing research in the space provided.

PERSON-LEVEL MECHANISMS

Poverty affects the healthy development of very young children through a wide variety of immediate deterrents to good physical health—from malnutrition and iron deficiency (Brown & Pollitt, 1996; Pollitt, 1994) to deficits in visual function and perceptual–motor development (Solan & Mozlin, 1997). Despite this wide variety, effects most often addressed in the research literature are low birthweight, increased infant mortality, jeopardized early brain development, increased illnesses, and increased injury due to accidents (see, e.g., Aber et al., 1997; Kopp & Kaler, 1989; Gunnar & Barr, 1998; Shore, 1997; Landrigan et al., 1998; Klerman, 1991; Klerman & Parker, 1991).

Following our developmental contextual and systems theory approach to understanding the impact of poverty on infant development, these person-level mechanisms can be conceptualized as (1) short-term biological outcomes, (2) longer-term mediators and moderators of the impact of poverty on outcomes in early childhood and the preschool years, and (3) risks associated with family processes and subsequent later outcomes. In this section, we address those studies in which these person characteristics are examined as short-term outcomes. Studies in which the person characteristics are examined as longer-term mediators, moderators, or risks associated with family processes are generally described in the section "Family-Level Mechanisms."

Low Birthweight and Infant Mortality

A comprehensive review of the literature describing the relationship between poverty and increased risk of low birthweight and high infant mortality rates can be found in Aber et al. (1997; see also Paneth, 1995). One early study stands out in particular. Gortmaker (1979), using data from the National Natality and National Infant Mortality Surveys, found that poverty status, net of other family demographic factors and pregnancy and hospitalization factors, significantly increased the risk of neonatal and postneonatal mortality, both directly and via their impact on low birthweight (Gortmaker, 1979). In contrast, more recent work has illustrated how the specific relationships between poverty and birthweight are less clear. For example, after controlling for individual-level factors, Roberts (1997) found that although community-level indicators of economic hardship and housing costs were associated with increased low birthweight, indicators of community socioeconomic status, crowded housing, and percentage of young African American residents were associated with reduced risk of low birthweight. Here, it appears that different community-level indicators of poverty (economic hardship vs. socioeconomic status) are differentially related to low birthweight.

Aber et al. (1997) described several barriers to understanding the link between poverty and these particular biological outcomes that may help us reconcile some of these inconsistencies in the literature. Specifically, the profound racial differences in incidence of low birthweight and its highly associated risk of infant mortality combined with racial differences in poverty rates in the United States complicate these relationships (Shiono & Behrman, 1995). According to the National Center for Health Statistics, infant mortality rates were highest for infants born to black mothers (14.6%) (MacDorman & Atkinson, 1998).

For example, researchers have shown that race is related to low birthweight *through* its association with poverty (Shiono, Rauh, Park, Lederman, & Zuskar, 1997). In contrast, as described in Aber et al. (1997), Starfield found that poverty increases the incidence of low birthweight for whites but not for blacks, though blacks have significantly higher low birthweight rates across socioeconomic levels (Starfield et al., 1991). Furthermore, researchers have found that Mexican Americans of low socioeconomic status have comparable low birthweight rates to whites and significantly lower rates than similar low-income populations of black Americans (Dowling & Fischer, 1987). Similarly, Bird (1995) describes different relationships between state structural variables and black and white infant mortality models. For example, only the percentage of individuals with a bachelor's degree or higher is significant for both whites and blacks, whereas the percentage of black individuals and urban residential segregation and the *low* percentage of individuals below the poverty level is significant in predicting infant mortality for blacks (Bird, 1995). These studies clearly indicate that there may be additional sociocultural and historical factors operating individually or in a synergistic fashion with poverty to affect birthweight outcomes for these populations. Furthermore, in the majority of the studies described earlier, poverty is operationalized in terms of global census-level indicators, which does not allow for the teasing apart of contributions due to individual or family-level factors.

In addition, the mechanisms through which poverty affects low birthweight and infant mortality are not well understood (Aber et al., 1997). Research has shown that poverty may affect low birthweight (and subsequent infant mortality) via multiple factors (Klerman, 1991). Some factors described in the literature are tobacco, alcohol, and drug use (Hofkosh et al., 1995; Abel, 1985; Abel & Skokol, 1987), poor maternal psychological well-being and physical health (Hughes & Simpson, 1995), inadequate access to prenatal care (Shiono & Behrman, 1995), and increased environmental toxins (Bearer, 1995).

Early Brain Development

Considerable attention has been paid recently to the impact of early disadvantage and poor stimulation on the developing brain by the general public, policymakers, and researchers alike; for example see the special reports in both *Time* and *Newsweek* in the spring of 1997, and multiple conferences and research reports ("Early childhood development and learning," 1997; Shore, 1997; National Center for Children in Poverty, 1997; Gunnar & Barr, 1998). Although much of this research is still in the early stages, some clear patterns have emerged.

Research with a wide variety of animals has indicated that repeated exposure to negative pre- and postnatal experiences (e.g., environmental stressors such as extreme early deprivation) adversely affects the number of cortisol receptors in the brain. Put simply, the number of cortisol receptors in the brain affects its ability to modulate future cortisol levels and, in turn, subsequent abilities to regulate stress responses (for a comprehensive review, see Benes, 1994; Gunnar & Barr, 1998). Much of this work has been conducted with animal populations, but there are a growing number of studies that focus on the relationship between early stress and brain development in human populations. For example, researchers have found higher cortisol levels to be related to poor attentional focus and self-control in preschoolers (Gunnar, Tout, deHann, Pierce, & Stansbury, 1997) and the use of a disorganized or avoidant attachment strategy in infancy and toddlerhood (Nachmias, Gunnar, Mangelsdorf, & Parritz, 1996; Spangler & Grossmann, 1993; Dawson, Klinger, Panagiotides, Spieker, & Frey, 1992). Although these studies do not implicate poverty per se, such potential environmental stressors as low stimulation in the home environment (Watson, Kirby, Kelleher, & Bradley, 1996), harsh punitive or neglectful parenting (McLoyd, 1998; Pianta & Egeland, 1990), and exposure to chronic community violence (Aber, 1994; Coulton, Korbin, Su, & Chow, 1995) have been associated with both family- and neighborhood-level indicators of poverty and in some cases, directly with an impact on the developing brain (e.g., Perry, 1997; Kaufman et al., 1997; Kaufman & Henrich, Chapter 11, this volume).

Another line of research on early brain development has focused on synaptogenesis, synapse elimination, and later development (Huttenlocher, 1994). The first years of life are characterized by dramatic growth in synapse formation and dendritic density in the developing brain. Continued activation of newly formed synapses due primarily to experience during these early years drives a pruning or selective retention process in which both the density and structure of synapses are altered and/or reduced (Dawson & Fischer, 1994; Greenough, Black, & Wallace, 1987; Huttenlocher, 1994). The early work of Hubel and Wiesel with cats demonstrated very clearly the negative impact of *early* deprivation on vision (Wiesel, 1982), and more recent work has made similar contributions and has supported the relationship between early deprivation and synaptic density and structure (e.g., Kemperman, Kuhn, & Gage, 1997, with mice).

Poverty also has been found to place developing fetuses at risk for congenital malformations. For example, Wasserman, Shaw, Selvin, Gould, and Syme (1998) found that after adjusting for relevant demographic variables, both maternal socioeconomic status (SES) and neighborhood social conditions (residence in a less educated neighborhood, residence in a neighborhood in which at least 20% of residents were living below the federal poverty level, residence in neighborhood characterized primarily by low occupational status, and residence in a crowded neighborhood) increased the odds of a pregnancy involving a neural tube defect. Furthermore, when these indicators of family and neighborhood SES were examined as an index, risk of neural tube defect increased as the number of low SES indicators increased (Wasserman, Shaw, et al., 1998).

Thus, recent research indicates that poverty, both directly and via its association with severe and chronic strain in the environment, affects at least two critical facets of the developing brain. In addition, poverty has an impact on the developing brain by increasing risk factors which, in turn, are related to a range of potential brain outcomes for young children. For example, poverty has been related to increased prenatal exposure to illicit substances, which has been linked to stunted neurons in the brain and a lack of brain cells in crucial developmental stages, causing serious neurological disorders (Mayes, 1996).

Children who are poor are more likely to be in poor-quality day care, which may hinder a child's brain activity and impede development by discouraging interaction and limiting environmental stimulation. Compared to those who were not in day care, studies show that high-quality day care can, in fact, enhance the intellectual development of poor children (Burchinal, Lee, & Ramey, 1989; Cost, Quality, & Child Outcomes Study Team, 1995).

Illnesses and Other Morbidities

In addition to increasing risk for low birthweight, infant mortality, and compromised brain development, poverty has been related to increased incidence of illnesses such as asthma (Malveaux & Fletcher-Vincent, 1995; Gottlieb, Beiser, & O'Connor, 1995), upper respiratory infection (Margolis et al., 1992), tuberculosis (Reinhard, Paul, & McAuley, 1997; Drucker, Alcabes, Bosworth, & Sckell, 1994), and pediatric AIDS (Klerman, 1991; Klerman & Parker, 1991). For example, Halfon and Newacheck (1993), using the data from the 1988 National Health Interview Survey on Child Health, reported a significantly higher prevalence of asthma for children whose families had incomes below the federal poverty level. Furthermore, the differential in prevalence of asthma between poor and nonpoor families was greatest for children under 6 years of age. These authors also found more debilitating effects of asthma on poor children, such as more days in bed and higher rates of hospitalization (Halfon & Newacheck, 1993). Other researchers have linked the high rates of asthma in poor, inner-city children to higher sensitivity and exposure to cockroach allergen (Rosenstreich et al., 1997).

FAMILY-LEVEL MECHANISMS

There are two primary ways in which poverty indirectly interferes with the family-level processes necessary to promote optimal mental health and cognitive development in infants. First, the financial and emotional stressors associated with poverty negatively affect parenting behaviors and the early caregiving relationship, thus having an impact on infant attachment strategies and leading to cognitive and behavioral disorders in preschool and school-age children (Lyons-Ruth, Alpern, & Repacholi, 1993; Lyons-Ruth, Easterbrooks, & Cibelli, 1997; McLeod & Shanahan, 1993; Shaw & Vondra, 1995). Second, the deleterious affect of poverty on parental ability to provide a

supportive and stimulating early home learning environment leads to problems with subsequent school readiness and cognitive achievement in children (Brooks-Gunn, Klebanov, & Liaw, 1995; Duncan et al., 1994; Klebanov, Brooks-Gunn, McCarton, & McCormick, 1998). This section highlights research that identifies some of the specific mechanisms by which poverty affects the quality of parenting behaviors and the early home learning environment, underscoring the multiple ways in which poverty inhibits child development through indirect family processes.

Poverty, Quality of Parenting, Quality of Attachment, and Behavioral Problems

Our first area of focus is on how poverty affects parenting behavior and, hence, mother–infant attachment and subsequent infant development. Mothers who are poor have been observed to have interactions with their infants that are characterized by lower overall ratings of maternal sensitivity and by more hostile, intrusive, and erratic responses (Pianta & Egeland, 1990; Shaw & Vondra, 1995). Such parenting styles in turn place infants at risk for the development of insecure or disorganized/disoriented attachment strategies (Lyons-Ruth, Connell, Grunebaum, & Botein, 1990; Lyons-Ruth et al., 1997; Zeanah, Boris, & Larrieu, 1997), as well as at heightened risk for maltreatment (Cicchetti & Toth, 1995; Crittenden & Ainsworth, 1989). Furthermore, the existing attachment literature has documented higher rates of insecure or disorganized/disoriented attachment in families at social risk, where low income is included as an index of risk (Lyons-Ruth, Repacholi, McLeod, & Silva, 1991).

Indeed, researchers have established a direct link between problematic mother–infant attachment styles and the development of subsequent behavioral problems in a number of low-income samples. Shaw and Vondra (1995) found in their sample of low-income mother–infant dyads that attachment insecurity observed at both 12 and 18 months was related to behavioral problems at age 3. This association was most strongly apparent when all subtypes of insecure attachment—avoidant, resistant, and disorganized styles—were combined. In addition, Lyons-Ruth et al. (1997) found, in their longitudinal study of low-income families, a striking association between disorganized/disoriented attachment and externalizing difficulties at age 7. In their sample, approximately 83% of the children age 7, who were identified by teachers as having problematic externalizing behaviors were observed to have a disorganized/disoriented attachment relationship during infancy and to have been below the national mean in mental development scores at 18 months.

This high incidence of negative parent–infant interactions, which compromise the development of secure attachments in young children, may be linked to a variety of maternal difficulties associated with poverty status. The stressors of living in poverty may severely tax and limit parents' emotional and coping resources when interacting with their infants (Halpern, 1993; McLeod & Shanahan, 1993; Watson et al., 1996). The most notable of these stressors include psychological distress as a result of "financial insecurity, or interruption of employment or perceived or actual lack of social support, either financially or emotionally" (Aber et al., 1997, p. 476). Stress associated with poverty has been shown to result from increased rates of negative life events, a higher incidence of single-mother and teenage parenting, marital conflicts, and increased rates of overall stress in dual-parent homes (Lempers, Clark-Lempers, & Simons, 1989; McLoyd, 1990). Furthermore, a number of studies have demonstrated a positive relationship between social support and the ability to parent effectively (Bendersky & Lewis, 1994; Hashima & Amato, 1994). Parents living in poverty have also been found to have higher rates of mental health difficulties, including depression, alcohol, and substance abuse (McLeod & Shanahan, 1993), all of which can severely interfere with parenting quality and infant development.

If we look specifically at the associations between poverty and parenting quality, we find studies that emphasize the indirect influence of maternal psychological distress on mother–infant interactions. Results of the Mother–Infant Project (Pianta & Egeland, 1990), a longitudinal study of high-risk disadvantaged families, indicated a significant relationship between maternal "personal stress" (i.e., stress in interpersonal relationships) and the quality of mother-child interactions observed when infants were 6 and 42 months. Mothers who experienced higher levels of personal stress were observed with their infants during free play and structured tasks to have lower scores on a measure of overall sensitivity at 6 and 42 months, marked by a less cooperative, more hostile, and intrusive parenting style. These associations were most strongly related for girls than for boys. Daughters were observed in a problem-solving task to demonstrate a "lack of persistence, low enthusiasm for the task, noncompliance, and negativity toward and avoidance of their mothers" (Pianta & Egeland, 1990, p. 334). Most striking was the disengaged or avoidant strategy of the daughters in response to maternal insensitivity, which places infants at increased risk for these strategies in subsequent years, as well as at-risk for emotional, behavioral, and cognitive difficulties.

Maternal depression, another factor leading to poor parenting, has been found to co-occur with poverty status at elevated rates and may be the "single most important mediator" of the quality of mother–infant interactions observed in infancy. Similarly, in middle-class samples, maternal depression during infancy has also been documented to be one of the greatest risks for both internalizing and externalizing problems among preschool and school-age children (Cicchetti, Rogosch, & Toth, 1998; Weissman, Warner, Wickramaratne, Moreau, & Olfson, 1997). In a study that provided intervention services to a subgroup of low-income, high-risk mother–infant dyads, Lyons-Ruth et al. (1990) found maternal depression to be the most powerful and specific predictor of lower cognitive attainment and attachment insecurity. Rates of child maltreatment were also elevated in the subgroup of mothers who were depressed. Infants of depressed mothers who did not receive intervention services performed on the Bayley Mental Developmental Index 10 points below the mean of the depressed mother–infant dyads who received intervention services and were more likely to have insecure attachment styles by a factor of 2 to 1. In contrast, infants of nondepressed mothers who received no intervention services and who were matched according to SES with the at-risk group achieved cognitive levels consistent with national norms and evidenced higher rates of secure attachment. Thus, these results further underscore the importance of considering the associated indirect effects that family-level processes have on infant development, above and beyond the influences of poverty, per se.

Alpern and Lyons-Ruth (1993) similarly examined the relationship between poverty status and maternal depression, as well as identifying associated links with behavioral problems among children ages 4 to 6. Findings indicated that maternal depression, occurring during both infancy and preschool age, increased the risk that children would display hostile–aggressive behaviors in the preschool period when assessed both at home and at school. Furthermore, Lyons-Ruth et al. (1997) found that high levels of maternal depressive symptoms during the first 5 years most strongly predicted children's internalizing symptoms as reported by both mothers and teachers at age 7. Results indicated that maternal depressive symptoms were "the best overall index linking a family climate of adversity to later internalizing symptoms, capturing variance shared with cumulative demographic risk scores and lowered infant MDI scores" (Lyons-Ruth et al., 1997, p. 689).

Yet maternal stress and depression are not the only relevant factors. The parent–infant interaction can also entail a negative circular relationship. Parenting difficulties may result from the fact that poverty increases the risk that infants will have a difficult temperament, thus compounding the potential stressors experienced by a parent (Halpern, 1993). Infants born in poverty have been documented to be at greater risk for temperaments in which they have difficulties with affect regulation, are more easily distracted and labile, and display less task persistence (Brooks-Gunn et al., 1995). And as described earlier, poverty also increases the risk that infants will be born with low birthweight (LBW) and experience medical illnesses during early infancy, which, when combined with poverty status, places them in "double jeopardy" for developing cognitive and behavioral problems (Parker, Greer, & Zuckerman, 1988; Escalona, 1982). This combination of risks poses further challenges to maternal psychological distress and mother–infant interactions.

Poverty, Early Home Learning Environment, and Diminished School Readiness

Turning to poverty's effect on the early home learning environment, we see an equally negative influence on child development. Indeed, the quality of the early home learning environment has been found to partially mediate the effects of poverty on the development of young children's cognitive attainment. Specifically, a number of studies of low birthweight premature (LBWPT) infants, born in poverty that were part of the Infant Health and Development Program (1990) found a strong association between a parent's ability to provide developmentally appropriate and stimulating activities in infancy and cognitive achievement in the first 3 to 5 years of life. These studies used the Home Observation for Measurement of the Environment (HOME) Scale to assess these factors, as well as the quality of emotional support provided to the infant (Caldwell & Bradley, 1984). Furthermore, the HOME scale "is highly related to a variety of child outcomes, often being a more potent predictor of cognitive and school academic readiness than maternal education" (Brooks-Gunn et al., 1995 p. 252; Bradley et al., 1989).

Brooks-Gunn et al. (1995) and Brooks-Gunn, Duncan, Klebanov, and Sealand (1993) found in their analyses that the HOME learning environment score most strongly predicted the association between the home environment and age 3 IQ score when considering multiple risks together. They found that the home learning environment is more predictive of IQ than are other aspects of the home environment (physical environment and warmth and responsiveness of the mother) and family structural characteristics (female headship), net of family income, ethnicity, and maternal education. Using the Infant Health and Development Program data, Duncan et al. (1994) found the quality of the home learning environment associated with poverty to also most clearly predict lower cognitive attainment at age 5. They found that maternal risk factors such as maternal depression and coping mediate children's behavioral problems at age 5.

Similarly, Klebanov et al. (1998) also found the presence of cumulative family risk factors (defined by the HOME scale as economic, family structure, social support, and maternal characteristics and responsiveness) in early infancy to be associated with lower cognitive achievement in the first 3 years of life. At age 1, they found no main effect for family poverty but, rather, a significant interaction between family poverty and family risk, where poor children's IQ scores were more negatively affected by the accumulation of family risk factors than those of nonpoor children. By age 2, they found family poverty as well as number of family risk factors to be associated with lower IQ scores. It was not until age 3 that neighborhood influences contributed to developmental test score outcome. Specifically, after controlling for the independent effects of aspects of the HOME environment on IQ scores, analyses "reveal[ed] the mediation by the HOME scale primarily operates through the learning environment inside the home . . ." (Klebanov et al., 1998, p. 1431). Klebanov et al. (1998) suggest that this is due, in part, to parents' ability to purchase stimulating experiences for their children, but more significantly related to the fact that "it is likely that poor parents, given the stresses in their lives, spend less time in provision of so-called learning experiences" (p. 1431). Therefore, these studies on the early home environment suggest that family-level mechanisms may be the first level of environmental effect on the cognitive development of children up to age 3.

Thus, a comprehensive review of the literature clearly illustrates the importance of examining the family-level processes by which poverty indirectly affects the developmental outcomes of very young children. It is thus important, when parceling out family effects on infant development, to consider specific mechanisms such as factors that contribute to parenting quality and the ability to provide a supportive and stimulating early home learning environment. Traditional measures of family poverty that consider SES and maternal education alone fail to illuminate the complexities of the interaction between family processes and infant development and reveal very little about the crucial effects that family-level variables have on child development. Furthermore, Bendersky and Lewis (1994), in their longitudinal study of premature infants, found that identifying family risk factors at 12 and 18 months (e.g., social support, parent–child interaction, stressful events, and organization of the environment) more strongly predicted 2-year-old child development outcome than did social risk factors comprising SES measures of parental education and occupation. In fact, their results highlight the critical impact that indirect family-level mechanisms have on infant development, determining these factors to be "about as powerful a predictor of overall two-year outcome for these high risk preterm children as measures of early medical compromise" (Bendersky & Lewis, 1994, p. 492).

It is, however, equally important to note that although the existing literature documents numerous family risks and subsequent behavioral and emotional difficulties in young children growing up in poverty, there is also much heterogeneity in parenting styles and child outcomes (Werner, 1989). Many infants born in poverty evidence resilient outcomes in childhood (Bradley et al., 1994) and adulthood (Werner, 1989), and do not display difficulties in cognitive attainment and emotional adjustment.

In addition, many parents who are poor provide family climates for their children that protect infants from the enduring effects of poverty and its associated risks on development.

ENVIRONMENTAL-LEVEL MECHANISMS

Poverty also affects young children via its impact on their immediate environment both directly through physical characteristics, such as increased risk of lead exposure and illnesses associated with crowded household conditions, for example, and indirectly through social characteristics, such as the chronic strain imposed on families by community disorganization and violence. Thus, such characteristics of the immediate environment operate both directly (via physical characteristics) and indirectly as moderators (via social characteristics) of the impact of risks (poverty and its correlates) on outcomes for very young children.

Physical Characteristics

Exposure to environmental lead and elevated blood lead levels has an impact on children of varying income levels but is most prevalent for low-income children, and in particular for those living in large urban centers. The National Center for Health Statistics (1998) has reported that children ages 1 to 5 years, living in low-income families, are more than seven times as likely to have elevated blood lead levels than those living in high-income families. However, as with the low-birthweight findings, this effect varies significantly by race/ethnicity with non-Hispanic black children having the highest blood lead levels (National Center for Health Statistics, 1998; "Update: Blood Levels," 1997).

Research indicates that even a relatively small or low level of exposure to lead in early childhood has a potential negative impact on both early brain development (Boivin & Giordani, 1995) and cognitive development (Tong, 1998) and is related to lower scores on the Emotional Regulation and Engagement/Orientation factors of the Behavior Rating Scale and the Destructive and Withdrawn subscales of the Child Behavior Checklist (Mendelsohn et al., 1998; Wasserman, Staghezza-Jaramillo, Shrout, Popovac, & Graziano, 1998). Furthermore, research has suggested that whereas exposure to lead is significantly related to such cognitive and behavioral problems, poverty places children at increased risk for both and thus may operate in a synergistic fashion, increasing the likelihood of exposure as well as exacerbating its negative impact.

Social Characteristics

In addition to the relationship between poverty and increased lead exposure in the environment, poor infants and children are more likely to be exposed to community and interpersonal violence than are nonpoor children (Aber, 1994; Garbarino, Dubrow, Kostelny, & Pardo, 1992; Korbin, Coulton, Chard, Platt-Houston, & Su, 1998; Pynoos & Nader, 1988). Building on Bronfenbrenner's (1979) seminal ecological theory of human development and drawing on the ecological/transactional framework proposed by Cicchetti and Lynch (1993; Lynch & Cicchetti, 1998), the impact of community disorganization and violence on infants and young children is viewed in terms of its impact on systems closer to the developing child (e.g., the caregiving system and immediate home environment). The impact of exposure to community violence and disorganization is, therefore, viewed as a moderator of the impact of risks on key mediating mechanisms, in particular parenting practices and subsequent child outcomes. The implication is not that infants and young children are not exposed directly to violence in their homes and communities (the incidence of pediatric homicides tripled between 1985 and 1992, a stark example described in Cristoffel, 1997, and more than 1 million children in the United States today are victims of child abuse and neglect) but, instead, that the ongoing experience of exposure to violence is processed through increased stress and strain placed on caregivers and the home environment.

Zeanah and Scheeringa (1997) described two major impacts of exposure to community violence on aspects of infant development: high levels of posttraumatic stress symptoms (e.g., reexperiencing the traumatic event, hyperarousal, and numbing of responsiveness) and serious disturbances of attachment. For example, infant exposure to partner violence in impoverished families has been linked to the development of disorganized/disoriented attachment behavior (Zeanah et al., 1999), perhaps due to frightened or frightening behavior of caregivers (Main & Hesse, 1990). These and other results support the notion that exposure to community violence does affect young children primarily by negatively influencing the emo-

tional availability and sensitivity of parents (Osofsky, 1995).

Furthermore, although relatively little research addresses the direct impact of exposure to community violence on *infant* development, considerable recent attention has been paid to the impact of neighborhood-level indicators of disorganization and violence on family processes and later child development, particularly adolescent development (see, e.g., Aber, 1994; Brooks-Gunn et al., 1997; Duncan et al., 1994; Klebanov et al., 1998; Lynch & Cicchetti, 1998; Coulton et al., 1995).

Other Contextual Characteristics

Major welfare-to-work policy and other large-scale social experiments indirectly affect the development of infants and young children via their impact on the economic security and support networks of families, as well as on the psychological well-being of participating mothers. Recent results from several large-scale social experiments have revealed that participation in a welfare-to-work program could have negative consequences for young children via increased parental stress and depression (Moore, Zaslow, Coiro, Miller, & Magenheim, 1995; Zaslow & Emig, 1997; Granger & Cytron, 1997) or participation in poor-quality child care (National Institute of Child Health and Human Development Early Child Care Research Network, 1997). In contrast, results from some evaluations indicate positive, however inconsistent, findings for parenting behavior (Zaslow, Tout, Botsko, & Moore, 1998). While the results of many of these experiments continue to filter in, poor families with young children face additional challenges as the "zeitgeist" surrounding welfare and family support changes from the "war on poverty" and the Family Support Act to "welfare to work" and the Personal Responsibility and Work Opportunity and Reconciliation Act of 1996. Poor mothers and their young children will increasingly face increased stress and upheaval associated with moving to work and finding adequate child care, both of which have clear consequences for the healthy development of very young children.

RESEARCH IMPLICATIONS

As this selective review documents, much progress has been made over the last decade in nonexperimental studies of the impact of poverty on the mental health and development of very young children. Several interrelated factors account for most of this progress. Studies have moved beyond cross-sectional, between-group differences designs (in which developmental outcomes for poor and nonpoor young children are measured and differences are attributed to poverty) to longitudinal, within-group differences designs that attempt to analytically identify the mechanisms by which poverty affects infant mental health and development. This has required conceptualizing and measuring the right mechanisms (e.g., maternal depression, insensitive parenting) and measuring and controlling for poverty cofactors (such as parental marital status, education, and employment status). In addition, the embedded nature of early child development in which infants and toddlers are viewed as developing within a nested set of interacting contexts means that poverty can exist on several levels (e.g., family and community) and have effects via processes on several levels (e.g., personal, familial, neighborhood, societal). All these changes in research design have led to a more dynamic, nuanced understanding of the effects of poverty on development.

But controversies about the proper interpretation of current "facts" and major gaps in knowledge both remain. For example, thoughtful scholars like Susan Mayer on the one hand (Mayer, 1997) and Greg Duncan and Jeanne Brooks-Gunn on the other (Duncan & Brooks-Gunn, 1997) come to significantly different interpretations of the extant research on the causal impact of income poverty per se on child development. Mayer believes that prior estimates of the impact of income poverty on child development derived from nonexperimental studies were inflated because of selection bias. She reasons that parents who are income poor are poor on other "unobserved" dimensions that are important to child development as well, such as moral development, future planning, and impulse control. She argues that unless studies account for those processes by which parents "select into" poverty, then they are really assessing the combined effects of poverty and unidentified cofactors on child development. When Mayer (1997) conducts a series of ingenious exercises to try to better account for selection bias, she does indeed reduce the estimated size of the impact of poverty on development. (But she rarely reduces the impact to zero. Income poverty does appear to have some effects.) Duncan and Brooks-Gunn share Mayer's concern to control for selection bias, but they believe that other features of nonexperimental research practice have served to inappropriately deflate estimates of the impact of income poverty on child development.

These debates will continue to be fought in research for some time to come. Better measures of important characteristics of poor parents and better ways to account for selection bias will lead to a new understanding of why the infants of poor parents face such challenges to their mental health and development.

Because of the limits of nonexperimental designs in supporting strong conclusions about causal factors, there will also continue to be the need for experimental studies to complement nonexperimental studies. Experimental studies are dependent in part on nonexperimental studies to identify potential targets of intervention, which could be subjected to evaluation by a randomized experiment. Several major social experiments such as the New Chance demonstration, the Teen Parent demonstration, and New Hope have relied on theory and measures developed from nonexperimental research to help design true experiments. And the two-year results from the New Hope experiment offer the clearest rebuttal to Mayer's claim that income poverty is not as important as we thought. Results suggest that wage supplements and/or a guaranteed public service job, plus health care and child care benefits can reduce family welfare dependence, increase parents' earnings and income, and enhance children's social development and academic achievement. An experiment carefully designed to reduce poverty improved parenting characteristics and child development (Duncan, McLoyd, & Granger, 1999). There are numerous other experimental and quasi-experimental evaluations of welfare reform and other social experiments in the field today that will drastically improve our understanding of the causal impact of poverty on infant and child mental health and development over the next decade. Summaries of most of these studies are available on a website run by the National Center for Children in Poverty (*www.researchforum.org*).

PROGRAM AND POLICY IMPLICATIONS

We should not wait until the absolutely definitive research on the impact of poverty on infant mental health and development is completed before we draw on the extant research to inform program and policy efforts. Indeed, there has been a complex and vital dialectic between research and policy/practice in early development and early intervention for over 40 years here in the United States. What has the last decade's research on the impact of poverty on child mental health and development contributed to this dialectic and to the improvement of program and/or policy? We believe it has begun to show us the larger picture made of the many smaller pieces of the puzzle. At the risk of oversimplification, we outline in Figure 6.1 the three major lines of influence of poverty on infant health and development, which we described in more detail above. If the figure is an accurate depiction of part of what has been learned, it has several implications for program and policy. First, there is no single causal process by which poverty effects child development. Indeed, this may be the reason both for the power of its effect and the relative difficulty of protecting children from the negative effects of poverty. Second, each of the mediating processes are potential targets for secondary prevention/early intervention (and, indeed, each have been targeted by an array of early intervention efforts; see Shonkoff & Meisels, 2000). For some of the targets, we already have effective program models (e.g., provision of high-quality early learning experiences); but for other targets, we are still searching for adequately effective program models (e.g., how can we powerfully reduce parental stress or improve parental sensitivity of care?). And while the field has assumed that comprehensive approaches aimed at multiple targets are more effective intervention strategies than more focused intervention approaches, the recent evaluations of programs like Comprehensive Child Development Program (CCDP) (St. Pierre, Layzer, & Barnes, 1995) and New Chance (Quint, Polit, Bos, & Cave, 1994) do not support this assumption. When one compares the results of programs that combined family support with early education back in the 1970s and 1980s (Yoshikawa, 1995) to the results of more recent efforts like CCDP and New Chance, we are left to wonder whether in our efforts to be more comprehensive, we have watered down the quality or intensity of individual program components. If so, then the next decade should be devoted to devising and testing more strategically targeted interventions that try to do a few key things targeted on key processes very well. These are some of the program implications we draw from the new research that has emerged over the last decade.

We turn now to policy implications. First, we will note that even for program models with considerable evidence of effectiveness and public support (e.g., Head Start), our nation is still not investing adequately to serve all eligible children. So one major issue is how to develop the political will needed to act on the emerging research base and invest in programs that work.

No doubt the biggest policy challenge is the reduction of child poverty itself. Over one-fifth of the country's young children live in families with incomes below the poverty line. This is a moral scandal in one of the most prosperous nations in the world. Other Western industrial-

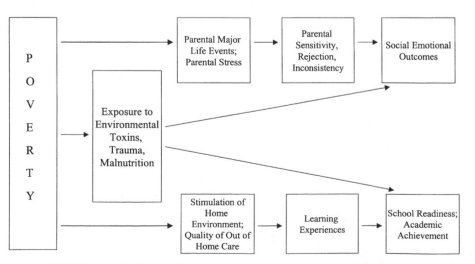

FIGURE 6.1. Influence of poverty on infant mental health and development.

ized democracies have achieved lower young child poverty rates through a variety of efforts that support low-wage work (child care, health care) and that provide families with a child allowance that recognizes the families' contribution to the nation by raising the next generation. These policies are responsible for child poverty rates that are between one eighth and one half of our country's rate.

While robust economic growth over the 1990s and an expansion of the Earned Income Tax Credit have combined to reduce child poverty somewhat in recent years, we can and must do more as a nation. Without public and private sector commitment to reducing child poverty, the enormous impact of poverty on infant mental health and development cannot be reversed.

REFERENCES

Abel, E. L. (1985). *Fetal alcohol exposure and effects.* Westport, CT: Greenwood Press.

Abel, E. L., & Skokol, R. J. (1987). Incidence of fetal alcohol syndrome and economic impact of FAS-related anomolies. *Drug and Alcohol Dependence, 19,* 51–70.

Aber, J. L. (1994). Poverty, violence, and child development: Untangling family and community level effects. In C. A. Nelson (Ed.), *Threats to optimal development: Integrating biological, psychological, and social risk factors* (pp. 229–272). Hillsdale, NJ: Erlbaum.

Aber, J. L. (1997). Measuring child poverty for use in comparative policy analysis. In A. Ben-Arieh & H. Wintersberger (Eds.), *Monitoring and measuring the state of children: Beyond survival* (pp. 193–208). Vienna: European Centre for Social Welfare Policy and Research.

Aber, J. L., Bennett, N. G., Conley, D. C., & Li, J. (1997). The effects of poverty on child health and development. *Annual Review of Public Health, 18,* 463–483.

Alpern, L., & Lyons-Ruth, K. (1993). Preschool children at social risk: Chronicity and timing of maternal depressive symptoms and child behavior problems at school and at home. *Development and Psychopathology, 5*(3), 371–387.

Bearer, C. F. (1995). Environmental health hazards: How children are different from adults. *Future of Children, 5*(2), 11–26.

Bendersky, M., & Lewis, M. (1994). Environmental risk, biological risk, and developmental outcome. *Developmental Psychology, 30*(4), 484–494.

Benes, F. M. (1994). Developmental changes in stress adaptation in relation to psychopathology. *Development and Psychopathology, 6*(4), 723–739.

Bird, S. T. (1995). Separate black and white infant mortality models: Differences in the importance of structural variables. *Social Science Medicine, 41*(11), 1507–1512.

Boivin, M., & Giordani, B. (1995). A risk evaluation of the neuropsychological effects of childhood lead toxicity. *Developmental Neuropsychology, 11*(2), 157–180.

Bradley, R. H., Caldwell, B. M., Rock, S. L., Ramey, C. T., Barnard, K. E., Gary, C., Hammond, M. A., Mitchell, S., Gottfried, A. W., Siegel, L., & Johnson, D. L. (1989). Home environment and cognitive development in the first three years of life: A collaborative study including six sites and three ethnic groups in North America. *Developmental Psychology, 25,* 217–235.

Bradley, R. H., Whiteside, L., Mundfrom, D. J., Casey, P. H., Kelleher, K. J., & Pope, S. K. (1994). Early indications of resilience and their relation to experiences in the home environments of low birth weight, premature children living in poverty. *Child Development, 65,* 880–888.

Brofenbrenner, U. (1979). *The ecology of human development: Experiments by nature and design.* Cambridge, MA: Harvard University Press.

Brooks-Gunn, J., Duncan, G. J., & Aber, J. L. (Eds.). (1997). *Neighborhood poverty: Context and consequences for children* (Vols. 1, 2). New York: Russell Sage.

Brooks-Gunn, J. B., Klebanov, P. K., & Liaw, F. (1995). The learning, physical, and emotional environment of the home in the context of poverty: The infant health and development program. *Children and Youth Services Review, 17*(1/2), 251–276.

Brooks-Gunn, J., Duncan, G. J., Klebanov, P. K., & Sealand, N. (1993). Do neighborhoods influence child development and adolescent development? *American Journal of Sociology, 99,* 353–395.

Brown, J. L., & Pollitt, E. (1996, February). Malnutrition, poverty and intellectual development. *Scientific American,* pp. 38–43.

Burchinal, M., Lee, M., & Ramey, C. T. (1989). Type of day-care and preschool intellectual development in disadvantaged children. *Child Development, 60*(1), 128–137.

Caldwell, B. M., & Bradley, R. H. (1984). *Home Observation for Measurement of the Environment.* Little Rock: University of Arkansas at Little Rock.

Cicchetti, D., & Aber, J. L. (Eds.). (1998). Contextualism and developmental psychopathology. *Development and Psychopathology, 10*(2), 137–141.

Cicchetti, D., & Lynch, M. (1993). Toward an ecological/transactional model of community violence and child maltreatment: Consequences for children's development. *Psychiatry, 56*(2), 96–118.

Cicchetti, D., Rogosch, F. A., & Toth, S. L. (1998). Maternal depressive disorder and contextual risk: Contributions to the development of attachment insecurity and behavior problems in toddlerhood. *Development and Psychopathology, 10,* 283–300.

Cicchetti, D., & Toth, S. L. (1995). Child maltreatment and attachment organization: Implications for intervention. In S. Goldberg, R. Muir, & J. Kerr (Eds.), *Attachment theory: Social developmental and clinical perspectives* (pp. 279–308). Hillsdale, NJ: Analytic Press.

Citro, C. F., & Michael, R. T. (Eds.). (1995). *Measuring poverty: A new approach.* Washington, DC: National Academy Press.

Cost, Quality, & Child Outcomes Study Team. (1995). *Cost, quality, and child outcomes in child care centers.* Denver: Department of Economics, University of Colorado at Denver.

Coulton, C., Korbin, J., Su, M., & Chow, J. (1995). Community level factors and child maltreatment rates. *Child Development, 66,* 1262–1276.

Cristoffel, K. K. (1997). Firearm injuries affecting U. S. children and adolescents. In J. D. Osofsky (Ed.), *Children in a violent society* (pp. 42–71). New York: Guilford Press.

Crittenden, P. M., & Ainsworth, M. D. S. (1989). Child maltreatment and attachment theory. In D. Cicchetti & V. Carlson (Eds.), *Child maltreatment: Theory and research on the causes and consequences of child abuse and neglect* (pp. 432–463). New York: Cambridge University Press.

Dawson, G., & Fischer, K. W. (Eds.). (1994). *Human behavior and the developing brain.* New York: Guilford Press.

Dawson, G., Klinger, L. G., Panagiotides, H., Spieker, S., & Frey, K. (1992). Infants of mothers with depressive symptoms: Electroencephalographic and behavioral findings related to attachment status. *Development and Psychopathology, 4*(1), 67–80.

Dowling, P. T., & Fischer, M. (1987). Maternal factors and low birthweight infants: A comparison of blacks with Mexican-Americans. *Journal of Family Practice, 25*(2), 153–158.

Drucker, E., Alcabes, P., Bosworth, W., & Sckell, B. (1994). Childhood tuberculosis in the Bronx, New York. *Lancet, 345*(8911), 1482–1485.

Duncan, G. J., & Brooks-Gunn, J. (Eds.). (1997). *Consequences of growing up poor.* New York: Russell Sage Foundation.

Duncan, G. J., Brooks-Gunn, J., & Klebanov, P. K. (1994). Economic deprivation and early childhood development. *Child Development, 65,* 296–318.

Duncan, G. J., McLoyd, V. C., & Granger, R. C. (1999, April). *New Hope impacts on families and children.* Paper presented at the Biennial Meeting of the Society for Research in Child Development, Albuquerque, NM.

Early childhood development and learning: What new research on the brain tells us about our youngest children. (1997, April 17). White House Conference, Washington, DC.

Escalona, S. (1982). Babies at double hazard: Early development of infants at biologic and social risk. *Pediatrics, 70*(5), 670–676.

Ford, D. H., & Lerner, R. M. (1992). *Developmental systems theory: An integrative approach.* Newbury Park, CA: Sage.

Garbarino, J., Dubrow, N., Kostelny, K., & Pardo, C. (1992). *Children in danger: Coping with the consequences of community violence.* San Francisco: Jossey-Bass.

Gortmaker, S. L. (1979). Poverty and infant mortality in the United States. *American Society Review, 44,* 280–297.

Gottlieb, D. J., Beiser, A. S., & O'Connor, G. T. (1995). Poverty, race, and medication use are correlates of asthma hospitalization rates: A small area analysis in Boston. *Chest, 108*(1), 28–35.

Granger, R. C., & Cytron, R. (1997, November 7). *A synthesis of the long-term effects of the New Chance Demonstration, Ohio's Learning, Earning, and Parenting (LEAP) Program and the Teenage Parent Demonstration.* Paper presented at the annual meeting of the Association for Public Policy Analysis and Management; Washington, DC.

Greenough, W. T., Black, J. E., & Wallace, C. S. (1987). Experience and brain development. *Child Development, 58,* 539–559.

Gunnar, M. R., & Barr, R. G. (1998). Stress, early brain development, and behavior. *Infants and Young Children, 1*(1), 1–14.

Gunnar, M. R., Tout, K., deHaan, M., Pierce, S., & Stansbury, K. (1997). Temperament, social competence, and adrenocortical activity in preschoolers. *Developmental Psychology, 31*(1), 65–85.

Halfon, N., & Newacheck, P. W. (1993). Childhood asthma and poverty: Differential impacts and utilization of health services. *Pediatrics, 91*(1), 56–61.

Halpern, R. (1993). Poverty and infant development. In C. H. Zeanah, Jr. (Ed.), *Handbook of infant mental health* (pp. 73–86). New York: Guilford Press.

Hashima, P. Y., & Amato, P. R. (1994). Poverty, social support and parental behavior. *Child Development, 65*(2), 394–403.

Hofkosh, D., Pringle, J. L., Wald, H. P., Switala, J., Hinderliter, S. A., & Hamel, S. C. (1995). Early interactions between drug involved mothers and infants: Within-group differences. *Archives of Pediatric and Adolescent Medicine, 149*(6), 665–672.

Hughes, D., & Simpson, L. (1995). The role of social change in preventing low birthweight. *Future of Children, 5*(1), 87–120.

Huston, A. (Ed.). (1991). *Children in poverty: Child development and public policy.* New York: Cambridge University Press.

Huttenlocher, P. R. (1994). Synaptogenesis, synapse elimination, and neural plasticity in human cerebral cortex. In C. A. Nelson (Ed.), *Threats to optimal development: Integrating biological, psychological, and social risk factors* (Vol. 27, pp. 35–54). Hillsdale, NJ: Erlbaum.

Infant Health and Development Program. (1990). Enhancing the outcomes of low-birth-weight, premature infants. *Journal of the American Medical Association, 263,* 3035–3042.

Kaufman, J., Birmaher, B., Perel, J., Dahl, R. E., Moreci, P., Nelson, B., Wells, W., & Ryan, N. D. (1997). The corticotropin-releasing hormone challenge in depressed abused, depressed nonabused, and normal control children. *Biological Psychiatry, 42,* 669–697.

Kemperman, G., Kuhn, H. G., & Gage, F. H. (1997). More hippocampal neurons in adult mice living in an enriched environment. *Nature, 386,* 493–495.

Klebanov, P. K., Brooks-Gunn, J., McCarton, C., & McCormick, M. (1998). The contribution of neighborhood and family income to developmental test scores over the first three years of life. *Child Development, 69*(5), 1420–1436.

Klerman, L. V. (1991). The health of poor children. In A. Huston (Ed.), *Children in poverty: Child development and public policy* (pp. 137–157). New York: Cambridge University Press.

Klerman, L. V., & Parker, M. (1991). *Alive and well? A research and policy review of health programs for poor young children.* New York: National Center for Children in Poverty, Joseph L. Mailman School of Public Health, Columbia University.

Kopp, C. B., & Kaler, S. (1989). Risk in infancy: Origins and implications [Special issue]. *American Psychologist, 44*(2), 224–230.

Korbin, J. E., Coulton, C. L., Chard, S., Platt-Houston, C., & Su, M. (1998). Impoverishment and child maltreatment in African American and European American neighborhoods. *Development and Psychopathology, 10,*(2), 215–233.

Landrigan, P. J., Carlson, J. E., Bearer, C. F., Cranmer, J. S., Bullard, R. D., Etzel, R. A., Groopman, J., McLachlan, J. A., Perera, F. P., Reigart, J. R., Robison, L., Schell, L., & Suk, W. A. (1998). Children's health and the environment: A new agenda for prevention research. *Environmental Health Perspectives, 106*(Suppl. 3), 787–794.

Lempers, J., Clark-Lempers, D., & Simons, R. (1989). Economic hardship, parenting, and distress in adolescence. *Child Development, 60*(1), 25–49.

Lynch, M., & Cicchetti, D. (1998). An ecological–transactional analysis of children and contexts: The longitudinal interplay among child maltreatment, community violence, and children's symptomatology. *Development and Psychopathology, 10*(2), 235–257.

Lyons-Ruth, K., Alpern, L., & Repacholi, B. (1993). Disorganized infant attachment classification and maternal psychosocial problems as predictors of hostile–aggressive behavior in the preschool classroom. *Child Development, 64*(2), 572–585.

Lyons-Ruth, K., Connell, D. B., Grunebaum, H. U., & Botein, S. (1990). Infants at social risk: Maternal depression and family support services as mediators of infant development and security of attachment. *Child Development, 61*(1) 85–98.

Lyons-Ruth, K., Easterbrooks, M. A., & Cibelli, C. D. (1997). Infant attachment strategies, infant mental lag, and maternal depressive symptoms: Predictors of internalizing and externalizing problems at age 7. *Developmental Psychology, 33*(4), 681–692.

Lyons-Ruth, K., Repacholi, B., McLeod, S., & Silva, E. (1991). Disorganized attachment behavior in infancy: Short-term stability, maternal and infant correlates and risk-related subtypes. *Development and Psychopathology, 3*(4), 377–398.

MacDorman, M. F., & Atkinson, J. O. (1998). Infant mortality statistics from the period linked birth/infant death data set. *Monthly Vital Statistics Report, 42*(Suppl. 12).

Main, M., & Hesse, E. (1990). Adult lack of resolution of attachment-related trauma related to infant disorganized–disoriented behavior in the Ainsworth Strange Situation: Linking parental states of mind to infant behavior in a stressful situation. In M. T. Greenberg, D. Cicchetti, & M. Cummings (Eds.), *Attachment in the preschool years: Theory, research and intevention* (pp. 339–426). Chicago: University of Chicago Press.

Malveaux, F. J., & Fletcher-Vincent, S. A. (1995). Environmental risk factors of childhood asthma in urban centers. *Environmental Health Persceptives, 103*(6), 59–62.

Margolis, P. A., Greenberg, R. A., Keyes, L. L., LaVange, L. M., Chapman, R. S., Denny, F. W., Bauman, K. E., & Boat, B. W. (1992). Lower respiratory illness in infants and low socio-economic status. *American Journal of Public Health, 82*(8), 1119–1126.

Mayer, S. E. (1997). *What money can't buy: Family income and children's life chances.* Cambridge, MA: Harvard University Press.

Mayes, L. (1996, June 13–14). *Early experience and the developing brain: The model of prenatal cocaine exposure.* Paper presented at the invitational conference, Brain Development in Young Children: New Frontiers for Research, Policy and Practice, University of Chicago.

McLeod, J. D., & Shanahan, M. (1993). Poverty, parenting and children's mental health. *American Sociologic Review, 58*(3), 351–366.

McLoyd, V. C. (1990). The impact of economic hardship on black families and children: Psychological distress, parenting, and socioemotional development. *Child Development, 61*(2), 311–346.

McLoyd, V. (1998). Socioeconomic disadvantage and child development. *American Psychologist, 53*(2), 185–204.

Mendelsohn, A. L., Dreyer, B. P., Fierman, A. H., Rosen, C. M., Legano, L. A., Kruger, H. A., Lim, S. W., & Courtland, C. D. (1998). Law-level lead exposure and behavior in early childhood. *Pediatrics, 101*(3), 101–107.

Moore, K. A., Zaslow, M. J., Coiro, M. J., Miller, S. M., & Magenheim, E. B. (1995). *The JOBS evaluation: How well are they faring? AFDC families with preschool-aged children in Atlanta at the outset of the JOBS evaluation.* Washington, DC: Department of Health and Human Services, Office of the Assistant Secretary for Planning and Evaluation.

Nachmias, M., Gunnar, M., Mangelsdorf, S., & Parritz, R. (1996). Behavioral inhibition and stress reactivity: Moderating role of attachment security. *Child Development, 67*, 508–522.

National Center for Children in Poverty. (1997). *Poverty and brain development in early childhood.* New York: Author.

National Center for Health Statistics. (1998). *Health, United States, 1998 with socioeconomic status and health chartbook.* Hyattsville, MD: Author.

National Institute of Child Health and Human Development Early Child Care Research Network. (1997). The effects of infant child care on infant–mother attachment security: Results of the NICHHD Study of Early Child Care. *Child Development, 68*, 860–879.

Osofsky, J. D. (1995). The effects of violence exposure on young children. *American Psychologist, 50*, 782–788.

Paneth, N. S. (1995). The problem of low birthweight. *Future of Children, 5*(1), 19–34.

Parker, S., Greer, S., & Zuckerman, B. (1988). Double jeopardy: The impact of poverty on early child development. *Pediatric Clinics of North America, 35*, 1227–1239.

Perry, B. D. (1997). Incubated in terror: Neurodevelopmental factors in the "cycle of violence." In J. D. Osofsky (Ed.), *Children in a violent society* (pp. 124–149). New York: Guilford Press.

Pianta, R. C., & Egeland, B. (1990). Life stress and parenting outcomes in a disadvantaged sample: Results of the mother-child interaction project. *Journal of Clinical Child Psychology, 19*(4), 329–336.

Pollitt, E. (1994). Poverty and child development: Relevance of research in developing countries to the United States. *Child Development, 65*, 283–295.

Pynoos, R., & Nader, K. (1988). Psychological first aid and treatment approach to children exposed to community violence: Research implications. *Journal of Traumatic Stress, 1*(4), 445–473.

Quint, J., Polit, D., Bos, H., & Cave, G. (1994). *New Chance: Interim findings on a comprehensive program for disadvantaged young mothers and their children.* New York: Manpower Demonstration Research Corporation.

Rainwater, L., & Smeeding. T. M. (1995). U. S. doing poorly compared to others. *News and Issues, 5*(3), 4–5.

The Random House Dictionary of the English Language. (1967). New York: Author.

Reinhard, C., Paul, W. S., & McAuley, J. B. (1997). Epidemiology of pediatric tuberculosis in Chicago, 1974 to 1994: A continuing public health problem. *American Journal of Medical Sciences, 313*(6), 336–340.

Roberts, E. M. (1997). Neighborhood social environments and the distribution of low birthweight in Chicago. *American Journal of Public Health, 87*, 4, 597–603.

Rosenstreich, D.L., Eggleston, P., Kattan, M., Baker, D., Slavin, R. G., Gergen, P., Mitchell, H., McNiff-Mortimer, K., Lynn, H., Ownby, D., & Malveaux, F. (1997). The role of cockroach allergy and exposure to cockroach allergen in causing morbidity among inner city children with asthma. *New England Journal of Medicine, 336*, 1356–1362.

Sameroff, A. J. (1983). Developmental systems: Contexts and evolution. In W. Kessen (Ed.), P. H. Mussen (Series Ed.), *Handbook of child psychology: Vol. 1. History, theories and methods* (pp. 237–294). New York: Wiley.

Shaw, D. S., & Vondra, J. I. (1995). Infant attachment security and maternal predictors of early behavior problems: A longitudinal study of low-income families. *Journal of Abnormal Child Psychology, 23*, 335–357.

Shiono, P. H., & Behrman, R. E. (1995). Low birthweight: Analysis and recommendations. *Future of Children, 5*(1), 4–18.

Shiono, P. H., Rauh, V. A., Park, M., Lederman, S. A., & Zuskar, D. (1997). Ethnic differences in birthweight: The role of lifestyle and other factors. *American Journal of Public Health, 87*(5), 787–793.

Shirk, M., Bennett, N., & Aber, J. L. (1999). *Living on the line: American families and the struggle to make ends meet.* New York: Westview Press.

Shonkoff, J. P., & Meisels, S. J. (Eds.) (2000). *Handbook of early childhood intervention* (2nd ed.). New York: Cambridge University Press.

Shore, R. (1997). *Rethinking the brain: New insights into early development.* New York: Families and Work Institute.

Solan, H. A., & Mozlin, R. (1997). Biosocial consequences of poverty: Associated visual problems. *Optometry and Visual Science, 74*(4), 185–189.

Spangler, G., & Grossmann, K. E. (1993). Biobehavioral organization in securely and insecurely attached infants. *Child Development, 64*, 1439–1450.

Starfield, B., Shapiro, S., Weiss, J., Liang, K. Y., Ra, K., Paige, D., & Wang, X. B. (1991). Race, family income, and low birth weight. *American Journal of Epidemiology, 134*, 1167–1174.

St. Pierre, R. G., Layzer, J. I., & Barnes, H. V. (1995). Two-generation programs: Design, cost, and short-term effectiveness. *Future of Children, 5*(3), 76–93.

Tong, S. (1998). Lead exposure and cognitive development: Persistence and a dynamic pattern. *Journal of Pediatrics and Child Health, 34*(2), 114–118.

Update: Blood lead levels—United States 1991–1994. (1997). *Morbidity and Mortality Weekly Report, 46*(7), 141–146.

Wasserman, C. R., Shaw, G. M., Selvin, S., Gould, J., & Syme, S. L. (1998). Socioeconomic status, neighborhood social conditions, and neural tube defects. *American Journal of Public Health, 88*(11), 1674–1680.

Wasserman, G. A., Staghezza-Jarmillo, B., Shrout, P., Popovac, D., & Graziano, J. (1998). The effect of lead exposure on behavior problems in preschool children. *American Journal of Public Health, 88*(3), 481–486.

Watson, J. E., Kirby, R. S., Kelleher, K. J., & Bradley, R. H. (1996). Effects of poverty on home environment: an analysis of three-year outcome data for low birth weight premature infants. *Journal of Pediatric Psychology, 21*(3), 419–431.

Weissman, M. M., Warner, V., Wickramaratne, P., Moreau, D., & Olfson, M. (1997). Offspring of depressed parents: 10 years later. *Archives of General Psychiatry, 54*(10), 932–940.

Werner, E. E. (1989). High risk children in young adulthood: A longitudinal study from birth to 32 years. *American Journal of Orthopsychiatry, 59*(1), 72–81.

Wiesel, T. (1982). Postnatal development of the visual cortex and the influence of environment. *Nature, 299*, 583–591.

Yoshikawa, H. (1995). Long-term effects of early childhood programs on social outcomes and delinquency. *Future of Children, 5*(3), 51–75.

Zaslow, M., & Emig, C. A. (1997). When low-income mothers go to work: Implications for children. *Future of Children, 7*(1), 110–115.

Zaslow, M., Tout, K., Botsko, C., & Moore K. (1998). *Welfare reform and children: Potential implications* (New federalism: Issues and options for states, No. 23). Washington, DC: The Urban Institute.

Zeanah, C. H., Boris, N. W., & Larrieu, J. A. (1997). Infant development and developmental risk: A review of the past 10 years. *Journal of the American Academy of Child and Adolescent Psychiatry, 36*(2), 165–178.

Zeanah, C. H., Danis, B., Hirshberg, L., Benoit, D., Miller, D., & Heller, S. S. (1999). Disorganized attachment associated with partner violence: A research note. *Infant Mental Health Journal, 20*, 77–86.

Zeanah, C. H., & Scheeringa, M. S. (1997). The experience and effects of violence in infancy. In J. D. Osofsky (Ed.), *Children in a violent society* (pp. 97–123). New York: Guilford Press.

7

Early Parenthood in Context: Implications for Development and Intervention

❖

LAUREN S. WAKSCHLAG
SYDNEY L. HANS

An early transition to parenthood has long been viewed as a social problem that poses risks for both young mothers and their offspring. The United States has the highest teenage birth rate of any Western industrialized nation (61 births each year for every 1,000 females ages 15–19), with more than 500,000 children born to mothers under age 20 annually (McElroy & Moore, 1997). Early childbearing often interferes with young mothers' educational attainment and economic self sufficiency and is associated with difficulties in parenting and poor developmental outcomes for offspring. Compared to older mothers, younger mothers have been shown to be less responsive to their children, to engage in harsher discipline, and to be more depressed (Smith & Brooks-Gunn, 1997; Zeanah, Boris, & Larrieu, 1997). In contrast to the children of older mothers, the children of adolescent mothers are more likely to have pre- and perinatal difficulties, to exhibit developmental and behavioral problems during early childhood and beyond, and to become teenage parents themselves (Furstenberg, Brooks-Gunn, & Morgan, 1987; Shapiro & Mangelsdorf, 1994).

Although it is well established that adolescent parenthood presents substantial risk for the teenagers themselves and their offspring (see Brooks-Gunn & Furstenberg, 1986; Coley &

Chase-Lansdale, 1998; Maynard, 1997; Osofsky, Hann, & Peebles, 1993, for reviews), early parenthood is often embedded in a broader context of risk including poverty, single parenthood, low educational attainment, and engagement in other risky behaviors, making it difficult to disentangle unique effects of maternal age per se. In fact, the social ecology of parenting for adolescent mothers is quite similar to the social context of young adult mothers living in disadvantaged circumstances (Chase-Lansdale, Brooks-Gunn, & Zamsky, 1994; Geronimus, 1991). It is also clear that, even though problematic outcomes are associated with early parenthood, there is considerable variability in the developmental pathways of adolescent mothers and their children (Furstenberg et al., 1987). Relatively little is known about processes which may explain such individual differences in outcome (Shapiro & Mangelsdorf, 1994). Individual differences may be a function of social and individual conditions that lead up to the adolescent pregnancy, social and developmental processes that serve a protective function once the child is born, or the interaction of these and other factors. Clearly, adolescent mothers are not a homogeneous group; in fact, there may be qualitatively different subgroups of young mothers. For example, for some young women early sexual activity and pregnancy may reflect the mothers' engagement in a broader group of risky behaviors (Ketterlinus, Lamb, & Nitz, 1994). In contrast, for other adolescents, early childbearing may represent an adaptive strategy within a context of limited opportunities (Burton, 1990).

This chapter examines within-group variation in adolescent mothers' parenting and in factors affecting the development of their children during the early years of life. We take an individual-differences approach to shed light on protective processes that help some young mothers make a successful adaptation to parenting and risk factors that interfere with this adaptation for others (for comparative findings, see the reviews cited previously). Reflecting current theory and research we place particular emphasis on the social context of adolescent parenting and the role that family relationship processes play in supporting competent parenting and child development. The "effect of relationships on relationships" (Emde, 1991) is a central tenet of the infant mental health perspective and is well illustrated in the literature on early parenthood. Developmental, sociodemographic, and mental health factors are also examined as contributors to the diversity of developmental pathways taken by young mothers and their children. Finally, implications for future research and intervention are discussed.

SOCIAL CONTEXT OF ADOLESCENT PARENTHOOD

Young mothers face numerous challenges and changes in their social role and relationships. They are learning to accept the responsibilities of motherhood at the same time that their own mothers and their partners are learning the interrelated roles of grandmotherhood and fatherhood, often as "off-time" events. They must redefine their sense of themselves in relation to their infants during a developmental period in which they also have to redefine their relationships with their families of origin and their male partners. They are expected to shoulder the independent responsibilities of motherhood at the same time they find themselves with an increased dependence on others' assistance. Understanding how young mothers and their families negotiate these challenges is critical for understanding individual differences in outcome for young mothers and their children

(Wakschlag, Chase-Lansdale, & Brooks-Gunn, 1996).

Factors in the social environment may affect infant developmental outcomes both directly (e.g., grandmother serves as an additional source of affection and stimulation for the infant) and indirectly (e.g., partner support enhances maternal sense of well-being, which in turn increases her emotional availability to her infant). Studying such processes in the families of young mothers is complex and involves recognition of varied family structures and household compositions, the prominent role that nonresidential family may play in child rearing, the level of harmony and conflict present in family relationships, and the extent to which residential patterns and family processes mutually influence each other (Rhodes, Ebert, & Fischer, 1992; Wilson & Tolson, 1988). In addition, family processes do not necessarily have uniformly positive or negative effects on outcome: protective factors for the mother may serve as risk factors for her child and vice versa. For example, high levels of grandmother involvement in child care have been associated with both higher grade completion by teen mothers *and* child behavior problems (Unger & Cooley, 1992). The effect of family processes on adaptation in young-mother families may also vary as a function of ethnicity and social class. (Although a comprehensive review of this important issue is not possible here, see, for example, Field, Widmayer, Adler, & De Cubas, 1990; Luster & Mittelstaedt, 1993.)

Multigenerational Family Relationships

Limited economic resources require most young mothers to live in households with members of their family of origin or with a male partner. Although in the past young American mothers often were married and living in households with their husbands, increasingly teenage mothers do not marry and continue to live with extended family members, particularly their own mothers, after their infants are born (Coley & Chase-Lansdale, 1998; Taylor, Chatters, & Jackson, 1993). According to the 1990 U.S. census, 58% of mothers under the age of 18 receiving public aid lived with their parents, 18% lived alone with their children, 12% lived with their husbands, and 12% lived with other adults (including male partners other than husbands). A larger percentage of 18- and

19-year-old mothers (46%) lived alone with their children (Sonenstein & Gregory, 1995). Recent federal welfare reform legislation mandating that minor mothers must live with a parent or guardian and stay in school will further increase the proportion of poor mothers under the age of 18 who live with their families (Child Welfare League of America, 1996).

The birth of a child involves significant adjustment and acceptance of many new demands. (Michaels & Goldberg, 1988). For adolescent mothers, the birth of an infant may be particularly disruptive because it is an "off-time," usually unplanned event that may completely alter the young mother's expectations for her future. In addition, parenting responsibilities are generally incompatible with the culturally normative adolescent activities of attending school and engaging in an active social life with peers. Young mothers, when confronted by the heavy demands of parenthood, often struggle with their loss of freedom and opportunity to engage in normal adolescent activities.

Adolescent parenthood is also a "counter-transition" (i.e., a life transition caused by someone else's life event) for grandmothers (Burton & Bengston, 1985). Grandmothers often share caregiving burdens, disrupting their own life plans and expectations. Mothers of teen parents are often relatively young women themselves who may still have young children at home or who may be anticipating a stage of life, after having raised their children, during which they have greater freedom to pursue their own educational and career goals. As Burton and colleagues have noted, particular strains may occur in age-condensed families where both mother and grandmother entered parenthood at an early age (Obeidallah & Burton, 1998).

At the same time that the new infant's needs must be addressed, young mothers continue to have their own developmental needs. Viewed from a developmental perspective, one of the problematic aspects of adolescent motherhood is that it complicates the resolution of the central developmental task of adolescence, achieving a balance of individuality and connectedness within the context of the family of origin (Cooper, Grotevant, & Condon, 1983). Adolescent mothers must negotiate issues of autonomy at the same time that their dependence on their mothers for assistance with child rearing has increased. If grandmothers do not help with the care of grandchildren, teenage mothers may

not have the opportunity to complete normative tasks such as completing school and preparing for employment as well as developing new types of relationships with peers (Coley & Chase-Lansdale, 1998). In fact, considerable evidence suggests that adolescent mothers who live in multigenerational households are more likely to remain in school and graduate (Spieker & Bensley, 1994; Testa, 1992). On the other hand, if grandmothers are too active in the parenting role, this may interfere with young mothers becoming competent and confident as parents. The challenge for families is to find a balance between providing assistance and encouraging the young mother's autonomy and competence. Empirical evidence suggests that many families do find such a balance, enhancing the mothers' well-being and commitment to the parenting role. For example, when grandmothers both encourage independence and provide support, teen mothers are less likely to be depressed (Leadbeater & Linares, 1992) and are more likely to be primary caregivers of their children at age 6 (Apfel & Seitz, 1997).

The burdens involved in caring for a new baby, the strains involved in negotiating roles between grandmother and mothers, and the challenges of balancing the varied developmental needs of the mother are great and may lead to stress and conflict in families. Such strains are likely exacerbated by poverty where all resources are scarce and a new "mouth to feed" leads to further depletion of resources. Strains are also likely to be exacerbated by coresidence between young mothers and their families, particularly if coresidency continues beyond infancy (Burton, 1990; Chase-Lansdale et al., 1994; Unger & Cooley, 1992). Coresiding may create household crowding, require ongoing negotiation of household and child-care responsibilities and roles, and lead to competition for resources, all of which are likely to result in tension and conflict.

Partners of Adolescent Mothers

Despite considerable research and public policy attention to adolescent mothers, relatively little attention has been given to the fathers of their children. Perhaps surprisingly, it appears that only 20–40% of the partners of adolescent mothers are themselves adolescents (Landry & Forrest, 1995; Males & Chew, 1996). Recently warnings have been sounded that large age discrepancies between teen mothers and their partners sometimes indicate abuse of the young women (Boyer & Fine, 1992; Butler & Burton, 1990).

Most adolescent mothers in the United States do not marry the fathers of their infants, and the proportion of adolescents giving birth out of wedlock is increasing dramatically, from only 15% in 1955 to 76% in 1994 (McElroy & Moore, 1997). There are large cultural differences in rates of marriage for adolescent mothers. In 1994, 95% of births to African American adolescents were outside marriage, compared to two-thirds of births to white and Latina adolescents, respectively (McElroy & Moore, 1997). Even for those young couples who do marry, the divorce rate is many times higher than that for older couples. Marriage is only one demographic indicator of the level of commitment and involvement of a father to the mother of his child. Although nonmarital childbearing suggests a lack of paternal commitment, other indicators of paternal involvement paint a more complex picture. Young mothers and their partners typically know each other for a period of many months before the pregnancy (East & Felice, 1996; Barret & Robinson, 1986; Redmond, 1985). During pregnancy most young fathers express a desire to be involved in the birth and child rearing (Elster, 1988; Hendricks & Montgomery, 1983; Rivara, Sweeney, & Henderson, 1986). Data from the National Longitudinal Study of Youth indicate that paternal involvement is most intensive soon after the birth. For young unwed fathers, nearly half visited their children weekly and nearly one-quarter had daily contact after the birth (Lerman, 1993). However, by the time children were 7 years old, less than a quarter had even weekly contact. Other studies also show a dramatic decline in father involvement after birth. In a study of adolescent mothers receiving public assistance with children under the age of 2 (Danziger & Radin, 1990), 39% of mothers indicated that quality of the fathers' relationship with the child was poor, but 31% indicated that it was very good. Child's age was correlated with mothers' ratings of the fathers' relationship with the child—with mothers' ratings becoming more negative as the infants became older. In a racially diverse sample of adolescent mothers (East & Felice, 1996), relationships between unmarried teenage mothers and their partners deteriorated over time so that by 3 years postpartum the couples rarely saw one another. Quality of the relationship be-

tween the young father and mother is an important factor in determining the level of involvement between the young father and his child (Amato & Rezac, 1994; Furstenberg, 1995). When the relationship between the father and mother becomes distant or strained, the father's involvement with the infant diminishes.

Fathers' involvement with children is also closely related to employment issues. Young fathers who are working are more likely to maintain involvement with their children than those who are not able to contribute financially (Chase-Lansdale, Gordon, Coley, Wakschlag, & Brooks-Gunn, 1999; Danziger & Radin, 1990). Stresses surrounding their abilities to provide for their families are felt strongly by young fathers (Elster & Hendricks, 1986). Fathers who are unable to provide financially for their children experience role strain that may lead to disengagement from other aspects of the paternal role (Bowman, 1989). Similarly, young mothers, acting as gatekeepers between fathers and their children, may limit access to fathers who are not good providers (Ray & Hans, 1997).

Father participation must be considered within the broader family system that includes the mother's kin. For example, the role of the father as a support may be particularly important in family systems in which the young mother's relations to her own kin are strained (Crockenberg, 1987a). In addition, because most young mothers remain unwed and need to rely heavily on their families for support, the role played by the father may depend on the mother's family of origin (Furstenberg, 1980). In some families, the father may be perceived as an outsider and as a threat to family closeness (Cervera, 1991). However, the support of a strongly involved grandmother can also foster father involvement with the child (Chase-Lansdale et al., 1999).

YOUNG MOTHERS' PARENTING

A large body of literature comparing the parenting of teenage and adult mothers has demonstrated that, in general, teenage mothers are less responsive and verbally stimulating, have less realistic developmental expectations, and are more restrictive with their children than are older mothers (Osofsky et al., 1993; Zeanah et al., 1997). However, maternal age is confounded with a constellation of risk factors associated with problematic parenting such as low education, poverty, and unmarried status (Wakschlag et al., 1999). In fact, studies that have examined age effects when comparing the parenting of teenage and adult mothers in similar sociodemographic circumstances have found fewer differences (Chase-Lansdale et al., 1994; Geronimus, 1991).

Despite the predominance of a comparative approach in research on adolescent mothers, an emerging body of literature has focused on factors associated with individual differences in parenting competence in young mothers. These factors may be broadly grouped into four categories: (1) relationship factors and coresidence, (2) mothers' personal resources and adjustment, (3) sociodemographic factors, and (4) child characteristics.

Relationship Factors and Coresidence

Young mothers clearly need the support of a social network as they begin caring for a new baby. Bolton (1990) found that young mothers who raise their children in social isolation are at risk for maltreating their children. Numerous studies have examined how social context factors such as coresidence, social support, and quality of relationships are associated with young mothers' parenting competence.

Psychological theory and research suggest that the quality of mothers' relationships with their own mothers has a central influence on parenting (Vondra & Belsky, 1993). Studies have shown links between adolescent mothers' histories of parental rejection or problematic attachment to parents and higher levels of depression and harsh, punitive parenting (Crockenberg, 1987a; Leadbeater & Linares, 1992; Ward & Carlson, 1995).

Concurrent relationships young mothers have with their own mothers have also been found to influence parenting. Some studies indicate that social support and instrumental assistance from grandmothers are associated with more responsive adolescent parenting (Crockenberg, 1987b; Davis, Rhodes, & Hamilton-Leaks, 1997; Voight, Hans, & Bernstein, 1996). However, other studies have also shown negative effects of grandmother social support on young mothers' parenting (East & Felice, 1996; Oyserman, Radin, & Saltz, 1994), and others have found that, under coresiding conditions, mothers' parenting is less warm and stimulat-ing, even for very young mothers (Black & Nitz, 1995; Spieker & Bensley, 1994). A closer look suggests, however, that these conflicting results may be understood by the varying effects of social support as a function of contextual factors. In three independent studies, closeness and support from grandmother predicted positive outcomes (i.e., competent parenting, infant attachment security, and lower levels of toddler aggression) but only when mother and grandmother live apart (East & Felice, 1996; Spieker & Bensley, 1994; Wakschlag et al., 1996). Under coresiding conditions, support may not always facilitate competence. For example, support that is accompanied by high levels of conflict or demands for reciprocal support by other family members may not foster competent parenting in the young mother (Davis et al., 1997; Voight et al., 1996).

It is important to go beyond whether or not grandmothers provide support to examine multigenerational relationship processes as contributors to young mothers' parenting competence. In the Baltimore Multigenerational Family Study (BMFS), the Scale of Intergenerational Relationship Quality was used to rate videotaped observations of adolescent mother–grandmother discussions of disagreements in terms of emotional closeness, positive affect, grandmother directness, and adolescent individuation (Wakschlag et al., 1996). Individuation was the most salient predictor of young mothers' parenting competence. Young mothers whose discussions with their mothers combined self-assertion with the ability to stay connected despite differences were significantly more likely to parent their preschoolers in a manner that balanced responsiveness and appropriate control (Wakschlag et al., 1996). Individuation was not merely a function of age, and, in fact, it appeared to exert strongest effects for young mothers living on their own.

When individuation is fostered within the family of origin, young mothers may be "primed" to provide appropriate parenting to their young children because they have acquired relationship skills which are readily transferable (Wakschlag et al., in press). Interestingly, in the BMFS, the preschool-age children of individuated mothers were also significantly more likely to function autonomously, suggesting that relational patterns that foster competence in young mothers may have long-term intergenerational implications (Wakschlag et al., in press).

Several studies which have compared the effects of living with a partner versus multigenerational coresidence on mothers' parenting have shown that mothers who live with partners feel more effective and provide higher-quality home environments for their children than do those living with grandmothers (Shapiro & Mangelsdorf, 1994; Wasserman, Brunelli, & Rauh, 1990). Although intriguing, these results should not be overinterpreted to mean that living with a male partner in and of itself causes young mothers to provide better rearing environments for their children. At present, a variety of social and economic factors make it relatively unusual for young parents to establish residence together, and those who do may be a highly motivated, competent subgroup of young parents with better than average economic and social resources. Although father involvement as measured by residential status is associated with mothers' parenting competence (Luster & Dubow, 1990; Wasserman et al., 1990), little is known about mother–partner relationship processes as an influence on parenting. Studies have found that partner support reduces stress in adolescent mothers (Lamb & Elster, 1985; Thompson & Peebles-Wilkins, 1992) and increases maternal psychosocial adjustment (Crockenberg, 1987b) and self-esteem (Unger & Wandersman, 1988). There is some evidence that adolescent mothers with supportive male partners are more responsive mothers (Unger & Wandersman, 1988). Yet other studies have failed to find relations between support from partner and maternal well-being or mothering, presumably because fathers are often a mixed blessing for mothers, providing them with not only support but stress (Musick, 1994; Voight et al., 1996). On the other hand, a supportive relationship with a partner appears to reduce the risk that young mothers who have had problematic developmental histories themselves will provide angry, punitive parenting (Crockenberg, 1987a).

The effectiveness of support from family members and partners may vary not only by coresidence issues but by other factors such as mothers' age, level of stress, and child health. There is some evidence for positive effects of social support for younger but not older mothers (East & Felice, 1996) and particularly for younger mothers under noncoresiding conditions (Spieker & Bensley, 1994; Wakschlag et al., 1996). In addition, social support seems to be especially important as a protective factor for mothers' parenting when there is a high level of conflict within mothers' social network (Nitz, Ketterlinus, & Brandt, 1995), but not if the providers of support are also a source of conflict (Voight et al., 1996). Support and coresidence also appear to exert favorable effects under particularly high-risk conditions, such as for mothers with low-birthweight infants and when mothers are depressed (Leadbeater & Linares, 1992; Pope et al., 1993).

As reviewed earlier, coresidence with grandmothers often appears to be negatively associated with mothers' parenting competence. Much remains to be learned about a variety of relevant issues such as the dynamics within coresiding families, the stresses they experience, the transitions they undergo over time, and how cultural context and socioeconomic factors may be related to these dynamics.

Personal Resources and Adjustment

Dimensions of maternal personal resources and adjustment that have been examined as predictors of young mothers' parenting include intellectual resources, maternal attitudes and commitment, overall adjustment (including self-esteem and feelings of well-being), and mental health.

A number of studies have identified an association between maternal intelligence and mothers' parenting (Luster & Dubow, 1990; Mylod, Whitman, & Borkowski, 1997; Whiteside-Mansell, Pope, & Bradley, 1996). In one of the few studies that have examined patterns of adolescent mothers parenting over time, maternal intelligence was the single factor that best discriminated mothers who had a consistently positive parenting style versus those mothers whose parenting was problematic or unstable (Whiteside-Mansell et al., 1996). One pathway by which intelligence and parenting may be linked is via mothers' "cognitive readiness" to parent (Miller, Miceli, Whitman, & Borkowski, 1996). Cognitive readiness includes mothers' knowledge and expectations about child development and attitudes and commitment toward child rearing, as well as ability to assimilate knowledge and apply it flexibly in a child-rearing context (Borkowski et al., 1992). Maternal cognitive readiness has been associated in young mothers with better maternal coping skills, more positive perceptions of the infant, and more responsive parenting (East & Felice, 1996; Luster & Rhoades, 1989; Miller et al., 1996). Accuracy of maternal perceptions of infant emotional cues has also been associated with more competent parenting (Shapiro & Mangelsdorf, 1994).

Mothers' mental health and adjustment have also been linked to parenting competence. Maternal social competence has been linked to higher levels of responsiveness and lower abuse potential in adolescent mothers (Mylod et al., 1997; Spieker & Bensley, 1994). Maternal self-confidence, sense of effectance, and self-esteem have also been linked to higher-quality parenting (East & Felice, 1996; Luster & Mittelstaedt, 1993).

Studies examining the relation of adolescent mothers' mental health and parenting have focused in large part on the effects of maternal depression. In general, depression in adolescent mothers has been linked to a less responsive parenting style during infancy (Osofsky et al., 1993). The relation of adolescent mothers' depression to parenting beyond infancy has not been as well established. There is some evidence that depressed adolescent mothers are less contingently responsive to their preschoolers (Leadbeater, Bishop, & Raver, 1996). Other types of internalizing problems, including maternal anxiety and social withdrawal, have also been linked to parenting difficulties in adolescent mothers (Serbin, Peters, McAffer, & Schwartzman, 1991; Zeanah, Keener, Anders, & Vieira-Baker, 1987).

The relation of adolescents' history of externalizing problems and their parenting has received surprisingly little attention, even though a history of behavior problems significantly increases the risk of early pregnancy (Kessler et al., 1997; Maughan & Lindelow, 1997). However, several studies have documented links between young mothers' history of aggression and conduct problems and unresponsiveness to their infants (Cassidy, Zoccolillo, & Hughes, 1996; Serbin et al., 1991).

A history of maltreatment also increases the risk of parenting problems in young mothers. A significant proportion of young women who become pregnant as teenagers have a history of sexual abuse and victimization which increases their risk for mental health problems as well as difficulties maintaining stable relationships with partners and establishing appropriate boundaries with their young children (Stevens-Simon & Reichert, 1994; Sroufe, Jacobvitz, Mangelsdorf, DeAngelo, & Ward, 1985). Teenage mothers with histories of exposure to violence are significantly more likely to engage in maltreatment of their own children (Bolton, 1990). One particularly high-risk group among victims of maltreatment is teenage mothers who are themselves in foster care, but to our knowledge this particular subgroup of mothers has not been systematically studied (but see Musick, 1993, for a clinical discussion).

High levels of contemporaneous environmental stress have also been repeatedly associated with poorer psychological functioning in adolescent mothers, including increased rates of depression and substance use and more problematic parenting (Barnet, Duggan, Wilson, & Joffee, 1995; Leadbeater & Linares, 1992). Under high levels of stress, adolescent mothers are less sensitive and responsive to their infants (Crockenberg, 1987b). It is difficult, however, to determine whether stress is a cause or a consequence of poorer adjustment in these mothers.

Sociodemographic Factors

Sociodemographic factors that have been examined as predictors of young mothers' parenting competence include mothers' age and education, socioeconomic status, and family size. Although it has been suggested that the youngest adolescents are at highest risk for poor parenting outcomes, the empirical evidence for this is equivocal (Luster & Mittelstaedt, 1993). Some studies have shown an inverse relation between maternal age and parenting competence (East & Felice, 1996; Luster & Dubow, 1990), but others have not (Shapiro & Mangelsdorf, 1994; Whiteside-Mansell et al., 1996). Similarly, a positive association between maternal education level and parenting quality has been established in some studies (Spieker & Bensley, 1994) but not others (Wakschlag et al., 1996). Family size and rapid subsequent fertility, in turn, are associated with poorer-quality parenting, including an increased risk of child maltreatment, perhaps due to the extent to which the demands of multiple, closely spaced young children reduce maternal emotional availability (Luster & Mittelstaedt, 1993; Miller & Moore, 1990). Cumulative demographic risk has also been associated with poorer-quality parenting in young mothers (Hann, Osofsky, & Culp, 1996).

Child Characteristics

Child characteristics that have been associated with variations in young mothers' parenting include child age and developmental vulnerability. Children who are vulnerable because of medical risk, developmental delays, or difficult temperament appear to be at higher risk of receiving poor parenting by young mothers (Bolton, 1990; Luster & Mittelstaedt, 1993). Variations in young mothers' parenting as a function of child age have not been studied extensively and what studies there are reveal a mixed picture. One study has reported that young mothers hold particularly harsh attitudes toward discipline when their children are toddlers (East & Felice, 1996); another has shown that young mothers of infants are more likely to demonstrate negativity (Nitz et al., 1995).

CHILD OUTCOME

A substantial body of research suggests that early motherhood is associated with a variety of adverse long-term outcomes for offspring including poor school achievement and completion, lowered intelligence, delinquent behavior, becoming a parent in adolescence, and lack of self-sufficiency during adulthood (Furstenberg et al., 1987; Moore, Morrison, & Greene, 1997; Hardy et al., 1997; Osofsky et al., 1993; Wakschlag et al., 1999). Disadvantage for the offspring of young mothers appears to worsen over time. During infancy, children of young mothers appear to make normal developmental progress (for reviews, see Brooks-Gunn & Furstenberg, 1986; Coley & Chase-Lansdale, 1998). Delays in cognitive development emerge by the preschool years (Furstenberg et al., 1987; Moore et al., 1997), as do overactivity, undercontrol, and behavior problems (e.g., Leadbeater et al., 1996; Wadsworth, Taylor, Osborn, & Butler, 1984).

Although offspring of adolescent mothers appear to be at high risk, it is also notable that there is considerable variability in their developmental outcome at all ages (Borkowski et al., 1992; Coley & Chase-Lansdale, 1998; Roosa & Vaughan, 1984). Factors associated with variability in child development are reviewed in four categories: (1) relationship factors and coresidence, (2) mothers' personal resources and adjustment, (3) sociodemographic factors, and (4) parenting characteristics.

Relationship Factors and Coresidence

Most investigations of adolescent parenthood have found that variables related to social support, coresidence, and family relationship patterns are among the strongest predictors of child development outcomes (but see Stoiber & Houghton, 1993). Studies of family systems and support variables are complicated, however, by the fact that support may have different meanings depending on residence patterns and age of child.

Most studies have suggested that father involvement is positively related to child outcomes. Father support and involvement have been linked to better cognitive and achievement outcomes in middle childhood (Unger & Cooley, 1992; Cooley & Unger, 1991; Dubow & Luster, 1990). In the BMFS, amount of father involvement was unrelated to adolescent academic achievement and psychosocial adjustment, although strength of the bond between father and child was predictive of outcome (Furstenberg & Harris, 1993). Several studies of infants of adolescent mothers suggest that father involvement is related to greater infant responsiveness (Unger & Wandersman, 1985) and father coresidence is related to more infant vocalizing, smiling, and exploration of toys (Field et al., 1990). Whereas father involvement may increase positive infant behaviors, it may not reduce problematic ones. One study, for example, found that partner support did not reduce the risk of problematic behavior in toddlers (Crockenberg, 1987a).

The role of involvement from the young mother's own mother is somewhat more complex. Support from the grandmother has been related to better performance on infant developmental tests (Unger & Wandersman, 1985), to security of infant attachment and infant persistence (Frodi et al., 1984), and to fewer preschool behavior problems (Leadbeater & Bishop, 1994). Still other studies suggest that support may be a mixed blessing. In one study, high levels of grandmother involvement in child care was associated with poor developmental outcomes for children of adolescent mothers, particularly for white families and particularly when sustained over time into middle childhood (Cooley & Unger, 1991). More recently, two studies have suggested that grandmother assistance must be understood in terms of residential findings. Optimal child outcomes in terms of attachment security (Spieker & Bensley, 1994) and preschool child's behavioral adjustment (East & Felice, 1996) occur when the young mother does not coreside with her mother but nevertheless receives assistance from her.

Personal Resources and Adjustment

Just as maternal cognitive readiness to parent has been associated with parental responsiveness, it has also been linked to improved child outcome. For example, young mothers' positive, realistic, and mature expectations of parenting have been linked to more adaptive and effective coping strategies in offspring during infancy and toddlerhood (Stoiber & Houghton, 1993), better intellectual development (Miller et al., 1996), and fewer internalizing and externalizing behavior problems at 3 years of age (Miller et al., 1996; East & Felice, 1996). Similarly, in a sample of adolescent mothers of preterm infants, those mothers with less realistic developmental expectations and child-rearing attitudes were more likely to describe their infants as having difficult temperaments (Field, Widmayer, Stringer, & Ignatoff, 1980). Young mothers' emotional readiness to parent may also have an effect on their children's development. Adolescent mothers who have not resolved attachment issues from their own childhoods are more likely to have insecurely attached infants (Ward & Carlson, 1995).

Maternal mental health and adjustment have also been linked to offspring outcomes. Self-esteem in young mothers has been related to fewer behavior problems in their children at school age and better reading achievement (Dubow & Luster, 1990). Young mothers' depressive symptoms have also been linked to infant difficultness (Cassidy et al., 1996), behavior problems in toddlers (Leadbeater et al., 1996), and externalizing problems in preschool-age children (Hubbs-Tait et al., 1996). Maternal antisocial history has been related to infant passivity (Cassidy et al., 1996).

Sociodemographic Factors

Variables reflecting socioeconomic status explain little variation in the development of children of adolescent mothers during infancy. By early childhood, however, they begin to account for variation in children's developmental outcome (Hann et al., 1996). Indices of family poverty have been associated with behavior problems in early childhood and adolescence in the offspring of teenage mothers (Dubow & Luster, 1990; Furstenberg et al., 1987). Offspring academic performance has been linked to maternal educational achievement (Cooley & Unger, 1991; Dubow & Luster, 1990;

Furstenberg et al., 1987) as well as grandparent educational achievement (Moore et al., 1997). However, the relationship between maternal and child educational achievement is complex because the living circumstances that seem to foster educational attainment in young mothers (e.g., coresidence) may carry costs for their children.

Delay of subsequent childbearing, following an early birth, also appears to be a protective factor for children born to teenage mothers. Young children born to teenage mothers who remain only children through preschool age fare better in higher academic achievement through age 12 (Apfel & Seitz, 1997).

Parenting Characteristics

For infants and young children, the impact of sociodemographic risk factors may largely be experienced through the type of parenting they receive, and much of the research focus on young children of adolescent mothers has focused on the linkages between quality of parenting by young mothers and child outcome. Children's cognitive outcomes during early elementary school have been related to concurrent measures of their young mothers' responsiveness (Cooley & Unger, 1991) and during infancy to maternal demonstration of toys and engagement with the child (Field et al., 1990). Children's externalizing and internalizing problems during preschool have been negatively associated with concurrent measures of mothers' and grandmothers' competent parenting (Pittman, Chase-Lansdale, McHale, & Brooks-Gunn, 1998).

Problems in parenting and parent–child relationships during infancy and toddlerhood may lay the groundwork for nonoptimal development. In a sample of young mothers, lack of dyadic engagement was related to insecure infant attachment (Lamb, Hopps, & Elster, 1987). Young mothers who directed angry punitive behavior toward their infants were more likely to have toddlers who displayed angry and noncompliant behavior (Crockenberg, 1987a). Characteristics of mother–infant interaction, particularly maternal affect and dyadic verbal reciprocity were related to their children's cognitive–linguistic development at preschool age (Hann et al., 1996). Conflict between young mothers and their toddlers was also related to behavior problems at preschool age (Leadbeater et al., 1996).

IMPLICATIONS FOR FUTURE RESEARCH AND INTERVENTION

This chapter suggests a high degree of variability in the resources young mothers bring to bear on the parenting enterprise and in the extent to which being born to an adolescent mother places young children's development at risk. Not surprisingly, mothers with greater personal resources, including both psychological well-being and cognitive preparedness for parenting, fare better, as do their children. The role of relationships in promoting young parent and child competence is clearly critical yet somewhat counterintuitive at times. It appears that family processes that support the successful resolution of the developmental processes of adolescence—achieving autonomy within a context of support and relatedness—are associated with higher-quality parenting and positive socioemotional outcomes in children. Although it is important that a young mother receive support, grandmother involvement can be "too much of a good thing" by interfering with the young mother's development of parenting skills and sense of competence as a mother as well as with the quality of the parent–child relationship.

We must go beyond structural variables such as coresidence with grandmothers or father absence to shed light on the complex processes that influence developmental outcome for young mothers and their children. Although there is increasing evidence that the problematic consequences of being born to a young mother can be far reaching, we still know far too little about how various associated factors fit together in influencing the long-term trajectories of the offspring of young mothers. For example, although both theory and practice suggest that many of the risks of young motherhood affect infant outcome via their impact on the quality of parenting (e.g., Osofsky et al., 1993), this has generally not been validated in studies that have attempted to demonstrate that parenting mediates other risks such as cognitive readiness or depression (e.g., Leadbeater et al., 1996; Miller et al., 1996).

Studies are needed that rigorously test integrated models of development and empirically demonstrate how risk and protective factors—at individual, dyadic, family, and social–contextual levels—interact in determining the developmental trajectories of young mothers and their infants. In particular, the convergence of evidence of the negative effects of coresidence

on parenting and socioemotional development requires further "unpacking." This will entail gaining a better understanding of the relation of coresidence and quality of family interactions, exploring why families choose particular residential patterns, understanding sources of stress and processes of coping and conflict resolution in multigenerational families, examining how grandmothers' own life-course issues and feelings about coresidence influence this process, and understanding how these issues vary by ethnicity.

At a clinical level, it seems clear that "universal" interventions for teenage mothers and their babies are likely to fall short. Musick and colleagues have suggested that interventions must be qualitatively different for young mothers who are "detoured" versus those who are "derailed" (Quint, Musick, & Ladner, 1994). These categories are similar to the two primary subgroups we have suggested here based on previous research; young women for whom adolescent pregnancy is an adaptive life course choice versus those for whom it is a manifestation of broader involvement in problem behavior and problematic relationships.

We would suggest that the mothers' relationships with families and partners, their psychological preparedness for parenting, and their mental health are critical variables by which intervention strategies should be guided, and that these two subgroups of mothers will vary systematically along these dimensions (see Table 7.1). We note as well that these domains are generally areas that can be assessed during pregnancy so that young women could be directed to appropriate interventions prior to the infants' birth and, most important, for those mothers at highest risk for parenting problems, *well before problematic mother–infant interaction patterns have been established.*

For example, the offspring of teenage mothers who have a history of conduct problems are at particular risk of emotional and behavioral problems because of the combination of increased familial risk and the likelihood that their mothers have experienced disrupted relationship histories themselves and are unlikely to receive high-quality family support (Osofsky, Eberhart-Wright, Ware, & Hann, 1992). Such dyads may need intensive therapeutic intervention focusing on treatment of both the young mothers' mental health needs and building a secure and stable relationship between mother and infant.

TABLE 7.1. Critical Domains for Consideration in Planning Mental Health Interventions for Young Mothers and Their Infants

Domains of risk factors	Possible impact on parenting and parent–infant relationship	Examples of possible interventions
Multigenerational • Coresidence with grandmother • Inadequate mentoring for parenting • Grandmother involvement that interferes with individuation and learning of parenting competence • Grandmother burden • Conflictual family relationships	• Grandmother involvement may undermine mother's parenting confidence • Strains of coresidence may lead to chronic family conflict • Lack of grandmother support may leave young mother without adequate mentorship for parenting	• Multigenerational intervention to facilitate mother–grandmother negotiation of respective roles/responsibilities • Guidance to grandmother on providing developmentally supportive assistance to daughter • Support and respite opportunities for grandmothers designed to reduce role strain
Partner relationship • Father uninvolvement with child • Father unemployment	• Fathers unable to provide financially will withdraw involvement or be excluded from the family	• Couples' intervention which emphasizes importance of father's stable involvement for infant emotional growth and maternal social support, regardless of his financial contribution • Father support groups emphasizing the importance of varied facets of fatherhood and the "manliness" of fathering
Maternal mental health • History of victimization • Depression • Conduct problems	• Mother's ongoing emotional and behavioral difficulties may interfere with her ability to read and empathize with her infant's cues • Mother may be uncomfortable with the intimacy and emotional intensity of the parent–infant relationship • Heightened negative affect and assertions of autonomy during toddler period may be particularly challenging for mothers with a history of difficulty modulating aggression and negotiating conflict adaptively	• Mental health interventions for mother to help her make links between past and present and to develop more adaptive relationship patterns • Dyadic mother–infant treatment to foster responsive caregiving and secure attachment • Therapeutic nursery • Parenting intervention during toddlerhood that fosters autonomy support combined with firm limit setting
Maternal personal resources • Limited knowledge of child development • Poor self-esteem • Limited intelligence	• Mother may have unrealistic expectations that may interfere with her capacity to understand her baby's needs and to respond in a developmentally appropriate fashion • Mother may lack self-confidence in her parenting and withdraw from child • Mother may not understand that she "makes a difference" for child • Mother may not understand the role that cognitive stimulation plays in learning	• Developmental guidance and parenting education • Interactional intervention that focuses on understanding how babies signal their needs • Programs to help mothers learn how to enrich their children's home learning environments • Developmental day care to allow mother to complete her education and provide child learning opporunities

Young women for whom early childbearing is an "alternative life course strategy" under circumstances of limited social and economic opportunities (Burton, 1990) may require less intensive intervention. These young women may also be more likely to receive high-quality support from their families. In this context, prevention of rapid subsequent fertility interventions that help mothers stay on track with their own life-course goals and brief multigenerational interventions may be sufficient to promote healthy outcomes (e.g., Apfel & Seitz, 1997).

The contrasting "profiles" of these young mothers and research findings suggest that the intensity, emphasis, and therapeutic nature of intervention needed by adolescent mothers and babies to support healthy development will vary widely. The majority of programs for adolescent mothers which have been evaluated have emphasized job training, contraceptive counseling, and staying in school. It appears that the assumption has been that such "successes" will trickle down to the children, but there is little evidence that this is so (but see Apfel & Seitz, 1997). This assumption is particularly problematic for dyads where the young mother's difficulties have preceded her transition to parenthood. Recently, the two-generation approach to intervention which combines parent self-sufficiency *and* child development services in one comprehensive program has held forth promise (Smith, 1995). However, although these integrated intervention programs are a major step forward, mental health and family interactions have generally not been a direct focus of intervention (but see Quint & Egeland, 1995). Based on the findings reviewed here, we would also suggest that the two-generation approach might need to be expanded to three generations, involving grandmothers as well as adolescent mothers and their children. Interventions need to be made available for adolescent parents, their parents, their partners, their children, and combinations of family members. This is particularly relevant in light of new welfare reform legislation which mandates coresidence for adolescent mothers (see Coley & Chase-Lansdale, 1998) and the substantial evidence that coresidence is not protective and may even have negative developmental consequences. Table 7.1 illustrates domains of risk from an infant mental health perspective, their implications for the parent–infant relationship, and proposed strategies for intervention. The development of universal screening techniques linked to targeted services based on assessment of high-risk status in these key domains would inform prevention efforts.

ACKNOWLEDGMENTS

We gratefully acknowledge the ongoing support of the Walden and Jean Young Shaw Foundation and the Irving B. Harris Center for Developmental Studies. We also thank Linda Henson and Holly Furdyna for their thoughtful comments on earlier versions of this chapter.

REFERENCES

Amato, P. R., & Rezac, S. J. (1994). Contact with nonresidential parents, interparental conflict, and children's behavior. *Journal of Family Issues, 15,* 191–207.

Apfel, N., & Seitz, V. (1997). The firstborn sons of African-American teenage mothers: Perspectives on risk and resilience. In S. Luthar, J. Burack, D. Cicchetti, & J. Weisz (Eds.), *Developmental psychopathology: Perspectives on adjustment, risk and disorder* (pp. 486–506). New York: Cambridge University Press.

Barnet, B., Duggan, A., Wilson, M., & Joffe, A. (1995). Association between postpartum substance use and depressive symptoms, stress and social support in adolescent mothers. *Pediatrics, 96,* 659–666.

Barret, R., & Robinson, B. (1986). Adolescent fathers: Often forgotten parents. *Pediatric Nursing, 12,* 273–277.

Black, M. M., & Nitz, K. (1995). Grandmother co-residence, parenting, and child development among low income, urban teen mothers. *Journal of Adolescent Health, 16,* 1–9.

Bolton, F. (1990). The risk of child maltreatment in adolescent parenting. In A. Stiffman & R. Feldman (Eds.), *Contraception, pregnancy and parenting* (Vol. 4, pp. 223–237). London, England: Kingsley.

Borkowski, J. G., Whitman, T. L., Passino, A. W., Rellinger, E. A., Sommer, K., & Keogh, D. (1992). Unraveling the "New Morbidity": Adolescent parenting and developmental delays. *International Review of Research in Mental Retardation, 18,* 159–196.

Bowman, P. J. (1989). Research perspectives on black men: Role strain and adaptation across the adult life cycle. In R. L. Jones (Ed.), *Black adult development and aging* (pp. 117–150). Berkeley, CA: Cobbs & Henry.

Boyer, D., & Fine, D. (1992). Sexual abuse as a factor in adolescent pregnancy and child maltreatment. *Family Planning Perspectives, 24,* 4–11.

Brooks-Gunn, J., & Furstenberg, F. (1986). The children of adolescent mothers: Physical, academic and psychological outcomes. *Developmental Review, 6,* 224–251.

Burton, L. (1990). Teenage childbearing as an alternative life-course strategy in multi-generation black families. *Human Nature, 1*, 123–143.

Burton, L., & Bengston, V. (1985). Black grandmothers: Issues of timing and continuity of roles. In V. Bengston & J. Robertson (Eds.), *Grandparenthood* (pp. 61–78). Beverly Hills, CA: Sage.

Butler, J. R., & Burton, L. M. (1990). Rethinking teenage childbearing: Is sexual abuse a missing link? *Family Relations, 39*, 73–80.

Cassidy, B., Zoccolillo, M., & Hughes, S. (1996). Psychopathology in adolescent mothers and its effects on mother–infant interactions: A pilot study. *Canadian Journal of Psychiatry, 41*, 379–384.

Cervera, N. (1991). Unwed teenage pregnancy: Family relationships with the father of the baby. *Families in Society, 72*, 29–37.

Chase-Lansdale, P. L., Brooks-Gunn, J., & Zamsky, E. (1994). Young African-American multigenerational families in poverty: Quality of mothering and grandmothering. *Child Development, 65*, 373–393.

Chase-Lansdale, P. L., Gordon, R., Coley, R., Wakschlag, L., & Brooks-Gunn, J. (1999). Young African-American multigenerational families in poverty: The contexts, exchanges and processes of their lives. In E. M. Hetherington (Ed.), *Coping with divorce, single parenting and remarriage: A risk and resilience perspective* (pp. 165–192). Mahwah, NJ: Erlbaum.

Child Welfare League of America. (1996). *Welfare reform and teen parents: An issue brief*. Washington, DC: CWLA Press.

Coley, R. L., & Chase-Lansdale, P. L. (1998). Adolescent pregnancy and parenthood: Recent evidence and future directions. *American Psychologist, 53*(2), 152–166.

Cooley, M. L., & Unger, D. G. (1991). The role of family support in determining developmental outcomes in children of teen mothers. *Child Psychiatry and Human Development, 21*, 217–234.

Cooper, C., Grotevant, G., & Condon, S. (1983). Individuality and connectedness in the family as a context for adolescent identity formation and role-taking skill. In H. Grotevant & C. Cooper (Eds.), *New directions for child development* (Vol. 22, pp. 43–59). San Francisco: Jossey-Bass.

Crockenberg, S. B. (1987a). Predictors and correlates of anger toward and punitive control of toddlers by adolescent mothers. *Child Development, 58*, 964–975.

Crockenberg, S. B. (1987b). Support for adolescent mothers during the postnatal period: Theory and research. C. F. Z. Boukydis (Ed.), *Research on support for parents and infants in the postnatal period* (pp. 3–24). Norwood, NJ: Ablex.

Danziger, S. K., & Radin, N. (1990). Absent does not equal uninvolved: Predictors of fathering in teen mother families. *Journal of Marriage and the Family, 52*, 636–642.

Davis, A., Rhodes, J., & Hamilton-Leaks, J. (1997). When both parents may be a source of support and problems: An analysis of pregnant and parenting female African-American adolescents' relationships with their mothers and fathers. *Journal of Adolescent Research, 7*, 331–348.

Dubow, E., & Luster, T. (1990). Adjustment of children born to teenage mothers: The contribution of risk and protective factors. *Journal of Marriage and the Family, 52*, 393–404.

East, P., & Felice, M. (1996). *Adolescent pregnancy and parenting: Findings from a racially diverse sample*. Mahwah, NJ: Erlbaum.

Elster, A. B. (1988). *Adolescent fathers: Fact, fiction, and implications for federal policy*. Washington, DC: U.S. Government Printing Office.

Elster, A. B., & Hendricks, L. (1986). Stresses and coping strategies of adolescent fathers. In B. Elster, & M. E. Lamb (Eds.), *Adolescent fatherhood* (pp. 55–65). Hillsdale, NJ: Erlbaum.

Emde, R. (1991). The wonder of our complex enterprise: Steps enabled by attachment and the effects of relationships on relationships. *Infant Mental Health Journal, 12*, 164–173.

Field, T. M., Widmayer, S., Adler, S., & De Cubas, M. (1990). Teenage parenting in different cultures, family constellations, and caregiving environments: Effects on infant development. *Infant Mental Health Journal, 11*, 158–174.

Field, T. M., Widmayer, S. M., Stringer, S., & Ignatoff, E. (1980). Teenage, lower-class, black mothers and their preterm infants: An intervention and developmental follow-up. *Child Development, 51*, 426–436.

Frodi, A., Keller, B., Foye, H., Liptak, G., Bridges, L., Grolnick, W., Berko, J., McAnarney, E., & Lawrence, R. (1984). Determinants of attachment and mastery motivation in infants born to adolescent mothers. *Infant Mental Health Journal, 5*, 15–23.

Furstenberg, F. F., Jr. (1980). Burden and benefits: The impact of early childbearing on the family. *Journal of Social Issues, 36*, 64–87.

Furstenberg, F. F., Jr. (1995). Fathering in the inner city: Paternal participation and public policy. In W. Marsiglio (Ed.), *Fatherhood: Contemporary theory, research, and social policy* (pp. 119–147). Thousand Oaks, CA: Sage.

Furstenberg, F. F., Jr., Brooks-Gunn, J., & Morgan, S. P. (1987). *Adolescent mothers in later life*. Cambridge, MA: Cambridge University Press.

Furstenberg, F. F., Jr., & Harris, K. M. (1993). When and why fathers matter: Impacts of father involvement on children of adolescent mothers. In R. I. Lerman & T. J. Ooms (Eds.), *Young unwed fathers* (pp. 117–138). Philadelphia: Temple University Press.

Geronimus, A. T. (1991). Teenage childbearing and social and reproductive disadvantage: The evolution of complex questions and the demise of simple answers. *Family Relations, 40*, 463–471.

Hann, D., Osofsky, J., & Culp, A. (1996). Relating the adolescent mother–child relationship to preschool outcomes. *Infant Mental Health Journal, 17*, 302–309.

Hardy, J., Shapiro, S., Astone, N., Miller, T., Brooks-Gunn, J., & Hilton, S. (1997). Adolescent childbearing revisited: The age of inner-city mothers at delivery is a determinant of their children's self-sufficiency at age 27–33. *Pediatrics, 100*, 802–809.

Hendricks, L. E., & Montgomery, T. (1983). A limited population of unmarried adolescent fathers: A preliminary report of their views of fatherhood and the relationship with the mothers of their children. *Adolescence, 18,* 201–210.

Hubbs-Tait, L., Pond-Hughes, K., Culp, A. M., Osofsky, J. D., Hann, D. M., Eberhart-Wright, A., & Ware, L. M. (1996). Children of adolescent mothers: Attachment representation, maternal depression, and later behavior problems. *American Journal of Orthopsychiatry, 66,* 416–426.

Kessler, R., Berglund, P., Foster, C., Saunders, W., Stang, P., & Walters, E. (1997). Social consequences of psychiatric disorders: II. Teenage parenthood. *American Journal of Psychiatry, 154,* 1405–1411.

Ketterlinus, R., Lamb, M., & Nitz, K. (1994). Adolescent nonsexual and sex-related problem behaviors: Their prevalence, consequences and co-occurrence. In R. Ketterlinus & M. Lamb (Eds.), *Adolescent problem behaviors: Issues and research* (pp. 17–40). Hillsdale, N.J.: Erlbaum.

Lamb, M. E., & Elster, A. B. (1985). Adolescent mother–infant–father relationships. *Developmental Psychology, 21,* 768–773.

Lamb, M. E., Hopps, K., & Elster, A. B. (1987). Strange situation behavior of infants with adolescent mothers. *Infant Behavior and Development, 10,* 39–48.

Landry, D. J., & Forrest, J. D. (1995). How old are U.S. fathers? *Family Planning Perspectives,* 27, 159–165.

Leadbeater, B. J., & Bishop, S. J. (1994). Predictors of behavior problems in preschool children of inner-city Afro-American and Puerto Rican adolescent mothers. *Child Development, 65,* 638–648.

Leadbeater, B., Bishop, S., & Raver, C. C. (1996). Quality of mother–child interactions, maternal depressive symptoms, and behavior problems in preschoolers of adolescent mothers. *Developmental Psychology, 32,* 280–288.

Leadbeater, B. J., & Linares, O. (1992). Depressive symptoms in black and Puerto Rican adolescent mothers in the first 3 years postpartum. *Development and Psychopathology, 4,* 451–468.

Lerman, R. I. (1993). A national profile of young unwed fathers. In R. I. Lerman & T. J. Ooms (Eds.), *Young unwed fathers* (pp. 27–51). Philadelphia: Temple University Press.

Luster, T., & Dubow, E. (1990). Predictors of the quality of the home environment that adolescent mothers provide for their school-aged children. *Journal of Youth and Adolescence, 19,* 475–494.

Luster, T., & Mittelstaedt, M. (1993). Adolescent mothers. In T. Luster & L. Okagaki (Eds.), *Parenting: An ecological perspective* (pp. 35–68). Hillsdale, NJ: Erlbaum.

Luster, T., & Rhoades, K. (1989). The relation between child-rearing beliefs and the home environment in a sample of adolescent mothers. *Family Relations, 38,* 317–322.

Males, M., & Chew, K. S. Y. (1996). The ages of fathers in California, adolescent births, 1993. *American Journal of Public Health, 86,* 565–568.

Maughan, B., & Lindelow, M. (1997). Secular change in psychosocial risks: the case of teenage motherhood. *Psychological Medicine, 27,* 1129–1144.

Maynard, R. (1997). The study, the context and the findings in brief. In R. Maynard (Ed.), *Kids having kids: Economic costs and social consequences of teen pregnancy* (pp. 1–22). Washington, DC: Urban Institute Press.

McElroy, S., & Moore, K. (1997). Trends over time in teenage pregnancy and childbearing: The critical changes. In R. Maynard (Ed.), *Kids having kids: Economic costs and social consequences of teen pregnancy* (pp. 23–53). Washington, DC: Urban Institute.

Michaels, G., & Goldberg, A. (Eds.). (1988). *The transition to parenthood: Current theory and research.* New York: Cambridge University Press.

Miller, B., & Moore, A. (1990). Adolescent sexual behavior, pregnancy, and parenting: Research through the 1980s. *Journal of Marriage and the Family, 52,* 1025–1044.

Miller, C., Miceli, P., Whitman, T., & Borkowski, J. (1996). Cognitive readiness to parent and intellectual–emotional development in children of adolescent mothers. *Developmental Psychology, 32,* 533–541.

Moore, K. A., Morrison, D. R., & Greene, A. D. (1997). Effects on the children born to adolescent mothers. In R. A. Maynard (Ed.), *Kids having kids: Economic costs and social consequences of teen pregnancy* (pp. 145–180). Washington, DC: Urban Institute Press.

Musick, J. S. (1993). *Young, poor and pregnant: The psychology of teenage motherhood.* New Haven, CT: Yale University Press.

Musick, J. S. (1994). Grandmothers and grandmothers-to-be: Effects on adolescent mothers and adolescent mothering. *Infants and Young Children, 6,* 1–9.

Mylod, D., Whitman, T., & Borkowski, B. (1997). Predicting adolescent mothers' transition to adulthood. *Journal of Research on Adolescence, 7,* 457–478.

Nitz, K., Ketterlinus, R., & Brandt, L. (1995). The role of stress, social support, and family environment in adolescent mothers' parenting. *Journal of Adolescent Research, 10,* 358–382.

Obeidallah, D., & Burton, L. (1998). Affective ties between mothers and daughters. In M. Cox & J. Brooks-Gunn (Eds.), *Conflict and cohesion in families: Causes and consequences* (pp. 37–49). Mahwah, NJ: Erlbaum.

Osofsky, J., Eberhart-Wright, A., Ware, L., & Hann, D. (1992). Children of adolescent mothers: A group at risk for psychopathology. *Infant Mental Health Journal, 13,* 119–131.

Osofsky, J. D., Hann, D. M., & Peebles, C. (1993). Adolescent parenthood: Risks and opportunities for mothers and infants. In C. H. Zeanah, Jr. (Ed.), *Handbook of infant mental health* (pp. 106–119). New York: Guilford Press.

Oyserman, D., Radin, N., & Saltz, E. (1994). Predictors of nurturant parenting in teen mothers living in three generational families. *Child Psychiatry and Human Development, 24,* 215–230.

Pittman, L., Chase-Lansdale, P. L., McHale, J., & Brooks-Gunn, J. (1998). *The influence of grandmothers on children of young mothers.* Manuscript in preparation.

Pope, S., Whiteside, L., Brooks-Gunn, J., Kelleher, K., Rickert, V., Bradley, R., & Casey, P. (1993). Low birth weight infants born to adolescent mothers: Effects of coresidency with grandmother on child development. *Journal of the American Medical Association, 269,* 1396–1400.

Quint, J., & Egeland, B. (1995). New Chance: Comprehensive services for disadvantaged families. In S. Smith (Ed.), *Advances in applied developmental psychology: Vol 9. Two generation programs for families in poverty: A new intervention strategy* (pp. 91–134). Norwood, NJ: Ablex.

Quint, J., Musick, J., & Ladner, J. (1994). *Lives of promise, lives of pain: Young mothers after New Chance.* San Francisco: Manpower Demonstration Research.

Ray, A., & Hans, S. L. (1997). *Fathers past and present: African-American women's views of their fathers and the paternal role of their children's fathers.* Paper presented at the meetings of the American Psychological Association, Chicago.

Redmond, M. A. (1985). Attitudes of adolescent males toward adolescent pregnancy and fatherhood. *Family Relations, 34,* 337–342.

Rhodes, J., Ebert, L., & Fischer, K. (1992). Natural mentors: An overlooked resource in the social networks of young, African-American mothers. *American Journal of Community Psychology, 20,* 445–461.

Rivara, F. P., Sweeney, P. J., & Henderson, B. F. (1986). Black teenage fathers: What happens when the child is born? *Pediatrics, 78,* 151–158.

Roosa, M. W., & Vaughan, L. (1984). A comparison of teenage and older mothers with preschool age children. *Family Relations, 33,* 259–265.

Serbin, L., Peters, P., McAffer, V., & Schwartzman, A. (1991). Childhood aggression and withdrawal as predictors of adolescent pregnancy, early parenthood and environmental risk for the next generation. *Canadian Journal of Behavioral Science, 23,* 313–331.

Shapiro, J. R., & Mangelsdorf, S. C. (1994). The determinants of parenting competence in adolescent mothers. *Journal of Youth and Adolescence, 23,* 621–641.

Smith, J., & Brooks-Gunn, J. (1997). Correlates and consequences of harsh discipline for young children. *Archives of Pediatric and Adolescent Medicine, 151,* 777–786.

Smith, S. (Ed.). (1995). *Two generation programs for families in poverty: A new intervention strategy. Advances in applied developmental psychology* (Vol. 9). Norwood, NJ: Ablex.

Sonenstein, F., & Gregory, A. (1995). Teenage childbearing: The trends and their implications. In I. Sawhill (Ed.), *Welfare reform: An analysis of the issues* (pp. 47–50). Washington, DC: The Urban Institute.

Spieker, S., & Bensley, L. (1994). Roles of living arrangements and grandmother social support in adolescent mothering and infant attachment. *Developmental Psychology, 30,* 102–111.

Sroufe, L. A., Jacobvitz, D., Mangelsdorf, S., DeAngelo, E., & Ward, M. J. (1985). Generational boundary dissolution between mothers and their preschool children: A relationship systems approach. *Child Development, 56,* 317–325.

Stevens-Simon, C., & Reichert, S. (1994). Sexual abuse, adolescent pregnancy, and child abuse: A developmental approach to an intergenerational cycle.

Archives of Pediatric and Adolescent Medicine, 148, 23–27.

Stoiber, K. C., & Houghton, T. G. (1993). The relationship of adolescent mothers' expectations, knowledge, and beliefs to their young children's coping behavior. *Infant Mental Health Journal, 14,* 61–70.

Taylor, R. T., Chatters, L. M., & Jackson, J. S. (1993). A profile of familial relations among three-generation black families. *Family Relations, 42,* 332–341.

Testa, M. F. (1992). Racial and ethnic variation in the early life course of adolescent welfare mothers. In M. K. Rosenheim & M. F. Testa (Eds.), *Early parenthood and coming of age in the 1990s* (pp. 89–112). New Brunswick, NJ: Rutgers University Press.

Thompson, M. S., & Peebles-Wilkins, W. (1992). The impact of formal, informal, and societal support networks on the psychological well-being of black adolescent mothers. *Social Work, 37,* 322–327.

Unger, D. G., & Cooley, M. (1992). Partner and grandmother contact in black and white teen parent families. *Journal of Adolescent Health, 13,* 546–552.

Unger, D. G., & Wandersman, L. P. (1985). Social support and adolescent mothers: Action research contributions to theory and application. *Journal of Social Issues, 41,* 29–45.

Unger, D. G., & Wandersman, L. P. (1988). The relation of family and partner support to the adjustment of adolescent mothers. *Child Development, 59,* 1056–1060.

Voight, J., Hans, S., & Bernstein, V. (1996). Support networks of adolescent mothers: Effects on parenting experience and behavior. *Infant Mental Health Journal, 17,* 58–73.

Vondra, J., & Belsky, J. (1993). Developmental origins of parenting: Personality and relationship factors. In T. Luster & L. Okagaki (Eds.), *Parenting: An ecological perspective* (pp. 1–33). Hillsdale, NJ: Erlbaum.

Wadsworth, J., Taylor, B., Osborn, A., & Butler, N. (1984). Teenage mothering: Child development at five years. *Journal of Child Psychology and Psychiatry, 25,* 305–313.

Wakschlag, L., Chase-Landsdale, P. L., & Brooks-Gunn, J. (1996). Not just "Ghosts in the Nursery": Contemporaneous intergenerational relationships and parenting in African-American families. *Child Development, 67,* 2132–2147.

Wakschlag, L., Gordon, R., Lahey, B., Loeber, R., Green, S., & Leventhal, B. (1999). *Maternal age at first birth as a risk factor for conduct disorder in clinic-referred boys.* Manuscript under review.

Wakschlag, L., Pittman, L., Chase-Landsdale, P. L., & Brooks-Gunn, J. (in press). "Mama, I'm a person, too": Individuation and young African-American mothers' parenting competence. In A. M. Cauce & S. Hauser (Eds.), *Adolescence and beyond: Family processes and development.* Mahwah, NJ: Erlbaum.

Ward, M., & Carlson, E. (1995). Associations among adult attachment representations, maternal sensitivity and infant–mother attachment in a sample of adolescent mothers. *Child Development, 66,* 69–79.

Wasserman, G., Brunelli, S., & Rauh, V. (1990). Social supports and living arrangements of adolescent and adult mothers. *Journal of Adolescent Research, 5,* 54–66.

Whiteside-Mansell, L., Pope, S., & Bradley, R. (1996).

Patterns of parenting in young mothers. *Family Relations, 45*, 273–281.

Wilson, M. N., & Tolson, T. F. J. (1988). Single parenting in the context of three-generational black families. In E. M. Hetherington & J. D. Arasteh (Eds.), *Impact of divorce, single parenting, and stepparenting on children* (pp. 213–241). Hillsdale, NJ: Erlbaum.

Zeanah, C. H., Boris, N., & Larrieu, J. (1997). Infant development and developmental risk: A review of the past 10 years. *Journal of the American Academy of Child and Adolescent Psychiatry, 36*, 165–178.

Zeanah, C. H., Keener, M. A., Anders, T. F., & Vieira-Baker, C. C. (1987). Adolescent mothers' perceptions of their infants before and after birth. *American Journal of Orthopsychiatry, 57*, 351–360.

8

Parental Mental Illness and Infant Development

❖

RONALD SEIFER
SUSAN DICKSTEIN

Children whose parents have mental illness are at risk for mental illness and other behavioral problems. This well-known epidemiological phenomenon originally led to studies of children whose parents had mental illness in order to gather evidence regarding the etiology of serious mental disorders (Mednick & McNeil, 1968). The initial work was not satisfying to some developmentalists as the attempts to disentangle influences of constitution and context began with examination of children after several years of developing in disordered family contexts. As the initial blush of enthusiasm for uncovering etiological factors in mental illness has worn off, attention has turned more and more to the interesting developmental processes that high-risk studies might reveal. It has become clear that there are no simple solutions to the problems of understanding the etiology of mental disorder, as high-risk studies have probably raised more questions than they have answered (Watt, Anthony, Wynne, & Rolf, 1984). However, a body of knowledge is emerging regarding differences in development associated with parental mental illness that may have an impact on understanding normative development as well as the development of pathology (Cicchetti, 1984; Sroufe & Rutter, 1984).

In this chapter we review existing knowledge about the development of infants whose parents have mental illness. We begin with a brief re-

view of the general long-term consequences of having a parent with mental disorder. Included in this discussion are theoretical models of intergenerational transmission of illness, identification of parents, and general methodological issues in this area of research. The main sections of the chapter review major developmental processes in infancy with findings specific to children born to mentally ill women. A summary and integration conclude the chapter.

EXAMINING THE CONSEQUENCES OF PARENTAL MENTAL DISORDER FOR INFANT DEVELOPMENT

The most straightforward hypothesis regarding mental illness in parents is that it results in mental illness in their children. There is ample epidemiological evidence to suggest that mental illness does indeed run in families (Weissman et al., 1987; Beardslee, Bemporad, Keller, & Klerman, 1983; Kendler, Neale, Kessler, Heath, & Eaves, 1992). In addition, there is also substantial evidence that parental mental illness is related to other types of negative outcomes in offspring, such as delinquency, poor social adaptations, or cognitive deficits (Watt et al., 1984; Shaw, Owens, Vondra, Keenan, & Winslow, 1996).

Given this range of potential outcomes, researchers are faced with the task of identifying these conditions, or their precursors, during the first years of life. However, application of diagnoses according to the fourth edtition of the *Diagnositc and Statistical Manual of Mental Disorders* (DSM-IV; American Psychiatric Association, 1994) is not useful with infants, with perhaps only one or two diagnoses (such as autism) possible in this age range. Similarly, assessing cognitive status that is predictive of later development is difficult until the end of the second year of life; delinquency will not be manifest until much later in development; social relationships with peers are poorly developed. Thus, when studying the effects of parental mental illness in infants, one is left with the need to study interim outcomes that may be predictive of later dysfunction (Seifer, 1995). Such interim outcomes include parent–child interaction, attachment relationships, developmental quotient, language achievements, temperament, developmental milestones, and biobehavioral regulation (e.g., eating and sleeping).

Unfortunately, little is known about the relation of such interim status variables and the development of later dysfunctional behavior. Most important, it is not clear whether there are specific developmental paths from single interim markers to individual outcomes (e.g., whether nonsecure attachment is related to a diagnosis of depression later in life) (Shaw et al., 1996). Alternatively, developmental relations may be nonspecific and predictive of many possible negative outcomes. For example, nonsecure attachment may predict later problems in a variety of domains, such as mental health, peer relations, and family functioning.

The product of this uncertainty has been to study development of at-risk infants by conducting state-of-the-art assessments of infant status focusing on those domains that have the best chance of predicting later developmental problems. We hope that by demonstrating associations between parental status and patterns of infant development, we also identify key constructs that illuminate the processes of intergenerational transmission of illness and incompetence.

Models of Transmission

Evidence of familial clustering of mental disorder has inevitably led to genetic hypotheses regarding the mechanism of intergenerational transmission (Rosenthal, Wender, Kety, Welner, & Schulsinger, 1971; Kendler et al., 1992). Epidemiological studies routinely demonstrate that mental illness runs in families, with demonstrable clustering according to specific diagnoses or groups of diagnoses, such as depressive disorders or schizophrenic spectrum disorders (Watt, 1984). Further, adoption and cross-fostering studies show that there are rates of disorder among adopted-away offspring of ill parents and adopted children reared by ill parents that relate more to biological parentage than to the context in which the children are reared (Rosenthal et al., 1971).

Despite the wealth of evidence supporting genetic models, it is also clear that these models may explain only a small portion of variance in the development of mental illness. The genetics of mental illness are not simple—the presumed genetic action is polygenic with complex patterns of inheritance (Kendler et al., 1992). To date, any specific markers identified by DNA sequencing studies for mental disorders have not withstood the test of replication (Hodgkinson et al., 1987; Holden, 1991). Although many more children with family history of mental disorder than expected will, themselves, develop mental illness, the vast majority of individuals with mental disorder (including the serious disorders of depression and schizophrenia) do not have a demonstrable family history of the illness. Further, even though there is some tendency for particular disorders to run in families, many, if not most, of the offspring of ill parents have disorders *different* from those of their parents (Downey & Coyne, 1990).

Environmental models posit that differences in the developmental context of children account for the incidence of mental disorder later in life. Factors such as parental disparagement or abuse, family composition, parenting behavior, or social networks have been invoked as explanations (e.g., Downey & Coyne, 1990). Related models identify specific environmental risk factors but indicate that the number of risks is the operative factor rather than the specific type of risk (Sameroff, Seifer, Zax, & Barocas, 1987; Shaw, Keenan, & Vondra, 1994; Walker, Downey, & Bergman, 1989).

The developmental psychopathology model attempts to integrate constitutional and environmental models (Cicchetti & Toth, 1998). Children are viewed as one aspect of a developing system that can be examined at different levels of complexity (biological, individual, social, cultural). In addition, the system is assumed to be dynamic and developing, so that change may be found at any of these levels of analysis. This approach attempts to encompass findings consistent with the other models discussed previously, yet reconcile the fact that none of those models accounts for large portions of variance in predicting the incidence of mental disorders.

Maternal Diagnosis

The vast majority of studies examining infant development in relation to parental mental illness have focused on mothers identified with disorders. This reflects the traditional economies associated with studying mothers versus fathers in developmental research. Most children in single-parent households live with their mothers. Mothers more frequently are responsible for caregiving (especially during the first years of life); they are more accessible to researchers, and perhaps more influential in determining the development of their children. Existing literature has focused on mothers and provides an important reference for replication. An additional factor in the field of transmission of mental illness is also an issue—when genetic models are important to consider, identifying with certainty the biological parentage of mothers is easier than with fathers. Although this list of reasons explains *why* mothers are routinely the focus of these studies, it is not an *endorsement* of that bias.

Whatever position one holds about the emphasis on mothers in this area of research, the fact remains that a review of the literature will focus on *maternal* diagnosis. It should be noted that two areas in which fathers *have* received attention in the offspring of mental illness literature are alcohol abuse and delinquency. However, little effort has been devoted to studying infant offspring of these men, and this is not a focus in this chapter.

One clear pattern in existing studies is that two diagnoses have dominated the field: schizophrenia and depression. This state of affairs is understandable. Schizophrenia, although affecting only 1% of the population, is an enormous public health problem in terms of the suffering of affected individuals, cost to the health care system, and other social implications such as homelessness. Likewise, depression, with its growing incidence, is also a major public health

concern with devastating impact on affected individuals.

Postpartum Depression

Of particular importance in the infancy period is the issue of postpartum depression. Although this diagnosis does not appear in DSM-IV, there is much active research studying the phenomenon as well as its effects on young infants (Murray & Cooper, 1996). Many women (perhaps 50–80% of new mothers) experience dysphoria following childbirth ("baby blues"); about 15% will have postpartum depression. As such, the postpartum period may be especially sensitive for disruptions in mother–infant relationship formation and adequate transition to parenthood (Campbell, Cohn, Flanagan, Popper, & Meyers, 1992). Depression during the postpartum period can best be considered an accident of timing—rates, antecedents, course, and quality of depression during the postpartum period are similar to episodes experienced at other times in a woman's life, perhaps related to negative life events during pregnancy and following delivery (e.g., financial difficulties, unemployment, and poor marital adjustment). The clearest risk factor for postpartum depression is a prior history of major depressive episodes (O'Hara, 1996).

The postpartum period is a time of unrivaled demands and challenges. Even during a normative postpartum experience there are often heightened family and family-of-origin issues associated with the transition to parenthood (Cowan & Cowan, 1992). Adjustments usually need to be made in areas such as sleep schedules, employment, and role allocation. And, even for seasoned parents, there is the adventure of understanding the particular infant's unique style, needs, vulnerabilities, and strengths. The experience of depression during the postpartum period transforms an already challenging process into a potentially overwhelming one. Normative change associated with the postpartum period and the challenges faced by families, including marital discord, may produce difficulty in negotiating this transition. Within this context, many families face the additional risk of postpartum depression.

Interestingly, no studies have focused on fathers' internal experiences during the postpartum transition. It is possible that in typical families, in which new fathers do not significantly alter work schedules, men may experience feelings of exclusion from the initial bonding process, inadequacy regarding caregiving, and distractibility at the workplace. Pruett (1987), in fact, anecdotally described "paternity blues" occurring in the first 3 months postpartum, involving feelings ranging from inadequacy to frustration related to the new paternal role.

Generic Methodological Issues

Before reviewing specific research, it is important to note methodological issues that greatly influence the interpretation of data from these high-risk studies (Seifer, 1995). Unfortunately, because of the difficulty of identifying and studying these families in cross-sectional and longitudinal studies, many suffer from methodological shortcomings that limit interpretation of results. Some of these problems are discussed in the next sections.

Identification of Disorders

The first choice one must make in this research area is the identification of families that will participate in studies. Ascertainment from clinical populations (e.g., clinics and hospital records) and advertising may yield different types of participants based on the details of the recruitment. Variation may be introduced regarding accuracy of diagnosis (when there is reliance on clinical records versus direct assessment of disorder), timing of illness based on when identified episodes occurred, and differences in phenomenology of illness if there is identification of individuals who have never sought treatment.

A related issue is whether diagnosis should be the sole identifier in these high-risk studies. The use of diagnosis as the marker for parental illness presupposes a model of specifically transmitted disorders. Studies that have examined categorical diagnostic descriptions of illness with dimensional symptom-based or severity assessments have found these latter factors useful in predicting additional variance in child development (Sameroff, Seifer, & Zax, 1982; Watt, 1984). From a theoretical perspective, the experience of the infant with a caregiver expressing specific symptoms may be more important (in some circumstances) than whether specific syndromal criteria have been met, although this has not been empirically verified.

Age of Children

Because it is difficult to identify large numbers of families for these high-risk studies, it is sometimes useful to examine children in a wider age range as opposed to children at a single fixed point in development. The obvious advantage of this approach is to maximize the available samples for study. The disadvantage, especially as the age of the children decreases, is that level of development will be a covariate that must be examined consistently and, perhaps, must qualify interpretations. There is also difficulty in generalizing information gained at one assessment age to other ages of interest.

Control Groups

Many studies examine only a group of families where parents have mental illness. Alternatively, studies may have a single control group of families with no illness. Both of the strategies are flawed. In the first case, there is no good way to compare rates of problems found in an identified group with any particular reference. Because researchers are aware of the nature of their population, thresholds for identifying disorder are often set very low, and rates appear high. However, when a no-illness control group is employed, comparably elevated rates are generally found among the control families as well (e.g., Beardslee et al., 1983).

No-illness control groups do not solve all design problems, however. Many factors are associated with specific mental illness diagnoses—chronicity of illness, severity of illness, and specific symptom dimensions (Sameroff et al., 1982; Seifer, 1995). As noted above, there is evidence that the nonspecific illness factors have a strong influence on development in addition to specific diagnostic factors. Finally, in addition to confounded factors of mental illness, many nonillness factors are confounded, such as socioeconomic status (SES), social support, stability of family life, or neighborhood quality. These contextual factors must also be considered (see discussion of multiple risk models in the "Conclusions" section).

Longitudinal Designs

Many high-risk studies follow families over extended periods. This brings up two important interpretation issues. The first involves the analysis and understanding of change or developmental growth. There is increasing realization that models of change over time are relatively primitive in human development research, and that research design and data analysis have not kept pace with theory and model building (Burchinal & Appelbaum, 1991; Willett, 1988). Thus, statements about change over time or causal relations must be accepted with the highest degree of caution. The second issue involves replication of findings. In many instances, replication of a phenomenon occurs in the same study using the same sample at different points in development. Although this evidence is important, it must be interpreted with the understanding that there may be sample specific characteristics driving the finding at both time points, which may not generalize to other samples.

STUDIES OF CHILDREN BORN TO MENTALLY ILL PARENTS

In the last two decades, the impact of parental psychopathology on child outcome has received much attention from researchers in a variety of disciplines. Recent reviews and empirical work (Downey & Coyne, 1990; Cummings & Davies, 1994) provide evidence for the increased risk of child disturbance and parenting difficulty associated with parental psychopathology, especially focusing on maternal depression. These reviews highlight the need to attend to contextual factors (such as psychosocial stress and family relationships) and to carefully assess diagnostic criteria given the heterogeneity of expression of depressive disorder. In this chapter, we focus on the impact of maternal psychopathology during *infancy and early childhood*, emphasizing (1) the impact of pathology on normative developmental processes within the first year of life and (2) its effects in the context of the unique transitions faced by families during this time (i.e., transition to parenthood, change in parental role functioning, and marital relationship changes).

Our bias in organizing the material in this chapter is consistent with a developmental systems perspective on the origins and maintenance of individual pathology. Two basic assumptions are operative. First, early parent–infant interactions are social in nature and provide the primary context in which generalized social skills are learned. Second, infants maintain affective interactions from their earliest

contacts with caregivers, which foster component skills necessary for later, more externally oriented social interactions (Sroufe & Waters, 1977). Four broad domains are reviewed: individual functioning, dyadic interaction, social interaction beyond the dyad, and family context.

Individual Functioning

Although relatively little can be discerned about very young children that is independent of their social contexts, two major domains of individual functioning addressed in the high-risk literature have been developmental status and temperament. In older children, developmental status is typically measured using IQ tests. With younger children, developmental quotients (DQ) are often assessed, even though the correlation with later IQ is relatively low. Temperament also is widely used to assess individual behavior in infants and young children. Both poor performance on DQ tests and difficult temperament are related to adjustment difficulties later in life, although there is little evidence that either is related in important etiological ways to serious mental disorder (Thomas & Chess, 1977; Worland, Edenhart-Pepe, Wecks, & Konnen, 1984).

Related to the temperament domain, children of depressed mothers show evidence of differential emotion processing. Field, Fox, Pickens, and Nawrocki (1995) found right frontal EEG (electroencephalogram) asymmetry during baseline recording, and Dawson, Klinger, Panagiotides, Hill, & Spieker (1992) found similar patterns during mother–infant interaction when compared with children of nondepressed mothers. These findings parallel their own mothers (who varied in a similar manner as a function of depressive symptoms) and other findings with depressed adults (Davidson, Schaefer, & Sron, 1985).

Dyadic Interaction

Human infants engage in species-typical behavior that involves communication with others. Infants, from birth, demonstrate perceptual sensitivities especially oriented toward human stimulation and response organization designed to facilitate contact with people (Newson, 1977). From very early on, parents and infants interact in ways that not only serve to regulate biological functions (e.g., state regulation and feeding) but support social and emotional learning as well (Brazelton, 1979). By the first year of life, organized attachment relationships are an integral part of the dyadic developmental process.

Individual State and Developmental Regulation

One of the fundamental qualities of social interactions is that each participant must be available for social discourse. An important component of this availability in infants is their ability to regulate their own states of arousal and attention. However, if the infant has particular difficulty with internal state regulation, there may be serious consequences for social interaction if the dyad does not adapt well to these state changes. Further, when there is a lack of synchrony in developmental achievements, parents' expectations may be disconfirmed, again resulting in interaction difficulties if the dyad does not adapt well.

Fish (1957, 1971), studying children of schizophrenic mothers, found disturbances of timing and integration of neurological maturation during the infancy period and shifts in periods of acceleration and retardation of motor skills. Marcus, Auerbach, Wilkinson, and Burack (1981) found that infants born to schizophrenic mothers (as compared with mothers with affective disorders, personality disorders, and controls) showed neurointegrative deficits rendering them especially vulnerable to external insults. These infant findings may best be understood when placed in the context of research with older children, which found offspring of schizophrenics to be more impaired by distraction, to have more difficulty paying attention (Harvey, Weintraub, & Neale, 1985), and to have hyperlabile and hypersensitive autonomic functioning (Mednick, Schulsinger, & Venables, 1981). Taken together, the offspring of schizophrenic parents have been shown to have vulnerabilities (which may be biological and/or environmental), affecting their ability to attend to, control, and regulate their social surround.

Interaction Style

Most infants engage in face-to-face interaction by about 6 weeks of age (Trevarthen, 1984). Parents can vary in their sensitivity to the implicit format and rules of the interaction script

and can regulate their rhythm of movement so it is contingent upon the infant's own temporal patterning. Furthermore, they can repeat activity to sustain infant gaze and present information at levels commensurate with the infant's capacities (Fogel, 1977; Trevarthen, 1984; Tronick, Als, & Brazelton, 1980).

Numerous studies have documented that depressed mothers are less contingently responsive, more disengaged, and more negative during dyadic interactions with their infants. In turn, the infants are also less positive and more negative. However, results are not entirely uniform, with some evidence that schizophrenic mothers may have even more distorted interaction patterns.

Many studies with depressed mothers have used the face-to-face paradigm (Tronick, Als, Adamson, Wise, & Brazelton, 1978). This structured interaction involves several 2-minute episodes of free play, "still-face" behavior by the mothers, and free play "reunion." When mothers' behavior was altered systematically by having them maintain a still-faced pose, withhold communication, or present only their profile, infants evidenced distress by looking to their mothers less often and for shorter intervals, frowning, grimacing, pouting, gaze averting, or making strong bids for mothers' attention (Cohn & Tronick, 1983). Infants whose mothers scored high on the Beck Depression Inventory had uniformly lower rates of positive behavior (and higher rates of negative behavior) in face-to-face interaction with their 3- to 6-month-old infants (Field et al., 1988; Field, 1984). The range of behavior included physical activity, head orientation, gaze, facial expression, vocalization, and fussiness. Mothers' physical activity, vocalization, responsivity, and game playing also were different. When examined with a nondepressed caregiver, infant behavior is more normative (Hossain, Field, Gonzalez, Malphurs, & del Valle, 1994).

Among mothers with postpartum depression, many effects have been noted, including decreased eye gaze during feeding, less playfulness and reciprocity, and perception of their infants as more bothersome and troubling with respect to infant care (Field, 1984; Field et al., 1985; Livingood, Daen, & Smith, 1983; Whiffen & Gotlib, 1989). In other studies, depressed mothers and their infants spent more time in matched negative behavior states and less time in matched positive behavior states, when compared with dyads in which the mother was not depressed (Field, Healy, Goldstein, & Guthertz, 1990). Cohn, Campbell, Matias, and Hopkins (1990) confirmed only some of the previous results. Specifically, depressed mothers had higher rates of negative behavior overall. However, lower rates of positive maternal behaviors were found with sons only; no differences in infant behavior were found. In studying the contour of mother vocalization (i.e., the adaptation for young children commonly called motherese), Bettes (1988) found that depressed mothers were less able to adapt their interaction style according to this cultural norm.

In more free-ranging interactions, the impact of maternal depression is less clear. Seifer, Sameroff, Anagnostopolou, and Elias (1992) did not find differences among schizophrenic, depressed, personality disordered, and well mothers on many indices of mother and infant behavior—including spontaneous, responsive, and negative—at both 4 and 12 months of age. In contrast to the lack of mental health effects, SES produced large group effects, and large differences in behavior were observed depending on the situation in which the behavior occurred (caretaking, close, distant). The reports of McNeil, Persson-Blennow, and colleagues describe many comparisons of schizophrenic, affect disordered, and well mothers at six points across the first year of life. Variables examined include positive and negative behaviors, amount of contact, and responsiveness to infant needs. Although there are many significant findings reported for the large variable sets, the number of such findings is about at levels expected by chance. There was little consistency of which variables were significant at different points during the first year. The only consistency was that the schizophrenic group differed from controls more often than other diagnostic groups (bipolar, affective, atypical psychosis) (McNeil, Naslund, Persson-Blennow, & Kaij, 1985; Person-Blennow, Naslund, McNeil, Kaij, & Malmquist-Larsson, 1984; Persson-Blennow, Naslund, McNeil, & Kaij, 1986). Goodman and Brumley (1990), in contrast, found significant differences between schizophrenic and well groups (with depressed generally midway between), indicating less affection, greater anger/hostility, and poorer home environment (as measured by the HOME Inventory). Campbell, Cohn, and Myers (1995) found that disruptions in interaction were associated with chronicity of maternal depression across the first year. In sum, when nonstructured observations are employed, there is only sporadic evidence that children of ill parents have substantially different interaction experiences, compared with children of well parents, during the early years of life. Perhaps the Campbell et al. (1995) finding will prove important in distinguishing those depressed mother–infant dyads that ultimately evidence social difficulties.

Attachment Relationships

One of the results of parent–child interaction during the first year of life is the development of attachment relationships. Using the Strange Situation procedure that includes a series of separations and reunions to activate the attachment system (Ainsworth, Blehar, Waters, & Wall, 1978), attachments are characterized as *secure* (the parent is a secure base for exploration and provides comfort and organization in the face of distress) or *insecure*, with subtypes of *avoidant* (infants actively avoid parents when stressed) and *resistant* (infants display active resistance to physical and social contact when stressed). Also, *disorganized* patterns of attachment have been noted (Main & Solomon, 1990).

Two studies completed by Naslund, Persson-Blennow, McNeil, Kaij, and Malmquist-Larsson (1984a, 1984b) found that infants and their schizophrenic mothers maintained insecure attachment relationships; in addition, these infants demonstrated virtually no fear of strangers (a usual reaction demonstrated by 8- to 12-month-olds). These findings suggest that from early on, infants of schizophrenics, indeed, demonstrate disrupted patterns of interaction with significant and social others.

In several studies, maternal depression has been related to higher rates of insecure attachment (Radke-Yarrow, Cummings, Kuczynski, & Chapman, 1985; Donovan & Leavitt, 1989; Teti, Gelfand, Messenger, & Isabella, 1995; Seifer et al., 1996). Attachment status also was evaluated in the Lyons-Ruth, Connell, Grunebaum, & Botein (1990) study, where three groups of multiple-risk families (treated, untreated, community) were subdivided on whether or not mothers were depressed. Children in the untreated-depressed group had the highest rates of insecure disorganized behavior. However, overall rates on insecure attachments were not markedly different among the groups. Perhaps more striking is the data available for children of bipolar parents. Although only a small number of children have been studied, rates of insecurity are 70–90% (Gaensbauer, Harmon, Cytryn, & McKnew, 1984; DeMulder & Radke-Yarrow, 1991).

Social Interaction beyond the Dyad

Parenting Perceptions and Beliefs

Closely related to how parents and infants behave with each other is how parents understand the meaning of those interactions. Early research on parental beliefs about child difficulties found that depressed mothers tended to overinterpret or distort child behavior as problematic (Rickard, Forehand, Wells, Griest, & McMahon, 1981). General parenting attitudes were also more negative in ill parents (i.e., more authoritarian, more hostile, and less democratic), although diagnostic groups of schizophrenia, depression, and personality disorder could not be distinguished (Sameroff et al., 1982). This study also found that ill mothers (but no specific diagnostic group) had lower expectations for their children's life-course achievement.

More recent work (with older children) has attempted to examine the interplay between maternal illness and child behavior. For example, Brody and Forehand (1986) replicated previous work, finding a main effect for parental illness in ratings of their children's maladjustment. However, they also found an interaction effect, indicating that this phenomenon was limited to those children who evidenced high levels of noncompliance. In a similar vein, Conrad and Hammen (1989) found that teacher- and child-reported child symptoms interacted with maternal symptoms in the prediction of maternal rated child maladjustment; that is, ill mothers with symptomatic children provided more negative assessments than did well mothers with equally problematic children. It is interesting to note that the well mothers did not differentiate among children with and without symptoms, as rated by the children and the teachers. Richters and Pelligrini (1989) compared maternal and teacher report of children in groups of well, depressed, and depressed–remitted mothers. They found differences between well and ill mothers in reports of child maladjustment, but this corresponded with teacher reports. Richters and Pelligrini (1989) argued that depressed mothers do indeed report more child problems but that most evidence supports the idea that these are appropriate (not

distorted) reports (see also Richters, 1992). In sum, the body of evidence regarding distortion in parental reports is small, with conflicting findings. Particularly in younger children, there appear to be consistent findings of some level of distortion that may prove important in understanding developmental outcomes.

From the perspective of maternal satisfaction and control in the role of parent, there are interesting differences among well and affective disordered mothers. Kochanska, Radke-Yarrow, Kuczynski, and Friedman (1987) found that overall satisfaction was equivalent among well, unipolar, and bipolar mothers, but that the unipolar mothers had a more selective pattern—they were more satisfied with cognitive development and less satisfied in the affective and social domains. When beliefs about control were examined, bipolar mothers more often endorsed notions of genetic control of their children's behavior. Also, both bipolar and unipolar mothers attributed uncontrollable causes to their children's behavior more than well mothers.

Despite these many findings, some investigators have indicated that maternal psychopathology is not important in determining links to maternal behavior at all, finding more association with demographic variables. For example, Sameroff et al. (1982) found no effects remaining for either diagnosis or severity of illness after social status was partialled. Teti, Gelfand, and Pompa (1990) examined parenting behaviors, mental health status, demographic factors, and psychosocial measures including stress and self-esteem; they found no evidence that mental health variables in mothers with major depression, dysthymia, and adjustment disorders had any predictive value, although there were no well mothers in this study. Conger, McCarty, Yang, Lahey, and Kropp (1984) also concluded that demographic factors play the dominant role in explaining parenting variables when emotional distress was indexed in abusive and nonabusive parents. Given the diversity of findings, it seems clear that there are no simple associations between maternal depression and parenting styles or beliefs, but, rather, it is likely that a variety of factors interact to produce outcomes. It is further likely that the nature (and number) of these factors will vary according to the developmental stage of the child and family and context within which particular behaviors are observed.

Conflict in Interactions

As infants grow older, one of the important social developmental processes is of separation individuation (Sander, 1980; Erikson, 1950). A common feature of this period, as the child asserts his or her independence, is the development of conflicted interactions between parents and their children, during which issues of parental control strategies are highlighted (Patterson, 1982). The manner in which these issues are negotiated between parents and their children relates to the development of patterns of social interaction, empathy, and aggression (Kochanska, Kuzcynski, & Radke-Yarrow, 1989). It is hypothesized that infants and affectively disordered parents may have special difficulty regulating these interactions due to decreased parental consistency in demands, expectations, and contingencies for behavior (see also Nolen-Hoeksma, Wolfson, Mumme, & Guskin, 1995 for related work with older children).

Kochanska et al. (1987) studied naturally occurring episodes of mother–child conflict in groups of well, unipolar depressed, and bipolar mothers. They found that affectively ill mothers tended to avoid confrontation and did not use compromise resolution strategies. Also, severity of the disorder was a critical factor within the unipolar depressed group—more seriously ill mothers were less likely to achieve compromise resolutions with their infants. On the other hand, more seriously impaired mothers with bipolar disorder were more likely to be nonconfrontational, to ultimately use enforcement rather than negotiated resolution strategies, to have less immediate success, and to initiate unresolvable conflict episodes. They also noted normative trends between 2 to 4 years of age, where mothers become increasingly successful, compromise more, and resort less to the use of power and control. Finally, Kuczynski and colleagues (e.g., Kuczynski, Kochanska, Radke-Yarrow, & Girnius-Brown, 1987; Kuczynski & Kochanska, 1990) have studied children through the preschool years and found trends suggesting that girls are generally more compliant and less defiant than boys, with maternal psychopathology not contributing significantly to group differences. Despite the lack of main effects for the diagnosis of depression, higher severity of depression was related to more child passive noncompliance (Kuczynski & Kochanska, 1990). Expressed emotion (Hooly & Teasdale, 1989) is another manifestation of conflict in family communication. Children who were identified during preschool years as having multiple-risk conditions (including parental mental illness) were more likely to have poor social–emotional outcomes at 13 years, when their mothers had high levels of negative expressed emotion (Seifer, Sameroff, Baldwin, & Baldwin, 1992).

Family Context

Thus far, we have reviewed developmental changes during the first year of life organized primarily around the milestones achieved by the infant. We next review the context within which this development occurs, namely, the family. Recent reports (e.g., Radke-Yarrow, Nottleman, Martinez, Fox, & Blemont, 1992) have stressed the need to be sensitive to factors that covary with a diagnosis of depression— such as marital discord, low SES, and increased psychosocial stress—that may contribute to poor child outcomes. Thus, when studying the effects of depression on young children's development, it is also necessary to consider the context in which this development occurs (Cummings & Davies, 1994). Many important stresses affect families, such as transition to parenthood, marital quality, and psychosocial pressures, all of which may exacerbate the effects of parental mental illness

The quality of the marriage has also been linked to etiology and maintenance of affective disorder (Barnett & Gotlib, 1988). This has been emphasized in treatment approaches to depression and has been considered predictive of relapse of depression, as difficulties in interpersonal interaction manifest as increased negative affect, inequality in decision making, and increased negative perceptions (Fincham, Beach, & Bradbury, 1989; Jacobson, Dobson, Fruzetti, Schmaling, & Salusky, 1991; Hooley & Teasdale, 1989).

The postpartum period is a time in the family's life during which they generally experience increased financial as well as other psychosocial stress or negative life events, which may play a major role in the experience of depression (Coyne & Downey, 1991; Hammen, 1991). Depressed women have ruminative styles of responding to their depression (perhaps prolonging the duration of episodes) and have confidants who displayed more negative speech content (Belsher & Costello, 1991; Nolen-Hoeksema, 1991).

As families with depression have more external stresses, these external stresses may lead to the onset of depressive symptoms. For example, mothers who preferred to be employed but, in fact, remained at home as a primary caregiver reported high rates of depressive symptoms (Hock & DeMeis, 1990). There is also evidence that women who have more parenting and marital stressors have increasing depressive symptoms during the first 6 months postpartum (Boyce, Hickie, & Parker, 1991; Cutrona & Troutman, 1986). To the extent that current illness is the operative factor in transmitting deleterious effects of parental illness to children, any factor that prolongs episodes or other aspects of family-related stress may have adverse consequences for young infants.

Although familial patterns of illness have spurred this general domain of inquiry, it is notable that few studies have examined cross-generation transmission of illness from a family perspective (Cummings & Davies, 1994). Our own work has more recently focused on overall family functioning. A wealth of evidence supports the assertion that family functioning is involved in the etiology and maintenance of depressive disorders in adults (Dickstein, Seifer, Hayden et al., 1998). Of further interest is that it appears to be an important contributor to overall risk in children of ill mothers (Seifer et al., 1996). In fact, in data yet to be published from our ongoing studies of children of ill mothers, family functioning is emerging as perhaps the strongest single predictor of child functioning. When compared in the same analyses with mental illness variables, family functioning has more unique predictive variance, which completely masks the effects of postpartum and lifetime history of depression (Dickstein, Seifer, Magee, & Mirsky, 1998).

SUMMARY AND INTEGRATION

The empirical literature on infants of mentally ill parents has provided many interesting clues to aid our understanding of the intergenerational transmission of illness. However, few domains of functioning have been systematically studied in a manner that yields firm conclusions. Perhaps the most thoroughly covered topic is the area of mother–infant interaction, yet many fundamental questions remain unanswered. Nevertheless, the data that have been accumulated suggest that different models of

family regulation are useful to consider. Models of goodness of fit, affect attunement, mutual regulation, and family transactions are useful in organizing the diversity of findings.

Goodness-of-Fit Model

The "goodness-of-fit" model (Thomas & Chess, 1977) stresses the nature of the temperament–environment interactive process (Radke-Yarrow, 1986). Goodness of fit involves concordance between the expectations of the environment (in this case, the parent) and the infant's abilities, characteristics, and style of behaving. Demands, stresses, and conflicts are inevitable concomitants of the developmental process that occur as new expectations and demands for change accompany progressively higher levels of functioning (Thomas & Chess, 1977). Childhood behavior disturbance is viewed as resulting from excessive stress or conflict involving dissonance between the environment and the child's capacities (Seifer, in press).

Early parent–infant interaction typically involves parental attempts to expand the infant's exposure to the social world. In this view, the infant comes to the world with his or her own level and range of tolerance for stimulation and arousal mechanisms. Thus, the parent (directed by his or her own beliefs, values, expectations, and behavior) "matches" his or her behavior to the infant's state of arousal. Stern (1985) cogently pointed out that mismatches between parent and infant facilitate the broadening of the infant's experience as long as it falls within a tolerated level for the infant. More extreme mismatches are detrimental to infant social and emotional learning.

As we reviewed previously, many of these disruptions in interactive sequences are manifest in dyads where the mother is depressed or otherwise ill. An infant who must consistently deal with social and emotional overstimulation by aversion and crying may, over time, learn a more extreme form of coping involving avoidance, withdrawal, and affective muting. Alternatively, when understimulated, infants must seek out experience and regulate the social–emotional world without requisite developmental skills. Stern (1985) proposed that this results in narrowing the infant's core self due to the decreased input from others. The goodness-of-fit model does not propose an all-or-nothing match between parents and infants. Rather, a parent may be unsympathetic to certain infant characteristics, restrictive about certain activities, and/or unsure with respect to certain child-care responsibilities. On the other hand, the same parent may be accepting, nonrestrictive, and self-confident with respect to other of their child's activities and characteristics. What is crucial in this formulation is the degree to which family systems adapt to the unique characteristics of individual children, and the degree to which flexible resources are appropriately applied to the many difficult developmental tasks, even if our understanding of some of the subtleties is still primitive (Seifer & Schiller, 1995).

Affect Attunement Model

The affect attunement model (e.g., Stern, 1985) builds on the goodness-of-fit model with more emphasis on the details of specific interactions. Attunement involves (1) parental matching (not necessarily imitating) of the infant's internal feeling state, (2) cross modal affective expression between parent and infant, and (3) demonstration of behaviors that express the quality of the shared affect state (Stern, Hofer, Haft, & Dore, 1985). For attunement to occur, the parent must be able to interpret the infant's feeling state from his or her overt behavior and then respond in such a way as to convey emotional resonance with the baby's feelings without directly imitating the baby's behaviors; the infant must be able to understand that the parental response is related to the infant's original feeling experience. Stern (1985) suggested that when the parent is attuned to the baby, behavior continues without disruption. However, if the parent's expressions are above or below the infant's level of intensity or rhythm, the infant will notice the discrepancy and briefly curtail activity. Interpersonal communication, as created by attunement, promotes infants coming to recognize shared internal feeling states and the rules of social discourse. The converse is also true; feeling states that are never attuned will not become part of the infant's developing repertoire.

In studies reviewed earlier, these qualities promoting affect attunement were apparently deficient in children with their ill parents. Dyadic interaction is distorted; conflicts in interactions are more common; parenting attitudes may be distorted; marital discord or psychosocial stressors may create a negative affective climate in which this attunement occurs. One especially intriguing finding was that the cultural norm of communicating with infants in "motherese" was less apparent in ill mothers.

Mutual Regulation Model

The mutual regulation model (Tronick, Cohn, & Shea, 1986) emphasizes infant initiation and regulation of the social interaction. The affect attunement and mutual regulation models are similar in the assumption that the infant's emotions serve to coordinate social communication; however, whereas the affect attunement model stresses parental matching of the infant's inner subjective state (independent of the infant's overt behavior); the mutual regulation model conceptualizes the infant's activity and affect as interdependent, with the infant as much in control of the social exchange as the parent. This model involves the infant acting to deploy emotional signals in an attempt to control the social environment. If the infant successfully controls the situation (i.e., gets the parent to interact reciprocally), positive emotions are generated and the infant gains a sense of effectance; if, however, the infant fails to control the situation, negative emotions are generated, and the infant experiences a sense of helplessness. The infant's success and failure depends, in part, on the cooperation, sensitivity, and responsiveness of the parent.

Both parents and infants experience social successes and failures. Whereas an infant's reactions are largely affected by immediate external and internal stimuli, a parent's reactions are more affected by historical and social factors that modify the parent's self-esteem and, thus, his or her interactions with the infant. When parents come to the interaction with positive historical social experiences, sensitivity to infants will likely be increased; when parents have had negative historical experiences, behavior is likely to be disorganized and less sensitive. Thus, the parent's reactions to the infant contribute to the infant's sense of effectance.

Similar to the goodness-of-fit model, this model of effectance (1) highlights the interdependence of the temperamental or personality factors of the parent and the infant and (2) predicts positive consequences for some amount of interactive dysyncrony between the parent and infant; that is, the infant is provided with an opportunity to renegotiate the interaction, from which renewed feelings of effectance can emerge.

We reviewed several studies that indicated that infants and young children of ill parents are compromised in their ability to regulate their own activity and regulate social interactions. Further, their developmental trajectories may not be as well regulated as those of children from nonill families. These deficits in regulatory processes in children with ill parents may serve as risks for less than optimal development. This lack of infant regulatory abilities may place extra, unrecognized burdens on the parents who may be least able to effectively adapt to those needs.

Transactions

The transactional model provides a broader framework within which to place the previously described family regulation models. A transactional model posits infants who actively work to regulate their social and emotional world, an environment in which these infants perform this work, and relationships of mutual influence and change between infants and their environments. Successful predictions regarding long-range (and more immediate) developmental outcomes cannot be made on the basis of a continuum of *reproductive* casualty alone (e.g., birth complications or potential genetic contribution of parental mental illness). An equally important continuum of *caretaking* casualty exists that moderates the reproductive casualty (Sameroff & Chandler, 1975). Thus, important aspects include (1) the degree of match between the infant and environment, in which the infant can restrict and/or expand his or her own boundaries, and (2) the extent to which interactions within the environment reflect versus contradict the infant's internal experiences.

Wynne (1968) stressed three important issues regarding the transactional viewpoint (also see Sameroff, 1980). First, behavior must be considered within the context in which it occurs. Second, internal change (within infant and parent) results from interchange with others; thus, both parents and infants exhibit behavioral and emotional responses that have emerged as an adaptation to their environment. Finally, the family system strives for homeostasis; if the transactions at any given developmental phase are distorted or omitted, all subsequent developmental phases are altered. The (mal)adaptive specificity of particular events or behaviors will vary with each individual developmental course (Wynne, 1968).

Multiple-Risk Models

An offshoot of the transactional approach is a model of risk that simultaneously considers multiple sources of risk and attends to the number, rather than specificity, of risk factors (Sameroff et al., 1987; Seifer et al., 1996). In the absence of the ability to actively trace the individual developments within dyads that a full implementation of the transactional model would involve, an interim prediction is that (1) more risk factors would increase the probability of the establishment of negative transactional processes and the inability to self-correct the developing system, (2) the nature of the risk is relatively unimportant because perturbation in relationships may be caused by many different events, (3) specific outcomes would be related to general (not specific) risk because families may adapt well to some perturbations but not to others, and (4) specific risks may be related to many different types of negative outcomes because of the individuality of transactional processes.

This model is consistent with the many qualifications attached to research findings reviewed in children of ill parents. Small portions of variance in child behavior or outcome are explained by any single risk factor. Instead, we propose that many risks must be considered simultaneously with the risk of parental illness. Such risks include, among others, interaction disturbances, parenting beliefs, marital conflict, or poverty. The cumulative nature of the risk will best explain the developmental outcomes of children at risk because of parental illness (Seifer 1995; Shaw et al., 1996; Teti et al., 1990)

Conclusions

To conclude, we summarize important findings that (1) have been established in high-quality studies and (2) have some degree of replication. We developed the list that follows for the first edition of this handbook—little substantive change has occurred in the field to warrant significant alteration of these assertions, beyond having a larger empirical base on which to base the claims. The major new addition to this list is the importance of overall family functioning.

- Children whose parents have mental illness are themselves at increased risk for mental health problems.

- Maternal depression and schizophrenia are associated with other risk factors (such as psychosocial stress, poverty, or marital difficulty), which heightens poor outcomes.
- Depressed mothers are less positive and more negative when interacting with their infants (at least in structured laboratory situations).
- Infants of depressed mothers are likewise less positive and more negative when interacting with their mothers in these laboratory protocols and, perhaps, when interacting with other adults.
- Insecure attachment is more common in children of ill parents.
- Conflict between parent and child is more prevalent in families in which a parent is ill.
- Overall family functioning may be an important moderator of intergenerational transmission of illness.
- Young children of depressed mothers tend to be more impulsive and have more difficult peer interactions.
- Depressed mothers view their children's behavior more negatively than do well mothers, but this may result from having children who, in fact, demonstrate more difficult behavior.

REFERENCES

Ainsworth, M. D. S., Blehar, M. C., Waters, E., & Wall, S. (1978). *Patterns of attachment: A psychological study of the strange situation.* Hillsdale, NJ: Erlbaum.

American Psychiatric Association. (1994). *Diagnostic and statistical manual of mental disorders* (4th ed.). Washington, DC: Author.

Barnett, P. A., & Gottlib, I. H. (1988). Psychosocial functioning and depression: Distinguishing among antecedents, concomitants, and consequences. *Psychological Bulletin, 104,* 97–126.

Beardslee, W. R., Bemporad, J., Keller, M. B., & Klerman, G. L. (1983). Children of parents with major affective disorder: A review. *American Journal of Psychiatry, 140,* 825–832.

Belsher, G., & Costello, C. G. (1991). Do confidants of depressed women provide less social support than confidants of nondepressed women? *Journal of Abnormal Psychology, 100,* 516–525.

Bettes, B. A. (1988). Maternal depression and motherese: Temporal and intonational features. *Child Development, 59,* 1089–1096.

Boyce, P., Hickie, I., & Parker, G. (1991). Parents, partners or personality? Risk factors for post-natal depression. *Journal of Affective Disorders, 21,* 245–255.

Brazelton, T. B. (1979). Evidence of communication in neonatal behavioral assessment. In M. Bullowa (Ed.),

Before speech: The beginning of interpersonal communication (pp. 79–88). Cambridge, UK: Cambridge University Press.

Brody, G. H., & Forehand, R. (1986). Maternal perceptions of child maladjustment as a function of the combined influence of child behavior and maternal depression. *Journal of Consulting and Clinical Psychology, 54,* 237–240.

Burchinal, M., & Appelbaum, M. I. (1991). Estimating individual developmental functions: Methods and their assumptions. *Child Development, 63,* 23–43.

Campbell, S. B., Cohn, J. F., Flanagan, C., Popper, S., & Meyers, T. (1992). Course and correlates of postpartum depression during the transition to parenthood. *Development and Psychopathology, 4,* 29–47.

Campbell, S. B., Cohn, J. F., & Meyers, T. (1995). Depression in first-time mothers: Mother-infant interaction and depression chronicity. *Developmental Psychology, 31,* 349–357.

Cicchetti, D. (1984). The emergence of developmental psychopathology. *Child Development, 55,* 1–8.

Cicchetti, D., & Toth, S. L. (1998). Perspectives on research and practice in developmental psychopathology. In W. Damon (Ed.), *Handbook of child psychology: Vol. 4. Child psychology in practice* (5th ed., pp. 479–584). New York: Wiley.

Cohn, J. F., Campbell, S. B., Matias, R., & Hopkins, J. (1990). Face-to-face interactions of postpartum depressed and nondepressed mother infant pairs at 2 months. *Developmental Psychology, 26,* 15–23.

Cohn, J. F., & Tronick, E. Z. (1983). Three-month-old infants' reaction to stimulated maternal depression. *Child Development, 54,* 185–193.

Conger, R. D., McCarty, J. A., Yang, R. K., Lahey, B. B., & Kropp, J. P. (1984). Perception of child, child-rearing values, and emotional distress as mediating links between environmental stressors and observed maternal behavior. *Child Development, 55,* 2234–3347.

Conrad, M., & Hammen, C. (1989). Role of maternal depression in perceptions of child maladjustment. *Journal of Consulting and Clinical Psychology, 57,* 633–667.

Cowan, C. P., & Cowan, P. A. (1992). *When partners become parents: The big life change for couples.* New York: Basic Books.

Coyne, J. C., & Downey, G. (1991). Social factors and psychopathology, stress, social support, and coping processes. *Annual Review of Psychology, 41,* 401–425.

Cummings, E. M., & Davies, P. T. (1994). Maternal depression and child development. *Journal of Child Psychology and Psychiatry, 35,* 73–112.

Cutrona, C. E., & Troutman, C. R. (1986). Social support, infant temperament, and parenting self-efficacy: A mediational model of postpartum depression. *Child Development, 75,* 1507–1518.

Davidson, R. J., Schaefer, C. E., & Sron, C. (1985). Effects of lateralized presentation of faces on self-reports of emotion and EEG asymmetry in depressed and non-depressed subjects. *Psychophysiology, 22,* 353–364.

Dawson, G., Klinger, L. G., Panagiotides, H., Hill, D., & Spieker, S. (1992). Frontal lobe activity and affective behavior of infants of mothers with depressive symptoms. *Child Development*, *63*, 725–737.

DeMulder, E. K., & Radke-Yarrow, M. (1991). Attachment with affectively ill and well mothers: Concurrent behavioral correlates. *Development and Psychopathology*, *3*, 227–242.

Dickstein, S., Seifer, R., Hayden, L. C., Schiller, M., Sameroff, A. J., Keitner, G., Miller, I., Rasmussen, S., Matzko, M., & Dodge-Magee, K. (1998). Levels of family assessment. II: Impact of maternal psychopathology on family functioning. *Journal of Family Psychology*, *12*(1), 23–40.

Dickstein, S., Seifer, R., Magee, K. D., & Mirsky, E. (1998, June). *Timing of maternal depression, family functioning, and child development (prospective view)*. Paper presented at the Biennial Meeting of the Marce Society, Iowa City, IA.

Donovan, W. L., & Leavitt, L. A. (1989). Maternal self-efficacy and infant attachment: Integrating physiology, perceptions, and behavior. *Child Development*, *60*, 460–472.

Downey, G., & Coyne, J. C. (1990). Children of depressed parents. *Psychological Bulletin*, *108*, 50–76.

Erikson, E. H. (1950). *Childhood and society*. New York: Norton.

Field, T. M. (1984). Early interactions between infants and their postpartum depressed mothers. *Infant Behavior and Development*, *7*, 517–522.

Field, T. M., Fox, N. A., Pickens, J., & Nawrocki, T. (1995). Relative right frontal EEG activation in 3- to 6-month-old infants of "depressed" mothers. *Developmental Psychology*, *31*, 358–363.

Field, T. M., Healy, B., Goldstein, S., & Guthertz, M. (1990). Behavior-state matching and synchrony in mother-infant interactions of nondepressed versus depressed dyads. *Development Psychology*, *26*, 7–14.

Field, T. M., Healy, B., Goldstein, S., Perry, S., Bendell, D., Schanberg, S., Zimmerman, E. A., & Kuhn, C. (1988). Infants of depressed mothers show "depressed" behavior even with nondepressed adults. *Child Development*, *59*, 1569–1579.

Field, T. M., Sandberg, D., Garcia, R., Vega-Lahr, N., Goldstein, S., & Guy, L. (1985). Pregnancy problems, postpartum depression, and early mother-infant interactions. *Developmental Psychology*, *21*, 1152–1156.

Fincham, F. D., Beach, S. R. H., & Bradbury, T. N. (1989). Marital distress, depression, and early mother-infant interactions. *Development Psychology*, *57*, 768–771.

Fish, B. (1957). The detection of schizophrenia in infancy. *Journal of Nervous and Mental Disease*, *125*, 1–24.

Fish, B. (1971). Contributions of developmental research to a theory of schizophrenia. In J. Hellmuth (Ed.), *Exceptional infant: Studies of abnormalities* (pp. 473–483). New York: Brunner/Mazel.

Fogel, A. (1977). Temporal organization in mother-infant face-to-face interaction. In H. R. Schaffer (Ed.), *Studies in mother-infant interaction* (pp. 119–152). New York: Academic Press.

Gaensbauer, T. J., Harmon, R. J., Cytryn, L., & McKnew, D. H. (1984). Social and affective development in infants with a manic-depressive parent. *American Journal of Psychiatry*, *141*(2), 223–229.

Goodman, S. H., & Brumley, H. E. (1990). Schizophrenic and depressed mothers: Relational deficits in parenting. *Developmental Psychology*, *26*, 31–39.

Hammen, C. (1991). Generalization of stress in the course of unipolar depression. *Journal of Abnormal Psychology*, *100*, 555–561.

Harvey, P. D., Weintraub, S., & Neale, J. M. (1985). Short report: Span of apprehension deficits in children vulnerable to psychopathology: A failure to replicate. *Journal of Abnormal Psychology*, *94*, 410–413.

Hock, E., & DeMeis, D. K. (1990). Depression in mothers of infants: The role of maternal employment. *Developmental Psychology*, *26*, 285–291.

Hodgkinson, S., Sherrington, R., Gurling, H., Marchbanks, R., Peeders, S., Mallet, J., McInnis, M., Petersson, H., & Brynjolfsson, J. (1987). Molecular genetic evidence for heterogeneity in manic depression. *Nature, 325*, 805–806.

Holden, C. (1991). Probing the complex genetics of alcoholism. *Science*, *251*, 163–164.

Hooley, J. M., & Teasdale, J. D. (1989). Predictors of relapse in unipolar depressives: Expressed emotion, marital distress, and perceived criticism. *Journal of Abnormal Psychology*, *98*, 229–235.

Hossain, Z., Field, T., Gonzalez, J., Malphurs, J. E., & del Valle, C. (1994). Infants of "depressed" mothers interact better with their nondepressed fathers. *Infant Mental Health Journal*, *15*, 348–357.

Jacobson, N. S., Dobson, K., Fruzzetti, A. E., Schmaling, K. B., & Salusky, S. (1991). Marital therapy as a treatment for depression. *Journal of Consulting and Clinical Psychology*, *59*, 547–557.

Kendler, K. S., Neale, M. C., Kessler, R. C., Heath, A. C., & Eaves, L. J. (1992). Major depression and generalized anxiety disorder: Same genes, (partly) different environments? *Archives of General Psychiatry*, *49*, 716–722.

Kochanska, G., Kuczynski, L., & Radke-Yarrow, M. (1989). Correspondence between mothers; self-reported and observed child-rearing practices. *Child Development*, *60*, 56–63.

Kochanska, G., Radke-Yarrow, M., Kuczynski, L., & Friedman, S. L. (1987). Normal and affectively ill mothers' beliefs about their children. *American Journal of Orthopsychiatry*, *57*, 345–350.

Kuczynski, L., & Kochanska, G. (1990). Development of children's noncompliance strategies from toddlerhood to age 5. *Developmental Psychology*, *26*, 398–408.

Kuczynski, L., Kochanska, G., Radke-Yarrow, M., & Girnius-Brown, O. (1987). A developmental interpretation of young children's noncompliance. *Developmental Psychology*, *23*, 799–806.

Livingood, A. B., Daen, P., & Smith, B. D. (1983). The depressed mother as a source of stimulation for her infant. *Journal of Clinical Psychology*, *39*, 369–375.

Lyons-Ruth, K., Connell, D. B., Grunebaum, H. U., & Botein, S. (1990). Infants at social risk: Maternal depression and family support services as mediators of infant developments and security of attachment. *Child Development*, *61*, 85–98.

Main, M., & Solomon, J. (1990). Procedures for identifying infants as disorganized/disoriented during the Ainsworth Strange Situation. In M. T. Greenberg, D. Cicchetti, & E. M. Cummings (Eds.), *Attachment in the preschool years: Theory, research, and intervention* (pp. 121–160). Chicago: University of Chicago Press.

Marcus, J., Auerbach, J., Wilkinson, L., & Burack, C. M. (1981). Infants at risk for schizophrenia. *Archives of General Psychiatry, 38*, 703–713.

McNeil, T. F., Naslund, B., Persson-Blennow, I., & Kaij, L. (1985). Offspring of women with nonorganic psychosis: Mother–infant interaction at three-and-a-half and six months of age. *Acta Psychiatrica Scandinavica, 71*, 551–558.

Mednick, S. A., & McNeil, T. F. (1968). Current methodology in research on the etiology of schizophrenia: Serious difficulties which suggest the use of the high-risk group method. *Psychological Bulletin, 70*, 681–693.

Mednick, S. A., Schulsinger, F., & Venables, P. H. (1981). A fifteen-year follow-up of children with schizophrenic mothers (Denmark). In S. A. Mednick & A. E. Baert (Eds.), *Prospective longitudinal research: An empirical basis for the primary prevention of psychosocial disorders* (pp. 286–295). Oxford, UK: Oxford University Press.

Murray, L., & Cooper, P. J. (Eds.). (1997). *Postpartum depression and child development*. New York: Guilford Press.

Naslund, B., Persson-Blennow, I., McNeil, T. F., Kaij, L., & Malmquist-Larsson, A. (1984a). Offspring of women with nonorganic psychosis: Fears of strangers during the first year of life. *Acta Psychiatrica Scandinavica, 69*, 435–444.

Naslund, B., Persson-Blennow, I., McNeil, T. F., Kaij, L., & Malmquist-Larsson, A. (1984b). Offspring of women with nonorganic psychosis: Infant attachment to the mother at one year of age. *Acta Psychiatrica Scandinavica, 69*, 231–241.

Newson, J. (1977). An inter-subjective approach to the description of mother–infant interaction. In H. R. Schaffer (Ed.), *Studies in mother–infant interaction* (pp. 47–61). London: Academic Press.

Nolen-Hoeksema, S. (1991). Responses to depression and their effects on the duration of depressive episodes. *Journal of Abnormal Psychology, 100*, 569–582.

Nolen-Hoeksema, S., Wolfson, A., Mumme, D., & Guskin, K. (1995). Helplessness in children of depressed and nondepressed mothers. *Developmental Psychology, 31*, 377–387.

O'Hara, M. W. (1996). The nature of postpartum depressive disorders. In L. Murray & P. J. Cooper (Eds.), *Postpartum depression and child development* (pp. 3–31). New York: Guilford Press.

Patterson, G. R. (1982). *A social learning approach to family intervention* (Vol. 3). Eugene, OR: Castalia.

Persson-Blennow, I., Naslund, B., McNeil, T. F., & Kaij, L. (1986). Offspring of women with nonorganic psychosis: Mother–infant interaction at one year of age. *Acta Psychiatrica Scandinavica, 73*, 207–213.

Persson-Blennow, I., Naslund, B., McNeil, T. F., Kaij, L., & Malmquist-Larsson, A. (1984). Offspring of women with nonorganic psychosis: Mother–infant interaction at three days of age. *Acta Psychiatrica Scandinavica, 70*, 149–159.

Pruett, K. D. (1987). *The nurturing father*. New York: Warner.

Radke-Yarrow, M. (1986). Affective development in young children. In T. B. Brazelton & M. W. Yogman (Eds.), *Affective development in infancy*. Norwood, NJ: Ablex.

Radke-Yarrow, M., Cummings, E. M., Kuczynski, L., & Chapman, M. (1985). Patterns of attachment in two- and three-year-olds in normal families and families with parental depression. *Child Development, 56*, 884–893.

Radke-Yarrow, M., Nottleman, E., Martinez, P., Fox, N. B., & Blemont, B. (1992). Young children of affectively ill parents: A longitudinal study of psychosocial development. *Journal of the American Academy of Child and Adolescent Psychiatry, 31*, 68–77.

Richters, J. (1992). Depressed mothers as informants about their children: A critical review of the evidence for distortion. *Psychological Bulletin, 11*(3), 485–499.

Richters, J., & Pellegrini, D. (1989). Depressed mothers' judgments about their children: An examination of the depression-distortion hypothesis. *Child Development, 60*, 1068–1075.

Rickard, K. M., Forehand, R., Wells, K. C., Griest, D. L., & McMahon, R. J. (1981). A comparison of mothers of clinic-referred deviant, clinic-referred non-deviant, and non-clinic children. *Behaviour Research and Therapy, 19*, 201–205.

Rosenthal, D., Wender, P. H., Kety, S. S., Welner, J., & Schulsinger, F. (1971). The adopted-away offspring of schizophrenics. *American Journal of Psychiatry, 123*, 307–311.

Sameroff, A. J. (1980). Issues in early reproductive and caretaking risk: Review and current status. In D. B. Sawin, R. C. Hawkins, L. O. Walker, & J. H. Penticuff (Eds.), *Exceptional infant: Psychosocial risks in infant–environment transactions* (Vol. 4, pp. 343–359). New York: Brunner/Mazel.

Sameroff, A. J., & Chandler, M. (1975). Reproductive risk and the continuum of caretaking casualty. In F. D. Horowitz, E. M. Hetherington, S. Scarr-Salapatek, & G. Siegel (Eds.), *Review of child development research* (vol. 4, pp. 187–244). Chicago: University of Chicago Press.

Sameroff, A. J., Seifer, R., & Zax, M. (1982). Early development of children at risk for emotional disorder. *Monographs of the Society for Research in Child Development, 47*(7, Serial No. 199).

Sameroff, A. J., Seifer, R., Zax, M., & Barocas, R. (1987). Early indicators of developmental risk: The Rochester Longitudinal Study. *Schizophrenia Bulletin, 13*, 383–394.

Sander, L. W. (1980). New knowledge about the infant from current research: Implications for psychoanalysis. *Journal of the American Psychoanalytic Association, 28*, 181–192.

Seifer, R. (1995). Perils and pitfalls of high risk research. *Developmental Psychology, 31*, 420–424.

Seifer, R. (in press). Temperament and goodness of fit: Implications for developmental psychopathology. In

M. Lewis & A. J. Sameroff (Eds.), *Handbook of developmental psychopathology*. New York: Plenum.

Seifer, R., Sameroff, A. J., Anagnostopolou, R., & Elias, P. K. (1992). Mother–infant interaction during the first year: Effects of situation, maternal mental illness and demographic factors. *Infant Behavior and Development, 15*, 405–426.

Seifer, R., Sameroff, A. J., Baldwin, C. P., & Baldwin, A. (1992). Child and family factors that ameliorate risk between 4 and 13 years of age. *Journal of the American Academy of Child and Adolescent Psychiatry, 31*, 893–903.

Seifer, R., Sameroff, A. J., Dickstein, S., Keitner, G., Miller, I., Rasmussen, S., & Hayden, L. C. (1996). Parental psychopathology, multiple contextual risks, and one-year outcomes in children. *Journal of Clinical Child Psychology, 25*, 423–435.

Seifer, R., & Schiller, M. (1995). The role of parenting sensitivity, infant temperament, and dyadic interaction in attachment theory and assessment. In E. Waters, B. E. Vaughn, G. Posada, & K. Kondo-Ikemura (Eds.), Caregiving, cultural, and cognitive perspective on secure-base behavior and working models: New growing points of attachment theory and research. *Monographs of the Society for Research in Child Development, 60,* (Serial No. 244) pp. 146–174.

Shaw, D. S., Keenan, K., & Vondra, J. I. (1994). Developmental precursors of externalizing behavior: Ages 1 to 3. *Developmental Psychology, 30*, 355–364.

Shaw, D. S., Owens, E. B., Vondra, J. I., Keenan, K., & Winslow, E. B. (1996). Early risk factors and pathways in the development of early disruptive behavior problems. *Development and Psychopathology, 8*, 679–699.

Sroufe, L. A., & Rutter, M. (1984). The domain of developmental psychopathology. *Child Development, 55,* 17–29.

Sroufe, L. A., & Waters, E. (1977). Attachment as an organizational construct. *Child Development, 48*, 1184–1199.

Stern, D. N. (1985). *The interpersonal world of the infant.* New York: Basic Books.

Stern, D. N., Hofer, L., Haft, W., & Dore, J. (1985). Affect attunement: The sharing of feeling states between mother and infant by means of inter-modal fluency. In T. M. Field & N. A. Fox (Eds.), *Social perception in infants* (pp. 249–268). Norwood, NJ: Ablex.

Teti, D. M., Gelfand, D. M., Messinger, D. S., & Isabella, R. (1995). Maternal depression and the quality of early attachment: An examination of infants, preschoolers, and their mothers. *Developmental Psychology, 31*, 364–376.

Teti, D., Gelfand, D. M., & Pompa, J. (1990, April). *Differences in depressed mothers' ability to parent: Maternal, infant and environmental correlates.* Poster presented at the Seventh International Conference on Infant Studies, Montreal.

Thomas, A., & Chess, S. (1977). *Temperament and development.* New York: Brunner/Mazel.

Trevarthen, C. (1984). Emotions in infancy: Regulators of contact and relationships with persons. In K. R. Scherer & P. Ekman (Eds), *Approaches to emotion* (pp. 129–157). Hillsdale, NJ: Lawrence Erlbaum.

Tronick, E. Z., Als, H., Adamson, L., Wise, S., & Brazelton, T. B. (1978). The infant's response to entrapment between contradictory messages in face-to-face interaction. *Journal of the American Academy of Child Psychiatry, 17,* 1–13.

Tronick, E. Z., Als, H., & Brazelton, T. B. (1980). Monadic phases: A structural descriptive analysis of infant–mother face-to-face interaction. *Merrill–Palmer Quarterly, 26*, 3–24.

Tronick, E. Z., Cohen, J., & Shea, E. (1986). The transfer of affect between mothers and infants. In T. B. Brazelton & M. W. Yogman (Eds.), *Affective development in infancy* (pp. 11–25). Norwood, NJ: Ablex.

Walker, E., Downey, G., & Bergman, A. (1989). The effects of parental psychopathology and maltreatment on child behavior: A test of the diathesis–stress model. *Child Development, 60*, 15–24.

Watt, N. F. (1984). In a nutshell: The first two decades of high-risk research in schizophrenia. In N. F. Watt, E. J. Anthony, L. C. Wynne, & J. Rolf (Eds.), *Children at risk for schizophrenia: A longitudinal perspective* (pp. 572–795). Cambridge, UK: Cambridge University Press.

Watt, N. F., Anthony, E. J., Wynne, L. C., & Rolf, J. (1984). *Children at risk for schizophrenia: A longitudinal perspective.* Cambridge, UK: Cambridge University Press.

Weissman, M. M., Gammon, G. D., John, K., Merikangas, K. R., Warner, V., Prusoff, B. A., & Sholomskas, D. (1987). Children of depressed parents. *Archives of General Psychiatry, 44*, 847–852.

Whiffen, V. E., & Gottlib, I. H. (1989). Infants of postpartum depressed mothers: Temperament and cognitive status. *Journal of Abnormal Psychology, 98*, 274–279.

Willett, J. B. (1988). Questions and answers in the measurement of change. In E. Z. Rothkopf (Ed.), *Review of research in education* (Vol. 15, pp. 345–422). Washington, DC: American Education Research Association.

Worland, J., Edenhart-Pepe, R., Weeks, D. G., & Konnen, P. M. (1984). Cognitive evaluation of children at risk: IQ, differentiation, and egocentricity. In N. F. Watt, E. J. Anthony, L. C. Wynne, & J. Rolf (Eds.), *Children at risk for schizophrenia: A longitudinal perspective* (pp. 148–159). Cambridge, UK: Cambridge University Press.

Wynne, L. C. (1968). Methodologic and conceptual issues in the study of schizophrenics and their families. In D. Rosenthal & S. S. Kety (Eds), *The transmission of schizophrenia* (pp. 185–199). Oxford, UK: Pergamon Press.

9

Maternal Substance Abuse and Child Outcome

❖

BARRY M. LESTER
C. F. ZACHARIAH BOUKYDIS
JEAN E. TWOMEY

INTRODUCTION

The problem of cocaine use by pregnant women gained national attention in the mid-1980s and was considered to be an epidemic with the expectation of devastating consequences for cocaine-exposed children. Early reports led to the fear that these children were brain damaged and intellectually and socially impaired. However, these early reports were exaggerated and led to a "rush to judgment" about the long-term outcome of these children (Mayes, Granger, Bornstein, & Zuckerman, 1992). The recent evidence has presented a different picture suggesting that the effects of cocaine are more subtle (Lester, 1998; Lester, LaGasse, & Brunner, 1997; Lester, LaGasse, & Seifer, 1998). This has led to a new controversy: that cocaine may not be as harmful as initially thought. This controversy has enormous implications for public policy and treatment as well as for our scientific understanding of the toxicity of cocaine.

EPIDEMIOLOGY

Although the use of cocaine by the general public may have decreased, estimates for pregnant women, especially poor, minority, inner-city pregnant women have not changed substantially since the mid-1980s. Current nationally cited estimates report that 5.5% of all pregnant women use an illicit drug during pregnancy (National Institute on Drug Abuse [NIDA], 1996). The prevalence rate for cocaine is approximately 1.1%, or 45,000 cocaine-exposed infants born per year. The U.S. General Accounting Office (GAO; 1990) reported to Congress that between 100,000 and 375,000 pregnant women use illicit drugs each year. Different estimates of the number of cocaine-using pregnant women are due, in part, to the methods used to identify drug use during pregnancy. The National Pregnancy and Health Study (NPHS) estimates that 45,000 cocaine-exposed children are born each year is based on maternal self-report. However, the NPHS also found significant underreporting in its sample when maternal self-report was compared with urine toxicology results. On the other hand, the GAO used reviewed hospital records, but the hospitals in that study were selected because of suspected high cocaine use. Estimates of opiate use during pregnancy indicate that as many as 10,000 children per year are affected (Bays, 1990).

Drug use is also related to demographic factors. Estimated use of illicit drugs during pregnancy is nearly three times higher among

161

African American women (12.6%) than it is among Hispanic (4.6%) and white women (4.4%). Specifically, cocaine use among African American women is estimated at 5.1%, compared to much lower rates for whites (0.4%) and Hispanics (0.7%) (NIDA, 1996).

In addition, there is increasing concern for children born into and raised in households where drug addiction is present (NIDA, 1996). The National Committee for the Prevention of Child Abuse (Bays, 1990) estimated that 10 million children in the United States are being raised by addicted parents. Also, according to this report, at least 675,000 children each year are seriously mistreated by a drug abusing or alcoholic caretaker.

DATABASE OF PUBLISHED STUDIES

It is well documented that the literature on the effects of prenatal cocaine exposure shows an inconsistent pattern of findings. There is inconsistency in reported findings between animal and human studies in maternal pregnancy effects, newborn medical effects, and developmental outcome. Some studies show effects of cocaine on child behavior and development, whereas other studies show no effects. As mentioned earlier, these inconsistencies can be attributed to overzealous interpretation of results based on few actual findings. Another interpretation is that studies are limited by methodological problems.

Concerns about the published literature on prenatal cocaine exposure and child outcome led us to develop a computerized database of characteristics and findings of past and current studies that provides an ongoing record of the literature (Lester et al., 1997). The database can be used to summarize and compare the literature, resulting in a more objective understanding of the findings, as well as to identify methodological problems in order to shape the direction of future studies.

Our most recent review includes 118 studies in the database published from 1985 through August 1997 (Lester et al., 1997). Another additional 52 studies were excluded for methodological reasons. The method includes a literature search from Medline and Psyclit. We reviewed each article to determine eligibility for inclusion in the final database contingent upon the inclusion criteria described below. We then abstracted, coded, and entered information from the articles into the database. We defined variables that represented either characteristics of the study, such as sample size, or method of drug detection or behavioral outcomes, such as IQ score. We then generated summary statistics across studies. We used seven criteria to identify studies to be included in the final database: (1) cocaine use during pregnancy, (2) human subjects, (3) neurobehavioral measures, (4) original research, (5) inclusion of control or comparison group, (6) statistical analysis of data, and (7) publication in a peer reviewed or refereed journal.

Confounding Factors

Cocaine use is often associated with three classes of potential confounding variables: other drugs, medical factors, and sociodemographic factors. These factors could provide alternative explanations for effects attributed to cocaine and therefore need to be controlled if cocaine effects are to be isolated. The initial problem of prenatal cocaine exposure has been redefined as a problem of polydrug exposure. Of the 118 studies, cocaine was reported as the only drug used in just 10 studies (8%). Alcohol (61%), marijuana (55%), and tobacco (58%) are the drugs most commonly used along with cocaine. Opiate use was reported in 19% of the studies.

History (including self-report) and/or toxicology analysis of urine, meconium, or hair are the methods used to detect maternal use of cocaine during pregnancy. Most studies do not rely on a single index; 90 (76%) used some combination of these methods. The most common indices were a combination of urine and self-report used in 77 studies (65% of the studies using multiple indices). The meconium assay provides a record of drug use from approximately 20 weeks gestational age in contrast to the urine assay that only provides a 72-hour record of drug use. However, most of these studies were conducted before the meconium assay was in widespread use. Meconium was used in 8 studies, 7 of which also used self-report. Similarly, most studies did not control for obstetrical and perinatal factors, including prenatal care, parity, and gravida. Factors such as birthweight, gestational age, and medical complications are potential mediator variables because they can be a consequence of prenatal drug exposure. Sociodemographic factors were not well controlled and may provide yet another set of explanations for effects attributed to cocaine. High rates of attrition and lack of control for examiner blindness affect the generalizability of findings. Finally, given the high-risk nature of this population, it would be reasonable to expect that many of the infants and mothers in these studies are receiving intervention services. Although intervention may affect the outcome of the child, information about intervention provided to the child or the mother was only mentioned in 28 (37%) of the studies.

Neurobehavioral Outcome

Table 9.1 shows the neurobehavioral measures used in the studies, including the number of times each measure was used, and if statistically significant cocaine effects were found. It is apparent from this table that a wide range of measures has been used, with few measures used across studies. The most frequently used measures, the Neonatal Behavioral Assessment Scale (NBAS), the Neonatal Intensive Care Unit (NICU) Network Neurobehavioral Scale (NNNS), and stress abstinence measures, as expected, pertain to early infancy. The NBAS/NNNS does show cocaine effects in 17 of 19 studies. Abstinence or withdrawal effects were reported in 12 of 21 studies and may be related to the additional effects of opiates as a confounding variable. It is also interesting that 6 of 12 studies using measures of developmental level, such as the Bayley scales, did not find

cocaine effects. By contrast, measures of more subtle function, such as temperament and attention, showed cocaine effects in 8 of 13 studies and in 7 of 8 studies, respectively. With older children, 4 of 9 language studies, and 3 of 7 IQ studies showed cocaine effects.

Arguably, the most important question about prenatal drug-exposed infants is their long-term developmental outcome. Yet, most of the published literature has not followed children beyond the infancy period. Of the 118 studies in the database, only 8 (7%) followed the children beyond 4 years of age. These findings are discussed later in the chapter.

Database Summary

To summarize, the initial outcry about the devastating effects of prenatal cocaine exposure on child development have now started to shift to proclamations about the benign effects of cocaine. However, we have seen from this review that our knowledge base is virtually confined to early infancy, with a striking absence of long-term follow-up studies. Findings are limited and compromised by methodological problems that mitigate any conclusions about whether or how prenatal cocaine exposure affects child outcome. Factors such as high attrition rates in longitudinal studies, failure to control for examiner blindness, and the effect of intervention further cloud interpretation of the findings. In

TABLE 9.1. Neurobehavioral Measures (*n* = 118)

	Significant	Not significant	Total[a]
Stress/abstinence/withdrawal	12	9	21 (18)
NBAS/NNNS	17	2	19 (16)
Cry	2	2	4 (3)
Feeding/sucking	2	2	4 (3)
Sleep	4	1	5 (4)
Temperament	8	5	13 (11)
Attention/information processing	7	1	8 (7)
Mother–child interaction	1	1	2 (2)
Developmental level	6	6	12 (10)
Motor assessment	1	2	3 (3)
Attachment	3	0	3 (3)
Play	3	1	4 (3)
Language	4	5	9 (8)
IQ	3	4	7 (6)
Caregiving environment	3	2	5 (4)

Note. From Lester (1998). Copyright 1998 by Annals of the New York Academy of Sciences. Reprinted by permission.
[a]Percentages given in parentheses.

an analysis of the sample sizes of the studies in the database, LaGasse, Seifer, and Lester (1999) found that the small sample sizes in these studies were problematic. Most studies did not have enough subjects to detect statistically small effects (less than one half of a standard deviation). Studies can detect large effects but, as we saw above, the effects that are being detected are subtle, that is statistically "small," suggesting that even if there are effects they are not observed.

The reliance on maternal self-report and urine assay to determine prenatal drug use increases the likelihood of drug-exposed infants being included in comparison or control groups. The frequency and timing of cocaine use during pregnancy may not be included in the data because the validity of relying on self-report has been questioned. Reliable frequency and timing of use data would enable computation of dose–response relationships. The results of meconium toxicology analysis generate values of the concentration of drug metabolites. However, these concentrations only represent the presence or absence of the drug; the value depends on factors such as when and how often the drug was used, transport mechanisms in the mother, and uptake mechanisms in the fetus. For example, two infants could have the same nanogram per gram level of a cocaine metabolite, with one fetus having a recent single exposure and the other fetus having continuous but earlier exposure. Therefore, these data are of questionable value for analysis of dose–response effects.

The neurobehavioral findings are scattered across a wide array of measures, most of which have been used in only a few studies. There is a clear need for measures to be used across studies to determine whether there is a consistent pattern of findings. There is also a question as to how measures are selected. Few appear to have been theoretically or hypothesis driven and some measures may be too gross to detect the more subtle effects that have been attributed to cocaine.

Lester and Tronick (1994) developed a theoretical model based on the hypothesis that cocaine affects neuroregulatory mechanisms, which in turn result in disorders of behavioral regulation. These disorders of behavioral regulation are manifest as the "four A's of infancy": attention, arousal, affect, and action. *Attention* refers to visual and auditory abilities that relate to the intake and processing of information

from the environment. *Arousal* includes control and modulation of behavioral states, from sleep to waking to crying, and the ability to display the entire range of states, from excitation to inhibition to incoming stimuli. *Affect* relates to the development of sociability and emotion, the mutual regulatory processes of social interaction and social relationships. Action indicates perceptual–motor function, the development of fine and gross motor skills, and the acquisition of knowledge and social exchange through motor patterns.

As shown in Table 9.1, these four areas do seem to be affected by prenatal drug exposure. However, the ability of the drug-exposed infant to recover from disorders in behavioral regulation will require regulatory input from the caregiving environment.

UNDERSTANDING SUBSTANCE-INVOLVED PREGNANT WOMEN

With our understanding of the limitations of the published data on prenatal cocaine exposure and child outcome has also come a closer look at substance-using pregnant women. The harm caused by substance abuse has particularly affected pregnant women and their children. There are reports that women who abuse substances have higher rates of mental health problems (Dansky et al., 1996); history of abuse (Gil-Rivas, Fiorentine, & Anglin, 1996); physical illness, family disorganization, and violence; and problems with parenting skills (Finkelstein, 1993). Their involvement with the illegal activity of drug taking decreases their contribution to society and makes higher demands on the legal system (Harrison, 1991). Children who have been exposed to substances *in utero* have increased the burden on the foster care system and are more likely to be victims of abuse and neglect (Bays, 1990; Brooks, Zuckerman, Bamforth, Cole, & Kaplan-Sanoff, 1994).

However, the complexities of understanding women who use drugs during pregnancy and their capacity for providing their infants with adequate caregiving are compounded by a host of factors that include a scarcity of empirical research and clinical material that are largely descriptive and lacking in a theoretical framework. Thus, an initial impediment in studying drug-using mothers is defining who they are.

Testing for perinatal substance abuse is usually performed when substance use is suspected. The factors typically used as criteria for screening include lack of prenatal care, premature labor, placental abruption, premature birth, and poor neonatal outcome. Women from lower socioeconomic backgrounds are more likely to be identified as perinatal substance users when these criteria are used (Behnke & Eyler 1994; Lester & Tronick, 1994). There is the additional concern that screening criteria may be based more on social factors, intuition, or bias than on objective criteria and sound scientific reasoning (Chasnoff, Landress, & Barrett, 1990; Mc-Calla, Minkoff, Feldman, Glass, & Valencia, 1992).

Stereotypical images of the woman who uses substances during pregnancy as a hardened addict, living in poverty and engaging in illicit activities to support her habit are prominent and may inadvertently influence decisions as to who gets selected for screening as well as reinforce the prototypical image. In actuality, substance abusers who become mothers are a diverse group of women who present with various risk factors as well as strengths (Lester & Fueyo, 1996). However, in part, because of the screening mechanisms used to identify perinatal substance users, much of what we know of this population is about women who live in poverty. Mothers who raise their children in poverty are confronted with a multitude of challenges that may contribute to the child's

poor developmental outcome. (See Aber, Jones, and Cohen, Chapter 6, this volume.) While the pharmacological effects of drugs on child outcome are being further investigated, the impact of issues related to poverty should not be underestimated. Much as health issues, such as poor prenatal care, inadequate nutrition, and lack of preventive medical care that are associated with drug using women may also be a function of being indigent, so too can the parenting difficulties faced by drug-using mothers be compounded by the effects of poverty. Much of the research that has been done on the effects of *in utero* drug exposure has not adequately addressed the impact of poverty on developmental outcome. This is a particularly striking omission given the powerful multiple health and social effects of poverty that may override the effects of all other risk factors on developmental outcome (Frank, Bresnahan, & Zuckerman, 1993).

To better understand how a woman who abuses substances will respond to the birth of a child and the attendant responsibilities of caring for her infant, a number of factors need to be considered. A focus that narrowly centers on her use of drugs disregards the influences of both the larger, external environment and the internal intrapsychic processes of the mother that are necessarily components of increasing our understanding of any parent–child relationship.

Figure 9.1 (Lester & Tronick, 1994) shows a

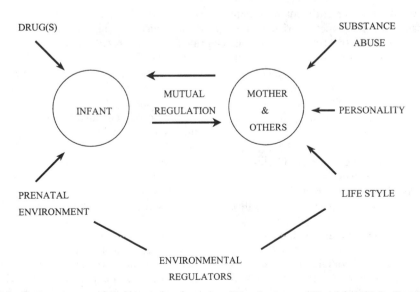

FIGURE 9.1. Systems approach to the study of cocaine. From Lester and Tronick (1994). Copyright 1994 by Michigan Association for Infant Mental Health. Reprinted by permission.

systems model approach that takes into account environmental or lifestyle issues that may mitigate or exacerbate the potential developmental outcomes of a child who is being raised by a mother who uses drugs. The model illustrates that the cocaine problem itself has been redefined in at least two ways. First, cocaine is a marker variable for a lifestyle that includes polydrug use. Second, cocaine is a marker variable for a lifestyle that includes caregiving environmental factors that have been shown to affect child development without drug exposure. The model shows that we need to study the psychological and social influences that contribute to a woman's taking drugs, as well as the nature of the community in which a child is being reared, to understand the factors that determine developmental outcome of prenatally drug-exposed infants.

Of particular concern in considering women who have used drugs during pregnancy is their ability to develop interactions with their infants that will promote the children's development. Lifestyle issues related to drug use are usually not conducive to providing a child with a consistent and secure caregiving environment. Basic parental functions, such as facilitating patterned sleeping and feeding routines, an ability to understand a child's developmental needs, and providing consistent limits and discipline, are often skills that drug-using parents lack. Some have contended that neglect is highly likely, if not inevitable, when a mother is a drug user (Bays, 1990; Black & Mayer, 1980; Kelley, 1992). Attributions for child maltreatment have been based on the perceived risk factors related to a drug-using lifestyle that includes expending considerable efforts in procuring illicit substances. The time and energy devoted to obtaining the money necessary to pay for drugs are viewed as taking away from time spent with children and further diminishing family resources. Although a causal effect between substance abuse and child abuse and neglect has not been empirically demonstrated, children whose mothers abuse drugs are considered to be at higher risk for maltreatment (Bays, 1990; Burns & Burns, 1988; Chasnoff, 1992; Kelley, 1992).

However, work with pregnant and postpartum addicts argues against acceptance of the stereotypical image of opiate addicts. Lief (1985) found that participation in a comprehensive parenting program led to these mothers being able to have positive interactions with their children and respond to them in a way that fostered the children's development. In a study comparing 17 methadone-exposed infants to 23 control infants, Jeremy and Bernstein (1984) took an approach that encompassed a variety of risk and protective factors that influenced maternal interactions with their infants. They found that the resources a mother had available to her were a greater predictor of maternal interactive performance than whether or not she used drugs.

Little is known about patterns of child neglect in women who use drugs. A small study of substance-using mothers with young children between the ages of 2 and 30 months found no differences on the HOME or Child Well-Being Scales between their caretaking abilities and those of a comparison group that was matched on race, education, and age of child (Harrington, Dubowitz, Black, & Binder, 1995). Another study compared 25 drug-addicted mothers with children under 6 years of age to a control group (Hawley, Halle, Drasin, & Thomas, 1995). Qualitative analysis of interviews pertaining to maternal perception of how drug use affected their ability to take care of their children showed that 60% of the drug-using mothers indicated they had emotionally neglected or abused their children, and 64% of the mothers indicated they had physically neglected their children. Interestingly, information regarding how the control group perceived their parenting abilities was not mentioned.

The literature is replete with assertions that women who have used drugs during pregnancy have experienced significant violence and trauma in their lives (Amaro, Fried, Cabral, & Zuckerman, 1990; Brooks et al., 1994; Davis, 1990; Raskin, 1993; Tracy & Williams, 1991). Recommendations have been made that addicted women routinely be screened for posttraumatic stress disorder because of high rates of sexual abuse and physical violence among this population (Frank et al., 1993; Raskin, 1993). It has been further suggested that the use of drugs and alcohol may be attempts at self-medication by women who have been traumatized by physical and/or sexual abuse (Brooks et al., 1994; Frank et al., 1993). In addition to childhoods that have been marked by sexual and physical abuse, substance-abusing women often continue to experience domestic violence by their partners in adulthood and become involved with men who are also using drugs (Hans, 1999).

In a large epidemiological study, more than

50% of substance-abusing individuals had major psychopathology (Regier et al., 1990). Anxiety disorders were most predominant, followed by affective disorders, antisocial disorders, and schizophrenia. Given the association between substance abuse and major psychiatric diagnoses, the presence of co-occurring mental health disorders found among drug-using mothers is another factor to be considered in assessing a woman's ability to adequately care for her child. Standardized psychological tests that were administered to 40 perinatal substance abusers found high comorbidity of psychiatric disorders, including depression, anxiety, and personality disorders among this population (Haller, Kniscly, Dawson, & Schnoll, 1993). Characteristics of the women who participated in this study included low socioeconomic status, low levels of education, histories of criminal behavior, and family histories of substance abuse, poverty, and violence. However, it is not clear how representative these mothers are of perinatal substance abusers, how their standardized scores compare to women who do not use substances matched on the above noted variables, and if the comorbid conditions found are a function of substance use or other complex psychosocial factors.

In a study of postpartum women from an urban high-risk clinic, results from the Brief Symptom Inventory (BSI) showed that women who used cocaine reported more phobic anxiety and paranoid ideational symptoms, as well as higher levels of personal inadequacy (Singer et al. 1995) than controls. No effects of cocaine using mothers were found on the Beck Depressive Inventory (BDI) (Singer et al., 1995). It was suggested that administering the BDI to the women immediately after they gave birth might have obscured differences between groups because depressive and somatic symptoms are often elevated after delivery.

Similar findings were reported in a study in which BDI scores in drug-using women and controls were comparable at 1 month postpartum after having been significantly higher in drug-using women following delivery (Woods, Eyler, Behnke, & Conlon, 1993). Higher scores among drug-using mothers after giving birth were possibly attributed to these women being investigated for child abuse because of state mandatory reporting laws. It was also suggested that depressive symptoms may have been related to the physiological effects of not using drugs while hospitalized for childbirth. The substance-using mothers may have been worried about the effects of drug use on their babies. Depressive symptomotology related to these issues may have diminished after caring for their infant for a month.

The claims that have been made about women who use drugs and their parenting abilities need to be further examined to better understand and conceptualize the strengths and deficits of these women as mothers. Maternal characteristics and environmental factors need to be delineated and analyzed in order to assess the risk and protective factors in the lives of children whose mothers use drugs.

Risk and Protective Factors

From the study of preterm and other at-risk populations, we have also developed multiple-risk models that should be useful in the study of drug-exposed infants. The study of risk factors has become an important part of our understanding of child development. A high-risk child is one who is at greater than average risk for later deviancies in behavior because of membership in some identifiable population (Sameroff & Seifer, 1983). Such populations could include infants with anomalous experiences, including medical conditions such as low birthweight, disordered parentage, disturbed family and child-rearing milieus, and disadvantaged environments. However, we also know that many children do not succumb to deprivation. Even in the face of disorganized, impoverished homes, many children appear to develop normally; these children are referred to as "resilient." (Anthony, 1987; Werner, 1986; Garmezy, 1981). This has led to the study of protective factors—dispositional attributes, environmental conditions, biological predispositions, and positive events that can act to contain the expression of deviance or pathology (Garmezy, Masten, & Tellegen, 1984; Fisher, Kokes, Cole, Perkins, & Wynee, 1987; Murphy, 1987). Our models of development are now enriched by the concepts of resilience and protective factors as the positive counterparts to the constructs of vulnerability and risk factors (Werner, 1986). These models have yet to be applied to the study of drug-exposed infants. The study of drug-exposed infants is probably best viewed as a special case of the infant at risk, and this suggests that we bring to the study of drug-exposed infants all that we have learned from the study of high-risk infants.

This includes the abandonment of preconceived biases about the infants and their caregivers.

Larger and more systematic studies are indicated if we are to more fully understand the parenting behaviors, capabilities, and deficits of drug-using women. Little explored areas that warrant closer examination are how drug-using mothers compare to mothers without a history of drug use when matched for a range of psychosocial factors, developmental outcomes of infants and children exposed to drugs *in utero* compared to those reared with their biological mothers and those who have been placed with alternative caregivers, and the impact of treatment intervention on improving parenting skills. Because competent caregiving is a critical aspect of child developmental outcome, it would be advantageous to better determine what factors predict parenting capabilities in this population.

TREATMENT

Overview of Drug Treatment Outcome

A recent national drug abuse treatment outcome study, the Drug Abuse Treatment Outcome Study (DATOS; Mueller & Wyman, 1997), examined treatment effects for participants in four types of treatment programs: (1) outpatient methadone ($n = 29$), (2) long-term residential ($n = 21$), (3) outpatient drug-free ($n = 32$), (4) short-term inpatient ($n = 14$). The DATOS study tracked more than 10,000 patients in the 96 programs in 11 cities in the United States for 3 years. Among the drug users studied, drug use dropped significantly from the 12 months before treatment to 12 months after treatment began. This was true for all four types of treatment and for each significant primary drug of choice (cocaine, heroin, and alcohol). In addition, significant depression and involvement in illegal acts also dropped significantly following all four types of treatment. Treatment retention was best predicted by high motivation, legal pressure to stay in treatment, no prior trouble with the law, receiving psychological counseling while in treatment, and lack of significant psychological problems, especially antisocial personality disorder.

Drug Abuse Treatment for Women

The DATOS study, compared with an earlier national study conducted by NIDA, the Treatment Outcome Prospective Study (TOPS, 1979–1981), indicated a greater percentage of women in outpatient methadone and long-term residential programs, with equal percentages of women in outpatient drug-free programs. In DATOS, women accounted for 37% of drug users admitted to short-term inpatient programs. These programs were not included in the TOPS study.

Prior to federal funding for women's treatment in the mid-1970s, there were few programs specifically for women, and fewer still for pregnant women (Reed, 1987; Finkelstein, 1990; Zweben & Brown, 1995). Many treatment programs that included women were based on recovery models oriented toward treatment of men and did not take into account women's recovery issues or women's status as parents (Lundy, Gottheil, Serota, & Weinstein, 1995; Kline, 1996). In the late 1980s, when concern increased about cocaine addiction in pregnant and parenting women, there was a substantial increase in publications on women's treatment (Davis, 1994), including the beginning development of new treatment models for drug-abusing women—among them pregnant and parenting women (Clayson, Berkowitz, & Brindis, 1995).

In response to federal initiatives to develop effective treatment for this population (Perinatal–20 Treatment Research Program; NIDA, 1996; CSAP Demonstration Projects), a new generation of treatment programs has been developed. One central component of these programs is keeping women and their infants together in either residential treatment for pregnant and postpartum women with their infant (and other children) or outpatient programs with a number of child and parenting services.

These programs, to various degrees, are responsive to the following issues in treatment for women:

1. Services are *family-centered*, recognizing that relationships are central in women's lives and that work with the family system is important in successful treatment (Finkelstein, 1993). This includes supporting and working with the *mother–child relationship* (Finnegan, 1988; Finkelstein, 1993).
2. Services promote *self-esteem, competence, self-control, and empowerment* (Egeland & Erikson, 1990).
3. Services are *coordinated to be maximally available* to each woman (Hutchins &

Alexander, 1990). A full range of services for a woman and her family (prenatal care, pediatric care, chemical dependency treatment, nutritional services, mental health services, social services, parenting education, and vocational/educational training) are part of a coordinated program (Kronstadt, 1990).

4. Services are *based in the community,* responsive to the cultural and linguistic needs of the neighborhoods served and easily accessible (Ewing, 1992).

5. *Children of mothers in treatment* are provided with services, including pediatric care, early stimulation and education, early intervention, and mental health services (Finkelstein, 1990, 1993; Brown, Huba, & Melchior, 1995).

6. *Services are responsive to individual needs* and change in type over time and are available in the long term (Brown, 1991).

7. Services address the *multiplicity of problems* with which women in treatment must deal (physical health, homelessness, unemployment, child care and custody, such psychosocial issues as depression and dual diagnosis, and issues of physical violence, sexual abuse, and incest; Amaro et al., 1990).

Treatment Models for Drug-Abusing Women

Recent publications on treatment for drug-abusing women (Haskett, Miller, Whitworth, & Huffman, 1992; Farkas & Parran, 1993; Clayson et al., 1995; Wald, Harvey, & Hibbard, 1995; Brown, 1995; Wallace, 1995; Committee on Opportunities in Drug Abuse Research, 1996; Clay, 1997; Coles, Russell, & Schuetze, 1997) have indicated two predominant models that have been developed or restructured to accommodate women in treatment and their children: (1) outpatient, including both hospital-based (Malow, Ireland, Halpert, & Szapocznik, 1994; Jansson et al., 1996) and community-based (Strantz & Welch, 1995; Ingala, 1996; Berkowitz, Brindis, Clayson, & Peterson, 1996; Laken & Ager, 1996), and (2) residential (Brow & Cripps, 1985; Comfort, Shipley, White, & Griffith, 1990; Lanehart, Clark, Kratochvil, & Rollings, 1994; Metsch et al., 1995), including therapeutic community (DeLeon & Jainchill, 1991; Brown, Sanchez, Zweben, & Aly, 1996; Coletti, Schinka, Hughes, & Hamilton, 1995; Stevens & Arbiter, 1995).

Issues of concern in treatment research for drug-abusing women include treatment needs of women (Comfort et al., 1990), comparing the effectiveness of different treatment models in maintaining retention in treatment (Roberts & Nishimoto, 1996), service components that predict substance-free time (Lanehart et al., 1994), characteristics of drug-abusing women who stay in treatment versus those who drop out (Chan, Wingert, Wachsman, Schultz, & Roberts, 1986; Stevens & Arbiter, 1995; Strantz & Welch, 1995; Ingersoll, Lu, & Haller, 1995), comparison of treated and untreated drug-abusing pregnant and postpartum women (Smith, Dent, Coles, & Falek, 1992), characteristics of drug-abusing women who use services in pregnancy (Messer, Clark, & Martin, 1996; Bendersky, Alessandri, Gilbert, & Lewis, 1996; Laken & Ager, 1996), effectiveness of treatment participation (Brow & Cripps, 1985), and mandatory versus voluntary participation in treatment (Berkowitz et al., 1996)

Research on Treatment for Drug-Abusing Women and Their Children: Programs with a Parenting Component

Research on new treatment options for drug-abusing women with their children is just beginning to be published in scientific peer-reviewed journals and federal publications (NIDA, 1996; Brindis, Clayson, & Berkowitz, 1997; Brindis, Berkowitz, Clayson, & Lamb, 1997). A recent study (Sweeney, Mattis, & Schwartz, 1997) examined the effects of prenatal versus postnatal enrollment in a treatment program on infant status. The evaluation indicated that women remained in treatment an average of 11 months. In a subset of 87 pregnant enrollees' newborns and 87 postpartum enrollees' newborns, the infants born to women who enrolled in the program during pregnancy fared better in birthweight (400 grams higher), gestational age (2 weeks later), length of hospital stay (6 days less), and confinement in the neonatal intensive care unit (8 days less). Hospital cost of the infants born to women who did not enroll in the program until after delivery were an average of $8,000 more than prenatally enrolled infants.

In addition to comprehensive services, effective case management, drug counseling, and school/job training (Uziel-Miller, Lyons, Kissiel, & Love, 1998), drug-abusing women in treatment indicate a high need for help with parenting skills and understanding and managing their children (Homan, Flick, Heaton, & Mayer, 1993; Davis, 1997). Two studies have compared women in treatment with their children versus those in treatment without their children (Hughes et al., 1995; Szuster, Chung, & Bisconer, 1996) and indicated that women stayed in treatment significantly longer when they had their children with them. Another study (Wobie, Eyler, Conlon, Clarke, & Behnke, 1997) indicated that the sooner an infant joined the mother in residential treatment, the longer her length of stay, with a significantly increased opportunity for program completion. Measures of depression were lower and self-esteem was higher for women who had reunited with their infant in the treatment program, compared with women who had not yet reunited with their infant.

Four studies include measures of women's parenting during treatment and measures of child developmental status (Cuskey, Watheg, & Richardson, 1980; Saunders, 1993; Shumacher, Siegel, Socol, Harkness, & Freeman, 1996; Wobie et al., 1997). One early study indicated improved ratings of the mother–child relationship, including more constructive discipline and less overindulgence and rejection (Cuskey et al., 1980). Another study found, on discharge, that after program participation, women were less distressed and had improved ratings of parenting skills, as well as positive changes in ratings of children's social functioning (Saunders, 1993). One study (Schumacher et al., 1996) included measures of women's functioning following treatment with children (increased length of stay; reduced severity of drug/alcohol use; less psychiatric, family/social, and legal problems); their parenting (less parenting stress); and child developmental outcome. They found that infants and toddlers scored in the average range on developmental screens and preschoolers showed improvement in development during treatment but still scored below average on developmental screens. All children improved in self-help and gross motor and language skills but declined in social functioning. The study of women in residential treatment cited previously (Wobie et al., 1997) also indicated that the development of infants living with their mothers was within normal limits on the Bayley Scales of Infant Development.

Another study examined the effectiveness of a parenting training program for women in residential drug treatment (Camp & Finkelstein, 1997). The parenting component consisted of multiple services for both women and their infants while they were in residential treatment, as well as aftercare services after discharge. Women made significant improvements in self-esteem and gains in parenting knowledge and attitudes.

PUBLIC POLICY

We have seen from this review that drug effects are subtle and not well understood, especially in terms of the role of the caregiving environment. There is also emerging evidence that treatment is effective, which raises important public policy issues. In this section, we discuss the implications of subtle effects for public policy.

Earlier in this chapter, we mentioned that only 8 studies have been completed with school-age children. IQ was measured in 5 studies, receptive language in 4 studies, and expressive language in 5 studies. Lester et al. (1998) conducted a meta-analysis of these findings to provide a better estimate of the long-term effects than can be determined by a single study. As shown in Table 9.2, the difference in IQ between cocaine-exposed and control groups across available studies is 3.26 IQ points. This difference, although small, is statistically significant and can have a substantial impact on society.

Early intervention and special education services are typically provided for children who score less than two standard deviations (SD) (or in some cases less than 1.5 SD) below the mean on standardized tests. This would correspond to IQ scores of < 70 or < 78. In a normal distribution (a good model for IQ scores), 2.28% of children will score < 70 (2 SD) and 6.68% of children will score < 78 (1.5 SD). When the IQ distribution is shifted downward by 3.26 IQ points, the number of children at the low end of the distribution will increase (see Table 9.2) to 3.75%. This results in a 1.6-fold increase in the number of children with IQs < 70 and to 10.03% or a 1.5-fold increase in the number of children with IQs < 78. These distributional changes then allow estimation of some of the costs to society associated with prenatal cocaine exposure. As mentioned earlier, estimates of the number of cocaine-exposed children born each year range from 45,000 (NIDA) to 375,000 (GAO). These figures predict that the number of children affected by this 3.26-point

TABLE 9.2. Societal Burden of Prenatal Cocaine Exposure

Measure	Effect (SEM)	% < 2 SD[a]	Increase	Additional affected children/yr (no.)	Additional cost for services (millions)	% < 1.5 SD[b]	Increase	Additional affected children/yr (no.)	Additional cost for services (millions)
IQ difference (n = 5)	3.26 (2.01) IQ points	3.75	1.6×	1,688–14,062	$4–35	10.03	1.5×	4,514–37,612	$10–80
IQ effect size (n = 5)	0.33 (0.13) SD units	4.75	2.0×	2,138–17,812	$7–59	12.10	1.8×	5,455–45,375	$15–129
Receptive language Effect size (n = 4)	0.71 (0.26) SD units	9.85	4.3×	4,432–36,938	$22–180	21.48	3.2×	9,666–80,550	$42–352
Expressive language Effect size (n = 5)	0.60 (0.29) SD units	8.08	3.5×	3,636–30,300	$17–138	18.14	2.7×	8,163–68,025	$33–272

Note. From Lester, LaGasse, and Seifer (1998). Copyright 1998 by American Association for the Advancement of Science. Reprinted by permission.
[a]Normal = 2.28%.
[b]Normal = 6.68%.

IQ difference is estimated to be between 1,688 and 14,062 at < 2 SD and between 4,514 and 37,612 for children < 1.5 SD. According to the U.S. National Center for Education Statistics (1996), special education services (additional services for special education) cost $6,335 per child per year. The added costs of these special educational services for the number of cocaine-exposed children with IQs less than 70, based on a 3.26 point IQ difference, is $4 to $35 million per year and $10 to $80 million per year for children with an IQ of < 78.

These IQ differences also may be thought of as an effect size, a useful construct because all measures are expressed in the same units (SD units). Effects on different tests can be compared even if they use different scales of measurement. As shown in Table 9.2, cocaine-exposed children had significantly lower scores on tests of IQ ($Z = 2.61, p < .01$), receptive language ($Z = 4.44, p < .001$), and expressive language ($Z = 3.99, p < .001$). The language studies showed a medium effect size, compared with the small effect size for the IQ studies. The effect size for receptive language was more than twice that of the effect size for IQ, and expressive language showed a 1.8 times greater effect size than IQ. Table 9.2 also shows the follow-up calculations for the percentage of children newly affected at < 2 SD and < 1.5 SD, the number of children newly affected each year, and the cost of added special education services for these children annually.

The moderate effect sizes in language result in a 2.7- to 4.3-fold increase in children who will be affected at clinically significant levels. For expressive language, this translates to be-

tween 3,636 and 68,025 children newly diagnosed annually who will need special education services, costing $17–$272 million per year. As these estimates are for additional costs due to cases newly diagnosed annually, the costs are underestimates, because the costs and burden would be accrued with the annual addition of children with the specific deficits identified.

The public health consequences of both of these effects are substantial, even if the effects themselves are subtle. Prenatal cocaine exposure may not cause devastating brain damage but will significantly increase the number of children who will fail in school and need special education services, at an estimated additional cost of up to $352 million per year. The "good news" is that these children are not hopelessly damaged and destined to become a burden to society. Instead, we can view them as children who can be helped to become productive members of society. Meanwhile, prevention efforts need to be directed toward ridding society of the cocaine problem and toward treatment programs for drug-using pregnant women to prevent the harm caused by cocaine use.

Instead of waiting until these children get to school, start to fail, and need special education services, we wonder whether it would not relieve suffering and be more cost-effective to start services early. If these funds were spent for early intervention, there is a high likelihood that we could prevent many of the later school-age deficits from even occurring. We would be able to take advantage of the plasticity and recovery capacity of the nervous system during the infancy period and of the special window of opportunity to engage the mother in drug treatment that is present following the delivery of a newborn baby. The mother's wish to be a good mother and help her child may increase her motivation to change, and we have intervention programs that have been found to be effective with these mothers.

If services were started during pregnancy, as we saw in some of the residential treatment programs, drug effects on the child could be eliminated altogether. This, too, is cost-effective. Hospital charges for both the cocaine-addicted mother and her newborn are much higher than in drug-free pregnancies. One study found that the average cost for the cocaine-exposed newborn was $13,222 compared with $1,297 for unexposed infants. In another study, hospital costs for newborn infants were $5,200 more for cocaine-exposed than for unexposed infants. The cost of an infant remaining in the nursery for social service evaluation if foster placement is needed adds another $3,500.

These policy changes will require a change in public perception. The punitive, reactive approach to drug-using mothers that currently predominates leads to our society spending more money on punishment than on prevention or treatment and fails to recognize that drug use is a complicated biopsychosocial problem. Tensions have been created between legalistic and psychological positions. We allow for relapse in the treatment of other problems, such as diabetes, cigarette smoking, and weight loss, but not with drug abuse. We all stand to benefit from a more humane, comprehensive approach to treating families affected by drug use, including the women who are struggling to raise their children, the children who have been exposed to drugs in the prenatal and postnatal environment and, ultimately, all of society, both in terms of cost effectiveness and assisting members of society in having productive lives. We have the knowledge to help these mothers and their babies, and we have empirical evidence that treatment works. It is sad and ironic, however, that it is not lack of knowledge that is preventing these mothers and their children from getting help but rather inappropriate societal attitudes and perceptions.

REFERENCES

Amaro, H., Fried, L., Cabral, H., & Zuckerman, B. (1990). Violence during pregnancy and substance abuse. *American Journal of Public Health, 80*(5), 575–579.

Anthony, E. J. (1987). Risk, vulnerability, and resilience: An overview. In E. F. Anthony & B. J. Cohler (Eds.), *The invulnerable child* (pp. 3–48). New York: Guilford Press.

Bays, J. (1990). Substance abuse and child abuse: Impact of addiction on the child. *Pediatric Clinics of North America, 37*, 881–903.

Behnke, M., & Eyler F. D. (1994). Issues in prenatal cocaine use research: Problems in identifying users and choosing an appropriate comparison group. *Infant Mental Health Journal, 15*, 146–157.

Bendersky, M., Alessandri, S., Gilbert, P., & Lewis, M. (1996). Characteristics of pregnant substance abusers in two cities in the northeast. *American Journal of Substance Abuse, 22*(3), 349–362.

Berkowitz, G., Brindis, C., Clayson, Z., & Peterson, S. (1996). Options for recovery: promoting success among women mandated to treatment. *Journal of Psychoactive Drugs, 28*(1), 31–38.

Black, R., & Mayer, J. (1980). Parents with special problems: Alcoholism and opiate addiction. *Child Abuse and Neglect, 4*, 45–54.

Brindis, C. D., Berkowitz, P. H., Clayson, Z., & Lamb, B. (1997). California's Approach to Perinatal Substance Abuse: Toward a model of comprehensive care. *Journal of Psychoactive Drugs, 29*(1), 113–121.

Brindis, C. D., Clayson, Z., & Berkowitz, G. (1997). Options for recovery: California's perinatal projects. *Journal of Psychoactive Drugs, 29*(1), 89–99.

Brooks, C., Zuckerman, B., Bamforth, A., Cole, J., & Kaplan-Sanoff, M. (1994). Clinical issues related to substance-involved mothers and their infants. *Infant Mental Health Journal, 15*(2), 202–217.

Brow, J., & Cripps, R. (1985). The Austin Family House program. *Journal of Substance Abuse Treatment, 2*(1), 63–67.

Brown, S. (1991) *Children and parental illicit drug use: Resarch, clinical and policy issues. Summary of a workshop*. Washington, DC: National Academy Press.

Brown, V. B. (1995). Interview with Maggie Willmore, Chief of Women & Children's Branch, Center for Substance Abuse Treatment. *Journal of Psychoactive Drugs, 27*(4), 321–323.

Brown, V. B., Huba, G. J., & Melchior, L. A. (1995). Level of burden: Women with more than one co-occurring disorder. *Journal of Psychoactive Drugs, 27*(4), 339–346.

Brown, V. B., Sanchez, S., Zweben, J. E., & Aly, T. (1996). Challenges in moving from a traditional therapeutic community to a women and children's TC model. *Journal of Psychoactive Drugs, 28*(1), 39–46.

Burns, W. J., & Burns, K. A. (1988). Parenting dysfunction in chemically dependent women. In I. J. Chasnoff (Ed.), *Drugs, alcohol, pregnancy, and parenting* (pp. 159–171). Boston: Kluwer Academic.

Camp, J. M., & Finkelstein, N. (1997). Parenting training for women in residential substance abuse treatment. Results of a demonstration project. *Journal of Susbstance Abuse Treatment, 14*(5), 411–422.

Chan, L. S., Wingert, W. A., Wachsman, L., Schuetz, S., & Rogers, C. (1986). Differences between dropouts and active participants in a pediatric clinic for substance abusing mothers. *American Journal of Drug and Alcohol Abuse, 12*(1–2), 89–99.

Chasnoff, I. J. (1992). Cocaine, pregnancy, and the growing child. *Current Problems in Pediatrics, 22*(7), 302–321.

Chasnoff, I. J., Landress, H. J., & Barrett, M. E. (1990). The prevalence of illicit drug or alcohol abuse during pregnancy and discrepancies in mandatory reporting in Pinellas County, Florida. *New England Journal of Medicine, 322*, 102–106.

Clay, R. A. (1997). How to build a perinatal addiction treatment program. *SAMSHA News, 5*(2), 1, 12–14.

Clayson, Z., Berkowitz, G., & Brindis, C. (1995). Themes and variations among seven comprehensive perinatal drug and alcohol abuse treatment models. *Health and Social Work, 20*(3), 234–238.

Coles, C. D., Russell, C. L., & Schuetze, P. (1997). Maternal substance use: Epidemiology, treatment outcome, and developmental effects: An annotated bibliography. *Substance Use and Misuse, 32*(2), 149–168.

Coletti, S. D., Schinka, J. A., Hughes, P. H., & Hamilton, N. L. (1995). PAR Village for chemically dependent women: Philosophy and program elements. *Journal of Substance Abuse Treatment, 12*(4), 289–296.

Comfort, M., Shipley, T. E., White, K., Griffith, E. M. (1990). Family treatment for homeless alcohol/drug-addicted women and their preschool children. Treating alcoholism and drug abuse among homeless men and women: Nine community demonstration grants [Special issue]. *Alcoholism Treatment Quarterly, 7*(1), 129–147.

Committee on Opportunities in Drug Abuse Research. (1996). Treatment. In *Pathways to addiction: Opportunities in drug abuse research*. Washington, DC: National Academy Press.

Cuskey,W. R., Watheg, R. B., & Richardson, A. (1980). Evaluation of a therapeutic community program for female addicts. *Journal of Addiction Health, 1*, 136–203.

Dansky, B. S., Brady, K. T., Saladin, M., Killeen, T., Becker, S., & Roitzch, J. (1996). *American Journal of Drug and Alcohol Abuse, 22*(1), 75–93.

Davis, S. K. (1990). Chemical dependency in women: A description of its effects and outcome on adequate parenting. *Journal of Substance Abuse Treatment, 7*, 225–232.

Davis, S. K. (1994). Effects of chemical dependency in parenting women. In R. R. Watson (Ed.), *Addiction behaviors in women*. Totowa, NJ: Humana Press.

Davis, S. K. (1997). Comprehensive interventions for affecting the parenting effectiveness of chemically dependent women. *Journal of Obstetrics, Gynecology, and Neonatal Nursing, 26*(5), 604–610.

DeLeon, G., & Jainchill, N. (1991). Residential therapeutic communities for female substance abusers. *Bulletin of the New York Academy of Medicine, 67*(3), 277–290.

Egeland, B., & Erikson, M. (1990) Rising above the past: Strategies for helping new mothers break the cycle of abuse and neglect. *Zero to Three, 11*(2), 29–35.

Ewing, H. H. (1992). Care of women and children in the perinatal period. In M. F. Fleming & K. L. Barry (Eds.), *Addictive disorders: A practical guide to treatment* (pp. 211–231). [Mosby-Year Book primary care series] St. Louis: Mosby Year Book.

Farkas, K. J., & Parran, Jr., T. V. (1993). Treatment of cocaine addiction during pregnancy. *Clinics in Perinatology, 20*(1), 29–45.

Finkelstein, N. (1990) *Treatment issues: Women and substance abuse*. Washington, DC: National Coalition on Alcohol and Drug Dependent Women and Their Children.

Finkelstein, N. (1993). Treatment programming for alcohol and drug-dependent pregnant women. *International Journal of the Addictions, 28*(13), 1275–1309.

Finnegan, L. (1988). Management of maternal and neonatal substance abuse problems. In L. Haeris (Ed.), *Problems of drug dependence* (pp. 177–182). Proceedings of the 50th Annual Scientific Meeting, Committee on Problems of Drug Dependence. Washington, DC: NIDA.

Fisher, L., Kokes, R. F., Cole, R. E., Perkins, P. M., & Wynne, L. C. (1987). Competent children at risk: A study of well-functioning offspring of disturbed parents. In E. J. Anthony & B. J. Cohler (Eds.), *The invulnerable child* (pp. 211–228). New York: Guilford Press.

Frank, D. A., Bresnahan, K., & Zuckerman, B. S. (1993). Maternal cocaine use: Impact on child health and development. *Advances in Pediatrics, 40*, 65–99.

Garmezy, N. (1981). Children under stress: Perspectives on antecedents and correlates of vulnerability and resistance to psychopathology: In A. I. Rabin, J. Aronoff, A. M. Barclay, & R. A. Zucker (Eds.), *Further explorations in personality* (pp. 196–269). New York: Wiley.

Garmezy, N., Masten, A., & Tellegen, A. (1984). The study of stress and competence in children: A building block for developmental psychopathology. *Child Development, 55*, 97–111.

Gil-Rivas, V., Fiorentine, R., & Anglin, M. (1996). Sexual abuse, physical abuse, and posttraumatic stress disorder among women participating in outpatient drug abuse treatment. *Journal of Psychoactive Drugs, 28*(1), 95–101.

Haller, H. L., Knisely, J. S., Dawson, K. S., & Schnoll, S. H. (1993). Perinatal substance abusers: Psychological and social characteristics. *Journal of Nervous and Mental Disease, 181*, 509–513.

Hans, S. L. (1999). Demographic and psychosocial characteristics of substance-abusing pregnant women. *Clinics in Perinatology, 26*(1), 55–74.

Harrington, D., Dubowitz, H., Black, M. M., & Binder, A. (1995). Maternal substance use and neglectful parenting: Relations with children's development. *Journal of Clinical Child Psychology, 24*, 258–263.

Harrison, M. (1991). Drug addiction in pregnancy: The interface of science, emotion, and social policy. *Journal of Substance Abuse Treatment, 8*, 261–268.

Haskett, M. E., Miller, J. W., Whitworth, J. M., & Huffman, J. M. (1992). Intervention with cocaine-abusing mothers. *Families in Society, 73*(8), 451–461.

Hawley, T. L., Halle, T. G., Drasin, R. E., & Thomas N. G. (1995). Children of addicted mothers: Effects of the "crack epidemic" on the caregiving environment and the development of preschoolers. *American Journal of Orthopsychiatry, 65*, 364–379.

Homan, S. M., Flick, L. H., Heaton, T. M., & Mayer, J. P. (1993). Reaching beyond crisis management: Design and implementation of extended shelter-based services for chemically dependent homeless women and their children [Special issue]. *Alcoholism Treatment Quarterly*, 10(3–4), 101–112.

Hughes, P. H., Coletti, S. D., Neri, R. L., Urmann, C. F., Stahl, S., Sicilian, D. M., & Anthony, J. C. (1995). Retaining cocaine-abusing women in a therapeutic community: The effect of a child live-in program. *American Journal of Public Health*, 85(8), 1149–1152.

Hutchins, E., & Alexander, G. (1990) *Substance use during pregnancy and its effects on the infant: A review of issues*. Baltimore: Johns Hopkins University Press.

Ingala, N. J. (1996). Under one roof. *Health Progress*, 77(5), 40–42.

Ingersoll, K. S., Lu, I. L., & Haller, D. L. (1995). Predictors of in-treatment relapse in perinatal substance abusers and impact on treatment retention: A prospective study. *Journal of Psychoactive Drugs*, 27(4), 375–387.

Jansson, L., Svikis, D., Lee, J., Paluzzi, P., Rutigliano, P., & Hackerman, F. (1996). Pregnancy and addiction: A comprehensive care model. *Journal of Substance Abuse Treatment*, 13(4), 321–329.

Jeremy, R. J., & Bernstein, V. J. (1984). Dyads at risk: Methadone-maintained women and their four-month-old infants. *Child Development*, 55, 1141–1154.

Kelley, S. J. (1992). Parenting stress and child maltreatment in drug-exposed children. *Child Abuse and Neglect*, 16, 317–328.

Kline, A. (1996). Pathways into drug user treatment: The influence of gender and racial/ethnic identity. *Substance Use and Misuse*, 31(3), 323–342.

Kronstadt, D. (1990). *Substance abuse during pregnancy—Impact on mothers and children: A guide to resources*. Washington, DC: CDM Group and Cosmos Corporation, OSAP, National Learning Community.

LaGasse, L. L., Seifer, R., & Lester, B. M. (1999) Interpreting research on prenatal substance exposure in the context of multiple confounding factors. *Clinics in Perinatology*, 26(1), 39–54.

Laken, M. P., & Ager, J. W. (1996). Effects of case management on retention in prenatal substance abuse treatment. *American Journal of Drug and Alcohol Abuse*, 22(3), 439–448.

Lanehart, R. E., Clark, H. B., Kratochvil, D., & Rollings, J. P. (1994). Case management of pregnant and parenting female crack and polydrug abusers. *Journal of Substance Abuse*, 6(4), 441–448.

Lester, B. M. (1998). The Maternal Lifestyles Study. *Cocaine: Effects on the developing brain, Annals of the New York Academy of Sciences*, 846, 296–305.

Lester, B. M., & Fueyo, M. (1996). Exposition prenatale a la cocaine: Environnement parental et impact sur l'enfant. *P.R.I.S.M.E.*, 6(1), 126–137.

Lester, B. M., LaGasse, L., & Brunner, S. (1997). Data base of studies on prenatal cocaine exposure and child outcome. *Journal of Drug Issues*, 27(2), 487–499.

Lester, B. M., LaGasse, L., & Seifer, R. (1998). Cocaine exposure and children: The meaning of subtle effects. *Science*, 282, 633–634.

Lester, B. M., & Tronick, E. Z. (1994). The effects of prenatal cocaine exposure and child outcome:

Lessons from the past. *Infant Mental Health Journal*, 15, 107–120.

Lief, N. R. (1985). The drug user as a parent. *International Journal of the Addictions*, 20, 63–97.

Lundy, A., Gottheil, E., Serota, R. D., & Weinstein, S. P. (1995). Gender differences and similarities in African-American crack cocaine abusers. *Journal of Nervous and Mental Disease*, 183(4), 260–266.

Malow, R. M., Ireland, S. J., Halpert, E. S., & Szapocznik, J. (1994). A description of the Maternal Addiction Program of the University of Miami/Jackson Memorial Medical Center. *Journal of Substance Abuse Treatment*, 11(1), 55–60.

Mayes, L. C., Granger, R. H., Bornstein, M. H., & Zuckerman, B. (1992) The problem of prenatal cocaine exposure: A rush to judgment. *Journal of the American Medical Association*, 267, 406–408.

McCalla, S., Minkoff, H. L., Feldman, J., Glass, L., & Valencia, G. (1992). Predictors of cocaine use in pregnancy. *Obstetrics and Gynecology*, 79, 641–644.

Messer, K., Clark, K. A., & Martin, S. L. (1996). Characteristics associated with pregnant women's utilization of substance abuse treatment services. *American Journal of Drug and Alcohol Abuse*, 22(3), 403–422.

Metsch, L. R., Rivers, J. E., Miller, M., Bohs, R., McCoy, C. B., Morrow, C. J., Bandstra, E. S., Jackson, V., & Gissen, M. (1995). Implementation of a family-centered treatment program for substance-abusing women and their children: barriers and resolutions. *Journal of Psychoactive Drugs*, 27(1), 73–83.

Mueller, M. D., & Wyman, J. R. (1997). Study sheds new light on the state of drug abuse treatment nationwide. *National Institute on Drug Abuse*, 12(5), 1.

Murphy, L. B. (1987). Further reflections on resilience. In E. J. Anthony & B. J. Cohler (Eds.), *The invulnerable child* (pp. 84–105). New York: Guilford Press.

National Institute on Drug Abuse. (1996). *National Pregnancy and Health Survey: Drug use among women delivering livebirths: 1992* (NIH, Publication No. 96–3819). Washington, DC: U.S. Department of Health and Human Services.

Raskin, V. D. (1993). Psychiatric aspects of substance use disorders in childbearing populations. *Psychiatric Clinics of North America*, 16, 157–165.

Reed, B. G. (1987). Developing women-sensitive drug dependence treatment services: Why so difficult? *Journal of Psychoactive Drugs*, 19(2), 151–164.

Regier, D. A., Farmer, M. E., Rae, D. S., Locke B. Z., Keith, S. J., Judd, L. L., & Goodwin, F. K. (1990). Comorbidity of mental disorders with alcohol and other drug abuse: Results from the epidemiological catchment area (ECA) study. *Journal of the American Medical Association*, 264, 2511–2518.

Roberts, A. C., & Nishimoto, R. H. (1996). Predicting treatment retention of women dependent on cocaine. *American Journal of Drug and Alcohol Abuse*, 22(3), 313–333.

Sameroff, A. J., & Seifer, R. (1983), Familial risk and child competence. *Child Development*, 54, 1254.

Saunders, E. J. (1993). A new model of residential care for substance-abusing women and their children. *Adult Residential Care Journal*, 7(2), 104–117.

Schumacher, J. E., Siegel, S. H., Socol, J. C., Harkness, S. & Freeman, K. (1996). Making evaluation work in a substance abuse treatment program for women with children: Olivia's house. *Journal of Psychoactive Drugs, 28*(1), 73–83.

Singer, L., Arendt, R., Minnes, S., Farkas, K., Yamashita, T., & Kliegman, R. (1995). Increased psychological distress in post-partum, cocaine-using mothers. *Journal of Substance Abuse, 7*, 165–174.

Smith, I. E., Dent, D. Z., Coles, C., & Falek, A. (1992). A comparison study of treated and untreated pregnant and postpartum cocaine-abusing women. *Journal of Substance Abuse Treatment, 9*, 343–348.

Stevens, S. J., & Arbiter, N. (1995). A therapeutic community for substance-abusing pregnant women and women with children: Process and outcome. *Journal of Psychoactive Drugs, 27*(1), 49–56.

Strantz, I. H., & Welch, S. P. (1995) Postpartum women in outpatient drug abuse treatment: Correlates of retention/completion. *Journal of Psychoactive Drugs, 27*(4), 357–373.

Sweeney, P. J., Mattis, N. G., & Schwartz, R. M. (1997). *Project LINK final report*. Unpublished report.

Szuster, R. R., Rich, L. L., Chung, A., & Bisconer, S. W. (1996). Treatment retention in women's residential chemical dependency treatment: The effect of admission with children. *Substance Use and Misuse, 31*(8), 1001–1013.

Tracy, C. E., & Williams, H. C. (1991). Social consequences of substance abuse among pregnant and parenting women. *Pediatric Annals, 20*, 548–553.

U.S. General Accounting Office. (1990). Report to the chairman, Committee on Finance, U.S. Senate, *Drug exposed infants, a generation at risk*. Washington, DC: U.S. General Accounting Office.

U.S. National Center for Educational Statistics. (1996). Digest of education statistics. Based on M. T. Moore, E. W. Strang, M. Schwartz, & M. Braddock. (1988). *Patterns in special education service delivery and cost*. Washington, DC: Decision Resources.

Uziel-Miller, N. D., Lyons, J. S., Kissiel, C., & Love, S. (1998). Treatment needs and initial outcomes of a residential recovery program for African-American women and their children. *American Journal of Addiction, 7*(1), 43–50.

Wald, R., Harvey, M., & Hibbard, J. (1995). A treatment model for women substance users. *International Journal of the Addictions, 30*(7), 881–888.

Wallace, B. C. (1995). Women and minorities in treatment. In A. M. Washton (Ed.), *Psychotherapy and substance abuse: A practitioner's handbook* (pp. 470–492). New York: Guilford Press.

Werner, E. E. (1986). Resilient offspring of alcoholics: A longitudinal study from birth to age 18. *Journal of Studies on Alcohol, 47*, 34–40.

Wobie, K., Eyler, F. D., Conlon, M., Clarke, L., & Behnke, M. (1997). Women and children in residential treatment: Outcomes for mothers and their infants. *Journal of Drug Issues, 27*(3), 585–606.

Woods, N. S., Eyler, F. D., Behnke, M., & Conlon, M. (1993). Cocaine use during pregnancy: Maternal depressive symptoms and infant neurobehavior over the first month. *Infant Behavior and Development, 16*, 83–98.

Zweben, J. E., & Brown, V. B. (1995). Current perspectives on substance abuse treatment for women. *Journal of Psychoactive Drugs, 27*(4), 319–320.

10

Prematurity and Serious Medical Conditions in Infancy: Implications for Development, Behavior, and Intervention

❖

KLAUS MINDE

Prematurity and serious medical illnesses that occur during infancy have long provided an opportunity to assess the potential role that biological adversities and the changes they may induce in parenting behaviors can play in the development of children. At the same time, such conditions also represent other complex variables. To take prematurity as an example, we know that despite the objective criteria defining this condition, prematurity is usually associated with other moderating factors such as multiple births, lower socioeconomic status, or particular emotional responses by parents. At the same time, the experience of the premature infant and his or her family in the hospital, as well as the medical and developmental outcome for the infant, will vary with the degree and type of complication as well as the technology available in different settings. Likewise, medical conditions caused by genetic defects or other medical complications may be associated with more or less frequent and extended hospitalizations in early life and can be precursors of a lifelong handicap or reflect a treatable abnormality. Different combinations of all these factors can influence in various ways both the future physical, emotional, and cognitive development of the affected children and the well-being of their families.

In addition, there is a debate whether only chronic but not acute medical conditions have an impact on later behavior. Most authors seem to assume this, although their definitions of a chronic illness vary. For example, some authors define a chronic illness by its severity; others by its duration (Perrin, Ayoub, & Willett, 1993). There is also a long-standing debate between those who claim that psychosocial concerns are specific to individual conditions such as asthma or diabetes (Lavigne & Faier-Routman, 1992) and others who maintain that such concerns are generalized and apply to all children and families coping with chronic conditions (Pless & Pinkerton, 1975).

The effects of an acute illness on later development and behavior are rarely evaluated. The exception is the substantial literature on the impact of prematurity on infants and their families (Minde, 1993). However, even these studies are generally unidimensional; that is, they discuss the effect a concrete event such as an intraventricular hemorrhage has on an infant's later intelligence, without factoring in the contribution of the associated medical conditions or the psychosocial risk factors of the family (Parmelee, 1995).

In this chapter, I first delineate the scope of

the problem; that is, examine the number of children who are affected by a severe medical condition and may spend a significant amount of time in hospitals during their first years of life. I then summarize data from a variety of studies as they relate to the biological and emotional risks premature and other medically compromised infants experience later in life. From the extensive literature on this topic, I selected primarily studies that have looked at small premature infants (i.e., children born weighing less 1,500 g) and infants who suffer from chronic health conditions. Finally, I discuss the practical implications of these data for the infant mental health practitioner and outline intervention strategies and programs that have demonstrated practical value for the development of these vulnerable infants and their families.

PREVALENCE AND SURVIVAL

Prematurity

About 1.1% of all annual live births in the United States and Canada are children weighing less than 1,500 g (Pharoah & Alberman, 1990). This means that there are about 36,000 such births per year in the United States and 3,900 in Canada (Statistics Canada, personal communication, 1997). Infants weighing less than 1,500 g at birth are at least 8 weeks premature and will normally remain in hospital until they have reached their expected date of birth. Survival of these babies has increased remarkably during the past 10 years. Although recent study reports are based mainly on well-equipped regional centers, findings show that survival is generally over 25% in infants weighing between 500 and 750 g, over 50% for those weighing 751 to 1,000 g (Bauchner, Brown, & Peskin, 1988), and 90% for babies with a birthweight between 1,001 and 1,500 g (Pharoah & Alberman, 1990). These data, which document the improved overall outcome, also suggest that more premature infants remain in hospitals for a longer time now than ever before.

Chronic Medical Conditions

The Committee on Children with Disabilities and the Committee on Psychosocial Aspects of Child and Family Health of the American Academy of Pediatrics (1993) have recently published new data about infants suffering from chronic health conditions. Both these committees defined a chronic condition as one that has lasted 3 months or longer. Severity is seen as the impact an illness has on a child's physical, intellectual, and psychological or social functioning (Stein et al., 1987). The impact may be a result of required treatments, persistent symptoms, limitations of activity or mobility, or interference with family activities.

The Committees estimated that 10–20 million children and adolescents in the United States have some type of chronic health condition or impairment. If one estimates the number of individuals under the age of 25 in the United States to be about 72 million, this comes to about 25% of this population. The committees furthermore estimated that about 10% of children with chronic conditions (i.e., about 1.5 to 2 million children and adolescents in the United States) have a chronic illness severe enough to affect their daily life. If these figures were extrapolated to the age group of infants and toddlers, we would expect approximately 250,000 infants in the United States and 3,000 in Canada to have handicaps that significantly affect their day-to-day activities.

Although these are substantial numbers, it must also be realized that the number of chronically ill children who show psychological symptoms is 20% (i.e., about twice as high as the number of children whose handicaps affect their daily lives) (Cadman, Boyle, Szatmari, & Offord, 1987; Gortmaker, Walker, Weitzman, & Sobol, 1990). Psychological symptoms seem less related to the severity of the chronic condition (Perrin, West, & Cylly, 1989) as to its duration. These figures suggest that there are approximately 500,000 infants and toddlers in the United States and 6,000 in Canada who suffer from chronic medical conditions and show behavioral or developmental difficulties.

If we include the approximately 20% prematurely born children who have behavioral or developmental difficulties without being chronically ill, we add another 1–1.5% of the infant population to the symptomatic group and come to about 650,000 American and 8,000 Canadian youngsters who require some form of mental health care during their first years of life.

Hospitalization

An additional psychosocial burden for premature and chronically ill infants is their high rate of hospitalization during their early years. Precise figures are difficult to obtain, but Canadian census data of 1991 indicate that 27% or 106,000 infants under 1 year were hospitalized in Canada in 1990. Of these children, some 2,500 had at least one hospital admission that lasted longer than 3 months during the first and second years of life (Statistics Canada, personal communication, 1991). Dusick (1997), in her discussion of the long-term sequelae of prematurity, states that bronchopulmonary dysplasia (BPD), the most common complication seen in small premature infants, is still present in 45% of these children at 24 months; 23% had more than two readmissions to hospital during that period. Readmission rates for all very-low-birthweight infants vary from 10 to 38%. This on average is two and a half times higher than seen in full-term infants (McCormick, McCarton, Tonascia, & Brooks-Gunn, 1993).

Although data for the early hospitalization of infants with chronic conditions are difficult to obtain, we reviewed the admission patterns for children ages 0 to 24 months at the Montreal Children's Hospital, the pediatric teaching hospital of McGill University, between April 1990 and March 1991. During that period, a total of 3,025 infants ages 0 to 24 months were admitted, making up 24% of all pediatric admissions. Of these infants, 101 stayed between 30 and 60 days, 33 between 61 and 90 days, 28 between 91 and 180 days, and 11 for more than 180 days (Mean = 349 days). This means that a total of 173 infants under two (i.e., 5.7% of all admissions for this age group) remained in hospital for longer than 1 month.

If one substracts all those children who were discharged before reaching 6 months—hence they did not remain in hospital during the ages of 6 to 24 months when hospitalization is most frequently associated with later behavioral problems—the number of long-staying children decreased from 173 to 71 (Direction Générale du Budget et de l'Administration Québécoise, 1992). However, these 71 children still made up about 3.5% of all the children hospitalized after 6 months of age. Furthermore, 96 of the 173 long-staying children had more than one hospital admission during the year of the census (mean = 4.4, *SE* = 3.0, range = 2–18) and may have had admissions in the preceding year as well. These children suffered primarily from cardiovascular diseases (10%), congenital abnormalities (25%), central nervous system (CNS) problems (9%), and infections (25%).

In summary, then, there is clear evidence that a substantial number of premature and chronically ill young children spend a significant part of their early life in hospitals. These children generally have serious physical disorders and their families must adjust to parenting their infants away from their homes. It is important for them to receive practical assistance and sensitive support.

DEVELOPMENTAL SEQUELAE

Biological Risk Factors

Improvements in prenatal care and neonatal medicine have resulted in increased survival of the very-low-birthweight (VLBW) (less than 1500 g) and extremely low-birthweight (ELBW) (less than 1,000 g) infants. This is most dramatic in the ELBW infants; 50 to 60 times more ELBW children survive today than they did 35 years ago (Wolke, 1998). Nevertheless, this increase in survival has been accompanied by a higher incidence of neuropsychiatric disorders in this population (Volpe, 1998; Lorenz, Wooliever, Jetton, & Paneth, 1998). In a recent review of 112 studies with 258 cohorts, Lorenz et al. (1998) examined the cognitive and behavioral outcome of extremely immature (EI) (gestational age of 23 to 26 weeks) and extremely small (ES) (birthweight between 501–800 g) infants. This group reported an increased survival rate of 2.2% per year, between 1980 and 1990, for this population. However, 12.2% of the EI and 7.5% of the ES babies at 24 months had cerebral palsy; 13.6% EI and 14.3% ES infants were mentally retarded (IQ less than 70); 7.5% versus 7.8% were blind and 2.6% vs. 2.9% were deaf. The authors furthermore suggest that each 1% increment in survival added 2% more disabled children to the population.

Although there has not been a parallel increment in developmental disorders in premature infants with a birthweight of more than 1,500 g, VLBW children on average still show a 5- to 7-point lower IQ than same-age controls and 25% exhibit significant abnormalities of cognition and/or behavior (Minde, Perrotta, & Hellmann, 1988; Sykes et al., 1997). This is probably a conservative figure as there is a good possibility that institutions with a poor cognitive and behavioral outcome of their premature population do not publish their follow-up data. Also, most reports to date are single-center studies which were conducted by those involved in the neonatal care of these children (Escobar, Littenberg, & Pettiti, 1991), resulting in a likely underestimation of the prevalence of developmental deficits (Ens-Dokkum et al., 1992).

The cognitive and behavioral sequelae of a chronic illness in early life obviously depend on the type and severity of the condition. For example, severely ill children will have more hospitalizations, which in turn may compromise their later behavior, than do those with less serious conditions (Quinton & Rutter, 1976). This has been well documented in a meta-analysis of 85 studies examining the behavior of children with chronic medical conditions by Lavigne and Faier-Routman (1992), which showed a doubling of both internalizing and externalizing symptoms in these youngsters over control populations up to age 12. However, some diseases seem to produce more consistent difficulties than do others. For example, children with chronic seizures, deafness, cardiac abnormalities, diabetes, and cystic fibrosis showed an effect size of at least 0.5 in five or more independent studies. Other conditions were not associated with an increase in behavioral problems (e.g., rheumatoid arthritis, cerebral palsy, or chronic renal problems). However, they might not have qualified because there were too few well-controlled studies in each category for a proper analysis. The data by Lavigne and Faier-Routman were based on symptoms on such behavior checklists as the Child Behavior Checklist (CBCL, Achenbach, 1991). Because the CBCL has not been standardized on children with chronic medical conditions, a shorter scale, specifically designed for medically compromised populations, was used in a study examining 3,924 children and their families (Offord et al., 1987). These authors found similar results to those described by Lavigne and Faier-Routman. Furthermore, Goldberg and her group, in a series of studies examining the families and the development and behavior of infants with cystic fibrosis (CF) and congenital heart disease (CHD) as well as a control group from age 3 months onward, report that children with CHD in general show more demanding behaviors, more negative mood, higher distractibility, and less acceptable behaviors, as rated by both parents, than do both control children and those affected by CF (Goldberg, Morris, Simmons, Fowler, & Levison, 1990). This finding suggests that precursors of the previously cited behavioral difficulties in children with medical conditions above age 4 can already be detected in infants and toddlers.

Behavioral Risk Factors

In addition to the biological consequences of prematurity, many other factors surrounding the birth of the low-birthweight infant potentially can influence the quality of this infant's later life. On the one hand, such an infant may have characteristics that can make parenting difficult. An example would be the comparatively high incidence of brain damage these children suffer, even in present-day high-technology nurseries. Children with neurological damage, in turn, show a two to three times higher incidence of behavioral disorders than do control populations (Rutter, 1981; Seidel, Chadwick, & Rutter, 1975; Minde, 1984). On the other hand, the long-term outcome of prematurity is, to a significant degree, also influenced by the particular responses each individual caretaker has to the early birth of such an infant and the effect these responses can have on the developing child's transaction with his or her family (Sameroff & Chandler, 1975; Sigman & Parmelee, 1979; Minde, 1980; Stern & Karraker, 1990).

Although details are discussed in the next section, the literature on VLBW infants later in life has long suggested that these children are at an increased risk for a variety of behavioral difficulties, including major and minor psychiatric disorders (Drillien, 1964). Sixty years ago prematurely born children were already described as suffering from "restlessness, nervousness, fatigueability which resulted in distractibility and disturbed concentration" (Benton, 1940, p. 737). However, research of this population has been rather unsystematic and decidedly atheoretical (Kopp, 1983).

Early hospitalization for nonpremature children has also been associated with adverse later emotional consequences (Douglas, 1975; Quinton & Rutter, 1976). However, here again it is not clear whether it is specific illnesses or particular family patterns that increase the vulnerability to later disorders.

Although such factors make comparisons of studies difficult, one can nevertheless distinguish between two general types of investigations that have examined these issues, best labeled the "outcome" and the "process" approaches.

OUTCOME STUDIES

Premature Infants

Most studies of premature infants are using the outcome approach. They focus on short- or long-term benefits of specific neonatal intensive care unit (NICU) treatment techniques or institutionalized psychosocial support programs such as liberal visiting hours. Percentages of disturbed children are tabulated and the children are categorized according to their particular neonatal complications or specific treatments they received. Studies using the outcome approach have come from Minde et al. (1989), Goldberg, Corter, Lojkasek, and Minde (1990), Szatmari, Seigal, Rosenbaum, and Campbell, (1993), Schothorst and van Engeland (1996), and Breslau et al. (1996).

Our own group followed 77 children, of whom 46 were twins, for 4 years (Minde et al., 1989). Youngsters in our study all had weighed less than 1,500 g at birth and been assessed at various times during their first year of life. At 48 months, the children and their families had a comprehensive evaluation, which included a clinical psychiatric interview as well as information on behavioral and cognitive functioning obtained from teachers, parents, and clinicians. Children with serious CNS damage were excluded from the evaluation.

At 4 years, all the children showed normal intelligence and good physical health. However, 43% of the youngsters scored within the abnormal range on the Richman Graham Behaviour Questionnaire (Richman & Graham, 1971), completed by the parents, who indicated a likelihood of a behavior disorder. This was four times higher than among a nonclinical preschool group examined by us earlier (Minde & Minde, 1977). The high-scoring children did not differ in their sex distribution, neonatal illness scores, or intellectual assessment at 12 and 48 months; however, more high scorers were reported by their mothers to have a difficult temperament than were children with low scores, both at 1 year (55% vs. 14%) and at 4 years (42% vs. 7%). Teacher ratings on the Preschool Behaviour Questionnaire (PBQ; Behar & Stringfield 1977) showed that 24% of the children scored in the abnormal range. As expected, that correlated poorly with the maternal ratings ($r = .17$).

An analysis of the individual items of the Richman Graham Behaviour Questionnaire scored by the parents indicated that the most frequently appearing problems (i.e., those oc-curring in more than 40% of all children) were associated with eating difficulties, settling, and overactivity as well as with temper tantrums, demanding attention, and general difficulties of control. Likewise, the PBQ items noted to be present most often by teachers were "being restless, solitary, inattentive, and showing poor concentration." One could conceptualize these symptoms to represent a general immaturity, possible hyperactivity, or an overall poor behavioral organization. This interpretation is supported by the results of our psychiatric evaluation of these children and their families. Only seven children (10.9%) warranted a psychiatric diagnosis using criteria according to the third edition of the *Diagnostic and Statistical Manual of Mental Disorders* (DSM-III; American Psychiatric Association, 1980). This is compatible with findings in other nonclinical populations (Offord et al. 1987).

Goldberg, Corter, et al. (1990) examined specific socioemotional factors in the same sample during infancy which predicted high scores on the behavior questionnaire filled out by parents and teachers at 4 years. Traditional attachment ratings obtained at age 12 months did not differentiate between high- and low-scoring children at 4 years of age on either questionnaire. However, 75% of the children who had disorganized attachment classifications (Main & Solomon 1986), which indicates lack of coherence in the strategies children use to respond to the separation from their attachment figure, were given a psychiatric diagnosis 3 years later. This suggests that the disorganized attachment classification may predict premature children's emotional disturbance.

Most predictive for teacher behavior ratings were scores on maternal responsiveness derived during mother–child observations and on a Family Rating Scale that assessed the emotional functioning of the family both at 12 months and 48 months. Specifically, it was found that the mother–child relationship and family rating accounted for 31% of the variance at age 12 months, whereas in year 4, when a stepwise regression analysis was performed, mother–child relationship and family functioning accounted for 55% of the variance of the behavioral problems score as rated by the teachers. As teachers are generally more objective in their assessment of emotional problems of children, this suggests that family and interactional variables significantly determine the emotional outcome even of medically highly compromised children.

Although our group looked at important variables and experienced no attrition in our sample, we did not follow the children into school age and hence could not explore their behavior with peers and the possible effects that minor cerebral dysfunctions may have had on their behavior.

Szatmari et al. (1993) addressed this issue when they compared 129 ELBW and 145 full-term infants on their psychopathology and impairments in adaptive functioning at ages 7 to 8. The authors used a thorough and valid assessment scheme and assessed three types of psychiatric problems: attention-deficit hyperactivity disorder (ADHD), conduct disorder, and emotional disorders. Parents' rating for ADHD were 9.7% for the ELBW children and 0.7% for the controls. Teachers rated 10.5% of ELBW and 5.6% of control children to have ADHD. Combined ratings signaled 18.3% of the ELBW and 5.7% of the control youngsters as having ADHD. ELBWs did not show an elevation in their rates of conduct and emotional disorders. However, they were judged to be significantly clumsier and less competent in sports, arts, and hobbies. They also had less self-esteem and poorer motor skills. However, a significant amount of the variance in all these behavioral difficulties was accounted for by the lower IQ of the ELBW group. This suggests that in children with birthweights from 501 to 1,000 g, ADHD reflects a neurodevelopmental impairment in brain maturation, resulting in several manifestations of immaturity. This is further supported by the observation that ADHD was diagnosed equally often among girls and boys.

Breslau et al. (1996) also followed a large cohort of low-birthweight (LBW) ($n = 473$) and normal-birthweight (NBW) children ($n = 350$) up to age 6. Their behavior assessment instrument, the National Institute of Mental Health Diagnostic Interview Schedule for Children—Parent Version (DISC-P), was more detailed than those used by other authors and allowed them to elicit information about all relevant DSM-III-R (American Psychiatric Association, 1987) diagnoses. ADHD was again the only diagnostic category associated with LBW status, a finding endorsed by the children's teachers. However, as the children in Breslau's study were only in first grade, the prognostic significance of this finding needs to be confirmed in a follow-up study.

In summary, then, there is evidence from outcome studies that a substantial number of premature infants score high on various behavioral checklists, primarily on symptoms denoting attention factors and impulsivity. These difficulties can be measured during the preschool years (Minde et al., 1989) and they remain quite stable, at least until early adolescence (Schothorst & van Engeland 1996). There is also some evidence that it is the ELBW and small for date children who most often show these difficulties. Nevertheless, it is possibile that most of these attention problems are reflections of a neurodevelopmental impairment in brain maturation, as was clinically documented in low IQ children (Szatmari et al., 1993). This suggests that there is no convincing evidence that prematurely born children, per se, have higher rates of psychiatric disturbances.

Hospitalized and Chronically Ill Infants

The behavioral outcome of children who are repeatedly hospitalized during their first 3 years of life was studied by Douglas (1975) and Quinton and Rutter (1976). Both investigations revealed that a single hospital admission of less than 1 week did not lead to later difficulties in children. However, multiple admissions, of which at least one had taken place between 6 and 60 months of age, were associated with a significant increase of both psychiatric disorder and delinquency at ages 12 to14. These findings suggest that young children are "sensitized" by their initial hospitalization. Because they are unable to conceptualize the nonpermanence of this experience, a second hospitalization and associated separation from their caretakers will then become a serious stress. Furthermore, even the much more liberal modern visiting practices do not seem to have significantly changed this pattern. Thus, Fahrenfort, Jacob, Miedena, and Schweizer (1996) assessed 40 children who had two or more hospitalizations before age 5 on the Behaviour Checklist developed by Rutter (1967). At age 7, they were compared to 73 control children who had not been hospitalized. The overall behavior rating of the clinical group was 50% higher than that of the controls (6.2 vs. 9.3), with children who experienced surgical procedures showing the most elevated scores. The study had a comparatively small sample and the children's actual experiences in hospital were assessed retrospectively. Nevertheless, it confirms the clinical impression that hospitalizations in children are traumatic to many young children even in contemporary institutions.

When we look at outcome studies of specific populations of chronically ill children who could be expected to have been hospitalized early on in life, the literature provides little guidance. Although many studies have examined the long-term psychological sequelae of specific medical conditions such as asthma, diabetes, or cancer (Lavigne & Faier-Routman, 1992), authors rarely specify the age of onset of the diseases in these children and never mention the number or length of hospitalizations these children experienced. Some reviews (Eiser, 1990; Pless & Nolan, 1991) nevertheless confirm that compared to physically well children, those with any type of chronic disorder have about twice the risk of developing a secondary emotional handicap. This is true for population-based studies (Offord et al., 1987) as well as for those referring to single disease groups. The exception, here again, are children who suffered CNS damage, of whom up to 35% show psychiatric disturbances (Breslau, 1985). Younger children seem to do much worse than older ones.

In other related work, Goldberg and colleagues followed a group of 26 children with CHD, 15 with CF, and 30 controls from 3 months onward and assessed their attachment patterns at 12 months. They report that among both controls and children with CF two-thirds were securely attached to their mothers (Fischer-Fay, Goldberg, Simmons, & Levison, 1988), while only 48% of the children with CHD were classified in this category (Goldberg, Fischer-Fay, Simmons, Fowler, & Levison, 1989). This may be related either to the more frequent hospitalizations in the CHD infants or to the stress reported by the parents of these children, which was significantly higher than the levels experienced by parents of children with CF (Goldberg, Morris, et al., 1990).

In summary, then, hospitalization is clearly upsetting to young children. Long-term detrimental effects have not been documented in children hospitalized during the last decade, when parents were actively encouraged to help care for their children in hospitals. Still, we have some indication that difficulties still occur at least up to age 7. Process studies may be helpful here because they attempt to discover the pathways which lead from event *A* to outcome *B*.

PROCESS STUDIES

In the process approach, investigators focus on small premature infants or chronically ill children as a prototype for studying how specific events and interactions may lead to normal or compromised psychosocial functioning. As will be appreciated, developmental pathways are generally complex and multifaceted. Process studies, therefore, do not always follow the rigorous criteria of traditional scientific inquiry but also include clinical data or individuals' reflections on how they have experienced specific events.

The model most commonly used to understand the complex interchanges between an infant and its caretakers is the transactional model, first described by Sameroff and Chandler (1975). These investigators saw the behavior of a child primarily to be the result of the ongoing changes and reassessments of behavior that take place between each child and those interacting with him within the context of their biological and social limitations. They also documented that the final intellectual and behavioral outcome of children who have experienced a biological insult early on in life depends far more on the care these children receive than on the severity of the injury. This theoretical model is an open one, suggesting that change can occur at any time and long-term predictions are difficult to make.

Another model that has been used to clarify these issues is based on the idea that children pass through specific "waystations," which can either ameliorate or compromise further development (Rutter, 1981). Rutter stresses that these waystations may be developmentally determined (e.g., include influences which come to bear when the child learns to talk or enters adolescence), or they can have primarily social or interpersonal determinants. For example, an infant may make his mother feel depressed, which in turn will lead her to become emotionally unavailable, leading to an insecure attachment of the infant.

It should be stressed that both these models encompass the notion that the interpretation of an individual's behavior can be based on observable interactions between the individual and others, as well as on the more or less idiosyncratic attributions the interactional partners may have regarding each others' behavior. Both models are, therefore, compatible with the increasing literature that suggests that our thoughts and fantasies about our children form an important matrix of these children's early emotional experiences, as they determine much of our early interactions with our children (Lebovici, 1983; Stern, 1985).

Premature Infants

What do we know about the impact of prematurity on the transactional system of an infant? A substantial body of descriptive research suggests that mothers of premature infants show continuing anxiety and low confidence in their caregiving competence, at least during the first year of their child's life (Crnic, Greenberg, Ragozin, Robinson, & Basham, 1983; Brooten et al., 1988; Corter & Minde, 1987). These concerns are thought to be related to specific interaction patterns that have been observed between premature infants and their caretakers. Briefly, it has been suggested that preterm infants have problems with information processing and are, therefore, easily disorganized in their overall behavior (Field, 1977). As this often makes them appear hypoactive to everyday stimuli or handling, mothers initially tend to compensate for this perceived deficit through excessive stimulation (Miles & Holditch-Davis, 1995). This, in turn, may have the unintended effect of derailing the infants' behavior even further. Consequently, the infants may abruptly shift from hypo- to hyperactivity, leaving the caregiver at a loss of how to appropriately stimulate such an infant (Beckwith & Cohen, 1983: Barnard, Bee, & Hammond, 1984).

Als (1992) has developed this thinking further. She has analyzed the NICU environment and its effect on infants who have suddenly been displaced from the econiche of the maternal womb, which is adapted to provide support and nurture neurodevelopmental progress, and developed the concept of "synaction." This concept incorporates a number of developmental principles (e.g., the principle of continuous organism–environment interaction) and explains many of the neurodevelopmental and parenting problems these infants experience. For example, in a recent paper, Als and Gilkerson (1997) report that the developing brain releases up to 100,000 cortical neurons per minute during the middle and later part of pregnancy. Premature exposure to an "unecological" environment obviously can have significant effects on neuronal release and, through it, on the infants' and parents' behavior.

Another suggested pathway to compromised parenting is thought to be the generally lower socioeconomic status of the parents of premature infants (Crnic et al., 1983). Poverty, among other things, is associated with (1) limited emotional support services for mothers and subsequent maternal insensitivity (Sameroff, 1986); (2) a lack or inconsistent stimulation for young children as parents lack the means to provide it; (3) poor child health and developmental problems, which affect parenting; and (4) economic life stresses to families, which decrease the parents' coping responses (Watson, Kirby, Kelleher, & Bradley, 1996). In fact, in a study of 159 poor and 437 nonpoor premature infants by Watson et al. (1996), density of living and poverty contributed 28% to the children's HOME scores (Bradley & Caldwell, 1984), ranging right after maternal intelligence.

Some authors also believe that an important aspect of our approach to these infants is based on stereotyped concepts we hold about prematurity. According to Stern and Karraker (1990), premature infants are generally seen as less physically developed, less cognitively competent, less behaviorally active, less sociable, and less likable than full-term infants. Interestingly, this is the opinion not only of women who have no personal experience in caring for a premature infant but also of actual mothers of premature infants. However, it should be stressed that mothers vary substantially in the extent to which they stereotype their infants, and no data show that these early misperceptions have a significant effect on the children's later development (Stern & Karraker 1990).

Still another set of events that typically affects the early interaction between caretakers and their small infants is linked to the disruption of some basic biological and social parameters associated with the pregnancy and delivery of these infants. Premature infants may be born only 3 to 4 weeks after their mothers have first felt the babies' movements. Experiencing a moving infant is an important step in the ongoing process of prenatal maternal preoccupation and attachment (Minde & Stewart, 1988; Brazelton & Cramer, 1990). If this process is suddenly interrupted, giving birth changes from the crowning event after a clearly marked preparation and waiting time to a crisis associated with anxiety and fear of losing this baby. In addition, mothers have usually not yet attended childbirth classes and, therefore, are often relatively poorly informed about the demands of early parenting. Often, they also experience a sense of failure and loss for having given birth to a less than perfect baby under difficult circumstances. An increasing number of premature twins and triplets are also the result of artificial insemination or drug-dependent fertility treatments. This often brings with it guilt and recrimination as parents feel that their powerful desire to have children may have compromised these babies' health and development. Added to this is the overwhelming technical environment of an NICU, the initial home of these tiny infants, and the mothers' fear that their infant may grow up with a developmental handicap.

Yet, after a premature delivery, there is little time to mourn the loss of the perfect baby before the demands of the new sick infant(s) must be met. Because they are so preoccupied with their own adjustment to this unforeseen event, it is often difficult for parents to obtain or comprehend appropriate information about their infant early on. Therefore, unreasonable expectations of the baby's future may develop. For example, many parents worry that their children will not be sufficiently attached to them because of the anomaly of their neonatal experience. In addition, mothers, even today, are frequently criticized by their relatives for having "failed" their families by giving birth to such tiny infants (Minde, 1984). The ensuing feelings of guilt, anger, and despair are exacerbated when mothers have given birth in an outside hospital (i.e., a hospital without an NICU) and are separated from their infants during the first days of their lives. The acute yearning for their infant that many mothers in outlying hospitals experience during this time was one of the reasons why some 10% of our mothers signed themselves out of the hospital before their obstetrician felt it to be appropriate (Minde, 1987). The father is often the only parent readily available to NICU staff as well as the conveyor of information to the mother of the infant. He, therefore, becomes a special source of comfort to the mother during this period. Nevertheless, a substantial number of fathers become so protective of their wives or partners at that time that they screen out information they feel the infant's mother should not hear yet (Marton, Minde, & Ogilvie, 1981).

These clinical data have been supplemented by work that has shown that a mother's representation and fantasy of her baby increase in richness between the fourth and seventh months of pregnancy. After that time, maternal thoughts about the growing infant become more vague. This is seen as a normal defensive phenomenon that allows the child to be born into a less predetermined set of expectations and thus to have a better chance to establish his or her unique characteristics within a more neutral environment (Ammaniti, 1989). These observations suggest a greater potential discordance between the imagined and real baby following a premature birth. This may add to the difficulties a mother may have in developing an easy and positive relationship with her newborn.

Another potential obstacle parents have to deal with is the NICU as an institution. As stated earlier, an intensive care unit invariably is a busy and highly technical space. However, such a unit also has a rather unique culture, based on myths and belief systems. For example, parents will usually be exposed to an ongoing split between the intimacy suggested by personalized namecards for their infants ("It is a boy") and the routine aspects of the almost robot-like care suggested by a respirator. This notion is further supported by the fact that the infants are fed at fixed intervals even if this means that they have to be aroused from a deep sleep. They are also subjected to some tough handling or even pain, all of which is contrary to the expected mother-mediated protection from environmental perturbations. Als et al. (1996) have convincingly documented that the traditionally practiced routine care of preterm infants deprives them of a steady supply of nutrients, temperature control, and hormone-regulating systems. This may have consequences for their future development. For example, there is increasing evidence that repetitive pain and stress may alter the neurological substrate associated with pain (Anand, 1998), and that this, in turn, can be implicated in the extension of early intraventricular hemorrhage to periventricular leukomalacia.

Many parents are instinctively aware of the physiological needs of their babies and feel frustrated that all through the hospital stay a truly intimate contact between them and their infant seems impossible. Thus, parents can make few decisions about their infants because virtually all routine caretaking tasks, such as feeding times, are determined by the medical establishment. As many mothers who give birth to a premature baby have had previous miscarriages and other serious obstetrical complications, they are especially sensitized to the potential loss of their infant. It is no wonder, therefore, that parents of premature infants often feel like visitors rather than parents to their newborns, which prevents them from having confidence in their own parenting skills (Freud, 1988; Minde & Stewart, 1988).

Concerns for the psychosocial welfare of infants and parents have led to many changes in the NICU scene in the last 30 years, best exemplified by the liberalization of visiting hours. Yet, parents continue to show differential behaviors toward their infants, and clinicians have long searched for explanations for such widely varying caretaking patterns. In our own studies, where we continuously recorded 10 discrete parent and 8 infant behaviors for 45 minutes twice a week, we found that mothers generally became more engaged with their infants during each successive visit. However, some mothers were consistently more engaged than others (Minde, Marton, Manning, & Hines, 1980). Not unexpectedly, we found that the quantity of interaction a mother showed during her visits was related to the frequency of her visits; mothers who showed little activity with their children visited infrequently. More significantly, we also found that the level of engagement with the infant in the hospital predicted how frequently mothers interacted with the infant at home at 3 months corrected age (i.e., the time at which the infant would have been 3 months of age had they been carried to term). The factors that most clearly distinguished between the high- and low-engagement groups was the strength of the relationships the mother reported with her own mother and with her husband rather than events occurring at the time of delivery.

The medical complications experienced by premature infants also appear to have a substantial impact on their parents' perception. Using an objective scale for measuring the 20 most common diseases or pathophysiological states encountered in premature infants every day, we reported on 20 infants with few and 20 infants with serious complications during their hospital stay (Minde, Whitelaw, Brown, & Fitzhardinge, 1983). Although the two groups did not differ on variables such as weight, gestational age, or socioeconomic status, there was a clear association between illness and mother–infant interaction. In a dyad with the sicker baby, the baby's level of motor activity and alertness and the mother's levels of smiling and touching were consistently lower both during nursery visits and during observations 6 and 12 weeks after discharge home. In a companion study that involved 14 infants with a long perinatal illness (more than 35 days) and 17 with a short perinatal illness (less than 17 days), we also found significant differences in infant and parental behaviors. In the case of infants who were sick for less than 17 days, both motor and social behaviors of the infant and mother rebounded quickly following recovery from the illness. However, in the case of infants who were sick for more than 35 days, the recovery of maternal behavior lagged behind the infant's recovery and could still be noted 3 months after discharge home. This means that even after the sick infant had recovered physically and reached healthy levels of activity with no sign of CNS damage, maternal behavior remained at a lower level.

One interpretation of these findings is that illness in infants leads mothers to view them as vulnerable, first described by Green and Solnit (1964) as the vulnerable child syndrome. This formulation is compatible with findings of Estroff, Yando, Burke, and Snyder (1994), who reported that 56% of 50 mothers of preschoolers who were born prematurely rated them as vulnerable at 36 months, using the Child Vulnerability Scale (Forsyth, McCue, Horwitz, Leventhal, & Burger, 1996). The vulnerable children also scored higher on social withdrawal and somatic problems and aggression on the CBCL (Achenbach, 1991), although their cognitive abilities and medical histories did not differentiate them from the controls.

In a subsequent study, Thomasgard and Metz (1996) provided 2-year follow-up data on 114 children some of whom had been rated as "vulnerable" 2 years earlier. Nineteen percent of these children had been born prematurely. The boys who had received high vulnerability ratings previously showed significantly increased externalizing problems on the CBCL at follow-up, while the vulnerable girls showed increased internalizing problems. Overall, there were three groups of children who were seen as more vulnerable by their mothers: (1) firstborn children ($p = .02$); (2) children who had a medical condition ($p = .003$); (3) children who had a previous life-threatening illness or injury ($p = .03$).

In summary, then, there is good evidence from process studies that the interactional difficulties between premature infants and their caretakers are reflections of the mother's insecurity and low self-esteem. These characteristics, in turn, may be related to the early relationships a mother had with her own mother, reinforced by the ecology of the NICU, an infant's initial medical status, the support available from the spouse and the rest of the family, and her conceptualization of the child as vulnerable.

Other Hospitalized Infants

When we look for data-based process studies to explain how early hospitalizations in nonpremature infants are translated into compromised behavior in later life, few such studies are available. There are multiple reasons for this. Authors studying the process of hospitalization have traditionally examined older children or looked at samples that included a wide age range of patients. They have also tried to substantiate associations between specific acute or chronic conditions, sociodemographic or personal factors, and children's psychological upsets. However, young children's concepts of hospitals or their prior personality are of little relevance in predicting the effects of hospitalization in them. Likewise, there is little evidence that specific procedures, such as an injection or a rectal temperature, which are frequently examined variables in past studies, will affect young children differentially.

In fact, our knowledge about development would indicate that the emotional stress experienced by hospitalized infants is primarily due both to the rupture of the infant's developing attachment with his or her caregivers and the parallel loss of habits or routines that help the young child organize his or her day-to-day life experiences. Young children's needs to be secure and concretely reassured about those ministering to them is clearly violated in a hospital. To give just some examples, a normal 36-month-old child on average has contacts with 6.6 different individuals a day and 8.4 individuals a week (Lewis, 1987). Hospitalized infants, on the other hand, have to cope with 40 and more different faces every day (Pinard & Minde, 1991). Young children require continuous and sensitive caretaking experiences as they develop patterns of trust to those important to them. However, nurses tend to have a more stereotyped way of acting than do parents and are involved in painful procedures as well as nurturing activities. This may be confusing and upsetting to young children.

Children also need routines to give them a sense of predictability and control over their lives, yet hospitals provide few such helpful structures. Thus, beds are used for playing as well as sleeping; lights may be on all through the night; comforting toys may not qualify for hygienic reasons; and the ever-changing scene of newly admitted or discharged patients does not allow easily for adaptation and the development of new structures.

In many ways, then, a normal hospital environment may present even the nonpremature infant and toddler with serious sensory overload. Because hospitalized young children usually battle an acute or chronic medical condition, their habitual coping abilities will already be compromised, and the lack of environmental familiarity will be perceived as that much more disruptive.

North American studies indicate that virtually all pediatric hospitals presently allow parents to visit their young children during the day (Hamlett, Walker, Evans, & Weise, 1994) and provide the possibility to room in on request (Alexander, Powell, Williams, White, & Conlon, 1988). However, mothers still show individualized visiting and rooming-in patterns. In a study by Knafl, Cavallari, and Dixon (1988), 62 families whose young children were hospitalized for up to 3 weeks were repeatedly interviewed. Among other things, parents were classified in terms of their participation in their children's day-to-day activities in hospital as level I or level II parents. Level I parents were more compliant toward the medical system and tried to look after their children by "being nice" to the hospital staff. They had less education and had experienced fewer hospitalizations within their families. Level II mothers more often brought along a sibling and were generally more critical of the nursing care (42% vs. 0%) and overall medical care (29% vs. 3%) their infants received.

The authors do not provide follow-up data on the infants but suggest that the more active behavior of level II parents, though creating more conflicts within the ward milieu, seemed to have been beneficial to the infants. Although they offered no reason for this conclusion, one may speculate that the 24 level II mothers (30% of the total sample) were generally more secure and autonomous in their mothering roles, and for that reason could model a more active form of support for their infants. Fathers of level II infants were also more involved with their infants; that is, they played and visited with them more often than did level I fathers.

Another area examined in a recent literature review on pediatric hospitalization (Thompson, 1985) suggests that mothers of young infants are much more committed to their infants if they had them home for 2 or more weeks during the first 3 months of life. In a study involving some 30 infants, Lampe, Trause, and Kennell (1977) found that only 16% of infants who had never been home were visited daily by their caretakers, whereas 70% of those who had been home had daily visits. As samples were matched for social class and illness, Lampe suggests that a relationship has to be sealed through total care provided at home before a mother can truly commit herself to her infant.

More recent work supports this notion. For example, Robinson, Rankin, and Drotar (1996) tested a comprehensive model of factors, which they hypothesized to predict maternal visitation and state anxiety, with 86 hospitalized children ages 10 months to 4 years. Factors included family resources, (e.g., socioeconomic status), proximity to hospital, family demands (e.g., number of children at home or duration of hospitalization), child characteristics (e.g., gender, age, and nature of illness), and parent–child relationship (e.g., security of attachment). The security of attachment, as measured by the Q-sort methodology of Waters (1991), was the only significant predictor variable of maternal visitation rate (R^2 change = .08). This confirms that the type of attachment is an important mediating variable in the parents' understanding of their children's needs. What is unexpected, however, is that it seems to override many of the practical parameters, such as financial resources or children at home, that have previously been accepted as valid predictors of parental visitation rates.

Even more striking, though also supported by attachment theory, are findings that maternal attachment security toward handicapped children are related to the way parents deal with the diagnosis of their chronically ill child (Pianta, Marvin, Britner, & Borowitz, 1996). Specifically, these authors objectively assessed the parents' resolution of their 91 infants' chronic medical conditions (epilepsy and cerebral palsy). Elements of resolution included the recognition that feelings had changed since the diagnosis; there was an assertion that life and activity continued; the search for "a reason" had been abandoned; and the child's abilities were accurately acknowledged. Marvin & Pianta (1996) found that 46% of mothers whose children suffered from these conditions had come to terms with their child's illness while 54% had not accepted it. The investigators found that parental resolution versus nonresolution of the child's diagnosis was more strongly associated with secure versus insecure child–parent attachment than with severity of child illness and type of illness (cerebral palsy vs. epilepsy) and age of child (Sheeran, Marvin, & Pianta, 1997). This suggests that some form of assessing attachment may be useful in predicting the acceptance, as well as the overall later parent–child relationship in medically high-risk dyads.

To summarize these data, there is much evidence that suggests that a stay in hospital is highly stressful for young children as well as for their families. Although no recent studies have delineated the possible consequences different durations of hospitalizations may have on the later psychosocial functioning of children, the present review indicates that hospital traditions are difficult to modify and require close monitoring by mental health professionals. Thus, the mission of hospitals even today is based on priorities other than those suggested by mental health principles. In effect, professionals in hospitals see themselves as diagnosticians and treaters of illness and disease and only secondarily as guardians for the psychosocial development of infants. In addition, hospitals have the task of catering to their long-staying employees while individual patients stay for comparatively brief periods. As a result, hospital organizations are serving two very different populations. This does not always lead to practices that are sensitive to children's developmental needs. Finally, we have to recognize that many young hospitalized children suffer from chronic illnesses that require further medical interventions, and that these illnesses may be associated with disruptions in the child's normal developmental pathway.

ROLES OF INFANT MENTAL HEALTH PROFESSIONALS IN HOSPITALS

Infant mental health specialists can have a significant role in providing "early intervention" to infants and their families (Zeanah & McDonough, 1989; Bromwich, 1990; Mahoney &

O'Sullivan, 1990). This term refers to the concept that the infant specialist "inter-venes" (i.e., "comes between") the components of a system early on to help those involved in the system to achieve a developmentally more appropriate functioning.

Using Bronfenbrenner's (1979) integrated approach to sources of social influence as a model, we postulate that such an intervention can take place on three distinct levels. The infant specialist can play a role in the assessment and treatment of emotional disturbances in infants and their families. This would reflect on Bronfenbrenner's "microsystem." However, a family also exists in the context of a "mesosystem," in which there are links between the child's microsystem settings. A good example here would be the effect a ward milieu might have on a child's behavior in hospital and later at home. Furthermore, policies and regulations on levels in which the child does not directly participate will also influence the child's behavior. Bronfenbrenner calls this the "exosystem." Relevant examples here would be the overall philosophy or ecology of an institution vis-à-vis parental involvement in the care of an infant and the support given to a family. Interventions may be necessary at this level as well.

Influencing Hospital Ecology

Although the last 20 years have seen great changes in the awareness administrators and clinicians have shown toward the needs of infants and their families, much can still be done to assist young children and their families in coping with the hospital experience. For example, our own studies, which took place in a 65-bed unit, showed that infants who stayed an average of 49 days in hospital were cared for by 72 different nurses (Marton, Dawson, & Minde, 1980). This does not help parents in their adjustment to their babies.

Infant mental health practitioners should attempt to participate actively and consult with hospital administrators and other interested groups to create a hospital milieu that furthers both the physical and psychological well-being of their infant patients. Although the approaches individual clinicians take in influencing their own institutions should respect local conditions, the following recommendations are designed to facilitate the attachment of parents to their infants through facilitating parental visiting.

1. A neonatal intensive care nursery should be limited to 30 beds, because larger units require so much personnel that meaningful personal interactions between staff, patients, and their families become very difficult.

2. Each intensive care nursery should have preventive intervention programs. In a recent annotation, Wolke (1991) points out that small and inexpensive changes in the physical and social environment and nursing care pattern help reduce unnecessary suffering of the smallest infants. These changes include the way small infants are handled (regular massages increase food intake and decrease apneas), the noise and light to which they are exposed, and how they are positioned in their incubators (they do better if they are put into a hammock). Als (1992) and Als, Duffy, and McAnulty (1996) have outlined methods by which these infants can be shielded against untoward stimulation. These include a review of the advisability of suctioning or chest physical therapy schedules as well as vital sign taking and other routine medical procedures. Suggestions also deal with positioning of the infant, specific holding techniques, and generally providing specific state regulatory and neurodevelopmentally supportive practices.

3. Each intensive care nursery should have facilities that make visiting a comfortable task for parents. For example, there should be rocking chairs, facilities for breastfeeding or pumping, and areas where parents can be alone with their infants.

4. The physician who provides care to the premature infant should be identified to the parents and he or she should actively approach the parents and tell them of their infant's progress. This is especially important for disadvantaged caregivers who often find it hard to advocate for their infants. Parents should also be told how to get in touch with the physician in charge of their infant (i.e., they should be given times of ward rounds or regular conferences).

5. Each infant should have a key nurse assigned to him or her for the entire hospitalization. This nurse would then be in a position to monitor the parents' visiting patterns and to find out details of their personal and social backgrounds. This knowledge may give important clues about the individuals' parenting abilities and may be used to alert other professionals if additional support is needed.

6. The parents should be given every opportunity to partake in the care of their infants. Thus, there should be no limits to parental and

sibling visits, and parents should be encouraged to get involved early on in the routine infant care. Breastfeeding should be encouraged and facilitated, and all parents should receive literature on prematurity as well as ward routines.

7. Parents of premature infants should have the opportunity to sleep at least one night with their infant in one room prior to the infant's discharge from hospital. This will familiarize the parents with the infant and alleviate potential fears or concerns.

Similar policies should be adopted on the regular infant ward. In addition, infants hospitalized there for any length of time need ongoing stimulation and care not usually provided by nurses. Child-life programs can be of great assistance, as can well-trained volunteers. Parents should also have the opportunity to stay with their infants for 24 hours a day; that is, there should be "adult" services such as showers, a place for clothes, or a place to get a snack on Sunday night.

The infant psychiatrist or mental health specialist, because of his or her intimate knowledge of child development and the psychosocial conditions necessary for optimizing the developmental process, can document the need for such services or assist others who attempt to obtain them.

Providing Consultation and Support for Staff and Families of Hospitalized Infants

In addition to helping create and maintain institutional developmental support structures for infants and their families, the infant psychiatrist or infant mental health specialist also can partake in the day-to-day activities of an NICU or regular infant ward. Such activities may include participating at regular staff ward rounds, psychosocial rounds, staff meetings, and/or in-service conferences. Joining members of the medical staff at their rounds is often especially beneficial, because medical problems can be linked with psychosocial concerns as they come up and possible interventions can be discussed immediately.

The role of the infant specialist in these situations may be as follows:

1. Helping parents and staff members to understand their different roles and needs vis-à-vis the infant and each other.

2. Serving as an advocate who is able to explain specific behaviors of a parent or staff person to others and thus facilitating communication between individuals or groups.

3. Assisting parents in understanding their feelings or actions and helping them regain control over their lives.

4. Teaching principles of child and family development. This may include lecturing about the possible detrimental consequences of hospitalization, developmental aberrations associated with repeated separation from primary caretakers, and post-traumatic stress disorder caused by specific traumatic medical or nursing procedures. It may also include discussions about ways the hospital staff can monitor the internal representations parents have of their children (i.e., pick out those who see their infants as perpetually helpless, vulnerable, ill, or handicapped or who have not come to terms with their condition).

It is clear that interventions by the infant specialist in any of these areas must be geared to the specific hospital milieu, the characteristics of parents and children, and the medical condition of the child in question. The roles of the infant specialist can also encourage such specific remedial or supportive activities as the following:

1. Setting up a hospitalwide program that identifies infants who may have to remain in hospital for more than 3 to 4 weeks. Staff members can then be educated to provide an environment for these infants that approximates their normal developmental needs as closely as possible. Such a schedule can assure the routines that are necessary to give young children a sense of mastery over their lives.

2. Encouraging members of the nursing staff to include parents in their team, perhaps by assessing the caretaker's strengths and limitations, after which their individual care commitment is negotiated. However, parental involvement can also be increased by giving parents exclusive caretaking tasks (e.g., bathing the child), which they must perform every day and are required to delegate to someone else, such as a nurse, if they cannot be present on a particular day. Such a task often gives the parents the sense that they are vital members of the treatment team and increases their visits and general involvement with their infant.

3. Helping to set up group meetings for par-

ents of premature infants. Such meetings are an effective way to increase the parents' feelings of competence. One way to structure such groups is to ask a parent who had such a small infant within the last 12 months to be the leader. These "veteran" parents invariably establish a good relationship with the new parents very quickly, which allows the latter to work through some of their own grief quite rapidly. Once this has been achieved, the new parents will feel that they are more active participants in the caregiving process, which leaves them in a better state to assimilate information on the treatment and care of their infants (Minde et al., 1980).

4. Encouraging the staff to provide flexible hospital arrangements for young children who stay in hospital for longer periods. Examples here may be to provide the child with two beds or a clearly divided crib where one side is the "sleeping" and the other the "play" or "eating" side. Such an arrangement supports the child's need for clearly demarcated structures in his or her day-to-day life. Parents may be encouraged to bring some special foods from home. It is also important to have the child sleep in a darkened room and provide sufficient space for parental rooming in.

5. Supporting arrangements that allow a child psychiatrist to join a multidisciplinary medical or surgical team whose members care for children who need organ transplants or suffer from specific serious disorders, such as cancer. Such teams often practice protocol-driven medical care and a psychosocial evaluation and possible treatment plan can easily be included in such protocols. This destigmatizes the role of the mental health specialist, and families are usually keen to being assisted in helping their young children to face and manage the challenges associated with such complex diseases (Pinard & Minde, 1991).

Providing Direct Treatment Services for Young Children and Their Parents

There is increasing evidence that the direct treatment of infants within the context of their families or other caregiving systems can have a significant impact on the psychological functioning of the infant (Cramer et al., 1990; Lieberman, Weston, & Pawl, 1991; Pinard & Minde 1991).

The principles of such treatment are to allow the hospitalized infant to experience the world

as predictable and to give the infant an opportunity to interact with an adult who permits him or her to experience some autonomy and mastery. This can be done by arranging a specific play time with the infant for 30 minutes, at the same time every day, in a private designated space. The therapist may use a small number of toys that are of interest to the child. During these sessions the therapist has the infant choose the activity or game and follows his or her interactive lead. Infants rapidly understand and appreciate the specialness of these time periods, as they provide the infants with an opportunity to experience a relationship whose intensity they can significantly modulate. As much as the hospitalized child's day-to-day activities are controlled from without, these islands of interactional mastery provide important nuclei for growing security and competence. After the infant has become familiar with the therapist, parents can be brought in to observe the interactions and to discuss their observations. This furthers their sensitive perception of the infant's behavior, including reciprocal communications and an awareness of the infant's sources of competence or stress. It can also demonstrate ways in which a particular behavior problem of a child may be solved. It is obvious that such a therapeutic regimen can only work within the context of a mutually supportive partnership among different hospital professionals, because both a private space and a regular, uninterrupted time period must be ensured to allow treatment to proceed.

Other types of interventions may focus on the parents and/or other family members because their behaviors are judged to be inappropriate by members of the staff. The aim here is often to learn more about the private associations the infant's illness has for the parents and to work on bringing these perceptions closer to the infant's actual developmental needs (Minde, 1999).

SUMMARY AND CONCLUSIONS

The data reviewed in this chapter document that the parenting of small premature infants is a highly complex process that defies easy generalization. However, they also suggest that these infants pass through specific "waystations," which may serve as important markers for their later development. For example, premature infants do show specific behavioral characteristics during their first year of life that make parenting more difficult and stressful. Mothers who rapidly engage themselves with their newborn infants in the hospital nursery also seem to be more sensitive to their behavioral cues and have a better relationship with these children during the ensuing years. There is also good evidence that interventions during the first months of life can modify the interactional patterns of the mother–child dyad quite significantly. Such interventions seem especially useful when they combine a supportive and educational component, and when they include other parents who have lived through the experience of having a premature infant in the recent past.

A further important theme of the reviewed studies is the repeated finding that children who are hospitalized early on in life, even within the context of present-day liberal visiting practices, are profoundly affected by this experience. In fact, it appears that the ecology of a hospital, which demands that the young child cope with many unfamiliar individuals and unpredictable challenges to his or her body, by its very nature does not foster normal development. Furthermore, there are caretakers who continue to perceive their children as vulnerable and fragile long after their medical recovery. Such a view can increase the emotional burden of these children and needs to be addressed by the mental health professional. As recent medical technology has made survival of many children with serious medical illnesses possible, we now see a parallel increase in the hospitalization rates of young children in our tertiary care institutions. This increase requires us to think about new ways of empowering families to participate in the care of their infants in hospitals. It also makes a reassessment of routine hospital practices desirable.

The infant psychiatrist who has an appreciation of the biological aspects of disease because of his training in medicine is also an expert on the developmental needs of infants, and following a systems approach such a professional can provide a helpful role in sensitizing the many players in this field to the best interest of the infant. Nevertheless, this chapter also shows that the work of establishing the developmental pathways that can guide the growth and development of these special infants has only begun and will provide many challenges for future generations of researchers and clinicians.

REFERENCES

Achenbach, T. M. (1991). *Manual for the Child Behavior Checklist and Revised Child Behavior Profile.* Burlington: Department of Psychiatry, University of Vermont.

Alexander D., Powell G. M., Williams, P., White, M., & Conlon, M. (1988). Anxiety levels of rooming-in and non-rooming-in parents of young hospitalized children. *Maternal Child Nursing Journal, 17,* 79–99.

Als H. (1992). Individualized, family-focused developmental care for the very low-birthweight preterm infant in the NICU. In S. L. Friedman & M. D. Sigman (Eds.), *The psychological development of low birthweight children* (pp. 341–388). Norwood, NJ: Ablex.

Als, H., Duffy, F. H., & McAnulty, G. B. (1996). Effectiveness of individualized neurodevelopmental care in the newborn intensive care unit (NICU). (1996). *Acta Paediatrica, 416,* 21–30.

Als, H., & Gilkerson, L. (1997). The role of relationship-based developmentally supportive newborn intensive care in strengthening outcome of preterm infants. *Seminars in Perinatology, 21,* 164–177.

American Psychiatric Association. (1980). *Diagnostic and statistical manual of mental disorders* (3rd ed.). Washington, DC: Author.

American Psychiatric Association. (1987). *Diagnostic and statistical manual of mental disorders* (3rd ed., rev.). Washington, DC: Author.

Ammaniti, M. (1989). *Symposium on maternal representations.* Paper presented at the Fourth World Congress of Infant Psychiatry and Allied Disciplines, Lugano, Switzerland.

Anand, K. J. (1998). Clinical importance of pain and stress in preterm neonates. *Biology of the Neonate, 73,* 1–9.

Barnard, K., Bee, H., & Hammond, M. (1984). Developmental changes in maternal interactions with term and preterm infants. *Infant Behavior and Development, 7,* 101–113.

Bauchner, H., Brown, E., & Peskin, J. (1988). Premature graduates of the newborn intensive care unit: A guide to follow-up. *Pediatric Clinics of North America, 35,* 1207–1225.

Beckwith, L., & Cohen, S. (1983, April). *Continuity of caregiving with preterm infants.* Paper presented at the Society for Research in Child Development, Detroit.

Behar, L., & Stringfield, S. (1977). The Preschool Behavior Questionnaire. *Journal of Abnormal Child Psycholology, 5,* 265–275

Benton, A. L. (1940). Mental development of prematurely born children. *American Journal of Orthopsychiatry, 10,* 719–746.

Bradley, R. H., & Caldwell, B. M. (1984). The HOME Inventory and family demographics. *Developmental Psychology, 20,* 315–320.

Brazelton, T. B., & Cramer, B. G. (1990). *The earliest relationship.* Reading, MA: Addison-Wesley.

Breslau, N. (1985). Psychiatric disorder in children with physical disabilities. *Journal of the American Academy of Child Psychiatry, 24,* 87–94.

Breslau, N., Brown, G. G., DelDotto, J. E., Kumar, S.,

Ezhuthachan, S., Andreski, P., & Hufnagle, K. G. (1996). Psychiatric sequelae of low birth weight at 6 years of age. *Journal of Abnormal Child Psychology, 24,* 385–400.

Bromwich, R. M. (1990). The interaction approach to early intervention. *Infant Mental Health Journal, 11,* 66–79.

Bronfenbrenner, U. (1979). *The ecology of human development.* Cambridge, MA: Harvard University Press.

Brooten, D., Gennaro, S., Brown, L., Butts, P., Gibbons, A., Bakewill–Sachs, S., & Kumar S. (1988). Anxiety, depression, and hostility in mothers of preterm infants. *Nursing Research, 37,* 213–216.

Cadman, D., Boyle, M., Szatmari, P., & Offord, D. R. (1987). Chronic illness, disability, and mental and social well-being: Findings of the Ontario Child Health Study. *Pediatrics, 79,* 805–812.

Committee on Children with Disabilities and Committee on Psychosocial Aspects of Child and Family Health. (1993). Psychosocial risks of chronic health conditions in childhood and adolescence. *Pediatrics, 92,* 876–878.

Corter, C., & Minde, K. (1987). Impact of infant prematurity on family systems. In M. Wolraich (Ed.), *Advances in Developmental Behavioral Pediatrics* (pp. 1–48). Greenwich, CT: JAI Press.

Cramer, B., Robert-Tissot, C., Stern, D. N., Serpa-Rusconi, S., De Muralt, M., Besson, G., Palacio-Espasa, F., Bachmann, J. P., Knauer, D., Berney, C., & D'Arcis, U. (1990). Outcome evaluation in brief mother-infant psychotherapy: A brief report. *Infant Mental Health Journal, 11,* 278–300.

Crnic, K. A., Greenberg, M. T., Ragozin, A. S., Robinson, N. M., & Basham, R. B. (1983). Effects of stress and social support on mothers and premature and full–term infants. *Child Development, 54,* 209–217.

Direction Générale du Budget de de l'Administration Québécoise. (1992). [Unpublished raw data]. Quebec City: Author. Service de la Gestion et de la Diffusion de l'Information Québec.

Douglas, J. W. B. (1975). Early hospital admissions and later disturbances of behavior and learning. *Developmental Medicine and Child Neurology, 17,* 456–480.

Drillien, C. M. (1964). *The growth and development of the prematurely born infant.* Edinburgh, Scotland: Livingstone.

Dusick, A. (1997). Medical outcomes in preterm infants. *Seminars in Perinatology, 21,* 164–177.

Eiser, C. (1990). Psychological effects of chronic disease. *Journal of Child Psychology and Psychiatry, 31,* 85–98.

Ens-Dokkum, M., Schreuder, A. M., Veen, S., Verloove-Vanhorick, S. P., Brand, R., & Ruys, J. H. (1992). Evaluation of care for the preterm infant: review of literature on follow-up of preterm and low birthweight infants. Report from the collaborative project on preterm and small for gestational age infants (POPS) in the Netherlands. *Paediatric Perinatal Epidemiology, 6,* 434–459.

Escobar, G. J., Littenberg, B., & Petitti, D. B. (1991). Outcome among surviving very low birthweight infants: a meta-analysis. *Archives of Disease in Childhood, 66,* 204–211.

Estroff, D. B., Yando, R., Burke, K., & Snyder, D. (1994). Perceptions of preschoolers' vulnerability by mothers who had delivered preterm. *Journal of Pediatric Psychology, 19,* 709–721.

Fahrenfort, J. J., Jacob, E. A., Miedena, S., & Schweizer, A. T. (1996). Signs of emotional disturbance 3 years after hospitalization. *Journal of Pediatric Psychology, 21,* 353–366.

Field, T. M. (1977). Effects of early separation, interactive deficits and experimental manipulations on mother–infant face–to–face interaction. *Child Development, 48,* 763–771.

Fischer-Fay, A., Goldberg, S., Simmons, R. J., & Levison, H. (1988). Chronic illness and infant-mother attachment. *Journal of Developmental and Behavioral Pediatrics, 9,* 266–270.

Forsyth, B. W. C., McCue Horwitz, S., Leventhal, J. M., & Burger, J. (1996). The child vulnerability scale: An instrument to measure parental perceptions of child vulnerability. *Journal of Pediatric Psychology, 21,* 89–101.

Freud, W. E. (1988). Prenatal attachment, the perinatal continuum and the psychological side of neonatal intensive care. In P. Fedor-Freybergh, V. M. Vogel (Eds.), *Prenatal and perinatal psychology and medicine* (pp. 217–234). Park-Ridge, NJ: Parthenon.

Goldberg, S., Corter, C., Lojkasek, M., & Minde, K. (1990). Prediction of behavior problems in 4–year–olds born prematurely. *Development and Psychopathology, 2,* 15–30.

Goldberg, S., Fischer-Fay, A., Simmons, R. J., Fowler, R. S., & Levison, H. (1989, April). *Effects of chronic illness on infant mother attachment.* Paper presented at Society for Research in Child Development, Kansas City, MO.

Goldberg, S., Morris, P., Simmons, R. J., Fowler, R. S., & Levison, H. (1990). Chronic illness in infancy and parenting stress: A comparison of three groups of parents. *Journal of Pediatric Psychology, 15,* 347–358.

Gortmaker, S. L., Walker, D. K., Weitzman, M., & Sobol, A. M. (1990). Chronic conditions, socioeconomic risks, and behavioral problems in children and adolescents. *Pediatrics, 85,* 267–276.

Green, M., & Solnit, A. J. (1964). Reactions to the threatened loss of a child: A vulnerable child syndrome. *Pediatrics, 34,* 58–66.

Hamlett, K. W., Walker, W., Evans, A., & Weise, K. (1994). Psychological development of technology-dependent children. *Journal of Pediatric Psychology, 19,* 493–503.

Knafl, K. A., Cavallari, K. A., & Dixon, D. M. (1988). *Pediatric hospitalization: Family and nurse perspectives.* Glenview IL : Scott, Foresman.

Kopp, C. B. (1983). Risk factors in development. In J. J. Campos & M. Haith (Eds.), *Handbook of Child Psychology* (Vol. 2, pp. 1081–1188). New York: Wiley.

Lampe, J., Trause, M. A., & Kennell, J. (1977). Parental visiting of sick infants: The effect of living at home prior to hospitalization. *Pediatrics, 59,* 294–296.

Lavigne, J. V., & Faier-Routman, J. (1992). Psychological adjustment to pediatric physical disorders: A meta-analytic review. *Journal of Pediatric Psychology, 17,* 133–157.

Lebovici, S. (1983). Le nourrisson, la mère et la psychanalyse. In *Collection paidos*. Paris: Le Centurion.

Lewis, M. (1987). Social development in infancy and early childhood. In J. D. Osofsky (Ed.), *Handbook of infant development* (2nd ed., pp. 419–493). New York: Wiley.

Lieberman, A. F., Weston, D., & Pawl, J. H. (1991). Preventive intervention and outcome with anxiously attached dyads. *Child Development, 62,* 199–209.

Lorenz, J. M., Wooliever, D. E., Jetton, J. R., & Paneth, N. (1998). A quantitative review of mortality and developmental disability in extremely premature newborns. *Archives of Pediatrics and Adolescent Medicine, 152,* 425–435.

Mahoney, G., & O'Sullivan, P. (1990). Early intervention practices with families of children with handicaps. *Mental Retardation, 28,* 169–176.

Main, M., & Solomon, J. (1986). Discovery of an insecure-disorganized/disoriented attachment pattern. In T. B. Brazelton & N. W. Yogman (Eds.), *Affective development in infancy*. Norwood, NJ: Ablex.

Marton, P., Dawson, H., & Minde, K. (1980). The interaction of ward personnel with infants in the premature nursery. *Infant Behavioral Development, 3,* 307–313.

Marton, P., Minde, K., & Ogilvie, J. (1981). Mother–infant interactions in the premature nursery: a sequential analysis. In S. Friedman & M. Sigman (Eds.), *Birth and psychological development* (pp. 179–205). New York: Academic Press.

Marvin, R. S., & Pianta, R. C. (1996). Mothers' reactions to their child's diagnosis: Relations with security of attachment. *Journal of Clinical Child Psychology, 25,* 436–445.

McCormick, M. C., McCarton, C., Tonascia, J., & Brooks-Gunn, J. (1993). Early educational intervention for very low birth weight infants: Results from the Infant Health and Development Program. *Journal of Pediatrics, 123,* 527–533.

Miles, M. S., & Holditch-Davis, D. (1995). Compensatory parenting: How mothers describe parenting their 3-year-old prematurely born children. *Journal of Pediatric Nursing, 10,* 243–253.

Minde, K. (1980). Bonding of parents to premature infants: Theory and practice. In P. Taylor (Ed.), *Monographs in neonatology series: Parent–infant relationships* (pp. 291–313). New York: Grune & Stratton.

Minde, K. (1984). The impact of prematurity on the later behavior of children and on their families. *Clinics in Perinatolology, 11,* 227–244

Minde, K. (1987). Parenting the premature infant: Problems and opportunities. In H. W. Taeusch & M. W. Yogman (Eds.), *Follow-up management of the high-risk infant* (pp. 315–322), Boston: Little, Brown.

Minde, K. (1993). The social and emotional development of low-birthweight infants and their families up to age 4. In S. Friedman & M. Sigman (Eds.), *The psychological development of low birth weight children. Advances in applied developmental psychology* (pp. 157–185). Norwood, NJ: Ablex.

Minde, K. (1999). Mediating attachment patterns during a serious medical illness. *Infant Mental Health Journal, 20,* 105–122.

Minde, K., Goldberg, S., Perrotta, M., Washington, J.,

Lojkasek, M., Corter, C., & Parker, K. (1989). Continuities and discontinuities in the development of 64 very small premature infants to 4 years of age. *Journal of Child Psychology and Psychiatry, 30,* 391–404.

Minde, K., Marton, P., Manning, P., & Hines, B. (1980). Some determinants of mother–infant interaction in the premature nursery. *Journal of the American Academy of Child Psychiatry, 19,* 139–164.

Minde, K., & Minde, R. (1977). Behavioral screening of preschool children: A new approach to mental health. In P. J. Graham (Ed.), *Epidemiological approaches in child psychiatry* (pp. 139–164). London: Academic Press.

Minde, K., Perrotta, M., & Hellmann, J. (1988). The impact of delayed development in premature infants on mother–infant interaction: a prospective investigation. *Journal of Pediatrics, 112,* 136–142.

Minde, K., Shosenberg, N., Marton, P., Thompson, J., Ripley, J., & Burns, S. (1980). Self-help groups in a premature nursery: A controlled evaluation. *Journal of Pediatrics, 96,* 933–940.

Minde, K., & Stewart, D. (1988). Psychiatric services in the neonatal intensive care unit. In R. Cohen (Ed.), *Psychiatric consultation in childbirth settings* (pp. 151–164). New York: Plenum.

Minde, K., Whitelaw, H., Brown, J., & Fitzhardinge, P. (1983). Effect of neonatal complications in premature infants on early parent–infant interaction. *Developmental Medicine and Child Neurology, 25,* 763–777.

Offord, D. R., Boyle, M. H., Szatmari, P., Rae–Grant, N., Links, P., Cadman, D. T., Byles, J. A., Crawford, J. W., Munroe–Blum, H., Bynne, C., Thomas, H., & Woodward, C. A. (1987). The Ontario Child Health Study: Prevalence of disorder and rates of service utilization. *Archives of General Psychiatry, 44,* 832–836.

Parmelee, A. H. Jr. (1995). Follow-up studies of preterm infants. *Journal of Developmental and Behavioral Pediatrics, 16,* 97.

Perrin, E. C., Ayoub, C. C., & Willett, J. B. (1993). In the eyes of the beholder: family and maternal influences on perceptions of adjustment of children with chronic illness. *Journal of Developmental and Behavioral Pediatrics, 14,* 94–105.

Perrin, E. C., West, P. D., & Culley, B. S. (1989). Is my child normal yet? Correlates of vulnerability. *Pediatrics, 83,* 355–363.

Pharoah, P. O. D., & Alberman, E. D. (1990). Annual statistical review. *Archives of Disease in Childhood, 65,* 147–151.

Pianta, R. C., Marvin, R. S., Britner, P. A., & Borowitz, K. C. (1996). Mothers' resolution of their children's diagnosis. Organized patterns of caregiving representations. *Infant Mental Health Journal, 17,* 239–256.

Pinard, L., & Minde, K. (1991). The infant psychiatrist and the transplant team. *Canadian Journal of Psychiatry, 36,* 442–446.

Pless, B., & Nolan, T. (1991). Revision, replication and neglect: Research on maladjustment in chronic illness. *Journal of Child Psychology and Psychiatry, 32,* 347–365.

Pless, I. B., & Pinkerton, P. (1975). *Chronic childhood disorder: Promoting patterns of adjustment*. London: Kimpton.

Quinton, D., & Rutter, M. (1976). Early hospital admissions and later disturbances of behaviors: An attempted replication of Douglas' findings. *Developmental Medicine and Child Neurology, 18,* 447–459.

Richman, N., & Graham, P. (1971). A behavioural screening questionnaire for use with three–year–old children: Preliminary findings. *Journal of Child Psychology and Psychiatry, 16,* 277–287.

Robinson, J. R., Rankin, J. L., & Drotar, D. (1996). Quality of attachment as a predictor of maternal visitation to young hospitalized children. *Journal of Pediatric Psychology, 21,* 401–417.

Rutter, M. (1967). A childrens' behaviour questionnaire for completion by teachers: Preliminary findings. *Journal of Child Psychology and Psychiatry, 8,* 1–11.

Rutter, M. (1981). Psychological sequelae of brain damage in children. *American Journal of Psychiatry, 138,* 1533–1544.

Sameroff, A. J. (1986). Environmental context of child development. *Journal of Pediatrics, 109,* 192–200.

Sameroff, A., & Chandler, M. (1975). Reproductive risk and the continuum of caretaking casualty. In F. D. Horowitz, M. Hetherington, S. Scarr–Salapatek, & G. Siegel (Eds.), *Review of child developmental research* (Vol. 4, pp. 187–244). Chicago: University of Chicago Press.

Schothorst, P. F., & van Engeland, H. (1996). Long-term behavioral sequelae of prematurity. *Journal of the American Academy of Child and Adolescent Psychiatry, 35,* 175–183.

Seidel, U. P., Chadwick, O., & Rutter, M. (1975). Psychological disorder in crippled children: A comparative study of children with and without brain damage. *Developmental Medicine and Child Neurology, 17,* 563–573.

Sheeran, T., Marvin, R. S., & Pianta, R. C. (1997). Mothers'resolution of their child's diagnosis and self-reported measures of parenting stress, marital relations and social support. *Journal of Pediatric Psychology, 22,* 197–212.

Sigman, M., & Parmelee, A. H. (1979). Longitudinal evaluation of the preterm infant. In T. M. Field, A. M. Sostek, S. Goldberg, & H. H. Shuman (Eds.), *Infants born at risk: Behavior and development.* (pp. 193–216). Jamaica, NY: Spectrum.

Stein, R. E., Gortmaker, S. L., Peril, E. C., Peril, J. M., Pless, I. B., Walker, D. K., & Weitzmann, M. (1987). Severity of illness: Concepts and measurements. *Lancet, 2,* 1506–1509.

Stern, D. (1985). *The interpersonal world of the child.* New York: Basic Books.

Stern, M., & Karraker, K. H. (1990). The prematurity stereotype: Empirical evidence and implications for practice. *Infant Mental Health Journal, 11,* 3–11.

Sykes, D. H., Hoy, E. A., Bill, J. M., Halliday, H. L., McClure, B. G., & Reid, M. M. (1997). Behavioural adjustment in school of very low birthweight children. *Journal of Child Psychology and Psychiatry, 38,* 315–326.

Szatmari, P., Saigal, S., Rosenbaum, P., & Campbell, D. (1993). Psychopathology and adaptive functioning among extremely low birthweight children at eight years of age. *Development and Psychopathology, 8,* 345–357.

Thomasgard, M., & Metz, W. P. (1996). The 2-year stability of parental perceptions of child vulnerability and parental overprotection. *Journal of Developmental and Behavioral Pediatrics, 17,* 222–228.

Thompson, R. H. (1985). *Psychosocial research on pediatric hospitalization and health care.* Springfield, IL: Charles C Thomas.

Volpe, J. J. (1998). Neurologic outcome of prematurity. *Archives of Neurology, 55,* 297–300.

Waters, E. (1991). *Attachment behavior Q-set, revision 3. 0.* New York: State University of New York at Stony Brook.

Watson, J. E., Kirby, R. S., Kelleher, K. J., & Bradley, R. H. (1996). Effects of poverty on home environment: an analysis of three-year outcome data for low birth weight premature infants. *Journal of Pediatric Psychology, 21,* 419–431.

Wolke, D. (1991). Annotation: Supporting the development of low birthweight infants. *Journal of Child Psychology and Psychiatry, 32,* 723–741.

Wolke, D. (1998). Psychological development of prematurely born children. *Archives of Disease in Childhood, 78,* 567–570.

Zeanah, C. H., & McDonough, S. (1989). Clinical approaches to families in early intervention. *Seminars in Perinatology, 13,* 513–522.

11

Exposure to Violence and Early Childhood Trauma

❖

JOAN KAUFMAN
CHRISTOPHER HENRICH

The first 3 years of life include significant trauma for an increasing number of children in this country. This chapter reviews estimates of the number of infants and toddlers who are victims of and witness to child abuse, spousal abuse, and community violence. The impact of early exposure to these various forms of trauma is discussed in relation to social and emotional development, the emergence of trauma specific diagnoses, alterations in biological stress systems and brain development, and later offending behavior. Mediating factors associated with variability in child outcome are also delineated, and treatment implications are briefly discussed.

It has been hypothesized that trauma that occurs during the first 3 years of life will have particularly pernicious effects, given the rapid changes that occur in brain architecture during this developmental period (Perry, Pollard, Blakey, Baker, & Vigilante, 1995). The data reviewed in this chapter provide preliminary support for this hypothesis. They also highlight considerable heterogeneity in the outcome of traumatized children. Numerous intrinsic and extrinsic risk and protective factors mediate children's response to trauma, and careful consideration of these and other developmental factors is essential to devise effective interventions for traumatized youth.

RATES OF TRAUMA EXPOSURE IN YOUNG CHILDREN

Among industrialized nations, the United States ranks last in protecting its children from violence (Children's Defense Fund, 1998). Infants and toddlers are frequent victims of—and witness to—child abuse, spousal abuse, and community violence. Moreover, children who experience any one of these forms of trauma are at increased risk of experiencing the other forms of trauma as well. As numerous studies have documented official and survey reports to underestimate the true rates of trauma experiences (Straus & Gelles, 1990), the statistics estimating rates of exposure in young children should be interpreted with caution.

In 1995 there were approximately 1 million substantiated reports of child maltreatment and 1,000 child fatalities due to abuse or neglect (U.S. Department of Health and Human Services, 1997). Children age 3 and younger comprised 26% of all indicated child maltreatment reports: 20% of physical abuse, 54% of medical neglect, 12% of sexual abuse, and 18% of all abandonment reports. In addition, children age 3 and under comprised the majority of all child fatalities. Seventy-seven percent of all reported child fatalities occurred to children in this age group. Consistent with this finding, nonaccidental injury is the leading cause of death for children this age (Carnegie Corporation of New York, 1994).

With regard to spousal abuse, surveys estimate that 3 million couples a year engage in severe violence, including kicking, punching, and stabbing one's partner (Straus & Gelles, 1990). Very young children are disproportionately present in homes with spousal abuse, with approximately 50% of the domestic violence cases that necessitate police involvement occurring in households with a child less than 5 years of age (Fantuzzo, Boruch, Beriama, Atkins, & Marcus, 1997). Among children who witness domestic violence, it is estimated that 37–63% are also victims of child abuse and/or neglect (Aron & Olsen, 1997).

As for figures on community violence, in 1995 more than 5,000 children died as a result of community related violence (Children's Defense Fund, 1998). Of children 1 to 5 years of age, it is estimated that 10% witnessed a shooting or stabbing, and 47% heard gunshots at some point in their lives (Taylor, Zuckerman, Harik, & Groves, 1994). However, rates of violence exposure in very young children have been derived only from maternal reports. In one study of 6- and 7-year-olds which collected trauma exposure data from both mothers and children, the child interview data generated estimates of violence exposure that were approximately four times greater than the estimates obtained from the mother interview data (Richters & Martinez, 1993). The epidemic of domestic and community violence affects not only children but their caregivers and the caregivers' capacity to nurture (Zeanah & Scheeringa, 1997). Growing evidence suggests that children's distress responses are strongly tied to caregivers' experiences, and parent and child distress following shared traumatic experiences are positively correlated (e.g., Pynoos, Steinberg, & Goenjian, 1996). As discussed later, this correlation is likely mediated by both intrinsic (e.g., inherent vulnerability to psychopathology) and extrinsic (e.g., social support) factors.

EFFECTS OF TRAUMA EXPOSURE

This section on the effects of trauma exposure in young children is divided into four parts. The first part examines core deficits that have been identified in trauma victims across the life cycle. The second part reviews trauma specific di-

agnoses assessed in early childhood. The third section reviews psychobiological sequelae of early trauma, and the last section discusses sexual acting out and sexual offending behavior in children abused during the first 3 years of life.

The majority of research on the effects of trauma during infancy and toddlerhood has been conducted in samples of maltreated children. Little empirical work exists documenting the effects of witnessing domestic and community violence on very young children. When younger children were included in empirical studies, the age range of subject participants tended to be quite broad. Studies conducted with school-age children suggest that a similar spectrum of difficulties are associated with child abuse, domestic violence, and community violence. In addition, the negative sequelae associated with domestic and community violence appear to be greatest in children who also experienced intrafamilial abuse (Hughes, Parkison, & Bargo, 1989; Martinez & Richters, 1993).

Core Deficits

Certain core deficits have been observed in trauma victims across the life cycle (Briere, Berliner, Bulkley, Jenny, & Reid, 1996; Cicchetti & Toth, 1995; Green, 1981). These include problems with (1) interpersonal relationships; (2) affect regulation; and (3) self-development. Whereas problems in these domains have been reported across the life cycle, their manifestations vary at different developmental levels. In addition, not all traumatized individuals experience difficulties in each of these areas. In one study that examined difficulties in maltreated children across three different domains of functioning (Kaufman, Cooke, Arny, Jones, & Pittinsky, 1994), 45% of the sample had problems in all three areas, 37% had difficulties in two areas, 13% only had problems in one area, and 5% of the sample were functioning competently in all domains assessed. As discussed later, there is considerable heterogeneity in adaptation and areas of problematic functioning within samples of trauma victims.

Interpersonal Relationships

In terms of the effects of trauma on interpersonal relationships, studies conducted with maltreated infants and toddlers report problems in relationships with primary caregivers and with peers. Numerous studies have documented that maltreated infants and toddlers are significantly more likely than controls to have insecure attachment relationships with their primary caregivers (Crittenden, 1981, 1992; Schneider-Rosen, Braunwald, Carlson, & Cicchetti, 1985). A number of investigators also observed that many maltreated children could not be classified using the traditional Strange Situation (Ainsworth, Blehar, Waters, & Wall, 1978) scoring procedures leading to Main and Solomon's (1990) description of the disorganized/disoriented (Type D) attachment classification. Children with disorganized/disoriented attachments lack an organized strategy for seeking proximity to caregivers following brief separations (Cicchetti & Toth, 1995). A child with a disorganized attachment to his mother may exhibit such bizarre behaviors as freezing or stereotypical rocking or may display such contradictory actions as running to the doorway when his mother calls his name, then screaming and pulling away from her after she reenters the room. In one study of 12-month-old maltreated infants (Carlson, Cicchetti, Barnett, & Braunwald, 1989), 81% were classified disorganized, compared to only 19% of the comparison children. In another study of 36-month-old maltreated children (Cicchetti & Barnett, 1991), only 28% were classified disorganized, suggesting that the proportion of disorganized attachment classifications may decrease significantly with age.

Problems in peer relationships have also been reported in several studies of young traumatized children. Maltreated toddlers tend to be more aggressive with their siblings than are controls (Crittenden, 1992) and to display more withdrawal and more aggressive behaviors when interacting with peers in a day-care setting (George & Main, 1979). They have also been found to have quite disturbing responses to witnessing a peer's distress (Main & George, 1985). Under these circumstances, when compared to controls, maltreated toddlers are less likely to show sadness or concern (0% vs. 56%) and more likely to become distressed (89% vs. 11%) and to threaten and/or assault the other child (33% vs. 0%). This behavior can be quite extreme, as illustrated below.

[In response to a peer's distress,] an abused boy of 32 months tried to take the hand of the crying other child, and when she resisted, he slapped her on the arm with his open hand. He then turned away from her to look at the ground and began vocalizing very strongly, "Cut it out! CUT IT OUT!," each time saying it a little faster and louder. He patted her, but when she became disturbed by his patting, he retreated, hissing at her and baring his teeth. He then began patting her on the back again, his patting became beating, and he continued beating her despite her screams. (Main & George, 1985, p. 410)

Affect Regulation

In addition to underscoring problems in peer relationships, the previous anecdote highlights the difficulties in affect regulation which are frequently reported in traumatized youth (Egeland & Sroufe, 1981; Fraiberg, 1982; Gaensbauer, 1982; Schneider-Rosen & Cicchetti, 1984, 1991). Overall, the affective responses of maltreated infants and toddlers tend to be less flexible, less responsive to environmental events, and skewed toward negative emotions (Gaensbauer, 1982). For example, maltreated toddlers have been found to display less pleasure and interest during free-play situations and less distress than controls when approached by a stranger or during maternal separation. This apparent emotional blunting, however, frequently gives way to extreme negative states, including tantrums in which the child throws himself on the floor and flails about until his or her screams become inconsolable sobs (Fraiberg, 1982). Significant negative states, including expressions of both sadness and anger, have been reported in maltreated toddlers during a range of experimental paradigms including free-play situations, problem-solving tasks, and mirror self-recognition testing (Egeland & Sroufe, 1981; Schneider-Rosen & Cicchetti, 1984; 1991). These early problems in affect regulation observed in clinical and experimental situations may represent beginning manifestations of later diagnosed mood and behavioral disorders.

Self-Development

Like deficits in interpersonal relationships and affect regulation, problems in self-development manifest early. Maltreated toddlers have been found to have problems in the development of self-understanding, self-esteem, and self-efficacy. For example, maltreated toddlers have been found to talk about themselves and their internal states less frequently than do controls, despite similarities in overall language development (Beeghly & Cicchetti, 1994; Gersten, Coster, Schneider-Rosen, Carlson, & Cicchetti, 1986). In addition, maltreated toddlers are significantly more likely than controls to display a neutral or negative response (e.g., frown or furrowed eyebrows) when observing themselves in the mirror (Schneider-Rosen & Cicchetti, 1984; 1991). They also show less self-efficacy (e.g., persistence) than do controls when confronted with a problem-solving situation, despite comparability in intellectual development (Egeland & Sroufe, 1981; Gaensbauer, 1982).

These disturbances in interpersonal relationships, affect regulation, and self-development represent core symptoms of disorders frequently diagnosed in older traumatized children (e.g., conduct, depression, and dissociation disorders). Early disturbances in these domains have proven to have predictive validity in the prospective longitudinal studies of Sroufe and colleagues who completed psychiatric interviews on 168 older adolescents followed prospectively from their mother's third trimester of pregnancy (Ogawa, Sroufe, Weinfeld, Carlson, & Egeland, 1997; Renken, Egeland, Marvinney, Mangelsdorf, & Sroufe, 1989; Warren, Huston, Egeland, & Sroufe, 1997). Attachment assessments were completed at 12 months of age, and a number of other assessments of affect regulation and self-development were completed at various intervals. The children were considered at risk for poor developmental outcomes at birth due to poverty, and a subset of the children were later found to have experienced significant abuse. Age of onset, chronicity, and severity of abuse were highly correlated with later assessments of psychopathology, as were both the avoidant and disorganized patterns of attachment.

The work of Sroufe and colleagues highlights the need for comprehensive interventions for young traumatized children, as few of those who grew up in chronically abusive and neglectful environments were emotionally healthy at follow-up (Farber & Egeland, 1987). One of the first steps toward this goal is the proper identification and assessment of children at risk. One component of the assessment of the treatment needs of traumatized infants and toddlers is psychiatric diagnoses. In the next section, we briefly discuss the diagnoses most relevant to children this age. Later in the chapter we delineate additional child and family treatment foci, as interventions with traumatized infants and toddlers require comprehensive multidisciplinary approaches.

Trauma Specific Diagnoses

The two most relevant psychiatric diagnoses used with traumatized infants and toddlers are reactive attachment disorder (RAD) and posttraumatic stress disorder (PTSD). The fourth edition of the *Diagnostic and Statistical Manual of Mental Disorders* (DSM-IV; American Psychiatric Association, 1994), is primarily symptom focused, atheoretical, and nonetiologically based. The criteria for RAD and PTSD diverge from this tradition, and include particular experiences presumed to be of etiologic significance in the criteria for the diagnoses. Specifically, a history of pathogenic care is required for the diagnosis RAD, and exposure to a traumatic event is necessary for the diagnosis PTSD. Although the data base supporting the validity of these diagnoses in very young children is extremely limited, both diagnoses are briefly discussed given their clinical relevance.

Reactive Attachment Disorder

According to DSM-IV diagnostic criteria, RAD is characterized by a prominent disturbance in social relatedness evident early in life and in association with a history of pathogenic care (for further discussion see Scheeringa & Gaensbauer, Chapter 23, this volume). This disturbance can be predominantly "inhibited," marked by an inability to attach positively to primary caregivers, or "disinhibited," marked by a history of indiscriminate sociability with caregivers and others, including strangers. In addition to the inhibited and disinhibited subtypes of RAD included in the DSM-IV (American Psychiatric Association, 1994), Zeanah, Boris, Bakshi, & Lieberman, (in press) developed criteria for additional attachment disorder subtypes: self-endangering, inhibited, vigilant/hypercompliant, and role reversed, as well as disrupted attachment disorder.

Although the diagnosis RAD is not synonymous with the insecure attachment classifications generated using the Strange Situation experimental paradigm (Zeanah, Mammen, & Lieberman, 1993), no data are available to estimate the proportion of children with insecure attachments (e.g., A, C, or D classification) who meet diagnostic criteria for RAD. RAD differs from the insecure attachment classifications in that the diagnosis is believed to describe something that resides within the child and generalizes across social situations. In contrast, the insecure attachment classifications are believed to describe the quality of a specific dyadic relationship. In very young children this distinction may be moot, however, as in the first 3 years of life disturbances in attachment are most often relationship specific (Zeanah et al., 1993).

RAD describes a pattern of disturbances not encompassed by other existing diagnostic categories in the DSM-IV (Richters & Volkmar, 1994). In addition, RAD helps define and highlight an important foci for intervention when working with traumatized children. As delineated further in the section on "Interventions," the relationship-focused work, however, is best accomplished when integrated into a comprehensive, multifaceted treatment effort (Larrieu & Zeanah, 1998).

Posttraumatic Stress Disorder

It is only within the past few years that the diagnosis PTSD has been used with infants and toddlers (for further discussion see Luby, Chapter 24, this volume). In a recent study (Scheeringa, Zeanah, Drell, & Larrieu, 1995), the reliability and validity of the DSM-IV and an alternate set of criteria for PTSD were examined in a cohort of infants and young children less than 4 years of age. The criteria for PTSD in both systems comprise three core types of symptoms: reexperiencing, avoidance or numbing, and increased arousal. DSM-IV items that require reports of subjective experience were eliminated from the alternate criteria, and all remaining items were behaviorally anchored. In addition, a category of symptoms describing new onset of fears and aggression following exposure to the traumatic event was incorporated into the alternate PTSD criteria for very young children. When both the DSM-IV and the alternate criteria were applied to 12 children less than 4 years of age, none of the 12 children met DSM-IV criteria for PTSD (Scheeringa et al., 1995). In contrast, 9 of the 12 children met the alternate criteria. In addition, the interrater reliability for the assignment of diagnoses and the rating of individual symptom clusters was excellent with the alternate criteria but not with the DSM-IV criteria.

There is a growing literature on PTSD in children, and an increasing awareness of the importance of understanding not just the effects of trauma on the development of PTSD but also the impact of PTSD on overall development (Pynoos, Steinberg, & Wraith, 1995). Further study of the onset and course of PTSD symptomatology in very young children is clearly warranted. The development of these alternate criteria will greatly help to promote the completion of systematic studies of PTSD symptomatology in traumatized infants and toddlers. Such criteria will also help to facilitate psychobiological studies of well-characterized clinical samples of very young children.

Psychobiological Sequelae

Studies conducted with children, adolescents, and young adults suggest that experiences of significant trauma during childhood are associated with long-term changes in the biological stress systems and alterations in brain development (DeBellis et al., 1999a, 1999b; Kaufman, Birmaher, Perel, 1997; Perry, Pollard, et al., 1995). Preliminary studies of very young children likewise suggest that early trauma may promote long-term changes in resting levels of stress (e.g., cortisol) hormones (Gunnar, 1998). As there has been little work on the psychobiological sequelae of trauma in very young children, the remainder of this section discusses research with older children.

Overall, the emerging data examining the psychobiological sequelae of trauma in children have been contradictory (Kaufman, 1996). Investigators have reported both increases and decreases in urinary catecholamine secretion (DeBellis et al., 1999b; Rogeness, 1991), heart rate in response to a stressor (Perry, Vigilinte, et al., 1995), corticotropin secretion in response to exogenous corticotropin releasing hormone (DeBellis et al., 1994; Kaufman et al., 1993; Kaufman, Birmaher, Perel, et al., 1997), and basal cortisol secretion (DeBellis et al., 1999b; Goenjian et al., 1996). In addition, hippocampal brain volume reductions have not been consistently reported across investigations (DeBellis et al., 1999a).

Preliminary evidence suggests that some of the heterogeneity in the psychobiological sequelae of trauma is related to inherent vulnerability factors. For example, in one study that administered the serotonin precursor L-5-hydroxytryptophan (L-5-HTP) to a cohort of depressed abused, depressed nonabused, and normal control elementary school-age children

(Kaufman et al., 1998), the importance of family history of psychopathology was demonstrated in explaining variance in neuroendocrine responses. Consistent with prior human (Pine et al., 1997) and nonhuman (Rosenblum et al., 1994) primate studies showing serotonergic system alterations in association with early adverse rearing conditions, the depressed abused children secreted significantly more prolactin post-L-5-HTP than did the depressed nonabused and normal control children. In addition to the association between abuse experiences and prolactin response to L-5-HTP challenge, however, family history of suicide attempt in first- and second-degree relatives was also significantly correlated with subjects' responses to the neuroendocrine challenge.

Variability in psychobiological correlates of trauma appear related to differences in clinical picture, which are likely also mediated by inherent vulnerability factors. For example, the investigation that reported significantly increased urinary catecholamines studied traumatized elementary school-age children with PTSD (DeBellis et al., 1999b). The investigation that reported reduced urinary catecholamines in traumatized children was conducted with boys who met criteria for conduct disorder (Rogeness, 1991). Just as evidence suggests that neurobiological alterations associated with a history of trauma are related to family history of psychopathology, there are likewise data that suggest that the type of symptomatology traumatized children manifest is related to family predisposition factors. For example, the first-degree relatives of depressed abused children are nine times more likely to have a lifetime history of major depression than are the first-degree relatives of normal control children (Kaufman et al., 1998).

Data also suggest that heterogeneity in the psychobiological correlates of trauma is related to current psychosocial stressors and availability of social supports. For example, in one study (Kaufman, Birmaher, Perel, et al., 1997), although depressed abused children had significantly greater corticotropin secretion post-corticotropin releasing hormone than did controls, the increased corticotropin secretion was *only* observed in depressed abused children experiencing ongoing chronic adversity (marital violence, emotional abuse, poverty, lack of supports). The corticotropin secretion of depressed abused children living in stable home environments was comparable to that of the nonabused

children. These results are consistent with the findings of another study that reported greater dysregulation in cortisol diurnal secretion patterns in maltreated children with fewer available supports and a history of more out-of-home foster placements, than maltreated children living in more stable and supportive families (Kaufman, 1991).

Developmental factors also appear important in mediating the psychobiological sequelae of early trauma. For example, when compared to children abused later in life and normal controls, children physically abused during the first 3 years of life have been found to have reduced catecholamine function as measured by dopamine beta hydroxylase activity (Galvin, Stilwell, Shekhar, Kopta, & Goldfarb, 1997). Lower enzyme activity was also associated with greater deficits in conscience development. In another study (DeBellis et al., 1999a), earlier onset abuse was associated with greater reduction in total brain volume and region 4 of the corpus callosum. In addition, greater reductions in corpus callosum volume were associated with more severe avoidant and hyperarousal PTSD symptoms, and higher scores on the Child Dissociation Checklist. As preclinical studies suggest that some of the stress system and brain development changes associated with early stress can be reversed with psychopharmacological interventions (P. M. Plotsky, personal communication, February, 1999), longitudinal clinical and psychobiological follow-up of traumatized children is clearly warranted.

More research is needed, however, to understand how inherent vulnerability and developmental factors interact with experiences of abuse and other psychosocial stressors to produce psychopathology in traumatized children. Better understanding of the interactions among these factors and psychobiological parameters will (1) enhance understandings of the neurobiological mechanisms that mediate the development of specific symptomatology and (2) promote the development of more effective multimodal interventions for traumatized children.

Sexual Acting Out and Sexual Offending Behavior

Most negative sequelae of trauma are nonspecific and found in association with a wide array of traumatic experiences. The development of sexual acting out and sexual offending behavior, however, is a relatively specific consequence of sexual abuse (Green, 1993). Moreover, emerging data suggest that these types of problems are most prevalent in children sexually abused during the first 3 years of life.

The topic of sexual abuse is not typically covered in chapters on the effects of early trauma, but children less than 7 years old comprise approximately 40% of all substantiated reports of child sexual abuse. In 1995, there were an estimated 15,128 substantiated cases of sexual abuse involving children less than 3 years old, and an estimated 36,559 substantiated cases of sexual abuse involving children 4 to 7 years old, with many of these children having experienced abuse from early in life (U.S. Department of Health and Human Services, 1997). Moreover, given the limited verbal capabilities of very young children, the sexual abuse of children less than age 3 is frequently quite severe, requiring positive medical findings to corroborate allegations.

McClellan et al. (1996) provide the most extensive data available examining the relationship between early child sexual abuse and the emergence of sexual acting-out behaviors. They reviewed 499 child and adolescent psychiatric inpatients' medical records and found that 55% had a history of child sexual abuse and 41% had a history of sexual-acting-out behaviors. Children who were sexually abused during the first 3 years of life ($n = 78$) were significantly more likely than children not abused and children abused later in life to have sexual acting-out problems. Eighty percent of the children sexually abused during the first few years of life had one or more types of sexual acting-out problems: 71% had problems with hypersexuality; 37% had a history of exposing their genitals, and 37% had victimized others. In contrast, rates of sexual-acting-out problems were significantly lower in children sexually abused between the ages of 7 and 12 ($n = 71$). Overall, 44% of these children had sexual acting-out problems: 32% had problems with hypersexuality, 10% had a history of exposing their genitals, and only 10% had victimized others. The rate of sexual behavior problems in the psychiatrically hospitalized children without a documented history of sexual abuse ($n = 226$) was 16%—a rate 80% lower than the rate reported in the children who were sexually abused during the first 3 years of life.

Children with the earliest sexual abuse experiences were at heightened risk for adverse outcomes due to other abuse-related factors (McClellan et al., 1996). When compared to the other sexually abused children, they had higher rates of physical abuse and neglect. In addition, their sexual abuse experiences were more likely to have been chronic and to have involved multiple perpetrators, one of whom was a parent or stepparent.

It is important to remember, of course, that psychiatrically hospitalized youth are not representative of all sexually abused children. In addition, although sexually abused children may be at increased risk of developing sexual acting-out behaviors, most sexually abused children do not engage in sexualized behavior (Friedrich, 1993).

While there are likely multiple possible mechanisms by which these very early sexual abuse experiences may lead to the development of persistent sexual acting-out behavior problems, there are some interesting psychobiological hypotheses worth brief discussion. Gonadotropin-releasing hormone inhibitor is one medication that is currently prescribed to adult sexual offenders (Rosler & Witztum, 1998). Interestingly, the first few years of life mark a period when gonadotropin-releasing hormone is normally secreted at very high levels. Gonadotropin-releasing hormone levels then fall quite dramatically and remain low until puberty (Neely et al., 1995). In addition, hormones (e.g., corticotropin-releasing hormone) and neurotransmitters (e.g., noradrenaline) released in response to stress increase gonadotropin-releasing hormone secretion (Herbison, 1997; Rivest & Rivier, 1995). Due to the normative elevations of gonadotropin-releasing hormone early in life, stressful sexual abuse experiences may be particularly pernicious during the first 3 years.

Sexual acting-out behaviors are frequently treatment resistant, although preliminary data does suggest they can be effectively targeted with cognitive behavioral interventions in preschool children (Cohen & Mannarino, 1996). In our specialty clinic for abused children and their families (Kaufman, Birmaher, Clayton, & Retano, 1997), we were referred several early school-age boys with a history of sexual abuse during the first 3 years of life. Their problems with persistent sexual acting-out behaviors were so severe they could not be left unsupervised with siblings or peers. As the majority of these children had comorbid attention-deficit/hyperactivity disorder, methyl-phenidate was prescribed as part of a multi-modal intervention. The combined methyl-phenidate and psychotherapeutic interventions had a positive effect on the sexual acting-out behavior symptoms in many of the children undergoing open trial treatments. Methyl-phenidate increases dopamine secretion (Greenhill, 1992), and dopamine decreases gonadotropin-releasing hormone secretion (Levavi-Sivan, Ofir, & Yaron, 1995), suggesting the need for more research to understand the gonadotropin system and its possible role in the development and maintenance of sexual acting-out behavior in children abused early in life. As discussed in the following section, many factors mediate the developmental trajectory of traumatized children. Better understanding of these factors will facilitate the development of more efficacious multimodal treatments.

MEDIATING FACTORS

Throughout the section on the impact of early trauma, we highlighted multiple factors that mediate children's outcomes. These factors interact in complex ways over time (Pynoos et al., 1995). Still, more research is needed to understand how inherent vulnerability and developmental factors interact with trauma and other psychosocial risk factors to produce variability in the developmental outcomes of traumatized children.

No one clinical profile characterizes traumatized children, and child outcomes are not static. They tend to change in predictable ways in response to alterations in different mediating factors (Farber & Egeland, 1987). In addition, not all traumatized children develop difficulties (Briere et al., 1996). In one review of the sequelae of child sexual abuse it was estimated that 40% of abused children were functioning well, with no significant trauma-related problems (Kendall-Tackett, Williams, & Finkelhor, 1993).

This section reviews child, family, social, and trauma-related factors that affect the outcome of traumatized children. For example, responses to trauma are influenced by children's age at the time of the event, temperament, history of preexisting psychopathology, IQ, coping styles, and cognitive appraisal of traumatic experiences (Briere et al., 1996; Kaufman & Mannarino, 1995; Okun, Parker, & Levendosky, 1994; Pynoos et al., 1996). They are also influenced

by numerous family factors including parental psychopathology, parental substance abuse, quality of spousal and parent–child relationship, family cohesion, and support received following the trauma (Cicchetti & Toth, 1995; Pynoos et al., 1995). The overall social context of development also influences child outcomes, with traumatic responses being affected by poverty status, community resources, psychotherapeutic interventions, and availability of extended social supports (Erikson & Egeland, 1996; Okun et al., 1994; Kaufman & Zigler, 1989). In addition, numerous trauma-related factors influence child outcome. These include level of traumatic exposure, number of traumatic stressors, duration of traumatic experiences, closeness of relationship with perpetrator, system responses (e.g., child protective services), the need to testify in court following a trauma, exposure to traumatic reminders, secondary adversities, and losses in association with trauma (Briere et al., 1996; Goodman et al., 1992; Kendall-Tackett et al., 1993; Pynoos et al., 1995; 1996).

Of the different mediating factors that have been identified, the availability of a supportive parent or alternate guardian has been demonstrated to be one of the most important factors that distinguishes traumatized children with good developmental outcomes from those with more deleterious outcomes (Pynoos et al., 1995). The importance of a positive support has been demonstrated in studies examining the intergenerational transmission of abuse (Egeland, Jacobvitz, & Sroufe, 1988; Kaufman & Zigler, 1989), the development of depressive disorders in maltreated children (Kaufman, 1991), the persistence of antisocial behavior from adolescence to adulthood in youth involved with protective services (Widom, 1991), and the severity of posttraumatic stress reactions in response to a wide array of stressors (Pynoos et al., 1995). In addition, as discussed previously, the availability of positive supports also appears to mediate some neurobiological alterations associated with trauma (Kaufman, 1991; Kaufman, Birmaher, Perel, 1997).

Whereas strengthening caregivers' capacity to support children is essential in work with traumatized populations, it is important to consider the full range of mediating factors in planning interventions. Although several of these factors cannot be modified, many of them can. We discuss these issues further in the following section.

INTERVENTIONS

In accordance with the data reviewed in the two prior sections, recommended foci for interventions with traumatized children are broad and comprehensive (Kaufman & Mannarino, 1995; Larrieu & Zeanah, 1998; Pynoos et al., 1995, 1996). They include (1) clinical symptomatology, with recognition that traumatized children present with a diverse range of problems necessitating the use of a wide variety of interventions; (2) developmental deficits, as improvements in interpersonal relationships and indices of adaptive functioning can greatly affect a child's long-term developmental trajectory; (3) parental problems, including spousal violence, substance abuse, and psychiatric disturbances; (4) social factors, including provision of concrete resources; and (5) trauma-specific interventions, with recognition that many traumatized children have experienced multiple forms of adversity. Trauma-specific interventions can include restructuring of cognitive appraisals of the trauma, survey and restriction of exposure to trauma-related triggers, interventions for secondary adversities, support through court proceedings, grief work for losses associated with the trauma, and facilitation of permanency planning efforts.

In recent years, a number of innovative interventions have been developed for victims of child abuse (Cohen & Mannarino, 1996; Finkelhor & Berliner, 1995; Larrieu & Zeanah, 1998; Wolfe & Wekerle, 1993), domestic violence (Miller & Krull, 1997), community violence (Marans, 1996; Murphy, Pynoos, & James, 1997; Osofsky, 1997a,b), and victims of a wide range of traumas who meet criteria for PTSD (van der Kolk, McFarlane, & Weisaeth, 1996). In addition, practice guidelines have been developed for interventions with infants and toddlers (American Academy of Child and Adolescent Psychiatry, 1997). As there is significant variation in the clinical, developmental, family, and social characteristics of trauma victims, it is, however, unlikely that any one intervention will be appropriate for all victims. In addition, for the children most severely traumatized, it is unlikely that short or single inoculation interventions will make significant impact on child outcome.

Of the different foci of intervention delineated, facilitating permanency planning efforts is one of the most important—particularly for victims of intrafamilial abuse (see Larrieu & Zeanah, 1998, for an excellent description of a permanency planning focused intervention program for maltreated infants and toddlers). Permanency planning involves the systematic implementation of interventions to secure a caring, legally recognized, and continuous family for traumatized children (Child Welfare League of America, 1985). The aim of these efforts is to maximize the likelihood of children having at least one adult whom they identify as a psychological parent (Goldstein, Solnit, Goldstein, & Freud, 1996). Permanency efforts can result in family reunification, placement with kin, or child adoption. The role of the clinician in this process is to complete assessments of child adaptation and family functioning, to communicate families' strengths and weaknesses to protective service workers, to conduct therapeutic interventions to alleviate weaknesses by building on child and family strengths, to facilitate referrals for additional services as necessary, to report changes in risk and new incidents of abuse, to evaluate child attachments over time, and to make recommendations for treatment and permanency determinations in juvenile court.

Last year there were slightly over 500,000 children in foster care (Children's Defense Fund, 1998). Children less than 5 years of age comprised more than one-third of all children in out-of-home care (Administration for Children and Families, 1996). While the average length of stay in foster care is estimated at 2 years (Administration for Children and Families, 1996), the range of time in care varies widely for children. In some states, up to one-third of all children who enter out-of-home care spend the majority of their lives in "foster-care drift"—moving from one home to the next without ever obtaining a permanent home (Kaufman & Zigler, 1996). In addition, the road to permanency can be quite drawn out. For example, in some states it is estimated to take 3 to 4 years from placement to the filing of a termination of parental rights (TPR) petition, 1 to 2 years from the filing of the petition until the date of the court hearing to determine the TPR ruling, and an additional 2 to 5 years to process appeals (Cahn & Johnson, 1993).

The Adoption and Safe Families Act (Public Law 105-89), passed in November 1997, was designed to facilitate permanency planning efforts on behalf of maltreated children. Mandates for achieving permanency within 15 months necessitates close clinical monitoring and careful case planning. The failure to allot significant resources within this legislation for services for traumatized children, birth parents, and foster parents, however, minimizes the likelihood that the permanency goals will be achieved.

Tragically, studies suggest that the majority of trauma victims receive no intervention. It has been estimated that less than half of all confirmed cases of child maltreatment receive any therapeutic or supportive services (McCurdy & Daro, 1992). Statistics for children who witness domestic and community violence are significantly worse. Consequently, consistent with the views of others (Dodson & Hardin, 1997; Hardin, 1992; Kaufman & Zigler, 1996), we believe systems changes are required to better meet the needs of traumatized children. Effective intervention, however, is within our reach.

CONCLUSION

The scope of the problem of childhood trauma is enormous. In this chapter, we discussed the effects of early trauma from multiple perspectives. The data reviewed highlight the particularly pernicious effects of trauma during the first few years of life. The results of preclinical and clinical studies suggest, however, that the negative effects of early trauma need not be irreversible. Unfortunately, far too few traumatized children are provided intervention services, and their traumas are frequently exacerbated by system failures. The cost of these system failures are great to the individual and to our society as a whole. Concerted, multidisciplinary efforts are required to minimize future traumatization of children and to alleviate its devastating effects when it does occur.

REFERENCES

Administration for Children and Families, Department of Health and Human Services (ACF). (1996). *Preliminary analysis of AFCARS data for children in foster care*. Washington, DC: U.S. Government Printing Office.

American Academy of Child and Adolescent Psychiatry (AACAP). (1997). Practice parameters for the psychiatric assessment of infants and toddlers (0–36 months). *Journal of the American Academy of Child and Adolescent Psychiatry, 36*(Suppl.), 21S–36S.

Adoption and Safe Families Act of 1997. Pub. L. No. 105–89. (1997).

Ainsworth, M. D., Blehar, M. C., Waters, E., & Wall, S. (1978). *Patterns of attachment: A psychological study of the strange situation*. Hillsdale, NJ: Erlbaum.

American Psychiatric Association. (1994). *Diagnostic and statistical manual of mental disorders* (4th ed.). Washington, DC: Author.

Aron, L. Y., & Olson, K. K. (1997, Summer). Efforts by child welfare agencies to address domestic violence. *Public Welfare*, 4–13.

Beeghly, M., & Cicchetti, D. (1994). Child maltreatment, attachment and the self system: Emergence of an internal state lexicon in toddlers at high social risk. *Development Pychopathology, 6,* 5–30.

Briere, J., Berliner, L., Bulkley, J. A., Jenny, C., & Reid, T. (1996). *The APSAC handbook on child maltreatment.* Thousand Oaks, CA: Sage.

Cahn, K., & Johnson, P. (1993). *Children can't wait: Reducing delays in out-of-home care*. Washington, DC: Child Welfare League of America.

Carlson, V., Cicchetti, D., Barnett, D., & Braunwald, K. (1989). Disorganized/disoriented relationships in maltreated children. *Development Psychology, 25,* 525–531.

Carnegie Corporation of New York. (1994). *Starting points: Meeting the needs of our youngest children* (Report of the Carnegie Task Force on Meeting the Needs of Young Children). New York: Author.

Children's Defense Fund. (1998). *The state of America's children: Yearbook 1998*. Washington, DC: Author.

Child Welfare League of America (CWLA). (1985). *Director's report, permanency report*. Washington, DC: Author.

Cicchetti, D., & Barnett, D. (1991). Attachment organization in maltreated preschoolers. *Development and Psychopathology, 3,* 397–411.

Cicchetti, D., & Toth, S. (1995). A developmental psychopathology perspective on child abuse and neglect. *Journal of the American Academy of Child and Adolescent Psychiatry, 34,* 541–565

Cohen, J., & Mannarino, A. (1996). A treatment outcome study for sexually abused preschool children. Initial findings. *Journal of the American Academy of Child and Adolescent Psychiatry, 35,* 42–50.

Crittenden, P. M. (1981). Abusing, neglecting, problematic, and adequate dyads: Differentiating by patterns of interaction. *Merrill–Palmer Quarterly, 27,* 201–218.

Crittenden, P. M. (1992). Children's strategies for coping with adverse home environments: An interpretation using attachment theory. *Child Abuse and Neglect, 16,* 329–343.

DeBellis, M. D., Baum, A., Birmaher, B., Keshavan, M., Eccard, C., Boring, A., Jenkins, F., & Ryan, N. (1999b). Developmental Traumatology, Part I: Biological Stress Systems. *Biological Psyciatry, 45,* 1259–1270.

DeBellis, M. D., Chrousos, G. P., Dorn, L. D., Burke, L., Helmers, K., Kling, M. A., Trickett, P. K., & Putnam, F. W. (1994). Hypothalamic–pituitary–adrenal axis dysregulation in sexually abused girls. *Journal of Clinical Endocrinology and Metabolism, 78,* 249–255.

DeBellis, M. D., Keshavan, M., Clark, D., Casey, B. J., Giedd, J., Boring, A., Frustaci, K., & Ryan, N.

(1999a). Developmental Traumatology, Part II: Brain Development. *Biological Psyciatry, 45,* 1271–1284.

Dodson, G. D., & Hardin, M. (1997). *On-time services to preserve families.* Washington, DC: American Bar Association.

Egeland, B., Jacobvitz, D., & Sroufe, L. A. (1988). Breaking the cycle of abuse. *Child Development, 59,* 1080–1088.

Egeland, B., & Sroufe, L. A. (1981). Developmental sequelae of maltreatment in infancy. *New Directions in Child Development, 11,* 77–92.

Erickson, M. F., & Egeland, B. (1996). Child neglect. In J. Briere, L. Berliner, J. Bulkey, C. Jenny, & T. Reid (Eds.), *The American Professional Society on the Abuse of Children (APSAC) handbook on child maltreatment* (pp. 4–20). Thousand Oaks, CA: Sage.

Farber, E. A., & Egeland, B. (1987). Invulnerability among abused and neglected children. In E. J. Anthony & B. J. Cohler (Eds.), *The invulnerable child* (pp. 253–288). New York: Guilford Press.

Fantuzza, J., Boruch, R., Bcriama, A., Atkins, M., & Marcus, S. (1997). Domestic violence and children: Prevalence and risk in five major U. S. cities. *Journal of the American Academy of Child and Adolescent Psychiatry, 36,* 116–122.

Finkelhor, D., & Berliner, L. (1995). Research on the treatment of sexually abused children: A review and recommendations. *Journal of the American Academy of Child and Adolescent Psychiatry, 34,* 1408–1423.

Fraiberg, S. (1982). Pathological defenses in infancy. *Psychoanalytic Quarterly, 51,* 612–635.

Friedrich, W. (1993). Sexual victimization and sexual behavior in children: A review of recent literature. *Child Abuse and Neglect, 17,* 59–66.

Gaensbauer, T. (1982). Regulation of emotional expression in infants from two contrasting caretaking environments. *Journal of the American Academy of Child Psychiatry, 21,* 163–171.

Galvin, M. R., Stilwell, B. M., Shekhar, A., Kopta, S. M., & Goldfarb, S. M. (1997). Maltreatment, conscience functioning and dopamine beta hydroxylase in emotionally disturbed boys. *Child Abuse and Neglect, 21,* 83–92.

George, C., & Main, M. (1979). Social interaction of young abused children: Approach, avoidance, and aggression. *Child Development, 50,* 306–318.

Gersten, M., Coster, W., Schneider-Rosen, K., Carlson, V., & Cicchetti, D. (1986). The socio-cmotional bascs of communicative functioning: Quality of attachment, language development, and early maltreatment. In M. E. Lamb, A. L. Brown, & B. Rogoff (Eds.), *Advances in developmental psychology* (Vol. 14, pp. 105–151). Hillsdale, NJ: Erlbaum.

Goenjian, A., Yehuda, R., Pynoos, R. S., Steinberg, A. M., Tashjian, M., Yang, R. K., Najarian, L. M., & Fairbanks, L. (1996). Basal cortisol, dexamethasone suppression of cortisol and MHPG among adolescents aftcr the 1988 earthquake in Armenia. *American Journal of Psychiatry, 154,* 536–542.

Goldstein, J., Solnit, A., Goldstein, S., & Freud, A. (1996). *The best interests of the child: The least detrimental alternative.* New York: Free Press.

Goodman, G., Taub, E., Jones, D., England, P., Port, L., Rud, L., & Pradp, L. (1992). Testifying in the criminal court: Emotional effects on child sexual assault victims. With Commentaries by J. Myers, GB Melton. *Monographs of the Society for Research in Child Development, 57*(Serial No. 5), 1 142.

Green, A. (1981). Core affective disturbances in abused children. *Journal of the American Academy of Psychoanalysis, 9,* 435–446.

Green, A. (1993). Child sexual abuse: Immediate and long-term effects and intervention. *Journal of the American Academy of Child and Adolescent Psychiatry, 32,* 890–902.

Greenhill, L. (1992). Pharmacologic treatment of attention deficit hyperactivity disorder. *Psychiatric Clinics of North America, 15,* 1–27.

Gunnar, M. (1998, March). *Bioprocesses in human development.* Presentation at the Canadian Institute for Advanced Research, Vancouver.

Hardin, M. (1992). *Establishing a core of services for families subject to state intervention.* Washington, DC: American Bar Association.

Herbison, A. E. (1997). Nonadrenergic regulation of cyclic GnRH secretion. *Reviews of Reproduction, 2,* 1–6.

Hughes, H., Parkison, D., & Bargo, M. (1989). Witnessing spouse abuse and experiencing physical abuse: A double whammy? *Journal of Family Violence, 4,* 197–209.

Kaufman, J. (1991). Depressive disorders in maltreated children. *Journal of the American Academy of Child and Adolescent Psychiatry, 30,* 257–265.

Kaufman J. (1996). Child abuse. *Current Opinion in Psychiatry, 9,* 251–256.

Kaufman, J., Birmaher, B., Brent, D., Dahl, R., Bridges, J., & Ryan, N. (1998). Psychopathology in the relatives of depressed-abused children. *Child Abuse and Neglect, 22,* 204–213.

Kaufman, J., Birmaher, B. Clayton, S., & Retano, A. (1997). Case study: Trauma related hallucinations in children. *Journal of the American Academy of Child and Adolescent Psychiatry, 36,* 1602–1605.

Kaufman, J., Birmaher, B., Perel, J., Dahl, R., Moreci, P., Nelson, B., Wells, W., & Ryan, N. (1997). The corticotropin releasing hormone challenge in depressed abused, depressed non-abused and normal control children. *Biological Psychiatry, 42,* 669–679.

Kaufman, J., Birmaher, B., Perel, J., Dahl, R., Stull, S., Brent, D., Trubnick, L., & Ryan, N. (1998). Serotonergic functioning in depressed abused children: Clinical and familial correlates. *Biological Psyciatry, 44,* 973–981.

Kaufman, J., Brent, D., Birmaher, B., Dahl, R., Perel, J., Ryan, N., Puig-Antich, J., & Williamson, D. (1993). *Measures of family adversity, clinical symptomatology, and cortisol secretion in a sample of preadolescent depressed children.* Paper presented at the annual meeting of the Society for Research in Child and Adolescent Psychopathology (SRCAP), Santa Fe, NM.

Kaufman, J., Cooke, A., Arny, L., Jones, B., & Pittinsky, T. (1994). Problems defining resiliency: Illustrations from the study of maltreated children [Special issue]. *Development and Psychopathology, 6,* 215–229.

Kaufman, J., & Mannarino, A. (1995). Evaluation of child maltreatment. In R. T. Ammerman & M. Hersen

(Eds.), *Handbook of child behavior therapy in the psychiatric setting* (pp. 73–92). New York: Wiley.

Kaufman, J., & Zigler, E. (1989). The intergenerational transmission of child abuse. In D. Cicchetti & V. Carlson (Eds.), *Child maltreatment: Theory and research on the causes and consequences of child abuse and neglect* (pp. 129–150). Cambridge, UK: Cambridge University Press.

Kaufman, J., & Zigler, E. (1996). Child abuse and social policy. In E. Zigler, S. L. Kagan, & N. Hall (Eds.), *Children, families, and government: Preparing for the twenty-first century* (pp. 233–255). Cambridge, UK: Cambridge University Press.

Kendall-Tackett, K. A., Williams, L. M., & Finkelhor, D. (1993). Impact of sexual abuse on children: A review and synthesis of recent empirical studies. *Psychology Bulletin, 113,* 164–180.

Larrieu, J., & Zeanah, C. (1998). Intensive intervention for maltreated infants and toddlers in foster care. *Child and Adolescent Psychiatric Clinics of North America, 7,* 33357–33371.

Levavi-Sivan, B., Ofir, M., & Yaron, Z. (1995). Possible sites of dopaminergic inhibition of gonadotropin release from the pituitary. *Molecular and Cellular Endocrinology, 109*(1), 87–95.

Main, M., & George, C. (1985). Responses of abused and disadvantaged toddlers to distress in agemates: A study in the day care setting. *Developmental Psychology, 21,* 407–412.

Main, M., & Solomon, J. (1990). Procedures for identifying infants as disorganized/disoriented during the Ainsworth Strange Situation. In M. Greenberg, D. Cicchetti, & E. M. Cummings (Eds.), *Attachment during the preschool years.* Chicago: University of Chicago Press.

Marans, S. (1996). Psychoanalysis on the beat. Children, police, and urban trauma. *Psychoanalytic Study of the Child, 51,* 522–541.

Martinez, P., & Richters, J. E. (1993). The NIMH community violence project: II. Children's distress symptoms associated with violence exposure. *Psychiatry, 56,* 22–35.

McClellan, J., McCurry, C., Ronnei, M., Adams, J., Eisner, A., & Storck, M. (1996). Age of onset of sexual abuse: Relationship to sexually inappropriate behaviors. *Journal of the American Academy of Child and Adolescent Psychiatry, 35,* 1375–1386.

McCurdy, K., & Daro, D. (1992). *Current trends in child abuse reporting and fatalities: The results of the 1992 annual fifth state survey Z.* Report of the National Center on Child Abuse Prevention Research. Chicago.

Miller, J., & Krull, A. (1997). Controlling Domestic Violence: Victim Resources and Police Intervention. In G. Kaufman Kantor & J. Jasinski (Eds.), *Out of the darkness: contemporary perspectives on family violence* (pp. 235–254). Thousand Oaks, CA: Sage Publications.

Murphy, L., Pynoos, R. S., & James, C. B. (1997). The trauma/grief-focused group psychotherapy module of an elementary school-based violence prevention/intervention program. In J. D. Osofsky (Ed.), *Children in a violent society* (pp. 223–255). New York: Guilford Press.

Neely, E. K., Hintz, R. L., Wilson, D. M., Lee, P. A.,

Gautier, T., Argente, J., & Stene, M. (1995). Normal ranges for immunochemiluminometric gonadotropin assays. *Journal of Pediatrics, 127,* 40–46.

Ogawa, J. R., Sroufe, L. A., Weinfeld, N. S., Carlson, E. A., & Egeland, B. (1997). Development and the fragmented self: Longitudinal study of dissociative symptomatology in a nonclinical sample. *Development and Psychopathology, 9,* 855–879.

Okun, A., Parker, J., & Levendosky, A. (1994). Distinct and interactive contributions of physical abuse, socioeconomic disadvantage and negative life events to children's social, cognitive and affective adjustment. *Developmental Psychopathology, 6,* 77–98.

Osofsky, J. D. (1997a). Prevention and policy: Directions for the future. In J. D. Osofsky (Ed.), *Children in a violent society* (pp. 323–328). New York: Guilford Press.

Osofsky, J. D. (1997b). The Violence Intervention Project for children and families. In J. Osofsky (Ed.), *Children in a violent society* (pp. 256–260). New York: Guilford Press.

Perry, B. D., Pollard, P., Blakey, T., Baker, W., & Vigilante, D. (1995). Childhood trauma, the neurobiology of adaption, and "use-dependent" development of the brain: How "states" become "traits." *Infant Mental Health Journal, 16,* 271–291.

Perry, B., Vigilante, D., Blakey, T., Baker, B., Withers, A., & Sturges, C. (1995, October). *Continuous heart rate monitoring in maltreated children.* Presented at the American Academy of Child and Adolescent Psychiatry, New Orleans.

Pine, D., Coplan, J., Wasserman, G., Miller, L., Fried, J., Davies, M., Cooper, T., Greenhill, L., Shaffer, D., & Parsons, B. (1997). Neuroendocrine response to fenfluramine challenge in boys. *Archives of General Psychiatry, 54,* 839–846.

Pynoos, R. S., Steinberg, A. M., & Goenjian, A. (1996). Traumatic stress in childhood and adolescence: Recent developments and current controversies. In B. A. van der Kolk, A. C. McFarlane, & L. Weisaeth (Eds.), *Traumatic stress: The effects of overwhelming experience on mind, body, and society* (pp. 331–358). New York: Guilford Press.

Pynoos, R., Steinberg, A., & Wraith, R. (1995). A developmental model of childhood traumatic stress. In D. Cicchetti & D. Cohen (Eds.), *Developmental psychopathology. Volume 2: Risk, disorder, and adaptation* (pp. 57–80). New York: Wiley.

Renken, B., Egeland, B., Marvinney, D., Mangelsdorf, S., & Sroufe, L. A. (1989). Early childhood antecedents of aggression and passive-withdrawal in early elementary school. *Journal of Personality, 57,* 257–281.

Richters J., & Martinez, P. (1993). The NIMH Community Violence Project: Children as victims of and witnesses to violence. *Psychiatry, 56,* 7–21.

Richters, M. M., & Volkmar, F. R. (1994). Reactive attachment disorder of infancy or early childhood. *Journal of the American Academy of Child and Adolescent Psychiatry, 33,* 328–332.

Rivest, S., & Rivier, C. (1995). The role of corticotropin-releasing factor and interleukin–1 in the regulation of neurons controlling reproductive functions. *Endocrine Reviews, 16,* 177–199.

Rogeness, G. A. (1991). Psychosocial factors and amine systems. *Psychiatric Research, 37,* 215–217.

Rosenblum, L., Coplan, J., Friedman, S., Bassoff, T., Gorman, J., & Andrews, M. (1994). Adverse early experiences affect noradrenergic and serotonergic functioning in adult primates. *Biological Psychiatry, 35,* 221–227.

Rosler, A., & Witztum, E. (1998). Treatment of men with paraphilia with a long-acting analogue of gonadotropin-releasing hormone. *New England Journal of Medicine, 338,* 416–422.

Scheeringa, M. S., Zeanah, C. H., Drell, M. J., & Larrieu, J. A. (1995). Two approaches to the diagnosis of posttraumatic stress disorder in infancy and early childhood. *Journal of the American Academy of Child and Adolescent Psychiatry, 34,* 191–200.

Schneider-Rosen, K., Braunwald, K., Carlson, V., & Cicchetti, D. (1985). Current perspectives in attachment theory: Illustration from the study of maltreated infants. *Monographs of the Society for Research in Child Development, 50*(Serial No. 1–2). 194–210.

Schneider-Rosen, K., & Cicchetti, D. (1984). The relationship between affect and cognition in maltreated infants: Quality of attachment and the development of visual self-recognition. *Child Development, 55,* 648–658.

Schneider-Rosen, K., & Cicchetti, D. (1991). Early self-knowledge and emotional development: Visual self-recognition and affective reactions to mirror self-images in maltreated and non-maltreated toddlers. *Developmental Psychology, 27,* 471–478.

Straus, M., & Gelles, R. (1990). How violent are American families: Estimates from the National Family Violence Resurvey and other studies. In M. A. Straus & R. J. Gelles (Eds.), *Physical violence in American Families: Risk factors and adaptations to violence in 8,145 families* (pp. 95 112). New Brunswick, NJ: Transaction.

Taylor, I., Zuckerman, B., Harik, V., & Groves, B. (1994). Witnessing violence by young children and their mothers. *Journal of Developmental Pediatrics, 15,* 120–123.

U.S. Department of Health and Human Services, National Center on Child Abuse and Neglect. (1997). *Child maltreatment 1995: Reports from the states to the national center on child abuse and neglect data system.* Washington, DC: U. S. Government Printing Office.

van der Kolk, B. A., McFarlane, A. C., & Weisaeth, L. (Eds.). (1996). *Traumatic stress: The effects of overwhelming experience on mind, body, and society.* New York: Guilford Press.

Warren, S. L., Huston, L., Egeland, B., & Sroufe, L. A. (1997). Child and adolescent anxiety disorders and early attachment. *Journal of the American Academy of Child and Adolescent Psychiatry, 36,* 637–644.

Widom, C. S. (1991). The role of placement experiences in mediating the criminal consequences of early childhood victimization. *American Journal of Orthopsychiatry, 61,* 195–209.

Wolfe, D., & Wekerle, C. (1993). Treatment strategies for child physical abuse and neglect: A critical progress report. *Clinical Psychology Review, 13,* 473–500.

Zeanah, C. H., Boris, N. W., Bakshi, S., & Lieberman, A. F. (in press). Disorders of attachment. In J. Osofsky & H. Fitzgerald (Eds.), *WAIMH handbook of infant mental health.* New York: Wiley.

Zeanah, C. H., Jr., Mammen, O. K., & Lieberman, A. F. (1993). Disorders of attachment. In C. H. Zeanah, Jr. (Ed.), *Handbook of infant mental health* (pp. 332–349). New York: Guilford Press.

Zeanah, C. H., & Scheeringa, M. S. (1997). The experience and effects of violence in infancy. In J. D. Osofsky (Ed.), *Children in a violent society* (pp. 97–123). New York: Guilford Press.

III

ASSESSMENT

❖

In the first edition of this handbook, Emde, Bingham, and Harmon (1993) noted the important distinction between the diagnosis of disorders and the assessment of individuals. An assessment may or may not lead to a diagnosis, and the assessment process must be concerned with strengths as well as weaknesses, with symptoms as well as disorders, with risks as well as established disturbances, and with deviations as well as delays. Assessment also must be concerned with the multilayered contexts in which infants develop. Part III considers a number of different types and methods of assessment.

Seligman begins a consideration of these contexts in Chapter 12 by describing an overview of the process and content of interviews with families of infants. He views the family interview as an opportunity to gather data from multiple perspectives simultaneously, and he highlights what sets the infant-with-family interview apart from other mental health assessments. When conducted properly, the family interview also provides the clinician with the most expedient and constructive way to establish and maintain a therapeutic alliance.

In Chapter 13, Zeanah, Larrieu, Heller, and Valliere present an approach to assessing infant–parent relationships. They suggest that the relationship is the appropriate unit of assessment because of its centrality in mediating and moderating intrinsic and extrinsic risk factors on infant development. They also describe an overall model of infant–parent relationship assessment and make explicit the basic premises that guide their approach. They indicate the dimensions of the relationship that seem important to measure and the process and methods they use to assess them. In addition to these components, they describe an approach to conceptualize the overall level of relationship adaptation/disturbance.

Gilliam and Mayes make clear that this relationship focus extends to a degree even into the area of developmental testing. In Chapter 14, they emphasize the importance of integrating information from a structured assessment with interviews and behavioral observations of infants and their caregivers to help ensure a more complete developmental evaluation. Although psychological assessments of individuals at any age require a synthesis of observations from both structured and nonstructured situations, the assessment of very young children demands this approach even more. The rapidly changing, growing systems represented by infants and their caregivers may be in or out of synchrony with one another, and this must influence choices of specific developmental assessment tools. Finally, they review available developmental tests, including their strengths and limitations.

In Chapter 15, Benham applies the time-honored method of the psychiatric mental status examination to the assessments of infants and toddlers. In so doing, she continues the emphasis of the preceding chapters on assessment of infants in context. She proposes that the mental status exam is a useful way of organizing observations of the infant and young child. Also in keeping with the other chapters in Part III, she emphasizes the importance of the role of the clinician in establishing a therapeutic relationship with infant and caregiver that facilitates assessment and treatment.

REFERENCE

Emde, R. N., Bingham, R. D., & Harmon, R. J. (1993). Classification and the diagnostic process. In C. H. Zeanah, Jr. (Ed.), *Handbook of infant mental health* (pp. 225–235). New York: Guilford Press.

12

Clinical Interviews with Families of Infants

❖

STEPHEN SELIGMAN

Infant mental health assessments are even more challenging than people commonly realize. They are clinically and interpersonally complex, with multiple purposes and data from an array of psychological, developmental, and cultural perspectives. Moreover, because infants' worlds are nonverbally and affectively organized, we cannot rely on verbal inquiries as we do with older children and adults. Even more daunting, infants' distress evokes extraordinary and often puzzling emotions, especially when parents are besieged by delicate and intense anxieties that are even more pervasive than those accompanying other mental health referrals. We are often pressed to respond to urgent demands, despite limited information and a meager collaboration with the family. In addition, the technical challenges of working with several family members, such as splitting one's clinical attention, may be especially exacting. Yet, offering emotional and developmental help to an infant's family can be among the most satisfying and effective of all mental health interventions. When it goes well, evaluating infants and parents offers both the intellectual appeal of sorting out complex diagnostic puzzles and the emotional gratification of providing sorely needed relief to distressed families, often with rapid and dramatic effects.

With such complex challenges in mind, this chapter presents a perspective on interviews with infants and their families that emphasizes the interplay of information gathering and relationship building. It begins with a conceptual framework, synthesizing basic mental health approaches with the broad psychodynamic relationship systems approach that has emerged from contemporary development research. Goals and practical guidelines for setting up the assessment phase of an infant mental health intervention are then presented. Specific content areas for organizing the multilayered assessment data and process are then described in some detail, with special reference to two unique aspects of the infant mental health process: the intertwined parent–infant and parent–therapist relationships. Finally, some specific techniques for approaching the interview process are offered.

CONCEPTUAL BASES OF THE CLINICAL INTERVIEWS

The Psychodynamic Relationship Systems Perspective

This chapter's approach to both evaluation and treatment rests on a psychodynamic relationship systems perspective. From this broad point of view, the interplay of actual relationships with internal representations of current and prior relationships is of special interest, along with the array of other hereditary, physiological, psychological, and sociocultural factors that determine development. Internal representations of relationships are understood as structuralized and expressed in powerful emotional and interactional formats, the nature and origins of which are often outside parents' or infants' full awareness. This approach is applied in tandem with specific disciplinary emphases that are especially relevant to the infant mental health enterprise, including the clinical psychological–psychiatric emphasis on assessment, diagnosis, prognosis, and treatment planning; the social work emphasis on the social surround, including family dynamics, institutional contexts, and mobilizing community resources; and the early interventionists' emphasis on evaluating and ameliorating specific deficits.

A corollary clinical feature of this approach is that the relationship between the therapist and the parents is a special focus for case formulation and intervention, with regard to both the overall formation of a supportive working relationship and attachment and specific parallels between parental transferences to the therapist and to the child—"the ghosts in the nursery" of which Fraiberg (1980) wrote.

The Transactional–Developmental Systems Model as a Clinical Perspective

The transactional systems model that has emerged in recent decades in varied fields, including developmental psychology, provides a fundamental orientation to conceptualizing both assessments and interventions. From this context-oriented perspective, the infant–family relationship is understood as a "transactional system" in which each element is viewed in relation to the other elements; no person or factor can be fully understood without reference to its effects on the others in the system (Sameroff & Emde, 1989; Sander, in press; Stern, 1995).

Normality and Pathology from a Transactional Perspective

From this point of view, the key issue in assessing parenting is whether the parents and infant are responding to each other so as to maximize whatever potentials exist for competent development in each member of the caregiving transaction. Alternatively, problem situations are often exacerbated when risk factors amplify one another, as in the case of the mother whose withdrawing from her weak-signaling infant leads to the infant's giving up, or that of the abused child who learns to provoke violence as the only way to gain any recognition from an otherwise unresponsive parent. In any case, although transactional outcomes vary in their desirability, each caregiver–infant relationship must be understood on its own terms and in the context of its own limitations and possibilities.

Similarly, particular factors that are liabilities in one relationship system may be assets in another. For example, one mother clung to her 2-year-old son, despite his normal strivings toward independence, as his autonomy evoked an ongoing fear of separation that was linked to being abandoned as an infant by her own mother. Her tendency toward clinginess, however, was beneficial with her second child, who was severely brain damaged, because it led her to be extraordinarily attentive.

The transactional model of the caregiver–infant relationship can also be applied to the network of societal and family relationships that surround the infant. Each member of a family affects and, in turn, is affected by the other members at multiple levels, including the internal representational world. Cultural attitudes and social policy toward infants and young children have a substantial and complex impact on the individual relationships between infants and their caregivers and should be considered in the assessment process.

GOALS OF THE CLINICAL INTERVIEW: THE INEXTRICABILITY OF INFORMATION GATHERING AND RELATIONSHIP BUILDING

The evaluation process should be approached as part of an ongoing, mutual negotiation aimed at finding a clinically effective and emotionally compelling picture of the family situation, the presenting problem, and the infant's and parents' experiences. The evaluation should also establish the basis for the all-important working alliance, on which the subsequent treatment will depend. Throughout the assessment and intervention process, diagnostic and therapeutic aims are inextricably intertwined: Even in the earliest stages of the evaluation, relationship building and information gathering are interdependent. In the final analysis, interventions should maximize whatever potentials for progressive development can be located within the caregiving system, rather than reaching some extrinsic criterion.

Case Formulation as a Relational Process

Citing Shevrin and Shechtman (1973), Hirshberg (1993) has described the goal of the clinical interviews as follows:

> not to gather objective data, but to form a personal relationship through which the assessor can elicit and observe in the family a range of psychological functioning on the basis of which the problem can be understood and a plan made cooperatively to solve it . . . what is learned about the infant and family is a picture or account that is constructed in the course of an active, dynamic exchange between family members and evaluator. (pp. 174–175)

Making this explicit to the family can be quite useful: I often tell the parents that a central goal of the assessment phase is to form a team on behalf of the infant, including getting to the point where we "see the same child." Such shared accounts are especially compelling, as they are rooted in the direct, evolving experience of the therapeutic inquiry. Progress in the clinical formulation and the evolving therapeutic relationship can be mutually reinforcing: To the extent that the parents feel that they have been collaborative partners in the assessment, they will be better able to embrace the treatment process. Rather than feeling blamed, intruded upon, or helpless, so as to recapitulate some of the difficulties that brought them to the assessment in the first place, the parents are more likely to feel that the therapeutic relationship will be responsive and flexible when their thinking about both the child and the evaluation process is given a central role.

Therapeutic Effects of the Evaluation Process

Under such congenial conditions, the assessment effort will be one of the cornerstones of the unfolding therapeutic process. The therapist's capacity to think through the family's problems offers a new vantage point from which the difficulties can be reviewed to yield new emotional understanding along with new interpersonal solutions. This is especially important in work with infants and parents when

things have begun to go badly, because such situations are often characterized by self-amplifying, pathogenic synergies in the infant–parent relationships. The calm but engaged reflective interest of the therapist can often serve to interrupt, or at least dampen, such "firestorms," to create space for at least a bit of reflective thinking, which can sometimes lead to some immediate reduction in distress and, at times, to new and more progressive solutions. Along related lines, the presence of the therapist can offer some hope, both in its promise of a clinical solution based on the intervenor's expertise and experience and through the evocation and ampification of whatever residues of helpful relationships lie within the parents' internal worlds.

In one case, for example, a mother whose son had a neurologically based hypersensitivity to novel stimuli became emotionally overwhelmed as he became inconsolable whenever she left him with a babysitter; this mother had also been left to cry herself to sleep as an infant, although she did not remember this at the beginning of the assessment. The clarification of the role of the son's sensory hypersensitivity freed the mother to think more emotionally about her early memories of abandonment, especially as she was beginning to trust her therapist. Once these synergistic processes were in process, the therapist and mother were able to add a behavioral strategy of gradually increasing the boy's time with new caretakers, in very gradual increments. The apparently overwhelming situation was obviated in the course of five weekly meetings.

Forming a Working Relationship through the Evaluation Process

The initial interviews, then, provide the basis from which the essential working relationship can proceed. Establishing a basic background of empathy, reciprocity, and support, to whatever extent possible, enhances the quality of both the initial interviews and whatever subsequent therapies are offered. Parents are more likely to offer information about themselves, especially their troubled histories and painful feelings, when they feel safe and accepted. At the same time, the family's strengths are more likely to emerge in a sympathetic atmosphere, which will allow for a more complete evaluation as well as providing a basis upon which subsequent intervention can draw. Overall, a therapeutic relationship can enhance the sense of being understood and supported, which can, in turn, lead to changes in the infant–parent relationship. (Seligman & Pawl, 1984)

Relationship-Oriented Diagnosis as an "Objective" Process

Becoming emotionally engaged while attending to the more "objective" questions of diagnosis and treatment planning is a crucial and uniquely demanding aspect of the intervention process. Building a working alliance and formulating the case are synergistic at every stage of the intervention process. Overall, such "split-mindedness" is one of the crucial skills of the infant intervenor, similar to the skill of splitting attention between various family members.

SETTING UP THE EVALUATION PROCESS: WHEN, WHERE, AND WITH WHOM

The Assessment Phase

From 4 to 6 weeks of once-weekly meetings seem to be a useful baseline time frame for the initial assessment process, although substantial conclusions can often be drawn more quickly in some cases, whereas others require an extended period of clinical involvement with the family before even basic issues become clarified. Offering an explicit explanation that there will be an assessment period is often quite useful. In general, the family should be informed about the assessment process so as to minimize mystifications and negative preconceptions.

Therapists should also realize that an agreement to proceed further with treatment can be made even though all the crucial assessment questions have not been answered. Families often benefit from partial problem formulations and may even be relieved that the apparently sophisticated and often idealized clinicians share some of their own uncertainty.

Home Visit versus Office Visit

Home visiting offers many advantages in both assessments and treatment, although it presents a number of logistical and technical challenges. Home visiting provides access to otherwise unavailable information about families' lives and reassures parents that the demands that come with the birth and development of a young child are being understood on a practical level. At times, concrete action is the only way the therapist can demonstrate his or her appreciation of the family's psychological and practical difficulties; this is especially true for families with histories of profound interpersonal insecurity and disappointment and for whom actions, rather than words, have been the most important carriers of meaning.

With these benefits, however, come a number of particular challenges. Home visits can be unpredictable and oversaturating to therapists. New strains are placed on the therapeutic "frame," and the usual clinical stance becomes even more difficult to maintain, as when a parent offers a meal (appetizing or otherwise) or asks the therapist's opinion of a racy television soap opera currently on the set. Concurrently, new configurations of transference and countertransference issues may arise, because some of the usual barriers that regulate both intimate and aversive reactions in the therapeutic relationship are now absent.

But in many cases, there may be no other way to reach the families that are most in need of treatment, and even in less challenging cases, the gains are quite substantial. When it is not possible to arrange a series of home visits, including one or two visits in the assessment plan is often worthwhile. Even when home visits are entirely precluded, naturalistic observation should not be abandoned. A playroom can be set up to provide a homelike environment, with the therapist following the family's leads to a greater extent than is typical in the usual clinical interview. Even when home visiting has been integrated into the assessment procedure, the clinic visit should always be offered as an alternative, both for the initial interviews and throughout the treatment.

Whom to Include: Noncustodial Parents and Others

Therapists often wonder whom to include in the evaluation, as so many people are involved in the care of infants, including noncustodial parents, extended family members, siblings, childcare providers, neighbors, and so on. Particularly vexing dilemmas emerge about fathers who live outside the infants' home or are otherwise not participating in the evaluation. Although eager to develop the fullest possible understanding of the infant's situation, they do not want to diffuse or undermine the relationship with the most important parent.

Because there are rarely simple answers to these quandaries, flexibility and inclusiveness are most helpful. Therapists sometimes underestimate the extent to which such dilemmas can be taken up with family members, often with startlingly useful outcomes; these difficulties reflect sensitive and problematic relationships that cannot be easily resolved and, instead, ought to be explored. Decisions might usefully be regarded as provisional, and discussed as such with the family; it is usually easier to include a new person if the possibility of doing so has been mentioned already.

In addition, therapists should realize that family structures vary widely along cultural and individual lines, as well as understanding that families with problems are often characterized by unstable and even porous boundaries. In one home visiting-based case, for example, the nonresident but involved father of two African-American daughters ages 1 and 4 would show up intermittently throughout the evaluation and treatment process. The therapist's willingness to engage with him when he was available without making either the unrealistic demand that he attend every meeting or excluding him because he would not do this enhanced the therapeutic alliance with him and with the children's mother (Seligman, 1994).

Special Issues

Including and Excluding the Older Infant

A complex issue arises with the older infant, both because the toddler's activity intensifies the already-challenging demand that the therapist and parent split attention between each other and the infant and because the linguistically competent toddler is even more likely than the younger infant to be disturbed by details of the discussions between the parents and therapist. It is sometimes useful, therefore, to schedule separate sessions for the older infant and the parents, along with the conjoint sessions. Individual child psychotherapy might be considered, often in conjunction with infant–parent psychotherapy.

Formal Testing and Videotape Review in the Relationship Context

Formal assessment instruments often play an important role in providing otherwise unavailable information and precision. But formal testing is most useful when integrated into the overall context of the dialogue-building evaluation process. Similar considerations apply to using videotape of infant interactions. Many intervenors have reported their essential value when reviewed and explored with the family, illustrating the crucial interplay of the therapeutic relationship with the information and insights yielded by this crucial source of information (McDonough, 1993).

When the Evaluator Cannot Be the Therapist

It is preferable for the professional who conducts the assessment to continue as the therapist. The beginnings of the working relationship are most likely to be sustained when continuity can be preserved. In some cases, a transfer will be experienced by parents as a repetition of early losses, and even the infant may be disturbed by the appearance of a new professional. When continuity is not practical, the attendant feelings should be discussed to the extent possible. Similar considerations should be included when cases must be transferred to new therapists because of the end of therapists' training courses.

THE "CONTENT" OF THE EVALUATION: ORGANIZING THE DATA

The specific information to be gathered differs widely from case to case, depending on the presenting problem, the family situation, and an array of other factors. In addition, the domains to be assessed can be organized along various lines. Generally, however, the evaluation should include the infant's affective and physiological development; the quality of the infant–parent relationship; the parents' mental status, personality, and other psychodynamic factors, especially as related to parenting; the parents' spousal relationship when there is one; the family's level of psychosocial and socioeconomic support, including the extended family and ethnic and cultural issues; and the parents' capacity to use infant mental health intervention. Following the transactional systems orientation, there should also be some effort to conceptualize, if only intuitively, how these different domains are interrelated.

In addition, special circumstances and their impact on the infant's development and the infant–family relationships should be evaluated. For example, in the midst of child custody disputes, or in those cases in which placing the child outside the home following allegations of abuse or neglect has occurred or is being contemplated, the legal situation should be considered, including in regard to cooperation with attorneys, courts, or child protective agencies. Similarly, assessments with infants with developmental disabilities require special attention to those issues, including collaboration with the appropriate professionals. Analogous considerations apply in cases with parental domestic violence, substance abuse, or psychopathology. Infant mental health evaluation is often best approached as a multidisciplinary process, with the possibility of building a multidisciplinary intervention team as the best outcome.

As the assessment unfolds, as well as in each clinical interview, there is an ongoing process of selection and emphasis with regard to which domains call for immediate attention; the therapist typically concludes that some are greater sources of distress and dysfunction than others, or that exploring certain difficulties must be deferred.

The Importance of Developmental Norms

As is well known, observers must always take the infant's age and developmental status into account, because affective and behavioral patterns that are appropriate at one age will be troubling at another. At the same time, norms must be applied flexibly and to reflect the family's specific situation rather than as abstract standards.

KEY AREAS FOR OBSERVATION

In the section that follows, I briefly outline nine areas to be assessed and then elaborate on two of them that play a unique role in the infant mental health process: the infant–parent and therapist–parent relationships. This list is meant as a guideline to use in connection with other orienting schemes rather than a firm set of comprehensive categories. The core areas to be assessed, then, can be organized as follows:

1. *The infant–parent relationships*, including microanalytic and macroanalytic perspectives. This is the single most essential area, including the quality of the infant–parent

interactions, security of attachment, and the particular meanings of the infant to the parents (see Zeanah, Larrieu, Heller, & Valliere, Chapter 13, this volume).

2. *The infant's individual psychological–developmental status*, including temperament and other aspects of constitutional endowment, progress toward developmental milestones and emerging psychological issues, including conflicts, self-esteem, and the array of psychological developmental issues that begin to emerge in the second and third years of life. More purely physiological factors—such as medical problems, neuropsychological deficits, developmental disabilities and other extraordinary factors, including special talents—should be considered (see Benham, Chapter 15, Gilliam & Mayes, Chapter 14, this volume).

3. *The parents' psychologies*, including psychopathology, psychiatric diagnoses and mental status, current and past substance abuse, overall level of personality development, and the history of early developmental experience as it affects parenting.

4. *The family as a caregiving system*, including the parental relationship, sibling and extended family relationships, friendships, work and community resources, and the overall level of social and economic support; particular cultural influences, including ethnicity, sexual orientation, and gender-based issues, should also be understood. The effect of medical problems should be assessed.

5. *The evolving therapist–parent relationship(s)*, including both the development of the working alliance and the complex transference relationship, with special reference to their interplay with the relationships within the family, including the parent–infant and mother–father relationships. This topic is elaborated in greater detail later.

6. *History of prior interventions*, including mental health, child protective services, criminal justice systems, and other agencies. This history is very important in understanding how the current offer of help will be experienced. Some parents come to infant mental health process with a "bureaucratic transference" (Seligman, 1994) reflecting prior experiences. Understanding such preconceptions can be crucial in evaluation and treatment.

7. *Current interventions*, such as other mental health treatment, child protective work, and special education, should be described and integrated into the diagnostic picture. Forming the

diagnostic picture often includes contact with other professionals and a plan for coordinating the various assessments into a more integrated and comprehensive picture that can be helpful to the family. Thus, the bases for future interdisciplinary collaboration, if indicated, should be established.

8. *The family's capacity to use interventions*, including some understanding of how they might make differential use of different interventions. Overall, monitoring and evaluating the development of the working relationship are crucial here, including identifying impediments to the working alliance (Seligman & Pawl, 1984). At the most basic level, one must assess whether the parents can maintain the practical arrangements necessary to collaborate with any intervention, such as keeping regular appointments and the like. With regard to psychotherapy, there is the question of whether the parents have enough "basic trust" to engage in a therapeutic relationship, along with, more ambitiously, the question of how psychologically minded the parents can be, including tolerating painful emotions. The assessment phase usually includes, in the course of its normal unfolding, trial interventions that provide very useful data about such questions.

9. *Developing a treatment plan* might include referrals for conjoint or individual psychotherapeutic or psychopharmacological treatment for family members (including child psychotherapy for older children). Treatment planning also includes an evaluation of whether non–mental health interventions are indicated or, at least, which non–mental health evaluations should now be undertaken as the psychotherapeutic work begins. As I described previously, treatment plans are most effective when parents feel included as partners in the evaluation process.

THE INFANT–PARENT RELATIONSHIP AS A SPECIAL FOCUS

The Observed Relationship: Infant–Parent Interaction

This aspect of the assessment draws on the broad array of observational descriptors that have evolved in the last decades, including attachment theory, infant–parent interaction research, and early affect development research

(e.g., Beebe & Lachmann, 1988; Bowlby, 1969; Stern, 1985). Although it is not possible to provide a complete account, several key points can be mentioned as a general orientation.

Interviewers should notice the overall affective tone of the infant–parent interactions, as well as characteristic rhythms and patterns of expectancy. Are the parents' responses to the baby appropriate and contingent upon the infant's cues? Are there characteristic affects in the interactions, and is there a comfortable emotional flow and sense of efficacy and coordination? Alternatively, are there, for example, frequent displays by infant or parents of negative and even out-of-control affects and/or pervasive senses of disruption, avoidance, freezing, ineffectuality, tension, and other dissonant affects (Fraiberg, 1982)?

Similarly, do the infant and parent(s) have a sense of shared predictable expectancies? Does the infant turn to the parents for comfort when distressed, and is the comfort forthcoming and effective? Do the parents protect the infant from dangerous situations, ideally "keeping a watchful eye out" while providing a background of safety for the baby to explore new situations? And, as a corollary, does the baby look to the parents for help with unfamiliar situations; that is, for social referencing (Sorce, Emde, Campos, & Klinnert, 1985)? Is there a sense of continuity and coherence to the family situation? With regard to this, differences between the affective tone of different meetings are often significant.

Such observations should also yield a sense of the overall quality of the infant's social and affective relatedness: How does the child relate to various people, including the therapist—is the child wary or withdrawing, for example, or, alternatively, overly quick to engage? Does the baby play coherently and age appropriately, and do the parents engage in play with responsive pleasure? Infants are especially sensitive to parents' emotions, including about the new intervenor, and such feelings should be taken into account because the infant often absorbs and communicates the parents' inner states. In one case, for example, a therapist noticed that the 3-month-old son of a mildly paranoid woman was regarding him carefully and said to the child's mother that he could imagine how the baby would want to "check him out" because he was unfamiliar.

Attachment researchers have called attention

to crucial aspects of the infant–parent relationship: the sense of felt security, as opposed to anxiety, ambivalence, and disorganzation; the infant's use of the parent as a secure base from which to explore; and behaviors and emotional displays on separation and reunion (Ainsworth, Blehar, Waters, & Wall, 1978; Bowlby, 1969). It is often possible to observe the infant's exploration (or its absence), including the extent to which the child can sustain appropriate interest and enthusiasm. Because it is often more difficult to observe a separation without orchestrating one or relying instead on the parents' accounts, it may be useful to inquire about the parents' experience of separations and reunions, including their understanding of the infant's experience. These accounts may be filtered through parents' own childhood experiences of separations, which are often evoked by current situations (Hirshberg, 1993).

The Represented Infant: Who Is the Baby for the Parents?

At another level, we are trying to understand "who the baby is to the parents," including which of the parents' childhood relationships are most prominently evoked by the baby, how the baby affects the overall family dynamics, and how the parents are experiencing the crucial developmental process of becoming a parent. Babies often evoke particular feelings and memories of the parent's childhood, and different babies sometimes evoke different representations from the past for the same parent. In one case, for example, the mother of two sons began to recall her own sexual abuse by an uncle when her first daughter was born; her identification with the girl baby was distinctively different from that with her boys.

Often, the infant will also play a particular role in the evolving marital relationship and in each parent's ongoing personality development. Commonly, this role will be constructive, if stressful, with the parents' alliance strengthened and differentiated. Nevertheless, at times, the infant's presence is disorganizing. In one case, for example, the mother of a 3-month-old was quite successful upon her return to her professional career, while her husband was left at home to care for the infant as his own business declined. This gender role reversal exacerbated existing tensions in the marriage, which led to further dissonance and an eventual divorce.

THE THERAPIST–FAMILY RELATIONSHIP SYSTEM AS A BASIC DATA SOURCE

This section discusses how the parent–provider relationship, including complex difficulties in those relationships, can become sources of data and therapeutic effect. This includes correlating affective–relational patterns in the infant–parent and therapist–parent relationships and the use of the therapist's own emotional reactions to enhance the assessment and treatment processes.

The Working Relationship

As the working relationship is the crucial locus for intervention, it also provides essential data. Because parents' relationships with providers often parallel their relationships with their children, observing the evolving therapeutic relationship can provide important information about parents' and infants' experiences of one another. As has been noted, these patterns often reflect the parents' childhood experiences of their own parents; although this is well acknowledged, the actuality of such stark repetitions can still be quite startling to clinicians. Understanding the evolving therapeutic relationship as a reflection of a complex interplay of past and present and internal and external realities is an essential part of both assessment and treatment, as well as providing a formidable guide for moment-to-moment formulation and intervention in the clinical interview. Such attention can be especially fruitful when the developments in therapeutic relationship are monitored in tandem with other information emerging in the ongoing assessment and treatment process, including the observation of the infant–parent relationships and parents' own direct accounts of their own developmental histories as well as their extratherapeutic relationships.

This was well illustrated in the early stages of the treatment of Harriet and her 7-month-old grandson, Jackson, for whom she was the primary caretaker. Increasingly, Harriet's daughter, Jennifer, had left Jackson's care to Harriet; this was consistent with her general pattern of unreliability and disappointing responses to her parents. In the face of Jennifer's absences, Harriet would make ever more strenuous efforts to gain her own daughter's loyalty by giving her gifts and extending other, self-sacrificing offers of support. Harriet had recently reported that her own mother had left her in the care of her grandaunt when Harriet's father died when she was 5 years old, in order to return to work in another city. Although Harriet had always known this fact, she felt little emotion about how it must have been. The therapist's suggestion that Harriet's relationship with Jennifer had evoked similar feelings was similarly met with assent but little emotion.

In one session, the therapist had announced that he would miss an upcoming session because of a commitment to speak in a distant city. Harriet began the meeting immediately preceding the cancellation by inquiring about the details of the talk, wishing him well, and saying how his mother, who lived nearby his destination, must be proud of him. After thanking Harriet for her kind words, the therapist wondered whether Harriet might be also preparing herself for his absence, because their work together had been growing quite important to her. Harriet agreed that this might be true, as she would indeed miss him. The therapist then wondered whether her kindness, too, might reflect a pattern of responding to inner disappointment with solicitousness, as with her daughter, and wondered whether that might distance her from the painful anticipation of his absence. He also added that he did not mean to devalue her good wishes about the talk.

Tearfully, Harriet talked about how she sometimes really worked hard, without realizing it, to avoid those feelings. She wondered whether something similar was at work with her efforts to think about what she felt when her father died. This led to a further elaboration of the feelings surrounding those early years and, more broadly, a more emotional elaboration of the themes of abandonment, disappointment, and the efforts to compensate for such distressing emotions by excessive attention to others' needs.

Parallels between the Infant–Parent and Therapist–Parent Relationships

Such processes can be further enhanced when observations about the infant–parent relationship are integrated into the emerging evaluation–intervention process. The infant–parent relationship and therapist–parent relationships often contain similar themes, although they may be managed and articulated in different ways. This was further illustrated in Harriet and Jackson's emerging relationship:

As Harriet became more involved as Jackson's primary caretaker, she began to feel that something was "not right" about him. After a neurological assessment confirmed that Jackson did, indeed, have a significant disability, Harriet devoted herself to finding the best interventions for her grandson. The therapist did not explicitly comment on how Harriet's zeal reflected her characterological pattern of sacrificing herself so as to sidestep inner distress, feeling that this mode might prove to be adaptive in this unusual situation.

However, when Harriet became irritably disappointed in the special educator, this understanding was crucial. Despite a growing sense of grievance, she could not talk directly with him and, instead, she began to skip appointments. As the evaluation became stalled, the therapist now spoke with Harriet about the abandonment themes that they had discussed earlier, saying, "It must be so difficult when someone from whom you had so much hoped for help appears not to care, nor to understand how crucial that care could be to you and your baby." Harriet wept and could now consider seeking another educator with very positive results.

Why How You Feel Matters: The Therapist's Reactions as Data Source

Clinical work with infants and parents is among the most evocative of all mental health interventions. The most basic psychological issues are at play in infancy, and affective and other nonverbal communications predominate such that therapists often respond with more raw and unmediated emotions than in other situations. In addition, the vulnerable and dependent state of the infant, combined with the sense of urgency that often accompanies infant mental health referrals, is especially evocative. Home visiting carries additional challenges, because the usual office routines are not structuring the therapist's responses. Sometimes, the specific relationship issues that families bring to the intervention situation evoke the therapist's deepest personal issues and conflicts.

Tolerating and reflecting on these feelings will generally prove more useful than succumbing to the pressure to respond or to prematurely act upon them. Such reactions should be treated as data for the assessment and for enhancing the intervention relationship. With Harriet, for example, the therapist felt uneasy with the compliment about his mother, experiencing a sense of intrusion and misrecognition at the same time that he appreciated the kindness that was conveyed. This helped sensitize him to the rich emotional complexity of the moment and helped him formulate his response (Seligman, 1993).

ORIENTING THE INTERVIEW TOWARD THE FAMILY'S SUBJECTIVE EXPERIENCE

Overall, then, the subjective experience of parents and infants should be the orienting hub of the therapeutic process. Eliciting parents' perceptions of their child's behavior and motivations can yield essential information about how they understand the child's behavior. The interview should be conducted to yield knowledge of the infant's and parents' interactions and personalities at the same time that it creates opportunities for discussing this knowledge with them. While observing and inquiring, the interviewer should convey a sense of appreciation of both parents' and children's experiences, especially the emotionally painful areas (Kalmanson & Seligman, 1992).

In addition to maintaining an empathic attitude, the therapist should speak in clear and simple terms, avoiding professional jargon. Parents should be invited to ask questions and ask for clarification. If therapists anticipate with the parents that what they say may not always be clear, parents will feel more able to express their feelings. Earning parents' trust and belief that they can be genuinely understood, especially in relation to their infant, is an essential element in the clinical process. With an interview style that follows the parents' and infant's lead, parents begin to sense that their own and their child's behavior and experience is more important than they had realized: Parents can thus be helped to feel that the baby's behavior and their reactions to it have meaning that can be interpreted and understood in collaborative efforts to enhance development.

History Taking in the Empathic–Observational Context

Historical and developmental information gathered as part of a relationship-building process will yield a richer and more affectively accurate reflection of the past and of the relationship of the past to the present. Information obtained from history taken in a question-and-answer or checklist format often feels sketchy and at times emotionally alienated; even formal assessment instruments, while sometimes yielding crucial findings, may present similar pitfalls. Attention to recurring feelings about the current situation that are associated with earlier experiences creates opportunities for reflection and allows freer access to the emotional underpinnings of the developmental data.

Reflecting on the Anxieties of the Intervention Process

The interviewer should be sensitive to the parents' emotions about the presenting problem and the intervention process. Assessments provoke substantial anxiety: Infant mental health evaluations are still uncommon, and parents are frequently worried that they have done something wrong, that they are inadequate parents, that their baby's development is jeopardized, and the like. Often, parents are intimidated or confused in the encounter with the professional. These problematic reactions can easily be overlooked; signs include parents' becoming subdued during sessions, avoiding obvious questions, or failing to follow through with recommendations with which they have appeared to agree.

Therapists should not underestimate the extent to which such concerns can be explored so as to bring some relief and even insight. Worries about the assessment often reflect the underlying concerns and personality problems that have led to the current problem, and a flexible, empathic interviewing style may allow for attention to the initial anxiety so as to yield more general psychological information.

The Tension between Intrusion and Support

Sometimes therapists fear that they will be seen as intruding on or criticizing the family if they ask questions. However, questions can be used nonjudgmentally and with a genuine interest in whatever response is forthcoming. At times, the interviewer's not asking questions will be interpreted as a condemnation, whereas genuine interest will move things forward. Similarly, directive and didactic approaches to helping parents with children's behavior often fall on deaf ears, experienced as criticism by already sensitive parents.

Tact is especially important in such situations. Sympathetic questions, such as those that allow the parents to say how they think the baby feels or to describe their own feelings, can yield both important data and therapeutic effects. Empathic, inquiring offers of developmental guidance are most effective when they acknowledge how puzzling the infant might be, find kernels of important data in parents' reports, and confirm them as experts about their own children. In the early stages of the assessment, such offers might be regarded as trial interventions whose outcome will yield important data about what works best with each family.

REFERENCES

Ainsworth, M., Blehar, M., Waters, E., & Wall, S. (1978). *Patterns of attachment: A psychological study of the strange situation*. Hillsdale: NJ: Erlbaum.

Beebe, B., & Lachmann, F. M. (1988). The contribution of mother–infant mutual influence to the origins of self- and object-representations. *Psychoanalytic Psychology, 5*, 305–337.

Bowlby, J. (1969). *Attachment and loss: Vol. 1. Attachment*. New York: Basic Books.

Fraiberg, S. (Ed.). (1980). *Clinical studies in infant mental health: The first year of life*. New York: Basic Books.

Fraiberg, S. (1982). Pathological defenses in infancy. *Psychoanalytic Quarterly, 51*, 612–635.

Hirshberg, L. M. (1993). Clinical interviews with infants and their families. In C. J. Zeanah, Jr. (Ed.), *Handbook of infant mental health*. New York: Guilford Press.

Kalmanson, B., & Seligman, S. (1992). Family–provider relationships: The basis of all interventions. *Infants and Young Children, 4*, 46–52.

McDonough, S. C. (1993). Interaction guidance: Understanding and treating early infant–caregiver relationship disturbances. In C. J. Zeanah, Jr. (Ed.), *Handbook of infant mental health*. New York: Guilford Press.

Sameroff, A. J., & Emde, R. N. (1989). *Relationship disturbances in early childhood: A developmental approach*. New York: Basic Books.

Sander, L. W. (in press). Thinking differently: Tasks and boundaries in constructing our pathway to the future. *Psychoanalytic Dialogues: A Journal of Relational Perspectives*.

Seligman, S. (1993). Why how you feel matters: Countertransference reactions in intervention relationships. *WAIMH Newsletter, 1*(2), 1–6.

Seligman, S. (1994). Applying psychoanalysis in an unconventional context: Adapting infant–parent psychotherapy to a changing population. *Psychoanalytic Study of the Child, 49*.

Seligman, S., & Pawl, J. (1984). Impediments to the formation of the working alliance in infant–parent psychotherapy. In J. D. Call, E. Galenson, & R. Tyson (Eds.), *Frontiers of infant psychiatry* (Vol. II). New York: Basic Books.

Shevrin, H., & Shechtman, F. (1973). *Bulletin of the Menninger Clinic, 37*, 451–494.

Sorce, J. F., Emde, R. N., Campos, J. J., & Klinnert, M. D. (1985). Maternal emotional signaling: Its effect on the visual cliff behavior of one year olds. *Developmental Psychology, 21*, 195–200.

Stern, D. N. (1985). *The interpersonal world of the infant*. New York: Basic Books.

Stern, D. N. (1995). *The motherhood constellation: A unified view of parent–infant psychotherapy*. New York: Basic Books.

13

Infant–Parent Relationship Assessment

❖

CHARLES H. ZEANAH, JR.
JULIE A. LARRIEU
SHERRYL SCOTT HELLER
JEAN VALLIERE

Over a decade ago, Sroufe (1989) boldly declared that most clinical disturbances in the first 3 years of life, although poignantly expressed as child behavioral problems, are more usefully conceptualized as relationship disturbances. In keeping with this emphasis, the infant–parent relationship is emerging as the target of most intervention and prevention efforts in infant mental health (Clark, Paulson, & Conlin, 1993; Cramer, 1987; Lieberman, 1993; Lieberman & Pawl, 1993; McDonough, 1993; Sameroff & Emde, 1989; Sroufe & Fleeson, 1988; Stern-Bruschweiler & Stern, 1989; Stern, 1995). That is, rather than assess the infant's behavior or the parent's behavior as potential foci of change, this approach involves understanding the organization of infant and parent behaviors as indices of the relationship *between* the two. For these reasons, a formal approach to assessing the infant–parent relationship is valuable for the infant mental health clinician.

Making infant–parent relationships the centerpiece of evaluation of infants and their families in clinical settings raises a number of challenging questions: Is assessing relationships more than assessing interactions? Do relationships exist between individuals, within individuals, or both? What are the crucial domains of infant–parent relationships that one ought to assess? What are the larger contexts in which infant–parent relationships ought to be assessed? How we answer these and related questions will determine our approaches to assessment and to treatment.

In this chapter, we present our approach to assessing infant–parent relationships. We begin by reviewing several areas of research that support a focus on relationships. We describe the overall model of infant–parent relationship assessment and elaborate the basic premises that guide our approach. Next, we describe the dimensions of the relationship that seem important to measure and the process and methods we employ to assess them. Finally, we describe an approach to conceptualize the overall level of relationship adaptation/disturbance.

EMPIRICAL BACKGROUND

An increasing amount of research supports changing the focus of assessment from the infant and parent to the infant with the parent. We highlight four of these areas.

222

Infant–Parent Relationships: Context for Infant Development

Several decades of research document the considerable power of parents to influence infant development. Synchrony and reciprocity in emotional interchanges between infants and parents have been demonstrated to be broadly predictive of subsequent adaptation in the young child (Crockenberg & Leerkes, Chapter 4, this volume; Zeanah, Boris, & Scheeringa, 1996). With few exceptions, as goes the relationship, so goes the infant's development. What is important about this influence, for our purposes, is that risk factors in the caregiving environment are transmitted through infants' experiences in their primary caregiving relationship. The infant–parent relationship effectively mediates environmental risk factors on infant development. Adolescent motherhood, maternal mental illness, or poverty, for example, mean nothing to a young infant except as they are experienced through the primary caregiving relationship. Even biological risk factors, such as prematurity or adverse temperamental characteristics, may be profoundly moderated by the effects of the infant–parent relationship (Minde, Chapter 10, this volume; Sameroff, 1997, Chapter 1, this volume).

Specificity of Infant–Parent Relationships

The pioneering research of Main and her colleagues on internal representational processes (Main, Kaplan, & Cassidy, 1985) has demonstrated that it is possible to describe different types of internal representations of attachment in adults through study of individual differences in narrative patterns. Further, Main reinterpreted research on infant attachment classifications as revealing types of internal representations in infants. This work provided the basis for a method of studying assertions about intergenerational transmission of relationship patterns. In dozens of investigations conducted around the world, this research has demonstrated convincingly that relationship patterns between infants and parents are transmitted intergenerationally (van IJzendoorn, 1995). Further, one of the most important and interesting findings has been the remarkable specificity of intergenerational transmission. For example, Benoit and Parker (1994) found concordance of attachment across three genera-

tions in a sample of grandmothers, mothers, and infants. More remarkably, Steele, Steele, and Fonagy (1996) showed that mothers' representations of attachment in pregnancy strongly predicted infants' patterns of attachment to them but only modestly to fathers over a year later. They also found that fathers' representations of attachment in pregnancy predicted infants' patterns of attachment to them but not to mothers 1 year later. These and similar findings emphasize that infants internalize specific relationship experiences with each of their parents and carry them forward into subsequent relationships (Sroufe & Fleeson, 1988; Zeanah, 1993).

Coherence of Infant–Parent Relationships

Patterns of attachment between infants and parents have proven to be one of the most robust predictors of subsequent development (Sroufe, 1988). Sroufe and Fleeson (1988) have argued eloquently that infant–parent relationships manifest coherence across developmental epochs and social contexts much as individuals do. That is, although specific interactive behaviors may change from setting to setting, the changes are predictable, and qualitative aspects of relationships are remarkably stable. Infant attachment classifications, for example, are stable over time and predictive of subsequent infant and parent behavior. Thus, 1-year-old infants who express distress directly to their mothers following a brief separation and who seek and obtain comfort directly from their mothers on reunion are more likely in the preschool years to be liked by and rated as competent by their teachers (Sroufe, 1988). These lawful transformations suggest that stability may be more apparent at the level of how behaviors are organized within a relationship across developmental epochs rather than at the level of discrete behaviors (Sroufe & Fleeson, 1988).

Relationship Context of Psychopathology in Infancy

Because of these and similar findings from infancy research, the infant–parent relationship is more often than not the target of intervention efforts and, therefore, of assessment. We have used this approach to assess infants and their parents in a number of different settings, including an interdisciplinary team evaluating maltreated infants and toddlers (Larrieu & Zeanah, 1998), in a hospital-based clinic setting, in a community-based clinic setting, in a consultation service to hospitalized infants, and in an infant–parent intervention program located in a homeless shelter (Valliere, 1994).

OVERALL MODEL

How do we approach a particular infant–parent relationship? Is the dyadic relationship more properly considered two relationships, one as perceived and experienced by the parent and one as perceived and experienced by the infant? Or, is the relationship an emergent property of the interaction and subjective experience of both partners that exists somehow *between* them? For purposes of assessment, we consider four major components of the infant–parent relationship.

Stern-Brushweiler and Stern (1989) provided the basic model for our approach to conceptualizing infant–parent relationships and their assessments (see Figure 13.1). As a way of defining commonalities among different psychotherapeutic approaches to mother–infant dyads, they asserted that the infant–parent relationship may be conceived as an open system of infant and parent interactive behaviors and infant and parent internal representations. An intervention aimed at one component of the system, they argued, will have an impact on the other components of the system, as well. Stern (1995) elaborated more completely the implications of this model for several different approaches to infant–parent interventions.

His model is also useful as a guide to infant–parent relationship assessment. It suggests that infant–parent relationships are more than interactions. Relationships also include the subjective experience of each partner, including

$$R_B \leftrightarrow I_B \leftrightarrow I_P \leftrightarrow R_P$$

FIGURE 13.1. Model of internal and external components of infant–parent relationships. R_B, baby's representational world; I_B, baby's interactive behavior; I_P, parent's interactive behavior; R_P, parent's representational world. Adapted from Stern-Brushweiler and Stern (1989). Copyright 1989 by Michigan Association for Infant Mental Health. Adapted by permission.

memories and representations of the history of interactions of the dyad. Interactive behaviors of infant and parent comprise the external, observable component of the relationship, whereas subjective experiences or representational processes of infant and parent comprise the internal component. Efforts to assess infant–parent relationships ought to include attention both to observable interactive behaviors and to internal subjective experiences. We discuss each of these components briefly before considering the specific relationship domains in which interactions and internal experience can be evaluated.

Interactive behaviors of infant and parent have been central to clinical infant work (Fraiberg, 1980; Lieberman & Pawl, 1988; Lieberman & Pawl, 1993; McDonough, 1993; Stern, 1995). Sroufe (1988) has emphasized that insight into the meaning of interactive behaviors may come from consideration of the *organization* of those behaviors. For this reason, clinicians routinely must account for the goals and contexts of the observed behaviors as a way of evaluating their meaning.

The meaning of interactive behaviors becomes clearer when we understand the next component in the model, the parent's internal subjective experience or representation of the infant and the relationship (Stern, 1991; Stern, 1995; Zeanah & Anders, 1987; Zeanah & Barton, 1989; Zeanah & Benoit, 1995). One of the most important developments in infancy research in the past 15 years has been the discovery that the subjective experience of parents may be systematically studied by attending to narrative patterns in their description of relationship experiences. Pioneered by Main and her colleagues (Main et al., 1985), this research has revealed that attention to the formal properties of parent narratives of their own childhood relationship experiences is remarkably and consistently predictive of attachment classifications in their infants (van IJzendoorn, 1995). From a clinical standpoint, these findings suggest that what parents say may be less important than how they say it, at least with regard to understanding the organization of different types of defensive processes (Zeanah, 1993).

Some have argued that the direct translation of research on narrative patterns into the clinical arena is problematic (Seligman, 1991). Nevertheless, we have argued that attention to narrative detail can be useful clinically (Boris, Fueyo, & Zeanah, 1997; Zeanah & Barton,

1991; Zeanah & Benoit, 1995), providing as it does another way of understanding the meaning of subjective experience. Further, specific links have been demonstrated between parents' representations of their infants, as measured by narrative patterns, and parent and infant interactive behaviors. Specifically, foster parents and biological parents were interviewed about and interacted with the same child. Although there was no concordance of their representations of the same child, both foster and biological parents' representations were specifically associated with their interactive behaviors with toddlers (Zeanah, Aoki, & Heller, 1998).

The final component of the model, infant subjective experience, is the most difficult to infer, despite its obvious importance. In fact, 30 years ago, Escalona (1967) anticipated Stern's (1985) focus on infant interpersonal experience when she asserted that when attempting to predict various outcomes what we really want to know about infant development is neither the infant's nor the environment's contributions but, rather, the infant's subjective experience of the world. Careful attention to infant and parent interactive behavior, coupled with systematic formal study of parent subjective experience, makes inferences about infant subjective experience possible. Throughout the process of assessment, we ask ourselves what it feels like to be this particular infant in this particular relationship with this particular parent at this particular time. Along these lines, a number of clinicians have advocated various forms of articulating the infant's perspective to the parent in the course of treatment (Carter, Osofsky, & Hann, 1991; Fraiberg, 1980; Lieberman & Pawl, 1993; Lieberman, Silverman, & Pawl, Chapter 30, this volume; McDonough, Chapter 31, this volume).

BASIC PREMISES

Before describing the content and process of relationship assessment, we must emphasize several fundamental assumptions of our approach. These concern context, the importance of identifying strengths, and the assumption that aspects of the therapist–family relationship may be used to change infant–parent relationships.

Context

Infant–parent relationships always are embedded in a complex hierarchical system of contexts (Sameroff, Chapter 1, this volume), from the network of family relationships beyond the dyad (Crockenberg, Lyons-Ruth, & Dickstein, 1993; Emde, 1991; Sroufe & Fleeson, 1988) to the social class of the family, to cultural belief systems (Garcia-Coll & Meyer, 1993; Lewis, Chapter 5, this volume), all of which regulate the infant–parent relationship in ways that are clinically salient. Appreciation of these larger contexts is vital to our efforts to understand and to change infant–parent relationships.

Nevertheless, one of the most consistent and striking findings in research designed to test models of genetic influence on individual children's development has been the importance of nonshared environmental influences (Plomin, 1995). Shared environmental influences include those factors that are presumed to affect all children within a family together, such as family social class or parental personality traits. Nonshared environmental factors are those comprising the unique, individual experiences of a child. Clearly in the first few years of life, one of the most crucial nonshared environmental influences is the infant–parent relationship. A meaningful proportion of the variance in the behavior of different children in the same family is due to the unique characteristics of the relationships between each young child and each parent. Simply put, no two children in the same family, even twins, grow up with the same environment.

Emde (1991) also reminded us that each important infant–parent relationship itself also will be influenced by other relationships in the family (see Crockenberg et al., 1993; Crockenberg & Leerkes, Chapter 4, this volume). Thus, the context in which each infant–parent relationship is embedded is vital to appreciate.

Strengths

Assessments must concern themselves with individual, dyadic, and family strengths and competencies as well as weaknesses. In fact, a focus on strengths is important to developing a therapeutic alliance that will permit a more productive examination of weaknesses. Beyond assaying strengths and weaknesses, of course, it is important to understand their interrelationships. Sometimes problems obscure or render strengths useless, and sometimes strengths provide the most promising approach to identified weaknesses.

As infant mental health clinicians, we must

avoid pathologizing and labeling infants at the same time we avoid idealizing them so much that we cannot consider their experiences of psychopathology. Similarly, we must avoid mother blaming and parent blaming but still be willing to assess and acknowledge serious shortcomings in parents. Learning to approach infant and/or parent shortcomings through identified strengths in fact defines the real value of the strengths perspective (Zeanah, 1998).

Clinician–Parent Relationship

The importance of the relationship between the primary clinician or therapist and family cannot be underemphasized. Many have asserted that it is through this relationship that the infant–parent relationship becomes available for change (Hirshberg, 1993; Lieberman & Pawl, 1993; Lieberman, Silverman, & Pawl, Chapter 30, this volume; McDonough, 1993; Seligman, Chapter 12, this volume). Stern (1995), in particular, has emphasized how both interactive behaviors and subjective experiences of infants and parents are modified by the presence of the clinician/evaluator. The clinician uses the therapeutic relationship to change the relationship between mother and infant. In fact, well-timed interpretations in infant–parent psychotherapy have been demonstrated to lead to immediately improved maternal interactive behaviors (Cramer & Stern, 1988).

RELATIONSHIP DOMAINS

Emde (1989) provided a basic outline of the salient functional domains of the infant–parent relationship. Our modifications of this outline, originally published in Zeanah et al. (1997), appear in Table 13.1. Despite some overlap, these seven parent and child domains provide a means of considering relationship adaptation and disturbances within specific areas. Several overall points about this conceptualization deserve special emphasis.

First, some of these domains of functioning are observable in brief clinic observations or home visits. These include play between infant and parent, parent emotional availability and infant emotion regulation, and parent warmth/nurturance/support and trust/security in the infant. Other domains may require specific probes in history taking, such as instrumental care/structure/ routines by the parent and self-regulation/response to structure in the infant or young child.

Second, the developmental level of the infant must be considered central to an assessment of a particular domain. We must account for differences in expected infant and parent behavior at different infant ages. For example, instrumental care of and provision for the newborn by the parent is closely tied to physiological regulation of sleep and feeding cycles and an appreciation of states and rhythmic processes (Anders, 1978). In toddlerhood, instrumental

TABLE 13.1. Domains of Infant–Parent Relationship and Relevant Crowell Episodes

Parent domains	Infant domains	Most relevant Crowell episodes
Emotional availability	Emotion regulation	All episodes are relevant
Nurturance/valuing/empathic responsiveness	Security/trust/self-esteem	All episodes are relevant
Protection	Vigilance/self-protection/safety	All episodes are potentially important, though none are definitely related
Comforting/response to distress	Comfort seeking	All, especially reunion
Teaching	Learning/curiosity/mastery	Teaching, play, cleanup
Play	Play/imagination	Play
Discipline/limit setting	Self-control/cooperation	All, especially cleanup
Instrumental care/structure/routines	Self-regulation/predictability	Limited opportunities, although how activities are structured may be useful

Note. Adapted from Sameroff and Emde (1989). Copyright 1989 by Basic Books, Inc. Adapted by permission of Basic Books, a member of Perseus Books, L.L.C.

care and provision of structure has a different function, that is, defining the predictability of the environment and allowing the young child to appreciate the necessity and the ubiquity of time-bounded activities and to develop the ability to manage transitions from one activity to another. The idea that relationships progress along developmental lines recalls Anna Freud's (1963) model, in which a developmental transformation occurs in the specific ways in which salient issues are manifest at different points in time, though there exists an overall coherence in each of the developmental lines as it develops over time.

Third, problems in the infant–parent relationship may derive from within the infant, the parent, or the unique fit between the two. One of the purposes of assessment is to attempt to understand the sources of relationship disturbance, if any, and to design interventions appropriate to the putative source of the disturbance. Infant mental health clinicians must be vigilant to avoid any tendency toward parent blaming for relationship disturbances. The goal should be understanding what is contributing to the disturbance, in what ways, and under what circumstances. Parents always will be scrutinized carefully by clinicians, in part because of the enormous influence they have on infant development and in part because of the repertoire of resources they have available for change. The key to success in this work is the therapeutic alliance that the clinician develops with parents, that is, the shared sense of working together in the best interest of the infant.

Next, we turn to assessing each of the components of the overall model. We begin by describing our assessment of infant–parent interactions, concentrating primarily on clinic-based assessments.

ASSESSMENT OF INFANT–PARENT INTERACTIONS

Our approach to the assessment of interactions follows the outline provided in Table 13.1 of the salient domains of interest. We attempt to make use of both naturalistic and clinic-based assessments because we believe that each has distinct advantages and disadvantages.

The major advantage of naturalistic (often home-based) assessments is that the dyad can be observed in a setting familiar to them. Therefore, they may be more likely to engage in routinized patterns of behavior that are of interest clinically. Although the clinician's presence is always a perturbation with definite (though often unknowable) effects on infant and parent behavior, naturalistic observations minimize the unfamiliarity of the setting and provide vivid images of the dyad in their familiar context. In our clinical program, we often find advantages in longer home observations, noting that in the first hour an observer's presence is often a focus of the young child, whereas in the second hour, more typical behavioral patterns often emerge, at least from the perspective of parents' reports.

On the other hand, clinic-based assessments may be quite useful in providing a standardized procedure in which to evaluate dyads, so that the dyad's negotiation of a fairly standard set of challenges can be observed. It is possible to take advantage of the inherently stressful nature of clinic settings by noting how the dyad manages stress. Further, it may be possible to elicit certain behaviors in infants and responses in parents, such as separation-induced distress, rather than waiting for them to occur in naturalistic observations. The concern about clinic-based assessments is that they are less standard than we presume, because of extraneous or contextual factors affecting infant and parent behavior (illness, recent external stressor, nervousness about being observed or videotaped, etc.). We make every effort to identify these factors, to reduce them when possible, and to consider them when drawing conclusions from our observations. Making multiple observations in the clinic across time mitigates against some of these concerns.

Because of these important but unavoidable influences, how we integrate clinic-based and more naturalistic observations is essential to making the most of each. Further, the process of relationship assessment always must include an active and ongoing dialogue with the parent about the representativeness of the behaviors observed and about potentially confounding factors. It is also important to determine whether what we observe represents the dyad's *typical* pattern of interaction or rather what the dyad is *capable* of enacting. Clearly, either can be useful clinically.

Once a dyad is engaged in a particular interactive pattern, it may be hard to determine the degree of contribution from each partner. For this reason, it is often useful to observe both partners as they interact in other important dyadic relationships to determine the relationship specificity of any problematic behaviors.

Clinical Problem-Solving Procedure (the Crowell Procedure)

The procedure we use routinely for clinic-based assessments was first described by Crowell and Feldman (1988) as an adaptation of the Matas, Arend, and Sroufe (1978) "tool use task," originally designed for 24-month-old children. Crowell and her colleagues modified the tasks involved to apply the procedure to children 24 to 54 months of age. Although clinical applicability of the procedure has been noted (Crowell & Fleischmann, 1993), it has been described primarily in studies of older toddlers (Crowell & Feldman, 1988; Crowell & Feldman, 1991; Crowell, Feldman & Ginsberg, 1988). Our group has extended the procedure downward, with only minor modifications, for use with children 12 months of age to 54 months of age (Zeanah et al., 1997; Zeanah et al., 1998).

The actual procedure involves nine separate episodes of varying lengths of time designed to elicit behaviors indicative of many of the different domains of infant–parent relationships described in Table 13.1. Parents are given a detailed visual and verbal orientation prior to the initiation of the procedure, and we make modifications through telephone calls during the procedure in rare instances when necessary. Transitions from one episode to another, which are especially important as indicators of how the child uses the parent for support, are controlled by the observing clinicians. Instructions about proceeding to the next episode are called in by telephone. Toys and tasks used in various episodes are kept in a locked cabinet, and the parent is given a key and the charge of selecting what is necessary for the next episode during telephone calls made between episodes. After the procedure has been explained carefully to the parent, and consent for videotaping has been obtained, each of the following episodes is conducted in order.

Free Play

Parent and child are instructed to play together "as you usually play together at home." A standard set of toys is provided in a large container. This episode is usually about 10 minutes in length, and we give no other instructions. This episode allows us to observe the dyad in the typically lower stress situation of unstructured time together, although some dyads seem more comfortable when activities are more structured. Many important observations are possible from observing free play, including the dyad's level of comfort with one another, the amount and kind of affection they share, their familiarity with play and having fun together, the dyad's use of the time as fun-oriented versus task-oriented, and their sense of partnership versus solitary play. Though this episode may be stressful for some dyads, more typically, it provides an opportunity for the dyad to relax in front of the camera, thereby diminishing any effects of parent anxiety about being videotaped.

Cleanup

The first transition observed is when the parent is called at the end of free play and told to instruct the child that it is time for "cleanup." The parent is instructed to have the child return all the toys to the large container and to help to the degree that the child needs assistance. Then, the parent is to set the toys outside the playroom (a clinician waits at the door to receive them). This episode pulls for evidence that the dyad can cooperate together sufficiently to complete a task which most toddlers (and young children) resist. It allows us to observe how the dyad negotiates this stressful situation, how they bargain (if at all) over conflicting agendas, how they express their feelings to one another, and how well they read and respond to one another.

Bubbles

After the container of toys is passed out of the room, the parent is called and instructed to get out the bubbles. The parent blows bubbles and the child is supposed to attempt to "pop" the bubbles. This episode is included as a way of attempting to elicit positive affect between children and parents. Degree of mutual enjoyment, pacing of the activity, turn taking, and so on are all apparent in this episode. Generally, this episode lasts for about 3 minutes.

Teaching Tasks 1–4

A series of four teaching tasks follows. These tasks are chosen a priori for inclusion in the cabinet based on a best guess by the primary clinician of the child's developmental level of functioning. The tasks are selected to move from age level (task 1) to significantly above age level (task 4), so that both the general stress level as well as the child's need to rely on the parent for help increase steadily. The tasks last generally 3 to 5 minutes for younger toddlers and 6 to 8 minutes for older toddlers and preschoolers. Again, the clinician directing the procedure controls when one episode ends and another begins to allow for flexibility in giving extra time (e.g., when the child is about to complete a task) or cutting it short (e.g., if the task is quickly and easily completed by the child).

We are less interested in the child's ability to complete the task than in the child's use of the parent in a stressful and structured activity. Again, how both partners handle transitions, and whether they can have fun in the face of a demanding situation is especially important. The parent's capacity to set limits, provide structure, teach effectively, provide encouragement, and maintain availability and support to the child all are important. The child's capacities for self-regulation, cooperation, showing affection, and learning style also are noted.

Separation

Following the fourth task, the clinician calls and asks the parent to leave the toy cabinet open and to leave the room as she might at home. Parents are given no specific instructions about preparing the child for their departure, and how they do this is considered useful information. Once outside the room, the parent either remains separated from the child for 3 minutes or returns sooner if the infant becomes significantly distressed. Separation provides a way of examining the child's proneness to distress but also specifically activates the young child's attachment system, as has been documented by research on attachment (Ainsworth, Blehar, Waters, & Wall, 1978; Cassidy & Marvin, 1992; Main & Cassidy, 1988).

Reunion

During the reunion, attachment behaviors such as proximity seeking, avoidance, controlling behavior, and clinging are noted, though we do not attempt to classify formally the child's attachment pattern (Boris et al., 1997; Zeanah, Mammen, & Lieberman, 1993). Disorganized attachment behaviors and breakdowns in a child's attachment strategies, as defined by Main and Solomon's (1990) criteria, are noted. The focus is on the dyad's way of reestablishing

contact after a brief separation and the congruence between the preseparation, separation and reunion behavior of the child in relation to the parent.

Summary of Crowell Procedure

The Crowell procedure is a helpful way of isolating the interaction of a particular dyad and attempting to probe many of its dimensions. The ecological validity of clinic-based assessments always should be an open question. Asking parents about the representativeness of the behaviors observed, as well as observing the dyad in more naturalistic settings, may add qualifiers to any conclusions about the interactions observed.

Infants in the First Year

Although the formal Crowell procedure as described earlier is not possible to administer to children less than 1 year of age, many of its components are. Play may be observed, but the emphasis is more on social play in the form of face-to-face interactions (especially for infants in the first 6 months) rather than on object play and mutual pretend play as with older toddlers. Teaching tasks may be used to observe many of the same types of interactions in parents and infants as with parents and toddlers. Different tasks may be selected for younger ages, and observers' expectations about the role of infant behaviors at different ages are considered in evaluating interactive patterns. Other procedures that may be used clinically in the first year are the still-face paradigm (Tronick, Cohn, & Shea, 1985) or structured observations of feeding (see Barnard, 1994).

ASSESSMENT OF PARENT SUBJECTIVE EXPERIENCE

To assess the degree that a particular problematic pattern of interaction is relationship specific, it is necessary to explore the meaning of the observed behaviors, especially from the parent's point of view. This is important because similar-appearing interactive behaviors may convey vastly different meanings in one or another dyad (Zeanah & Barton, 1989). Inquiring about the meaning of particular patterns of behavior to the parent may be accomplished in different ways at different points in the overall assessment. Linking this inquiry to observations from the outset is often informative (Hirshberg, 1993; Lieberman & Pawl, 1993). Alternatively, similar interchanges may come about during later review of videotapes of particular interactive sequences (McDonough, 1993), or they may be inquired about through systematic interviewing about a parent's perceptions of the infant (Zeanah & Benoit, 1995).

As with interactions, clinicians will observe many parental perceptions and attributions of the child expressed formally in response to query and informally in a variety of settings during the assessment. We regard all these potentially useful sources of data for the clinical task. Nevertheless, routinely we use a semistructured interview, the Working Model of the Child Interview (WMCI; Zeanah & Benoit, 1995), as a way of systematically examining and characterizing this component of the relationship.

Working Model of the Child Interview

The WMCI is an interview, typically administered and videotaped in the clinic, which we have found to be a useful way of eliciting the parent's story of the infant and the parent's relationship with the infant. Indeed, devoting an hour or more to this story in and of itself sends a message to the parent about the importance of the infant and the importance of the parent's thoughts and feelings about the infant. For this reason, the interviewer does not interrupt the story except to obtain clarifications or to probe further. The interviewer does not attempt to rephrase what a parent says or to make links between different thoughts or feelings that the parent expresses. At a later time, of course, the videotaped interview may be reviewed with the parent and further exploration of the attributions or stories may be pursued at that time.

The WMCI has been used in a number of investigations of infants and parents, and a formal scoring system exists. Nevertheless, when used for purposes of clinical assessment of the parent's representation of a child, the formal scoring system is not really necessary. Clinicians are encouraged to review the tape and to note the content and formal narrative features that seem clinically meaningful.

The interview requires roughly 1 hour of time, and we recommend videotaping it for later review. The interview begins with a developmental history of the infant and the parent's relationship with the infant. In contrast with the traditional history, however, the emphasis here is on the parent's experience of the child rather than on the details of what the child did or did not do at a given time. After this story of the baby is elicited, beginning with prepregnancy thoughts about the idea of children and continuing up through the present, a number of other specific questions are pursued. These include descriptions of the child's personality, of whom the child reminds the parent, how the child is like and unlike each parent, and what the child's behavior is like in general and in specific situations. We inquire about instances in which the child is upset or displays difficult behavior, and we pay careful attention to the feelings and thoughts elicited in the parent at these times. Parents describe their relationship with the child, what pleases or displeases them about that, and what they might change if they could. Parents also describe their anticipations about the child's future development and their hopes and fears about it.

Elsewhere, we have described in some detail the use of this measure in clinical settings (Zeanah & Benoit, 1995). Here, we review briefly some of the features of the measure that seem especially salient to infant–parent relationship assessment. We listen carefully for consistent themes of content in the interview. Nevertheless, the major areas that are important in our work beyond the content of the interview material are its narrative features, affective tones, and narrative organization, all of which we infer to be meaningful characteristics of the parent's representation of the child.

Narrative Features

We consider eight narrative features to be useful clinical indices to the nature of the parent's representation of the child: richness of perceptions, openness to change, coherence, intensity of involvement, caregiving sensitivity, acceptance/rejection, infant difficulty, and fear of loss. In keeping with the contemporary work on representations pioneered by Main et al. (1985), we attend not only to content but also to content-free aspects of the descriptions.

Richness of perceptions describes the relative richness or poverty of detail about the parent's description of the infant as an individual. Rather than the amount that a parent says about an infant, this feature refers to the way that the details are used to describe a clear sense of who the baby is. Succinct but vivid descriptions may be richer than lengthy descriptions that are unclear, inconsistent, or digressions from the topic of the child.

The degree to which the parent's narrative seems open to accommodate new information or insights about the child is regarded as its *openness to change* or flexibility. It is important to emphasize that openness to change is the opposite of rigidity as opposed to uncertainty. That is, narratives about the infant may be certain but still open to accommodate new information or insights.

The *coherence* of the narrative was highlighted by Main and her colleagues (Main et al., 1985) as a central feature of scoring the Adult Attachment Interview (George, Kaplan, & Main, 1984). We have also found this feature to be an extremely useful way of listening to the parent's story of the child. The clarity, consistency, and believability of the narrative all are elements of its coherence.

We attempt to understand also the *intensity of involvement* of the parent with the infant and the degree of the parent's psychological immersion in the relationship with the infant. Here, we are interested in the degree of psychological preoccupation with the infant, ranging from hardly noticing the infant to being so preoccupied that the parent thinks of little else.

We are interested in the degree to which parents accept the child as is versus the degree to which they reject the child or some aspect of the child's personality or behavior. In extreme cases, parents may even express an aversion to the infant, although this usually comes up indirectly. *Acceptance* by the parent also requires appreciating the sometimes delicate balance between the intense dependence of an infant or young child, on the one hand, and the ubiquitous pressure of development moving the child toward greater independence, on the other.

Another feature of importance is the degree to which the parent appreciates the child's own perspective. *Caregiving sensitivity* means appreciating the child as a unique individual and involves understanding, accepting, and even valuing the infant's needs and experiences, especially in the emotional realm. This requires, of course, being able to respond sensitively to infants' changing developmental needs over the course of the first several years of life, as well as recognizing the individuality and unique needs of the infant.

The parent's subjective responses to an *infant's degree of difficulty* or burdensomeness also is important. Although the clinician inevitably compares his or her perceptions of the infant to those of the parent, here we are concerned primarily with the parent's subjective experience of the infant's difficult behavior. Therefore, how well the parent is able to maintain a protective envelope around the infant and to modulate negative dispositional attributions also is important.

Finally, we attend carefully to any suggestions of an irrational *fear of loss* of the infant or young child. Following Main and Goldwyn (1991), excessive fears in the parent for the safety of the child or irrational fears of losing the child that are not consciously connected to their source appear to have important implications for the relationship and for the infant.

Affective Tones

A number of affective tones of the narrative are possible to note. Generally only one to three tones are prominent in a particular narrative. That is, a parent may become angry at some point in the interview, but for anger to reach the level of an overall affective tone of the narrative it would have to be prominent enough to be thematic. This feature of the narrative is usually best appreciated from consideration of the entire interview, and review of the interview through videotape may be helpful with this determination.

Narrative Organization or Classification

For research purposes, we have developed a typology of narrative organizations or classifications that are somewhat analogous to the Strange Situation (Ainsworth et al., 1978) and the Adult Attachment Interview (Main & Goldwyn, 1991) classifications. We do not recommend attempting to determine the formal classification of the representation when using the interview as part of a clinical assessment. Nevertheless, we present a brief description of each of the classifications because some of their features may be important clinically.

Narratives about the infant and the parent's relationship with the infant that are clear and straightforward, that convey a reasonably detailed sense of the infant as a unique individual, and that demonstrate an empathic appreciation for the infant's experience are classified as *balanced*. Usually, parents convey a sense of meaningful involvement with the child and a belief that their relationship with the child is important for the child's development. Joy and pride are the most common overall affective tones of these interviews.

Narratives that convey an emotional distance or coolness toward the infant and in which the infant is described in rather generic terms are likely to be classified as *disengaged*. Parents seem psychologically much less involved with the infant than in the balanced type, and indifference is likely to be a prominent emotional tone.

Other narratives, classified as *distorted*, are confused, inconsistent, or unrealistic. Parents seem to be struggling unsuccessfully to feel close to their infants but for one of several reasons do not. They may be preoccupied by other concerns and not know the infant as an individual, they may be self-preoccupied and unable to appreciate the infant as a distinct individual, they may look to the infant for developmentally inappropriate care and comfort, or they may find the infant confusing and bewildering. Sometimes, a combination of these distortions is present.

These WMCI classifications have been demonstrated to be associated with infant attachment classifications (Zeanah, Benoit, Hirschberg, Barton, & Kegan, 1994; Benoit, Parker, & Zeanah, 1997) and with mother and child interactive behavior (Zeanah et al., 1998). In fact, even when mothers described the baby they expected during pregnancy, classification of their narratives was strongly predictive of their infant's attachment to them more than 1 year later (Benoit, Parker, & Zeanah, 1997).

Summary of the WMCI

After completion of the interview, the clinician may profit from detailed review of the videotape. Important issues are the narrative features and affective tone of the representation and how they are organized. At times, it is useful to review the videotape with the parent for purposes of further exploration, or to highlight features of the infant–parent relationship as part of therapeutic intervention.

LEVEL OF RELATIONSHIP ADAPTATION/DISTURBANCE

Having assessed each component of the infant–parent relationship, the final step is to de-termine a level of relationship adaptation/disturbance for the dyad. The Parent–Infant Relationship Global Assessment Scale (PIRGAS; Zero to Three, 1994) provides a continuously distributed scale of infant–parent relationship functioning, ranging from "well adapted" to "dangerously impaired." This measure was derived from the model of relationship disturbances described by Anders (1989), which includes relationship perturbations, disturbances, and disorders. Because it covers the full range of relationship adaptation, it is intended to be used in a variety of settings, ranging from infant mental health programs and clinics to early education and child-care settings and to pediatric clinics of all types. As such, it is included in the *DC: 0–3* manual (Zero to Three, 1994) as an aid in the Axis II diagnosis of relationship disorders.

Preliminary validity data for the PIRGAS are accumulating. For example, Papousek and von Hofacker (1998) found that PIRGAS scores derived from observations of mother–infant interactions were lower in infants with regulatory difficulties than in those without such difficulties. PIRGAS scores in that study also were associated with maternal psychopathology and cumulative family risk scores. Boris, Zeanah, Larrieu, Scheeringa, and Heller (1998) found that clinic-referred toddlers diagnosed with attachment disorders had PIRGAS scores that were significantly lower than clinic-referred toddlers diagnosed with other disorders. Further, Aoki, Ruggieri, Bakshi, and Zeanah (1997) found that PIRGAS scores obtained from ratings of 10 minutes of laboratory-based free play between mothers and their 20-month-old infants were predictive of both interactive behavior and internalizing symptomatology in the infants at age 24 months. These data suggest that PIRGAS scores are lawfully related to infant and maternal behavior.

CONCLUSIONS

We have presented one approach to infant–parent relationship assessment based on a model that includes both interactive and subjective components of the relationship. To conclude, we emphasize that infant–parent relationships are wholes that cannot be reduced to the sum of characteristics of the partners (Sroufe & Fleeson, 1988). Individual characteristics of the partners derive their importance from their impact on the infant–parent relationship. Further, the components of the relationship, as we envision them, are relational rather than individual characteristics. Therefore, infants are assumed to be "oppositional" and parents to be "controlling" only with regard to the relationship in which these patterns are observed. We make no assumptions about the generalizability of interactive or representational patterns to other contemporaneous relationships, although in keeping with contemporary research findings, we believe that early relationship experiences are predictive of subsequent psychological adaptation in the child (Main et al., 1985; Suess, Grossmann, & Sroufe, 1992).

If we are correct that infant–parent relationships ought to be a central focus for assessment in infant mental health, we can anticipate the emergence of other methods of assessment that share broadly our underlying assumptions but with different approaches to content or process. Ideally, these efforts ultimately will lead to more effective interventions with infants and parents at risk for adverse outcomes.

ACKNOWLEDGMENT

This chapter was adapted from Zeanah et al. (1997). Copyright 1997 by Michigan Association for Infant Mental Health.

REFERENCES

Ainsworth, M. D. S., Blehar, M., Waters, E., & Wall, S. (1978). *Patterns of attachment: A psychological study of the strange situation*. Hillsdale, NJ: Erlbaum.

Anders, T. F. (1978). States and rhythmic processes. *Journal of the American Academy of Child Psychiatry, 17*, 401–420.

Anders, T. F. (1989). Clinical syndromes, relationship disturbances and their assessment. In A. J. Sameroff & R. N. Emde (Eds.), *Relationship disturbances in early childhood* (pp. 125–144). New York: Basic Books.

Aoki, Y., Ruggieri, C., Bakshi, S., & Zeanah, C. (1997, October). *Attachment and affiliation: Motivational systems in high-risk toddlers*. Paper presented at the annual meeting of the American Academy of Child and Adolescent Psychiatry, Toronto, Ontario, Canada.

Barnard, K. (1994). Feeding and teaching scales. In *Nursing child assessment satellite training program*. Seattle: University of Washington.

Benoit, D., & Parker, K. (1994). Stability and transmission of attachment across three generations. *Child Development, 65*, 1444–1457.

Benoit, D., Parker, K., & Zeanah, C. H. (1997). Mothers' representations of their infants assessed prenatally: Stability and association with infants' attachment

classifications. *Journal of Child Psychology, Psychiatry and Allied Disciplines, 38*, 307–313.

Boris, N. W., Fueyo, M., & Zeanah, C. H. (1997). Clinical assessment of attachment in the first five years of life. *Journal of the American Academy of Child and Adolescent Psychiatry, 36*, 291–293.

Boris, N., Zeanah, C. H., Larrieu, J., Scheeringa, M, & Heller, S. (1998). Attachment disorders in infancy and early childhood: A preliminary study of diagnostic criteria. *American Journal of Psychiatry, 155*, 295–297.

Carter, S. L., Osofsky, J., & Hann, D. (1991). Speaking for the baby: A therapeutic intervention for adolescent mothers and their infants. *Infant Mental Health Journal, 12*, 291–301.

Cassidy, J., & Marvin, R., with the Attachment Working Group of the John D. and Catherine T. MacArthur Foundation Network on Transition from Infancy to Early Childhood. (1992). *Attachment organization in preschool children: Procedure and coding manual*. Unpublished manual.

Clark, R., Paulson, A., & Conlin, S. (1993). Assessment of developmental status and parent–infant relationships: The therapeutic process of evaluation. In C. H. Zeanah, Jr. (Ed.), *Handbook of infant mental health* (pp. 191–209). New York: Guilford Press.

Cramer, B. (1987). Objective and subjective aspects of parent–infant relations: An attempt at correlation between infant studies and clinical work. In J. Osofsky (Ed.), *Handbook of infant development* (pp. 1037–1057). New York: Wiley.

Cramer, B., & Stern, D. N. (1988). Evaluation of changes in mother–infant brief psychotherapy: A single case study. *Infant Mental Health Journal, 9*, 20–45.

Crockenberg, S., Lyons-Ruth, K., & Dickstein, S. (1993). The family context of infant mental health: II. Infant development in multiple family relationships. In C. H. Zeanah, Jr. (Ed.), *Handbook of infant mental health* (pp. 38–55). New York: Guilford Press.

Crowell, J., & Feldman, S. (1988). The effects of mothers' internal working models of relationships and children's behavioral and developmental status on mother–child interaction. *Child Development, 59*, 1273–1285.

Crowell, J., & Feldman, S. (1991). Mothers' working models of attachment relationships and mother and child behavior during separation and reunion. *Developmental Psychology, 27*, 597–605.

Crowell, J., Feldman, S., & Ginsburg, N. (1988). Assessment of mother–child interaction in preschoolers with behavior problems. *Journal of the American Academy of Child and Adolescent Psychiatry, 27*, 303–311.

Crowell, J. A., & Fleischmann, M. A. (1993). Use of structured research procedures in clinical assessments of infants. In C. H. Zeanah, Jr. (Ed.), *Handbook of infant mental health* (pp. 210–221). New York: Guilford Press.

Emde, R. N. (1989). The infant's relationship experience: Developmental and clinical aspects. In A. J. Sameroff & R. N. Emde (Eds.), *Relationship disturbances in early childhood* (pp. 33–51). New York: Basic Books.

Emde, R. N. (1991). The wonder of our complex enterprise: Steps enabled by attachment and the effects of relationships on relationships. *Infant Mental Health Journal, 12,* 164–173.

Escalona, S. (1967). Patterns of infantile experience and the developmental process. *The Psychoanalytic Study of the Child, 22,* 197–244.

Fraiberg, S. (1980). *Clinical studies in infant mental health: The first year of life.* New York: Basic Books.

Freud, A. (1963). The concept of developmental lines. *The Psychoanalytic Study of the Child, 5,* 7–17.

Garcia-Coll, C. T., & Meyer, E. C. (1993). The sociocultural context of infant development. In C. H. Zeanah, Jr. (Ed.), *Handbook of infant mental health* (pp. 56–69). New York: Guilford Press.

George, C., Kaplan, N., & Main, M. (1984). *Adult attachment interview.* Unpublished manuscript, University of California at Berkeley.

Hirshberg, L. M. (1993). Clinical interviews with infants and their families. In C. H. Zeanah, Jr. (Ed.), *Handbook of infant mental health* (pp. 173–190). New York: Guilford Press.

Larrieu, J., & Zeanah, C. H. (1998). An intensive intervention for infants and toddlers in foster care. In K. Pruett & M. Pruett (Eds.), *Custody: Child and adolescent psychiatric clinics of North America* (pp. 357–371). Philadelphia: W. B. Saunders.

Lieberman, A. F. (1993). *The emotional life of the toddler.* New York: Free Press.

Lieberman, A. F., & Pawl, J. H. (1988). Clinical applications of attachment theory. In J. Belsky & T. Nezworski (Eds.), *Clinical implications of attachment* (pp. 327–351). Hillsdale, NJ: Erlbaum.

Lieberman, A. F., & Pawl, J. H. (1993). Infant–parent psychotherapy. In C. H. Zeanah, Jr. (Ed.), *Handbook of infant mental health* (pp. 427–442). New York: Guilford Press.

Main, M., & Cassidy, J. (1988). Categories of response to reunion with the parent at age 6: Predictable from infant attachment classifications and stable over a 1-month period. *Developmental Psychology, 24,* 415–426.

Main, M., & Goldwyn, R. (1991). *Adult attachment classification system.* Unpublished manuscript, University of California at Berkeley.

Main, M., Kaplan, N., & Cassidy, J. (1985). Security in infancy, childhood and adulthood: A move to the level of representation. *Monographs of the Society for Research in Child Development, 50*(Serial No. 209), 66–106.

Main, M., & Solomon, J. (1990). Procedures for identifying infants classified as disorganized/disoriented during the Ainsworth Strange Situation. In M. T. Greenburg, D. Cicchetti, & E. M. Cummings (Eds.), *Attachment in the preschool years* (pp. 121–160). Chicago: University of Chicago Press.

Matas, L., Arend, R. A., & Sroufe, L. A. (1978). Continuity of adaptation in the second year: the relationship between quality of attachment and later competence. *Child Development, 49,* 547–556.

McDonough, S. C. (1993). Interaction guidance: Understanding and treating early infant–caregiver relationship disturbances. In C. H. Zeanah, Jr. (Ed.), *Handbook of infant mental health* (pp. 414–426). New York: Guilford Press.

Papousek, M., & von Hofacker, N. (1998). Persistant crying in early infancy: A non-typical condition of risk for the developing mother–infant relationship. *Child Care and Health Development, 24,* 395–424.

Plomin, R. (1995). Genetics and children's experiences in the family. *Journal of Child Psychology, Psychiatry and Allied Disciplines, 36,* 33–68.

Sameroff, A. J. (1997). Understanding the social context of psychopathology in early childhood. In J. Noshpitz (Ed.), *Handbook of child and adolescent psychiatry* (pp. 224–236). New York: Basic Books.

Sameroff, A. J., & Emde, R. N. (Eds.). (1989). *Relationship disturbances in early childhood.* New York: Basic Books.

Seligman, S. (1991). Conceptual and methodological issues in the study of internal representation: A commentary on *Infant Mental Health Journal, Volume 10. 3. Infant Mental Health Journal, 12,* 126–129.

Sroufe, L. A. (1988). The role of infant–caregiver attachment in development. In J. Belsky & T. Nezworski (Eds.), *Clinical implications of attachment* (pp. 18–40). Hillsdale, NJ: Erlbaum.

Sroufe, L. A. (1989). Relationships, self and individual adaptation. In A. J. Sameroff & R. N. Emde (Eds.), *Relationship disturbances in early childhood* (pp. 70–94). New York: Basic Books.

Sroufe, L. A., & Fleeson, J. (1988). The coherence of family relationships. In R. Hinde & J. Stevenson-Hinde (Eds.), *Relationships within families: Mutual influences* (pp. 27–47). New York: Oxford University Press.

Steele, H., Steele, M., & Fonagy, P. (1996). Associations among attachment classifications of mothers, fathers and their infants: Evidence for a relationship-specific perspective. *Child Development, 67,* 541–555.

Stern, D. N. (1985). *The interpersonal world of the infant: Views from psychoanalysis and developmental psychology.* New York: Basic Books.

Stern, D. N. (1991). Maternal representations: A clinical and subjective phenomenological view. *Infant Mental Health Journal, 12,* 174–186.

Stern, D. N. (1995). *The motherhood constellation.* New York: Basic Books.

Stern-Brushweiler, N., & Stern, D. N. (1989). A model for conceptualizing the role of the mother's representational world in various mother–infant therapies. *Infant Mental Health Journal, 10,* 142–156.

Suess, G. J., Grossmann, K. E., & Sroufe, L. A. (1992). Effects of infant attachment to mother and father on quality of adaptation in preschool: From dyadic to individual organization of self. *International Journal of Behavioral Development, 15,* 43–65.

Tronick, E. Z., Cohn, J., & Shea, E. (1985). The transfer of affect between mothers and infants. In T. B. Brazelton & M. Yogman (Eds.), *Affective development in infancy* (pp. 11–25). Norwood, NJ: Ablex.

Valliere, J. (1994). Infant mental health: A consultation and treatment team for at-risk infants and toddlers. *Infants and Young Children, 6,* 46–53.

van IJzendoorn, M. (1995). Adult attachment representations, parental responsiveness, and infant attachment: A meta-analysis on the predictive validity of the adult attachment interview. *Psychological Bulletin, 117,* 387–403.

Zeanah, C. H. (1993). Subjectivity in infant–parent relationships: Contributions from attachment research. *Adolescent Psychiatry, 19*, 121–136.

Zeanah, C. H. (1998). Reflections on the strengths perspective. *The Signal, 6*, 11–12.

Zeanah C. H., & Anders T. F. (1987). Subjectivity in parent–infant relationships: A discussion of internal working models. *Infant Mental Health Journal, 8*, 237–250.

Zeanah, C. H., Aoki, Y., & Heller, S. S. (1998, October). *Relationship specificity in foster and birth parents' relationships with their children.* Paper presented at the annual meeting of the American Academy of Child and Adolescent Psychiatry, Anaheim, CA.

Zeanah C. H., & Barton M. L. (1989). Internal representations and parent–infant relationships. *Infant Mental Health Journal, 10*, 135–141.

Zeanah C. H., & Barton M. L. (1991). Representing the internal world. *Infant Mental Health Journal, 12*, 130–133.

Zeanah, C. H., & Benoit, D. (1995). Clinical applications of a parent perception interview. In K. Minde (Ed.), *Infant psychiatry: Child psychiatric clinics of North America* (pp. 539–554). Philadelphia: W. B. Saunders.

Zeanah, C. H., Benoit, D., Hirshberg, L., Barton, M. L., & Regan, C. (1994). Mothers' representations of their infants are concordant with infant attachment classifications. *Developmental Issues in Psychiatry and Psychology, 1*, 9–18.

Zeanah, C. H., Boris, N. W., Heller, S. S., Hinshaw-Fuselier, S., Larrieu, J., Lewis, M., Palomino, R., Rovaris, M., & Valliere, J. (1997). Relationship assessment in infant mental health. *Infant Mental Health Journal, 18*, 182–197.

Zeanah, C. H., Boris, N. W., & Scheeringa, M. S. (1996). Infant development: The first three years of life. In A. Tasman, J. Kay, & J. Lieberman (Eds.), *Psychiatry* (pp. 75–100). Philadelphia: W. B. Saunders.

Zeanah, C. H. Jr., Mammen, O. K., & Lieberman, A. F. (1993). Disorders of attachment. In C. H. Zeanah, Jr. (Ed.), *Handbook of infant mental health* (pp. 332–349). New York: Guilford Press.

Zero to Three, National Center for Clinical Infant Programs. (1994). *Diagnostic classification: 0–3 Diagnostic classification of mental health and developmental disorders of infancy and early childhood: 0–3.* Arlington, VA: Author.

14

Developmental Assessment of Infants and Toddlers

❖

WALTER S. GILLIAM
LINDA C. MAYES

The developmental evaluation of infants and toddlers should involve more than the simple administration of a set of developmental test protocols. Assessments performed in the first 3 years of life require the clinician to synthesize information gathered from parents, other relatives, and other professionals with data gathered through direct assessment and observation of the child. The full developmental assessment also requires observations from many different frames of reference. These include the child's responses to specific tasks included in the developmental protocols, how the child uses the developmental materials in "nonstandardized" but, nonetheless, individually informative ways, and inferences from spontaneous behavior during solitary play or interactions with parents. Whereas all thorough psychological assessments ideally require a synthesis of observations from both structured and nonstructured situations, the assessment of very young children demands this kind of scientist/clinician mix even more. All assessments of infants and toddlers are framed by the context of rapidly changing, growing systems that may be in or out of synchrony with one another. Infants and toddlers are preverbal or just beginning to use language, and their performance and comfort in a new situation are dependent on the presence of their parents or close guardians. Also, many of the most critical and informative developmental capacities, such as emerging language skills, are often more evident at home with familiar people

and may not be directly available to the clinician during a "formal assessment."

This chapter covers the following areas:

1. The importance of integrating information from a structured assessment with interviews and behavioral observations to help ensure a more complete developmental evaluation;
2. Considerations for selecting developmental assessment tools; and
3. A review of available developmental tests, including their strengths and limitations.

INTEGRATION OF INFORMATION FROM MULTIPLE SOURCES

In this section, we address the clinical aspects of an infant assessment (Mayes, 1991): how to augment the information gained from a structured developmental assessment with material from interviews with parents and behavioral observations. Clinicians evaluating infants and toddlers often need to synthesize knowledge from child psychiatry, pediatrics, neurology, developmental psychology, genetics, physical and occupational therapy, and speech/language therapy (Mayes & Gilliam, 1999). In addition, clinicians evaluating young children also need to know about early educational programs and laws about child abuse and neglect. Knowledge from these diverse fields allows a clinician to place the results of a developmental assessment

236

in a meaningful context for the individual child. For example, understanding the physiological effects of prolonged malnutrition helps the clinician evaluate the relatively pronounced gross motor delays of a child with failure to thrive who has no other neurological signs. Similarly, understanding the effects of a parent's affective disorder on a child's responsiveness to the external world adds another dimension to the clinician's understanding of that infant's muted or absent social interactiveness, babbling, and smiling.

Interviewing

Accomplished interviewing is central to a complete developmental assessment, because much of the information about infants' and toddlers' daily functioning and their relationship with their caregivers comes from interviews. Skillful interviewing techniques include allowing caregivers to begin their story wherever they choose; using directed, information-gathering questions in such a way as to clarify but not disrupt the caregivers' account; and listening for affect as well as content. Importantly, nearly every step of the assessment process requires an alliance between clinician and caregiver, because infants usually perform better when they are in the company of familiar adults, and the initial interview is crucial in setting the tone for such an alliance. Assessments of young children are quite compromised when there are no familiar adults available to meet with the clinician and be with the infant. Unfortunately, it is often in cases involving the most severe environmental disturbance that clinicians do not have caregivers available to describe the child's history.

When caregivers are available, skillful interviewing also is critical in helping caregivers follow through with the assessment process. Coming for a developmental evaluation or participating in one while their child is hospitalized is enormously stressful and often frightening for parents. Clinicians working with young children and their families need to recognize that regardless of what parents have been told about the assessment, parents' fears and fantasies about the process may be as potent as the facts of the presenting problem. Not uncommonly, parents have started to see their child as damaged or flawed in some way and are afraid and guilty about the effect of their own behavior on their child. They may express their fears of what the infant's problems signify in many ways. They may anticipate that their infant is developmentally retarded or will have serious emotional difficulties in school, or that they will be, or already are, inadequate parents. Evaluations are always a vulnerable time for parents, and clinicians should keep in mind that what seem inconsequential moments and statements to clinicians may be memorable and powerful for parents.

Furthermore, the stress of coming for an assessment affects the parents' abilities to report about the infant's development. When first interviewed, parents may be reluctant to be candid or may not themselves be fully aware of their own perceptions and beliefs about their child. Open-ended questions, allowing parents to begin their story wherever they feel most comfortable, and conveying a nonjudgmental attitude are crucial beginning points in establishing the working alliance with the parents.

Practically, the purpose of interviews with caregivers is to gather information about the infant. The important areas to cover in terms of the child's development are the medical history and major developmental milestones; the history of the mother's pregnancy, delivery, and immediate perinatal period; the number, ages, and health of family members; and how the infant fits in the family's daily life. Also, the meaning of the individual child for both parents may be an important window on the child's place in the family.

Specifically, the interviewer should develop a picture of the parents' perceptions of the child's level of functioning in several areas. These areas include motor development and activity level, speech and communication, problem-solving and play, self-regulation (e.g., ease of comforting and need for routines), relationships with others, and level of social responsiveness. Questions about whether the pregnancy was planned or came at a good time for the family and what expectations the parents had for the infant provide important information about perceptions, anticipations, disappointments, and stresses. Similarly, at some point, asking the parents whom the infant reminds them of or what traits they like best and least may be useful avenues for learning about how the parents view both the infant's difficulties and place within their family. The sessions with the child also provide an opportunity to gather more interview information, as other questions will occur in the context of the child's behavior and performance. For example, asking whether the child's response to a particular situation in the evaluation context is usual for him or her may open up another area of information from the parents.

Clinicians must sometimes conduct evaluations under less than ideal conditions. At times, the evaluation must be completed in one session; the clinician may have limited access to the child or no caregivers may be available. Situations of severe abuse, abandonment, multiple placements, or seriously ill parents are examples of times at which the clinician will not have access to critical sources of information. As in situations in which the time for the evaluation is brief, it is important for clinicians to be clear about the limitations of the evaluation and to place a "clinical confidence interval" around the findings from the structured assessment.

Observing

Every developmental evaluation must include descriptions of behavior and the qualitative aspects of the child's behavior in the structured setting. For example, how an infant responds to developmental tasks (e.g., with excitement, positive affect, and energy vs. slowly, deliberately, and with little affective response) is as important as the age appropriateness of the infant's response. Such qualitative observations are often the best descriptors of those capacities for which there are few standardized assessment techniques but which are fundamental for fueling the development of motor, language, and problem-solving skills. Through observing how infants and toddlers do what they do, the clinician gains information about how the infant copes with frustration and engages with the adult world, as well as his or her range of emotional expressiveness and capacity for persistence and sustained attention.

Observation is the fundamental skill needed for measuring infants' development. What distinguishes the observational skill necessary for developmental assessment from other diagnostic evaluations is that it occurs on many levels simultaneously. The observational skills basic to evaluations of younger children require a blend of free-floating attention bounded by the structure of the formal assessment. In other words, the clinician must be comfortable enough in the setting to attend to whatever occurs, but he or she must also have a mental framework by which to organize the observations collected during the session. Such a framework entails at least four broad areas: (1) predominant affective tone of the participants, (2) involvement in the situation (curiosity and interest), (3) use of others (child's use of the parents or examiner, or parents' of examiner), and (4) reactions to transitions (initial meetings, end of sessions, changes in amount of structure).

Using this framework, the clinician makes observations continuously on at least three levels. Perhaps the most obvious level is the observations of how the child responds to the structured assessment items administered during formal testing. Observations during formal testing should not be confined solely to whether the child passes or fails a given item but also to how the child approaches the task. The second level of observation is how the child reacts to the situation apart from the formal testing structure. Does the child approach toys, initiate interactions, or refer to the examiner or his parents? How does the child react in the beginning of the evaluation and later when the situation and the examiner are more familiar? The third observational level is a specific focus on the interactions between parent and infant. The clinician makes these observations throughout the evaluation process and revises his or her hypotheses as both parent and infant become familiar with the process.

Interpreting the behaviors one observes between parent and child in terms of their ongoing relationship partially requires experience and also time to gather many observational points. However, several general areas may provide important descriptive clues. Does the child refer to the parent for both help and reassurance? Similarly, does the child show his or her successes to the parent, and does the parent respond? Another important observation for toddlers is whether or not the child leaves his parent's immediate company to work with items or explore. For infants, how parents hold and soothe their baby may be a window to the relationship between the two. A caregiver participates with his or her child during structured testing situations in varying ways, and the clinician must judge continuously how intrusively involved, withdrawn, or comfortably facilitative a caregiver is. Adults may appear very different as individuals in their own right compared to when they are interacting with their children, and the very act of having one's child (and by implication, one's self) observed by another is anxiety provoking in varying degrees for all caregivers.

Synthesizing and Reporting Findings

The process of synthesizing all the data gathered from the different sources during a developmental assessment is a technique and skill unto itself. Moreover, how this synthesis, with its attendant recommendations, is conveyed to parents (and consultants) is another essential step in the assessment process, and the assessment is not complete until clinicians have worked with parents to help them understand the assessment findings. Also, assessments of young children often involve referring pediatricians and other clinicians, who need to be included individually in the clinician's data-gathering interviews and in the final synthesis of findings.

The synthesis of information from an infant assessment differs from the synthesis involved in other medical diagnostic processes in that there are few specific diagnostic categories that encapsulate all the findings of an assessment of a young child. Assigning a "mental age" or developmental quotient is often the least important goal of the assessment. The synthesis in an assessment of a young child involves bringing together all the data gathered from interviews, observations, and testing into a qualitative and quantitative description of the child's capacities in different functional areas (motor, problem-solving, language and communication, and social) and of the child's current strengths and weaknesses. It involves integrating the assessment information in the context of the child's individual environment. For example, an infant who has experienced multiple foster placements may be socially delayed, but such a finding assumes a different significance for a young child from a stable home environment.

Finally, it is often during the synthesis process that the assessment's therapeutic impact for the parents seems most evident. At the very least, parents often begin to revise or change their perceptions of their child's capacities. They may see strengths in their child they had not previously recognized or become deeply and painfully aware of weaknesses and vulnerabilities that they may or may not have feared before the assessment. Any of these changes in perceptions will affect the parents' view of themselves and of their role as parents. Emphasizing the potentially therapeutic value of an assessment with a young child underscores that the synthesis process is not simply wrapping up the assessment and conveying information but also a time to explore with the parents the meaning of the process for them.

CONSIDERATIONS FOR SELECTING A DEVELOPMENTAL TEST

Some considerations are presented in order to offer basic guidelines for choosing an infant developmental test that best meets the user's specific needs and to provide a framework for presenting some of the various tests currently in use. Four areas of consideration are presented: purpose, sources of data, standardization, and reliability and validity.

Purpose

Developmental testing may accomplish one or more of several different purposes: diagnostic, screening, and intervention planning. Tests designed for these three different purposes typically are quite different, and selecting the correct tests to match the stated purpose is essential. First, testing may be used to provide important information necessary for diagnostic purposes, either clinically or eligibility oriented. Clinically oriented diagnoses are used by clinicians to capture succinctly the infant's overall presentation and to provide a common nomenclature for communicating that information to other clinicians. Eligibility-oriented diagnoses, however, are quite different. Most programs that provide early intervention services, particularly in the public sector, prescribe certain criteria for eligibility. Often the infant must demonstrate a particular degree of developmental delay (e.g., performance that is two standard deviations below the mean) to "qualify" for services. Second, screening tests may be used when it is desirable to use a relatively brief instrument to identify infants who may be "at risk" for delayed development and would benefit from further diagnostic testing. Usually screening tests are used when relatively many children need to be assessed and a full diagnostic assessment for all children would be too costly or cumbersome. Third, additional testing for identified children may be used to plan an individualized early intervention program, by identifying important programmatic goals and objectives or to track an infant's achievement of these goals over time in order to document the effects of the program.

Sources of Data

All tests, including developmental assessment instruments, are methods of collecting and organizing data. Developmental tests for infants may use at least three different types of data: direct assessment, observational, and caregiver report. Indeed, many developmental tests use some combination of all three of these types of data. Some, however, use data from only one source. Each source of data has its own strengths and limitations. For instance, direct assessment has the strength of being potentially standard in its presentation, so that an infant's performance may be directly compared to other infants with the assumption that the material was presented in a similar standard method. The limitation of direct assessment, however, is that it represents only a small slice of the infant's life that will be influenced greatly by current issues regarding the infant's motivation, mood, comfort, and responsiveness to the examiner and the evaluative process. Although parent report surveys may be useful for screening purposes, to document behaviors that occur infrequently or are difficult to elicit in a structured assessment, to assess parents' perspectives of their children, or as a method of follow-up, one must be cautious in their interpretation (Meisels & Waskik, 1990) as caregiver reports are understandably biased by the caregiver's perceptions and feelings regarding the infant. For this reason, the results of assessment instruments that rely exclusively on caregiver report may be interpreted best as representing the caregiver's *perspective* of the infant's development or behavior, which may or may not be also indicative of the infant's actual developmental status. Given the strengths and limitations of each of these types of data, a comprehensive assessment should use multiple sources of data from multiple informants and contexts.

Standardization

Test standardization involves the process of collecting normative data regarding children's typical performance on the test. By using this normative data, experienced evaluators can determine a specific infant's standing relative to the normative group. This relative standing can be expressed in terms of percentile ranks, standard scores (typically expressed with a mean of 100 and a standard deviation of 15), or any of a number of other score systems. These standardized scores are often used with other information to determine the extent of any developmental delays and to decide whether early intervention services (in the case of a diagnostic test) or further assessment (in the case of a screening test) is warranted.

Test users, however, must decide whether a given test's standardization sample is representative of the type of infants the test user plans to assess. For instance, it clearly would be inappropriate to compare the developmental performance of an infant raised in a large city in a highly developed nation to a normative sample of infants living in a small village in a less developed nation, unless one knew a priori that infants from both of these settings scored similarly on the test. Most decisions regarding the representativeness of a test's standardization are not this apparent, however. Also, test users must realize that standardized scores are norm-sample dependent. Therefore, standard scores from a nationally standardized test indicate an infant's standing relative to other infants throughout that nation and not necessarily to other infants of the same specific locality, gender, ethnicity, or economic status. Some tests are normed on specific populations of children, such as children from a specific city or state or a particular economic status. The use of standard scores derived from these tests with infants from other localities or economic backgrounds, without specific empirical evidence to justify their generalization, may produce questionable results and is, therefore, generally not recommended.

In addition to representativeness, normative data should also be relatively recent. Research has indicated that since the 1930s, Americans have been scoring higher on IQ tests at a rate of about 3 standard score points per decade (Flynn, 1984). The Flynn Effect highlights the importance of periodic revision of normative data. For example, comparing a person's score on a test to normative data derived 10 years previous may result in a standard score that overestimates the person's true standing by about 3 points. Likewise, 20-year-old data may result in a 6-point overestimation, 30-year-old data may result in a 9-point overestimation, and so forth. Though these findings were documented for IQ tests, the effect may also be true for developmental tests. Such overestimation may lead to disqualifying infants erroneously for needed services.

Reliability and Validity

The soundness of a psychometric test is judged based on its reliability and validity. *Reliability* is a measure of a test's dependability, its ability to produce similar results under differing conditions (e.g., at different times or with different examiners). *Validity*, however, refers to a test's accuracy based on a collection of evidence that supports that it is measuring what it purports to do.

Several forms of reliability exist. *Test–retest reliability* is a measure of a test's temporal stability, obtained by correlating test scores obtained at one time with test scores of the same individuals taken at a later date, such as 2 weeks later. Test–retest reliability coefficients are often lower for infant tests as compared to tests designed for older children, possibly due in part to the rapidity of early development. *Interrater reliability* refers to the degree to which test scores are not dependent on individual differences between test examiners but, rather, reflect the infant's abilities regardless of who is administering the test. Finally, *internal consistency* refers to the correlation between various test items and provides evidence as to the degree to which a test measures a single unitary construct, as opposed to representing an unrelated collection of test items. As a guideline, Salvia and Ysseldyke (1991) recommend reliability coefficients of at least .90 for diagnostic tests and .80 for screening tests.

Besides its use in evaluating the psychometric soundness of a test, reliability coefficients serve a practical purpose, as well. Because no test can be completely reliable, scores are often presented with a given *confidence interval*. This confidence interval is based on the test's reliability coefficient and allows a test user to express a given score within a certain range of error (e.g., "Jane obtained a score of 100 ± 8."). This presentation more accurately represents the error inherent in all tests, as opposed to presenting a single score, as if it were an exact measurement.

In comparison to reliability, validity is even more multifaceted. There is no single or preferred way to establish a test's validity. Rather, validity represents an accumulation of evidence that together builds a case for the accuracy of that test. Infant developmental tests are expected to correlate significantly with other similar tests (concurrent validity) and to be at least somewhat predictive of future test results or some other criterion, such as success in school or absence of a diagnosable disorder (predictive validity). The prediction of subsequent IQ scores based on infant developmental test scores has not been supported (Honzik, 1983), however, and infant test scores are best interpreted as estimates of *current* functioning.

REVIEW OF DEVELOPMENTAL TESTS

A variety of representative developmental tests are presented here under three basic headings: neonatal, developmental, and screening.

Neonatal Assessment Tests

Before Dr. Virginia Apgar developed the well-known Apgar Screening Test (Apgar, 1953), few methods for assessing the conditions of newborns (birth to 4 weeks) existed. Although the Apgar proved to be predictive of infant mortality, studies have been inconsistent at best regarding its ability to predict subsequent infant development (Francis, Self, & Horowitz, 1987). Nonetheless, the Apgar helped pave the way for the two neonatal neurobehavioral assessment tests described below.

Graham–Rosenblith Behavioral Test for Neonates

The Graham–Rosenblith Behavioral Test for Neonates (Rosenblith, 1979) consists of five neurodevelopment scales: Motor, Tactile–Adaptive, Visual Responsiveness, Auditory Responsiveness, and Muscle Tone. Despite some encouraging early findings regarding the Graham–Rosenblith's reliability and predictive validity (Francis et al., 1987), it was never used extensively in research and appears to be seldom used today.

Brazelton Neonatal Behavioral Assessment Scale

The Neonatal Behavioral Assessment Scale (NBAS), currently in its second edition (Brazelton, 1984), is a popular test of the neonate's current organizational and coping capacities to respond to the stress of labor, delivery, and adjustment to the *ex utero* environment. The NBAS-2 is designed for use with neonates 37 to 44 weeks gestational age who are not currently needing mechanical supports or oxygen and takes about 20 to 30 minutes to administer, followed by about 15 minutes to record and score the baby's performance. Brazelton (1984) recommends that newborns ideally be assessed more than once beginning no earlier than 3 days old. Although the NBAS was originally designed for use with full-term healthy infants, it has been used extensively with premature and otherwise medically fragile infants.

Although interrater reliability for the NBAS is quite high, studies of the test–retest reliability of the NBAS suggest poor temporal stability for most items (Sameroff, 1979). Methods to derive factor or summary scores are complicated, requiring recoding items to a continuous scale in order to derive meaningful summative scores. The validity of the NBAS is supported by research that has demonstrated its ability to correctly identify neonates who are underweight or who have experienced *in utero* drug and alcohol exposure, maternal malnutrition, and gestational diabetes. Furthermore, the NBAS has been shown to predict infant–parent attachment and subsequent infant development. Unfortunately, research has not consistently shown the NBAS to be a good predictor of infant development much beyond the first year of life (Horowitz & Linn, 1982). Interestingly, the NBAS has been shown to be an effective intervention tool for increasing the maternal involvement and responsiveness of low-socioeconomic status and adolescent mothers (Worobey & Brazelton, 1990).

Infant/Toddler Development Tests

For the most part, tests that measure infant and toddler development can be grouped into one of three categories, each based on a different model: (1) multidomain developmental, (2) infant cognition, and (3) criterion-referenced assessment. Each of these models of assessment, as well as some selected instruments from each, are addressed here.

Multidomain Developmental Assessment Model

This model of infant/toddler assessment is arguably the oldest and most established. Based on the pioneering work of psychologist/physician Dr. Arnold Gesell at the Yale University Clinic of Child Development, now the Yale

Child Study Center, the multidomain model posits that child development is an interactively unfolding, continuous process that occurs in several distinct but interrelated domains (Gesell, 1940). Even today, many of the assessment techniques pioneered by Dr. Gesell can be found nearly unaltered in the modern assessment instruments described here.

Perhaps the most enduring contribution of this model is the concept of distinct but related domains of development. This model of development and assessment has been affirmed in recent early intervention legislation for children birth through 5 years old (Individuals with Disabilities Education Act Amendments of 1986 Public Law No. 99-457, passed in 1986), which mandates assessment in at least five areas of development in order to establish a young child's eligibility for public-funded early intervention programs. These areas include (1) Motor (fine and gross motor skills), (2) Communication (receptive and expressive language abilities), (3) Cognition (problem-solving skills), (4) Adaptive (self-help behaviors, such as dressing, eating, and toileting), and (5) Personal–Social (social competence, emotional regulation, and sense of self). Although these domains may appear distinct and separate, they are conceptualized as interrelated, and most are represented in the various multidomain instruments presented below. In addition to using multidomain assessment instruments, clinicians may augment their assessment by selecting from several existing tests that assess a particular domain of functioning, such as the Receptive–Expressive Emergent Language Scale—2 (Bzoch & League, 1991), the Peabody Developmental Motor Scale (Folio & Fewell, 1983), or the Vineland Social–Emotional Early Childhood Scales (Sparrow, Balla, & Cicchetti, 1998).

Bayley Scales of Infant Development—II. The Bayley Scales of Infant Development, currently in its second edition (BSID-II, Bayley, 1993), is arguably the most widely used measure of the development of infants and toddlers in both clinical and research settings. Also, it has the most extensive history of validation and is psychometrically quite sophisticated. The BSID-II is applicable to children from 1 through 42 months of age. Administration time is about 25 to 35 minutes for infants under 15 months old and up to 60 minutes for children over 15 months.

There are three main components of the BSID-II: the Mental Development Index (MDI), Psychomotor Development Index (PDI), and Behavior Rating Scale (BRS). The MDI provides information about the child's language development and problem-solving skills, whereas the PDI assesses the child's gross and fine motor development. The BRS is a form that evaluators may use to rate the child's behaviors during the assessment. Items assess attentional capacities, social engagement, affect and emotion, and the quality of the child's movement and motor control. The BSID-II provides a method for obtaining age equivalence scores for four facets of development: Cognitive, Language, Social, and Motor. Unfortunately, little empirical evidence exists to support the validity of these facet scores. Also, determining the correct facet age-equivalent score is often difficult, as several months of development are often determined on the basis of passing only one item. Considerably more research is needed before clinicians and researchers can have confidence in these facet scores.

The BSID-II is normed on 1,700 infants representative of 1988 U.S. Census data, an exceedingly large normative sample by infant assessment standards. Test–retest reliability for 1 to 16 days ranges from .83 to .91 for the MDI and from .77 to .79 for the PDI. Stability for the BRS varies greatly depending on the age of the child, ranging from .55 to .90. Interrater reliability for the BSID-II was reported to be .96 for the MDI, .75 for the PDI, and .70 for the total BRS. These stability coefficients approach adequacy for the MDI but fall somewhat short of optimal for a diagnostic test on the PDI (Salvia & Ysseldyke, 1991). Concurrent validity of the MDI, as compared to other measures of general cognitive ability, typically falls in the .70 range, whereas the PDI correlated best with the Motor score of the McCarthy at .59. In general, the BSID appears to have some ability to predict which infants will score very poorly on intelligence tests in their preschool years but shows limited ability to accurately predict specific IQ scores, especially in average developing infants (Gibbs, 1990; Whatley, 1987).

The BSID-II is administered in "item sets," that are determined based on the age of the infant. This represents a substantial revision from the original BSID, which used a continuous series of items. This change has created some confusion among infant examiners in terms of which "item set" to use for infants born prematurely (Ross & Lawson, 1997). For testers who use the corrected age procedure, the test developers recommend using the same item set that corresponds to the normative group used for determining that child's standard score. In other words, if an infant's performance will be compared to that of a typical 7-month-old, the examiner should administer the 7-month-old item set (Matula, Gyurke, & Aylward, 1997).

Griffiths Mental Development Scales. Though seldom used in the United States, the Griffiths Mental Development Scales warrants a brief description due to its continued use in Europe and its influence on extending infant developmental testing internationally. The Griffiths consists of two tests: The Abilities of Babies (Griffiths, 1954), designed for infants from birth to 24 months and The Abilities of Young Children (Griffiths, 1979), for children 24 months to 8 years old. The infant scale consists of five domains, modeled closely after Gesell's early work: Locomotor, Personal and Social, Hearing and Speech, Eye and Hand Coordination, and Performance. The test is normed on 571 infants from London, England, but strangely stratified to match the 1940 U.S. Census figures. Reliability studies for the Griffiths have yielded mixed results, and validity studies have indicated relatively weak predictive ability for later IQ test scores (Thomas, 1970). Despite its outdated and questionable standardization, the Griffiths is rather popular in Europe.

Battelle Developmental Inventory. The Battelle Developmental Inventory (BDI; Newborg, Stock, Wnek, Guidubaldi, & Svinicki, 1984) has quickly become an exceedingly popular developmental assessment tool for measuring development in children ages birth through 7 years old. The assessment time required by the BDI is quite long compared to other similar tests, ranging from about 1 to 2 hours depending on the age of the child. Five domains are measured by the BDI, including Personal–Social, Adaptive, Motor, Communication, and Cognitive. Each of the five domains of the BDI is divided into subdomains that finely assess the components of each domain. All domains contribute to a total developmental score.

The standardization sample for the BDI consisted of 800 children, stratified to match the 1980 U.S. Census data based on geographic region, race, and gender. In a review of the technical merits of the BDI, McLinden (1989) raised several concerns. First, although the test authors reported exceptionally strong test–retest and interrater reliability for the BDI, a general lack of procedural details in the manual makes it difficult to evaluate these data adequately. No information regarding the BDI's internal reliability is provided. Second, the concurrent validity of the various domains was established by statistically significant correlation with other assessment measures. These validity studies, however, were exceptionally small, ranging from only 10 to 37 subjects. Furthermore, correlations for the BDI Cognitive domain were much less than optimal ($r = .44$; $N = 13$ for the Full Scale IQ from the Wechsler Intelligence Scale for Children—Revised; $r = .50$; $N = 23$ for the Stanford–Binet Intelligence Scale) (Newborg et al., 1984).

A potentially more detrimental limitation of the BDI exists in its normative data (Boyd, 1989). For the first 2 years, normative data are presented in 6-month groups. Thereafter, normative data are provided in 12-month groups. Therefore, children's performance is compared to others that can be as many as 6 months older or younger for children under 24 months old, or as many as 12 months older or younger for children older than 24 months. Clearly, standard scores for children who are old for their normative group will be inflated, whereas standard scores for children who are young for their normative group will underestimate their true development. Due to these normative discontinuities, children could theoretically score in the average range just before their birthday (e.g., a standard score of 100) and a day or so later, with the exact same performance, score in the range suggestive of mental retardation (e.g., a standard score of 65). For this reason, age-equivalent score may be more stable on the BDI than are standard scores (Boyd, Welge, Sexton, & Miller, 1989). This limitation greatly reduces the diagnostic utility of the BDI and may even lead to grossly distorted results when BDI standard scores are used for longitudinal research or for tracking the development of individual children. For these reasons, diagnostic use of the BDI for infants and toddlers in general is not recommended.

Mullen Scales of Early Learning. A recent addition to the family of multidomain assessment instruments is the Mullen Scales of Early Learning (Mullen, 1995). This revision of the original Mullen Scales combined earlier versions of the test designed for infants and preschoolers into one test with continuous norms from birth through 68 months. The Mullen takes about 15 to 60 minutes to administer, depending on the age of the child (15 minutes at 1 year old, 30 minutes at 3 years, and 60 minutes at 5 years). The Mullen is based on a well-articulated model of infant neurodevelopment and assesses child development in five separate domains: Gross Motor, Visual Reception (primarily visual discrimination and memory), Fine Motor, Receptive Language, and Expressive Language. The Gross Motor scale is only applicable to children birth through 33 months old and does not contribute to the overall Early Learning Composite score.

Normative data for the Mullen are based on a sample of 1,849 children from across the United States, somewhat overrepresentative of children from the Northeast. Internal reliability ranges from .75 to .83 for Mullen subtests and is .91 for the Early Learning Composite. Median 1- to 2-week test–retest reliability ranges from .78 to .96 for subtests. Interrater reliability ranges from .94 to .98. The Mullen Receptive and Expressive Language scales showed acceptable correlation with similar scales from the Preschool Language Assessment Scale, .85 and .80, respectively. Gross Motor correlated with the Bayley Motor Scale at .76, and Fine Motor correlated with the Peabody Fine Motor Scale at .70. These correlations for the motor scales also are acceptable. Overall, these validation studies are quite promising. Additional studies, however, of the Mullen's concurrent and predictive validity are warranted.

Infant Cognition Model

In 1905, Alfred Binet and Theodore Simon introduced a test that could be used to identify French school children who were likely to experience difficulties learning due to mental retardation. So was born the tradition of intelligence testing, or IQ assessment. As opposed to the multidomain model, this model is based on the theory that a single factor of general cognitive ability exists, "g," that can be measured and used to predict subsequent performance.

The best example of a test that follows the infant cognition model is the Cattell Infant Intelligence Scale (Cattell, 1960). The Cattell was conceptualized as a downward extension of the 1937 Stanford–Binet Intelligence Scale, the much revised American version of the Binet–Simon test. The Cattell was designed to assess infants and toddlers from 2 through 30 months old, and it extensively "borrowed" items from Gesell's work. Items that addressed gross motor and personal–social development, however, were excluded in order to more closely resemble items from the IQ paradigm. Although reliability studies were encouraging, the ability of the Cattell to predict subsequent Stanford–Binet IQ scores at 36 months was weak. The Cattell demonstrates poor predictive validity for infants from birth to 2 years old but approaches acceptability for 24- to 30-month-olds (Thomas, 1970). Overall, the Cattell and other "infant IQ tests" appear unable to extend the IQ assessment model into infancy meaningfully and are used seldom today.

Criterion-Referenced Model

Typically, diagnostic and screening tests are used to compare an infant's current level of functioning to other infants and are, therefore, norm-referenced. Conversely, criterion-referenced tests are used to compare an infant's functioning to some set of standards or expected competencies. Though not typically useful for diagnostic or screening purposes, these tests are essential when planning intervention programs. To accomplish this, criterion-referenced tests are designed to sample extensively the universe of skills that a child is expected to have mastered at various ages. The infant's performance on these tests can then be translated directly into an individualized intervention plan by targeting those skills that the infant was expected to have mastered but as of yet had not.

One of the most popular criterion-referenced tests for use with young children is the Brigance Diagnostic Inventory of Early Development—Revised (Brigance, 1991). The Brigance is useful for children birth to 7 years old and surveys skills in 12 different developmental domains, including social and emotional, communicative, motor, and preacademic skills. Other similar tests specifically for infants include the Hawaii Early Learning Profile (HELP; Furuno et al., 1987) and the Early Learning Accomplishment Profile for Infants (Sanford, 1981). The Rossetti Infant–Toddler Language Scale (Rossetti, 1990) is also a criterion-referenced instrument but is specific to assessing an infant's verbal and nonverbal communication and parent–infant interaction. Some criterion-referenced tests for infants are based on the Piagetian, rather than psychoeducational, model of infant development. One of the most commonly used Piagetian model instruments is the Infant Psychological Developmental Scale (Uzgiris & Hunt, 1975), which assesses an infant's ability to grasp object permanence, understand means–ends and cause–effect relationships, imitate vocalizations and gestures, and manipulate objects in space.

Infant–Toddler Screening Tests

Screening tests are brief assessments of a child's current level of functioning, used to determine which children may be developmentally at risk and require further assessment. Therefore, scores on these instruments should be somewhat predictive of scores from more comprehensive assessments (e.g., the Bayley) but require substantially less time to administer and score. They are intended to be used routinely for large groups of children, when a comprehensive assessment for all children would be either too costly or unwarranted. Due largely to their brevity, these instruments usually are not as reliable or as valid as comprehensive assessment tools. The goal of all screening tests is to identify correctly those children who would likely score poorly on a more comprehensive assessment and to reduce two possible sources of error: false positives and false negatives. The ability of a screener to reduce false-negative rates is referred to as the test's *sensitivity*, its ability to accurately detect children with delays or disabilities. Conversely, the ability of a screener to reduce false positives is referred to as its *specificity*, its ability to avoid mislabeling a child as delayed or disabled when, in fact, that child is developmentally normal. Though it is desirable to reduce the percentage of both types of error, sensitivity is more important than specificity with tests designed to be used for screening purposes. This is because it is assumed that follow-up assessment will correct false positives, whereas false negatives usually will not be referred for further assessment. Meisels (1989) recommends that developmental screeners possess both sensitivity and specificity levels of at least 80%. Unfortunately, too many developmental screeners do not provide this data.

Table 14.1 presents information on a selected sample of developmental screeners current-

TABLE 14.1. Developmental Screening Tests

Screening test	Age	Domains[a]	Norm sample	Reliability/validity	Comments
Battelle Developmental Inventory Screening Test (Newborg, Stock, Wnek, Guidubaldi, & Svinicki, 1984)	6 mos–7 yr	PS, Ad; GM; FM; EC; RC; Cg	Representative but small	Strong correlation with full BDI	Suffers same limitations as full BDI
Bayley Infant Neurodevelopmental Screen (Aylward, 1995)	3–24 mo	N; RC; EC/M; Cg	Large; representative	Excellent reliability; promising validity	
Birth to Three Developmental Scale (Bangs & Dodson, 1979)	Birth–36 mo	EC/RC; Cg; PS; M	Small; questionable representation	Strong interrater reliability, but little evidence of validity	
Denver Developmental Screening Test—II (Frankenburg et al., 1990)	Birth–6 yr	GM; FM/Cg; PS; EC/RC	Large but all from Colorado	See text	See text
Developmental Activities Screening Inventory—II (Fewell & Langley, 1984)	Birth–60 mo	15 sensory and problem-solving areas	>200 disabled children	Little evidence of reliability; valid for severely delayed children	Can be used with language- and visually impaired children
Developmental Indicators for the Assessment of Learning—Revised (Mardell-Czudnowski & Goldenberg, 1990)	2–6 yr	M; AS; EC/RC; B	Large; representative	Acceptable reliability and validity	
Diagnostic Inventory for Screening Children—4 (Amdur, Mainland, & Parker, 1996)	Birth–60 mo	FM; GM; RC; EC; AM; VM; Ad; PS	Small; all from southwest Ontario	Excellent reliability; limited evidence of validity	
Developmental Observation Checklist System (Hrescko, Miguel, Sherbenou, & Burton, 1994)	Birth–6 yr	Cg; EC/RC; PS; FM/GM; Adj; PS&S	Adequate; representative	Sound reliability and concurrent validity	Parent report only
Developmental Profile—II (Alpern, Boll, & Shearer, 1986)	Birth–9½ yr	M; Ad; PS; AS; EC/RC	Large	Adequate reliability and validity	Parent report only
Early Screening Profile (Harrison, 1990)	2–6 yr	Cg; EC/RC; M; Ad/PS; Ar	Adequate; representative	Good reliability; exceptional validity	
Kent Infant Development Scales (Reuter & Bickett, 1985)	Birth–12 mo	Cg; M; EC/RC; Ad; PS	All from Northeast Ohio	Adequate reliability and validity	Primarily parent report
Child Development Inventory (Ireton, 1992)	15 mo–6 yr	GM; FM; EC; RC; Ad; PS; L; N	Small; from St. Paul, MN	Little evidence of reliability and validity	300 parent report items

[a]Adj, adjustment; Ad, adaptive, self-help or daily living; AM, auditory attention and memory; Ar, articulation; AS, academic or preacademic skills; B, behavior; Cg, cognitive or problem-solving; EC, expressive communication/language; FM, fine motor; GM, gross motor; L, letters; N, numbers; M, motor or physical; N, neurological intactness; PS, personal-social; PS&S, parental stress & support; RC, receptive communication/language; VM, visual attention and memory. A slash mark (/) indicates that multiple domains are assessed in the same scale or subtest.

ly available. All screening tests presented use direct assessment or observation of the child, unless otherwise stated. Most also allow for parent report of information in order to gain additional data about behaviors that may be difficult to elicit in the brief assessment period. Some, however, are based solely on parent re-

port (e.g., the Developmental Profile—II and the Developmental Observation Checklist System).

The Denver Developmental Screening Test—II (Frankenburg et al., 1990), one of the most popular developmental screening tests, warrants individual comment. The popularity of the

Denver, especially in medical settings, may be due at least in part to its brevity, as it can be administered in as little as 15 to 20 minutes. Items are scored based on parent report, direct assessment of the child, and observation. The Denver produces one overall score that places children in one of four descriptive categories: Pass, Questionable, Abnormal, or Untestable. As the Denver-II was normed exclusively on children living in Colorado, considerable caution should be used when using this screener outside of that state.

The original version of the Denver (Frankenburg, Dodds, & Fandal, 1975) was criticized for not being sensitive enough to identify correctly most children with developmental delays or disabilities, missing as many as 80% of children with delays or disabilities (Greer, Bauchner, & Zuckerman, 1989). Although the Denver-II is a clear improvement over the original Denver, there is evidence that it now significantly overidentifies children, often by as many as 72% of children (Glascoe & Byrne, 1993). As a result, child-find personnel in both Kentucky and Tennessee have reportedly requested that evaluators use a different screening instrument before referring children for developmental services in order to reduce costly false positives (Johnson, Ashford, Byrne, & Glascoe, 1992).

CONCLUSIONS

Assessments of infants and toddlers are clinical explorations involving a combination of structured and unstructured approaches. A range of structured developmental assessment instruments are reviewed, each with varying strengths and weaknesses in its ability to detect delays in development in specific functional areas. All structured developmental assessments with young children need to be supplemented with information from caregivers (and other professionals) and observations of the child's behavior during the evaluation sessions. The evaluation provides information for caregivers about their child's developmental strengths and weaknesses, but there also may be a potential therapeutic impact from the evaluation process itself. Assessments of young children are often the first step in facilitating referrals to appropriate educational or rehabilitative services and, as such, serve a critical role in making a bridge between diagnosis and intervention.

REFERENCES

Alpern, G. D., Boll, T. J., & Shearer, M. (1986). *Developmental profile—II*. Aspen, CO: Psychological Development Publications.

Amdur, J. R., Mainland, M. K., & Parker, K. C. H. (1996) *Diagnostic Inventory for Screening Children (DISC) manual* (4th ed.). Kitchner, Ontario: Kitchner-Waterloo Hospital.

Apgar, V. (1953). A proposal for a new method of evaluation of the newborn infant. *Anesthesia and Analgesia: Current Research, 32,* 260–267.

Aylward, G. P. (1995). *Bayley infant neurodevelopmental screener*. San Antonio, TX: Psychological Corporation.

Bangs, T. E., & Dodson, S. (1979). *Birth to three developmental scale*. Allen, TX: DLM Teaching Resources.

Bayley, N. (1993). *Bayley Scales of Infant Development* (2nd ed.). San Antonio, TX: Psychological Corporation.

Boyd, R. D. (1989). What a difference a day makes: Age-related discontinuities and the Battelle Developmental Inventory. *Journal of Early Intervention, 13,* 114–119.

Boyd, R. D., Welge, P., Sexton, D., & Miller, J. H. (1989). Concurrent validity of the Battelle Developmental Inventory: Relationship with the Bayley Scales in young children with known or suspected disabilities. *Journal of Early Intervention, 13,* 14–23.

Brazelton, T. B. (1984). *Neonatal Behavioral Assessment Scale* (2nd ed.). *Clinics in Developmental Medicine, 88.*

Brigance, A. H. (1991). *Brigance Diagnostic Inventory of Early Development: Revised.* North Billerica, MA: Curriculum Associates.

Bzoch, K., & League, R. (1991). *The Receptive–Expressive Emergent Language Scale (REEL)—2.* Austin, TX: Pro-Ed.

Cattell, P. (1960). *Cattell Infant Intelligence Scale.* Cleveland, OH: Psychological Corporation.

Fewell, R. R., & Langley, M. B. (1984). *Developmental Activities Screening Inventory—II.* Austin, TX: Pro-Ed.

Flynn, J. R. (1984). The mean IQ of Americans: Massive gains 1932 to 1978. *Psychological Bulletin, 95,* 29–51.

Folio, M. R., & Fewell, R. R. (1983). *Peabody Developmental Motor Scale and activity cards.* Allen, TX: Teaching Resources.

Francis, P. L., Self, P. A., & Horowitz, F. D. (1987). The behavioral assessment of the neonate: An overview. In J. D. Osofsky (Ed.), *Handbook of infant development.* New York: Wiley.

Frankenburg, W. K., Dodds, J., Archer, P., Bresnick, B., Maschka, P., Edelman, N., & Shapiro, H. (1990). *Denver II: Technical manual.* Denver, CO: Denver Developmental Materials.

Frankenburg, W. K., Dodds, J., & Fandal, A. (1975). *Denver Developmental Screening Test.* Denver, CO: LADOCA.

Furuno, S., O'Reilly, K. A., Hosaka, C. M., Inatsuka, T. T., Allman, T. L., & Zeisloft, B. (1987). *Hawaii Early*

Learning Profile (HELP): Activity guide. Palo Alto, CA: VORT.

Gesell, A. (1940). *The first five years of life: A guide to the study of the preschool child.* New York: Harper.

Gibbs, E. D. (1990). Assessment of infant mental ability: Conventional tests and issues of prediction. In E. D. Gibbs & D. Teti (Eds.), *Interdisciplinary assessment of infants: A guide for early intervention professionals* (pp. 77–90). Baltimore: Brookes.

Glascoe, F. P., & Byrne, K. E. (1993). The accuracy of three developmental screening tests. *Journal of Early Intervention, 17,* 368–379.

Greer, S., Bauchner, H., & Zuckerman, B. (1989). The Denver Developmental Screening Test: How good is its predictive validity? *Developmental Medicine and Child Neurology, 31,* 774–781.

Griffiths, R. (1954). *The Abilities of Babies.* London: University of London Press.

Griffiths, R. (1979). *The Abilities of Young Children.* London: Child Development Research Center.

Harrison, P. L. (1990). *Early Screening Profiles (ESP): Manual.* Circle Pines, MN: American Guidance Service.

Honzik, M. P. (1983). Measuring mental abilities in infancy: The value and limitations. In M. Lewis (Ed.), *Origins of intelligence in infancy and early childhood* (pp. 67–107). New York: McGraw-Hill.

Horowitz, F. D., & Linn, L. P. (1982). The Neonatal Behavioral Assessment Scale. In M. Wolraich & D. K. Routh (Eds.), *Advances in developmental pediatrics* (vol. 3, pp. 223–256). Greenwich, CT: JAI.

Hrescko, W. P., Miguel, S. A., Sherbenou, R. J., & Burton, S. D. (1994). *Developmental Observation Checklist System.* Austin, TX: Pro-Ed.

Individuals with Disabilities Education Act Amendments of 1986, Pub. L. No. 99-457, § 303 (1986).

Ireton, H. (1992). *Child Development Inventory.* Minneapolis: Behavior Science Systems.

Johnson, K. L., Ashford, L. G., Byrne, K. E., & Glascoe, F. P. (1992). Does Denver II produce meaningful results? [Letter to the editor]. *Pediatrics, 90,* 477–478.

Mardell-Czudnowski, C. D., & Goldenberg, D. (1990). *DIAL-R (Developmental Indicators for the Assessment of Learning—Revised).* Edison, NJ: Childcraft Education.

Matula, K., Gyurke, J. S., & Aylward, G. P. (1997). Response to commentary. Bayley Scales—II. *Developmental and Behavioral Pediatrics, 18,* 112–113.

Mayes, L. C. (1991). Infant assessment. In M. Lewis (Ed.), *Child and adolescent psychiatry* (pp. 431–439). New York: Williams & Wilkins.

Mayes, L. C., & Gilliam, W. S. (Eds.). (1999). Preface: Comprehensive psychiatric assessment of young children. *Child and Adolescent Psychiatric Clinics of North America, 8*(2), xiii–xiv.

McLinden, S. E. (1989). An evaluation of the Battelle Developmental Inventory for determining special education eligibility. *Journal of Psychoeducational Assessment, 7,* 66–73.

Meisels, S. J. (1989). Can developmental screening tests identify children who are developmentally at risk? *Pediatrics, 83,* 578–585.

Meisels, S. J., & Waskik, B. A. (1990). Who should be served? Identifying children in need of early intervention. In S. J. Meisels & J. P. Shonkoff (Eds.), *Handbook of early childhood intervention* (pp. 605–632). New York: Cambridge University Press.

Mullen, E. M. (1995). *Mullen Scales of Early Learning: AGS Edition.* Circle Pines, MN: American Guidance Service.

Newborg, J., Stock, J., Wnek, L., Guidubaldi, J., & Svinicki, J. S. (1984). *Battelle Developmental Inventory (BDI).* Allen, TX: DLM/Teaching Resources.

Reuter, J., & Bickett, L. (1985). *Kent Infant Development Scale (KIDS).* Kent, OH: Developmental Metrics.

Rosenblith, J. F. (1979). The Graham–Rosenblith behavioral examination for newborns: Prognostic value and procedural issues. In J. Osofsky (Ed.), *Handbook of infant development.* New York: Wiley.

Ross, G., & Lawson, K. (1997). Commentary. Using the Bayley—II: Unresolved issues in assessing the development of prematurely born children. *Developmental and Behavioral Pediatrics, 18,* 109–111.

Rossetti, L. M. (1990). *Infant–toddler assessment: An interdisciplinary approach.* Boston: College Hill.

Salvia, J., & Ysseldyke, J. E. (1991). *Assessment* (5th ed.). Boston: Houghton Mifflin.

Sameroff, A. J. (Ed.). (1979). Organization and stability of newborn behavior: A commentary on the Brazelton Neonatal Behavioral Assessment Scale. *Monographs of the Society for Research in Child Development, 43*(5–6).

Sanford, A. (1981). *Learning Accomplishment Profile for Infants (Early LAP).* Winston-Salem, NC: Kaplan School Supply.

Sparrow, S. S., Balla, D. A., & Cicchetti, D. V. (1998). *Vineland Social–Emotional Early Childhood Scales.* Circle Pines, MN: American Guidance Service.

Thomas, H. (1970). Psychological assessment instruments for use with human infants. *Merrill–Palmer Quarterly, 16,* 179–223.

Uzgiris, I., & Hunt, J. McV. (1975). *Assessment in infancy: Ordinal scales of psychological development.* Urbana: University of Illinois.

Whatley, J. (1987). Bayley Scales of Infant Development. In D. Keyser & R. Sweetland (Eds.), *Test critiques* (Vol. 6, pp. 38–47). Kansas City, MO: Westport.

Worobey, J., & Brazelton, T. B. (1990). Newborn assessment and support for parenting. In E. D. Gibbs & D. M. Teti (Eds.), *Interdisciplinary assessment of infants: A guide for early intervention professionals.* Baltimore: Brookes.

15

The Observation and Assessment of Young Children Including Use of the Infant–Toddler Mental Status Exam

❖

ANNE LELAND BENHAM

The process of an evaluation is shaped by certain underlying theoretical principles that point to important avenues for inquiry and assessment. For infant mental health evaluations, a key principle is the transactional model of development (see Sameroff & Chandler, 1975 and Sameroff & Fiese, Chapter 1, this volume). This model of development posits a constant, dynamic interaction between the child's innate characteristics and his caregiving and interpersonal environment. A transactional model demands of clinicians that we try to understand both infant and environment and that we examine how they are affecting each other in developmentally supportive or counterproductive ways.

Evaluations of young children integrate data from multiple sources. Information is gathered through questionnaires and interviews with the parents about the child, the child's history, and the family. Clinical assessment of the child may include observations in play settings, structured interactions and specific testing paradigms to assess the emotional, behavioral, developmental, and relational aspects of his functioning. Further information may be gathered from the child's physicians, teachers, or other caregivers. The clinician or clinical team then organizes the information into a formulation or under-

standing of the child, followed by a diagnosis and recommendations for additional intervention, if needed.

This chapter addresses one part of an evaluation, the clinical observation of the child. The Infant and Toddler Mental Status Exam (ITMSE; American Academy of Child and Adolescent Psychiatry, 1997), presented in this chapter, is a framework for organizing and communicating the clinician's observations. Babies and young children communicate through behavior, body language, facial expression, and play. Observing a young child playing with his parent, being fed, entering an unfamiliar playroom, or reacting to a minor bump or fall can provide the clinician rich information from which to infer the child's self-confidence, attention, curiosity, expectation of and interaction with the parent, as well as his developmental status. The evaluation attends to capabilities and areas of weakness and to protective factors and risk, both inherent to the child and in his environment. The evaluation unites history and observations into a shared effort by the clinician and the child's family to understand the child. There is no correct or necessary setting, timing, or set of equipment for such observations, as there is in structured, normed assessment protocols. Although an office-based model is described, this chapter aims to give clinicians portable tools to carry into any assessment situation.

The chapter addresses three topics: (1) the role of the clinician, (2) a way to organize and describe clinical observations using the ITMSE and (3) further discussion on what to look for and how to elicit and understand child behaviors in certain domains of functioning. Other chapters elaborate on other parts of the mental health assessment.

To avoid confusion, in this chapter clinicians are referred to as "she," infants are referred to as "he," and caregivers are called the "parent." In this chapter, infant refers to 0–1-year-olds, young toddlers to children 12–18 months, and older toddlers to children 18–36 months. Young preschooler refers to children 36–48 months and older preschooler to 4–5-year-olds. Clearly, these are somewhat arbitrary designations and for many discussions young children refers to the whole group. The approach to evaluation described in this chapter has been used for evaluation of children from 0 through 5 years.

THE ROLE OF THE CLINICIAN

Assessment is a complex process that asks the clinician to gather information, to create an atmosphere of comfort and safety for parents and child, and to observe in great detail. The clinician's capacity to analyze and to understand what she has seen and heard depends on the quality and variety of her observations and on the preservation of an open, questioning search for the meaning of the data.

Interviewing parents alone, prior to observing the child, allows the clinician to develop rapport and an alliance with parents. The clinician may become aware of both overt concerns and unspoken worries, and of parental tensions and divergent views of the child and of the issues, which will inform her observations. If there is parental psychopathology that affects the child, it may be identified. Toddlers and preschoolers, if present, may understand a significant amount of the content, and certainly the affective tone, of a history session. This may distress the child, especially if there is a focus on the child's "bad" behavior, and can negatively color his view of the clinician as a safe, friendly person. Attending to the child's physi-

cal and psychological comfort during the evaluation will allow the clinician to see the child's best functioning as well as his difficulties.

Parents are often relieved to hear, "I hope to see your child at his best and his worst times." They may be disappointed either if the child has acted almost perfectly or if they feel the clinician has focused only on problems and has not looked at the child's abilities, achievements in learning, or endearing qualities.

Observation

Observation is the primary tool of the clinician in the evaluation of young children. Observation includes watching how the child responds to new situations and new people and how his responses change over time. The clinician observes the role each parent plays in the child's regulation of his state, attention, behavior, and affect. The presence of a given child behavior or parent–child interaction is not as significant as its context and meaning in a wider fabric of multiple interactions and behaviors. It is the clinician's challenge to observe not only patterns of behavior, the tone of parent–child interaction, and the themes of the child's play but also the child's developmental skills as they emerge spontaneously in the playroom. These skills include the child's communication, movement and coordination, level of play, and self-regulation. The clinician can engage in three kinds of observation: quiet observation, directed observation, and participant observation.

Quiet Observation

Quiet observation is used first, so that the clinician can observe parent–child interaction with the least interference. An unstructured parent–child play session is a useful starting point, with minimal instruction such as "help him become comfortable in the playroom." The clinician can observe quietly and perhaps take notes in the room, behind a one-way mirror, or when reviewing a videotape at a later time. Parent or child may take the lead in unstructured play.

Directed Observation

After observing for some time, the clinician may structure activities to tap skills and functions not yet observed. This may include asking the parent to engage the child in certain activities or to offer a specific toy. For example, to evaluate fine motor skills, one might give a baby small objects to pick up and release, give a toddler some cubes to stack, and give an older toddler interlocking blocks, insert puzzles, or paper and pens. Some clinicians or teams observe a structured or semistructured play session with instructions to parents for the majority of their evaluation (see Crowell & Fleischman, 1993, for a review of such paradigms). This chapter describes a more "as needed" use of clinician-directed parent activity.

Participation Observation

Participant observation by the clinician is useful to probe areas of behavior not seen spontaneously, or behavior at the opposite pole of what has been seen, or behavior the parent may be hesitant to elicit. Such clinician activity should be thoughtful, have a purpose, test a hypothesis, or serve to make the session more fun and relaxed. Sections of this chapter that describe clinician activity with the child include those on assessing attention span, frustration tolerance, aggression, and play. The clinician is also active in trying to draw toddlers and preschoolers into fantasy play, often with toy people or animals. In this play, the clinician seeks to elicit the child's highest level of symbolic functioning and to expand on themes presented by the child or raised as concerns by the parents.

Structuring the Evaluation

The way a clinician structures the evaluation will greatly affect what she is privileged to observe. The young child will show different aspects of himself depending on whom he is with, where he is seen, the time of day, his state of hunger, rest and health, and other uncontrollable variables. It is important for the clinician to attempt to understand these effects and to see the child as many times as needed to observe a representative range of his behavior, affective states, and capacity for engagement with others. Several sessions in a clinical setting will allow the hesitant child to relax and the overactive, highly stimulated child to settle down.

Inclusion of Caregivers

Ideally, the young child is observed interacting with all the most important people in his daily life (see Zeanah, Larrieu, Heller, & Valliere,

Chapter 13, this volume). This includes parents, siblings, and other primary caregivers, such as grandparents or a primary babysitter. The child in foster care will be much better served if seen with biological parents as well as with foster parents. This can be scheduled as part of supervised visitation, if such supervision is legally mandated. The presence of siblings, either younger or older, often helps the child client relax and act more like himself at home. In addition, the content and quality of sibling rivalry may be revealed rapidly. Frequently, the index child's role in the family (e.g., as "good" or "bad" child) is represented vividly, as are the distortions and misrepresentations of such designated roles.

Occasionally, it is rarely preferable to see the child alone or without familiar caregivers. When abuse is suspected from the history or because the child appears to be afraid of the parent, a longer period of interaction between child and clinician alone may be useful in eliciting a wider range of behavior and interaction from the child. Generally, a brief separation experience provides important information about how the parent prepares the young child for separation and how the child copes with this stress. This is not the formalized Strange Situation procedure (Ainsworth, Blehar, Waters, & Wall, 1978), which is a research tool.

The Clinical Setting

An ideal clinical setting allows enough space for clinician and family to sit on the floor with accessible toys. A comfortable couch or chair allows for observation of the parents' soothing of the child. A one-way mirror and viewing room, if available, allow both clinician and parents the option of observing out of the child's view. Simple videotaping (a camera on a tripod) facilitates review by the clinician or with the parents.

It is helpful to have toys appropriate for the developmental age span of infants to preschoolers, because a child's play may be considerably behind or ahead of his chronological age. Both manipulative toys and those that stimulate "pretend" play may be important to elicit a full range of the child's functioning and issues. Toys engage young children and facilitate the demonstration of their attention, interest, language, motor skills, and cognitive capacities. The scenes and stories they create, with accompanying affect, give important clues about children's emotional life, their experiences, and their joys, fears, and preoccupations. "Manipulative" toys can be used to assess concentration, fine motor coordination, and frustration tolerance in the child and to observe parent–child interaction around a challenging activity. Almost any toy has many uses for both clinician and child, and one can make do with few toys. In addition, the child's use of his own body (e.g., covering his eyes for peek-a-boo) and of his parent as playmate are important foci for observation of play. The "Methods and Meaning of the ITMSE" section of this chapter expands on the use of play materials to address particular areas of the assessment.

Observation in Other Settings

Many toddlers and young preschoolers present with complaints about their behavior in out-of-home settings. Such behaviors range from withdrawal or distress to aggressiveness or tantrums. These complaints may stem from characteristics in the child, but they may also stem from unrealistic expectations, overcrowding, neglectful or harmful care, or a mismatch between child and setting. Observations in day care or preschool, as in the child's home, include assessment of the environment itself, including the adequacy of age-appropriate play materials and physical space. The personality and interactional style of his teachers and caregivers; the number, ages, and behavior of peers; and the structure of the child's day should all be noted as they appear to affect the child being observed. Observation of the child in more than one setting is often necessary to understand discrepancies in the child's reported behavior. These variations should be noted in the ITMSE whenever significant, as context often clarifies the etiology and meaning of behavior.

Case Example

Charlie, a bright 3-year-old boy with significant sensory hypersensitivities, was described by his parents as "gifted and highly creative" and by his preschool teacher as "perhaps autistic or retarded." Observation revealed that in his parents' quiet and supportive presence, he was highly verbal and creative in his symbolic play. At a normally noisy preschool, with a loud and directive teacher who excluded parents from the room, Charlie became shut down, withdrawn, and unwilling to participate in the struc-

tured activities. He sat watching as glue dripped from his brush. Indeed, he looked like the two different children who had been described. Charlie was placed in another busy, but more supportive and relaxed preschool, which allowed his mother to stay for the first 2 weeks. There, he became a shy, but fully participating member of the group.

THE ITMSE: ORGANIZING AND DESCRIBING CLINICAL OBSERVATIONS

I developed the ITMSE to help clinicians, from a variety of disciplines, organize observations of young children made across natural and clinical settings. It focuses on both individual and interactional behaviors and on the emotional and developmental functioning of the infant. The adult mental status exam is a central part of psychiatric evaluations. It is used to describe the examiner's observations and impressions of the adult client's appearance, speech, actions, and thoughts at the time of the interview (Kaplan & Sadock, 1988). To describe the mental status of a child, the clinician adds descriptions of play as a window to the child's thoughts and feelings and to understand mental organization (Simmons, 1985; American Academy of Child and Adolescent Psychiatry, 1995). The ITMSE describes ways in which the traditional categories of the mental status exam may be further adapted for use with infants and toddlers, age birth to 36 months. Play is even more central for evaluation in this age group. Categories have been added in the ITMSE, including sensory regulation and state regulation, which reflect important facets of infant development and of disorders in young children. A focus on parent–infant interaction reflects the primacy of those relationships in infancy. The ITMSE is not a rating scale, a behavior coding system, or a test with norms. It is a framework that may be used to describe observations from a brief session or piece of videotape or to pool data from many contacts with a child, across time and settings, to describe both constant and variable characteristics.

Developmental status in young children (both constitutional and maturational factors) may be characterized by age-expected skills, precociousness, delays, and deviations from the norm. Not every child needs or has access to developmental testing. The clinician must be sufficiently familiar with early child development to use this exam to guide clinical observations. The following sections of the ITMSE provide information most relevant to developmental status: III: Self-Regulation; IV: Motor; V: Speech and Language; VIII: Play; and IX: Cognition. Observations from the ITMSE, coupled with developmental questionnaires, will aid the clinician in making decisions about further evaluations.

When using the ITMSE, it is useful to describe the flow of the session, especially symbolic play, in a narrative form, as well as noting findings on each part of the ITMSE. Each piece of observational data can be looked at in context to evaluate its meaning. For example, a simple action, such as throwing a toy, if simply noted as aggressive behavior, could be seriously misunderstood or inadequately communicated. An 8-month-old often throws or drops toys as part of his exploration of them, because he is finished with them, or to get a parent's attention. A 2-year-old might throw a toy because it would not open or move. He might throw it angrily at his mother's face as she was talking about his faults or after she denied his request. Only the last instance would likely represent a focused aggressive act. This single piece of behavior also might be used for observations in other domains, such as the child's motor coordination, impulsivity, frustration tolerance, and the mother–child interactions. The ITMSE stands between raw data (i.e., frame by frame description or frequency counts of multiple aspects of behavior) and summary conclusions about broad constructs such as attachment. The nature of data in infant observation is complex, at times ambiguous, and often open to multiple interpretations. Clinical data may be used to generate new hypotheses, which can then be explored by structured testing, further history, or more clinical assessment.

The ITMSE was published by American Academy of Child and Adolescent Psychiatry (AACAP) as part of the "Practice Parameters for the Assessment of Infants and Toddlers (0–36 months)" (AACAP, 1997). (See Table 15.1.)

METHODS AND MEANING OF THE ITMSE

The presenting complaints for young child evaluations usually have many possible meanings. The clinician must make the most careful, complete observations she can given the limitations imposed by each evaluation. Then, using the history obtained, she must step back from her data and think critically, "What do my observations mean? What is explained by the child's culture, temperament, and family constellation? What represents normal variation versus developmental delay, psychopathology, or neurological impairment?"

To develop this formulation, the clinician needs data that tap the broad range of the child's functioning. This section expands on selected parts of the ITMSE to explain in more detail what to look for, how to elicit data if they do not emerge spontaneously, and how ITMSE observations may be used to address issues of differential diagnosis. For example, some sections of the ITMSE, which are very important, such as play and relatedness, are not singled out here but are discussed throughout the chapter and this section, as well as receiving fuller attention in the ITMSE itself. Affect and dyadic affect regulation are so important that they are discussed first. Aggression, which is in the ITMSE under Self-Regulation and Play, is given an extensive discussion for three reasons: First, it is the focus of referral for a great many older toddlers and preschoolers, especially from group care settings. Second, it is one of the least specific behaviors, which can have myriad meanings. Third, aggression is one aspect of evaluation where clinician activity may be especially useful. The subsections of Self-Regulation are given fuller discussion, both individually and in a subgroup. Certain aspects of developmental status are described more fully (motor, language, and cognition), but readers are directed to the chapters on developmental testing (Gilliam & Mayes, Chapter 14, this volume), disorders of communication (Prizant, Wetherby, & Roberts, Chapter 17, this volume), and mental retardation (Walters & Blane, Chapter 16, this volume) for further discussion.

Affect (ITMSE Section VII)

Our field has been confusing in its use of the words "affect," "emotion," and "mood." In the adult psychiatric mental status, emotion refers to a complex feeling state, with psychic, somatic, and behavioral components. Mood is a pervasive emotion experienced and reported by the person and observed by others. Affect refers to the expression of emotion as observed by oth-

TABLE 15.1. Infant and Toddler Mental Status Exam, by Anne L. Benham, MD

I. **Appearance**
Size; level of nourishment; dress and hygiene; apparent maturity compared with age; dysmorphic features, e.g., facies, eye and ear shape and placement, epicanthal folds, digits, etc.; abnormal head size; cutaneous lesions.

II. **Apparent Reaction to Situation**
Note where evaluation takes place and with whom.
   A. Initial reaction to setting and to strangers: explores; freezes; cries; hides face; acts curious, excited, apathetic, or anxious (describe).
   B. Adaptation.
      1. Exploration: when and how child begins exploring faces, toys, stranger.
      2. Reaction to transitions: from unstructured to structured activity; when examiner begins to play with infant; cleaning up; leaving.

III. **Self-Regulation**
   A. State regulation: an infant's state of consciousness ranges from deep sleep through alert stages to intense crying. Predominant state and range of states observed during session; patterns of transition, e.g., smooth versus abrupt; capacity for being soothed and self-soothing; capacity for quiet alert state. (Some of these categories also apply to toddlers.)
   B. Sensory regulation: reaction to sounds, sights, smells, light and firm touch; hyperresponsiveness or hyporesponsiveness (if observed) and type of response, including apathy, withdrawal, avoidance, fearfulness, excitability, aggression or marked behavioral change; excessive seeking of particular sensory input.
   C. Unusual behaviors: mouthing after 1 year of age; head banging; smelling objects, spinning; twirling; hand flapping; finger flicking; rocking; toe walking; staring at lights or spinning objects; repetitive, perseverative, or bizarre verbalizations or behaviors with objects or people; hair pulling; ruminating; or breath holding.
   D. Activity level: overall level and variability (note that toddlers are often incorrectly called hyperactive). Describe behavior, e.g., squirming constantly in parent's arms, sitting quietly on floor or in infant seat; constantly on the go; climbing on desk and cabinets; exploring the room; pausing to play with each of six to eight toys.
   E. Attention span: capacity to maintain attentiveness to an activity or interaction: longest and average length of sustained attention to a given toy or activity; distractibility. Infants: visual fixing and following at 1 month; tracking at 2 to 3 months; attention to own hands or feet and faces; duration of exploration of object with hands or mouth.
   F. Frustration tolerance: ability to persist in a difficult task, despite failure; capacity to delay reaction if easily frustrated, e.g., aggression crying, tantrums, withdrawal, avoidance.
   G. Aggression: modes of expression; degree of control of or preoccupation with aggression; appropriate assertiveness.

IV. **Motor**
Muscle tone and strength; mobility in different positions; unusual motor pattern, e.g., tics, seizure activity; intactness of cranial nerves, e.g., movement of face, mouth, tongue, and eyes, including feeding, swallowing, and gaze (note excessive drooling).
   A. Gross motor coordination. Infants: pushing up; head control; rolling; sitting; standing. Toddlers and preschoolers: walking; running; jumping; climbing; hopping; kicking; throwing and catching a ball. (It is useful to have something for the child to climb on, such as a chair.)
   B. Fine motor coordination. Infants: grasping and releasing; transferring from hand to hand; using pincer grasp; banging; throwing. Toddlers: using pincer grasp; stacking; scribbling; cutting. Both fine motor and visual–motor coordination can be screened by observing how the child handles puzzles, shape boxes, a ball and hammer toy, small cars, and toys with connecting parts.

V. **Speech and Language**
   A. Vocalization and speech production: quality, rate, rhythm, intonation, articulation, volume.
   B. Receptive language: comprehension of others' speech as seen in verbal or behavioral response, e.g., follows commands; points in response to "where is" questions; understands prepositions and pronouns. Include estimate of hearing, especially in child with language delay, e.g., response to loud sounds and voice; ability to localize sound.

TABLE 15.1. *Continued*

C. Expressive language: level of complexity, e.g., vocalization, jargon, number of single words, short phrases, full sentences; overgeneralization, e.g., uses "kitty" to refer to all animals: pronoun use including reversal; echolalia, either immediate or delayed; unusual or bizarre verbalizations. Preverbal children: communicative intent, e.g., vocalizations, babbling, imitation, gestures, such as head shaking and pointing; caregiver's ability to understand infant's communication; child's effectiveness in communication.

VI. Thought

The usual categories for thought disorder almost never apply to young children. Primary process thinking, as evidenced in verbalizations or play, is expected in this age group. The line between fantasy and reality is often blurred. Bizarre ideation; perseveration; apparent loose associations; and the persistence of pronoun reversals, jargon, and echolalia in an older toddler or preschooler may be noted in a variety of psychiatric disorders, including pervasive developmental disorders.

A. Specific fears: feared object; worry about being lost or separated from parent.

B. Dreams and nightmares: content is sometimes obtainable in children ages 2 to 3 years. Child does not always perceive it as a dream, e.g., "A monster came in the front door. "

C. Dissociative state: sudden episodes of withdrawal and inattention; eyes glazed: "tuned out"; failure to track ongoing social interaction. Dissociative state may be difficult to differentiate from an absence seizure, depression, autism, or deafness. The context may be helpful, e.g., child with a history of neglect freezes in a dissociative state as mother leaves room. Neurological or audiological evaluation may be warranted.

D. Hallucinations: extremely rare, except in the context of a toxic or organic disorder, then usually visual or tactile.

VII. Affect and Mood

The assessment of mood and affect may be more difficult in young children because of limited language, lack of vocabulary for emotions, and use of withdrawal in response to a variety of emotions from shyness and boredom to anxiety and depression.

A. Modes of expression: facial; verbal; body tone and positioning.

B. Range of expressed emotions, especially in parent–child relationship; predominant mood.

C. Responsiveness: to situation, content of discussion, play, and interpersonal engagement.

D. Duration of emotional state: need history or multiple observations; lability of affect.

E. Intensity of expressed affect, especially in parent–child relationship; affect regulation.

VIII. Play

Play is a primary mode of information gathering for all sections of the ITMSE. In very young children, play is especially useful in the evaluation of the child's cognitive and symbolic functioning, relatedness, and expression of affect. Themes of play are helpful in assessing older toddlers. The management and expression of aggression are assessed in play as in other areas of behavior. Play may be with toys or with the child's own or another's body, e.g., peek-a-boo, roughhousing; verbal, e.g., sound imitation games between mother and infant; interactional or solitary. It is important to note how the child's play varies with different familiar caregivers and with parents versus the examiner.

A. Structure of play (ages approximate).

  1. Sensorimotor play.

    a. (0–12 months): mouthing, banging, dropping and throwing toys or other objects.

    b. (6–12 months): exploring characteristics of objects, e.g., moving parts, poking, pulling.

  2. Functional play.

    a. (12–18 months): child's use of objects shows understanding and exploration of their use or function, e.g., pushes car, touches comb to hair, puts telephone to ear.

  3. Early symbolic play.

    a. (18 months and older): child pretends with increasing complexity; pretends with own body to eat or sleep; pretends with objects or other people, e.g., "feeds" mother; child uses one object to represent another, e.g., a block becomes a car; child pretends a sequence of activities, e.g., cooking and eating.

  4. Complex symbolic play.

    a. (30 months and older): child plans and acts out dramatic play sequences, uses imaginary objects. Later, child incorporates others into play with assigned roles.

  5. Imitation, turn taking, and problem solving as part of play.

(continued)

TABLE 15.1. *Continued*

VIII. Play (*cont.*)

B. Content of Play. The toddler's choice and use of toys often reflect emotional themes. It is desirable to have on hand toys that tap different developmental and emotional domains. An overfull playroom may be overwhelming or overstimulating and reduce meaningful observations. Young toddlers of both sexes often gravitate to dolls, dishes, animals, and moving toys, such as cars. The examiner's choice of specific materials may facilitate the expression of pertinent emotional themes. For example, a child traumatized by a dog bite may more likely reenact the trauma if a toy dog and doll figures are available. The child's reaction to scary toys, such as sharks, dinosaurs, or guns, should be noted, especially if they are avoided or dominate the session. Does aggressive pretend play become "real" and physically harmful? By age 2½ to 3 years, a child's animal or doll play can reveal important themes about family life, including reactions to separation, parent–child and sibling relationships, experiences at day care, quality of nurturance and discipline, and physical or sexual abuse. The examiner must use caution in interpreting play, viewing it as a possible combination of reenactment, fears, and fantasy.

IX. Cognition

Using information from all above areas, especially play, verbal and symbolic functioning, and problem solving, roughly assess child's cognitive level in terms of developmental intactness, delays, or precocity.

X. Relatedness

A. To parents: how "in tune" do the child and parent seem? Does the child make and maintain eye, verbal, or physical contact? Is there active avoidance by child? Note infant's level of comfort and relaxation being held, fed, "molding" into caregiver's body. Does toddler move away from caregiver and check back or bring toys to show, to put into his or her lap, to play with together or near caregiver? Comment on physical or verbal affection, hostility, reaction to separation and reunion, and use of transitional objects (blanket, toy, caregiver's possession). Describe differences in relating if more than one caregiver is present.

B. To examiner: young children normally show some hesitancy to engage with a stranger, especially after 6 to 8 months of age. Appropriate wariness in young children may result in a period of watching the examiner; staying physically close to a familiar caregiver before engaging; or showing some constriction of affect, vocalization or play. After initial wariness, does the child relate? Does the child engage too soon or not at all? How does relatedness with a stranger compare to that with a parent? Is the child friendly versus indiscriminately attention-seeking, guarded versus overanxious? Can examiner engage the child in play or structured activities to a degree not seen with caregiver? Does the child show pleasure in successes if the examiner shows approval?

C. Attachment behaviors: observe for showing affection, comfort seeking, asking for and accepting help, cooperating, exploring, controlling behavior, and reunion responses. Describe age-related disturbances in these normative behaviors. Disturbances often are seen in abused and neglected children, e.g., fearfulness, clinginess, overcompliance, hypervigilance, impulsive overactivity, and defiance: restricted or hyperactive and distractible exploratory behavior; and restricted or indiscriminate affection and comfort seeking.

Note. Adapted from American Academy of Child and Adolescent Psychiatry (1997). Copyright 1997 by the American Academy of Child and Adolescent Psychiatry. Adapted by permission from Lippincott Williams & Wilkins.

ers. Affect addresses qualitative aspects across different feeling states, such as appropriateness, depth or flatness, intensity, and lability of affect (Kaplan & Sadock, 1988). In the ITMSE, affect refers both to the qualitative properties of emotional expression and to specific emotions. In the examination of infants and young children, the clinician is usually describing the child's behavior and facial expressions and drawing inferences from the child's interactions and play themes to assess affect and mood. Only some young preschoolers can directly describe what

they are feeling. The clinician has an important role during play with 2- to 3-year-olds in asking how a given character is feeling. This is especially true during scenes in which dolls, animals, or puppets are interacting, but feelings can also be attributed to inanimate objects. For example, if a car is continually being crashed in a child's play, the clinician may ask, "How does that car feel?" The child may focus on angry or scared feelings, which can be explored further.

The clinician must be cautious when describing affect. The qualitative aspects of affective style can be described relatively clearly. Intensity of affective expression may reflect temperament and disposition, but it may be modified by the response from the caregiving environment. Inferences about specific emotions being experienced by the child should be linked to specific observations. For example, labeling a child "anxious" because he is overactive and distractible, and the clinician knows he has been experiencing escalating fighting between his parents, is an unsupported interpretation. The clinician must not describe the child as showing the affect the clinician thinks the child must be feeling. However, if this child becomes overactive and distractible when one parent is describing a recent altercation with the absent spouse, when tension between two parents obviously rises in the room, or when the child enacts a scene of fighting between family dolls, then the clinician can describe the basis for his inference of anxiety, even if the child appears excited and gleeful during this time.

Discrete Affects

Discrete affects are expressed and understood across cultures because of characteristic facial displays. Some affects can be observed in young infants, whose facial expressions include interest, joy, distress, disgust, and surprise (Izard, 1978). Early expressions of interest in sights, sounds, and people and of pleasure, including the social smile at 2 to 3 months, are usually balanced by expressions of distress. Over time, expressions of distress, initially read by caregivers in terms of specific needs (baby is hungry, wet, cold, tired, alone), become more clearly differentiated into expressions of the specific emotions of fear, anger, and sadness. Expressions of fear, for example, emerge in facial display only at 6 months (Cicchetti & Sroufe, 1978). Fearful expressions come to prominence at 6 to 9 months with the onset of stranger anxiety and separation anxiety. The clinician may invite the parents to join as coobservers of the infant's expressions, "wondering along" with parents about their meaning (Clark, Paulson, & Conlin, 1993). This may elicit parent representations of the child, as well as focusing attention on the infant's experience. It is my experience that parents of clinically referred young children often have difficulty differentiating the "negative" emotions of fear, anger, and sadness in their children. A fearful facial expression, if followed by aggressive behavior, is often missed, and the parent labels the child "angry." The clinician also should look at the clarity of the child's signaling of emotion in trying to tease out the intrinsic versus interactional aspects of disturbances in this area.

Affect in Relationships

Affect regulation is considered a central aspect of infant–parent relationships (Emde, 1989). "Affect regulation and sharing on the infant's side are enabled by empathic responsiveness on the caregiver's side . . . regulation of affect is especially important for adaptation; the infant must be guided to avoid the extremes of excitement, distress, and withdrawing" (Emde, 1989, p. 37). The clinician not only looks at how the infant's mood varies within a session but also at how interaction between infant and caregiver seems to help the infant in attaining a variety of positive emotional states (including interest and happiness) and in controlling or modulating the distressing affective states as they are triggered, as in separation and reunion. Sometimes infant–caregiver interaction seems to have little effect (the caregiver does not animate or soothe the infant) or to have a dysregulating effect (interactions are accompanied by rising distress in the infant).

The clinician may wish to take an active role in evaluation of affect regulation when the range of affect observed in the young child is narrow or when there is a predominantly negative affective state in the child. The clinician can ask the parent to "see if you can get your baby really excited and interested." A baby or toddler can also be wooed by the clinician using interesting toys or making funny faces or noises to elicit interest, pleasure, and brightness if this has not been seen. Affect regulation is a key part of parent–infant regulation, but Stern argues that affects also have invariant qualities that are part of the young infant's development of a sense of self. "Affects belong to the self, not to the person who may elicit them" (Stern, 1985, p. 90).

Appearance (ITMSE Section I)

Children with defects in single genes leading to metabolic disorders and those with chromosomal abnormalities often present with varying degrees of mental retardation. In addition, both groups may show physical abnormalities, including unusual head size and shape (usually microcephaly), cutaneous abnormalities, and dysmorphic features. The face itself or body parts such as eyes, nose, ears, hands, feet, fingers, and genitalia may be affected by having an unusual shape or position (e.g., low-set ears). Some genetic anomalies, such as Trisomy 21, and syndromes related to prenatal toxins such as fetal alcohol syndrome, have characteristic, well-known physical features. Many genetic abnormalities have a range of clinical presentations, and some syndromes have associated medical findings. Unusually small size, low weight, and/or low weight-to-height ratio should alert the clinician to consider failure to thrive or other medical conditions, in consultation with the child's pediatrician.

Apparent Reaction to Situation (ITMSE Sections IIA and IIB; XC)

The child's initial reactions provide an important window on aspects of normal variation such as temperament and secure-base behavior, as well as possible areas of disturbance. In an assessment, the child is exposed to a new setting, new people, and new toys. This mild stress often triggers attachment behaviors, such as going to the parent or clinging. Sometime later, with the reassurance of parental presence, the child usually feels safe enough to explore the environment. Exploration in a new setting is an important infant–toddler mechanism for learning and may be a sign of self-confidence or even recklessness. The balance between attachment behaviors and exploration in toddlers is key to understanding the child's ability to use the attachment figure as a "secure base" (Ainsworth, 1967) for exploration and a "safe haven" (Bretherton, 1980) for comfort and reassurance (Zeanah, Mamman, & Lieberman, 1993). Disturbances in "secure-base behavior" are one red flag to the clinician to assess further for an attachment disorder (see Zeanah & Boris, Chapter 22, this volume).

Temperament refers to individual differences in behavioral style, believed to be the product of constitutional variables in ongoing interaction with the child's environment (Chess & Thomas, 1989). This section of the ITMSE asks for observations about approach–withdrawal and adaptation, two of the nine dimensions of temperament studied by Chess and Thomas, which characterized the three most common types of child temperament in their sample.

"Easy" children showed predominantly approach to a new stimulus and adaptability. "Slow to warm up" children were both withdrawing and slow to adapt, and "Difficult" children showed withdrawal and did not adapt over time. Difficult children are highly represented in clinical samples. Slow-to-warm-up children, who may be misdiagnosed with an anxiety disorder, often cling to the parent initially and do little physical exploring. Such children often explore the playroom with visual scanning but may fuss and require soothing if pressed to interact too soon.

The child's reaction to a new environment can have many other explanations. The overtired or physically ill child may continue to be distressed and trying to leave throughout the first session yet look very different in subsequent visits. The child's behavior may turn out to be relationship mediated, if he presents differently when with another caregiver. A parent who is particularly anxious about the assessment of the child may communicate this nonverbally to an attuned child, who then reacts initially with withdrawal. This child may adapt well once he and the parent relax.

Self-Regulation (ITMSE Section III)

The ITMSE groups, under Self-Regulation, a wide variety of capacities that develop during early childhood. These capacities move the child toward greater self-control, organization of behavior, and engagement with the animate and inanimate world. They are both intrinsic to the child and subject to mediation or facilitation by the caregiving environment. One of the early manifestations of self-regulation is a baby's development of homeostasis in the first months of life. This involves modulation of physiological states, including sleep–wake and hunger–satiety cycles, and his learning of self-calming and emotional modulation. The infant must learn to take an interest in the world while simultaneously regulating his arousal and his responses to sensory stimulation (Greenspan, 1992; DeGangi & Breinbauer, 1997).

Self-regulation tasks move quickly beyond physiological stability to many other capacities as the infant learns to cope with and embrace stimulation through all senses and especially in human interaction. Areas such as activity level, attention span, frustration tolerance, and aggression are an increasing focus of parental attention through the first 2 to 3 years of a child's life. These capacities exhibit innate differences, a normal developmental trajectory toward greater self-regulation, and a vulnerability to disruption from both physical stressors (e.g., prematurity and prenatal cocaine exposure) and psychosocial ones (e.g., poor parent limit setting, abuse, trauma, or lack of parental engagement). This section of the ITMSE focuses the clinician's attention on observable behaviors in the infant which relate to regulation, without attempting to delineate etiology or the degree to which such capacities are interpersonally mediated.

State Regulation (Section IIIA)

State regulation is the newborn infant's ability to regulate his level of arousal in the face of internal and external stimulation. The clinician can often observe a young infant's state changes during a single session. The infant passes regularly through six "states," described as states of consciousness (Brazelton, 1973) and behavioral states (Needleman, 1996). These are quiet (deep) sleep, active (rapid-eye-movement) sleep, drowsy, alert, fussy (active), and crying. In the alert state, infants are best able to focus attention on a source of stimulation such as auditory and visual stimuli. The infant's availability for interpersonal interaction and for learning is maximal in the alert state. Thus, the baby's capacity to maintain an alert state in response to arousal and stimulation, without becoming distressed, is an important aspect of his readiness for social interaction. The ability to self-calm, to return from a state of higher arousal to quiet alertness, also involves state regulation.

A baby's degree of state lability reflects on his capacity for self-organization. Some parents report smooth and predictable state transitions, as when the child awakens from sleep. The baby who goes rapidly from deep sleep to a distressed state (crying) is much more stressful for the parent than the baby who moves slowly and smoothly from deep sleep to a quiet alert state and coos and smiles when he sees mom. The baby who spends much of his awake time fussing and crying has fewer opportunities to develop games that involve reciprocal smiling or imitation of sounds and facial expressions. Such games are important in cementing the parents' sense of specialness and connection with their baby. The clinician's observations, which identify difficult patterns of state regulation, can be used to reframe the parents' concerns from "what is wrong with my parenting," or "my baby is always angry (unhappy, dissatisfied)," toward mobilizing efforts to support the infant's development of homeostasis.

Sensory Regulation (ITMSE Section IIIB)

Sensory regulation is the infant's capacity to experience and process sensory input, at the same time maintaining a stable state and maintaining the capacity to be engaged and attentive. The clinician may easily miss disturbances in sensory regulation unless attuned to observe this area of functioning. Infants may be hypersensitive or hyposensitive to both physical and emotional stimulation. Physical stimulation occurs in the visual, auditory, tactile (both touch and texture), and temperature senses. Emotional stimuli can be both internal and external in origin. Some babies are easily overstimulated, perhaps because of temperament, from prematurity, or as the result of a prenatal influence such as maternal drug use. These infants are so overwhelmed by simultaneous holding, feeding, and making eye contact that they do not feed but cry instead, until the amount of stimulation is greatly decreased. There are many presumed mechanisms and etiologies of fussy babies, which are not reviewed here. One example, sensory hypersensitivity, can often be checked by the clinician by observing the changes in an irritable infant after lowering the lights and getting the parent to talk softly to the infant. The transformation of a fussy baby who has rejected all attempts to soothe, feed, or distract into a quiet, alert, observing baby is dramatic to parent and clinician. Sensory regulation can be further evaluated by a parent report checklist (DeGangi, Poisson, Sickel, & Wiener, 1995) and/or an examination of sensory functions (DeGangi & Greenspan, 1989).

Difficulty in sensory regulation is an important component of the regulatory disorders, a diverse group of clinical disturbances in infants, toddlers, and young prechoolers described in the *Diagnostic Classification: 0–3* (DC:0–3) (Zero to Three, 1994). Children with auditory hypersensitivity may be hyperalert to sounds outside the playroom (obviously here the category overlaps with distractibility) or may begin to cry when exposed to loud sounds. Hypersensitive children may cover their eyes or ears to ward off light or sounds that seem perfectly unremarkable to the clinician. In a busy child-care setting, the clinician may observe children with tactile hypersensitivity who try to shield themselves by withdrawal or by angry and aggressive pushing away of peers and adults who come too close. Hyposensitive children may crave sensory input and crash their bodies into people or objects or repeatedly jump on furniture. Disturbances presenting as disruptive behaviors in young children should alert the clinician to evaluate sensory regulation as a possible contributing factor (J. M. Thomas, 1995).

Activity Level, Attention Span, and Frustration Tolerance (ITMSE Sections IIID, IIIE, IIIF)

Observations of activity level, attention span, and frustration tolerance (or persistence) are useful both for assessing aspects of temperamental style (Thomas & Chess, 1977) and for delineating areas of difficulty seen in a variety of clinical syndromes. Difficulties with activity level, impulsivity, attention span, and frustration tolerance often cluster together but may exist separately.

Activity level refers to the child's general arousal as it is manifested in the motoric system (Goldsmith & Campos, 1982). Activity level shows wide variations in "normal" babies and toddlers (Brazelton, 1969; Lieberman, 1993). Although many parents describe their toddlers as "hyperactive," only some toddlers are constantly running, climbing, or moving from area to area. Constant "fidgity" movements of arms or legs may be observed when an overactive child is sitting at a table playing with an object. The hypoactive baby or toddler likewise stands out because he moves very little in space. Low activity level may be distinguished from weakness or low muscle tone by enticing the child to reach for an attractive object or to get up from the floor. True difficulty in movement is revealed once the child tries to move. Some children remain glued to their mother's side because of shyness and anxiety.

True hyperactivity, sometimes described as "bouncing off the walls," may suggest an early form of attention-deficit/hyperactivity disorder (ADHD) (American Psychiatric Association, 1994), especially when associated with short attention span, distractibility, and impulsivity, or it may be part of a regulatory disorder (Zero to Three, 1994). However, young children who have been traumatized may also exhibit high arousal with hyperactivity, poor attention span and concentration, and irritability with low frustration tolerance or impulsivity (J. M. Thomas, 1995; J. M. Thomas & Tidmarsh, 1997).

Attention span, or the child's ability to focus attention on a given activity, is revealed spontaneously by the child's pattern of focus across a session. There are no norms for "appropriate" attention span, which may vary with many factors including age, setting, time of the day, and type or intensity of stimuli (Linder, 1993). Attention span may refer to quiet watching (e.g., a baby watching a mobile) or active engagement in a form of play or tabletop activity. The clinician can sometimes elicit a much longer attention span by engaging the child using an interesting activity, toy, or interpersonal style. Blowing soap bubbles captures the attention of most children from a few months through preschool age, including shy and withdrawn children, highly active and distractible children, and avoidant or autistic children. The clinician may then be able to move to other toys or play activities. The child's ability to attend to structured tasks may be different from self-chosen activities or physical play. Attention span may also be interrupted by sensory stimuli in a hypersensitive child.

The setting may influence a child's behavior greatly in the areas of activity level, attention span, and distractibility. Large playrooms with a dazzling array of toys can elicit distractible "flitting" behavior from many normal children, especially those who do not have access to many toys. In a less stimulating environment the child may demonstrate a wider range of behavior, more meaningful interaction with both clinician and parent, and more sustained play sequences.

Frustration tolerance refers to the child's ability to persist at an activity that is difficult for him. Many children are referred for the behavioral *result* of low frustration tolerance (tantrums, crying, or aggressive acts). By close observation, the clinician should try to delineate the context and associated behaviors. A child can become frustrated as a result of the nature of the activity (e.g., taking off the lid of a container which is tightly attached), the child's own skill level in the motor domain, or his interactions with others. The highly reactive, easily frustrated child may be able to attend and persist in trying a task or completing a play activity if the clinician provides quiet support, structuring, and engagement. Conversely, the clinician can "test" for frustration tolerance, if stresses have not arisen spontaneously in parent–child play, by introducing periods of structured activity, such as puzzles or a shape-sorting box. Difficulties in communication may tax a child's frustration tolerance. Tantrums and irritability are often provoked by a child's inability to communicate his wishes or needs to a caregiver. Failures of communication may have components arising in child, caregiver, or both.

Aggression (ITMSE Sections III and VIII)

The clinician must be attuned to the wide cultural variations in what is considered acceptable, normal, or desirable in the range from assertive to aggressive behavior. Aggressive themes may be seen in the emerging symbolic play of the toddler or in the more complex symbolic play of the young preschooler. Toddlers and young preschoolers engage in a variety of behaviors which others interpret as aggressive, including biting, hitting, kicking, throwing, and grabbing. These behaviors may be evident in interactions with the parents and peers or may be seen in the child's use of play materials. Other young children show a marked lack of aggressive behavior or play. Much of this behavior is "normal." Aggressive behavior is a frequent complaint in the presentations of older toddlers and young preschoolers. The clinician looks for the types of aggression, context of aggressive behavior and fantasy, and the child's management of and reactions to internal and external aggressive stimuli. The clinician may need to take an active role with the child to explore this issue fully.

Types of Aggression

Clinically, we can think of young children's aggression as territorial, defensive, impulsive, or deliberate. Developmentally typical toddler behavior includes what might be called territorial aggression. The toddler grabs a toy he wants and he pushes away or hits another child or adult who seeks to take an object he prizes at that moment. Most parents see this as a stage in socialization to be worked through. Clinically relevant disturbances in the parent–child sphere can be observed (1) when the parent overinterprets malevolent intent in this normal period or reacts with aggression toward the child and (2) when the parent sets no limits or ineffective

limits on this behavior. Then, the clinician may see territorial aggression persisting in a 2- to 4-year-old who does not use verbal strategies, help seeking, or other forms of negotiation instead of striking out. Family sessions with siblings or preschool observations usually reveal the behavior of such children if it does not occur spontaneously in initial clinical contacts. Language or cognitive delays can be associated with such aggression, or the clinician may observe that a young child's usually adequate language "fails" him at moments of affective arousal.

A defensive form of aggression may be observed in children with sensory hypersensitivities. Children with tactile defensiveness often hit or push away peers when they come too close physically, which may occur in group transition times, circle time, or regular play. This pattern is often missed in a clinical evaluation setting but is revealed during observation in the child's day care or preschool. Some children who have been the target of frequent aggressive acts by adults or peers will strike out first in response to minor threats or provocations.

The impulsive, nonangry, hitting out by a young child with ADHD often looks like a mistake, whereas angry, focused, deliberate hurting behavior toward others looks quite different. With deliberate aggression, affect is intense and the child looks angry in a persistent or pervasive manner. Much of the child's play alone or with others is dominated by crashing, throwing, kicking down blocks (in a toddler), and/or by aggressive and destructive themes in the child with symbolic play. This group of children is of special clinical concern in their apparently deliberate, aggressive intent. Such children may appear to be flooded with aggressive fantasy.

Aggression in Play (ITMSE IIIG)

A majority of young children will gleefully knock down towers of blocks and make toy figures such as lions roar, dinosaurs attack, or soldiers go "bang bang." The child's degree of self control with such toys has a developmental progression. One expects the line between "make believe" and "real" to get blurry in this age group at times. The clinician observes several aspects of play: (1) Does such "aggressive" play predominate, constituting most of what the child chooses to do? (2) Do aggressive themes invade all kinds of play, (e.g., doctor play focuses only on jabbing with the needle, family doll or animal play involves fighting, building is only for the purpose of knocking down or "blowing up," feeding a doll becomes force feeding), or does the child show a range of play? (3) When using a clearly aggressive toy stimulus, such as a toy crocodile, wolf, or shark, does the child move from having it pretend to attack to actually hunting the examiner? Is the child unable to stop when reminded to "pretend?"

Aggressive Toys

The "aggressive" toy is an important piece of equipment for assessing young children. I recommend a soft puppet or stuffed animal with a big mouth and soft teeth as a useful but safe play stimulus. Recognizable "characters" from popular movies or television shows are less useful because they carry their own stories. The clinician can initiate play by showing the child the "aggressive" toy if he has not been drawn to it. While the clinician never wants to frighten the child or to become a threatening figure, 2- to 3-year-olds who have an idea of make-believe should have some coping mechanisms, including the use of the parent for reassurance. The child's use of the parent and the parent's response to such play is revealing.

The "aggressive" toy may elicit a wide range of the child's developing ego strengths and coping mechanisms. The child may declare that the crocodile "is really nice" or is going to make friends. He may put the aggressive animal under control in some way, giving it to an adult, putting it "in jail" or in "time out" if it has "bitten." He may lecture it on proper behavior. He may enact the powerful, scary animal himself. The clinician may invite the child to wonder about or explain what makes the alligator feel "bitey," angry, or sad and alone.

A Frightened Response to Aggression

A child may alternate between interest in aggressive-looking toys and sudden anxiety. Many young children in this age range identify a "toothy" puppet as "the monster." This opens up fruitful discussions with the child about "monsters" at home who make him afraid to go to bed or who awaken him at night. Parents who have discounted such fears may develop new insights and sensitivity into (1) the cause of sleep problems, (2) normal developmental stages, and (3) the effect of movies, TV, older siblings' scare tactics, or other environmental stressors from which the child needs protection or shielding. The clinician may want to explore questions of abuse when a child responds to an aggressive stimulus with intense fearfulness.

Developmental Status (Sections IV, V, VIII, and IX)

Although all areas of a young child's functioning are part of his developmental status, the areas of cognition, motor functioning, and speech and language have specific, widely accepted norms and structured assessment procedures. A child with clear developmental delays may benefit from such assessments to delineate delays, deficits, and disturbances in functioning for which specific therapies exist. Some publicly funded programs require such testing to qualify for intervention. Considerable controversy about the value of traditional norm-referenced testing and other structured tests for very young children (Meisels & Fenichel, 1996) has focused attention on the value of observation of the child in spontaneous interaction with his parent, and on the importance of eliciting the child's best functioning. The ITMSE addresses the areas to observe in clinical consideration of developmental status. The clinician should be sufficiently familiar with early child development to use this exam as a mental checklist in deciding whether a child is showing delays, unusual patterns, particular abilities, or wide variation in these skills. Clinicians may find Linder's *Transdisciplinary Play Based Assessment* (1993) useful for detailed age norms and observational strategies.

The infant mental health clinician is presented with a wide variety of children. Developmental status may be an overt concern. Developmental issues may also serve as a ticket of admission for parents who have wider underlying concerns. For example, a parent may bring his child for evaluation of delayed speech, when he is even more worried about his child's interpersonal avoidance and other signs of possible autism. Conversely, disruptive behavior, such as hitting or tantrums, may be the parent's dominant concern, whereas the clinician will note delayed language and the child's frustration in trying hard to communicate.

Cognition (ITMSE IX)

Cognitive development involves many domains. Some areas of cognitive development which can be observed in a play session with 0- to 3-year-olds include attention to the child's type and level of play, problem solving, and imitation. Categories of play develop both sequentially and as overlapping layers, in that earlier forms of play are often preserved even after the child develops more complex forms of play. Play generally moves developmentally from the concrete (e.g., exploration of objects with hands and mouth) to the abstract (symbolic or dramatic play in which the child pretends to do something or to be someone). Expressive language develops in a similar progression from the concrete (single nouns) to the abstract (concepts). Both language and play development reflect the child's increasing capacity to represent experience in a symbolic form. (see Section VIII, and Linder, 1993). Children with global delays tend to exhibit play which is at a level typical of a younger child. However, some children in the pervasive developmental disorder spectrum show a discrepancy, with level of play being lower than other cognitive skills.

Early problem solving, such as object permanence (knowing how to find an object when it is hidden from view), occurs in the sensorimotor stage of play, about 9 to 12 months. The young toddler's (12–18 months) use of problem-solving skills, which involve understanding the relationship between actions and consequences, can be observed in his play with objects such as pop-up boxes, which require the child to push a button or the lever to open a door on the toy.

Imitation is considered a cognitive skill because it is one of the primary means by which children learn. A baby's physical and vocal imitation can be observed in the first year, especially in parent–infant play. The child develops more facility for imitation in the second year. When he can perform the imitation mentally, the child has the capacity for deferred imitation, which is the basis of symbolic or dramatic play. The clinician can look at a child's play as it presents spontaneously first and then determine what can be elicited by imitation. This will capture not only his current functioning but also the child's emerging skills.

Motor (ITMSE IV)

The toddler's movement in space may occur spontaneously on or around the parent's body, as he crawls, climbs up to his mother's lap, runs away, and carries toys back to her. Little equipment is needed to elicit most of a young child's gross motor repertoire. Babies should be observed down on a blanket on the floor for part of the session.

Young children should be observed in spontaneous activities for basic muscle strength or weakness, left to right symmetry in movement and body appearance, and motor functioning, impairment, or paralysis. Depending on age, the child should be enticed to roll, crawl, walk, and climb onto or over an obstacle and up and down stairs to allow for such observations. Games of throwing or kicking a soft ball and jumping or hopping usually capture the cooperation of children of this age. The child's handling of all toys, but especially of small objects, "manipulatives," and a pen (for preschoolers), will demonstrate strengths and weaknesses in fine motor skills.

Speech and Language (ITMSE V)

Spontaneous interactions with the parent are the most likely to elicit both language and other communication strategies, such as gestures and vocalizations, from a young child. A child may be preverbal because of his age (under 12–18 months) or because of language delay or disturbance in older toddlers and preschoolers. Careful observations will reveal the infant's attempts to communicate with the caregiver in the preverbal stages through, for example, pointing, giving, reaching, head nods or shakes, and protesting (Wetherby & Prizant, 1996). Verbal children's language should be observed for its pragmatics, the useful and social aspects of language for communication (Bates, 1976; Linder, 1993). Paucity of communicative attempts in a preverbal child or poor pragmatics in a verbal child may suggest an autism spectrum disorder. A child with a more circumscribed communication disorder (American Psychiatric Association, 1994) usually shows more consistent efforts to communicate.

CLINICAL EXAMPLE

Mark, a 34-month-old child who was born prematurely at 26 weeks gestation, with many postnatal complications, showed excellent communication despite delayed speech with motor impairments. His mother's attentive facilitation supported his experience of successful conversation. Mark: "ow" (*pointing*)—Mom "you went outside?" Mark: "Da . . . d"—Mom "with daddy?" Mark:

"(*engine noise*)"—Mom: "you went out while Daddy mowed the lawn." Mark beamed. Each word or gesture was painfully slow or awkward, but turn-taking and nonverbal communication were intact. Mutual pleasure and feelings of success were evident.

Communication is a mutual process between parent and child. Unrecognized delays in receptive or expressive language may impair the child's ability to understand others and to make himself understood. Sometimes the parent has difficulty "reading" the child or is a poor communicative partner for the infant because of depression, preoccupation, withdrawal, or lack of attuned attention to the child. It is the clinician's role to identify the parent's difficulty for possible further evaluation and intervention. Evaluation by a speech and language pathologist is often needed to delineate communication delays and disturbances in the child for diagnosis and intervention planning. (see Prizant, Wetherby, & Roberts, Chapter 17, this volume).

CONCLUSION

Clinical assessment is a complex and creative process that links clinician and parents in a mutual search for understanding about a child and his family. The ITMSE is presented as a guide that may help the clinician to observe the young child carefully in multiple domains, to organize her observations, and to communicate those observations both to the family and to other professionals. The process of formulation is that part of assessment when history, observations, testing, and the clinician's judgment are all integrated into an understanding that makes sense to both family and professional. The "Methods and Meaning of the ITMSE" section attempts to aid clinicians both in the process of making useful observations and in weighing one piece of data against another to develop a formulation. When the clinician includes the parents in the process of observation and inquiry, the evaluation process becomes an opportunity to "co-construct" (Emde, 1994) new narratives, or understandings, of the child and his family.

ACKNOWLEDGMENTS

I wish to thank Carol Slotnick, PhD, for her invaluable help in the revisions of the Infant and Toddler Mental Status Exam and of this chapter, and Marina Zelenko, MD, and Caroline Wood, MSW, for their reviews of an earlier draft of this chapter.

REFERENCES

Ainsworth, M. D. S. (1967). *Infancy in Uganda: Infant care and the growth of love*. Baltimore: Johns Hopkins University Press.

Ainsworth, M. D. S., Blehar, M. C., Waters, E., & Wall, S. (1978). *Patterns of attachment: A psychological study of the strange situation*. Hillsdale, NJ: Erlbaum.

American Academy of Child and Adolescent Psychiatry. (1995). Practice parameters for the psychiatric assessment of children and adolescents. *Journal of the American Academy of Child and Adolescent Psychiatry, 34*, 1386–1402.

American Academy of Child and Adolescent Psychiatry (1997). Practice parameters for the psychiatric assessment of infants and toddlers (0–36 months). *Journal of the American Academy of Child and Adolescent Psychiatry, 36*, 215–365.

American Psychiatric Association. (1994). *Diagnostic and Statistical Manual of Mental Disorders* (4th ed.). Washington, DC: Author.

Bates, E. (1976). *Language and context: The acquisition of pragmatics*. New York: Academic Press.

Brazelton, T. B. (1969). *Infants and mothers: Differences in development*. New York: Dell.

Brazelton, T. B. (1973). Neonatal Behavioral Assessment Scale. *Clinics in Developmental Medicine, 50*.

Bretherton, I. (1980). Young children in stressful situations. In G. V. Coelho & P. Ahmed (Eds.), *Uprooting and development*. New York: Plenum.

Chess, S., & Thomas, A. (1989). Issues in the clinical application of temperament. In G. S. Kohnstamm, J. E. Bates, & M. K. Rothbart (Eds.), *Temperament in childhood*, (pp. 377–386). New York: Wiley.

Cicchetti, D., & Sroufe, L. A. (1978). An organizational view of affect: Illustration from the study of Down's Syndrome infants. In M. Lewis & L. Rosenblum (Eds.), *The development of affect*. New York: Plenum.

Clark, R., Paulson, A., & Conlin, S. (1993). Assessment of developmental status and parent–infant relationships: The therapeutic process of evaluation. In C. H. Zeanah, Jr. (Ed.), *Handbook of infant mental health* (pp. 191–209). New York: Guilford Press.

Crowell, J. A., & Fleischmann, M. A. (1993). Use of structured research procedures in clinical assessment of infants. In C. H. Zeanah, Jr. (Ed.), *Handbook of infant mental health* (pp. 210–221). New York: Guilford Press.

DeGangi, G. A., & Breinbauer, C. (1997). The symptomatology of infants and toddlers with regulatory disorders. *Journal of Developmental and Learning Disorders, 1(1)*, 183–215.

DeGangi, G. A., & Greenspan, S. I. (1989). *The test of sensory functions in infants*. Los Angeles, CA: Western Psychological Services.

DeGangi, G. A., Poisson, S., Sickel, R. Z., & Wiener, A. S. (1995). The Infant–Toddler Symptom Checklist. Tucson, AZ: Therapy Skill Builders.

Emde, R. N. (1989). The infant's relationship experience: Developmental and affective aspects. In A. J. Sameroff & R. N. Emde (Eds.), *Relationship disturbances in early childhood: A developmental approach* (pp. 33–52). New York: Basic Books.

Emde, R. N. (1994). Developing psychoanalytic representations of experience. *Infant Mental Health Journal, 15(1)*, 42–49.

Goldsmith, H., & Campos, J. (1982). Toward a theory of infant temperament. In R. M. Emde & R. J. Harmon (Eds.), *Advances in Infant Behavior and Development.* Hillsdale, NJ: Erlbaum.

Greenspan, S. I. (1992). *Infancy and early childhood: The practice of clinical assessment and intervention with emotional and developmental challenges.* Madison, CT: International Universities Press.

Izard, C. E. (1978). On the ontogenesis of emotions and emotion–cognition relationship in infancy. In M. Lewis & L. A. Rosenblum (Eds.), *The development of affect.* New York: Plenum.

Kaplan, H. I., & Sadock, B. J. (Eds.). (1988). *Synopsis of psychiatry: Behavioral sciences, clinical psychiatry* (6th ed.). Baltimore: Williams & Wilkins.

Lieberman, A. F. (1993). *The emotional life of the toddler.* New York: Free Press.

Linder, T. W. (1993). *Transdisciplinary play-based assessment: A functional approach to working with young children* (rev. ed.). Baltimore: Brookes.

Meisels, S. J., & Fenichel, E. (Eds.). (1996). *New visions for the developmental assessment of infants and young children.* Washington, DC: Zero to Three, National Center for Infants, Toddlers, and Families.

Needleman, R. D. (1996). The newborn. In R. E. Behrman, R. M. Kliegman, & A. M. Arvin (Eds.), *Textbook of pediatrics* (15th ed.). Philadelphia: W. B. Saunders.

Sameroff, A. J., & Chandler, M. J. (1975). Reproductive risk and the continuum of caretaking casualty. In F. D. Horowitz, E. M. Hetherington, S. Scarr-Salapatek, & G. Siegal (Eds.), *Review of child development research* (Vol. 4, pp. 187–244). Chicago: University of Chicago.

Simmons, J. E. (1985). *Psychiatric examination of children* (4th ed.). Philadelphia: Lea & Febiger.

Stern, D. N. (1985). *The interpersonal world of the infant.* New York: Basic Books.

Thomas, A., & Chess, S. (1977). *Temperament and development.* New York: Brunner/Mazel.

Thomas, J. M. (1995). Traumatic stress disorder presents as hyperactivity and disruptive behavior: Case presentation, diagnosis and treatment. *Infant Mental Health Journal, 16(4)*, 306–317.

Thomas, J. M., & Tidmarsh, L. (1997). Hyperactive and disruptive behaviors in very young children: Diagnosis and intervention. *Infants and Young Children, 9*, 46–55.

Wetherby, A. M., & Prizant, B. M. (1996). Toward earlier identification of communication and language problems in infants and young children. In S. J. Meisels & E. Fenichel (Eds.), *New visions for the developmental assessment of infants and young children* (pp. 289–312). Washington, DC: Zero to Three, National Center for Infants Clinical Programs.

Zeanah, C. H., Jr., Mamman, O. K., & Lieberman, A. F. (1993). Disorders of attachment. In C. H. Zeanah, Jr. (Ed.), *Handbook of infant mental health* (pp. 332–349). New York: Guilford Press.

Zero to Three, National Center for Clinical Infant Programs. (1994). *Diagnostic Classification: 0–3. Diagnostic classification of mental health and developmental disorders of infancy and early childhood.* Arlington, VA: Author.

IV

PSYCHOPATHOLOGY

❖

Psychopathology in infancy is a disturbing topic. Babies are designed to be appealing, typically conjuring up thoughts of renewed beginnings and hopes for the future. Associating serious psychiatric symptomatology with very young children runs counter to the images we typically generate. We wonder whether it is more useful to suppose that infants may be at risk for subsequent psychopathology rather than already experiencing it. Part II considered various risk factors of infancy related to subsequent adverse outcomes, whereas Part IV considers infants who are not merely at risk for subsequent difficulties but who already are manifesting them. In my experience, the discomfort that many of us feel in thinking about psychopathology in infancy often impedes recognition of serious problems and access to treatment for young children in need.

Still, given what we know about infancy, aren't there unique features of psychopathology in the first 3 years of life? Zeanah, Boris, and Scheeringa (1997) suggested several differences between psychopathology in the early years and later in childhood and adolescence. First, measurement problems are inherently more complex, because infants and toddlers cannot report on their own subjective experience. Second, infants are constantly changing, as development proceeds at a pace unprecedented in the life cycle. This constant change must be reconciled with the immutability of psychopathology and clearly affects how it is conceptualized. We do not yet have systems of classification that are sufficiently developmental in nature. Finally, infants develop in a relationship context, and this is inextricably linked with most forms of psychopathology in the early years. The primary caregiving relationship mediates and moderates the effects of risk factors on development even more profoundly in infancy than with older children or adolescents.

This volume, and particularly this section, takes a strong stand not only that psychopathology occurs in infancy but also that "disorders" are a useful way to conceptualize putative disturbances. Many of the disorders considered in this section are unproven, and the authors of the chapters are often circumspect about how useful the "disorder" approach is likely to prove. Of course, the same may be said about many of the disorders described in DSM-IV (American Psychiatric Association, 1994), ICD-10 (World Health Organization, 1992), and DC: 0–3 (Zero to Three, 1994) as they apply to young children. Nevertheless, the area of disorders of infancy is currently being actively investigated and discussed, and the authors and I hope these chapters will prove stimulating in that regard.

The first three chapters in Part IV cover the developmental disorders of infancy. In part because they have been extensively studied and in part because their symptoms are more readily described by quantitative tests, they are less controversial as disorders than others described in subsequent chapters in this section.

In Chapter 16, Walters and Blane provide an overview of many issues that arise in diagnosing and treating infants and young children with mental retardation. They emphasize a parent–professional partnership that begins with diagnosis in early childhood and continues through intervention efforts across the life span. They also note that intervention focuses on family understanding and acceptance, and they advocate for understanding the disorder in context.

Prizant, Wetherby, and Roberts note increasing opportunities for infant mental health clinicians and speech and language therapists to work collaboratively on issues related to early childhood communication disorders in Chapter 17. They begin by providing an overview of the development of language as it unfolds typically in the first 3 years of life. They identify precursors and sequella of communication problems in early childhood, and they enumerate essential principles of assessment and intervention. They conclude by describing implications of these principles for infant mental health.

In Chapter 18, Koenig, Rubin, Klin, and Volkmar provide an overview of the pervasive developmental disorders (PDDs). They begin by noting the essential features of this heterogeneous group of disorders united by the pervasiveness of disturbances in multiple domains of functioning. Given that these disorders are readily apparent in the first 3 years of life, the authors note the irony that our knowledge of autism and the PDDs in infants and very young children remains limited in important respects. Their review makes clear that studying infants and young children with autism has important implications not only for practice but also for our understanding the course of early child development.

Barton and Robins, in Chapter 19, describe the more controversial concept of regulatory disorders. This diagnostic construct, introduced by Greenspan and his colleagues (Greenspan & Weider, 1993), describes putative disorders involving difficulties in the regulation of affect and attention associated with irregularities in sensory processing. The latter are presumed to derive from individual differences in underlying neurobiological characteristics. Barton and Robins note that there is relatively little research on the construct of regulatory disorder itself, but they draw on emerging data on sensory processing and sensory integration that they believe may implicate sensory processing difficulties in the genesis of some behavioral problems in young children.

Continuing the theme of disturbances of regulation, Anders, Goodlin-Jones, and Sadeh, in Chapter 20, consider problems with sleep and rhythmic processes. After reviewing briefly the development of states in infants, they then review the presentation of infant and toddler sleep–wake disturbances. They conclude by proposing a new multiaxial scheme to classify sleep problems in infants and toddlers based on their own clinical and research experiences.

In Chapter 21, Benoit describes feeding disorders, failure to thrive, and obesity as other common regulatory problems of infancy. She notes that these problems are among the most common in young children presenting to primary health care settings. As her review makes clear, failure to thrive and feeding disorders may coexist, although they do not inevitably do so. She reviews the literature on these disorders, emphasizing research findings that have appeared in the past 10–15 years.

In the first edition of this handbook, disorders of attachment were described based on unsystematic clinical observations and developmental research on attachment. In the ensuing 7 years, a small but growing body of data on clinical disturbances and disorders of attachment has emerged. In Chapter 22, Zeanah and Boris review critically proposed models of attachment disorders and find them incompatible to varying degrees with extant research findings. They propose changes in the conceptualization of attachment disorders, primarily using a dimensional rather than a categorical approach to classify both traditional and proposed types of disturbances and disorders of attachment.

Also in the previous edition of the handbook, the chapter on posttraumatic stress disorder was the first review of this type of symptomatology in infants and toddlers. It concerned primarily whether or not the disorder existed in young children. An emerging literature has changed the question from "Does it exist?" to "How is it similar to and dissimilar from posttraumatic symptomatology/disorders later in the life cycle?" In Chapter 23, Scheeringa and Gaensbauer review preliminary systematic research findings on diagnostic validity, as well as case studies that have focused on assessment and treatment. Without minimizing the enormous gaps in our current knowledge about posttraumatic symptomatology in young children, the authors assert that sufficient advances already have been made such that it is now widely accepted that infants and toddlers can become functionally impaired due to life-threatening trauma. They emphasize that clinicians have potentially vital roles in helping them adapt.

Chapter 24 introduces the controversial notion of clinical depression in infancy. As Luby notes, the central question is whether very young children can experience clinically significant symptoms of depression or, instead, whether they experience more transient adverse mood disturbances associated with being reared by a depressed parent. Based on her review, it is clear that some infants and toddlers manifest depressive-like signs and symptoms. Using findings from child development and developmental psychopathology on emotion states and emotion regulation, Luby explores the question: Does a depressive disorder exist in infancy? She explores the uses and limitations of this model to explain extant findings and to guide subsequent research.

Shaw, Gilliom, and Giovannelli describe another new category in infancy, aggressive behavior disorders, in Chapter 25. The authors are well aware of the controversial nature of their topic, and they begin their chapter by cautiously weighing data supporting and failing to support use the of term "disorder" to describe children with significant levels of aggression in the second and third years of life. They conclude that there are significant limitations in infants' cognitive abilities to understand aggression and that aggressive behaviors are quite frequent in low-risk populations. Nevertheless, aggression during infancy shows comparable stability and has similar correlates to aggressive behavior in older children. They suggest that prevention and intervention efforts in the early years need to be directed at similar targets as they are for older children, with special attention to infant–parent relationships.

In Chapter 26, Zucker and Bradley consider the evidence supporting the inclusion of gender identity disorder as a clearly demarcated form of psychopathology in young children. They assert that gender is a substantive part of the emerging sense of self and that phenotypic expression of gender identity typically emerges between the ages of 2 and 3 years, if not earlier. They review the core phenomenology, associated features, and putative risk factors pertaining to gender identity disorder in young children, and they describe the complexities inherent in trying to address the etiological question of what specific factors are involved.

In the concluding chapter (Chapter 27), Mrazek proposes a new model of psychosomatic disorders. He suggests that abnormal gene expression, whose specifics are not as yet specified, is a core vulnerability that precedes physiological dysfunction. After an historical review, Mrazek describes three different illustrative clinical problems, infantile-onset obesity, early-onset asthma, and atopic dermatitis, all of which begin in the first year of life. He discusses these clinical conditions as they reflect an interaction between genetic vulnerability and early environmental stressors and suggest that all three diseases are candidates for early intervention strategies.

REFERENCES

American Psychiatric Association. (1994). *Diagnostic and statistical manual of mental disorders*, (4th ed.). Washington, DC: Author.

Greenspan, S., & Weider, S. (1993). Regulatory disorders. In C.H. Zeanah, Jr. (Ed.), *Handbook of infant mental health* (pp. 280–290). New York: Guilford Press.

World Health Organization. (1992). *The ICD-10 classification of mental and behavioral disorders: Clinical descriptions and diagnostic guidelines*. Geneva: Author.

Zeanah, C. H., Boris, N., & Scheeringa, M. (1997). Psychopathology in infancy. *Journal of Child Psychology, Psychiatry and Allied Disciplines, 38*, 81–99.

Zero-to-Three. (1994). *Diagnostic classification of mental health and developmental disorders of infancy and early childhood*. Arlington, VA: Zero-to-Three Task Force on Diagnostic Classification.

16

Mental Retardation

❖

ANNE S. WALTERS
KARYN KAUFMAN BLANE

Developmental delay is a frequent referral question for practitioners working in the area of infancy and early childhood. The term "developmental delay," though imprecise, is used deliberately in recognition of the changeability of early developmental trajectories as well as to highlight reluctance to apply the label of mental retardation to children in early stages of development. With current definitions of mental retardation stressing the notion of adaptation, resources, and support, concern about labels has perhaps become secondary to the emphasis on early intervention for children and their families, and to the goal of improving short- and long-term outcome through matching intensity of supports to the child and family level of need. For this reason, a thorough understanding of the field of developmental disabilities is essential for the clinician working in the area of infancy and early childhood. This chapter outlines the topics germane to an understanding of mental retardation in early childhood: definition, epidemiology, etiology, diagnosis, and treatment.

DEFINITION

There have been wide shifts in the definition of mental retardation over the past 50 years; these shifts have included and excluded large percentages of the population with each change in diagnostic criteria. The most recent definition of mental retardation was published by the American Association of Mental Retardation (AAMR) in 1992 (Luckasson et al., 1992). Although consistent with previous definitions in the sense that it includes deficits in both IQ and adaptive behavior, it constitutes a departure in that it allows increased flexibility with regard to the upper limit of mental retardation, as well as providing increased specificity to the area of adaptive behavior:

> Mental retardation refers to substantial limitations in present functioning. It is characterized by significantly subaverage functioning, existing concurrently with related impairments in two or more of the following applicable adaptive skill areas: communication, self care, home living, social skills, community use, self direction, health and safety, functional academics, leisure and work. Mental retardation manifests before age 18. (Luckasson et al., 1992, p. 1)

The new definition goes further to delineate the importance of assessing an individual's supports, capabilities, and environment, and it requires consideration of psychological and physical health and environmental skills. Assumptions considered crucial to the application of the definition include factors such as cultural and linguistic diversity, adaptive behavior in the context of the typical community environment for the child's age, coexistence of adaptive behavior deficits with strengths, and the notion that functioning improves over time with appropriate supports.

Clearly, this new perspective of mental retardation views the disability as the outcome of a complex and dynamic interaction between limitations in intellectual functioning and environmental supports or deficits. It emphasizes current level of functioning and, therefore, is not conceptualized as, necessarily, a permanent condition (Syzmanski & Kaplan, 1997). Perhaps most important, the model is less deficit based and more focused on the interplay between the strengths and weaknesses of the child and of the environment in which the child lives.

In contrast to the avoidance of specifying levels of retardation in the AAMR definition, the fourth edition of the *Diagnostic and Statistical Manual of Mental Disorders* (DSM-IV; American Psychiatric Association, 1994) has retained a delineation of severity that is based on IQ, though the overall definition does specify that deficits in adaptive behavior must be present. Separate codes are used for each of four levels of mental retardation, with one code delineated to describe unspecified mental retardation. The tenth edition of the *International Classification of Disorders* (ICD-10; World Health Organization, 1992) includes all the features outlined by the AAMR and DSM-IV and notes that assessment should be based on clinical findings, adaptive behavior, and psychometric performance. Levels are designated as cited previously, though they do not include the 5-point range specified by the AAMR.

ASSESSMENT

Common to all the diagnostic classification systems, then, is a two-pronged approach of assessing IQ and adaptive behavior. Assessing IQ is completed using standardized tests of intellectual functioning; for infants and preschoolers, examples of these are the Bayley Scales of Infant Development—Revised (Bayley, 1994) or the Wechsler Scales of Primary and Preschool Intelligence—Revised (Wechsler, 1989). Choice of the appropriate instrument is highly dependent on an estimate of level of functioning, existence of physical or sensory impairments, and cultural background. Further, several of the most widely used instruments have inadequate floors, meaning that they have a lower limit for IQ testing that does not yield a number beyond a certain point, for example, scores of 45–50 for several widely used instruments. For children functioning at a level lower than this (moderate–severe–profound mental retardation), clinicians typically are forced to use instruments that may yield an estimate of IQ and a picture of strengths and weaknesses but have norms and/or psychometric properties that are not adequate to give confidence to the stability and/or predictive validity of the assessment results.

This is less of an issue as the field moves away from reliance on IQ scores in identifying mental retardation and toward the use of adaptive behavior assessment and educational testing that is likely to be of assistance in specifying areas of need for remediation and education. Nonetheless, current best practice guidelines suggest that there is a need for special training for examiners of infants and preschoolers with developmental disabilities. These disabilities are frequently low incidence, and, therefore, many clinicians have not had the breadth of experience necessary to obtain an optimum assessment. Children with multiple handicaps and/or more severe levels of mental retardation are frequently labeled "untestable" when, in reality, the standardization of the assessment instruments makes the test challenging to administer to young children functioning in the extreme ranges of abilities and/or skills.

Ideally, young children are seen through multidisciplinary evaluations; these evaluations are completed by professionals from a range of disciplines including psychology, speech and language, education, occupational therapy, physical therapy, psychiatry, and sometimes neurology or pediatrics. Table 16.1 summarizes the assessment instruments used most often for cognitive evaluation.

Assessing adaptive behavior is important to ensure that children whose IQ scores have been affected by cultural deprivation or other factors are not diagnosed with mental retardation when their ability to function adaptively is intact across domains. The current definition specifies 10 adaptive behavior domains and requires impairment in 2 of the 10 to constitute mental retardation. For purposes of assessment in early childhood, some of these domains are not yet applicable. The advantage of instruments such as these are that they are directly applicable to the process of identifying a family service plan or an individual educational plan. Table 16.2 summarizes instruments most often used for adaptive behavior evaluation.

TABLE 16.1. Typically Used Assessment Instruments for the Early Childhood Period

Name of instrument	Age range	Advantages	Disadvantages
WPPSI-R (Wechsler, 1989)	3–7yr	Corresponds to WISC-III, excellent standardization, useful diagnostically	Limited floor for MR (IQ of 45), scoring difficult, long to administer
Stanford–Binet, 4th ed. (Thorndike, Hagan, & Sattler, 1986)	2 yr and up	Well standardized, low floor (into severe MR range), easy to administer and score	Area scores not supported by factor analysis, scores not comparable at all ages
Bayley Scales (Bayley, 1994)	1–42 mo	Good clinical utility; Good psychometric properties	Training and time to administer, IQ floor of 50
McCarthy Scales (McCarthy, 1978)	2.5–8.5 yr	Appealing tasks; well normed and constructed	Limited use with MR (IQ floor of 50), scoring cumbersome, no prorating
Kaufman Assessment Battery for Children (Kaufman & Kaufman, 1983)	2.5–12.5 yr	Easel construction assists administration	Difficult to use for preschool MR, sampling problems, ambiguous terms (sequential/simultaneous), no verbal comprehension items
Leiter—Revised (Royd & Miller, 1997)	3 yr and up	Not used in place of IQ, utility for estimate of functioning with nonverbal children	Norms and standardization are inadequate

EPIDEMIOLOGY

Mental retardation (MR) is thought to affect between 1 and 3% of the population. Specifying the exact numbers is made difficult by the shifts in definition, but predictions from a normal distribution of IQ scores yield estimates that 2–3% of the population have assessed IQs below 70. Inclusion of adaptive behavior deficits narrows the range considerably to 1% (Baroff, 1986), and most diagnostic classifications offer this as a prevalence estimate (American Psychiatric Association, 1994). The estimate of 1% was also recently supported by a federal survey of the metropolitan Atlanta area (Yeargin-Allsop, Murphy, Oakley, & Sikes, 1992).

Of this 1%, approximately 85–89% are thought to function in the mild range. For moderate MR, prevalence estimates are 2 per 1,000; for severe retardation, 1.3 per 1,000; for profound retardation, 0.4 per 1,000 (McLaren & Bryson, 1987). There is wide variability in overall rates per 1,000 by region of the United States, with an overall estimate of school-age children to be 11.4 per 1,000, with a range from

TABLE 16.2. Typically Used Adaptive Behavior Instruments for Early Childhood Period

Name of instrument	Age range	Advantages	Disadvantages
Vineland Scales (Sparrow, Balla, & Cicchetti, 1984)	Birth and up	School, survey, and expanded forms, useful for assessing several areas of adaptive behavior	Difficult to administer, few items for young ages
Scales of Independent Behavior—Revised (Bruininks, Woodcock, Weatherman, & Hill, 1996)	2.5 yr and up	Scales for early development and severe–profound MR	Additional research needed
AAMR Adaptive Behavior Scale (Nihira, Foster, Schellhaus, & Loland, 1974)	3–69 yr	Clinically useful scale	Standardization and psychometrics are questionable

3.2 to 31.4 (King, State, Shah, Davanzo, & Dykens, 1997). Clearly, fewer children are identified with MR in the infancy or preschool range, though exact numbers are difficult to ascertain. In a comprehensive paper summarizing recent work on epidemiology and etiology, Murphy, Boyle, Schendel, Decoufle, and Yeargin-Allsop (1998) note that prevalence estimates are considerably lower in the range of children from 0–4 years, at 1 per 1,000 children. However, the population of children with IQs in the range below 50 is more stable across ages, at 2–4 per 1,000 (Murphy et al., 1998).

Higher prevalence rates of MR have been reported in boys than girls; with a ratio of 1.4:1. The association of MR with socioeconomic factors is clear and inverse. This has held true across developed countries and preliminary data support the relationship even in less developed nations (Murphy et al., 1998). Importantly, children from consistently impoverished families have an IQ that is a mean of 9 points lower than those in more advantaged families (Murphy et al., 1998). Any variance attributed to race appears in fact to be primarily related to socioeconomic status (Murphy et al., 1998).

ETIOLOGY

Assessing etiology has importance for several reasons: Some causes of MR are curable; etiology provides a way of grouping children with MR for purposes of intervention and/or research; some etiologies have associated medical conditions that require treatment; and an understanding of etiologies can inform prevention (Stone, MacLean, & Hogan, 1995). Previous conceptualizations of the etiology of MR held that there were two subgroups: organic and cultural–familial (Zigler, Balla, & Hodapp, 1984). The former included children with identifiable pre-, peri-, and postnatal insults such as substance exposure, hypoxia, or meningitis, whereas the latter referred to those children with less than optimum social, familial, or environmental circumstances and no identifiable cause for their impairment. Recently, it has become clearer that these two groups are not at all distinct. Many children with mild MR actually have a biological substrate for their conditions (Murphy et al., 1998).

Current views of etiology emphasize the multifactorial nature of MR, though most often the cause of MR is unknown. Luckasson et al.

(1992) noted that a recent review found 30% of cases of severe MR and 50% of cases of mild MR had unknown etiology, and that as many as 50% of cases of MR have more than one causal factor whose effects are cumulative or interactive. To phrase it slightly differently, Murphy et al. (1998) noted that 43–70% of children with severe MR have a known cause, compared with 20–24% of those with mild MR. Bregman and Harris (1995) report slightly higher numbers of known causes for mild MR, at 30–45%.

Multiple risk factors interact to cause MR; these may be psychosocial, genetic, and/or organic. Correspondingly, both the types of the predisposing factors and the timing of these factors in development are crucial to specify; Luckasson et al. (1992) identifies four groupings: biomedical factors such as genetic disorders, social factors such as family interaction, behavioral factors such as substance abuse, and educational factors including supports that under ideal circumstances will advance development. The timing of these factors in development refers to pre-, peri-, and postnatal events that influence the outcome of development and that are relevant to prevention and intervention efforts. Even within these periods of development, the same risk factor can have different effects at varying points; for example, rubella has devastating effects on the fetus during the first trimester of pregnancy, but it is much less likely to cause significant damage in the third trimester.

Genetic causes make up the largest proportion of etiologies, comprising 7–15% of all cases of MR, and 30–40% of cases with an identifiable etiology (Murphy et al., 1998). More than 500 genetic disorders are linked to mental retardation (Bregman & Harris, 1995), and the mechanisms of some of the more common ones are gradually being delineated (for a discussion of genetics and behavioral phenotypes, see State, King, & Dykens, 1997, or see Bregman & Harris, 1995, for an in-depth discussion of etiologies).

Prenatal events in general are reported to be a cause of severe MR in 25–55% of cases, and a cause of mild MR in 7–23% of cases (Murphy et al., 1998). This includes MR that is linked to chromosomal anomalies, syndromes, inborn errors of metabolism, and brain malformation, as well as environmental influences such as maternal substance abuse. Perinatal etiologies are reported in 10–15% of severe MR and 4–18% of mild MR (Murphy et al., 1998) and include obstetrical complications such as hypoxia. Postnatal events are causal in 7–10% of cases of severe MR, and 2–4% of cases of mild MR (Murphy et al., 1998). Examples include head injury, disease (meningitis, encephalitis), seizure disorder, malnutrition, or lead exposure (see Luckasson et al., 1992, for a complete listing of MR with etiologies).

In terms of associated conditions, children with severe impairment frequently have other neurosensory impairments as well, including seizure disorders in 20–32% of children with severe MR and 4–7% percent of children with mild MR. Cerebral palsy exists in 30% of children with severe MR and 6–8% of children with mild MR (Murphy et al., 1998). Autism and pervasive developmental disorder occurs in 9–20% of children with MR, whereas sensory impairment occurs in 2% of children with mild MR and 11% of children with severe MR (Murphy et al., 1998).

DIAGNOSIS

The diagnostic process begins when a child is brought to see a medical or mental health professional because the parents are concerned about the child's development. Discussion of developmental and family history reveals early indicators and potential family causes of MR, a review of the child's developmental skill acquisition, and an opportunity to forge a relationship with parents that can lead to a parent–professional partnership to meet the child's needs. Pediatric evaluation is an important part of the evaluation, though it often yields unremarkable results. However, when atypical physical features are present, this may indicate a specific disorder that can be treated medically. Consistent with this, laboratory studies should be conducted to rule out any organic etiology for the infant's difficulties. These include, but are not limited to, metabolic evaluation with blood and urine screens, chromosomal analysis, and audiological evaluation (see Accardo & Capute, 1998).

Language milestones are expected to be achieved within certain ages; when these are not met, concern arises. In the infant, these milestones begin with the newborn's reflexive auditory alerting and expressive (guttural) noises exhibited during certain physiological responses, such as belching, coughing, and crying (Capute & Accardo, 1991). Research supports an expected path in language acquisition (Zeanah, Boris, & Larrieu, 1997). As the infant grows, cooing occurs at approximately 6–8 weeks, with increased verbalizations (e.g., "ah-goo" and a wet raspberry sound) at 4 months and babbling beginning at approximately 6 months. Indiscriminate sounds (e.g., "dada" and "mama") are expected at 8 months, with discrimination beginning at approximately 10–11 months of age. The first word is anticipated at 11 months, and vocabulary is expected to gradually increase to approximately 20 words and beginning two-word phrases at the 18-month level. At 21 months, a 50-word minimum is typical, along with complete two-word sentences, and at 36 months, almost all personal pronouns are used appropriately. Capute and Accardo (1991) denote three other milestones achieved by 3 years of age: at least a 250-word vocabulary, three-word sentences, and use of plurals.

Gross motor skill levels, although comprising the weakest correlation with general functional ability (intelligence or global developmental level), nevertheless, are part of the evaluation of the infant and young child (Capute & Accardo, 1991). Infant scales also tend to be highly motor dependent. Developmental expectations include rolling at 3–4 months, sitting unsupported by 6–7 months, crawling at 7–8 months, cruising at 8–9 months, walking at 11–12 months, and running at 15 months. Fine motor skills require eye–hand coordination and manipulative abilities, and expectations include a neat pincer grasp at 10 months, marking with a pencil by 12 months, building a tower of three cubes at 21 months, copying shapes by 36 months, and drawing a square by 4 years.

The first 3 years of life is a time of rapid changes in social development, during which time infants and young children who have MR may respond inconsistently to their parents, display limited attachment behaviors, and appear to be inactive and inattentive (Syzmanski & Kaplan, 1997). Difficulties are evident in early peer interactions, communication skills, and self-help skills. Because atypical physical features are not consistently present in children with MR, and children's attainment of developmental milestones varies widely across the cognitively intact population, diagnoses are best made with multiple data points over time. Specific delays in language skills or motor skills do not necessitate the diagnosis of MR (Gemelli,

1996). Rather, a consistent pattern of developmental delays across skill areas and over time results in the confirmation of the diagnosis.

AGE OF IDENTIFICATION AND LEVELS OF MENTAL RETARDATION

Classification of *mild* MR may result from evidence of minor delays during the preschool years but is not typically identified until academic and behavioral problems appear in school (Editorial Board, 1996). Early developmental achievements include expressive language of two- to three-word sentences and ability to develop social interactive play; ultimately understanding beginning money concepts and vocational skills are expected. Classification of *moderate* MR generally occurs in preschool years and yields consistent delays in attainment of language facility and social play (Editorial Board, 1996). Children show poor social awareness, generally fair motor development, and initially poor self-help skills. They begin with single words and gestures to communicate and ultimately use simple sentences to communicate and may develop basic self-help skills and beginning reading and writing abilities. Classification of *severe* MR generally occurs during infancy due to significant impairment in development. Poor motor development is notable, along with minimal speech skills. Self-help skills are delayed and may not be evident until latency age. Future expectations vary from single-word communication to two- to three-word phrases, with ability to master self-help skills under complete supervision. Classification of *profound* MR also typically occurs in infancy, with a minimal capacity for functioning in sensorimotor areas and a need for complete supervision and care. Infants may sit alone, imitate simple sounds, understand simple words, and recognize familiar people (Editorial Board, 1996). Some motor development occurs as the child ages, but complete care and supervision are necessary for daily living.

DIFFERENTIAL DIAGNOSIS

Mental retardation is often an associated feature of autism and pervasive developmental disorders (PDD). In fact, 50–75% of children with autism also are diagnosed with MR (American Psychiatric Association, 1994; Farber, 1991), but most children with MR do not meet criteria for the PDD diagnoses. For instance, children diagnosed solely with MR demonstrate social relatedness and functional use of objects, whereas PDD is characterized by qualitative and pervasive impairment in the areas of social communication, social interaction, and play or interests. In addition, children with autism and PDD often achieve developmental motor milestones within normal limits and may show beginning language skills through the first 12–18 months, followed by regression, as opposed to the overall delays demonstrated by children with mental retardation.

Most important to differential diagnosis is a thorough assessment of social interactive abilities, as well as play skills, and a well-established "map" of development in these areas and the ages at which they most typically emerge. The child with MR, as compared to PDD, typically presents delay without qualitative impairment; that is, with the sociability, communication, and play skills of a younger child.

Communication disorders are defined by language skills that are significantly impaired (generally 15 IQ points below or more), as compared with other cognitive abilities. These include impaired articulation or expressive/receptive deficits. Global communication disorders are defined when both expressive and receptive language skills are found to be significantly below nonverbal skills. When expressive language skills are significantly below receptive language and nonverbal skills, then an expressive language disorder is identified. An apparent receptive language delay often indicates a global communication deficit; the expressive use of language is typically rote and repetitive in manner, whereas understanding of the functional use of language is absent (Farber, 1991). If there is a significant discrepancy between language and nonverbal skills but both sets of skills are found to be two or more standard deviations below the population mean, then diagnoses of both communication disorder and MR are given. The provision of both diagnoses indicates that the area of impaired functioning is in excess of what would be attributable to MR (American Psychiatric Association, 1994). However, if the criteria are met for autism or a PDD, then a diagnosis of a communication disorder is not given. In infants, the diagnosis of a communication disorder may be done through informal assessment, developmental history, and observation, as well as through standard-ized testing procedures.

FAMILY SUPPORTS

Despite the lack of a documented "cure" for mental retardation, the disability can be managed effectively using a combination of behavioral and educational intervention in conjunction with family support services. Hodapp and Kasari (1997) note that almost every technique used with developmentally intact children has been attempted with children with MR. Research supports a comprehensive approach to understanding and assisting families and children with disabilities. Consistent communication among different systems (families, professionals, schools, and communities) can serve to further the developmental process (Hodapp & Zigler, 1995).

In keeping with the emphasis in the new definition on supports, current focus on treatment is aimed at applying the dimensions of support to improve capabilities of children with MR. Supports are defined as "resources and strategies that promote the interests and causes of individuals with or without disabilities; that enable them to access resources, information, and relationships inherent within integrated work and living environments; and that result in their enhanced independence/interdependence, productivity, community integration, and satisfaction" (Luckasson et al., 1992, p. 101). Dimensions of supports are noted to be resources, functions, intensities, and desired outcomes. During the preschool period, examples of resources are technology that improves quality of life, networks of assistance, or services such as counseling or schooling. Examples of functions are in-home programming or behavioral support; intensity can range from intermittent to pervasive. Finally, desired outcomes include contributions to personal development or strengthening family coping or individual self-esteem. Ideally, supports are conceptualized as fluctuating across developmental stages, as occurring in as natural a setting as possible, and as highly individualized. Future planning is highly emphasized.

Family Acceptance

The initial reactions to the birth of a child with a disability are characterized by sociological variables, such as the timing of the diagnosis and the support system the family has in place (Seligman & Darling, 1997). Providing diagnostic feedback to parents should be interactive, incorporating the child's current level of functioning, expectations for later development, prognosis and etiology of the disability (if known), recommendations for services, and a sensitivity to parental response that may require modification of the feedback process to allow plenty of time for questions and discussion of concerns.

The security of early attachment for an infant born with MR may be jeopardized by family stress and grief in adjusting to the diagnosis. Grief reactions may last for variable amounts of time during the early years or may reoccur repeatedly as the child reaches or does not reach developmental milestones (Hodapp & Zigler, 1995). Parents can display decreased emotional availability to the child, as well as to each other and to the rest of the family, at various times during the lifespan, which will in turn shape the developmental pathway (Frazier, Barrett, Feinstein, & Walters, 1997). These observations speak to the importance of intervention at these nodal points in child and family development.

In defining models of family adjustment, there is controversy with regard to whether a process of normalization takes place, in which the family accepts the diagnosis of MR and feels comfortable with school placements, social relationships, and financial resources (Seligman & Darling, 1997), or whether parents of disabled children never feel their lives become normal but learn to accommodate to their child's special needs (Gemelli, 1996). Likely, family responses are grounded in individual differences, and defining an absolute family response to MR is neither possible nor productive. Floyd, Singer, Powers, and Costigan (1996) note that most often, parents move through this initial period successfully and caution clinicians against presuming maladaptation.

There is a trend in the research to focus on the positive aspects of having a disabled child in the home rather than emphasizing the negative impact of childhood disability on the family system (Gemelli, 1996; Seligman & Darling, 1997). Although it is difficult to make generalizations with regard to sibling relationships, benefits in terms of pride in assisting a sibling, and increased awareness and tolerance of disabilities are apparent in siblings of children with disabilities (Lobato, 1983).

Cultural Context

Culture plays a significant role in the family approach to a child with a disability and the providers' approach to intervention (Coates & Vietze, 1996; Seligman & Darling, 1997). Awareness of cultural biases of the family and of the provider are necessary in order to forge a parent–professional partnership for successful intervention. Contrary to the historical notion that parents are uninformed and in need of help, parents and parent groups are clearly essential sources of community awareness, professional activism, social change, and mutual support. Coates and Vietze (1996) explain that being a member of a particular social group may influence the importance of schooling and community, the response to children's transgressions and requests for help, and the expectations for children with mental retardation. Professionals must be aware of the impact of cultural values and barriers in assessment, diagnosis, and treatment.

Legal Mandates

Attitudes toward MR have evolved from a focus on an incurable defect and a need to protect society to the current recognition and implementation of the rights of all people to education and treatment, and a concept of adaptation, regardless of disability. Legal guidelines, such as Public Law No. 94-142 (Education for All Handicapped Children Act of 1975; Federal Register, 1975), have ensured that mentally retarded individuals have access to special education. However, the degree to which these services meet a child's specific needs varies considerably across communities and school districts (Borden, Walters, & Barrett, 1995). Subsequent to Public Law No. 92–142, services were extended to the 0- to 3-year period through the passage of Public Law No. 99-457 (U.S. House of Representatives, 1986), now Individuals with Disabilities Education Act (Federal Register, 1997), which provides federal legislation to intervene during the early years (0 to 5 years).

EARLY INTERVENTION

Early intervention is a widespread and commonly accepted service for at-risk children and those with mental retardation (Hodapp & Kasari, 1997). As discussed previously, Public Laws No. 92-142 and No. 99-457 have provided services for infants and toddlers through federal legislation and have also mandated service coordination and case management to assist families. These mandates not only translate into professional services but also necessitate a family focus by requiring the development of a individual family service plan.

Short-term effects of early intervention have been noted by authors such as Guralnick (1998), but long-term benefits are less reliable, with rapid decrease of gains noted to the point that control and intervention groups are ultimately indistinguishable. Longitudinal concerns are addressed by pointing to the necessity for comprehensive services provided with the intensity and specificity warranted to meet and maintain the child and family needs (Guralnick, 1998; Singh, Osborne, & Huguenin, 1996).

Special Education

School services for children with developmental delays, under current laws, typically begin with the transition from early intervention at age 3. Special education planning begins with initial referral and completion of any outstanding assessment procedures and is followed by the convening of the parents and multidisciplinary team to develop an individualized educational plan (IEP) that will establish the child's goals and objectives for the learning process that will begin with entry into a preschool program. Options for programming vary with the school district and with the strengths and weaknesses of the child; dimensions that are relevant are full-day versus half-day programming, in-district or out-of-district (usually private) placement, and the level of inclusion with non–special education identified peers. In keeping with the mandate by law to provide the least restrictive environment, children are placed with the highest level of inclusion that allows them to make progress at an optimal rate.

Parent Training

Depending on the family, levels of assistance are necessary to manage the child's behavior, determine financial services and support networks, and navigate educational and therapeutic services. Parent training refers to the teaching of interventions to parents that will be helpful in addressing the needs of their children. Parent training programs have evolved from an historically narrow focus on specific behavioral intervention to the current emphasis on education and overall family functioning. Contrary to managing children with behavior or conduct problems, parent training with children with MR focuses on skill acquisition, lifelong support issues, and reduction of maladaptive behavior. Skills necessary to implement behavioral change are taught in a systematic manner to improve child and family functioning. Behavioral management techniques, including positive reinforcement, punishment, shaping, prompting, fading, chaining, and generalization to various settings, are often employed. Self-help skills as well as behavioral concerns can be addressed. Parent training is most effective within a supportive atmosphere, where parents are able to discuss concerns, learn and practice techniques, and receive constructive feedback; and professionals are able to assist families as their needs evolve over time.

Behavioral Intervention

Behavioral intervention is based on principles of behavioral psychology, with a primary premise being that behavior that is consistently rewarded when it occurs will increase in frequency (reinforcement), and that which is consistently ignored or consequated will decrease in frequency (punishment). Singh et al. (1996) cite that "the application of behavioral procedures has improved the quality of life of people with mental retardation in ways that range from the teaching of basic living skills to the elimination of responses that may result in death" (p. 344).

Children with MR reportedly fail more often than do typically developing children (Hodapp & Zigler, 1995). This leads to a belief that they will not succeed when given difficult problems and, ultimately, to a pattern of learned helplessness. Provision of applied behavioral interventions, including positive reinforcement and prompting to ensure success with gradual generalization of skills (Singh et al., 1996), improves the child's expectancy of success and helps to develop a more active, capable style of problem solving.

PSYCHIATRIC DISORDERS AND DUAL DIAGNOSIS

Though confounded by differing methodologies that make comparisons across prevalence studies problematic, the rate of psychiatric disorders in children with developmental disabilities has been cited to be four to six times greater than for children without developmental disabilities (Matson & Barrett, 1993). Agreement has gradually grown over time that children with MR can demonstrate the full range of psychiatric diagnoses and, further, that children with MR have a high rate of behavioral disorders and are at high risk for development of serious mental illness (Kobe & Mulick, 1995). This increased risk is related to psychosocial experiences associated with MR, as well as with physiological factors such as brain damage, sensory impairment, seizure disorders, and behavioral manifestations of genetic syndromes (Stone et al., 1995).

Diagnoses of psychiatric disorder in this population, particularly in the severe to profound ranges, is complicated by the lack of diagnostic instruments that are normed on this population, and by the fact that many children at this level of functioning are nonverbal or minimally verbal. Diagnosis is further complicated by the empirically documented phenomenon termed "diagnostic overshadowing" (Reiss, Levitan, & Szysko, 1982). This term refers to the tendency to view maladaptive behavior in the child with MR as secondary to the MR itself. As awareness of both the mental health needs and the complex mental and affective life of these children grows, failure to diagnose and treat comorbid psychiatric disorder is less common.

For the early childhood population, many of the same array of psychosocial stressors that can be associated with growing up with MR are beginning to exert effects in early childhood. Most prevalence studies, however, sample older children and/or adults, and an estimate of the presence of psychiatric disorders in early childhood is lacking. Mental retardation does not in any way serve as a buffer against the effects of psychosocial neglect or abuse, and clearly, a child with cognitive and constitutional vulnerabilities is at high risk for posttraumatic stress disorder and/or reactive attachment disorder. Other risk factors have been identified as family stressors—low socioeconomic status, communicative disorders, and seizures, as well as the etiology of MR—with some syndromes showing comorbidity with certain psychiatric diagnoses (examples are tuberous sclerosis and autism, fragile-X, and attention-deficit/hyperactivity disorder symptomatology) (Hodapp & Kasari, 1997).

PSYCHOPHARMACOLOGY

As discussed earlier, diagnosis and treatment are comprehensive processes that need to incorporate the many facets of cognitive and behavioral difficulties, family relationships, peer interactions, cultural biases, self-help skills, and academic abilities. For infants and preschoolers, psychopharmacology is rarely the first line of treatment; rather, treatment generally centers around educational and behavioral interventions, including parent training and improving parent–child interactions.

CONCLUSION

Being aware of the many issues that arise in diagnosing and treating infants and preschool-age children with MR is as imperative as knowing the myriad resources available for assistance. Intervention focuses on family understanding and acceptance, as well as cognitive evaluation and assessment of adaptive functioning. Identification of potential barriers to successful adaptation and of supports that will enhance it takes place in the context of a parent–professional partnership that begins with diagnosis in early childhood and continues through intervention efforts across the lifespan. A thorough understanding of the definition, epidemiology, etiology, diagnosis, and treatment methods is essential to this process.

REFERENCES

Accardo, P. J., & Capute, A. J. (1998). Mental retardations. *Mental Retardation and Developmental Disabilities Research Reviews, 4,* 2–5.

American Psychiatric Association. (1994). *Diagnostic and statistical manual of mental disorders* (4th ed.). Washington, DC: Author.

Baroff, G. S. (1986). *Mental retardation: Nature, causes, and management* (2nd ed.). Washington, DC: Hemisphere.

Bayley, N. (1994). *Bayley Scales of Infant Development,* (2nd ed.). New Psychological Corporation.

Borden, M. C., Walters, A. S., & Barrett, R. P. (1995). Mental retardation and developmental disabilities. In V. B. Van Hassett & M. Hersen (Eds.), *Handbook of adolescent psychopathology: A guide to diagnosis and treatment* (pp. 497–524). New York: Lexington Books.

Bregman, J. D., & Harris, J. C. (1995). Mental retardation. In H. I. Kaplan & B. J. Saddock (Eds.), *Comprehensive textbook of psychiatry* (6th ed., Vol. 2, pp. 2207–2241). Baltimore: Williams & Wilkins.

Bruininks, R. H., Woodcock, R. W., Weatherman, R. A., & Hill, B. K. (1996). *Scales of Independent Behavior—Revised.* New York: Riverside.

Capute, A. J., & Accardo, P. J. (1991). Language assessment. In A. J. Capute & P. J. Accardo (Eds.), *Developmental disabilities in infancy and childhood* (pp. 165–179). Baltimore: Brookes.

Coates, D. L., & Vietze, P. M. (1996). Cultural considerations in assessment, diagnosis, and intervention. In J. W. Jacobson & J. A. Mulick (Eds.), *Manual of diagnosis and professional practice in mental retardation* (pp. 243–256). Washington, DC: American Psychological Association.

Editorial Board. (1996). Definition of mental retardation. In J. W. Jacobson & J. A. Mulick (Eds.), *Manual of diagnosis and professional practice in mental retardation* (pp. 13–53). Washington, DC: American Psychological Association.

Farber, J. M. (1991). Autism and other communication disorders. In A. J. Capute & P. J. Accardo (Eds.), *Developmental disabilities in infancy and childhood* (pp. 305–323). Baltimore: Brookes.

Federal Register. (1975). Education for All Handicapped Act of 1975. Public Law 94-142.

Federal Register. (1997). The Individual with Disabilities Act Amendments of 1997. Public Law 105-17, § 300.24(b)(3).

Floyd, F. J., Singer, G. H. S., Powers, L. E., & Costigan, C. L. (1996). Families coping with mental retardation: Assessment and therapy. In J. W. Jacobson & J. A. Mulick (Eds.), *Manual of diagnosis and professional practice in mental retardation* (pp. 277–288). Washington, DC: American Psychological Association.

Frazier, J. A., Barrett, R. P., Feinstein, C. B., & Walters, A. S. (1997). Moderate to profound mental retardation. In J. Noshpitz & N. E. Alessi (Eds.), *Handbook of child and adolescent psychiatry* (Vol. 4, pp. 397–408). New York: Basic Books.

Gemelli, R. (1996). *Normal child and adolescent development.* Washington, DC: American Psychiatric Press.

Guralnick, M. J. (1998). Effectiveness of early intervention for vulnerable children: A developmental perspective. *American Journal on Mental Retardation, 102*(4), 319–345.

Hodapp, R., & Kasari, C. (1997). The child with mental retardation. In S. Greenspan, S. Wieder, & J. Osofsky (Eds.), *Handbook of child and adolescent psychiatry* (pp. 414–427). New York: Wiley.

Hodapp, R. M., & Zigler, E. (1995). Past, present, and future issues in the developmental approach to mental retardation and developmental disabilities. In D. Cicchetti & D. Cohen (Eds.), *Developmental psychopathology, Vol. II: Risk, disorder, and adaptation* (pp. 299–331). New York: Wiley.

Kaufman, A. S., & Kaufman, N. L. (1983). *Kaufman assessment battery for children.* Circle Pines, MN: American Guidance Service.

King, B. H., State, M. W., Shah, B., Davanzo, P., & Dykens, E. (1997). Mental retardation: A review of the past ten years, pt. I. *Journal of the American Academy of Child and Adolescent Psychiatry, 36*(12), 1656–1671.

Kobe, F. H., & Mulick, J. A. (1995). Mental retardation.

In R. T. Ammerman & M. Hersen (Eds.), *Handbook of child behavior therapy in the psychiatric setting: Wiley series on personality processes* (pp. 153–180). New York: Wiley.

Lobato, D. (1983). Siblings of handicapped children: A review. *Journal of Autism and Developmental Disorders, 13*, 347–364.

Luckasson, R., Coulter, D. L., Polloway, E. A., Reiss, S., Schalock, R. L., Snell, M. E., Spitalnik, D. M., & Stark, J. A. (1992). *Mental retardation: Definition, classification, and systems of support* (9th ed.). Washington, DC: American Association on Mental Retardation.

Matson, J. L., & Barrett, R. P. (Eds.). (1993). *Psychopathology in the mentally retarded* (2nd ed.). Boston: Allyn & Bacon.

McCarthy, D. A. (1978). *The McCarthy screening test.* New York: Psychological Corporation.

McLaren, J., & Bryson, S. E. (1987). Review of recent epidemiological studies of mental retardation: Prevalence, associated disorder, and etiology. *American Journal of Mental Retardation, 92*(3), 243–254.

Murphy, C. C., Boyle, C., Schendel, D., Decoufle, P., & Yeargin-Allsop, M. (1998). Epidemiology of mental retardation in children. *Mental Retardation and Developmental Disabilities Research Reviews, 4*, 6–13.

Nihira, K., Foster, R., Schellhaus, N., & Loland, H. (1974). *AAMR Adaptive Behavior Scale manual.* Austin, TX: Pro-Ed.

Reiss, S., Levitan, G. W., & Szysko, J. (1982). Emotional disturbance and mental retardation: Diagnostic overshadowing. *American Journal of Mental Deficiency, 86*, 567–574.

Royd, G. H., & Miller, L. J. (1997). *Leiter International Performance Scale—Revised.* Wood Dale, IL: Stoelting.

Seligman, M., & Darling, R. B. (1997). *Ordinary families, special children.* New York: Guilford Press.

Singh, N. N., Osborne, J. G., & Huguenin, N. H. (1996). Applied behavioral interventions. In J. W. Jacobson & J. A. Mulick (Eds.), *Manual of diagnosis and professional practice in mental retardation* (pp. 341–353). Washington, DC: American Psychological Association.

Sparrow, S., Balla, D. A., & Cicchetti, D. V. (1984). *Vineland adaptive behavior scales.* Circle Pines, MN: American Guidance Service.

State, M. W., King, B. H., & Dykens, E. (1997). Mental retardation: A review of the past ten years, pt. II. *Journal of American Academy of Child and Adolescent Psychiatry, 36*(12), 1664–1671.

Stone, W., MacLean, W. E., & Hogan, K. L. (1995). Autism and mental retardation. In M. C. Roberts (Ed.), *Handbook of pediatric psychology* (2nd ed., pp. 655–675). New York: Guilford Press.

Syzmanski, L. S., & Kaplan, L. C. (1997). Mental retardation. In J. M. Wiener (Ed.), *Textbook of child and adolescent psychiatry* (pp. 183–218). Washington, DC: American Psychiatric Press.

Thorndike, R. L., Hagan, E. P., & Sattler, J. M. (1986). *Stanford–Binet intelligence scale: Guide for administering and scoring the fourth edition.* Chicago: Riverside.

U.S. House of Representatives. (1986). *Education of the Handicapped Act Amendments of 1986* (Report No. 99-860). Washington, DC: U.S. Government Printing Office.

Wechsler, D. (1989). *Manual for the Wechsler preschool and primary test of intelligence—revised.* New York: Psychological Corporation.

World Health Organization. (1992). *The ICD-10 classification of mental and behavioral disorders: Clinical descriptions and diagnostic guidelines.* Geneva, Switzerland: Author.

Yeargin-Allsop, M., Murphy, C. C., Oakley, G. P., & Sikes, R. P. (1992). A multiple source method of studying the prevalence of developmental disabilities in children: The metropolitan Atlanta developmental disabilities study. *Pediatrics, 18*(4), 624–630.

Zeanah, C. H., Boris, N. W., & Larrieu, J. A. (1997). Infant development and developmental risk: A review of the last ten years. *Journal of the American Academy of Child and Adolescent Psychiatry, 36*(2), 165–178.

Zigler, E., Balla, D., & Hodapp, R. (1984). On the definition and classification of mental retardation. *American Journal of Mental Deficiency, 89*, 215–230.

17

Communication Problems

❖

BARRY M. PRIZANT
AMY M. WETHERBY
JOANNE E. ROBERTS

One of the most complex, amazing and engrossing developments of the first 3 years of life is the transformation of newborns who communicate through vocalizations and body language into 3-year-olds who communicate through multiword utterances about their imaginations, their emotions, their memories, and their desires. To be sure, newborns communicate powerfully and effectively with their caregivers, but the reciprocal partnership in which complex symbolic ideas are exchanged, conflicting agendas are negotiated, and feeling states shared must await a series of developmental advances. These developmental advances depend in part on hard wiring in the central nervous system and in part on young children's experiences with their caregivers. Problems in either or both can lead to clinically significant communication problems. In this chapter, we begin by defining terms and describing frameworks. Next, we consider the development of language as it unfolds typically in the first 3 years of life. Then we consider the precursors and sequelae of communication problems. We also consider principles of assessment and intervention that we believe are essential. We conclude by describing implications for infant mental health.

TERMINOLOGY AND DEFINITIONS

In considering communication problems in young children, distinctions have to be made among the terms "communication," "language," and "speech." *Communication* is the broadest construct and includes any behavioral act, whether intentional or unintentional, that influences the behavior, ideas, or attitudes of another person. *Language* is a complex, conventional system of arbitrary symbols that are combined and used in a rule-governed manner for communication. The acquisition of language involves learning rules of four dimensions of language: (1) *pragmatics*, or the rules governing language use in social contexts; (2) *semantics*, or the rules governing the meanings of words and word classes; (3) *morphology and syntax*, or the grammatical rules for combining morphemes (i.e., units of meaning) and words into sentences; and (4) *phonology*, or the rules governing the allowable sounds and sound combinations within a specific language system. Speech is one mode for the expression of language based on vocal output and auditory input. A second important distinction is between expressive ability, or the ability to produce vocalizations, gestures, and/or speech, and receptive ability, or the ability to receive and/or comprehend the communicative signals of others. Both receptive and expressive skills are essential for successful communication.

A communication disorder is an impairment in the ability to (1) receive and/or process a symbol system, (2) represent concepts or symbol systems, and/or (3) transmit or use symbol systems (American Speech–Language–Hearing Association, 1982). Communication disorders typically are diagnosed and treated by speech–language pathologists and audiologists. For children birth to 3 years of age, early intervention legislation requires that concerns about a child's development, including communication development, be addressed through a multidisciplinary process, and that an individualized family service plan be developed to address child and family needs.

Childhood communication disorders have traditionally been classified into mutually exclusive categories using a diagnostic model based on etiological factors; however, this model has several limitations including the high frequency of problems associated with idiopathic (i.e., unknown) or multiple etiologies and the great variability in behavioral presentation even when a common etiological factor is known. Impairments of communication, language, or speech development are best understood by considering a child's profile of abilities and disabilities across communicative, linguistic, cognitive, and social–affective domains of development. It is useful to conceive of the spectrum of childhood disorders ranging along a continuum from specific speech and language delays to more pervasive social–communicative and/or cognitive impairments. Profiling a child's language, cognitive, and social abilities and disabilities provides direct information for intervention planning and may contribute to early identification (Prizant & Wetherby, 1993).

Different categorical frameworks for diagnosing speech, language and communication disorders have been developed by the American Speech–Language–Hearing Association (1982), and the American Psychiatric Association (1994). These frameworks have been developed for older children and adults; currently, there is a paucity of information regarding the validity of applying these frameworks to very young children. Table 17.1 contrasts the frameworks.

Speech, language, and communication disorders in young children are relatively common with reported prevalence rate as high as 11% in kindergartners (Beitchman, Nair, Clegg, & Patel, 1986). Of all identified preschool children with disabilities in the 3- to 5-year-old range, 70% have speech and language impairments (U.S. Department of Education, 1987). Although communication disorders are among the most prevalent disabilities in early childhood, they are typically not identified until after 2 years of age except when associated with severe developmental disabilities or other impairments that can be identified early in life (Wetherby & Prizant, 1996). The early identification of a primary language and communication impairment traditionally has posed a dilemma. The first evident symptom of a communication impairment attended to by parents and most professionals is a delay in language development when other significant disabilities do not co-occur with the communication prob-

TABLE 17.1. Diagnostic Frameworks of ASHA (1982) and APA (1994)

ASHA	APA
A. Speech disorder	
1. Voice disorder	1. Coded on Axis III[a]
2. Articulation disorder	2. Coded on Axis III[a]
3. Fluency disorder	3. Stuttering (Axis I) Cluttering (Axis I)
B. Language disorder	
1. Phonology	1. Developmental phonological disorder (Axis II)
2. Morphology or Syntax	2. Developmental expressive or mixed receptive–expressive language disorder (Axis II)
3. Semantics	3. Developmental expressive or mixed receptive–expressive language disorder (Axis II)
4. Pragmatics	4. Addressed only in pervasive developmental disorder (Axis II)
C. Hearing disorder	1. Coded on Axis III[a]

[a]Physical condition causing disorder is specified.

lem. Because the normal range of first-word acquisition is between 12 and 20 months of age (Bates, O'Connell, & Shore, 1987), a child typically is not referred for a language delay until at best, 20–24 months, but more commonly after 30–36 months.

LANGUAGE AND COMMUNICATION DEVELOPMENT: AN OVERVIEW

A large body of research has described the sequences through which children develop various communication abilities (see Bates et al., 1987; McLean, 1990, for reviews). This research has documented that communication development is closely related to social–cognitive development, communication abilities are first expressed in nonverbal behavior and then in verbal (symbolic) behavior, and the complexity and variety of communicative behavior increase as children grow older. The social–affective exchange occurring between infants and caregivers provides the foundation for the social or pragmatic aspects of communication (McLean, 1990). Interrelationships between communication and socioemotional development have received increased attention in recent years (see Prizant & Wetherby, 1990b; Prizant & Meyer, 1993, for further discussion).

From birth, and in the first few months of life, an infant's facial expressions, body posture, vocalizations, and even skin color communicate a great deal of information to caregivers. The information communicated includes a child's state of comfort, discomfort or distress, readiness to engage in interaction, and interest in objects or events. In these early months, caregivers respond to infant cues to help regulate the child's level of physiological and emotional arousal. Thus, an infant's behavior serves communicative functions when adults interpret and respond to the behavior. Responses may include efforts to comfort the child, provide appropriate levels of stimulation, and provide for tangible needs such as feeding or changing the child. Caregivers speak in a tone of voice that heightens the child's attention and elicits sustained face to face contact. Infants may quiet to a caregiver's voice and touch and focus on the caregiver's face, creating early joint attentional states and a transactional pattern of cycles of affective engagement and disengagement (Brazelton & Cramer, 1991).

Between 3 and 8 months, a child makes significant social, cognitive, and motoric gains providing the foundation for further communicative growth. Social–affective development is characterized by increased engagement with caregivers, production of more varied and readable behavioral signals, and increased ability to participate in reciprocal vocal and action-based turn-taking sequences, which are thought to be precursory to later communicative reciprocity (Bruner, 1981). With a child's increased mobility and interest in exploration of the immediate environment, many opportunities are provided for adults to engage in teaching interactions involving language modeling and mutual engagement with toys. During this period, caregivers continue to respond to their child's behavior as if it was intentionally communicative, and such contingent responding leads to children's intentional use of signals to affect the behavior of others (McLean, 1990).

The last 3 months of the first year are characterized by a major shift in communication development; the intentional use of communicative signals to have specific preplanned effects on the behavior of others (Wetherby, Reichle, & Pierce, 1998). Initially, primitive gestures and vocalizations are used to communicate intentions, but by 12 months and continuing into the second year, the prelinguistic communicative means or behaviors become more sophisticated and conventionalized. Stern (1985) noted, however, that infants are far more adept at communicating emotions than specific intentions by the end of the first year. Bruner (1981) indicated that children communicate for three major purposes by the end of the first year. These communicative intentions are initially expressed through preverbal means and later are expressed through language as it emerges:

1. *Behavioral regulation*, including signals to regulate another person's behavior for purposes of requesting objects or actions, rejecting objects, or protesting another person's behavior (e.g., pointing to request food and pushing object away to reject it);
2. *Social interaction*, including signals to attract and maintain another's attention to oneself for affiliative purposes such as greeting, calling, requesting social routines, and requesting comfort (e.g., waving "bye-bye" and reaching to be comforted); and
3. *Joint attention*, including signals used to direct another's attention to interesting objects

and events for the purpose of sharing the experience with others (e.g., showing interesting objects to others and pointing at an object to bring it to someone's attention).

Later in development, children share information about topics by providing and requesting information through language.

The roots of receptive communication development also are apparent from birth. Early in development, infants orient to sounds and speech in the environment and recognize familiar voices and by approximately 4 months become proficient at localizing auditory stimulation. There is increasing evidence that the infant's auditory system is especially attuned to perceive acoustic features of oral language, especially intonational patterns that aid in recognition of familiar voices (Leonard, 1991). By the last few months of the first year, children respond to many nonlinguistic cues such as gestures, situational routines, and commonly used ritualized language (e.g., "peek-a-boo") and single words in familiar routines which may give the appearance of fairly sophisticated comprehension (Wetherby et al., 1998).

The second year is marked by the acquisition of language, and children's communicative signaling becomes more consistent, explicit, readable, and sophisticated in form, resulting in greater success in communicating intentions and in regulating interactions. There also is a dramatic increase in rate of communication (Wetherby, Cain, Yonclas, & Walker, 1988) between 12 and 24 months. Early in the single-word stage, between 12 and 18 months, new word acquisition is slow and unstable; words may be used inconsistently and may drop out of a child's vocabulary as new words are acquired. Gestures and vocalization still comprise a large proportion of communicative behaviors. Vocabulary increases slowly and steadily until about 18 months, when two major shifts begin to occur (see Wetherby et al., 1998). First, vocabulary begins to expand at a dramatic rate. Second, children begin to combine two or more words that express more complex meanings. Throughout this period, there is much continuity in the meanings that children communicate in the transition from prelinguistic to linguistic communication. Children's emerging words, which begin to appear during the first half of the second year, express similar meanings that were initially expressed through nonverbal behavior. These meanings include recognition of the existence, disappearance, and recurrence of objects and events and statements of desire and rejection. During this period, language use still refers primarily to immediately observable events.

Throughout the second year, children typically comprehend more language than they can produce. By about 1 year, consistent responses to inhibitions (i.e., "no") and simple familiar actions are observed. By 18 months, children can locate familiar objects, identify body parts, and follow simple directions. By 24 months, comprehension of vocabulary has expanded greatly, and children are able to respond to words referring to object or persons not in the immediate environment. Thus, children's receptive development is characterized by more consistent responding to language directed to them with less need for contextual or environmental support.

Between 24 and 36 months, the basics of sentence grammar, including morphology or word organization and syntax or sentence organization, are acquired by children. Children move from a semantic or meaning base to sentence grammar. Grammatical knowledge and forms that serve to fine-tune meanings are acquired. Due to an ever-expanding vocabulary, use of language is more precise, explicit, and descriptive. A variety of sentence modalities appears, allowing for more conventional grammatical means for asking questions and expressing negation. Communication about future and past events, and about emotional states increases substantially throughout this period, and connected narrative discourse emerges as children begin to relate logical sequences of events across many utterances. Advances in comprehension typically predate achievements in production. Children are increasingly able to understand language pertaining to past and future events and are capable of responding to a much wider range of vocabulary. Children's greater comprehension and increased ability to follow meaning in narrative discourse (e.g., stories) play a major role in their emergence as conversational partners.

RISK FACTORS ASSOCIATED WITH COMMUNICATION DISORDERS

Both biological conditions and environmental circumstances are believed to put children at risk for the development of communication dis-

TABLE 17.2. Risk Factors Associated with Communication Disorders in Young Children

Biological factors	Environmental factors
Genetic/metabolic	Poverty
Down syndrome	
Fragile X	
PKU	
Histidinemia	
Prenatal acquired/congenital	Interactional
Prenatal infections (e.g.,	disturbances
rubella)	
Fetal alcohol syndrome	
Prenatal toxins	
Low birthweight	
Anoxia	
Hearing loss	
Cognitive impairment due	
to idiopathic etiology	
Postnatal	Child abuse/neglect
Otitis media with effusions	
Environmental toxins	
(e.g., lead)	
Other (multiple etiology)	
Pervasive developmental	
disorder	

Note. Although this table isolates risk factors, the developmental outcome of young children is clearly influenced by an interaction of biological and environmental factors (Sameroff & Fiese, 1990).

orders. As shown in Table 17.2, biological conditions affecting communication disorders can be categorized as genetic (hereditary), congenital (attributable to insults during the prenatal or perinatal periods that are not hereditary), or postnatal. Many characteristics of the child-rearing environment also increase the risk for communication disorders.

SEQUELAE OF PRESCHOOL LANGUAGE AND COMMUNICATION DISORDERS

The far-reaching effects of early childhood communication disorders are apparent in the problems experienced by children and their families. First, a significant body of research has demonstrated a high co-occurrence of communication and emotional and behavioral disorders in preschool and school-age children. Various studies have documented co-occurrence rates of 50–60% of language and communication disorders and emotional–behavioral

disorders in children and adolescents (Prizant et al., 1990). There are differing opinions regarding causal relationships between communication and emotional–behavioral disorders; however, there is general agreement that intervention programs must address young children's communication problems. Cantwell and Baker (1991) noted that early intervention for speech and language difficulties may prevent the development of psychiatric disorders.

Second, a significant relationship has been found between a history of preschool language disorders and later learning problems. Howlin and Rutter (1987) noted that "studies of language and speech disordered children have consistently found a high incidence of learning disorders and educational problems" (p. 277). It has been suggested that language intervention at an early age may prevent learning problems at school age (Guralnick & Bennett, 1987). Third, it also has been found that children with communication disorders may be more likely to experience problems in peer relationships than other children (Redmond & Rice, 1998). Communication difficulties may place a child at a disadvantage in participating in the social exchange and negotiation inherent in play. Furthermore, because of the important role played by language in behavioral and emotional self-regulation (Prizant & Meyer, 1993), children with language disorders may behave in inappropriate or impulsive ways and thus may be less desirable as playmates.

Finally, families of children with communication problems may experience stress related to problems in early identification and problems in managing their children's behavior. Difficulties in early identification of communication disorders may occur due to the lack of clearly defined criteria for determining communication problems in young children and the resulting lack of appropriate referrals when a problem is suspected by caregivers (Wetherby & Prizant, 1996). Thus, parents of children with communication disorders may experience significant stress due to potential spousal conflict over whether a problem exists and whether professional guidance should be sought. This problem is more likely to occur when communication and language delays do not coexist with significant physical, sensory, or cognitive disabilities, any of which may lead to earlier identification and more definitive diagnosis. The behavior of young children with communication difficulties also may pose significant challenges for parents (Bristol & Schopler, 1984).

Although conclusive data are not yet available, it is likely that early identification and intervention that address family concerns about a child's communication difficulties would serve to alleviate stress for caregivers and may prevent or mitigate later learning problems and emotional or behavioral disturbances (McLean & Cripe, 1997; Wetherby & Prizant, 1996). Therefore, efforts directed toward communication enhancement may have far-reaching positive and preventive effects for both children and families (Prizant et al., 1990), underscoring the need for early identification and referral (Wetherby & Prizant, 1996).

ASSESSMENT ISSUES

The most obvious goal of a comprehensive assessment for a young child is to determine whether a problem exists. Children who are suspected of having delays in communication development and/or co-occurring emotional and behavioral difficulties should be referred for a comprehensive evaluation addressing communication and socioemotional dimensions of development. Establishing a child's developmental level of communicative, language, and socioemotional functioning is an important component of determining both whether a problem exists and eligibility for services. However, although determining developmental levels and extent of delay helps to verify eligibility for services, this type of information in and of itself provides minimal specific direction for intervention planning or for working with caregivers. In this discussion, the focus is on those aspects of assessment that contribute most directly to intervention planning and the intervention process (see Crais, 1995, for a critical review of communication assessment instruments used with young children, and Meisels & Fenichel, 1996, for detailed consideration of "state-of-the-art" practices in assessment of young children).

Early Identification

Literature on prelinguistic and early language assessment suggests that early identification of communication disorders in children can begin prior to the expected acquisition of first words. Wetherby and Prizant (1996) have advocated

for the assessment of prelinguistic communicative behaviors known to be predictive of later language acquisition to ascertain the presence or absence of a communication delay. Research has delineated specific high-risk indicators that are associated with social–communicative disorders (see Table 17.3) (Wetherby & Prizant, 1996). Thus, an attitude of "let's wait and see" is no longer acceptable for very young children suspected of having a communication impair-

TABLE 17.3. High-Risk Indicators for Persisting Language Disabilities in Young Children

Emotion and use of eye gaze

Limited ability to share attention and affective states with eye gaze and facial expression

Limited use of gaze shifts between people and objects

Delay in comprehending and following others' points and eye gaze

Use of communication

Low rate of communicating with gestures and/or vocalizations

Limited range of communicative functions, particularly lacking in the joint attention function

Use of gestures

Limited repertoire of conventional gestures (i.e., giving, showing, reaching, pointing)

Limited use of symbolic gestures (i.e., waving, nodding head, depictive gestures)

Reliance on gestures and a limited use of vocalizations to communicate

Use of sounds

Limited consonant inventory
Immature syllable structure

Understanding and use of words

Delay in both language comprehension and production

Use of objects

A delay in the spontaneous use of action schemes in symbolic play

Limited ability to imitate actions on objects

Note. Adapted from Kasari, Sigman, Mundy, and Yirmiya (1990); Mundy, Sigman, and Kasari (1990); Paul (1991); Paul, Looney, and Dahm (1991); Rescorla and Goosens (1992); Terrell and Schwartz (1988); Thal and Tobias (1992); Thal, Tobias, and Morrison (1991); Wetherby and Prizant (1993); Wetherby and Prizant (1996); Wetherby and Prutting (1984); Wetherby, Yonclas, and Bryan (1989); Wetherby, Prizant, and Hutchinson (1998).

ment, especially considering recent efforts to provide services for the 0–2 population who are disabled or are at risk as outlined in early intervention legislation.

A comprehensive assessment is an essential component in planning appropriate early intervention for young at-risk and disabled children and their families. At least 70% of preschool children with disabilities have identified speech, language, and communication impairments (McLean & Cripe, 1997; Wetherby & Prizant, 1996). Furthermore, the degree of successful communication in caregiver–child relationships has a great impact on the emotional well-being of the child and family (Prizant & Meyer, 1993; Prizant & Wetherby, 1990a). Therefore, clinicians and educators need to be familiar with state-of-the-art practices in early assessment of communication and related abilities (Meisels & Fenichel, 1996).

Principles of Assessment

Communication and language assessment should be guided by a number of basic principles or underlying assumptions (Prizant & Bailey, 1992). These principles reflect the fact that communication is first and foremost a social activity that occurs in virtually all environments a child and his or her family encounters.

Principle 1

Assessment involves gathering information about a child's communication and socioemotional functioning across situational contexts over time. Communicative and socioemotional abilities vary greatly as a function of many factors including, but not limited to, the environment or setting in which a child is observed, the persons interacting with the child, and the familiarity of the situation (Greenspan & Wieder, 1998; Lund & Duchan, 1993). Thus, communication assessment should account for the normal variability observed in young children across contexts. This requires that assessment be an ongoing process, for the picture of a child's abilities and needs will not be complete, and, indeed, may change significantly as information from different sources help to complete the picture.

Principle 2

A variety of strategies should be used for collecting information. To ascertain a child's strengths and needs, as well as determine the learning opportunities available to a child, strategies including direct assessment, naturalistic observation, and interviewing significant others may be utilized (Prizant & Wetherby, 1993). The use of a variety of strategies reflects currently recognized "best practices" in early intervention for all assessment domains (Crais, 1995; Prizant & Wetherby, 1993). Each of these strategies has the potential to provide qualitatively different information about a child's communicative and socioemotional abilities that may ultimately be integrated to construct a more holistic picture.

Principle 3

Assessment must account for conventional as well as unconventional communicative behavior. For some young children, the acquisition of conventional verbal or nonverbal means of communication is especially difficult or challenging. Due to their disability, some children may develop idiosyncratic and even socially unacceptable means to communicate their intentions, which may be viewed in terms of a primary behavior disorder. Idiosyncratic means may include subtle or difficult-to-read behaviors that can only be understood by those who know a child well. Such behavior has been documented in children with multiple handicaps (Yoder, 1989) and children with social–communicative disorders such as autism (Prizant & Wetherby, 1993). Socially unacceptable forms of communication including aggression (e.g., biting and scratching) and tantruming have been documented as forms of intentional communication in children with developmental disabilities (Carr & Durand, 1985; Reichle & Wacker, 1993; Wetherby & Prutting, 1984).

Principle 4

Parents or primary caregivers should be considered expert informants about their child's communicative and socioemotional competence. Caregivers have opportunities to observe and interact with their child far more frequently in more familiar and emotionally secure situations than do professionals. Professionals must refine their interviewing skills (see Westby, 1990) and must use culturally appropriate information-gathering strategies to tap into such knowledge (Lynch & Hanson, 1998).

Principle 5

Assessment should always provide direct implications and directions for intervention and should be viewed as a potential form of intervention. Intervention planning should be based on ongoing assessment documenting changes in a child's communication, language, and socioemotional functioning. Such documentation provides feedback in evaluating the effectiveness of approaches to enhance communicative competence. In addition, caregivers' active involvement and participation in assessment activities may contribute significantly to their understanding of their child's communicative and socioemotional strengths and needs. Thus, assessment may serve as a form of intervention. For example, caregivers may become more aware of their child's subtle or difficult-to-read communicative signals, and as a result, develop strategies that are conducive to supporting their child's development.

Domains of Assessment

Current best practice in early childhood assessment recognizes that communication and socioemotional development are transactional processes, thus requiring that a child's typical interactions with communicative partners be addressed (McLean, 1990; Sameroff, 1987). Thus, a comprehensive assessment should address child abilities in communicative interactions as well as identify aspects of communicative partner behavior and learning environments that support, or limit, successful communicative exchange.

Assessment of Child Abilities

The following section presents a framework delineating content areas in assessment that address communicative, socioemotional, and related abilities. The information gathered for each domain may be collected through one or more of the assessment strategies discussed earlier. The major domains include the following.

Expressive Language and Communication. The primary focus in this domain is documentation of (1) communicative means, or the behaviors by which a child expresses emotions, physiological states, or intentions, and (2) communicative functions, or the purposes for which a child communicates (Prizant & Wetherby, 1993). For developmentally young, preintentional children, communicative means may include nonverbal and vocal behaviors (e.g., body posture and movement, facial expression, hand gestures, directed gaze and gaze aversion, and vocalizations). These signals may function to inform a receiver of the child's physiological and emotional state, level of alertness, focus of attention, interest in interacting or receiving comfort, interest in obtaining objects, or desire to have events continue or cease.

For developmentally more advanced children who communicate through prelinguistic means, intentional use of idiosyncratic and conventional gestures, as well as vocalizations and emerging word forms, should be documented. For children using language-based systems including speech, sign language, or graphic systems (e.g., communication boards); range of vocabulary; and semantic and syntactic complexity as well as communicative functions should be documented. In addition, the rate of communicative acts and a child's ability to persist in repairing communication breakdowns should also be documented.

Speech Production. Many young at-risk or developmentally delayed children may not be able to acquire and use speech as a primary mode of communication, due to severity of cognitive impairment or severe to profound hearing loss, or specific neuromotor speech disorders, including (1) dysarthria, a paralysis or paresis (i.e., weakness) in the oral musculature often observed in children with cerebral palsy or other identified neurological disorders, or (2) developmental dyspraxia, a dysfunction in the ability to plan the coordinated movements to produce intelligible sequences of speech sounds. Assessment should address the status of speech and vocal production to determine whether an augmentative nonspeech mode of communication may be beneficial.

Receptive Language and Communication. A child's ability to receive, comprehend, and respond to others' communicative signals is a crucial and often overestimated ability for children with communication and socioemotional difficulties. Clinical experience suggests that periodically, caregivers and/or professionals may assume a child understands others' communicative signals and may interpret a lack of response to gestures and/or speech as noncompliant or uncooperative behavior. Such negative attributions may significantly affect the success of interactions with a child, especially when lack of response is due to significant comprehension difficulties. A child's hearing status should always be assessed by a thorough audiological evaluation. In addition, the types of informal observations that are relevant for assessing awareness of environmental sounds include whether a child shows any startle response to loud environmental sounds, localizes or orients to speech or environmental sounds, or can be soothed or comforted by a caregiver's voice.

At higher levels of ability, children's ability to respond to communicative gestures and vocalizations of others, with and without the support of gestural and situational cues, should be documented. True linguistic comprehension is evidenced when children can comprehend words without situational or nonverbal cues, especially when words refer to persons, objects, and events outside the immediate environment. Lund and Duchan (1993) and Miller and Paul (1995) provided guidelines and procedures for more in-depth assessment of comprehension.

Language-Related Cognitive Abilities. Communication, language, and socioemotional abilities should always be considered in the context of a child's cognitive abilities. By profiling a young child's communicative and socioemotional abilities relative to nonverbal cognitive abilities and capacities, relevant information is provided about the nature of a communication or language delay and for differential diagnosis. Guidelines for assessing language-related cognitive abilities through observing play and problem solving in young children are available (Linder 1990; Westby, 1988).

Social–Affective Signaling and Socioemotional Functioning. Communicative interactions are regulated, to a great extent, by social–affective signals. These signals include facial expression, vocalizations, gaze, and other behaviors reflecting attentional, emotional, and physiological states. Some children with socioemotional and communicative impairments may demonstrate limited use of gaze shifts to regulate interactions, and their emotional states may be difficult to read due to a limited range of affect expression (Prizant & Wetherby, 1990b). Because these signals influence communicative interactions, assessment should go

beyond consideration of intentional nonverbal and verbal behaviors to include social–affective signals.

For young children, a number of additional socioemotional dimensions may be addressed in initial and ongoing assessment through both naturalistic and informal observation (Greenspan, 1996; Prizant & Meyer, 1993; Rogers, 1991) and more structured observations (e.g., Prizant & Wetherby, 1990b). These dimensions include social relatedness, emotional expression and relatedness, sociability in communication, emotion regulation and communicative competence, and expression of emotion in language and play. Greenspan (1996), Linder (1990), and Prizant and Meyer (1993) provide guidelines for addressing socioemotional dimensions in early childhood assessment.

Family-Centered Assessment Issues

Early childhood professionals need to be cognizant of the full range of possible responses that family members may experience in raising a child with communication and socioemotional difficulties, and that most often, such responses are natural, not maladaptive, and not evidence of pathology (Trout & Foley, 1989). Clinicians should inquire about caregiver perceptions of their child's developmental difficulties, including how these perceptions have evolved over time. It is important to ask caregivers to discuss their child's strengths and difficulties and to articulate their primary concerns and expectations regarding the child's development. Caregivers may be provided with the opportunity to discuss their understanding of their child's disability, how the disability impacts on their interactions and relationship with the child, and whether and how the child's disability affects family life.

Assessing the Behavior of Communicative Partners

Communicative partners may include parents, other caregivers, educators, therapists, or any others who interact with a child on a regular basis. Partners demonstrate a wide range of strategies and behavior that may serve to support and facilitate a child's communicative growth or, in some cases, may hinder communicative transactions and possibly constrain growth. In extreme cases, some partners may develop maladaptive interactive styles that are thought to be detrimental to a child's communicative and socioemotional development (Barnett, 1997). For very young children, caregivers' style and the degree of match or mismatch with a child's abilities are of primary interest.

Partners' strengths and weaknesses in supporting communicative interactions may be observed and documented during observations of familiar daily living and play activities. Dimensions of partner style that may be documented include degree of acceptance or rejection of a child's communicative attempts (Duchan, 1989), use of directive versus facilitative styles of interaction (Duchan, 1989), and use of specific interactive strategies such as responding contingently to child behavior, providing developmentally appropriate communicative models, maintaining topic of child initiations, and expanding or elaborating on communicative attempts (Duchan, 1989; Peck, 1989). The primary purpose of assessing partner style is to help partners develop an awareness of strategies they are using that appear to facilitate successful and positive interactions and help them recognize and modify interactive styles that may limit successful communicative exchange. A partner's level of comfort using a particular style and cultural influences on interactions with young children also must be considered. Child-rearing practices may vary significantly with families of diverse cultural backgrounds, and such differences must be taken into account in both assessment and intervention efforts (Garcia Coll & Meyer, 1993; Van Kleeck, 1994). Literature on approaches and strategies for assessing different dimensions of partner–child interaction is available (Duchan 1989; McCollom & Hemmeter, 1997; Peck, 1989; Wilcox, 1989).

From Assessment to Intervention

Once a child's profile of developmental strengths and needs has been documented and caregiver priorities and needs have been determined, an intervention plan and specific goals may be derived with caregivers. Goals should address the specific communicative means and functions to be targeted and modifications in partner behavior and social–communicative contexts that would be most facilitative of communication and socioemotional development. In addition, strategies to deal with challenging aspects of a child's socioemotional functioning

should be addressed (Reichle & Wacker, 1993). As with assessment, caregivers would ideally play an active and significant role in these efforts. Such efforts may occur within regularly occurring caregiving and play routines within the family context, in addition to services provided by professionals.

INTERVENTION ISSUES

In planning intervention for young children and their families, it is assumed all efforts will be made to involve caregivers directly and, when relevant, brothers, sisters, and playmates as equal-status partners (Prizant, Meyer, & Lobato, 1997; Prizant & Bailey, 1992). Information about a child and family's strengths and needs and family priorities, as gathered in assessment, should be the basis on which specific goals are derived. As caregivers are primary intervention agents, they must develop confidence in facilitating communication skills

Principles of Intervention

After an extensive review of research on early intervention with young children with communication disorders, McLean and Cripe (1997) concluded that that no one model of treatment is the best choice for all young children. Specific strategies and procedures to enhance communication, language, and socioemotional abilities of young children will vary depending on a child's chronological age, developmental status in areas of communicative, socioemotional, and cognitive functioning, motor abilities, and a child's unique learning style. Other significant factors include family priorities and routines, family supports, and caregivers' motivation and ability to make modifications on daily activities and environments, if necessary, to support their child's communicative and socioemotional growth. Service delivery options available (e.g., home- or center-based services) also influence the types of services provided and the frequency and duration of services.

Despite the myriad factors that need to be considered, recent literature and clinical consensus suggest several fundamental principles underlying communication and language enhancement for young children (Bricker & Cripe, 1992; Dunst, Lowe, & Bartholomew, 1990; MacDonald, 1989; Prizant & Bailey 1992; Prizant & Meyer 1993).

Principle 1

Communication enhancement should be one dimension of an integrated intervention plan for a child and his or her family. The most critical social–communicative and social–affective experiences for most children occur in their interactions with family members, both when young children are learning to communicate and as they expand their communicative mastery. When designing intervention strategies to be used by family members and integrated into daily family routines, it is critical that recommendations be compatible with the family's belief systems and sociocultural characteristics (Garcia Coll & Meyer, 1993; Lund, 1986).

Principle 2

Successful approaches to communication enhancement are achieved through caregiver–professional partnerships. Given the prominence of a child's early family relationships and family environment, early childhood professionals need to work closely with families in promoting communicative and socioemotional competence and fostering healthy social and emotional development. Coordination is needed in the use of an interactive style most conducive to a child's active participation and communicative growth, in developing strategies for arranging learning environments, and in using specific approaches to help a child develop more effective and sophisticated means of communication.

In some cases, caregivers' perceptions of their child's communication abilities may be skewed toward attributing lesser or greater competence than is observed by an educator or clinician. In these situations, an important goal is to help caregivers develop more accurate perceptions or redefine their perceptions (Theadore, Maher, & Prizant, 1990) of their child's abilities in a supportive and collaborative problem-solving climate.

Principle 3

Caregivers should be viewed as primary intervention agents. Whether services are provided in a home- or center-based program, caregivers possess the greatest potential for actuating positive change in their child's communicative abilities (Girolametto, Verbey, & Tannock, 1994; MacDonald, 1989). However, caregivers

must be willing and voluntary participants in such endeavors, requiring that they be respected and supported in setting communication priorities and goals that they value.

Principle 4

A child's motivations and preferences should be documented and taken into account in planning activities and strategies for communication enhancement. Social motivation is a major factor in a child's growing communicative competence (Mahoney, 1988; Prizant & Meyer, 1993). Some children with delays or disabilities may find social interaction and communication to be difficult or even stressful, and they may communicate only during times of need or during a limited number of favorite activities. Observation of a child in natural routines and regularly scheduled activities provides important information about motivations and preferences.

Principle 5

Activities should be identified and designed to address a child's developmental strengths and learning style. Many children with language, communication, and socioemotional needs have uneven profiles of abilities and disabilities (Prizant & Wetherby, 1993) and may demonstrate unique learning styles. In planning communication enhancement activities that foster socioemotional growth, learning strengths and styles should be taken into account in structuring learning environments, choosing materials and activities, and, when needed, selecting augmentative communication systems.

Principle 6

Communication enhancement efforts should be embedded in naturally occurring events and routines. Communication enhancement efforts can be targeted in a wide variety of daily routines, as well as in the context of activities addressing other developmental needs of a child. Daily routines and family events provide the experiential opportunities in which children learn and practice their communicative abilities. The value of using naturally occurring events for communication enhancement has been demonstrated repeatedly. Kaiser and Hester (1994) reviewed research literature on milieu and enhanced milieu approaches, a category of intervention strategies that use naturally occurring events as contexts for communication enhancement.

Principle 7

As communication enhancement approaches have become more focused on interactional and relationship variables, rather than child variables alone, the modification of partners' interactive style to be facilitative of a child's communicative growth becomes a primary intervention goal (Duchan, 1986; Giralametto, Greenberg, & Manolson, 1986; Girolametto et al., 1994; MacDonald, 1989; McCollom & Hemmeter, 1997; Wilcox, 1989). Clinicians must work closely with caregivers to discover interactive styles and strategies that will best support a child's communicative development and socioemotional competence and enable a child to communicate intentions as independently as possible. Effective approaches are available to support clinicians' efforts in working with caregivers (e.g., Manolson, 1992; McCollom & Hemmeter, 1997; MacDonald, 1989).

Contexts of Intervention

Characteristics of relationship and situational contexts can have a profound effect on children's ability to participate and communicate actively and confidently. The following guidelines should be considered in planning intervention contexts (Prizant & Meyer, 1993).

1. *Intervention contexts should be safe and predictable, and thus allow young children to expend greater "energy" on exploration, play, and communication.* The importance of predictability for young children with communication and socioemotional difficulties has been emphasized for children with a variety of developmental challenges (Crittenden, 1989; Prizant & Bailey, 1992). The cognitive and emotional comfort afforded by familiar routines in the physical environment, in the activity schedule, and within caregiver–child interactions fosters children's sense of security and thus contributes to communicative competence and socioemotional well-being.

2. *Contexts should support children's development of mastery motivation and a proactive sense of self.* Mastery motivation, or children's developing capacity to enjoy persisting and succeeding in mastering tasks (Brockman, Morgan, & Harmon, 1991), may be enhanced by introducing activities that are challenging but within children's developmental grasp or "zone of proximal development." Opportunities for choice making and decision making (Ostrosky & Kaiser, 1991) foster development of a sense of self as children come to learn that their preferences can be communicated and respected. Therefore, frequent opportunities should be made available for children to indicate or state preferences, whether at a preverbal or verbal level, and activities selected for intervention should reflect children's motivations and developmental strengths.

3. *Preferred relationships with peers, siblings, and adults should be taken into account.* Young children need to develop secure attachments to feel safe in participating in and exploring unfamiliar activities and contexts. Special relationships allow for intervention contexts where emerging communication skills can be learned and practiced with responsive partners.

Models of Service Provision

Interventions designed for specific populations of children who are at risk or disabled, and their caregivers, may be appropriate as preventive or remedial approaches for communication and socioemotional difficulties. Different models for providing intervention services to caregivers have been reviewed for biologically at-risk infants and toddlers (Barnard, 1997; Feldman, 1997; Olson & Burgess, 1997; Seitz & Provence, 1990), for children with identified developmental disabilities (Dawson & Osterling, 1997; McCollum & Hemmeter, 1997; McLean & Cripe; 1997; Spiker & Hopmann; 1997), for children at environmental risk (Barnett, 1997), and for children with identified emotional or behavioral disorders (Webster-Stratton, 1997).

The most typical model is direct individual caregiver–child therapy. In this model, professionals work directly with a caregiver and his or her child, often interacting directly with a child and asking caregivers to observe and eventually to emulate the style modeled by the teacher or clinician (MacDonald, 1989; MacDonald & Gillette, 1988; MacDonald & Carroll, 1992; Mahoney, 1988; Mahoney & Powell, 1988; Greenspan & Wieder, 1998). MacDonald's and Mahoney's programs are based on the concepts of balanced turn taking and developmental matching in teaching parents' interactional strategies to support their children's communication development. Greenspan's approach (Greenspan, 1992; Greenspan & Wieder, 1998), referred to as "floor time," encompasses a broad range of strategies to support children's development in a variety of domains, with the primary focus being on socioemotional and related capacities. In this approach, educators/therapists provide guidance and/or literally get down on the floor with parents and a child to help parents engage the child in developmentally appropriate and affectively charged play interactions designed to foster development in core socioemotional processes.

Interaction guidance (McDonough, Chapter 31, this volume) is an additional strategy used in caregiver–child therapy, which involves reinforcing desirable caregiver behaviors through the use of videotape replay. The emphasis is on changing caregiver–child interactions during regular routines or play activities to improve communicative and caregiving interactions through a focus on strengths rather than on liabilities.

Another model of providing services to young children and caregivers is caregiver–toddler groups, which may be designed to address many of the goals discussed previously, but in a group format. Small groups (three to five caregiver–toddler pairs) may meet for one to three sessions a week, and they involve direct work with caregivers and children. During a predictable schedule of activities appropriate for the children's abilities (e.g., music, circle time, snack time, and gross motor), clinicians/educators model facilitative communicative interactions and strategies to foster each child's socioemotional capacities. Individual therapy and caregiver support meetings occur in coordination with the groups to more specifically address challenges faced by each child and caregiver. The additional benefits of this group model include the opportunity for caregivers to observe other children with communication and socioemotional difficulties, develop strategies that may be helpful for their child, and benefit from a support network with other caregivers to preclude feelings of isolation.

IMPLICATIONS FOR MENTAL HEALTH PROFESSIONALS

Mental health professionals working with very young children and their families need to be aware of issues related to early identification, assessment, and intervention for communication disorders due to their high co-occurrence with socioemotional difficulties and their transactional impact on the emotional well-being of the family. It is likely that a significant proportion of young children first seen by mental health professionals will either have or be at risk for communication disorders. Intervention studies have documented the beneficial effects of early intervention for children younger than age 3 (McLean & Cripe, 1997; Shonkoff & Hauser-Cram, 1987), and early identification, differential diagnosis, and provision of appropriate services may significantly reduce stress on families (Theadore, Maher, & Prizant, 1990) and may be an important preventive measure to preclude the development of secondary emotional, behavioral, and learning problems.

Speech–language pathologists and mental health professionals traditionally have had limited opportunities to work collaboratively on issues related to early childhood communication disorders. Different diagnostic frameworks and terminology, different models of development, and relatively isolated training at preservice levels have perpetuated this lack of integration (Prizant et al., 1990). Early intervention legislation and its mandate for interdisciplinary cooperation within a family-centered framework holds great promise for making this fragmentation a thing of the past, which can only benefit young children and their families.

REFERENCES

American Psychiatric Association. (1994). *Diagnostic and statistical manual of mental disorders.* (4th ed.). Washington, DC: Author.

American Speech–Language–Hearing Association. (1982). Definitions: Communicative *disorders and variations.* ASHA, *24*, 949–950.

Barnard, K. (1997). Influencing parent–child interactions for children at-risk. In M. Guralnick (Ed.), *The effectiveness of early intervention* (pp. 249–270). Baltimore: Brookes.

Barnett, D. (1997). The effectiveness of early intervention on maltreating parents and their children. In M. Guralnick (Ed.), *The effectiveness of early intervention* (pp. 147–170). Baltimore: Brookes.

Bates, E., O'Connell, B., & Shore, C. (1987). Language and communication in infancy. In J. Osofsky (Ed.), *Handbook of infant development* (2nd ed., pp. 149–203). New York: Wiley

Beitchman, J., Nair, R., Clegg, M. & Patel, P. (1986). Prevalence of speech and language disorders in five year old kindergarten children in the Ottawa–Carlton region. *Journal of Speech and Hearing Disorders, 51,* 98–110.

Brazelton, T. B., & Cramer, B. G. (1991). *The earliest relationship.* New York: Addison Wesley.

Bricker, D., & Cripe, J. (1992). *An activity-based approach to early intervention.* Baltimore: Brookes.

Bristol, M., & Schopler, E. (1984). A developmental perspective on stress and coping in families of autistic children. In J. Blacher (Ed.), *Families of severely handicapped children* (pp. 91–134). New York: Academic Press.

Brockman, L., Morgan, G., & Harmon, R. (1991). Mastery motivation and developmental delay. In T. Wachs & R. Sheehan (Eds.), *Assessment of young developmentally disabled children.* New York: Plenum.

Bruner, J. (1981). The social context of language acquisition. *Language and Communication, 1,* 155–178.

Cantwell, D., & Baker, L. (1991). *Psychiatric and developmental disorder in children with communication disorder.* Washington, DC: American Psychiatric Press.

Carr, E., & Durand, V. (1985). The social communicative basis of severe behavior problems in children. In S. Reiss & R. Bootzin (Eds.), *Theoretical issues in behavior therapy* (pp. 219–254). New York: Academic Press.

Crais, E. (1995). Expanding the repertoire of tools and techniques for assessing the communication skills of infants and toddlers. *American Journal of Speech–Language Pathology, 4,* 47–59.

Crittenden, P. (1989). Teaching maltreated children in the preschool. *Topics in Early Childhood Special Education, 9,* 16–32.

Dawson, G., & Osterling, J. (1997). Early intervention in autism. In M. Guralnick (Ed.), *The effectiveness of early intervention* (pp. 307–326). Baltimore: Brookes.

Duchan, J. (1986). Language intervention through sensemaking and fine tuning. In R. Schiefelbusch (Ed.), *Language competence: Assessment and intervention* (pp. 182–212). Austin, TX: Pro-Ed.

Duchan, J. (1989). Evaluating adults' talk to children: Assessing adult attunement. *Seminars in Speech and Language, 10,* 17–27.

Dunst, C., Lowe, L., & Bartholomew, P., (1990). Contingent social responsiveness, family ecology and and infant communicative competence. *National Student Speech–Language–Hearing Association Journal, 17,* 39–49.

Feldman, M. (1997). The effectiveness of early intervention for children of parents with mental retardation. In M. Guralnick (Ed.), *The effectiveness of early intervention* (pp. 171–191). Baltimore: Brookes.

Garcia Coll, C. T., & Meyer, E. C. (1993). The sociocultural context of infant development. In C. Zeanah, Jr. (Ed.), *The handbook of infant mental health* (pp. 56–69). New York: Guilford Press.

Girolametto, L., Greenberg, J., & Manolson, H. A. (1986). Developing dialogue skills: The Hanen early language parent program. *Seminars in Speech and Language, 7,* 367–382.

Girolametto, L., Verbey, M., Tannock, R. (1994). Improving joint engagement in parent–child interaction: An intervention study. *Journal of Early Intervention, 18,* 155–167.

Greenspan, S. I. (1992). *Infancy and early childhood: The practice of clinical assessment and intervention with emotional and developmental challenges.* Madison, CT: International Universities Press.

Greenspan, S. I. (1996). Assessing the emotional and social functioning of infants and young children. In S. Meisels, & E. Fenichel (Ed.), *New visions for the developmental assessment of infants and young children* (pp. 231–266). Washington, DC: National Center for Infants, Toddlers & Families.

Greenspan, S. I., & Wieder, S. (1998). *The child with special needs: Encouraging intellectual and emotional growth.* Reading, MA: Addison Wesley.

Guralnick, M., & Bennett, F., (1987). *The effectiveness of early intervention for at-risk and handicapped children.* New York: Academic Press.

Howlin, P., & Rutter, M. (1987). The consequences of language delay for other aspects of development. In W. Yule & M. Rutter (Eds.), *Language development and language disorders.* Philadelphia: Lippincott.

Kaiser, A., & Hester, P. (1994). Generalized effects of enhanced milieu teaching. *Journal of Speech and Hearing Research, 37,* 63–92

Kasari, C., Sigman, M., Mundy, P., & Yirmiya, N. (1990). Affective sharing in the context of joint attention. *Journal of Autism and Developmental Disorders, 20,* 87–100.

Leonard, L. (1991). New trends in the study of early language acquisition. *ASHA, 33,* 43–44.

Linder, T. (1990). *Transdisciplinary play-based assessment.* Baltimore: Brookes.

Lund, N. J. (1986). Family events and relationships: Implications for language assessment and intervention. *Seminars in Speech and Language, 7,* 415–431.

Lund, N., & Duchan, J. (1993). *Assessing children's language in naturalistic contexts. 3rd Edition.* Englewood Cliffs, NJ: Prentice Hall.

Lynch, E., & Hanson, M. (1998). *Developing cross-cultural competence: A guide for working with young children and their families* (2nd ed.). Baltimore: Brookes.

MacDonald, J. (1989). *Becoming partners with children.* San Antonio: Special Press.

MacDonald, J., & Carroll, J. (1992). Communicating with young children: An ecological model for clinicians, parents, and collaborative professionals. *American Journal of Speech–Language Pathology, 1,* 39–48.

MacDonald, J., & Gillette, Y. (1988). Communicating partners: A conversational model for building parent–child relationships with handicapped children. In K. Marfo (Ed.), *Parent–child interaction and developmental disabilities.* New York: Praeger.

Mahoney, G. (1988). Enhancing the developmental competence of handicapped infants. In K. Marfo (Ed.), *Parent–child interaction and developmental disabilities.* New York: Praeger.

Mahoney, G., & Powell, A. (1988). Modifying parent–child interaction: Enhancing the development of handicapped children. *Journal of Special Education, 22,* 82–96.

Manolson, H. A. (1992). *It takes two to talk* (2nd ed.). Toronto: Hanen Early Language Resource Centre.

McCollum, J., & Hemmeter, M. (1997). Parent–child

interaction intervention when children have disabilities. In M. Guralnick (Ed.), *The effectiveness of early intervention* (pp. 549–578). Baltimore: Brookes.

McLean, L. (1990). Communication development in the first two years of life: A transactional process. *Zero to Three, 11*, 13–19.

McLean, L., & Cripe, J. (1997). The effectiveness of early intervention for children with communication disorders. In M. Guralnick (Ed.), *The effectiveness of early intervention* (pp. 349–428). Baltimore: Brookes.

Meisels, S., & Fenichel, E. (Eds.) (1996) *New visions for developmental assessment.* Arlington, VA: Zero to Three, National Center for Clinical Infant Programs.

Miller, J., & Paul, R. (1995). *The clinical assessment of language comprehension.* Baltimore: Brookes.

Mundy, P., Sigman, M., & Kasari, C. (1990). A longitudinal study of joint attention and language development in autistic children. *Journal of Autism and Developmental Disorders, 20*, 115–128.

Olson, H., & Burgess, D. (1997). Early intervention for children prenatally exposed to alcohol and other drugs. In M. Guralnick (Ed.), *The effectiveness of early intervention* (pp. 109–146). Baltimore: Brookes.

Ostrosky, M., & Kaiser, A. (1991). Preschool classroom environments that promote communication. *Teaching Exceptional Children, 23*, 6–10.

Paul, R. (1991). Profiles of toddlers with slow expressive language development. *Topics in Language Disorders, 11*, 1–13.

Paul, R., Looney, S., & Dahm, P. (1991). Communication and socialization skills at ages 2 and 3 in "late-talking" young children. *Journal of Speech and Hearing Research, 34*, 858–865.

Peck, C. (1989). Assessment of social communicative competence: Evaluating environments. *Seminars in Speech and Language, 10*, 1–15.

Prizant, B., Audet, L., Burke, G., Hummel, L., Maher, S., & Theadore, G. (1990). Communication disorders and emotional/behavioral disorders in children. *Journal of Speech and Hearing Disorders, 55*, 179–192.

Prizant, B., & Bailey, D. (1992). Facilitating acquisition and use of communication skills. In D. Bailey & M. Wolery (Eds.), *Teaching infants and preschoolers with handicaps* (pp. 299–361). Columbus, OH: Merrill.

Prizant, B., & Meyer, E. (1993). Socioemotional aspects of language and social-communication disorders in young children. *American Journal of Speech–Language Pathology, 2*, 56–81.

Prizant, B., Meyer, E., & Lobato, D. (1997). Brothers and sisters of young children with communication disorders. *Seminars in Speech and Language, 18*, 263–282.

Prizant, B., & Wetherby, A. (1990a). Assessing the communication of infants and toddlers: Integrating a socioemotional perspective. *Zero to Three, 11*, 1–12.

Prizant, B., & Wetherby, A. (1990b). Toward an integrated view of language and socioemotional development in children. *Topics in Language Disorders, 10*, 1–16.

Prizant, B., & Wetherby, A. (1993). Communication in preschool autistic children. In E. Schopler, M. Van-Bourgondien, & M. Bristol (Eds.), *Preschool issues in autism* (pp. 95–128). New York: Plenum.

Redmond, S., & Rice, M. (1998). The socioemotional behaviors of children with SLI: Social adaptation or social deviance. *Journal of Speech and Hearing Research, 41*, 688–700.

Reichle, J., & Wacker, D. (Eds). (1993). *Communicative alternatives to challenging behavior.* Baltimore: Brookes.

Rescorla, L., & Goosens, M. (1992). Symbolic play development in toddlers with expressive specific language impairment. *Journal of Speech and Hearing Research, 35*, 1290–1302.

Rogers, S. (1991). Observation of emotional functioning in young handicapped children. *Child: Care, Health and Development, 17*, 303–312.

Sameroff, A. (1987). The social context of development. In N. Eisenburg (Ed.), *Contemporary topics in development* (pp. 273–291). New York: Wiley.

Sameroff, A., & Fiese, B. (1990). Transactional regulation and early intervention. In S. Meisels & J. Shonkoff (Eds.), *Handbook of early childhood intervention* (pp. 119–149). New York: Cambridge University Press.

Seitz, V., & Provence, S. (1990). Caregiver-focused models of early intervention. In S. Meisels & J. Shonkoff (Eds.), *Handbook of early childhood intervention* (pp. 400–427). Cambridge: Cambridge University Press.

Shonkoff, J., & Hauser-Cram, P. (1987). Early intervention for disabled infants and their families: A quantitative analysis. *Pediatrics, 80*, 650–658.

Spiker, D., & Hopmann, M. (1997). The effectiveness of early intervention for children with down syndrome. In M. Guralnick (Ed.), *The effectiveness of early intervention* (pp. 271–306). Baltimore: Brookes.

Stern, D. (1985). *The interpersonal world of the infant.* New York: Basic Books.

Terrell, B. Y., & Schwartz, R. G. (1988). Object transformations in the play of language-impaired children. *Journal of Speech and Hearing Disorders, 53*, 459–466.

Thal, D., & Tobias, S. (1992). Communicative gestures in children with delayed onset of oral expressive vocabulary. *Journal of Speech and Hearing Research, 35*, 1281–1289.

Thal, D., Tobias, S., & Morrison, D. (1991). Language and gesture in late talkers: A 1-year follow-up. *Journal of Speech and Hearing Research, 34*, 604–612.

Theadore, G., Maher, S., & Prizant, B. (1990). Early assessment and intervention with emotional and behavioral disorders and communication disorders. *Topics in Language Disorders, 10*, 42–56.

Trout, M., & Foley, G. (1989). Working with families of handicapped infants and toddlers. *Topics in Language Disorders, 10*, 57–67.

U.S. Department of Education. (1987). *Ninth annual report to congress on the implementation of the Education of the Handicapped Act.* Washington, DC: U.S. Department of Education.

Van Kleeck, A. (1994). Potential cultural bias in training parents as conversational partners with their children who have delays in language development. *American Journal of Speech-Language Pathology, 3*, 67–78.

Webster-Stratton, C. (1997). Early intervention for families of preschool children with conduct problems. In M. Guralnick (Ed.), *The effectiveness of early intervention* (pp. 429–454). Baltimore: Brookes.

Westby, C. (1988). Children's play: Reflections of social competence. *Seminars in Speech and Language, 9,* 1–13.

Westby, C. (1990). Ethnographic interviewing: Asking the right questions to the right people in the right ways. *Journal of Childhood Communication Disorders, 13,* 101–111.

Wetherby, A., Cain, D., Yonclas, D., & Walker, V. (1988). Analysis of intentional communication of normal children from the prelinguistic to the multiword stage. *Journal of Speech and Hearing Research, 31,* 240–252.

Wetherby, A., & Prizant, B. (1993). Profiling communication and symbolic abilities in young children. *Journal of Childhood Communication Disorders, 15,* 23–32.

Wetherby, A., & Prizant, B. (1996). Toward earlier identification of communication and language problems in infants and young children. In S. Meisels & E. Fenichel (Eds.), *New visions for developmental assessment* (pp. 289–312), Arlington, VA: Zero to Three, National Center for Clinical Infant Programs.

Wetherby, A., Prizant, B., & Hutchinson, T. (1998). Communicative, social/affective and symbolic profiles of young children with autism and pervasive developmental disorders. *American Journal of Speech–Language Pathology, 7,* 79–91.

Wetherby, A., & Prutting, C. (1984). Profiles of communicative and cognitive social abilities in autistic children. *Journal of Speech and Hearing Research, 27,* 364–377.

Wetherby, A., Reichle, J., & Pierce, P. (1998). The transition to symbolic communication. In A.M. Wetherby, S. F. Warren, & J. Reichle (Eds.), *Transitions in prelinguistic communication: preintentional to intentional and presymbolic to symbolic* (pp. 197–230). Baltimore: Brookes.

Wetherby, A., Yonclas, D., & Bryan, A. (1989). Communicative profiles of handicapped preschool children: Implications for early identification. *Journal of Speech and Hearing Disorders, 54,* 148–158.

Wilcox, M. J. (1989). Delivering communication-based services to infants, toddlers, and their families: Approaches and models. *Topics in Language Disorders, 10,* 68–79.

Yoder, P. (1989). Relationship between degree of infant handicap and clarity of infant cues. *American Journal of Mental Deficiency, 91,* 639–641.

18

Autism and the Pervasive Developmental Disorders

❖

KATHLEEN KOENIG
EMILY RUBIN
AMI KLIN
FRED R. VOLKMAR

The pervasive developmental disorders (PDDs) are a group of conditions that share some general clinical features but likely reflect diverse etiologies. The conditions have their onset in infancy or early childhood and are associated with characteristic patterns of delay and deviance in the development of basic social, communicative, and cognitive skills. Of the various conditions sometimes included within the overarching PDD class, infantile autism, or as it more recently has been termed, "autistic disorder" (American Psychiatric Association, 1994) has been the most intensively studied and will be discussed in greatest detail in this chapter. The convergence of diagnostic criteria in the tenth edition of the *International Classification of Disorders* (ICD-10; World Health Organization, 1992) and the fourth edition of the *Diagnostic and Statistical Manual of Mental Disorders* (DSM-IV; American Psychiatric Association, 1994) have allowed for international diagnostic consensus in autism and other conditions within the PDD class. In general, the PDDs are associated with some degree of mental retardation, although the pattern of developmental and behavioral features differs from that seen in children with primary mental retardation. The term "pervasive developmental disorder" emphasizes the pervasiveness of difficulties across various domains of development as well as the important developmental aspects of these conditions.

DIAGNOSTIC CONCEPTS

Historical Background

Over the past century, a major point of debate has been the relationship of the severe psychiatric disturbances of childhood to adult psychoses. The concept of childhood "psychosis" became more or less synonymous with the term "childhood schizophrenia"; an assumption based on the severity of the conditions (Volkmar & Cohen, 1988). However, various lines of evidence (e.g., Kolvin, 1971; Rutter, 1972; Volkmar, Cohen, Hoshino, Rende, & Paul, 1988) now suggest that autism differs from schizophrenia in a number of ways, and the term "psychosis" has seemed less appropriate, in general, to apply to children, particularly to younger and lower-functioning children. Other diagnostic concepts have proven more enduring, and still others (e.g., multisystem developmental disorder) await verification. The "nonautistic PDDs," such as childhood disintegrative disorder (CDD), Rett's syndrome, and PDD-NOS, have been less commonly studied than autism. These disorders have been included in both DSM-IV and ICD–10. In many instances, modifications in the original description of the concept have been made based on research.

Autism

Of all the diagnostic concepts proposed, Leo Kanner's (1943) description of early infantile autism has proven to be remarkably enduring. He described children with a congenital inability to relate to other people (autism), which was in striking contrast to their relatedness to the inanimate environment. These children also exhibited a number of unusual developmental and behavioral features (e.g., insistence on sameness and resistance to change, stereotyped mannerisms, and when it developed at all, unusual language characterized by echolalia, pronoun reversal, and extreme literalness).

Although Kanner's phenomenological description of the condition has been enduring, certain aspects of his original report were mistaken; for example, he suggested that autism was not associated with mental retardation, that autistic children were more likely to come from more educated families, and that the condition was not associated with other "organic" conditions. It is clear that most autistic children are also mentally retarded; the condition can be observed in association with a host of medical conditions, for example, tuberous sclerosis, congenital rubella, and fragile-X syndrome (Dykens & Volkmar, 1997), although medical conditions are most likely to be associated with more severe impairment (Rutter, Bailey, Bolton, & LeCouteur, 1994). In some cases, children with autism develop seizure disorders, with peak onset in early childhood and adolescence (Volkmar & Nelson, 1990). Other neurobiological abnormalities are also frequently observed and consistent with an as yet unspecified underlying "organic" etiology (Minshew, Sweeney, & Bauman, 1997).

Kanner's initial observation of deviance in parent–child interaction was taken by some to suggest a role of parental psychopathology in syndrome pathogenesis. It now appears that deviant patterns of parent–child interaction stem primarily from the disturbance in the child and that parental psychopathology is no more frequent in parents of autistic children than those of children with other developmental disorders (DeMyer, Hingtgen, & Jackson, 1981).

Nonautistic PDDs

Childhood Disintegrative Disorder

Theodor Heller, a Viennese educator, described a condition in which young children who had previously developed normally exhibited marked developmental and behavioral deterioration with only minimal subsequent recovery. In the years subsequent to Heller's description, perhaps 100 cases of the condition have appeared in the world literature (Volkmar, Klin, Marans, & Cohen, 1997). Generally, early development is entirely normal, and the child progresses to the point of using language prior to the onset of a profound developmental regression; once established, the condition behaviorally resembles autism, although the prognosis may be somewhat worse (Volkmar & Cohen, 1989). In some instances, the condition has been reported in association with a specific disease process, for example, a progressive neurological condition. However, it is clear that such a medical condition is observed only in a minority of cases. The validity of CDD apart from autism was supported through comparison of onset data during DSM-IV field trials for autistic disorder (Volkmar & Rutter, 1995). Patients with CDD are more likely to be mute, with profound mental retardation, and have a worse prognosis.

Asperger's Syndrome

In 1944, Hans Asperger, an Austrian pediatrician with interest in special education, described four children who had difficulty integrating into groups. Despite preserved intellectual skills, the children showed marked paucity of nonverbal communication involving both gestures and affective tone of voice, poor empathy and a tendency to intellectualize emotions, an inclination to engage long-winded, one-sided, and sometimes pedantic speech; rather formalistic, all-absorbing interests involving unusual topics which dominated their conversation; and motoric clumsiness (Klin, 1997). Unlike Kanner's patients, these children were not as withdrawn or as aloof; they also developed, sometimes precociously, highly grammatical speech, and their difficulties were not diagnosed in the first years of life. Discarding the possibility of a psychogenic origin, Asperger highlighted the familial nature of the condition and even hypothesized that the personality traits were primarily male transmitted. Asperger's work, originally published in German, became widely known to the English-speaking world only in 1981, when Lorna Wing published a series of cases showing similar symptoms. Since then, several studies have attempted to validate Asperger syndrome (AS) as distinct from autism without mental retardation; analysis of neuropsychological characteristics is consistent with a nonverbal learning disability profile rather than high-functioning autism (Volkmar et al., 1996; Klin, Volkmar, Sparrow, Cicchetti, & Rourke, 1995). Additionally, AS individuals are likely to show interest but little facility in social relationships.

Rett's Syndrome

Andreas Rett (1966) described the syndrome now commonly referred to as Rett's syndrome. Although exhibiting some "autistic-like" features, particularly during the preschool years, this syndrome appears to differ from autism in several ways: It is reported only in females, the "autistic-like" phase is relatively brief, it is associated with characteristic motor behaviors (stereotyped hand "washing" or "wringing" movements), abnormalities in gait or trunk movement (e.g., apraxia or gait scoliosis), and breath-holding spells. Early growth and development are normal but followed shortly by developmental regression, relative failure of head growth, loss of acquired speech, and loss of purposeful hand movements. Loss of interest in people and decreased interpersonal contact occur but eye contact is maintained. This deterioration occurs usually within 1 year (Van Acker, 1997). Eventual mental retardation is even more severe than in autism.

PDD-NOS

The term "PDD-NOS" is used in DSM-IV (American Psychiatric Association, 1994) to describe children with some, but not all, features of autism. These children exhibit patterns of unusual sensitivities and difficulties in social interaction, but not sufficient for a diagnosis of autism. The term "PDD-NOS" is problematic in several respects. The definition is essentially a negative one. The lack of an explicit definition means that it is used rather inconsistently (Towbin, 1997). Research on the condition has been uncommon. More commonly, PDD-NOS has been used for children with better cognitive and communicative skills, and the most common reasons for referral in such cases include concerns of parents about the child's emotional and social development rather than, as in autism, the failure to develop language.

CLINICAL DESCRIPTION OF AUTISM

Onset and Characteristics of Early Development

Kanner (1943) originally suggested that autism was present from birth. Subsequent research has suggested that the condition is usually apparent within the first year of life but sometimes appears to have its onset within the second or third year of life (Short & Schopler, 1988; Volkmar, Stier, & Cohen, 1985). Age and type of onset have some value in the differential diagnosis of autism, although various extraneous factors may act to delay case detection (e.g., as parental sophistication or denial and level of associated mental retardation in the child).

Most studies of early development in autism rely on parental retrospection or, less frequently, contemporaneous videotapes or movies of the child (Stone, 1997). Although parents often have concerns from the first months of life, they may seek guidance from health professionals only when the child is 18–24 months and still not speaking. The parents may report concern that the child might be deaf, although they paradoxically often note that the child is exquisitely sensitive to certain sounds in the inanimate environment (e.g., the noise of the vacuum cleaner).

The child may not respond differentially to parents but may be particularly attached to a highly unusual object. The young autistic child may also have interest in nonfunctional aspects of objects (e.g., their smell or taste), and normal use of materials for play is typically absent. Younger autistic children often exhibit unusual stereotyped behaviors or motor mannerisms, such as hand flapping or toe walking, and seem to prefer such activities to those involving social interaction, although such behaviors become more prominent as the child becomes older. Bizarre affective responses may be observed; for example, the child may become highly agitated if the same route or routine is not precisely followed.

Some behaviors have been shown to discriminate autistic from nonautistic children at 2 and 3 years of age. Lord (1995) studied 30 children referred for autism at age 2 and followed-up at age 3. Not raising arms to be lifted, directing attention, and not attending to voice discriminated 2-year-olds with autism. At age 3, failing to share enjoyment, use of another's body to have needs met, absence of pointing, and repetitive hand and finger mannerisms were strongly associated with autism. Differences in social interaction, expression and understanding of emotion, and joint attention have been noted (Adrien et al., 1993; Osterling & Dawson, 1994).

Delays in case detection and referral in autism are common and reflect more general problems: primary care providers' general lack of awareness of mental health problems in childhood and lack of familiarity with autism. These delays are unfortunate because there is some suggestion that early intervention may reduce subsequent morbidity (Dawson & Osterling, 1996; Lovaas, 1987), and it is clear that developmental skills at age 5 predict subsequent outcome. The issue of early case detection and intervention has assumed increasing importance in light of recent federal mandates for extension of services to young children.

Social Development

Autism was initially described as a disturbance of affective contact (Kanner, 1943), and social deviance is the major defining feature of the condition. Most recently, research into social development in autism has supported the notion that social criteria tend to be the most potent predictors of diagnosis (Volkmar, Carter, Grossman, & Klin, 1997; Lord, 1995). Social development in autistic children does occur but is qualitatively different from that of typical children, and syndromic behavior is expressed differently at each developmental level. Relative to nonautistic developmentally delayed children, autistic children tend to be significantly more delayed in the domain of social behavior and social skills (Klin, Volkmar, & Sparrow, 1992).

For normally developing infants, social stimuli are particularly interesting; the predisposition to form social relationships appears to be an important foundation for the development of other skills. In contrast, for autistic infants and young children, the human face holds little interest, and lack of eye contact, lack of prefer-

ence for speech sounds, poor attachments, and a general lack of social interest are typical (Volkmar, Carter, et al., 1997; Klin, 1992).

Although some evidence of differentiated social responsiveness may be observed in young autistic children (Sigman & Ungerer, 1984), the usual robust patterns of attachment do not develop, and autistic children may not respond differentially to their parents until the elementary school years. Deficits in social interaction remain a source of marked disability even for the highest intellectually functioning autistic adults (Volkmar, Klin, & Cohen, 1997) and may include difficulty dealing with social rules, social interchange, and the pragmatics of social communication.

Communicative Development

Qualitative differences in communication are present in all children with autism. One of the first notable differences in development is often a delayed onset of intentional communication (both nonverbal and verbal) (Schuler, Prizant, & Wetherby, 1997). Children with autism may be less motivated to communicate at an early age and typically exhibit delays in the acquisition of conventional nonverbal gestures, speech, and language (Wetherby & Prutting, 1984). As infants, children with autism have been found to use a lower frequency of pointing and showing gestures, head shakes, and head nods and may use idiosyncratic behaviors to have their needs met (Schuler et al., 1997). Approximately half of children with autism never gain useful communicative speech, and those who do frequently use immediate and delayed echolalia (e.g., repetition of words and phrases) for communicative purposes (Prizant & Rydell, 1984). Qualitative differences in language acquisition may also include delays in syntactic development, abnormal use of words and phrases, pronoun reversal, and the use of unusual intonation patterns (Lord & Paul, 1997).

Although linguistic form and speech development are often affected, it is the social use of language (i.e., pragmatics) that differentiates children with autism from those with a more circumscribed language disorder. Autistic children who develop intentional communication may communicate less for social purposes than do typically developing children; they may have difficulty monitoring the appropriateness of their discourse and may communicate at a reduced rate (Lord & Paul, 1997). Wetherby

(1986) found that while typically developing children engage in reciprocal interactions for a variety of purposes (e.g., requesting, social interaction, and commenting), children with autism may communicate primarily for instrumental purposes (e.g., requesting and/or protesting activities). In particular, joint attention skills or the ability to establish and maintain a common focus of attention on an entity or event are often restricted in young children with autism (Mundy, Sigman, & Kasari, 1990; Wetherby & Prutting, 1984). Likewise, older children with autism have been found to exhibit difficulty with maintaining conversations and inferring the implicit intentions of their communicative partner (Lord & Paul, 1997). For example, children with high-functioning autism or AS may use unusual discourse (e.g., pedantic speech) and may have difficulty providing relevant and coherent information (Volden & Lord, 1991).

Cognitive Development

Approximately 75–80% are mentally retarded, with about 30% falling within the mild to moderate range and about 45% falling within the severe to profoundly mentally retarded range. Mental retardation is not simply a consequence of negativism while taking intelligence tests, lack of motivation, or oversensitivity to being tested. The typical profile on psychological testing is one marked by significant deficits in abstract reasoning, verbal concept formation, and integration skills and on tasks requiring a degree of social understanding. In contrast, relative strengths are usually observed in the areas of rote learning and memory skills and visual–spatial problem solving, particularly if the task can be completed "piecemeal," that is, without having to infer the context or "Gestalt" of the task.

Developmental and psychological testing of infants and young autistic children can be challenging but often reveals difficulties with tasks that require more verbal language (either receptive or expressive), symbolic thinking, or social interaction (e.g., tasks that involved imitation). Nonverbal problem-solving abilities, such as matching shapes and solving simple inset puzzles, is closer to age-expected levels (Klin & Shepard, 1994). Deficits in sensorimotor skills, as opposed to more symbolic or verbal skills, are more variably noted (Curcio, 1978; Morgan, Curtrer, Coplin, & Rodrique, 1989).

Based on the unusual neuropsychological profile in individuals with autism and two decades of cognitive experiments, several influential cognitive theories of the social dysfunction in autism have been proposed. One hypothesis posits that there is a lack of a central drive for coherence, with the consequent focus on dissociated fragments rather than integrated "wholes," leading to a fragmentary and overly concrete experience of the world. Another hypothesis posits that the commonly found difficulties in abstracting rules, inhibiting irrelevant responses, shifting attention, and profiting from feedback, as well as maintaining "on line" different pieces of information while a decision is made—the so-called executive functions—underlie the social, communicative, and behavioral aspects of autism. As executive functions are thought to be mediated by frontal areas, this hypothesis highlights the similarities between autism and conditions resulting from frontal lobe lesions.

Yet another hypothesis, so far the most influential, posits that autism is caused by the child's inability to attribute mental states such as beliefs and intentions to others. Devoid of a "theory of mind," individuals with autism are thought to be unable to infer their thoughts and motivations, thus failing to predict their behavior and adjust accordingly, resulting in lack of reciprocity in communication and social contact (Baron-Cohen, 1989). This line of research is of considerable interest in that it more parsimoniously accounts for observed deficits in social interaction and play in autistic children. However, the theory is limited in several important respects. The theory is highly cognitive, and the social deficits in autism are viewed as secondary to an essentially cognitive deficit. Because theory-of-mind capacities are not apparently exhibited much before 1 year of age, at the earliest, the theory does not account for the very early onset of the condition. Comparison of preverbal social behavior in autistic and nonautistic children showed that autistic children lacked early emerging social behaviors that would predate the emergence of the cognitive capacity to appreciate other's minds (Klin et al., 1992). Moreover, experimental work using the theory has tended to focus on verbal subjects, and it is quite unclear how or whether the theory has applicability to lower-functioning subjects (Klin & Volkmar, 1993). At least some work has suggested that apparent theory-of-mind problems are more a function of verbal ability and developmental level than of diagnostic category (Prior, Dahlstrom, & Squires, 1990; Tager-Flusberg & Sullivan, 1994).

Neurobiological Studies

Considerable evidence suggests the operation of some as yet unspecified neurobiological factor in pathogenesis. For example, autistic children are more likely to exhibit physical anomalies, persistent primitive reflexes, various neurological "soft" signs, and abnormalities on electroencephalogram computed tomography, or magnetic resonance imaging scans (Minshew et al., 1997). As many as 25% of autistic individuals develop seizure disorders (Volkmar & Nelson, 1990). There is some suggestion of reduced obstetrical and neonatal optimality, although this may reflect problems in the fetus rather than the pregnancy per se (Tsai, 1987).

There is now evidence suggesting the operation of genetic mechanisms in at least some cases (International Molecular Genetic Study of Autism Consortium, 1998; Rutter et al., 1994). Recent research suggests that siblings of autistic children are at significantly greater risk for also exhibiting autism and other developmental difficulties, and that monozygotic twins are more likely than fraternal twins to be concordant for the disorder (Folstein & Rutter, 1977; Rutter, Bailey, Simonoff, & Pickles, 1997). In addition, a recent study of families with more than one child on the autism/PDD spectrum showed preliminary evidence of chromosomal abnormalities (International Molecular Genetic Study of Autism Consortium, 1998).

Unfortunately, neurobiological findings vary considerably and findings are often subtle. Neuroanatomical models of the disorder have placed the "site" of the lesion at various points on the neuraxis from brain stem to cerebellum to cortex. Autistic children exhibit elevated peripheral levels of serotonin, a central nervous system neurotransmitter, yet the significance of this observation is unclear (Anderson & Hoshino, 1997). Also, elevated levels of plasma beta-endorphin, and ACTH found in autistic children suggest abnormal functioning within the hypothalamic–pituitary–adrenal axis (Tordjman et al., 1997). This suggests a biochemical abnormality in association with autistic individuals' heightened response to stress, and stands in contrast to prior studies of cortisol or ACTH secretion, which have not shown significant and robust differences when compared with nonautistics.

Epidemiology

Various problems complicate epidemiological studies, including the relative infrequency of the conditions, difficulties in case identification, sampling techniques, changes in diagnostic criteria, and scope of syndrome definition. Over 20 epidemiological studies worldwide have been conducted (Forbonne, 1998). Prevalence rates ranged from 0.7 per 10,000 to 21.1 per 10,000. The median value of prevalence estimates is 4–5 per 10,000. Since the mid-1980s, a series of studies have reported higher prevalence rates, although it is still unclear whether these reports provide evidence for either a more accurate (and higher) prevalence rate of autism or for an increase in prevalence of autism in the past decade. Possible reasons for the increased rates are (1) the adoption of broader definitions of autism; (2) the inclusion of smaller size target populations, given that in general, smaller studies have yielded the higher rates; and (3) better detection of cases in the extreme ranges, that is, the severely mentally retarded and the nonretarded individuals with autism. Most studies suggest that autism is more frequent in males, usually four or five times as common as in females. When girls are affected, however, they are more severely affected, particularly in terms of lower IQ. The significance of the observed sex difference is unclear but may reflect the operation of underlying genetic mechanisms (Bryson, 1997).

Epidemiological information on other "nonautistic" PDDs is more limited. It does, however, appear that PDD–NOS is much more common than more strictly defined autism. The other PDDs are apparently less common than autism. For example, CDD is perhaps 10 times less common than more strictly defined autism. Although the reliability for diagnostic ascertainment of these autistic-like conditions is still questionable, there is compelling evidence to suggest that perhaps one in every 1,000 children exhibits social disabilities consistent with the autistic spectrum of disorders.

Course and Prognosis

Younger children more typically display the "pervasive" unrelatedness alluded to in DSM-IV (American Psychiatric Association, 1994) criteria for the condition. Although some evidence of differentiated responsiveness to parents may be observed as the child reaches the elementary school years, patterns of social interaction remain quite deviant, and the child's behavior can be quite problematic. Often, some gains in communicative and social skills are observed during the elementary school years. During adolescence, some autistic children exhibit behavioral deterioration, and a smaller number improve (Rutter, 1970). As adults, even the highest-functioning individuals exhibit marked difficulties in social interaction (Volkmar & Cohen, 1988). Various interactional styles can be observed in the autistic child, ranging from aloof to passive and to eccentric; these styles appear to be closely related to developmental level (Wing, 1997).

Available data suggest that the outcome for autistic children is quite poor, with perhaps only one-third able to achieve some degree of personal independence and self-sufficiency as adults (DeMyer et al., 1981). In general, two major factors appear predictive of ultimate outcome: the acquisition of truly communicative speech by age 5 and IQ. However, much of the available outcome information is based on samples collected during the 1960s and 1970s. During this period, fewer services were available, and services provided were often not provided until the school years. There is some reason to hope that over the past decade, the mandates for earlier intervention, earlier recognition of the disorder, and more intensive behavioral and social–communicative interventions (Lovaas, 1987; Wetherby, Schuler, & Prizant, 1997) have improved the long-term outcome for the disorder. Research in this area is critically needed.

DIAGNOSIS OF AUTISM

Categorical Definitions

Categorical definitions of autism typically have emphasized four features essential for diagnosis (1) early onset, (2) social dysfunction, (3) communicative dysfunction, and (4) various unusual behaviors, such as stereotypies and resistance to change, which are typically subsumed under the term "insistence on sameness." Most categorical definitions emphasize that deviance in social and communicative development is not just a function of developmental level. During field trials for the DSM-IV, ef-

forts were made to make diagnostic criteria convergent with ICD–10 definitions (Volkmar et al., 1997).

Dimensional Definitions

Dimensional approaches also have been used in the diagnosis of autism. These methods attempt to assess dimensions of function/dysfunction that are relevant to the diagnosis. Most dimensional assessment instruments are designed for school-age children. These instruments rely either on parental or teacher report or on direct observation in structured settings; in most instances highly deviant behaviors are rated or sampled. Reliance on parental retrospection brings attendant issues of reliability; direct observational procedures may prove less useful for sampling low-frequency behaviors. In typically developing infants and young children, the frequency of apparently "autistic-like" behaviors raises particular problems for most "deviance model" assessment instruments.

Another approach relies on dimensional assessment instruments that are more truly developmental in nature. The utility of normative assessments of cognitive or communicative ability is well established (Lord, 1997; Lord & Paul, 1997; Sparrow, 1997). The availability of an instrument that normatively assesses social skills, the Revised Vineland Adaptive Behavior Scales (Sparrow, Balla, & Cicchetti, 1984), offers considerable potential in this regard.

CLINICAL ASSESSMENT

The clinical assessment of a child with autism or another PDD is most effective when carried out by an experienced interdisciplinary team. Two fundamental considerations should guide the assessment process: (1) an awareness of the challenges that autistic children pose for usual assessment methods and (2) an awareness that some modifications in more usual assessment procedures may be helpful to parents (Klin & Shepard, 1994). For example, to the extent possible, parents should be encouraged to observe the evaluation of the child. This procedure helps to demystify assessment procedures, provides a common set of observations for subsequent discussion, and helps to establish a long-term collaborative relationship.

A careful history should be obtained, including information related to the pregnancy and neonatal period, early development and characteristics of development, and medical and family history. Information on the nature and age at apparent onset of the condition can provide important information relevant to differential diagnosis. Questions about development can sometimes be helpful if framed for parents around a specific time or event (e.g., the first birthday).

Assessment of the child should include both psychological and communication assessments which aim to establish levels of functioning. Instruments should be selected with consideration of the child's apparent developmental levels. For cognitive assessment, tests that are not highly dependent on verbal abilities should be used, for example, the Bayley Scales (Bayley, 1969), the Uzgiris–Hunt Scales (Uzgiris & Hunt, 1975; Dunst, 1980), the Leiter International Performance Scale—Revised (Roid & Miller, 1997), and the Kaufman Assessment Battery for Children (Kaufman & Kaufman, 1983). For children with nonverbal mental ages over 2 years, several nonverbal tests are available (see Sparrow, 1997, for a discussion of assessment procedures and instruments). When direct assessment of the child is difficult, results of the Revised Vineland (Sparrow et al., 1984) may be helpful. Relative to developmentally disordered, non-PDD comparison groups, the social development of autistic children, as assessed by the Vineland, is lower than expected given the child's overall developmental level (Volkmar, Carter, et al., 1997).

Several instruments are available for assessing communicative skills in young children with autism. Tools that appear to be the most successful involve the use of objects rather than picture stimuli. The Reynell Developmental Language Scales—U.S. edition (Reynell & Gruber, 1990), for example, provides a measure of formal aspects of language comprehension and expression (e.g., vocabulary and syntax) using a variety of miniature objects and figurines. The Communication and Symbolic Behavior Scales—Normed edition (Wetherby & Prizant, 1993) incorporates motivating toys and "communicative temptations," which are useful for providing a profile of a child's communicative skills (e.g., nonverbal and verbal communicative means, communicative functions, and reciprocity), as well as a child's social–affective and symbolic behavior.

Psychiatric examination of the child should include observation during more and less structured periods. Areas for assessment, observation, and inquiry include social development (interest in social interaction, patterns of gaze and eye contact, differential attachments, style of social interaction), communication (receptive and expressive language, nonverbal and pragmatic communication, communicative intents, echolalia), responses to the environment (motor stereotypies, idiosyncratic responses, resistance to change), and play skills (nonfunctional or idiosyncratic uses of play materials, developmental level of play). The child's capacities for self-awareness (e.g., interest in mirror image and awareness of his or her own body) and motor skills should be observed. Problem behaviors that are likely to interfere with remedial programming should also be noted (e.g., marked aggression or problems in attention).

Given the difficulties in assessing infants and younger children, several assessment sessions may be required. If a multidisciplinary treatment team is providing the evaluation, it is important that team members maintain close communication with each other to avoid fragmentation and duplication of effort. When possible, the evaluation should be sufficiently integrated so that parents receive a single coherent picture of the child and his or her difficulties; such a report also has the practical advantage of facilitating discussion between team members who must be able to reconcile, or understand, apparent discrepancies in the results.

For younger children, consultations with other medical professionals, such as pediatric neurologists or geneticists, may be indicated. History or examination may suggest the need for specific laboratory studies or medical procedures. For example, a family history of mental retardation, severe mental retardation, or dysmorphic features in the child suggest the need for genetic screening and chromosome analysis (including screening for fragile X); symptoms suggestive of seizures (apparent periodic unresponsiveness) suggest the need for an electroencephalogram and possible neurological consultation. Computed tomography or magnetic resonance imaging scans sometimes reveal disorders such as tuberous sclerosis or degenerative central nervous system disease. A careful history of the pregnancy and neonatal period should be obtained to ascertain possible pre- or postnatal infections such as congenital rubella.

Usually the child's hearing has been tested prior to comprehensive evaluation. If this has not been done, or if it was not possible to elicit the child's cooperation, brainstem auditory-evoked response procedures should be used. In most instances, extensive medical evaluations fail to reveal an associated medical condition; this suggests reasonable care in obtaining additional assessments. On the other hand, certain features may suggest the importance of extensive medical investigations, for example, the abrupt behavioral and developmental deterioration of a child who was previously developing normally.

The differential diagnosis of autism and other PDDs includes language and other specific developmental disorders, mental retardation, sensory impairments (particularly deafness), and reactive attachment disorders. Usually children with language disorders do not exhibit the pattern of serious social deviance and deficit exhibited in autism; nonverbal communicative abilities are an area of evident strength. In mental retardation, social and communicative skills are usually on a par with overall cognitive skills. Deaf children may exhibit some difficulties in social interaction and repetitive activities; however, they are usually interested in social interaction and may make use of gesture for communicative purposes. Children with reactive attachment disorders have, by definition, experienced marked psychosocial deprivation, which results in deficits in social interaction (most notably in attachment). However, the quality of social deficit is different than in autism; the child may be withdrawn or indiscriminantly attached to others. The disturbance tends to improve relatively quickly after an appropriately responsive psychosocial environment is provided.

In young children, the task of differential diagnosis is complicated by the inherent difficulties in child assessment, the frequency of autistic-like behaviors in other conditions, and the fact that autism can be associated with deafness and with mental retardation as well as with other medical conditions. Differential diagnosis is often most complicated in young children without expressive language, odd social behavior, and some apparent degree of cognitive delay. Consideration of the pattern of developmental deviance is often helpful in such instances. The assessment of relative levels of sensorimotor and cognitive skills in relation to communication and social ones is important. In general, the presence of both communication for more social purposes and of some evidence of differential social responsiveness argues against the diagnosis of autism. Often the issue of diagnosis in such cases is clarified with certainty only over time. It is appropriate to share with parents a sense of the clinician's degree of confidence in the diagnosis. It is also important to realize that the diagnosis may have important, if not necessarily intended, implications for other purposes, such as educational programming, special services in the community, and so forth. It is critical that the importance of educational and other interventions be emphasized regardless of how "classically" autistic the child appears to be.

INTERVENTIONS

In the absence of a definitive cure there are a thousand treatments. Essentially, every conceivable treatment has been used for autism. With the exception of a few areas (notably behavior modification and pharmacological intervention and, to a lesser extent, educational interventions), most proposed interventions have not been rigorously studied, and it has been difficult to assess treatment effects systematically. This poses difficulties for professionals who are asked by parents to recommend or evaluate a therapy. Unfortunately, short-term changes readily occur when treaters and/or evaluators are not blind to the hypothesis under study; short-term changes may be neither sustained nor clinically meaningful.

In some instances, particularly with single case reports demonstrating improvement, it is unclear whether the individual was autistic and which specific factors are responsible for improvement. The observation that a few autistic individuals achieve relatively good outcomes is gratifying but also complicates the interpretation of single case studies. To further compound the problem, there is no "untreated" autistic child; that is, even by the time the diagnosis is definitively made, parents often have tried multiple interventions.

The available evidence suggests the importance of appropriate, intensive educational interventions to foster the acquisition of basic social, cognitive, and communicative skills (Schuler, Prizant, & Wetherby, 1997; Olley & Stevenson, 1989), which are, in turn, related to outcome. Behavior modification techniques can be quite helpful. Early and continuous intervention is highly desirable (Rogers, 1996).

Some reports have suggested marked improvement following early, intensive intervention, such as Applied Behavioral Analysis (Lovaas, 1987). However, questions have been raised about the methodological weaknesses of the research supporting this approach (Gresham & MacMillan, 1998), casting doubt on the high rate of "recovery" of lower-functioning autistic children. Although behavioral approaches have the advantage of addressing a range of behaviors in autism, they should not be considered a comprehensive program to the exclusion of other developmentally based communicative strategies.

Dawson and Osterling (1996) identified several common elements of appropriate early intervention programs designed for young children with autism. The first of these elements, curriculum, included the facilitation of basic skills such as attending to social cues within the environment, imitation, spontaneous communicative intent, symbolic play, and social interaction with both adults and peers. The second element emphasized the need for balancing highly structured teaching environments with conscious efforts to support generalization of those skills to more natural environments. In addition to teacher-directed therapy sessions, a child's motivation and/or ability to initiate communication spontaneously throughout his or her daily schedule should be targeted in order to foster communicative skills within naturally occurring contexts (Prizant & Wetherby, 1993; Schreibman & Pierce, 1993). Dawson and Osterling (1996) also emphasized the need for predictability and routine, family involvement, and intensive service delivery (especially in the early years).

Educational programs should be highly structured and oriented around the individual needs of the child. Intervention programs should be comprehensive and include the services of various professionals including special educators, speech pathologists, occupational therapists, and so forth. Parental involvement should be encouraged to enhance consistency in approaches at home and in school and to facilitate generalization of skills across settings. Professionals should work with parents to obtain appropriate educational placement and help parents become aware of other community resources, such as respite care.

A marked shift in social policy has resulted in most state agencies attempting to maintain children in their families and communities. Unfortunately, many necessary services may not be provided as a result of this trend. A similar issue has arisen with regard to the integration of autistic children into regular classroom settings. Given the nature of social deficits in autism, there is considerable reason to worry that autistic children may not be as able as mentally retarded, nonautistic, children to profit from such an approach. In considering various alternative educational placements, the individual needs of the child should be paramount. Competency in social skills is as important as level of cognitive functioning when considering the appropriate setting.

In general, pharmacological interventions with infants and young autistic children are best avoided. The best studied agents (i.e., the major tranquilizers) have some limited utility in selected cases, but their many side effects (particularly sedation) may prove problematic (Campbell, Anderson, Green, & Deutsch, 1987). The newer "atypical" neuroleptics may hold some promise for treating specific symptom clusters (McDougle et al., 1997), but efficacy has not been established through controlled trials as of yet. These agents may be indicated in some situations but are typically used in older children and, even then, at the lowest effective dose for the shortest period. Although stimulants have been used to treat inattention and hyperactivity in children with PDDs, they have no demonstrable effect on the "core" symptoms of autism (McDougle, 1997). Their use is entirely empirical, and often they cause serious adverse effects in austistic children. They should not be a first-line pharmacological intervention. The efficacy of other pharmacological agents has not been clearly established.

Many nontraditional treatments are presently available. In discussing such treatments with parents, it is helpful to explore the rationale for the proposed treatment, the evidence (if any) of efficacy, and its potential costs (in both financial and human terms) to the child and family. Treatments that are minimally disruptive of the child's educational program and that represent little apparent risk to the child are of less concern than those that entail considerable disruption of the child's educational program or the family's life.

In the clinical management of the autistic child, it is important not to lose sight of the needs of the family. Mothers of autistic children show high levels of stress and reactive depression, and the marriage may suffer as well

(Siegel, 1997). The adaptation of parents, siblings, and other family members often varies over time, both as a result of the normative stress and transitions inherent in family life and as a result of the special needs of the autistic child. Parental and family isolation, "burnout," and marital disharmony may be observed, and the increased demands on parents may be experienced negatively by siblings. On the other hand, many families cope well. Support for the family may take various forms depending on the specific needs of the family and the special characteristics of the autistic child; such support is best delivered in the context of an ongoing relationship. It is important to emphasize that the need for intervention in the family does not imply that parents are responsible for the affected child's autism.

IMPLICATIONS

Considerable progress in understanding the nature of autism and related disorders has been made over the past 50 years. Given the early onset of the condition, it is somewhat paradoxical that our knowledge of autism in infants and very young children remains limited in important respects. Knowledge of the other PDDs in infancy and early childhood is even more limited. Mental health professionals have important roles to play in evaluation and provision of remedial programming. Although it now appears that these conditions arise as the result of some insult to the developing central nervous system, precise and testable pathophysiological mechanisms remain to be identified. The study of infants and young children with autism may have important implications for both clinical service and our understanding of the course of early child development.

REFERENCES

Adrien, J. L., Lenoir, P., Martineau, J., Perrot, A., Hameury, L., Larmande, D., & Sauvage, D. (1993). Blind ratings of early symptoms of autism based upon family home movies. *Journal of the American Academy of Child and Adolescent Psychiatry, 33,* 617–626.

American Psychiatric Association. (1994). *Diagnostic and statistical manual of mental disorders* (4th ed). Washington, DC: Author.

Anderson, G. M., & Hoshino, Y. (1997). Neurochemical studies of autism. In D. Cohen & F. Volkmar (Eds.), *Handbook of autism and pervasive developmental disorders* (2nd ed., pp. 166–191). New York: Wiley.

Asperger, H. (1944). Die 'autistichen Psychopathen' im Kindersalter. *Archiv für psychiatrie und Nervenkrankheiten, 117,* 76–136.

Baron-Cohen, S. (1989). The autistic child's theory of mind: a case of specific developmental delay. *Journal of Child Psychology and Psychiatry, 30,* 285–297.

Bayley, N. (1969). *Bayley Scales of Infant Development.* New York: Psychological Corporation.

Bryson, S. (1997). Epidemiology of Autism: Overview and issues outstanding. In D. Cohen & F. R. Volkmar (Eds.), *Handbook of autism and pervasive developmental disorders,* (2nd ed., pp. 41–46). New York: Wiley.

Campbell M., Anderson L. T., Green W. H., & Deutsch S. I. (1987). Psychopharmacology. In D. Cohen & A. Donnellan (Eds.), *Handbook of Autism and Pervasive Developmental Disorders* (pp. 545–565). New York: Wiley.

Curcio, F. (1978). Sensorimotor functioning and communication in mute autistic children. *Journal of Autism and Childhood Schizophrenia, 8,* 281–292.

Dawson, G., & Osterling, J. (1996). Early intervention in autism. In M. J. Guralnick (Ed.), *The effectiveness of early intervention.* Baltimore: Brookes.

DeMyer M. K., Hingtgen J. N., & Jackson R. K. (1981). Infantile autism reviewed: A decade of research. *Schizophrenia Bulletin, 7,* 388–451.

Dunst, C. (1980). *A clinical and educational manual for use with the Uzgiriz and Hunt Scales.* Baltimore: University Park Press.

Dykens, E., & Volkmar, F. R. (1997). Medical conditions associated with autism. In D. Cohen & F. R. Volkmar (Eds.), *Handbook of autism and pervasive developmental disorders* (2nd ed., pp. 388–410). New York: Wiley.

Folstein, S., & Rutter, M. (1977). Infantile autism: A genetic study of 21 twin pairs. *Journal of Child Psychology and Psychiatry, 18,* 297–321.

Forbonne, E. (1998). The epidemiology of child and adolescent psychiatric disorders: Recent developments and issues. *Epidemiologia E Psichiatria Sociale, 7,* 161–166.

Gresham, F. M., & MacMillan, D. L. (1998). Early Intervention Project: Can its claims be substantiated and its effects replicated? *Journal of Autism and Developmental Disorders, 28*(1), 5–13.

International Molecular Genetic Study of Autism Consortium. (1998). A full genome screen for autism with evidence for linkage to a region on chromosome 7q. *Human Molecular Genetics, 7*(3), 571–578.

Kanner L. (1943). Autistic disturbances of affective contact. *Nervous Child, 2,* 217–250.

Kaufman, A., & Kaufman, N. (1983). *Kaufman Assessment Battery for Children.* Circle Pines, MN: American Guidance Service.

Klin, A. (1992). Listening preferences in regard to speech in four children with developmental disabilities. *Journal of Child Psychology and Psychiatry, 33*(4), 763–769.

Klin, A. (1997). Aperger's syndrome. In D. Cohen & F. R. Volkmar (Eds.), *Handbook of autism and pervasive developmental disorders* (2nd ed., pp. 94–122). New York: Wiley.

Klin, A., & Shepard, B. (1994). Psychological assessment of autistic children. *Child and Adolescent Psychiatric Clinics of North America, 3*(1), 53–69.

Klin, A., & Volkmar, F. R. (1993). The development of individuals with autism: Some implications for the theory of mind hypothesis. In S. Baron-Cohen, H. Tager-Flusberg, & D. Cohen (Eds.), *Understanding other minds: Perspectives from autism* (pp. 317–334). Oxford, UK: Oxford University Press.

Klin, A., Volkmar, F. R., & Sparrow, S. (1992). Autistic social dysfunction: Some limitations of the theory of mind hypothesis. *Journal of Child Psychology and Psychiatry, 33*(5), 861–876.

Klin, A., Volkmar, F. R., Sparrow, S., Cicchetti, D. V., & Rourke, B. P. (1995). Validity and neuropsychological characterization of Asperger syndrome: Convergence with nonverbal learning disabilities syndrome. *Journal of Child Psychology and Psychiatry, 36*(7), 1127–1140.

Kolvin I. (1971). Studies in the childhood psychoses: I. Diagnostic criteria and classification. *British Journal of Psychiatry, 118*, 381–384.

Lord, C. (1995). Follow-up of two year olds referred for possible autism. *Journal of Child Psychology and Psychiatry, 36*(8), 1365–1382.

Lord, C. (1997). Diagnostic instruments in autism spectrum disorders. In D. Cohen & F. Volkmar (Eds.), *Handbook of autism and pervasive developmental disorders* (2nd ed., pp. 460–483). New York: Wiley.

Lord, C., & Paul, R. (1997). Language and communication in autism. In D. Cohen & F. Volkmar (Eds.), *Handbook of autism and pervasive developmental disorders* (2nd ed., pp. 195–225). New York: Wiley.

Lovass, O. I. (1987). Behavioral treatment and normal educational and intellectual functioning in young autistic children. *Journal of Consulting and Clinical Psychology, 55*, 3–9.

McDougle, C. (1997). Psychopharmacology. In D. Cohen & F. Volkmar (Eds.), *Handbook of autism and pervasive developmental disorders* (2nd ed., pp. 707–729). New York: Wiley.

McDougle, C., Holmes, J. P., Bronson, M. R., Anderson, G. M., Volkmar, F. R., Price, L. H., & Cohen, D. J. (1997). Respiridone treatment of children and adolescents with pervasive developmental disorders: a prospective, open label study. *Journal of the American Academy of Child and Adolescent Psychiatry, 36*, 685–693.

Minshew, N., Sweeney, P. J., & Bauman, M. (1997). Neurological aspects of autism. In D. Cohen & F. R. Volkmar (Eds.), *Handbook of autism and pervasive developmental disorders* (2nd ed., pp. 344–369). New York: Wiley.

Morgan, S., Curtrer, P. S., Coplin, J. W., & Rodrique, J. R. (1989). Do autistic children differ from retarded and normal children in Piagetian sensorimotor functioning? *Journal of Child Psychology and Psychiatry, 30*, 857–864.

Mundy, P., Sigman, M., & Kasari, C. (1990). A longitudinal study of joint attention and language development in autistic children. *Journal of Autism and Developmental Disorders, 20, 1*, 115–128.

Olley, J. G., & Stevenson, S. E. (1989). Preschool curriculum for children with autism: Addressing early social skills. In G. Dawson (Ed.), *Autism: Nature, diagnosis, and treatment* (pp. 346–366). New York: Guilford Press.

Osterling, J., & Dawson, G. (1994). Early recognition of children with autism: A study of first birthday home videotapes. *Journal of Autism and Developmental Disorders, 24*, 247–257.

Prior, M., Dahlstrom, B., & Squires, T. (1990). Autistic children's knowledge of thinking and feeling states in other people. *Journal of Child Psychology and Psychiatry, 31*, 587–601.

Prizant, B., & Rydell, P. (1984). An analysis of the functions of delayed echolalia in autistic children. *Journal of Speech and Hearing Research, 27*, 183–192.

Prizant, B., & Wetherby, A. (1993). Communication in preschool autistic children. In E. Schopler, M. Van Bourgondien, & M. Bristol (Eds.), *Preschool issues in autism* (pp. 95–128). New York: Plenum.

Rett, A. (1966). Uber ein eigenartiges hirntophiscес Syndrome bei Hyperammonie im Kindersalter. *Wein Medizinische Wochenschrift, 118*, 723–726.

Reynell, J., & Gruber, C. (1990). *Reynell Developmental Language Scales—U.S. edition*, Los Angeles: Western Psychological Services.

Rogers, S. (1996). Brief report: early intervention in autism. *Journal of Autism and Developmental Disorders, 26*(2), 243–246.

Roid, G. H., & Miller, L. J. (1997). *Leiter International Performance Scale—Revised.* Wood Dale, IL: Stoelting.

Rutter M. (1970). Autistic children: Infancy to adulthood. *Seminars in Psychiatry, 2*, 435–450.

Rutter, M. (1972). Childhood schizophrenia reconsidered. *Journal of Autism and Childhood Schizophrenia, 2*, 315–338.

Rutter, M., Bailey, A., Bolton, P., & LeCouteur, A. (1994). Autism and known medical conditions: Myth and substance. *Journal of Child Psychology and Psychiatry, 35*(2), 311–322.

Rutter, M., Bailey, A., Simonoff, E., & Pickles, A. (1997). Genetic influences in autism. In D. Cohen & F. Volkmar (Eds.), *Handbook of autism and pervasive developmental disorders* (2nd ed., pp. 370–387). New York: Wiley.

Schreibman, L., & Pierce, K. (1993). Achieving greater generalization of treatment effects in children with autism: Pivotal response training and self management. *The Clinical Psychologist, 46*, 184–191.

Schuler, A., Prizant, B., & Wetherby, A. (1997). Enhancing language and communication development: Prelinguistic approaches. In D. Cohen & F. Volkmar (Eds.), *Handbook of autism and pervasive developmental disorders* (2nd ed., pp. 539–571), New York: Wiley.

Short, A. B., & Schopler, E., (1988). Factors relating to age of onset in autism. *Journal of Autism and Developmental Disorders, 18*, 207–216.

Siegel, B. (1997). Coping with the diagnosis of autism. In D. Cohen & F. R. Volkmar (Eds.), *Handbook of autism and pervasive developmental disorders* (2nd ed., pp. 745–766). New York: Wiley.

Sigman, M., & Ungerer, J. (1984). Attachment behaviors in autistic children. *Journal of Autism & Developmental Disorders, 14*, 231–244.

Sparrow, S. (1997). Developmentally based assessments. In D. Cohen & F. R. Volkmar (Eds.), *Handbook of autism and pervasive developmental disorders* (2nd ed., pp. 411–447). New York: Wiley.

Sparrow, S., Balla, D., & Ciccheti, D. (1984). *Vineland Adaptive Behavior Scales*. Circle Pines, MN: American Guidance Service.

Stone, W. (1997). Autism in infancy and early childhood. In D. Cohen & F. R. Volkmar (Eds.), *Handbook of autism and pervasive developmental disorders* (2nd ed., pp. 266–282). New York: Wiley.

Tager-Flusberg, H., & Sullivan, K. (1994). Predicting and explaining behavior: A comparison of autistic, mentally retarded and normal children. *Journal of Child Psychology and Psychiatry, 35*(6), 1059–1075.

Tordjman, S., Anderson, G., McBride, P. A., Hertzig, M. E., Snow, M. E., Hall, L. M., Thompson, S. M., Ferrari, P., & Cohen, D. J. (1997). Plasma β-Endorphin, Adrenocorticotropin hormone, and cortisol in autism. *Journal of Child Psychiatry and Psychology, 38*(6), 705–715.

Towbin, K. (1997). Pervasive developmental disorders not otherwise specified. In D. Cohen & F. R. Volkmar (Eds.), *Handbook of autism and pervasive developmental disorders* (2nd ed., pp. 123–147). New York: Wiley.

Tsai, L. Y. (1987). Pre–, peri–, and neonatal factors in autism. In E. Schopler & G. B. Mesibov (Eds.), *Neurobiological issues in autism* (pp. 180–187). New York: Plenum.

Uzgiris, I. C., & Hunt, J. McV. (1975). *Assessment in infancy: Ordinal scales of psychological development*. Urbana: University of Illinois Press.

Van Acker, R. (1997). Rett's syndrome. In D. Cohen & F. Volkmar (Eds.), *Handbook of autism and pervasive developmental disorders* (2nd ed., pp. 60–93). New York: Wiley.

Volden, J., & Lord, C. (1991). Neologisms and idiosyncratic language in autistic speakers. *Journal of Autism and Developmental Disorders, 21,* 109–130.

Volkmar, F. R., Carter, A., Grossman, J., & Klin, A. (1997). Social development in autism. In D. Cohen & F. Volkmar, (Eds.), *Handbook of autism and pervasive developmental disorders* (2nd ed., pp. 173–194). New York: Wiley.

Volkmar, F. R., & Cohen D. J. (1988). Diagnosis of pervasive developmental disorders. In B. Lahey & A. Kazdin (Eds.), *Advances in clinical child psychology* (vol. 11, pp. 249–284). New York: Plenum.

Volkmar, F. R., & Cohen, D. J. (1989). Disintegrative disorder of "late onset" autism. *Journal of Child Psychology and Psychiatry and Allied Disciplines, 30*(5), 717–724.

Volkmar, F. R., Cohen, D. J., Hoshino, Y., Rende, R., &

Paul, R. (1988). Phenomenology and classification of the childhood psychoses. *Psychological Medicine, 18,* 191–201.

Volkmar, F. R., Klin, A., & Cohen, D. (1997). Diagnosis and classification of autism and related conditions: Consensus and Issues. In D. Cohen & F. R. Volkmar (Eds.), *Handbook of autism and pervasive developmental disorders* (2nd ed., pp. 5–40). New York: Wiley.

Volkmar, F. R., Klin, A., Marans, W., & Cohen, D. J. (1997). Childhood disintegrative disorder. In D. J. Cohen & F. R. Volkmar (Eds.), *Handbook of autism and pervasive developmental disorders* (2nd ed., pp. 47–59). New York: Wiley.

Volkmar, F. R., Klin, A., Schultz, R., Bronen, R., Marans, W., Sparrow, S., & Cohen, D. J. (1996). Asperger syndrome. *Journal of the American Academy of Child and Adolescent Psychiatry, 35*(1), 118–123.

Volkmar, F. R., & Nelson, D. S. (1990). Seizure disorders in autism. *Journal of the American Academy of Child and Adolescent Psychiatry, 29*(19), 127–129.

Volkmar, F. R., & Rutter, M. (1995). Childhood disintegrative disorder: results of the DSM-IV autism field trial. *Journal of the American Academy of Child and Adolescent Psychiatry, 34,* 1092–1095.

Volkmar, F. R., Stier, D. M., & Cohen, D. J. (1985). Age of recognition of pervasive developmental disorder. *American Journal of Psychiatry, 142,* 1450–1452.

Wetherby, A. (1986). The ontogeny of communicative functions in autism. *Journal of Autism and Developmental Disorders, 16,* 295–316.

Wetherby, A., & Prizant, B. (1993). *Communication and Symbolic Behavior Scales—Normed edition*. Chicago: Riverside.

Wetherby, A., & Prutting, C. (1984). Profiles of communicative and cognitive–social abilities in autistic children. *Journal of Speech and Hearing Research, 27,* 364–377.

Wetherby, A., Schuler, A., & Prizant, B. (1997). Enhancing language and communication development: Theoretical foundation. In D. Cohen & F. R. Volkmar (Eds.), *Handbook of autism and pervasive developmental disorders* (2nd ed., pp. 513–538). New York: Wiley.

Wing, L. (1997). Syndromes of autism and atypical development. In D. Cohen & F. R. Volkmar (Eds.), *Handbook of Autism and Pervasive Developmental Disorders* (2nd ed., pp. 148–170). New York: Wiley.

World Health Organization. (1992). *The ICD-10 classification of mental and behavioral disorders: Clinical descriptions and diagnostic guidelines*. Geneva, Switzerland: Author.

19

Regulatory Disorders

❖

MARIANNE L. BARTON
DIANA ROBINS

In recent years the concept of emotion regulation has emerged as central to a contemporary understanding of emotional development in young children. The development of characteristic patterns of behavior in early childhood is believed to be rooted in the developing child's ability to regulate emotional state and to organize a behavioral response to experience. Characteristic patterns of regulating state and organizing experience are presumed to develop from repeated interactions between infant and caregiver around the achievement of physical, and later, emotional homeostasis (Sroufe, 1995). The establishment of such patterns early in life also is believed to affect the development of neuronal pathways in the brain, encouraging the elaboration of those circuits that are activated repeatedly in infancy (Schore, 1994).

The behavior of caregivers is clearly central to this process, as it is the caregiver who provides strategies for state regulation which are subsequently internalized by the developing child (Stern, 1985; Sroufe, 1995). These strategies generalize over time to include the regulation of affective states, arousal, attention, and the organization of complex behaviors including social interaction. Failures in the development of self-regulatory capacities are believed to underlie a variety of behavioral problems, including attention deficits, oppositional behavior, tantrumming, and some forms of social isolation. Although the child's contribution to this process has long been recognized (e.g. Sameroff & Chandler, 1975), it is often lumped

under such poorly defined categories as biological vulnerability or temperament. Equally important, as Greenspan and Weider (1993) point out, theory regarding intrinsic individual differences in the capacity for self-regulation has not been integrated into a sophisticated understanding of behavioral problems in young children.

The construct of regulatory disorders was initially proposed by Greenspan and his colleagues (Greenspan, 1992; Greenspan & Weider, 1993; Zero to Three, 1994) in an effort to address this deficit and to describe a group of children observed in clinical settings who present specific behavioral patterns coupled with clear difficulties in sensory processing or motor planning. The construct has been quite useful clinically because it provides a novel understanding of a common clinical picture and offers some suggestions for new intervention models. Empirical investigations of the construct have been slow to follow, although recent work in the field of occupational therapy is beginning to provide some measure of empirical support.

THE CONSTRUCT OF REGULATORY DISORDERS

Regulatory Disorders are defined as distinct patterns of atypical behaviors coupled with specific difficulties in sensory, sensory–motor, or organizational processing (Zero to Three, 1994). The latter may include atypical patterns of sensory reactivity, including both hyper- and hyposensitivity, as well as difficulties with the organization of motor activity and the modulation of affect. Difficulties with information processing in various sensory modalities are common. These difficulties are presumed to be constitutional in origin. They compromise the infant's ability to establish comfortable interactive patterns with the external world, including caregivers, and are believed to have significant implications for long-term development. Infants with regulatory disorders may have difficulty achieving a quiet, alert state or an affectively positive state. They may have difficulty sustaining attention at developmentally appropriate levels and may be excessively aroused by routine environmental stimulation. Often they are described as fussy, irritable, or prone to excessive crying (Maldonado-Duran & Sauceda-Garcia, 1996). All these patterns are presumed to reflect behavioral efforts to accommodate sensory processing difficulties. Greenspan and his colleagues (Greenspan, 1992; Greenspan & Weider, 1993) have described infants with regulatory disorders as having significant difficulty organizing their physiology, their sensory responses, and their behavioral state. They note that to be considered a regulatory disorder, distinct behavioral patterns must be accompanied by difficulties in underlying sensory or information-processing capacities, and that these difficulties must be significant enough to affect daily adaptation and relationships. At least one of the following sensory, sensory–motor, or processing difficulties must be observed to make the diagnosis of regulatory disorder: over- or underreactivity to sound, lights or visual images, odors, or temperature; tactile defensiveness, oral motor difficulties or incoordination influenced by poor muscle tone, motor planning problems or oral–motor hypersensitivities; underreactivity to touch or pain; gravitational insecurity; poor muscle tone and muscle stability, or qualitative deficits in motor planning skills; ability to modulate motor activity; fine motor skills; articulation; visual–spatial processing skills; or the capacity to attend and focus.

The *Diagnostic Classification: 0–3* (DC: 0–3; Zero to Three, 1994) for children from birth to age 3 includes four subtypes of regulatory disorders. Three of these are characterized by one predominant pattern of behavior and sensory functioning. The remaining subtype is a mixed category which is used to classify those children who do not fit into the first three classes. The primary subtypes include the *hypersensitive* type, the *underreactive* type, and the *motorically disorganized/impulsive* type.

Children classified as Type I: Hypersensitive are highly reactive to sensory input, although their level of sensitivity may vary across sensory modalities and/or over the course of a day. Two behavioral patterns are associated with this subtype: the fearful, cautious pattern and the negative and defiant pattern. Children who exhibit the former pattern are highly fearful and inhibited. They tend to dislike changes in routine and may cling to caregivers excessively in new situations. Such children tend to be easily upset and have difficulty self-soothing. They are slow to recover from disappointment or frustration. Associated sensory patterns include sensitivity to touch, noises, and bright lights. These children may also have difficulties with visuospatial processing and may present motor planning problems.

Children classified as negative and defiant tend to be controlling, stubborn, and defiant in interaction with others. They have difficulty making transitions and prefer repetition or slow, gradual change. As infants they may be fussy and difficult, whereas preschoolers may be angry and negativistic, as well as perfectionistic and compulsive. At times, it appears that the negative and defiant child achieves some form of internal organization through negative interactive patterns; in contrast, the fearful child appears to be unable to impose any organization upon his or her internal world. The child classified as defiant is likely to be overreactive to touch and sound, with some difficulties in motor planning or fine motor coordination.

The child with Type II: Underreactive regulatory disorder may be described as exhibiting one of two behavioral patterns: The child is either withdrawn and difficult to engage, or self-absorbed. Children in the former category appear disinterested in exploring social relationships or the environment. Their play is impoverished and may include a limited range of ideas and diminished verbalization. Their sensory patterns are characterized by underreactivity to sound and movement but either under- or overreactivity to touch. Auditory processing problems and poor motor planning are also commonly observed.

Children described as self-absorbed present more creative and imaginative activity, but they may prefer to attend exclusively to their own ideas and activities. Infants may appear self-absorbed, whereas older children may seem inattentive or preoccupied. Some children may show difficulties with auditory processing.

The Type III: Motorically disorganized/impulsive regulatory disorder is characterized by high activity levels and reckless, impulsive behavior. These children seem to seek sensory input. Often their behavior is viewed as aggressive, although their difficulties appear to be rooted in excitability, impulsivity, and poor motor planning rather than in any aggressive intent. These children frequently exhibit sensory underreactivity and disorganized motor activity. They frequently have poor motor modulation and motor planning and have difficulty maintaining focused attention.

Although the broad category of regulatory disorders has preliminary support from clinical experience and an emerging research base, the subtypes are ambiguous, confusing, and not well supported. Some behaviors are intended to distinguish one subtype from another (e.g., sensory reactivity to input in one sensory modality); however, other difficulties, such as motor planning, are observed in children in nearly every subtype. Even the notion that children may be classified by modality specific sensitivities is suspect, as some studies have suggested that reactivity in one sensory modality may be highly correlated with sensitivity in other modalities (Miller et al., in press). At present, it seems that the classification of children with regulatory disorders into meaningful and reliable subtypes awaits more careful specification of patterns of sensory reactivity and associated behavior and empirical data supporting the reliability of subtypes.

EMPIRICAL INVESTIGATIONS OF REGULATORY DISORDERS

Empirical investigations of the construct of regulatory disorders have been extremely limited. To date, no data have been published on the temporal stability of the diagnosis of regulatory disorder, nor of the various subtypes. Although the Zero to Three Task Force continues to collect data regarding the diagnostic categories described in the DC:0–3, no data are available regarding either the reliability or the validity of new diagnostic entities such as regulatory disorder. Nor are data available on the extent to which independent evaluators can agree on the diagnosis or can be readily trained to do so. The criteria in the *DC: 0–3* system provide no specific guidelines for cutoff, leaving unclear who does not have a regulatory disorder.

DeGangi and her colleagues (DeGangi, DiPietro, Greenspan, & Porges, 1991; DeGangi, Porges, Sickel, & Greenspan, 1993) have reported on two pilot studies of a sample of 11 infants with regulatory disorder. The authors report that infants were diagnosed with regulatory disorder on the basis of independent diagnostic observations made by a nurse practitioner and a clinical psychologist, but no index of agreement was provided. DeGangi et al. (1991) required that children present difficulties in at least two of the following areas to qualify for a diagnosis of regulatory disorder: sleep disturbance, difficulties self-soothing, feeding difficulties, emotional lability, or distress with changes in routine, routine caregiving, and play experiences that offer a sensory challenge.

DeGangi et al. (1991) attempted to identify physiological correlates of regulatory disorder by comparing the cardiac vagal tone of infants with regulatory disorder to a small sample of typically developing children. Vagal tone and reactivity are presumed to measure activity in the autonomic nervous system that underlies movement and emotional regulation. The authors reported no differences in baseline vagal tone between their groups, but children with regulatory disorders showed much greater variability in their capacity to suppress vagal tone during a cognitive challenge. The researchers suggest that these data reflect the difficulty experienced by infants with regulatory disorder in modulating the autonomic nervous system to permit more focused attention and efficient information processing during the administration of a cognitive test. Although the sample size was quite small, and the study has not been replicated, it nonetheless suggests some link between the behaviors characterized by regulatory disorder and the function of the autonomic nervous system.

DeGangi et al. (1993) provided data on the long-term follow-up of 9 of the 11 youngsters in the original sample. Eight of the nine children exhibited regulatory, developmental, and/or sensorimotor deficits at age 4. One child appeared to fall within normal limits all measures but exhibited wide variation in his development across cognitive areas. Four of the children presented with hyperactivity and short attention span, and more than half had behavioral or emotional regulation problems, tactile defensiveness, sensory integration deficits, or poor motor planning. Five of the nine youngsters with regulatory disorder also presented delays in motor development or cognitive development. The authors noted the significant limitations imposed by their small sample, and the fact that eight of the nine children in the regulatory-disordered group were boys. They also noted methodological problems, including the fact that the evaluators at follow-up were not blind to the children's initial group membership. Nonetheless, they suggest that the study offers preliminary evidence that untreated regulatory disorders may persist into the preschool years.

To date there have been no other empirical studies describing the use of the regulatory disorder classification. Maldonado-Duran and Sauceda-Garcia (1996) described their use of the construct in a clinical setting and reported on a series of case vignettes. They also noted the lack of clear specification of the number and severity of atypical sensitivities required for the diagnosis. They proposed that the diagnosis of regulatory disorder be reserved for those infants with several abnormal sensitivities (more than two), and that they should be "severe enough to cause dysfunction in the infant and concern in the parent" (p. 67).

REGULATORY DISORDERS AND SENSORY REGULATION

Perhaps the best evidence for the validity of the construct of regulatory disorders comes from the work of occupational therapists interested in the concept of sensory modulation. Sensory modulation has been defined as "the ability to react to sensory stimulation in a manner appropriate to task demands, environmental context, social supports and cultural expectations" (Shyu, Miller, McIntosh, & Dunn, 1999). Individuals who experience difficulty with sensory modulation may be hyperreactive or hyporeactive to sensory input, or they may fluctuate between the two extremes (Dunn, 1997). Sensory modulation disruptions (SMD) may be distinguished from the concept of regulatory disorder because the former refers specifically to variations in an individual's sensory reactivity. Regulatory disorders include distinctive behavioral patterns which are presumed to accompany variations in sensory reactivity. Regulatory disorders also include the regulation of affective state and attention, which some measures of SMD exclude. Ayres (1972, 1979) initially described children with sensory integration difficulties and proposed sensory integration training as a variant of occupational therapy. Her methods have been widely adopted in the occupational therapy of young children with a variety of sensory difficulties. Some data suggest that sensory integration training is helpful in reducing sensory sensitivity, but there is very little evidence linking sensory integration training to broader changes in behavior. In addition, many of the studies assessing the efficacy of sensory integration training have serious methodological limitations (see Miller & Kinnealey, 1993; Deams, 1994 for reviews).

Occupational therapists rely on two broad approaches to the assessment of sensory irregularities. A number of published tests provide a series of structured activities to which children respond. Therapists then can observe directly the child's capacity to regulate sensory input and respond to different stimuli. The Sensory Integration and Praxis Tests (SIPT; Ayres, 1989) are a more recent version of the Southern California Sensory Integration Tests (Ayres, 1972) and the Southern California Postrotary Nystagmus Test (Ayres, 1975). The SIPT evaluates sensory processing in different modalities (e.g., visual, tactile, and vestibular) and has been standardized on children between 4 and 9 years old. Another standardized measure is the DeGangi–Berk Test of Sensory Integration (TSI; DeGangi & Berk, 1983). Normed on children between the ages of 3 and 5, the TSI assesses primarily proprioceptive and vestibular functioning. These measures are limited by the fact that they sample a small subset of a child's behavior and have numerous constraints imposed upon their validity by the artificial nature of the setting in which they are administered. Nonetheless, they are useful because they avoid some of the subjectivity inherent in parental report.

The second approach to the assessment of sensory irregularities relies on parental report of the frequency with which a child engages in a variety of sensory behaviors in natural settings. This method provides for a broader sample of behavior and has the benefit of caregiver observations across time and across settings. Its primary disadvantage lies in the fact that it may be biased by parental perception and expectations. This concern has been ameliorated to some degree by the use of specific descriptions of behavior instead of more global rating scales, and by the use of multiple informants including parents, teachers, and children themselves (e.g., DeGangi, Poisson, Sickel, & Wiener, 1998). There are a small number of scales available to rate sensory processing, and few have been subjected to any analysis of their psychometric properties.

One exception is the Sensory Profile (Dunn & Westman, 1997), developed and studied by Dunn and her colleagues. The Sensory Profile consists of 125 items originally derived from interviews with the parents of children who had disabilities (Dunn, 1997). These items are divided into eight areas of sensory processing: (1) auditory, (2) visual, (3) taste/smell, (4) movement, (5) touch, (6) activity level, (7) body position, and (8) emotional/social. Each subscale consists of three to 21 items which parents endorse by rating the frequency with which their child displays each behavior on a 5-point Likert scale. Parents rate their children as (1) always engaging in the behavior; (2) frequently engaging in the behavior, or at least 75% of the time; (3) occasionally exhibiting the behavior, approximately 50% of the time; (4) seldom exhibiting the behavior, or 25% of the time; and (5) never exhibiting the behavior.

Dunn and her colleagues conducted a series of studies to ascertain the presence of sensory processing concerns in a normative sample and to identify items that might discriminate between groups of children with varying disabilities. In a national study of 1,115 children, ages 3 to 10 years, without disabilities, Dunn and Westman (1997) found no age or gender differences among their items. More significantly, they report that more than two-thirds of their items were rarely or never observed in typical children.

Dunn and Brown (1997) completed a principal component factor analysis of the items on the Sensory Profile using the same data set. They identified nine factors that accounted for 47% of the variance and included 78 items from the original pool. Most items loaded on only one factor because item loadings below .40 were dropped from the analysis. The factors are interpreted as follows: (1) sensory seeking, (2) emotionally reactive, (3) low endurance/tone, (4) oral sensory sensitivity, (5) inattention/distractibility (6) poor registration, (7) sensory sensitivity, (8) sedentary, and (9) fine motor/perceptual. The authors hypothesize that although their sample included only children without disabilities, many of the factors represent areas of difficulty for children with a variety of disabilities. The authors suggest that their data provide preliminary evidence regarding the nature of sensory processing in all children and, furthermore, that children with various disabilities may differ in the rate or intensity of sensory processing patterns, or in the extent to which these patterns interfere with daily life. The data also reveal that factors emerged based on children's sensitivity and reactivity to sensory input *overall* rather than on which sensory modality was being assessed. This may suggest reframing the way in which sensory regulation is assessed, since it may be more important to know if a child is primarily underreactive or overreactive to stimuli across sensory modalities, rather than whether he or she responds differently to input in different modalities. A related study used electrodermal responses to assess sensory reactivity in a sample of children with fragile-X syndrome (Miller et al., in press). These data also reveal a high degree of consistency in reactivity across sensory modalities and lend support to the reconceptualization of sensory disregulation suggested by Dunn and Brown (1997).

Ermer and Dunn (1998) compared sensory profiles obtained from 679 typical children, 61 children diagnosed with attention-deficit/hyperactivity disorder (ADHD), and 38 children diagnosed with autistic disorder. The children in both of the clinical samples had significantly higher rates of behaviors reported on the Sensory Profile than did children in the typical group, but children in the two clinical groups had higher frequencies of behaviors on different items. A discriminant function analysis using the nine factors led to the correct diagnosis for 89% of the children in the study. Four factors contributed to the discrimination between groups: sensory seeking, oral sensory sensitivity, inattention/distractibility, and fine motor/perceptual. Children with autism displayed a pattern of behavior very different from that of children without disabilities. They exhibited high levels of oral sensitivity, inattention/distractibility, and fine motor or perceptual problems and lower than normal levels of sensory seeking. Children with ADHD displayed high levels of sensory seeking and distractibility but lower levels of oral sensitivity and fine motor/perceptual problems. The finding that autistic children showed low levels of sensory-seeking behaviors may seem counterintuitive at first. However, the sensory-seeking factor combines healthy sensory-seeking behaviors (e.g., seeking out movement and enjoying strange noises) with atypical sensory responses (e.g., twirls self frequently and takes excessive risks during play), and it may be that if the autistic children were not exhibiting sufficient healthy sensory-seeking behaviors, they obtained a lower factor score.

A shorter version of the Sensory Profile has been developed (McIntosh, Miller, & Shyu, in press). The Short Sensory Profile (SSP) consists of 38 items from the Sensory Profile which were specifically selected to discriminate children with sensory modulation disruptions from typical children. It is psychometrically sound and has excellent reliability and validity. The SSP contains seven factors that relate closely to seven of the nine factors from the Sensory Profile. These new factors are (1) tactile sensitivity, (2) taste/smell sensitivity, (3) visual/auditory sensitivity, (4) movement sensitivity, (5) underresponsive/seeks sensation, (6) auditory filtering, and (7) low energy/weak. Reliability was found to be greater than .90 for the entire scale, and the reliability for the subscales ranged from .70 to .93. The SSP demonstrates moderate intercorrelations between the subscales. Convergent validity was found by comparing SSP responses to electrodermal responses (EDR) following a sensory challenge (during which participants' responses to repeated sensory stimulation were recorded). EDR are viewed as an indirect measure of the activity of the sympathetic nervous system, which varies in response to sensory stimulation. Children who scored in the lower range of the SSP (more abnormal sensory responses) had abnormal EDR (either too high or too low). Children who had normal EDR had significantly higher scores on each subscale of the SSP (Miller et al., in press).

Based on her data from studies of the Sensory Profile, Dunn (1997) proposed a model for the integration of concepts from neuroscience and behavior that fits easily with the continuum of regulatory disorders described by Greenspan and his colleagues. Dunn suggests a four-celled model which describes the interaction between a child's sensory threshold, that is, the amount of stimulation needed for the nervous system to notice and respond, and the child's behavioral response repertoire, that is, the manner in which the young child responds to his sensory experience. The vertical axis in her model reflects the neurological threshold continuum which varies from high thresholds characterized by habituation to incoming stimuli to low thresholds evidenced by high sensitivity to sensory input. The horizontal axis reflects the child's potential behavioral response continuum and varies between responses in accord with his or her threshold (the child makes no effort to compensate for threshold irregularities) and responses that seek to counteract the threshold (the child attempts to compensate behaviorally for either high or low sensory thresholds). The resulting cells of the model reflect the interaction of the neurological threshold and the behavioral response: *poor registration, sensitivity to stimuli, sensation seeking*, and *sensation avoiding*.

Children who exhibit poor registration have high neurological thresholds and behave in accord with those thresholds. They may appear dull or disinterested because sensory experiences are slow to register, and they do little to augment their experience. Dunn (1997) proposed that this category of her model is analogous to the Type II: Underreactive child described by the Zero to Three Task Force (Zero to Three, 1994).

Children who fall in the sensitivity to stimuli quadrant have low sensory thresholds. They are highly sensitive to sensory input and they act in accord with their sensory threshold. They may appear inattentive and unable to organize their behavior. They are viewed as similar to children with a Type I: Hypersensitive regulatory disorder.

Children who have high sensory thresholds and are, therefore, slow to register sensory input may develop behavioral strategies, such as high activity levels and risk-taking behavior, to counteract those thresholds. These children are labeled sensation seeking in Dunn's model and appear similar to children with a Type III: Motorically disorganized/impulsive regulatory disorder.

Finally, children who have low sensory thresholds and are, therefore, highly sensitive to sensory stimulation may also develop behavioral patterns, such as reducing their activity and withdrawing from interaction, to counteract their sensory threshold. These children are called sensation avoiding. They are viewed as similar to children with two types of regulatory disorders, dependent on the nature of the behaviors they use to counteract their threshold. Children who rely on stubborn and controlling behaviors might be classified as negative and defiant Type I: Hypersensitive regulatory disorder. Children who exhibit more inattention to stimuli, narrowing of focus to solitary pursuits, and preoccupation with certain stimuli may appear more consistent with the self-absorbed type of the Type II: Underreactive regulatory disorder. Dunn (1997) noted that her model is a working hypothesis which requires further testing and elaboration.

Studies comparing the Zero to Three regulatory disorder subtypes with Dunn's classification schema, and with parental report on the Sensory Profile and the SSP, have not been published yet. Evidence of some convergence between the two systems would provide preliminary evidence for the validity of the construct of regulatory disorders. The fact that two groups of researchers working with relative independence have structured their observations of difficulties associated with sensory processing in ways that are broadly similar suggests that there may be validity to their observations. At the very least, both models are deserving of further investigation.

Data from the study of sensory modulation disruptions have led to good theories but insufficient empirical support for those hypotheses. The Sensory Profile (Dunn & Westman, 1997) is one of the first attempts to standardize the measurement of sensory irregularities through parent report. It is extremely valuable, although it has several limitations. The Sensory Profile lacks strong reliability and validity data, and the factor structure is not very clear (e.g., although items are said to load on only one factor, the temper tantrum item loads on both fine motor/perceptual and emotionally reactive factors), and there is little explanation about items that load on seemingly unrelated factors. The SSP (McIntosh et al., in press) is more psychometrically sound, although the validity studies will be stronger once larger sample sizes are included and a clearer measure of discriminant validity is studied. In addition, the seven factors make more sense intuitively than the nine factors of the Sensory Profile, and each item loads on only one factor. However, the authors of the SSP eliminated all items that did not pertain directly to sensory reactivity, which included all items from the emotional/social area of sensory processing (and the emotional reactivity factor). Difficulty regulating emotion is one of the

diagnostic criteria for regulatory disorder (Zero to Three, 1994); without the emotion/social subscale from the original Sensory Profile, the SSP is lacking items to measure emotional reactivity, making comparison with measures of regulatory disorder less meaningful.

TEMPERAMENT AND REGULATORY DISORDERS

Infants' biologically determined contribution to the construction of early caregiver–infant interaction has long been studied under the rubric of infant temperament. Temperament has been defined in a variety of ways since the pioneering work of Thomas, Chess, and their colleagues (Thomas, Chess, Birch, Hertzig, & Korn, 1963; see Lyons-Ruth & Zeanah, 1993, for a review). All current conceptualizations of temperament have in common an assumption that infants have biologically based predispositions to react to environmental events and affective experience in unique ways, and that these intrinsic differences affect the development of relatively stable patterns of interpersonal behavior. At the same time, temperamental variations are assumed to be influenced and altered by the caregiving matrix, and infant interactive experience is now assumed to affect the biology of ongoing development. There is little dispute about the influence of temperament or intrinsic infant characteristics on behavior; however, there is considerable debate about the measurement of the construct and about its relative contribution to infant development. Chiefly, debate has centered on the fact that temperament is most often measured by parental report and, thus, reflects parental perceptions of their infant as much as the unique characteristics of the child (Zeanah, Keener, & Anders, 1986; Seifer, Sameroff, Barrett, & Krafchuk, 1994). Although recent efforts to measure temperament independent of parental report have been fruitful (Seifer et al., 1994), they are not without controversy and questions regarding the measurement of the construct persist. This is an issue that affects the assessment of regulatory disorders as well. While parental report is clearly extremely important to the clinical assessment process, the assumption that parental report accurately reflects a biologically based problem must be questioned.

New conceptualizations of temperament have defined the construct in ways that make it highly relevant to the study of regulatory disorders. Rothbart and colleagues (Rothbart & Dayberry, 1981; Rothbart, Ahadi, & Hershey, 1994) posit that temperament refers to biologically based differences in the reactivity of the central nervous system and in the individual's capacity for self-regulation. Although their work has based the assessment of temperament primarily on parent report, Buss and Goldsmith (1998) has developed a laboratory-based assessment of temperament that appears to be quite promising. The studies by DeGangi et al. (1993), and Miller et al. (in press) offer some suggestion of a link between atypical central nervous system functioning and regulatory disorder and between atypical central nervous system responses and sensory modulation disruptions. The DeGangi et al. (1993) study also revealed that seven of nine infants diagnosed with regulatory disorder were rated by their mothers as difficult on the fussy–difficult scale of the Infant Characteristics Questionnaire (Bates, 1984), suggesting some overlap between the diagnosis of regulatory disorder and maternal assessment of difficult temperament. That does not imply, however, that regulatory disorders are synonymous with difficult temperament. Difficult temperament, as it is typically defined, is found in approximately 10% of infants and represents a normal variation in development (Barr, 1990). Regulatory disorder, by definition, describes a more rarely seen pathological state. Regulatory disorders may represent the atypical extreme of normal variations in temperament or central nervous system reactivity; however, that hypothesis is by no means certain given the present state of knowledge.

Similarly, regulatory disorders are distinguished from infant colic by the fact that the latter is a self-limiting condition which disappears at approximately 4 months (Maldonado-Duran & Sauceda-Garcia, 1996). Although some infants with colic may also demonstrate sensory irregularities similar to those described in children with regulatory disorders, those are not typically considered part of the diagnosis or clinical picture of colic. Furthermore, it is unclear whether those infants with colic who also present sensory irregularities outgrow them with the colic, or whether those infants develop more persistent difficulties similar to regulatory disorders.

The view of regulatory disorders presented here focuses heavily on the uniqueness of the individual child and his or her specific biologically based vulnerabilities. The contribution of the interpersonal relationships in which the child is embedded cannot be overlooked. As Greenspan (1992) and others (Maldonado-Duran & Saceda-Garcia, 1996) have noted, different caregiving relationships will have a dramatic impact on the child's ability to modulate sensory input, to maintain a positive and calm affective state, and to develop the ability to regulate affect and behavior. It is assumed that patterns of fussiness and reactivity are modifiable, to some extent at least, by a sensitive caregiving relationship, and successful experiences of other-directed regulation affect brain development as well as personality. Conversely, an infant's emotional equilibrium may be disturbed by negative caregiving experiences, and intrinsic difficulties may be exacerbated by nonempathic caregiving experiences. What is made critically apparent in the construct of regulatory disorders is the realization that some babies tax their caregiving environment in ways that are severely challenging, due to their unique sensory processing patterns. In these circumstances, the successful caregiver must identify those atypical demands and create an interactive matrix where they can be managed with greater comfort.

DIRECTIONS FOR RESEARCH

Numerous questions remain about the definition of the construct of regulatory disorders. Is regulatory disorder truly a disorder itself, or might it represent an early risk factor for later developing pathologies? How malleable are characteristic behavioral patterns to the influence of the caregiving environment? To what extent does the tolerance level of the caregiver contribute to the assignment of a diagnostic label? Some caregivers experience a fussy baby as difficult but normal, whereas another caregiver might find the same baby's behavior intolerable and pathological. How strongly do sensory processing abnormalities and emotion regulation difficulties cluster? In the absence of clear data about the incidence of the condition, the reliability of the diagnosis, and the long-term outcome, it seems that the term "disorder" should be used with caution.

Alternatively, regulatory disorders may represent the earliest manifestations of other disorders related to the modulation of attention, affect, and behavior. For example, the view that regulatory disorders reflect an inability to modulate one's reaction to sensory stimulation seems quite consistent with a recent conceptualization of attention-deficit disorder as a difficulty inhibiting reaction to sensory input (Barkley, 1997). Although some data suggest an association between early diagnosis of regulatory disorder and later attention problems (DeGangi et al., 1993), that is likely true only for a subset of children diagnosed with regulatory disorder. Who those children are and how they might be identified or treated early in development remain unclear.

Given the present state of knowledge, a certain measure of skepticism seems warranted until further research can either elaborate or repudiate the construct. Research should begin with an effort to specify the nature of sensory processing problems and to measure them quantitatively. The Sensory Profile and the SSP are important contributions to this effort, but they need more normative data, a more detailed scoring system, and greater evidence of reliability and validity. Given such data, either measure might be useful in delineating the severity of variations in sensory processing. A similar measure or a modification of one of the current ones should be developed for use with children under 3. The diagnostic criteria for regulatory disorder should include much greater specificity in the definition of the behavior patterns associated with sensory processing problems and the role of emotion regulation in conceptualizing the disorder. Data regarding the reliability of the diagnosis using the current system are also needed. Once reliability is established, the incidence of regulatory disorders in the general population can be assessed. Similarly, data are needed regarding the long-term follow-up of children diagnosed with regulatory disorder and their response to intervention. Further studies of the relationship of regulatory disorder to physiological measures of reactivity of the central nervous system are also important. Finally, the subtypes of regulatory disorder should be subjected to a similar set of empirical investigations to determine their reliability, validity, and clinical utility. The publication *DC: 0–3* (Zero to Three, 1994) may permit this research process to begin in earnest, as clinicians begin to use and modify diagnostic constructs.

All these empirical concerns notwithstanding, the diagnostic category of regulatory disorder already has demonstrated enormous clinical utility. The notion that children bring their own sensitivities and patterns of emotional regulation to the caregiving matrix, and that these require empathic recognition and differential responses from caregivers, has already been influential in the practice of early intervention and in the popular press (e.g., Kurcinka, 1992; Greenspan, 1995; Kranowitz, 1998). The model offers the clinician working with infants and their families a way to articulate the interplay between sensory processes and behavioral patterns. In doing so, it draws attention to the central role of sensory processing in the daily lives of infants and young children and challenges caregivers and service providers to examine this often overlooked component of experience with greater sensitivity.

Equally important, the theory of regulatory disorders permits parents to label and begin to understand the challenges presented by these difficult children. That recognition alone is sometimes sufficient to alter a negative interactive cycle and prevent the reification of negative representations of a child in the mind of his caregiver. When the child can be redefined to caregivers as struggling with reaction patterns beyond his control, rather than as willfully noncompliant, fussy, or insatiable, there is room in the relationship for new problem-solving strategies, greater flexibility, and a fresh perspective. Finally, the recognition of the role of sensory processing problems in the genesis of negative behavioral patterns suggests intervention strategies aimed at altering the underlying sensitivities or adjusting the environment to better support the child.

INTERVENTION STRATEGIES

Intervention strategies used with children with regulatory disorders reflect an amalgam of approaches borrowed from the work of occupational therapists and infant–parent psychotherapists. The therapist, often in consultation with other professionals, moves flexibly between a focus on the sensory processing challenges presented by the child and the broader social and emotional context in which the child lives.

The idea that behavioral problems may reflect underlying sensory irregularities immediately suggests changes in parental responses to children's difficult behavior. Parents are encouraged to look for children's atypical reactions to various sensory input and to attempt to alter the environment as much as possible to limit children's exposure to stimulation they find excessive. Thus, infants who are hyperreactive to sensory input should be protected from loud, noisy environments, which are likely to include big family gatherings and busy, crowded settings. Such infants also may benefit from efforts to reduce the amount of sensory input in the home, especially in their bedrooms (e.g., keeping lights low, providing soft, soothing music, avoiding extremes of temperature, and avoiding rapid changes in sensory stimulation of any sort). Children who are underreactive may benefit from the provision of sensory information in multiple modalities; nearly all children with processing problems will benefit from adults' efforts to slow down the rate at which information is communicated in any modality.

Infants with sensory irregularities also may benefit from increased exposure to certain kinds of sensory experiences, which are thought to provide them with sensory input they can process and use adaptively. Young infants may be calmed by being held or even swaddled, or by rhythmic vestibular stimulation such as swinging or rocking; older children as well as infants appear to respond positively to massage and other forms of firm touch. Occupational therapists often prescribe a sensory "diet," or a program that includes a variety of activities designed to help children with processing problems focus their attention, adapt to their environment, and improve their processing skills. These may include alerting activities to encourage the underresponsive child to attend more actively, organizing activities to help focus attention and direct action and calming activities to help the overresponsive child diminish their reactivity (Kranowitz, 1998). All these strategies represent a continued phase of assessment during which caregivers and professionals experiment with variations in sensory input until they find strategies that are effective in soothing a child, preventing overarousal, and encouraging comfortable engagement with the environment. Greenspan and Weider (1993) point out that the successful identification of sensory processing issues permits caregivers to sidestep obstacles to relatedness and begin the process of helping children engage and attend to the external environment, thus putting developmental processes back on a typical course. These strategies are crucial to the initial goal of restoring some equilibrium to a relationship upset by the disorganizing effect of atypical sensory responses.

Greenspan (1992) outlined a series of strategies designed to remediate sensory irregularities, or at least reduce their impact on a child's functioning, consistent with his broader model of development. Once sensory sensitivities are identified, children can be encouraged to develop a problem-solving orientation to the frustration that often accompanies their efforts to negotiate typical environments. Rather than being overwhelmed by sensory experiences, children can be encouraged to practice graduated exposure to those experiences they find most stressful. A child who is particularly sensitive to noise, for example, may benefit from the opportunity to play with toys that make noise in ways he or she can initially control and then become more random. If the child can be encouraged to approach such a toy in a setting that feels comfortable and safe, and at a pace he determines, he or she may be willing to experiment with the object and slowly increase his or her tolerance for stimulation that was previously quite threatening. Greenspan (1992) argues that children with regulatory disorders require extra practice and opportunities for anticipation in precisely those areas in which they have atypical sensitivities.

As children become verbal, caregivers can begin to encourage them to use language to anticipate and describe their reactions to sensory input. The experience of manageable levels of practice and anticipation permit the child to develop a more functional approach to regulatory issues and move slowly toward experiences with more challenging stimuli. Greenspan (1992) asserts that it is the task of parents and educators to help the child identify a series of small steps which permit him or her to move forward, however slowly, in pursuit of the mastery of sensory experiences and their own developmental agenda.

Young children can use a variety of cognitive behavioral strategies, including graduated exposure to stimulating activities, behavioral rehearsal strategies, and practice to help cope with situations they find overwhelming. Verbal rehearsal strategies, such as social stories, can be helpful both in mastering the anxiety associated with situations children experience as overwhelming and in preparing children for graduated practice. Occupational therapists can suggest a variety of specific interventions to help children improve their sensory processing (e.g., Poisson, DeGangi, & Nathanson, 1991; Wilbarger & Wilbarger, 1991; Trott, 1993).

The second set of intervention strategies helpful in the treatment of young children with regulatory issues is borrowed from the work of parent–infant psychotherapists. These strategies are designed to help parents enrich their internal model of their child by incorporating information regarding the child's sensory processing problems. Parents' revised understanding of their children's motivation for problematic behavior can lead to increased empathy for their children's experience and decreased guilt and anxiety about its causes. Therapists attempt to reframe behavioral problems and interactive difficulties as reflective of parents' and children's response to the challenges posed by sensory irregularities.

Therapists must begin with an empathic understanding of parents' experience in caring for a difficult and demanding child and use that as a basis for challenging parents' affective and cognitive constructions of that experience. Many parents of difficult infants, especially young parents, must feel that their own distress is heard and acknowledged before they can muster the additional resources necessary to care for a particularly challenging child. It is only when these parents experience themselves as valued partners in a problem-solving process that they can begin to entertain new visions of their children and new hopes for their future. In some cases, parenting difficulties reflect much more than frustration and disappointment in response to a particularly challenging infant, such as parents' own difficulties in the modulation or control of emotional responses. In those cases, more in-depth exploration of parents' subjective experience and personal histories may be required.

Once parents can consider an alternative view of their child, they can begin to experiment with strategies for altering sensory reactivity. At the same time, they must begin to impose limits for behavioral responses to sensory difficulties in a fashion that encourages the modulation, rather than the escalation, of emotional reactions. That will include maintaining one's own emotional equilibrium and modeling effective emotional regulation.

Children with regulatory disorder are often calmed by the security afforded by structure and consistency and by the provision of clear limits, within which they can begin to organize their behavior. Nonetheless, they require flexibility in rule setting so that behavioral standards do not exceed their capabilities. Parents often find it helpful to observe children's behavior closely for several weeks and complete a functional analysis of problem behaviors. That process permits them to observe patterns in the child's behavior, and identify precipitants and reinforcers for specific behavioral sequences. Most important, it permits parents to discover the function served by a given behavior. For many children the function of negative behavior is related to the control or avoidance of sensory input. Armed with that information, parents can make choices about the battles they choose to fight and the concessions they can make to sensory processing concerns. Parents can then select one or two behavioral sequences to target for change, either by imposing new limits or by altering contingencies.

Children with poor motor planning and high levels of impulsivity may benefit from a relatively structured routine that imposes order on their day but permits time for active and relatively less structured pursuits. Most children with regulatory issues will benefit from a structure that permits a variety of sensory experiences, some of which will be comfortable and others more challenging. Greenspan (1992) argues that the imposition of limits should be carefully balanced with playtime in which an adult follows a child's lead in order to prevent the escalation of continuous power struggles between parent and child.

Although research data on the efficacy of treatment efforts for children with regulatory disorder are lacking, clinical experience suggests that many families find considerable relief in the diagnostic process itself and the strategies that follow from a different understanding of their children. Many children appear to experience marked changes in their sensory profiles in response to treatment efforts; others continue to have marked sensory irregularities but develop a variety of strategies for coping with those more comfortably. Progress in altering sensory processing may be slow, but the benefits that accrue from developing a richer understanding of the impact of those difficulties on the developing child are only beginning to be appreciated.

Case Illustration

Carl was the son of a young, single mother who was unable to care for her newborn child. Carl's mother had received little prenatal care and was suspected of substance abuse during pregnancy, although no definitive information was available. Carl was placed in a highly stable foster family within days of his birth, with the likelihood of his placement becoming an adoptive home. Carl's foster mother, Lisa, and her husband, David, had one child of their own, age 6 years, and had cared for numerous foster children in the past.

Lisa described Carl as an extremely difficult infant from the very beginning. As a newborn, he screamed and arched his back for hours at a time, and he was unresponsive to virtually any effort to soothe him. He had feeding problems and vomited frequently. He was extremely reactive to any form of sensory stimulation and quickly became agitated and behaviorally disorganized. At times, Carl was soothed by being held and carried; more often, touch seemed aversive to him and increased his discontent. Sometimes, Carl seemed able to soothe himself if placed in a very quiet, dimly lit room, but that was not consistently helpful either.

Carl was referred for physical therapy services as an infant due to low motor tone and delayed motor development. He was slow to develop postural control and seemed lethargic and nonresponsive when he was not agitated and upset. At approximately 8 months, Carl began to sit independently, and he became much more interested in social interaction. He engaged in a variety of social games with Lisa and other familiar adults, and he began to make rapid developmental gains in all areas. Nonetheless, he continued to have frequent episodes of intense agitation. At those times, he would become distressed without apparent provocation, and he would scream, flail his arms and legs, and cry. Sometimes he would appear to lose motor skills and would drop items he was holding. During these episodes, Carl was completely intolerant of any physical contact. Eventually, he would wear himself out and either permit himself to be distracted or fall asleep.

Carl's physical therapy services were terminated before his first birthday because he had attained appropriate motor milestones. His foster mother sought early intervention services again when he was 14 months old because of his persistent crying, oppositionality, and tantrumming. Evaluation of Carl's difficulties included a request that Lisa keep detailed records of his behavior over a period of several weeks. Those data revealed enormous variabili-

ty in Carl's functioning. One some days, Carl seemed happy and content for much of the day. On other days he exhibited prolonged periods of fussiness. He was unable to engage in sustained activity, but he presented no significant behavioral problems. On still other days, Carl would have repeated tantrums, some lasting for 2 hours or more. During those times, he might throw himself on the floor, throw himself at windows, or bang his head on a variety of surfaces. Lisa felt helpless to alter Carl's behavior, although she felt she could predict what kind of day he would have on the basis of his mood when he woke up in the morning.

Further inspection of Carl's behavioral patterns revealed that he had great difficulty adjusting to minor variations in sensory input across modalities. In addition, when he was tired or otherwise stressed, his tolerance for any kind of sensory stimulation decreased markedly. When Carl was unable to moderate his response to sensory stimulation, he became so intensely agitated that he was unable to calm himself despite Lisa's heroic efforts to help him do so. Carl exhibited a second pattern which seemed less related to environmental stimulation. At times he seemed to awaken from sleep in an agitated state and immediately began tantrumming without any apparent provocation. At these times, Carl clearly wanted to be held by Lisa, but even physical contact was inconsistently successful in helping Carl calm down. Finally, it was clear that some of Carl's negative behaviors had achieved functional autonomy as successful strategies for controlling Lisa's behavior. His tantrums and, especially, his head banging were at least intermittently successful in securing his escape from activities he disliked and in obtaining objects he desired.

Carl was diagnosed with a Type I: Hypersensitive regulatory disorder, with negative and defiant behavioral patterns. It was hypothesized that his negative behavior helped to organize Carl's experience of intense disorganization attendant upon even mild sensory input. The association between episodes of intense disorganization following the transition from sleep to waking led to speculation about the neurological basis of Carl's problems. Although there had been some suggestion of neurological problems in early infancy, repeated neurological examinations revealed no clear evidence of abnormality.

Carl and his foster mother began to attend a parent–toddler nursery on a weekly basis. The intervention program included graduated exposure and practice with a variety of sensory activities, as well as a parent support group and parental guidance regarding behavior management. Initially, Carl was readily overstimulated by a variety of sensory and motor games (e.g., rolling on a large ball), but he learned quickly to move away from those activities for a brief period and then rejoin them. He was quick to model the movements of other children, but he had great difficulty modulating his activity sufficiently to take turns or to wait at all. Slowly, with adult support, Carl's behavioral modulation skills improved. Although he continued to have episodes of intense disorganization and upset, they decreased in frequency, duration, and severity.

At the same time, Lisa made a concerted effort to reduce the level of sensory stimulation in the home and to impose clearer limits on Carl's behavior. She declined to accept more foster children when several children left the home, and the decreased level of noise and activity seemed to help Carl a great deal. Lisa then began to challenge him to comply with routine directives for brief periods. Simultaneously, she became more attentive to Carl's early signs of distress and permitted his escape from structured activities when his tolerance level was reached but before his behavior deteriorated. For example, when Carl was approaching his second birthday, he began to refuse to eat at mealtimes. Instead he would play with his food, smear it, pour it, and otherwise experiment with its sensory properties. Although he enjoyed that sensory exploration, Carl became increasingly hungry and cranky but was unable to interrupt his activity long enough to eat. After several days of control battles, Lisa agreed to feed Carl at mealtimes and then permit him to play with his food. Immediately, the control battles ended. Carl ate the food Lisa offered, and his interest in playing with food waned on its own.

Carl's tantrums continued to diminish until they became relatively rare. He continued to have an exaggerated startle response to rapid changes in sensory input, and he looked to Lisa immediately for comfort and reassurance, but he was most often able to negotiate changes and transitions comfortably. Lisa noted that he had an occasional "bad day," but she learned to interrupt his negativistic bouts by engaging him in some structured activity in a novel environment (e.g., a special game outside or a brief trip to visit a relative.) As Carl's language increased, it became a critical tool in his effort to develop self-regulatory skills. He commented frequently on his own activity and attempted to use language and familiar routines to inhibit negative behavior. For example, he was heard saying, "Carl, no more crying" to himself and to Lisa, as he attempted to recover from a momentary upset. As his regulatory difficulties abated, Carl's mood brightened. He became a delightfully inquisitive toddler with impressive motor skills and precocious language abilities. He was remarkably persistent at new tasks, a trait Lisa attributed to the remarkable struggles he experienced.

Despite these many gains, Carl continues to experience periods of significant regression, which seem to accompany developmental spurts, the acquisition of new skills or environmental changes. Shortly after his second birthday, for example, Carl became much more adept at unlocking doors, climbing, and gaining access to places he could not formerly reach. At the same time, he grew confident in exploring his house away from adults. Lisa reported that his behavior became increasingly frenzied and disorganized as his activity level increased, and he got into everything. His negativity also increased as she attempted to set limits on his behavior. Lisa responded to these changes by aggressively childproofing the house to diminish the incidence of control battles and by attempting to help Carl anticipate verbally which behaviors were permitted and which were not. She reported that he responded readily to her interventions and returned to his former level of modulation and behavioral control.

Although the changes in Carl's presentation were impressive, changes in Lisa's view of him were important as well. She was no longer overwhelmed by a child whose behavior she neither understood nor felt she influenced. She no longer sought a variety of medical evaluations of everything from allergies to arthritis to explain Carl's behavior. She did not question her ability to respond to him and care for him, and she looked to his future with promise. Shortly before Carl's second birthday, Lisa and her husband adopted him formally. They did so well aware of the fact that parenting Carl may require a different level of energy, persistence, and patience than other children. They also were aware that in spite of his difficulties, and to some extent because of them, he brought unique gifts to their family.

SUMMARY

The diagnostic construct of regulatory disorder reflects an attempt to link specific patterns of behavior, including difficulties in the regulation of affect and attention, with irregularities in sensory processing. The sensory processing problems are presumed to be rooted in biological factors and are hypothesized to underlie the behavioral difficulties described. Although there is relatively little research on the construct of regulatory disorder itself, data from the related fields of sensory processing and sensory integration lend helpful insights. Clinical experience also suggests that the recognition of the role of sensory processing difficulties in the genesis of behavioral problems in young children is of critical importance. It is hoped that as clinicians grow more familiar with the manifestations of regulatory disorder, they will spur research efforts to refine the construct and objectify its measurement, even as they use the imperfect tools currently available to guide their efforts to help these challenging children and their families.

REFERENCES

Ayres, A. J. (1972). *Sensory integration and learning disorders*. Los Angeles: Western Psychological Services.

Ayres, A. J. (1975). *Southern California Postrotary Nystagmus Test manual*. Los Angeles: Western Psychological Services.

Ayres, A. J. (1979). *Sensory integration and the child*. Los Angeles: Western Psychological Services.

Ayres, A. J. (1989). *Sensory integration and praxis tests*. Los Angeles: Western Psychological Services.

Barkley, R. A. (1997). *ADHD and the nature of self-control*. New York: Guilford Press.

Barr, R. G. (1990). The "colic" enigma: Prolonged episodes of a normal predisposition to cry. *Infant Mental Health Journal, 11*, 340–348.

Bates, J. E. (1984). *Infant Characteristics Questionnaire, revised*. Bloomington: Indiana University Press.

Buss, K. A., & Goldsmith, H. H. (1998). Fear and anger regulation in infancy: Effects on the temporal dynamics of affective expression. *Child Development, 69*, 359–374.

Deams, J. (Ed.). (1994). *Reviews of research in sensory integration*. Torrance, CA: Sensory Integration International.

DeGangi, G., & Berk, R. (1983). *DeGangi–Berk Test of Sensory Integration (TSI)*. Los Angeles: Western Psychological Services.

DeGangi, G., DiPietro, J., Greenspan, S., & Porges, S. (1991). Psychophysiological characteristics of the regulatory disordered infant. *Infant Behavior and Development, 14,* 37–50.

DeGangi, G., Poisson, S., Sickel, R., & Weiner, A. (1998). *Infant–Toddler Symptom Checklist*. San Antonio, TX: Psychological Corporation.

DeGangi, G., Porges, S., Sickel, R., & Greenspan, S. (1993). Four year follow-up of a sample of regulatory disordered infants. *Infant Mental Health Journal, 14*(4), 330–343.

Dunn, W. (1997). The impact of sensory processing abilities on the daily lives of young children and their families: A conceptual model. *Infants and Young Children, 9*(4), 23–35.

Dunn, W., & Brown, C. (1997). Factor analysis of the sensory profile from a national sample of children without disabilities. *American Journal of Occupational Therapy, 51*(7), 490–495.

Dunn, W., & Westman, K. (1997). The Sensory Profile: The performance of a national sample of children without disabilities. *American Journal of Occupational Therapy, 51*(1), 25–34.

Ermer, J., & Dunn, W. (1998). The sensory Profile: a discriminant analysis of children with and without disabilities. *American Journal of Occupational Therapy, 52*(4), 283–289.

Greenspan, S. (1992). *Regulatory disorders. Infancy and early childhood: The practice of clinical assessment and intervention with emotional and developmental challenges*. Madison, CT: International Universities Press.

Greenspan, S. (1995). *The challenging child*. Reading, MS: Addison Wesley.

Greenspan, S., & Weider, S. (1993). Regulatory Disorders. In C. H. Zeanah, Jr. (Ed.). *Handbook of infant mental health*. New York: Guilford Press.

Kranowitz, C. S. (1998). *The out-of-sync child*. New York: Penguin Putnam.

Kurcinka, M. S. (1992). *Raising your spirited child*. New York: Harper

Lyons-Ruth, K., & Zeanah. C. H. (1993). The family context of infant mental health: I. Affective development in the primary caregiving relationship. In C. H. Zeanah, Jr. (Ed.). *Handbook of infant mental health*. New York: Guilford Press.

Maldonado-Duran, M., & Sauceda-Garcia, J. (1996). Excessive crying in infants with regulatory disorders. *Bulletin of the Menninger Clinic, 60*(1), 62–78.

McIntosh, D., Miller, L. J., & Shyu, V. (in press). Development and validation of the Short Sensory Profile. In W. Dunn, *The Sensory Profile Examiner's Manual*. San Antonio, TX: Psychological Corporation.

Miller, L. J., & Kinnealey, M. (1993). Researching the effectiveness of sensory integration. *Sensory Integration Quarterly, 21*, 2.

Miller, L. J., McIntosh, D., McGrath, J., Shyu, V., Lampe, M., Taylor, A., Tassone, F., Neitzel, K., Stackhouse, T., & Hagerman, R. J. (in press). Electrodermal responses to sensory stimuli in individuals with Fragile X Syndrome: A preliminary report. *American Journal of Medical Genetics*.

Poisson, S., DeGangi, G., & Nathanson, B. (1991). *Emotional and sensory processing problems: Assessment and treatment approaches for young children and their families*. Rockville, MD: Reginald S. Lourie Center for Infants and Children.

Rothbart, M. K., Ahadi, S. A., & Hershey, K. I. (1994). Temperament and social behavior in childhood. *Merrill–Palmer Quarterly, 40*, 21–39.

Rothbart, M. K., & Dayberry, D. (1981). Development of individual differences in temperament. In M. E. Lamb & A. L. Brown (Eds.), *Advances in developmental psychology* (Vol. 1). Hillsdale, NJ: Erlbaum.

Sameroff, A. J., & Chandler, M. J. (1975). Reproductive risk and the continuum of caretaking casualty. In F. D. Horowitz, E. M. Hetherington, S. Scarr-Salapatek, & G. M. Seigel, (Eds.), *Review of child development research* (Vol. 4). Chicago: University of Chicago Press.

Schore, A. M. (1994). *Affect regulation and the origins of the self*. Hillsdale, NJ: Erlbaum.

Seifer, R., Sameroff, A. J., Barrett, L. C., & Krafchuk, E. (1994). Infant temperament measured by multiple observations and mother report. *Child Development, 65*(5), 1478–1490.

Shyu, V., Miller, L. J., McIntosh, D., & Dunn, W. (1999). Identification of disruptions in sensory modulation using a parent report measure: The Short Sensory Profile. Manuscript submitted for publication.

Sroufe, L. A. (1995). *Emotional development: The organization of emotional life in the early years*. Cambridge: Cambridge University Press.

Stern, D. (1985). *The interpersonal world of the infant*. New York: Basic Books.

Thomas, A., Chess, S., Birch, H. G., Hertzig, M. E., & Korn, S. (1963). *Behavioral individuality in early childhood*. New York: New York University Press.

Trott, M. C. (1993). *SenseAbilities: Understanding sensory integration*. Tucson, AZ: Therapy Skill Builders.

Wilbarger, P., & Wilbarger, J. L. (1991). *Sensory defensiveness in children aged 2–12: An intervention guide for parents and other caretakers*. Santa Barbara, CA: Avanti Educational Programs.

Zeanah, C. H., Keener, M. A., & Anders, T. F. (1986). Developing perceptions of temperament and their relation to mother and infant behavior. *Journal of Child Psychology and Psychiatry, 27*, 499–512.

Zero to Three, National Center for Clinical Infant Programs. (1994). *Diagnostic classification: 0–3. Diagnostic classification of mental health and developmental disorders of infancy and early childhood*. Washington, DC: Author.

20

Sleep Disorders

❖

THOMAS ANDERS
BETH GOODLIN-JONES
AVI SADEH

The first edition of the *Handbook of Infant Mental Health* (Zeanah, 1993) described sleep disorders from a developmental perspective. We suggested that a reliable diagnostic classification scheme for infant sleep disorders was not yet available (Sadeh & Anders, 1993). Since then, two new nosologies, *Diagnostic and Statistical Manual of Mental Disorders* (DSM-IV; American Psychiatric Association, 1994) and *Diagnostic Classification of Mental Health and Developmental Disorders of Infancy and Early Childhood* (DC: 0–3; Zero to Three, 1994), have been published. In this chapter, we again begin by reviewing briefly the development of sleep and waking states in infants. We then review the presentation of infant and toddler sleep–wake disturbances. A discussion follows of possible etiologies, treatments, and assessment of sleep problems. Finally, we preview DC: 0–3, as it pertains to sleep disorders, and compare it to DSM-IV (1994) and the *International Classification of Sleep Disorders: Diagnostic Coding Manual* (ICSD: DCM; American Sleep Disorders Association, 1990). We propose a new multiaxial scheme to classify sleep problems in infants and toddlers, based on our own clinical and research experience, which provides clinicians and researchers with a more objective and quantifiable framework. Our conclusions include recommendations from a recent National Institute of Mental Health consensus conference that suggests directions for future infancy research.

We want to acknowledge at the outset our own bias. We believe that sleep and waking state organization in the first 3 years of life depends largely on the "relationship context" in which it develops. Transitions between sleep and waking occur many times during each 24-hour day and provide regular opportunities for homeostatic (hunger, temperature, dryness) and social/affective (separation, reunion, comfort, security) regulation. The repeated sleep–wake transitions involve parent–infant separations and reunions, mimicking the Strange Situation paradigm that tests the attachment system (Ainsworth, Blehar, Waters, & Wall, 1978). Through consistent and predictable recurring social interactions, the primary caregiver (most often the mother) and infant form an enduring relationship that fosters biological and social regulation (Anders, 1994). Failure to develop such a secure relationship leads to dysregulation. Thus, we believe that the development of sleep–wake organization is intimately involved in the emerging attachment relationship and the process of self-regulation.

DEVELOPMENT OF SLEEP–WAKE STATES

The maturation of two related chronobiological processes during the first 6 months of life influence sleep–wake organization in human infants. Diurnal organization refers to the circadian (about 24–hour) periodicity of the sleep–wake cycle that becomes associated with the light–dark cycle. Ultradian organization refers to a shorter (60- to 90-minute) intrasleep cycle of rapid-eye-movement and non-rapid-eye-movement (REM–NREM) sleep states.

Diurnal Organization: The Sleep–Wake Cycle

Normal, full–term newborns spend approximately 18 of the 24 hours asleep with short periods of wakefulness interrupting sleep every 3 to 4 hours. That is, there are six to eight regularly occurring sleep periods in a 24-hour day, with as much wakefulness at night as sleep during the day (Coons & Guilleminault, 1982). Significant variability exists, however, so that some newborns, for the first few days after birth, sleep for 22 hours while others sleep for only 10 hours in a 24-hour period (Sadeh, Dark, & Vohr, 1996). Within the first month following birth, sleep–wake state organization begins to adapt to the light–dark cycle and to social cues. By 6 months of age, the longest continuous sleep period has lengthened from 4 hours to 6 hours, and several of these longer sleep periods coalesce at night, interrupted by one or two brief awakenings. The wakeful periods similarly consolidate, lengthen, and shift to the daytime, interrupted by briefer periods of napping sleep. Gradually, the total number of sleep–wake cycles in a 24-hour period decreases as periods of sleep and wakefulness shift to a diurnal pattern of expression.

Thus, by 1 year of age, there are one to two long periods of sleep at night (8–12 hours), and 2 shorter sleep periods of approximately two hours each during the day. The infant still sleeps 16 hours, on average, in the 24-hour period, but diurnal organization of sleep and waking is clearly evident. The process of day–night consolidation seems psychobiological in origin, related to the maturation of the pineal gland and the establishment of a diurnal secretion pattern for melatonin (Sadeh, 1997). In the second year, one of the daytime naps disappears and sleep becomes restricted to two clock times—one long episode during the night and one brief nap during the afternoon (Weissbluth, 1995). In the preschool years, depending on social expectations, many children give up the remaining daytime nap and sleep becomes truly

monotonic, although a tendency for afternoon naps remains throughout the life cycle (Lavie, 1986).

Ultradian Organization: The REM–NREM Cycle

During the first 3 months of life, when asleep, infants spend 50% of their sleep time in REM sleep (also known as "dreaming sleep," "active sleep," and "paradoxical sleep") and the other 50% in NREM sleep (also known as "quiet sleep" and "slow–wave sleep"). With increasing maturity, the proportionate amount of time in REM sleep diminishes. The 2- to 3-year-old child spends approximately 35% of sleep time in REM sleep, while the adult spends about 20% in REM sleep (Louis, Cannard, Bastuji, & Challamel, 1997). When the young infant falls asleep, the initial sleep episode is typically a sleep onset REM period. In the neonatal period, REM and NREM sleep periods alternate with each other in 50- to 60-minute sleep cycles. In each sleep cycle during the sleep period, there is as much REM sleep as NREM sleep. After 3 months of age, REM periods continue to recur with a periodicity of 50–60 minutes; however, the amount of REM sleep in each cycle begins to shift. REM sleep predominates in the later sleep cycles of the night and NREM sleep predominates during the earlier cycles, especially NREM Stage 4 sleep. By 3 years of age, the temporal organization of sleep during the night resembles that of adult sleep except for the sleep cycle periodicity, which does not lengthen to the 90-minute periodicity of adults until adolescence. Interested readers are referred to Anders and Eiben (1997) and to Louis et al. (1997) for more detailed descriptions of sleep–wake state maturation.

COMMON SLEEP PROBLEMS OF INFANCY AND EARLY CHILDHOOD

Parental concerns about infant sleep problems are common during the first 3 years of life. Surveys of pediatricians indicate that questions about sleep are among the most frequently posed by parents (Wolfson, Lacks, & Futterman, 1992). Often, there are close associations between family stress, parental depression, and infant sleep problems, although which is etiologically salient remains unclear. The problems that parents report most frequently are night waking and sleep-onset difficulties.

Night Waking Problems

Reports about the frequency of night waking in older infants have typically been derived from parent surveys or as part of complaints to professionals (Wolfson et al., 1992). During early infancy, night waking is frequent, as the young infant awakens during both the day and night for a feeding. Both the frequency and length of awakenings at night tend to decrease with age. During the first few months of life, 95% of infants cry (signal) after an awakening and require a parental response before returning to sleep. By 8 months of age, 60–70% of infants are able to self-soothe after a nighttime awakening, as measured by parental report (Anders, Halpern, & Hua, 1992). A Finnish study using parental report also found that 35% of 3-month-olds and 72% of 9- to 12-month-olds were sleeping uninterrupted for at least 6 hours at night (Michelsson, Rinne, & Paajanen, 1990). Moore and Ucko (1957) noted that 50% of 1-year-old infants who had previously "slept through the night" again began to awaken. During the second year of life, they reported a further transient increase in problematic night awakenings. In other studies, using parental reports, approximately 20–30% of toddlers were described as night wakers (Bernal, 1973; Jenkins, Owen, Bax, & Hart, 1984).

Videosomnography and actigraphy, two objective sleep recording methods, have demonstrated that nighttime awakenings in early childhood are actually more prevalent than parents report (Anders, 1978; Minde et al., 1993; Sadeh, Lavie, Scher, Tirosh, & Epstein, 1991). These methods indicate that most infants wake up one or more times during the night, although only briefly for 1 to 5 minutes. Parents are often unaware of these awakenings because the child does not cry out.

Studies using the activity monitor have reported that in the age range of 9–24 months, nonproblem sleepers woke up twice nightly on average. Most of these infants were able to soothe themselves and return to sleep without signaling (Sadeh et al., 1991). Videosomnography, like actigraphy, also demonstrates significantly more nighttime awakenings than that reported by the parents (Gaylor, Goodlin-Jones, Burnham, & Anders, 1998). In fact, the actual frequency of nighttime awakenings at 3, 6, 9,

and 12 months of age in solitary sleeping infants, coded from videosomnography, averaged 2.3 at each age. However, when mothers were asked the following morning about the number of waking bouts their infant experienced during the previous videotaped night, they consistently underreported this frequency. By 12 months of age, self-soothing behavior occurred approximately 70% of the time after an awakening. Thus, more objective methods of assessing sleep have established that "sleeping through the night" as a developmental achievement is a misnomer, and night waking as a problem is more appropriately defined as infant signaling rather than awakening per se (Anders, 1994; Messer & Richards, 1993; Sadeh, 1996).

Sleep-Onset Problems

Problems at sleep onset focus on both going to bed (leaving or separating from the caregiver) and falling asleep. From a developmental perspective, problems with falling asleep precede problems with going to bed. At young ages, falling asleep often occurs outside the bed. Feeding, rocking, and being held are commonly associated with falling asleep, even though newborns are able to fall asleep on their own and do not need these soothing interventions to help them. This pattern of rocking or holding at bedtime until sleep onset occurs in approximately 15–20% of children ages 6 months to 3 years (Mindell, 1993). Fewer than 50% of 3- and 6-month olds are placed in their cribs awake. By 12 months of age, approximately 70% of infants enter the crib awake at the beginning of the night (Burnham, Anders, Gaylor, & Goodlin-Jones, 1998). Being placed in the crib awake at the beginning of the night affords infants the opportunity to learn to fall asleep on their own.

In the second year of life, falling asleep may not be problematic per se; however, children may protest vigorously when put into their bed and refuse to remain recumbent. Bedtime may elicit worry about separation from the parent, as separation anxiety becomes prominent after 12 months of age. Stalling at bedtime or refusing to go to bed occur in 5–10% of children. The presence of the primary caregiver becomes necessary for some toddlers to remain in bed. Because separation problems are often dyadic in origin, the parent may experience feelings of separation anxiety as well. In families in which both parents work all day, the evening may be the primary time for family interaction. Both the children and their parents need this family time, and bedtimes may be delayed as a result. In other circumstances maternal depression, anxiety, and decreased marital satisfaction have been reported in parents of children with bedtime struggles, although it is not clear which comes first (Durand & Mindell, 1990).

Difficulty in returning to sleep following a nighttime awakening often repeats the difficulty at bedtime. The wakeful infant usually demands the same pattern of parental soothing in the middle of the night that was used when he or she was put to bed at the beginning of the night. When assessing night waking problems in a clinical setting, it is important to obtain a detailed history of bedtime interactions that occur at the beginning of the night. Assessment of falling asleep at naptime also may shed light on the middle-of-the-night problem. At older ages, some children may exhibit nonspecific anxiety, or they may show specific fears of the dark or of being alone. When transient, such common fears benefit from reassurances from parents and the use of night lights.

Parasomnias in Early Childhood

Parasomnias are sleep disorders in which behaviors involving motor and autonomic activation intrude on ongoing sleep. Night terrors and nightmares are two of the more common parasomnias and may begin during the toddler–preschool period. Parasomnias are more common in males than in females, and children with symptoms often have a positive family history for parasomnias. Night terror attacks are a type of arousal disorder and are usually frightening to parents. During a night terror attack, the child "wakes up" screaming and appears extremely frightened and agitated. In fact, the child is not awake, but deep in Stage 4 NREM sleep. The child is difficult to soothe, is unaware of his or her surroundings, and may fight with the person who is trying to console him or her. Night terrors are considered to be atypical arousals from these deep sleep stages and typically occur during the first few hours of sleep. Unless the problem is intractable in terms of frequency and persistence, there is no need for special intervention; children normally "outgrow" their attacks as they mature. In contrast, nightmares are arousals from REM sleep, usually occurring during the last few hours of the night, which are associated with frightening dream reports involving anxiety or fears. Whereas night terrors are difficult to recall the next morning and usually are without any mental imagery, nightmares are often remembered the next day. Immediate reassurance by the caregiver at the time of the nightmare and lessening stress during the day is the most effective treatment.

Other common bedtime behaviors that concern parents of toddlers are the repetitive rhythmic behaviors at sleep onset, which may include self-rocking and head banging. These behaviors, usually observed while an infant is trying to fall asleep, have been classified as parasomnias in ICSD: DCM (American Sleep Disorders Association, 1990). Klackenberg (1987) reported that at 9 months of age, 58% of infants exhibited at least one of these repetitive behaviors (head turning, head banging, or rocking). The prevalence of these activities decreased to 33% by 18 months of age and to 22% by 2 years of age. When intense rocking or head banging persists and is disruptive, parents may view the behavior as a problem. Most often, guidance and support for the parents suffice; the only concern should be in ensuring the child's safety from self-injury.

Sleep Apnea Syndromes

The most common intrinsic (biologically based) sleep disorder in young children is sleep apnea, the failure to breathe during sleep. Two distinct central nervous system mechanisms control breathing in humans. A voluntary cortical mechanism functions during wakefulness and provides control of breathing during vocalization; an involuntary subcortical mechanism maintains oxygen saturation during sleep. When the involuntary system fails during sleep, blood and brain oxygen saturation fall to dangerous levels. Self-preservation is achieved by a brief arousal, which is sufficient to return control of breathing to the voluntary system. Once the "central" sleep apnea episode has ended with an awakening, the subject returns to sleep. The awakening during sleep is most often a microarousal unknown to the sleeper. The sequence of apnea, arousal, and return to sleep may recur many times during the night.

There are also peripheral causes of sleep apnea in young children. Sleep apnea may result from mechanical obstruction of the upper airway secondary to anatomical factors, such as enlarged tonsils and adenoids or excessive obesity, which closes the airway during sleep. Again, only an arousal restores breathing. "Obstructive" sleep apnea is characterized by expiratory snoring or mouth breathing. Sleep apnea can also result from neurological conditions or medical conditions of the cardiopulmonary system or from combinations of central and peripheral mechanisms.

Both obstructive and central sleep apnea syndromes can produce chronic sleep loss. Consequently, such children may present with symptoms of daytime sleepiness and chronic fatigue. If the awakenings also interrupt the secretion of growth hormone, which normally occurs during NREM Stage 4 sleep, the child may present with mild growth retardation or, in extreme cases, a full-blown failure-to-thrive syndrome. Sleep apnea should be investigated by polysomnographic technology in a sleep laboratory in order to identify its specific cause and prescribe the appropriate intervention.

ETIOLOGIES OF SLEEP PROBLEMS

A number of studies have attempted to determine the causes of night waking and sleep-onset problems in infancy and early childhood. Perhaps the most consistent research finding is the association of sleep problems with parent–infant bedtime interaction. Van Tassel (1985) found that bedtime interactions were the best predictors of sleep problems in both early and late infancy. Adair, Bauchner, Philipp, Levenson, and Zuckerman (1991) reported that infants whose parents were present while the infants were falling asleep were significantly more likely to wake at night than were infants whose parents were not present. Johnson (1991) also found highly significant differences between night wakers and good sleepers in bedtime routines. Infants who were actively soothed by their parents (nursed, rocked, or comforted) were more likely to be night wakers. Because these studies are correlational in design, causal relationships should be interpreted cautiously. It is equally plausible to assume that infants who have difficulty in falling asleep or who have a propensity for night waking and signaling "push" their parents to become more involved at bedtime, compared to infants who "teach" their parents that their presence is not necessary.

In the first few months of life, nutritional factors and states of physical discomfort may influence sleep patterns. Because young infants need physiological regulation from caregivers, sleep difficulties may arise from insufficient or inadequate regulation (Kraemer, 1992; McKenna et al., 1993). For example, Kahn, Mozin, Rebuffat, Sottiaux, and Muller (1989) identified allergy to cow's milk in a group of infants with persistent sleep problems who did not benefit from behavioral interventions. Kahn et al. (1991) have also demonstrated that proximal esophageal reflux can induce arousals in infants. In a recent review of extant literature, Breakey (1997) found that diet changes could improve sleep disturbances and other behaviors in some children. It has also been reported that infants with colic sleep less than infants without colic (Weissbluth, 1987; White, Gunnar, Larson, Donzella, & Barr, 1998). In contrast, two other studies have found no significant relationship between colicky infants, or "high fussers," and concurrent sleep patterns (Lehtonen, Korhonen, & Korvenranta, 1994; St. James-Roberts & Plewis, 1996). However, follow-up with one of these study's sample 3 years later described a significant relationship: Parents of colicky infants reported that when their children were preschoolers, they felt more distress with parenting tasks, and their children had more sleep problems (Rautava, Lehtonen, Helenius, & Sillanpaa, 1995).

Specific infant characteristics, such as sensitivity, activity, responsivity, and persistence, referred to in the aggregate as infant temperament or behavioral style, also may affect sleep–wake organization. Carey (1974) found in a pediatric clinic sample that according to parental report, infants with sleep problems had lower sensory thresholds than did infants in the clinic without sleep problems. In support of this hypothesis, Weissbluth and Liu (1983) found that children with difficult temperaments slept less than children with "easy" temperaments, and Schaefer (1990) found a higher-than-expected incidence of difficult temperament in young children referred for night awakenings. Infants with night waking patterns have also been rated by their mothers as being less adaptive, more distractible, and more demanding, compared to controls (Sadeh, Lavie, & Scher, 1994). A recent study conducted in a pediatric sleep clinic with preschoolers and kindergartners found a similar temperamental profile (more negativity, irritability, low sensory threshold) in those preschoolers with a behavioral sleep disorder (Owens-Stively et al.,

1997). In contrast, other researchers have found no relationship between parental reports of temperament and sleep patterns (St. James-Roberts & Plewis, 1996).

"Co-sleeping" (i.e., a parent's sleeping with an infant in the same bed) at an early age has been reported to affect sleep–wake state regulation and organization. The age of the infant seems relevant to whether or not co-sleeping is associated with sleep problems (Stein, Colarusso, McKenna, & Powers, 1997). In the first 6 months of life, the physiological adaptation of infants may benefit from co-sleeping as the best approximation to prenatal mother–infant physiological unity (McKenna, Mosko, Dungy, & McAninch, 1990). Recent research on co-sleeping 3-month-olds suggests the presence of more arousals and greater synchrony in infant and maternal arousals (Mosko, Richard, & McKenna, 1997). In these co-sleeping infants, breastfeeding was more frequent than in solitary sleep infants but of shorter duration, yielding less actual wakefulness and more sleep time in mothers and infants. Also, newborns who co-sleep with their mothers spend more time in quiet sleep and less time in crying and indeterminate sleep than do newborns who sleep in a separate room (Keffe, 1987). McKenna and his colleagues (McKenna et al., 1990; McKenna et al., 1993; Mosko et al., 1997) have suggested that co-sleeping during the first few months of life increases the number of brief, spontaneous arousals from sleep, which may in turn reduce the opportunity for the occurrence of sudden infant death syndrome (SIDS).

Cultural practices may determine whether co-sleeping is associated with sleep problems. Lozoff, Wolf, and Davis (1985) found a threefold increase in sleep problems in preschool children who were co-sleeping with their parents. However, it was not clear that co-sleeping caused the sleep problem. It may be that co-sleeping in this age group was reactive to prior existing sleep problems. Zuckerman, Stevenson, and Baily (1987) reported an even higher rate in respect to the co-sleeping partner's sleep problems. Other studies in Western cultures also suggest relationships between co-sleeping and sleep problems (Kataria, Swanson, & Trevathan, 1987; Schacter, Fuchs, Bijur, & Stone, 1989). The important dimension may not be co-sleeping per se but rather the psychosocial meaning of (and cultural sanctions in regard to) co-sleeping.

Parental conflict, maternal psychopathology,

and family stress have also been identified as possible contributors to infants' sleep problems (Sadeh, 1996). Richman (1981) reported that mothers of 1- to 2-year-old sleep disturbed infants exhibited more psychopathology than mothers of control infants. These mothers tended to be nervous, to lose control more often, and to have less trusting, supportive relationships with their husbands. Zuckerman et al., (1987) reported that maternal depression was the only measure of maternal psychopathology that was significantly more common in children with persistent sleep problems from the age of 8 months to 3 years. Guedeney and Kreisler (1987) also reported a relationship between sleep problems in the first 18 months of life and traumatic events, maternal depression, and maternal anxiety during pregnancy. In addition, dysregulation of sleep–awake cycles has been described in infants of depressed and emotionally unavailable mothers (Field, 1994) and in toddlers of depressed and anxious mothers (Minde et al., 1993). Recent results from our ongoing research showed that maternal levels of depressive feelings were negatively correlated with self-soothing by infants in the middle of the night at 6 and 12 months of age (Goodlin-Jones, Eiben, & Anders, 1997). Finally, mothers of infants with sleep disorders were more likely to have distorted or disengaged representations of their infants (Benoit, Zeanah, Parker, Nicholson, & Coolbear, 1997) and to have insecure attachment classifications themselves (Benoit, Zeanah, Boucher, & Minde, 1992).

Studies refute the myth that children outgrow their "trivial" developmental sleep problems. Several investigators have followed infants longitudinally into the childhood years and observed that almost half of infants with sleep problems continue to exhibit those problems later (Kataria et al., 1987; Zuckerman et al., 1987). However, a recent longitudinal study reported less stability and found that 30% of full-term night wakers at 5 months were also night wakers at 20 months. Only 17% of these night wakers were reported to be night wakers at 56 months (Wolke, Meyer, Ohrt, & Riegel, 1995).

ASSESSMENT OF SLEEP IN INFANCY

As part of every routine health check, clinicians should screen with questions about regularity of sleep–wake schedules (American Academy of Child and Adolescent Psychiatry, 1997). Does an infant's schedule conform to the family's schedule in a socially appropriate way, and does it meet the infant's need for sleep? How many hours of sleep does the child get each day? How regular is this pattern? How regular are daytime naps? Screening also should inquire about any potential sleep concerns such as difficulty in falling asleep at bedtime, waking in the middle of the night, and behaviors that interrupt sleep. Are there symptoms of asthma, mouth breathing, or snoring during sleep? Finally, screening should assess daytime functioning in regard to sleep. Does the child appear to be too irritable or sleepy during the day?

When a sleep problem is the presenting complaint, a more detailed history needs to be obtained. Specific diaries completed by the caregivers need to be reviewed. These diaries record the periods of sleep and waking around the 24-hour clock, the presence and nature of bedtime routines, sleeping arrangements, family history of sleep problems, sibling relationships, and current environmental stresses. For a few problems in infancy, mostly related to sleep apnea, laboratory assessments are important. Alternative methods for objectively recording infant sleep in the home include structured questionnaires, ambulatory monitoring instruments, and video recording. Unfortunately, agreement on the classification of problems and knowledge of base rates in community samples of sleep-onset and night waking problems at different ages, which take into account sleeping contexts and cultural practices, are nonexistent. There have been few large sample studies using double-blind, randomized treatment trials. Follow-up studies of treatment outcomes are too short in duration to answer questions of effectiveness.

APPROACHES TO TREATMENT

Approaches to treatment for managing sleep problems have included pharmacological, behavioral, and psychotherapeutic regimens, alone or in combination. Most are reported as successful. It still is not clear whether some treatments are better than others, or whether some treatments are better for some families than for others (treatment matching) (Robert-Tissot et al., 1996). The central hypothesis that

underlies most behavioral interventions is that sleep-onset difficulties result from learned interaction patterns between a child and caregiver (France, Henderson, & Hudson, 1996; Mindell, 1993). Behavioral techniques usually focus on teaching children to fall asleep by themselves in their own beds, with minimal parental interaction. Several techniques have been described and encourage parents to manage their children's bedtime behavior more effectively (Ferber, 1985; France et al., 1996; Minde et al., 1993; Richman, Douglas, Hunt, Lansdown, & Levene, 1985; Weissbluth, 1987).

In contrast to the behavioral methods, structured parent–infant guidance (McDonough 1993) and psychodynamic approaches that focus on the meanings and motivations of parents' behavior in the context of their child's sleep behavior (Daws, 1989; van Hofacker & Papousek, 1998) have been used. Viewing an infant's pattern of sleep as being influenced by maternal well-being and other contextual variables supports a relational perspective in the development of sleep–wake consolidation (Minde et al., 1993). The success of the different dynamic and dyadic psychotherapies, which repeatedly have been shown to improve sleep in infants, support the hypothesis of a strong relational component in the development of sleep disturbances (Robert-Tissot et al., 1996).

Sleep aids also have been used. At young ages, infants use fingers or pacifiers and other soft objects. As infants mature, some continue to use such objects, although this varies by culture and socioeconomic class. At the point at which an infant selects a "special" object, the sleep aid becomes imbued with the properties of an attachment or "transitional" object (Winnicott, 1965). Research on the relationship between sleep and transitional objects has provided support for their utility. Paret (1983), using time-lapse video recordings, found that 9-month-old infants who slept uninterruptedly without signaling were more likely to suck their fingers or use transitional objects than infants who were night wakers. Wolf and Lozoff (1989) found that children who fell asleep in the absence of their parents were more likely to use transitional objects than were children who tended to fall asleep in the presence of their parents. Interestingly, in a sample of older children (ages 4 to 14 years), no significant relationships were found between the use of transitional objects and sleep problems (Klackenberg, 1987). Sadeh (1994) has noted that a brief period of a parent sleeping in the same room with the infant is also effective.

CLASSIFICATION OF SLEEP DISORDERS

For clinicians and researchers alike, a reliable, valid diagnostic nosology is critical. It should be based on data and developmentally appropriate. Several competing nosologies for classifying sleep disorders are currently available, but they don't meet these criteria for infants and toddlers. They are the ICSD: DCM (American Sleep Disorders Association, 1990), DSM-IV (American Psychiatric Association, 1994), and DC: 0–3 (Zero to Three, 1994). Table 20.1 portrays some of their principal similarities and differences.

The *International Classification of Sleep Disorders: Diagnostic and Coding Manual* (American Sleep Disorders Association, 1990) defines three major categories of disordered sleep: (1) dyssomnias, (2) parasomnias, and (3) sleep disorders associated with medical/psychiatric conditions. Because the most common sleep problems of infants and young children are characterized by night waking, difficulty in falling asleep, or both, these problems are classified in this nosology as dyssomnias. More specific subclasses suggested in ICSD-DCM, such as limit-setting sleep disorder, sleep-onset association disorder, or food allergy insomnia, point to possible etiologies. Unfortunately, few studies support these sub-categories. The distinction between disorder and normal variation is not clearly specified, especially as it pertains to changing developmental norms. The labels for the subcategories are largely derived from clinical impressions related to case reports.

DSM-IV (American Psychiatric Association, 1994) categorizes sleep disorders somewhat similarly to ICSD: DCM. Primary sleep disorders include both the dyssomnias and parasomnias of ICSD: DCM. Secondary sleep disorders include sleep disorders related to another mental condition, to a general medical condition or induced by substances. Although DSM-IV provides detailed phenomenological criteria required to make a diagnosis of disorder, a similar lack of developmental norms makes DSM-IV difficult to apply to disturbances in infants and toddlers. Moreover, diagnoses in DSM-IV require functional impairment, which is difficult to define at young ages. The only specific reference to childhood sleep disorders in DSM-IV is found in primary sleep disorders, parasomnias, where nightmare disorder, sleep terror disorder, and sleep walking disorder are described.

DC: 0–3 (Zero to Three, 1994) is a new, multiaxial classification system developed specifically for use in infancy and early childhood. DC: 0–3 was designed to complement DSM-IV in terms of an extension downward to younger ages, and by focusing on problems and behaviors not addressed adequately in DSM-IV. Like DSM-IV, Axis 1 in DC: 0–3 identifies primary diagnoses that reflect the most prominent features of the disorder. Axis 2 presents an opportunity to classify the characteristics of the primary relationship in which the symptoms arise. Axis 3 addresses medical and developmental issues, and Axis 4 focuses on the adequacy of the parent–infant relationship. The last axis,

TABLE 20.1. The Classification of Sleep Disorders

	ICSD: DCM	DSM-IV	DC: 0–3
Dyssomnias	Intrinsic disorders Extrinsic disorders Circadian disorders	Primary insomnia Primary hypersomnia Narcolepsy Breathing related Circadian rhythm	Sleep-behavior disorder
Parasomnias	Arousal disorders Sleep–wake transition disorder REM parasomnias	Nightmare disorder Sleep terror disorder Sleep walking disorder	Sleep-behavior disorder
Medical/psychiatric disorders	Mental disorders Neurological disorders Other medical disorders	Mental disorders General medical disorders Substance-induced	Regulatory disorder with sleep problems

Axis 5, includes the child's developmental level.

DC: 0–3 provides several opportunities to classify sleep problems, either as a primary entity or as a symptom of another Axis 1 disorder, such as traumatic stress disorder, adjustment disorder, regulatory disorder, anxiety disorder, or mood disorder. The primary sleep disorder is called sleep-behavior disorder. This diagnosis is suggested when a sleep disturbance is the only presenting problem in a child younger than 3 years of age. Unfortunately, this single diagnosis does not effectively differentiate between the several types of sleep problems that have been described previously. According to DC: 0–3, a diagnosis of sleep-behavior disorder should not be used when the sleep problem is secondary to anxiety, developmental delay, transient adjustment problems, or traumatic stress disorder. Whereas it is critically important to diagnose these other syndromes when they are present and to consider that the sleep disruption may be secondary, it is often not possible to distinguish what is primary in infants and pre-schoolers. Moreover, it is not clear why DC: 0–3 lumps multiple presentations of sleep disorder under one category.

Another problematic area in DC: 0–3 pertains to the diagnosis of "regulatory disorder," on Axis 1, and "relationship disturbance," on Axis 2. For infants and toddlers, the caregiving relationship represents a "holding environment" (a system) that serves a regulatory function (Anders, 1994; Sadeh & Anders, 1993). That is, parent and infant interactions comprise a dynamic system that mutually regulates each partner's sense of well-being. As described in the introduction, our bias is that sleep–wake state development occurs in the context of these regulatory interactions and becomes an important substrate of the emerging attachment relationship. The dyadic interactions serve both homeostatic and social/affective regulatory functions. According to our theoretical perspective, then, the presence of sleep-behavior disorder indicates a type of dysregulation in this dynamic system. DC: 0–3 confuses the constructs of relationship, regulation, and sleep disorder by separately diagnosing a relationship disorder on Axis 2, and on Axis 1, forcing a distinction between regulatory disorder and sleep-behavior disorder. In our view, sleep-behavior disorder most often is associated with disturbed regulation, which is often causally related to an insecure attachment relationship or a relationship disorder.

Alternative Classification

In an attempt to improve the classification of infant sleep disorders, we propose a new research-based, clinically relevant, diagnostic scheme for classifying sleep problems in young infants and toddlers. We distinguish between night waking protodysomnia (Table 20.2) and sleep-onset protodysomnia (Table 20.3) Our proposal's strength is that it is amenable to objective measurement. Because the problems can be described as problems in initiating or maintaining sleep, they fall in the general DSM-IV class of primary sleep disorders and in the ICSD: DCM class of dysomnias. However, because they do not meet full adult criteria of DSM-IV functional impairment, we refer to them as protodysomnias. Our classification scheme is derived largely from clinical experience, from developmental sleep–wake data from studies of objectively recorded nighttime sleep and waking, and from

TABLE 20.2. Night Waking Protodysomnia

Age (mo)	Perturbation (1 night/wk; 2–4 wk duration)	Disturbance (2–4 nights/wk; 2–4+ wk duration)	Disorder (5–7 nights/wk; >4 wk duration)
12–24	2 AW/night and/or >10 min AW	2 AW/night and/or >10 min AW	2 AW/night and/or >10 min AW
24–36	1–2 AW/night and/or >20 min AW	1–2 AW/night and/or >20 min AW	1–2 AW/night and/or >20 min AW
>36	1 AW/night and/or >30 min AW	1 AW/night and/or >30 min AW	1 AW/night and/or >30 min AW

Note. Occurs after infant has been asleep for > 10 minutes. AW, awakenings from sleep that are accompanied by signaling (crying or calling).

TABLE 20.3. Sleep-Onset Protodysomnia

Age (mo)	Perturbation (1 night/wk; 2–4 wk duration)	Disturbance (2–4 nights/wk; 2–4+ wk duration)	Disorder (5–7 nights/wk; >4 wk duration)
12–24	>30 min to fall asleep and/or parent remains in room for sleep onset and/or more than 1 reunion[a]	>30 min to fall asleep and/or parent remains in room for sleep onset and/or more than 1 reunion	>30 min to fall asleep and/or parent remains in room for sleep onset and/or more than 1 reunion
>24	>20 min to fall asleep and/or parent remains in room for sleep onset and/or more than 1 reunion	>20 min to fall asleep and/or parent remains in room for sleep onset and/or more than 1 reunion	>20 min to fall asleep and/or parent remains in room for sleep onset and/or more than 1 reunion

Note. Occurs at bedtime or nap time.
[a]Reunions refer to resistances to going to sleep. Reunions may differ in style: (1) repeated bids (kisses, hugs, glasses of water), or (2) struggles (crying, screaming, physical resistance), or (3) mixed. Reunions should be subclassified as to type.

reviewing the literature. It provides a framework by which to track sleep behaviors. A quantitative tool such as this is valuable for clinicians making an individual diagnosis, as well as for epidemiological researchers attempting to study the prevalence and course of these problems in community samples.

Three underlying assumptions define the applicability of our system. First, we do not classify sleep problems before 12 months of age. Prior to that age, sleep patterns continue to change at such a rapid rate that it is difficult to classify disorder. Second, it is applicable only when the infant sleeps in his or her own bed rather than a family bed. Third, the infant is being reared in a diurnal environment, with more sleep expected at night and more waking during the day.

We grade a sleep problem objectively and on the basis of its severity. A problem is graded from mild (perturbation, variant of normal) to moderate (disturbance, risk of disorder, likely to benefit from preventive intervention) to significant (disorder requiring intervention) (Anders, 1989). Measurement of symptoms should be as objective as possible, using standardized instruments, such as sleep diaries, actigraphy or videosomnography, and not relying on the severity of the parental complaint. Retrospective parental reports should be discouraged.

Perturbations are short-term disruptions that fall within normal developmental boundaries for a particular age. Professional reassurance with information should suffice. Disturbances are viewed as potential risk situations which, if unattended, may lead to a more protracted disorder. Parent education and guidance with a child health professional should suffice to ameliorate the problem. A disorder is more severe and prolonged. More intensive treatment, individualized to the particular problem, is usually necessary.

We propose four axes:

Axis I—*Perturbation/disturbance/disorder*
    Night waking protodysomnia*
    Sleep-onset protodysomnia
    Schedule disruption protodysomnia
Axis II—*Parent–child interaction styles*
    Balanced/synchronous
    Overregulating/controlling
    Underregulating/distant
    Inconsistent/unpredictable
Axis III—*Infant factors*
    Temperament
    Developmental quotient
    Medical illnesses
Axis IV—*Context factors*
    Family/marital stress
    Parenting stress/hassle
    Family psychopathology
    Family trauma/violence

Notes: Code protodysomnias as a perturbation, disturbance, or disorder. If daytime napping is disturbed, diagnose a schedule disruption protodysomnia. Diagnose more than one Axis I condition if criteria for several protodysomnias are met. The parasomnias and sleep apnea syndromes are also diagnosed on Axis 1.

SUMMARY AND CONCLUSIONS

We have reviewed sleep–wake state development and the common sleep disorders that affect human infants and young children through the first 3 years of life. We have emphasized the importance of taking a developmental perspective in making a diagnosis. We have reviewed a diverse set of treatments and have recommended that treatment strategies be individualized to match the child's age, developmental needs, and family circumstances. We have emphasized the psychological issues of separation and autonomy as they relate to sleep and parent–infant nighttime interactions during this age period. We have presented a diagnostic scheme that quantitatively classifies symptoms and that should be useful for clinicians and researchers alike.

Before settling on a final classification system for any group of infancy disorders, a number of areas need more investigation. We use the sleep disorders as an example of how further infancy research should proceed.

1. *Development (biology and context)*. We need better explanations about the origins, natural history, and long–term sequellae of sleep problems. We need further investigation on how infant temperament interacts with parenting practices and early experience to impact sleep.

2. *Classification and symptoms*. Night waking that is problematic (signaling) needs to be differentiated from night waking that is not detected or that does not cause troublesome caregiver–infant interaction (self-soothing). Defining what is acceptable and "normal" in large community samples and in multiethnic populations requires more research.

3. *Methods*. Sleep studies should be standardized, using multiple data gathering techniques that combine surveys (questionnaires and sleep diaries), observations (videosomnography, actigraphy, etc.), and physiological recording (polygraphy).

4. *Sampling*. Population-based samples should be studied in addition to clinic-based samples, and subjects should be followed longitudinally to assess the severity, stability, and outcome of sleep problems.

5. *Context*. Psychosocial contexts should be measured systematically. Parental well being, family stress, and cultural values need to be controlled statistically when studying infant sleep disturbances. Infants who sleep in their own rooms, in their own cribs in their parent's room, or in bed with their parents organize their sleep–wake patterns differently and sleep prob-

lems are reported at different rates. Each of these contexts requires special study.

To fully apply a transactional, relationship-based model (Sameroff & Emde, 1989) to the development of sleep and waking states and the emergence of infant sleep disorders requires a better understanding of the biological basis of regulation. We need more knowledge about the roles of internal clocks and pacemakers and of the neurophysiological processes that activate and inhibit the synchronization of systems. We need to integrate knowledge of cellular regulation with a better understanding of the varied responses of the environment and the emerging social and emotional regulatory needs of the infant. In summary, future researchers need to incorporate developmental, multimethod and multifactor transactional approaches to better understand and more precisely define infant and toddler sleep disorders.

REFERENCES

Adair, R., Bauchner, H., Philipp, B., Levenson, S., & Zuckerman, B. (1991). Night waking during infancy: Role of parental presence at bedtime. *Pediatrics, 87*(4), 500–504.

Ainsworth, M. D. S., Blehar, M. C., Waters, E., & Wall, S. (1978). *Patterns of attachment: A psychological study of the strange situation*. Hillsdale, NJ: Erlbaum.

American Academy of Child and Adolescent Psychiatry (1997). Practice parameters for the psychiatric assessment of infants and toddlers (0–36 months). *Journal of the American Academy of Child and Adolescent Psychiatry, 36*(10), S21–S36.

American Sleep Disorders Association. (1990). *The international classification of sleep disorders: Diagnostic and coding manual (ICSD: DSM)*. Kansas City, KS: Allen Press.

American Psychiatric Association. (1994). *Diagnostic and statistical manual of mental disorders* (4th ed.). Washington, DC: Author.

Anders, T. F. (1978). Home recorded sleep in two and nine month old infants. *Journal of the American Academy of Child Psychiatry*, 17, 421–432.

Anders, T. F. (1989). Clinical syndromes, relationship disturbances and their assessment. In A. Sameroff & R. Emde (Eds.), *Relationship disturbances in early childhood: A developmental approach* (pp. 145–165). New York: Basic Books.

Anders, T. (1994). Infant sleep, night time relationships and attachment. *Psychiatry, 57*, 11–21.

Anders, T. F., & Eiben, L. A. (1997). Pediatric sleep disorders: A review of the past 10 years. *Journal of the American Academy of Child and Adolescent Psychiatry, 36*, 1–12.

Anders, T. F., Halpern, L., & Hua, J. (1992). Sleeping

through the night: A developmental perspective. *Pediatrics, 90,* 554–560.

Benoit, D., Zeanah, C. H., Boucher, C., & Minde, K. K. (1992). Sleep disorders in early childhood: Association with insecure maternal attachment. *Journal of the American Academy of Child & Adolescent Psychiatry, 31,* 86–93.

Benoit, D., Zeanah, C. H., Parker, K. C., Nicholson, E., & Coolbear, J. (1997). "Working model of the child interview": Infant clinical status related to maternal perceptions. *Infant Mental Health Journal, 18,* 107–121.

Bernal, J. (1973). Night waking in infants during the first 14 months. *Developmental Medicine and Child Neurology, 14,* 362–372.

Breakey, J. (1997). The role of diet and behaviour in childhood. *Journal of Paediatrics and Child Health, 33*(3), 190–194.

Burnham, M., Anders, T., Gaylor, E., & Goodlin-Jones, B. (1998). *Night-to night consistency of sleep variables over the first year: A preliminary analysis.* Poster presented at the International Conference of Infant Studies, Atlanta.

Carey, W. B. (1974). Night waking and temperament in infancy. *Journal of Pediatrics, 84,* 756–758.

Coons, S., & Guilleminault, C. (1982). Development of sleep wake patterns and non-rapid eye movement sleep stages during the first six months of life in normal infants. *Pediatrics, 69*(6), 793–798.

Daws, D. (1989). *Through the night: Helping parents and sleepless infants.* London: Free Association Books.

Durand, V. M., & Mindell, J. A. (1990). Behavioral treatment of multiple childhood sleep disorders: Effects on child and family. *Behavior Modification, 14,* 37–49.

Ferber, R. (1985). *Solve your child's sleep problems.* New York: Simon & Schuster.

Field, T. (1994). Infants of depressed mothers. *Infant Behavior and Development, 18,* 1–13.

France, K. G., Henderson, J. M., & Hudson, S. M. (1996). Fact, act, and tact: A three-stage approach to treating the sleep problems of infants and young children. *Child and Adolescent Psychiatric Clinics of North America, 5*(3), 581–599.

Gaylor, E. E., Goodlin-Jones, B. L., Burnham, M. M., & Anders, T. F. (1998, April). *Maternal perception of night awakenings and infant self-soothing behavior during the first year of life.* Poster presented at the International Conference of Infant Studies, Atlanta, GA.

Goodlin-Jones, B. L., Eiben, L. A., & Anders, T. F. (1997). Maternal well-being and sleep–wake behaviors in infants: An intervention using maternal odor. *Infant Mental Health Journal, 18*(4), 378–393.

Guedeney, A., & Kreisler, L. (1987). Sleep disorders in the first 18 months of life: Hypothesis on the role of mother–child emotional exchanges. *Infant Mental Health Journal, 8*(3), 307–318.

Jenkins, S., Owen, C., Bax, M., & Hart, H. (1984). Continuities of common behavior problems in pre-school children. *Journal of Child Psychology and Psychiatry, 25,* 75–89.

Johnson, M. C. (1991). Infant and toddler sleep: A telephone survey of parents in one community. *Journal of Developmental and Behavioral Pediatrics, 12*(2), 108–114.

Kahn, A., Mozin, M. J., Rebuffat, E., Sottiaux, M., & Muller, M. F. (1989). Milk intolerance in children with persistent sleeplessness: A prospective double-blind crossover evaluation. *Pediatrics, 84,* 595–603.

Kahn, A., Rebuffat, E., Sottiaux, M., Dufour, D., Cadranel, S., & Reiterer, F. (1991). Arousals induced by proximal esophageal reflux in infants. *Sleep, 14*(1), 39–42.

Kataria, S., Swanson, M. S., & Trevathan, G. E. (1987). Persistence of sleep disturbances in preschool children. *Journal of Pediatrics, 110,* 642–646.

Keffe, M. R. (1987). Comparison of neonatal nighttime sleep–wake patterns in nursery versus rooming-in environments. *Nursery Research, 36,* 140–144.

Klackenberg, G. (1987). Incidence of parasomnias in children in a general population. In C. Guilleminault (Ed.), *Sleep and its disorders in children.* New York: Raven Press.

Kraemer, G. W. (1992). A psychological theory of attachment. *Behavioral and Brain Sciences, 15,* 493–541.

Lavie, P. (1986). Ultrashort sleep-waking schedule: III. "Gates" and "forbidden zones" for sleep. *Electroencephalography and Clinical Neurophysiology, 63,* 414–425.

Lehtonen, L., Korhonen, T., & Korvenranta, H. (1994). Temperament and sleeping patterns in colicky infants during the first year of life. *Journal of Developmental and Behavioral Pediatrics, 15,* 416–420.

Louis, J., Cannard, C., Bastuji, H., & Challamel, M-J. (1997). Sleep ontogenesis revisited: A longitudinal 24-hour home polygraphic study on 15 normal infants during the first two years of life. *Sleep, 20*(5), 323–333.

Lozoff, B., Wolf, A. W., & Davis, N. S. (1985). Sleep problems seen in pediatric practice. *Pediatrics, 75,* 477–483.

McDonough, S. C. (1993). Interaction guidance: Understanding and treating early infant–caregiver relationship disturbances. In C. H. Zeanah, Jr. (Ed.), *Handbook of infant mental health* (pp. 414–426). New York: Guilford Press.

McKenna, J. J., Mosko, S., Dungy, C., & McAninch, J. (1990). Sleep and arousal patterns of co–sleeping human mother/infant pairs: A preliminary physiological study with implication for the study of sudden infant death syndrome (SIDS). *American Journal of Physical Anthropology, 83,* 331–347.

McKenna, J. J., Thoman, E. B., Anders, T. F., Sadeh, A., Schechtman, V. L., & Glotzbach, S. F. (1993). Infant–parent co-sleeping in an evolutionary perspective: Implications for understanding infant sleep development and the sudden infant death syndrome. *Sleep, 16,* 263–282.

Messer, D., & Richards, M. (1993). The development of sleeping difficulties. In I. St. James-Roberts, G. Harris, & D. Messer (Eds.), *Infant crying, feeding, and sleeping* (pp. 150–173). New York: Harvester Wheatsheaf.

Michelsson, K., Rinne, A., & Paajanen, S. (1990). Crying, feeding, and sleeping patterns in 1 to 12-month-old infants. *Child: Care, Health, and Development, 16,* 99–111.

Minde, K., Popiel, K., Leos, N., Falkner, S., Parker, K., & Handley-Derry, M. (1993). The evaluation and treatment of sleep disturbances in young children. *Journal of Child Psychology and Psychiatry, 34,* 521–533.

Mindell, J. (1993). Sleep disorders in children. *Health Psychology, 12,* 151–162.

Moore, T., & Ucko, L. E. (1957). Night waking in early infancy. *Archives of Disease in Childhood, 32,* 333–342.

Mosko, S., Richard, C., & McKenna, J. (1997). Maternal sleep and arousals during bed sharing with infants. *Sleep, 20*(2), 142–150.

Owens-Stively, J., Frank, N., Smith, A., Hagino, O., Spirito, A., Arrigan, M., & Alario, A. J. (1997). Child temperament, parenting discipline style, and daytime behavior in childhood sleep disorders. *Developmental and Behavioral Pediatrics, 18,* 314–321.

Paret, I. (1983). Night waking and its relation to mother–infant interaction in nine month old infants. In J. D. Call, E. Galenson, & R. L. Tyson (Eds.), *Frontiers of infant psychiatry* (pp. 171–177). New York: Basic Books.

Rautava, P., Lehtonen, L., Helenius, H., & Sillanpaa, M. (1995). Infantile colic: Child and family three years later. *Pediatrics, 96,* 43–47.

Richman, N. (1981). A community survey of characteristics of one to two year olds with sleep disruptions. *Journal of the American Academy of Child Psychiatry, 20,* 281–291.

Richman, N., Douglas, J. W. B., Hunt, H., Lansdown, R., & Levene, R. (1985). Behavioural methods in the treatment of sleep disorders: A pilot study. *Journal of Child Psychology and Psychiatry, 26,* 581–590.

Robert-Tissot, C., Cramer, B., Stern, D. N., Serpa, S. R., Bachmann, J., Palacio-Epasa, F., Knauer, D., DeMuralt, M., Berney, C., & Mendiguren, G. (1996). Outcome evaluations in brief mother–infant psychotherapies: Report on 75 cases. *Infant Mental Health Journal, 17,* 97–114.

Sadeh, A. (1994). Assessment of intervention for infant night waking: Parental reports and activity-based home monitoring. *Journal of Consulting and Clinical Psychology, 62,* 63–98.

Sadeh, A. (1996). Stress, trauma, and sleep in children. *Child and Adolescent Psychiatric Clinics of North America, 5,* 685–700.

Sadeh, A. (1997). Melatonin and sleep in infants: A preliminary study. *Sleep, 20,* 185–191.

Sadeh, A., & Anders, T. (1993). Infant sleep problems: Origins, assessment, and intervention. *Infant Mental Health Journal, 14,* 17–34.

Sadeh, A., Dark, I., & Vohr, B. (1996). Newborns' sleep–wake patterns: The role of maternal, delivery, and infant factors. *Early Human Development, 44,* 113–126.

Sadeh, A., Lavie, P., & Scher, A. (1994). Sleep and temperament: Maternal perceptions of temperament of sleep-disturbed toddlers. *Early Education and Development, 5,* 311–322.

Sadeh, A., Lavie, P., Scher, A., Tirosh, E., & Epstein, R. (1991). Actigraphic home monitoring of sleep-disturbed and control infants and young children: A new method for pediatric assessment of sleep–wake patterns. *Pediatrics, 87*(4), 494–499.

Sameroff, A. J., & Emde, R. N. (Eds.). (1989). *Relationship disturbances in early childhood: A developmental approach.* New York: Basic Books.

Schacter, F. F., Fuchs, M. L., Bijur, P. E., & Stone, R. K. (1989). Cosleeping and sleep problems in Hispanic American urban young children. *Pediatrics, 84,* 522–530.

Schaefer, C. E. (1990). Night waking and temperament in early childhood. *Psychological Report, 67,* 192–194.

St. James-Roberts, I., & Plewis, I. (1996). Individual differences, daily fluctuations, and developmental changes in amounts of infant waking, crying, fussing, and sleeping. *Child Development, 67,* 2527–2540.

Stein, M., Colarusso, C., McKenna, J., & Powers, N. (1997). Cosleeping (bedsharing) among infants and toddlers. *Developmental and Behavioral Pediatrics, 18*(6), 408–412.

van Hofacker, N., & Papousek, M. (1998). Disorders of excessive crying, feeding, and sleeping: The Munich Interdisciplinary Research and Intervention Program. *Infant Mental Health Journal, 19,* 180–210.

Van Tassel, E. B. (1985). The relative influence of child and environmental characteristics on sleep disturbances in the first and second year of life. *Journal of Developmental and Behavioral Pediatrics, 6,* 81–86.

Weissbluth, M. (1987). *Sleep well: Peaceful nights for your child and you.* London: Unwin Hyman.

Weissbluth, M. (1995). Naps in children: 6 months–7 years. *Sleep, 18,* 82–87.

Weissbluth, M., & Liu, K. (1983). Sleep patterns, attention span and infant temperament. *Journal of Developmental and Behavioral Pediatrics, 4,* 34–36.

White, B., Gunnar, M., Larson, M., Donzella, B., & Barr, R. (1998). Behavioral and physiological responsivity and patterns of sleep and daily salivary cortisol in infants with and without colic. Manuscript submitted for publication.

Winnicott, D. W. (1965). The capacity to be alone. In D. W. Winnicott, *The maturational processes and the facilitating environment.* New York: International Universities Press.

Wolf, A. W., & Lozoff, B. (1989). Object attachment, thumbsucking, and the passage to sleep. *Journal of the American Academy of Child and Adolescent Psychiatry, 28*(2), 287–292.

Wolfson, A., Lacks, P., & Futterman, A. (1992). Effects of parent training on infant sleeping patterns, parents' stress, and perceived parental competence. *Journal of Counseling and Clinical Psychology, 60,* 41–48.

Wolke, D., Meyer, R., Ohrt, B., & Riegel, K. (1995). The incidence of sleeping problems in preterm and fullterm infants discharged from neonatal special care units: An epidemiological investigation. *Journal of Child Psychology and Psychiatry, 36,* 203–223.

Zeanah, C. H., Jr. (Ed.). (1993). *Handbook of infant mental health.* New York: Guilford Press.

Zero to Three, National Center for Clinical Infant Programs. (1994). *Diagnostic classification:* (DC: 0–3), Arlington, VA: Author.

Zuckerman, B., Stevenson, J., & Baily, V. (1987). Sleep problems in early childhood: Continuities, predictive factors, and behavioral correlates. *Pediatrics, 80,* 664–671.

21

Feeding Disorders, Failure to Thrive, and Obesity

❖

DIANE BENOIT

Feeding disorders (FDs), failure to thrive (FTT), and obesity are common problems of infancy. Specifically, FDs affect up to 25% of infants developing normally and up to 35% of those with developmental handicaps (Lindberg, Bohlin, & Hagekull, 1991; Wolke, Meyer, Ohrt, & Riegel, 1995). In the United States, FTT affects up to 30% of infants seen in ambulatory care and inner-city emergency room settings, 22% of those born prematurely with low birthweight, 1–5% of those hospitalized, and 10% of those living below the poverty level in rural and urban areas (Casey et al., 1994; Frank & Zeisel, 1988; Powell, Low, & Speers, 1987). In Britain, 1.8% of all infants in the community (inner city) and 3.3% of those born full-term and appropriate for gestational age are affected, although as few as 28% of those are referred to hospital services (Skuse, Gill, Reilly, Wolke, & Lynch, 1995; Skuse, Wolke, & Reilly, 1992). British children from lower socioeconomic backgrounds are two to three times more likely than children from more affluent backgrounds to have FTT (Wright, Waterston, & Aynsley-Green, 1994). In Israel, 3.9% of full-term infants in the community develop FTT (Wilensky et al., 1996). Although FTT and FDs may coexist, the frequency of association has not yet been firmly determined. Obesity affects about 10% of U.S. infants (Whitaker, Wright, Pepe, Seidel, & Dietz, 1997). Each of these problems (FDs, FTT, and obesity) is reviewed in this chapter, with an emphasis on research findings since 1987.

FEEDING DISORDERS

Definition, Classification, and Etiology

There are no universally accepted definitions or validated classifications of common FDs of infancy (Arts-Rodas & Benoit, 1998; Kerwin & Berkowitz, 1996; Lindberg, Bohlin, Hagekull, & Palmerus, 1996; Skuse, 1993; Skuse & Wolke, 1992), although rare FDs have been extensively studied, including rumination disorder (or merycism), pica (or ingestion of nonnutritive substance), and psychosocial dwarfism. One general definition of FD is the inability or unwillingness to eat certain foods (Arts-Rodas & Benoit, 1998; Babbitt et al., 1994; Wolke & Skuse, 1992), although this definition does not include problems related to overeating. Further, there are no universally accepted guidelines to determine when a feeding *problem* becomes a *disorder* (transient feeding problems are common during infancy and do not necessarily constitute a FD). A long list of symptoms have been described in infants with FD and reflect the heterogeneous nature of feeding problems in infancy. Some of these symptoms relate directly to feeding skills and behaviors exhibited by the infant when food is offered (e.g., partial to total food refusal, quick loss of interest, oral motor, oral sensory and oropharyngeal difficulties, vomiting, inability to graduate to textured foods, gagging, coughing, ingestion of nonnutritive substances [pica], and tantrums) whereas others are vague and nonspecific (e.g., colic, flatulence, diarrhea, and constipation) (Arts-Rodas & Benoit, 1998; Chatoor et al., 1992; Dahl, 1987; Lindberg et al., 1991; Lindberg et al., 1996; Turner, Sanders, & Wall, 1994; Wolke et al., 1995).

Thus far, studies on FDs have been limited by serious methodological problems, including inconsistent and questionable definitions and determination of the presence and severity of feeding problems often based on parental report only (Lindberg et al., 1991; Wolke et al., 1995). These problems make a comparison among studies difficult and raise questions about the validity of the definitions used in some studies (e.g., Are colic, flatulence, vomiting, diarrhea, and constipation truly symptoms of FD and are they comparable to oropharyngeal dysfunction, refusal to open the mouth, refusal to swallow, spitting food out, crying, and tantruming when food is offered?). Future research should address such questions.

Despite the various problems with definition and methodology, there is a growing awareness of the interplay among various physiological and environmental contributors to a child's "normal" (Skuse & Wolke, 1992; Wolke & Skuse, 1992) and abnormal swallowing and eating skills and behaviors (Arts-Rodas & Benoit, 1998; Jolley, McClelland, & Mosesso-Rousseau, 1995; Lindberg et al., 1991; Skuse & Wolke, 1992). Various infant characteristics have been identified as contributing to feeding problems and reflect the heterogeneous nature of feeding problems in infancy. Such characteristics include (1) capacity to self-regulate, including the ability to experience hunger/thirst and satiety (Benoit, in press; Jolley et al., 1995; Lindberg et al., 1991; Skuse, 1993; Wolke et al., 1995); (2) oral–motor, oral–sensory, and oropharyngeal functioning (Bazyk, 1990; Mathisen, Skuse, Wolke, & Reilly, 1989); (3) developmental readiness (Arts-Rodas & Benoit, 1998; Skuse, 1993); (4) health history (Arts-Rodas & Benoit, 1998; Bazyk, 1990); and (5) past feeding and "oral" experiences (Arts-Rodas & Benoit, 1998; Bazyk, 1990; Benoit, Green, & Arts-Rodas, 1997; Chatoor, Conley, & Dickson, 1988; Skuse & Wolke, 1992; Wolke & Skuse, 1992).

Various environmental factors have been identified as contributing to FDs. For instance, during feeding and/or play interactions, infants with FD reject food more often and exhibit less clear signals than infants without FD, whereas their parents are more controlling, more insensitive, and less cooperative than parents of infants without FD (Chatoor, Egan, Getson, Menvielle, & O'Donnell, 1987; Chatoor et al., 1997; Lindberg et al., 1996; Sanders, Patel, Le Grice, & Shepherd, 1993). Lindberg et al. (1996) also found no significant differences in attachment classifications between infants with food refusal and those without. However, the disorganized/disoriented classification was not used, representing a potentially serious limitation. Future research is needed to assess the contribution of attachment to infant FD.

Associated Features and Outcome

There is some evidence (albeit controversial) for comorbidity, in particular with FTT, sleep problems, and various regulatory difficulties and health problems (Benoit, in press; Budd et al., 1992; Heptinstall et al., 1987; Lindberg, Bohlin, Hagekull, & Thunstrom, 1994; Raynor & Rudolf, 1996; Wolke et al., 1995). In addition, food refusal has been related to weaning problems, breastfeeding, low food and calorie consumption, frequent meals, family problems, and parents' less positive perceptions of parenting and infant behaviors (Linscheid, 1992; Lindberg et al., 1994).

In two large Swedish samples of 841 (Sample A) and 567 infants (Sample B) between the ages of 30 and 71 weeks, Lindberg et al. (1991) examined factors associated with feeding problems (defined as colic, vomiting, poor appetite, refusal to eat, difficulty to swallow, refusal of solids, and other). In Sample B, compared to subjects in the no-problem group: (1) more girls had feeding problems; (2) more affected infants had siblings; (3) infants with colic showed less concentration during the meal, and (4) mothers had higher occupational level (no significant differences on these variables were found for Sample A). In both samples, the following events were more commonly reported by parents of infants with feeding problems than parents in the no-problem group: (1) previous feeding problems in members of the family; (2) physical problems during the pregnancy for mothers in the colic and refusal-to-eat groups; (3) severe breastfeeding problems for infants with vomiting; (4) severe and enduring breastfeeding problems, irritability during meals, and diarrhea in the colic group; (5) tendency for lower weight for infants with vomiting and refusal to eat; (6) "other diseases" in the refusal-to-eat group; and (7) worries and anxiety about infant health. There were no significant differences in prematurity, birthweight, body mass index, maternal anxiety, and duration of sick leave during pregnancy between the FD and non-FD groups.

Dahl (1987) demonstrated that not only do 50% of infants with feeding problems in the first year continue to show significant feeding problems at age 2, but they also have significantly more infections and behavioral problems than infants who do not have early feeding problems. Other researchers have documented associations between early FD and negative nutritional, developmental, and psychological sequelae (Dahl, 1987; Dahl & Sundelin, 1992; Marchi & Cohen 1990) and between severity of sequelae and age of onset, duration, and degree of the feeding problem (Skuse, 1993). Thus, the early identification and treatment of FDs is important.

Assessment of Feeding Problems

To begin to address the problems with definition and to assist in the early identification of feeding problems, several researchers have provided guidelines to assess feeding problems in infancy. Instruments have also been developed (e.g., parent and observer rating scales) to assess the presence, nature, and/or severity of FD, based on specific skills and behaviors exhibited by the infant when food is offered during a meal (e.g., Arts-Rodas & Benoit, 1998; Benoit & Green, 1995; Mathisen et al., 1989; Turner et al., 1994).

A comprehensive assessment should include a review of the child's health, developmental, feeding, regulatory, and growth history, measurement of growth parameters, parental report of mealtime behaviors and nutrient intake, and observation of meals with primary feeders (ideally both at the office and in the home—live or via videotapes; Arts-Rodas & Benoit, 1998). A comprehensive assessment of an infant with feeding and/or swallowing problems should answer questions about whether or not (1) the child has growth failure, (2) the child is safe to feed (If so, is the child anatomically and developmentally able to feed? If so, is the child will-

ing to eat?), and (3) there are caregiver–infant relationship problems or other environmental problems. Based on the answer to these various questions, the next level of intervention can then be determined; for example, no oral feeding because it is unsafe to feed; occupational therapy and/or speech and language assessment and/or therapy when oral–motor, oropharyngeal, oral–sensory dysfunction, or neurologically based swallowing difficulties are suspected; pediatrics and/or nutrition when growth failure is present; parent–infant psychotherapy when parent–infant relationship problems are present; behavior therapy when food refusal/aversion is present; and combined treatment modalities when multiple problems are present (Arts-Rodas & Benoit, 1998; Linscheid, Tarnowski, Rasnake, & Brams, 1987; Luiselli, 1994; Skuse, 1993; Turner et al., 1994; Werle, Murphy, & Budd, 1993). The next sections examine some recently described FDs characterized by undereating (and excluding FDs characterized by overeating and those that have a strong neurodevelopmental component such as cerebral palsy as a significant contributor).

Conditioned Dysphagia (or Food Aversion/Phobia or Posttraumatic Feeding Disorder)

This FD is characterized by partial to total food refusal, acceptance of the "feared" food only when in a drowsy state, and/or anxious/fearful anticipation of mealtimes as evidenced by escape behaviors, crying, coughing, gagging, vomiting at the sight of food or objects or events associated with feeding such as putting a bib on, high chair, or the "beeping" sound of a microwave oven. DiScipio, Kaslon, and Ruben (1978) and Griffin (1979) identified aspects of this FD, which were later termed "posttraumatic eating disorder" by Chatoor et al. (1988). Essentially, this FD occurs when infants undergo painful or frightening medical procedures (e.g., suctioning, intubation, and nasogastric tube feeding) or experience painful or frightening events (e.g., forced feeding, esophagitis, gastroesophageal reflux, and choking). In this FD, it seems that infants become unwilling to eat because they associate swallowing with pain and discomfort (Arts-Rodas & Benoit, 1998; Benoit, Green, et al., 1997; Chatoor et al., 1988) and/or because they may develop visceral hyperalgesia, a neuropathic condition in which prior experience changes sensory nerves so that previously innocuous stimuli are perceived as painful (Hyman, 1994). Conditioned dysphagia may affect 4% of infants with gastroesophageal reflux who do not have an underlying neurological or craniofacial problem or a history of esophageal surgery (Dellert, Hyams, Treem, & Geertsma, 1993) and up to 40% of children who undergo esophageal surgery (DiScipio et al., 1978). Conditioned dysphagia may be increasingly common as advances in medical technology allow very ill infants to survive. In a case series of 24 infants with conditioned dysphagia, a three-component treatment program was found to be effective in almost half to three quarters of cases, depending on predetermined criteria for success versus failure of treatment (Benoit, Green, et al., 1997). In a randomized clinical trial comparing the effectiveness of two interventions in the treatment of infants with conditioned dysphagia who were fed by gastrostomy or gastrojejunostomy tubes, Benoit, Zlotkin, and Wang (1999) showed that flooding techniques were more effective than traditional nutritional counseling in eliminating the need for tube feedings and getting infants to eat and drink. Recent studies have focused on identifying factors influencing the effectiveness of flooding in the treatment of conditioned dysphagia (Benoit & Coolbear, 1998; Benoit et al., 1999).

Infantile Anorexia

This FD has been described as a disorder of separation and individuation characterized by FTT, food refusal, a failure to achieve somatopsychological differentiation, and conflicts between feeder and infant during play and feeding interactions (Chatoor, 1989; Chatoor et al., 1987; Chatoor et al., 1997). There are no data on the prevalence of this FD or whether it is a diagnostic entity separate from FTT. Chatoor (1989) argues that the treatment of infantile anorexia should consist of a combination of (1) structured feeding schedules and routines, (2) firm and consistent limit setting, and (3) a cognitive-behavioral approach (to formulate the conflicts in the infant and the infant–parent relationship around autonomy and somatopsychological differentiation). Nevertheless, no data have been published to document the effectiveness of this or other approaches in the treatment of infantile anorexia.

Picky Eating (or Choosiness or Faddiness)

This FD is characterized by selective food refusal, disinterest in specific foods or inadequate intake (Rydell, Dahl, & Sundelin, 1995; Wolke & Skuse, 1992). The prevalence, specificity, and validity of this FD have not been established. There is some evidence that choosy behavior (food refusal) in infancy has long-term consequences, including emotional and behavioral problems, persistent lower relative weight compared to controls, and persistent eating problems (Dahl, 1987; Dahl & Sundelin, 1992; Lindberg et al., 1994; Marchi & Cohen, 1990; Rydell et al., 1995). In a randomized clinical trial examining the effectiveness of two interventions in the treatment of picky eating, Turner et al. (1994) found that both behavioral parent training and dietary education (1) diminished food refusal and disruptive behavior at mealtimes and (2) increased the variety of foods eaten by 3 to 4 months follow-up. More positive mother–child interactions during mealtimes and more satisfaction with treatment were associated with the behavioral parent training. Generally, behavioral management is recommended for the treatment of picky eating and food refusal, providing the child has the skills to eat and it is safe to do so (Arts-Rodas & Benoit, 1998; Babbitt et al., 1994; Linscheid et al., 1987; Luiselli, 1994; Werle et al., 1993). Still, more research is needed to refine the concept of this FD and assess the efficacy of various treatments.

FAILURE TO THRIVE

Definition, Classification, and Etiology

FTT is a multifactorial problem involving biological, nutritional, and environmental factors (Pollitt, 1987; Pollitt et al., 1996). Although there is no agreement on a definition for FTT, many clinicians and researchers agree that FTT is present when there is at least a 1-month history of (1) weight below the fifth percentile for age on standardized growth charts and/or (2) deceleration in the rate of weight from birth to the present (downward crossing of at least two major percentiles on standardized growth charts), and (3) weight for height age less than 90%. However, researchers have used different criteria for FTT (e.g., some use weight and/or length below the 10th percentile for age without any criteria related to deceleration in rate of weight gain over time or weight for length ratio). The inconsistent diagnostic criteria likely account for the conflicting results in the literature regarding various aspects of FTT, especially when combined with the different recruitment strategies (e.g., samples recruited from the community vs. hospital wards vs. hospital outpatient clinics vs. specialized FTT or psychiatric clinics vs. pediatric clinics in the community; Drotar, 1990; Puckering et al., 1995; Wolke, 1996).

FTT continues to be referred to as organic when an underlying medical problem contributing to FTT is present (~25% of cases), nonorganic when no contributing medical problem is present, and mixed when both organic and nonorganic factors are present (~20% of cases). Whereas all infants with FTT end up with an organic problem (undernutrition), a minority have an organic problem as a precipitant of FTT (Drotar, 1990). Yet, infants with FTT often undergo expensive medical work-ups, usually to rule out an organic cause to the FTT (Fryer, 1988; Singer, 1987). On the one hand, some studies have documented associations (*not* causal links) between FTT and various "nonorganic" factors, including characteristics of infants (e.g., temperament), caregivers (e.g., mental illness), caregiver–infant relationship (e.g., insecure attachment and neglect), and family environment (e.g., poverty, isolation, violence, and family dysfunction). On the other hand, many studies have failed to identify such associations. The next sections examine the conflicting findings pertaining to nonorganic factors.

Characteristics of Infants and Outcome

Given that brain growth is rapid for infants under age 2, permanent damage to the developing central nervous system may occur if severe undernutrition goes uncorrected (Bithoney et al., 1991; Casey et al., 1994). Malnutrition in early life also is associated with an impairment of defenses against disease, reduced neural cell growth, and delayed neural maturation. Thus, infants with FTT not only may have developmental delays but they may be ill more often (and when they are ill, they are more ill and stay ill longer) than those without FTT. In fact, infants with FTT recruited in the community

are twice as likely to be admitted to hospital in the first year of life than infants without FTT (Wilensky et al., 1996).

With respect to developmental delays and delayed neural maturation, infants with FTT recruited from the community samples have been found to be more likely than controls to have lower birthweights and hypotonia in the first year (Wilensky et al., 1996). Further, in a small study of nine infants with FTT "nominated" by home visitors to be recruited as study participants, Mathisen et al. (1989) found more oral motor problems and hypotonia in infants with FTT than in controls. Controlled and noncontrolled studies of infants with FTT recruited from hospital outpatient clinics (Coolbear, personal communication, September, 1998) and specialized FTT clinics (Raynor & Rudolf, 1996), or the community (Black, Dubowitz, Hutcheson, Berenson-Howard, & Starr, 1995; Dowdney, Skuse, Heptinstall, Puckering, & Zur-Szpiro, 1987; Puckering et al., 1995; Wilensky et al., 1996; Wolke, Skuse, & Mathisen, 1990) document developmental delays in all areas of development (Black et al., 1995; Dowdney et al. 1987; Puckering et al., 1995; Raynor & Rudolf, 1996; Wilensky et al., 1996; Wolke et al., 1990), with almost one third of infants with FTT being severely delayed (Raynor & Rudolf, 1996). The only study that has not found developmental delays at the time of study enrollment was a noncontrolled study of hospitalized infants with FTT who were tested at an average age of about 5 months (Drotar & Sturm, 1988). However, when retested at age 36 months, a significant decrease in developmental scores was documented.

Many studies also have identified serious long-term (from 1 to more than 10 years after the onset of FTT) developmental problems associated with FTT. For instance, compared to norms for the general population, children with FTT (irrespective of the presence of prematurity and of whether they are recruited from the community, pediatric primary care clinics, or hospitals) have lower intelligence and show declines in their reading and language skills and in their cognitive and intellectual functioning over time (Black et al., 1995; Dowdney et al., 1987; Drotar & Sturm, 1988; Kristiansson & Fallstrom, 1987; Pollitt et al., 1996; Puckering et al., 1995), including one third who were "seriously retarded" at age 4 (Dowdney et al., 1987).

Studies have shown that although short-term

nutritional status may improve with increased nutrient intake (Black et al., 1995), children with FTT generally remain shorter and lighter than other children as they get older, whether they are hospitalized at the time of recruitment (Kristiansson & Fallstrom, 1987) or are recruited from the community (Puckering et al., 1995). In a noncontrolled study, Sturm and Drotar (1989) pointed out that shorter duration of FTT prior to diagnosis (made at an average age of 5 months in this hospitalized sample of FTT infants) and greater rate of weight gain immediately following hospitalization predict weight for height at 36 months.

Behavioral and socioemotional problems at the time of diagnosis and in the long term have been described in infants with FTT (Pollitt, 1987; Pollitt et al., 1996), irrespective of whether they are recruited from hospital wards (Powell et al., 1987) or outpatient and/or FTT clinics (Berkowitz & Senter, 1987; Polan, Leon, et al., 1991; Raynor & Rudolf, 1996), or the community (Crittenden, 1987; Valenzuela, 1990; Wilensky et al., 1996; Wolke et al., 1990). Behavioral and emotional problems described in a small group of 12-month-old infants with FTT recruited in a community sample include more demanding, fussy, and unsociable behaviors and less task-oriented and persistent behavioral style, compared to 12-month-old infants without FTT (Wolke et al., 1990). Three- to 24-month-old infants with "nonorganic" FTT recruited from hospital wards exhibited several problem behaviors (both spontaneously or during interactions with examiner) more frequently than did infants with "organic" FTT and controls who thrived normally (Powell et al., 1987). The problematic spontaneous behaviors included general inactivity, flexed hips, expressionless face, infantile posture, rumination, thumb sucking, disproportionate hand and finger activity, and lack of vocalization. The problematic interactive behaviors included gaze abnormality (hyperalertness, not directed eyes, avoidance, disinterest) and abnormal response to interactive stimulus (lack of smile, motor activity, or vocalization).

Other behavioral characteristics identified in infants with FTT recruited from a hospital outpatient clinic include less positive affect during meals and play (Polan, Leon, et al., 1991). Also, compared with infants without FTT, infants with FTT identified in the community (Wilensky et al., 1996) have been described as less sociable and showing more fearful responses toward examiners. In addition, findings from a noncontrolled study of infants referred to an FTT clinic (Raynor & Rudolf, 1996) and a controlled study of infants with FTT recruited in the community (Wilensky et al., 1996) indicate that feeding problems (often starting early in life) are common. Although sleep and regulatory problems have also been described in infants with FTT referred to specialized FTT clinics (Benoit, in press; Raynor & Rudolf, 1996), the two studies that examined temperamental characteristics of infants with FTT (measured by parental report) showed conflicting results. In one study (subjects recruited from a community sample) no differences in temperament between infants with FTT and controls were identified (Wilensky et al., 1996). In another controlled study, infants with FTT who were recruited from hospital clinics, including an FTT clinic, were rated as having more difficult temperament than were infants without FTT (Gorman, Leifer, & Grossman, 1993). Whether the developmental, behavioral, and emotional problems reported in infants with FTT precede the onset of FTT or are a consequence of it is still unanswered.

Characteristics of Environment and Parents of Infants with FTT

Controlled and noncontrolled studies, irrespective of recruitment strategies, have documented that families of infants with FTT are highly stressed with poverty, violence, substance abuse, criminality, and dysfunctional relationships (Crittenden, 1987; Drotar & Eckerle, 1989; Gorman et al., 1993; Kristiansson & Fallstrom, 1987; Raynor & Rudolf, 1996; Wolke, 1996; Wright et al., 1994). Whether mothers of infants with FTT have more mental illness than do mothers of thriving infants is controversial. On the one hand, studies that recruited subjects from hospital outpatient clinics and used operationalized diagnostic criteria for psychopathology and a control group (Polan, Kaplan, et al., 1991) or from the community (Crittenden, 1987; Wolke, 1996) have shown that mothers of infants with FTT have more mental illness (anxiety, depression, and co-occurrence of both disorders) than do mothers of thriving infants. In addition, in one noncontrolled study of mothers of infants with FTT recruited from a specialized FTT clinic, more than four fifths were found to have symptoms consistent with clinical depression, and almost one in five had symptoms consistent with severe anxiety (Raynor & Rudolf, 1996). On the other hand, other controlled studies of infants hospitalized (Benoit, Zeanah, & Barton, 1989) or recruited in the community (Wilensky et al., 1996) have failed to document more mental illness in mothers of infants with FTT.

Compared to their matched counterparts, mothers of infants with FTT recruited from hospital wards or outpatient clinics have (1) been childhood victims of sexual and physical abuse and neglect more often (Weston et al., 1993), (2) more often experienced abuse in general and sexual abuse in particular as adults (Weston et al., 1993), (3) experienced more caregiver instability and crises during childhood (Gorman et al., 1993), (4) more life stresses and less optimal social support (Benoit et al., 1989; Gorman et al., 1993; Ward, Kessler, & Altman, 1993), (5) more negative perceptions of their infants with FTT (Benoit, Zeanah, Parker, Nicholson, & Coolbear, 1997; Coolbear & Benoit, 1999; Gorman et al., 1993), and (6) more insecure attachment as assessed by the Adult Attachment Interview (Benoit et al., 1989; Coolbear & Benoit, 1999).

Characteristics of the Parent–Infant Relationship

One of the most studied and controversial nonorganic factors in FTT is disturbed parent–infant relationships. With respect to play interactions, mothers of infants with FTT have been shown to have more conflicted interactions with their FTT infants, compared to matched counterparts who were also recruited in the community (Hepstinstall et al., 1987). Wolke (1996) also reported that in the community-based sample he studied, only small differences between groups of FTT and non-FTT were identified during play interactions, with mothers of infants with FTT being more controlling and infants mouthing objects more often and communicating their needs less efficiently than controls. In another controlled, community-based study of 4-year-old children with histories of FTT, Puckering et al. (1987) found that compared to matched controls, mothers of children with FTT were less positive when interacting with their child. However, the group differences were markedly reduced when measures took into account the child's contribution to the disturbed interaction. One controlled study of infants with FTT recruited in hospital

outpatient clinics has failed to document significant differences between groups during play (Coolbear & Benoit, 1999). Finally, findings from numerous studies of subjects recruited from hospital wards or outpatient clinics, psychiatric clinics, or the community suggest that compared with mothers of infants without FTT, mothers of infants or toddlers with FTT are less responsive, less flexible, more controlling, more intrusive, overstimulating, less affectionate, less accepting, less sensitive, use more physical punishment, and express more negative (hostile, angry) emotion during interactions with their infants (Chatoor et al., 1987; Crittenden, 1987; Drotar, Eckerle, Satola, Pallotta, & Wyatt, 1990; Hutcheson, Black, & Starr, 1993; Black et al., 1993; Ward et al., 1993; Wolke et al., 1990).

With respect to mealtimes, more disturbed feeding habits and interactions have been identified in groups of infants with FTT and their caregivers recruited in the community (Mathisen et al., 1989), compared to matched controls. However, other controlled studies of infants with FTT recruited in the community (Wolke, 1996), primary health care clinics in the community (Hutcheson et al., 1993), and hospital outpatient clinics (Coolbear & Benoit, 1999) have failed to document significant differences between groups during feeding interactions (Hutcheson et al., 1993; Wolke, 1996). Further, after controlling for severity and chronicity of FTT, Hutcheson et al. (1993) found that mothers of toddlers with FTT (13½ to 26 months old) were more cold, hostile, intrusive, and inflexible than mothers of infants with FTT (8 to 13.4 months old). Similarly, in a study of toddlers with infantile anorexia nervosa (and associated FTT) who were referred to a psychiatrist for assessment of feeding problems and FTT, Chatoor et al. (1987) found that during feeding interactions, mothers of infants with FTT positioned their infants poorly, handled them excessively and roughly, missed their cues, forced food into their mouths, and were more erratic compared with mothers of thriving infants. In their community-based study, Mathisen et al. (1989) also found that, compared to their matched counterparts, mothers of infants with FTT fed their infants in less appropriate surroundings and for much briefer periods and positioned them poorly during the meal. In a controlled study of subjects recruited from hospital outpatient clinics, Polan and Ward (1994) found that compared to controls, mothers of infants with FTT provided

less matter-of fact touch during feeding and unintentional touch during play, and that within the
FTT group, cases of extreme touch aversion can
be identified.

In summary, the long-held belief that FTT is
caused by parenting problems, neglect, parental
psychopathology, and conflicted family relationships has recently been challenged (Boddy
& Skuse, 1994; Skuse et al., 1995; Wachs et al.,
1992; Wolke, 1996), as a growing number of
studies fail to show differences in parent–infant
interaction during feeding and play between
FTT and non-FTT groups. Possible explanations for the conflicted results include (1) inconsistent definitions of FTT, (2) inclusion of
groups of infants with FTT that may not be comparable across studies (e.g., community samples
vs. infants hospitalized vs. referred to mental
health professionals), (3) different methodologies (and specifically, instruments used to assess
interaction), and (4) failure to examine both internal (perceptions and subjective experience)
and external (observable interactions) components of the caregiver–infant relationship.

Infants' internal representation of their attachment relationship with the primary caregiver has been studied in FTT. Table 21.1 lists
studies that have used the most up-to-date classification system of the Strange Situation (i.e.,
including the disorganized/disoriented or
equivalent insecure classification in addition to
the secure, avoidant, and resistant classifications). There is an overrepresentation of insecure attachment in infants with FTT recruited
from high-risk community samples (Crittenden, 1987; Valenzuela, 1990) and hospital outpatient clinics (Ward et al., 1993). This suggests that many infants with FTT may

experience their caregiver as rejecting, angry,
or unpredictable. Valenzuela (1990) reported
that in her study, infants classified as both
avoidant and ambivalent (one type of disorga-
nized/disoriented classification) in the Strange
Situation presented the most serious weight
deficits within the underweight group. Infants
with FTT who are classified as insecurely attached at 12 months are more rigid under stress
and less competent, skillful, and creative and
were rehospitalized twice as often between time
of diagnosis and age 42 months, compared to
infants with FTT classified as insecurely attached (Brinich, Drotar, & Brinich, 1989).

Management/Treatment

By and large, the focus of intervention in FTT
has been on treating the physical/nutritional
symptoms of FTT to improve growth and developmental outcome. Medical treatments of
FTT have included tube feeding, gastric proki-
netic drugs (e.g., Domperidone), zinc supplementation, in addition to the specific treatment
of underlying "organic" problems contributing
to the FTT. Other treatments have included hospitalization, various types of psychotherapy,
and various forms of outpatient treatment, often
delivered by multidisciplinary teams (Babbitt et
al., 1994; Bithoney et al., 1991; Black et al.,
1995; Casey et al., 1994; Chatoor et al., 1992;
Fryer, 1988; Hobbs & Hanks, 1996; Larson,
Ayllon, & Barrett, 1987; Singer, 1987).

Randomized clinical trials and other studies
from developing and developed countries show
that increased caloric intake usually leads to
improved growth (Bithoney et al., 1991; Black
et al., 1995; Casey et al., 1994; Drotar & Sturm,

TABLE 21.1. Cross-Sectional Studies of Attachment in Failure to Thrive Using SSP-4

Study	n	% Disorganized/ disoriented per group	% Insecure per group	p
Crittenden (1987)	18 FTT 21 controls	45% FTT [b]	92% FTT 33% controls	[a]
Valenzuela (1990)	42 FTT 43 controls	32% FTT 5% controls	93% FTT 50% controls	<.0001
Ward, Kessler, & Altman (1993)	26 FTT 28 controls	46% FTT 7% controls	65% FTT 36% controls	<.01

Note. FTT, failure to thrive; SSP-4, Strange Situation using three-way classification (secure, avoidant, resistant) in addition to the disorganized/disoriented or equivalent classification.
[a]p value not given.
[b]Not mentioned for control group.

1988; Grantham-McGregor, Schonfield, & Powell, 1987; Sturm & Drotar, 1989; Super, Herrera, & Mora, 1990). Although noncontrolled studies often have claimed dramatic results for multidisciplinary interventions in FTT (Bithoney et al., 1991), randomized trials show mixed, non-specific, and generally disappointing effects on nutritional, developmental and socioemotional outcomes (see Table 21.2).

In summary, FTT is common, multifactorial, and associated with serious sequelae in growth, health, development, and socioemotional functioning. Treatments of FTT that are lengthy, intense, and broad based may help to improve nu-

TABLE 21.2. Randomized Trials of Interventions for Failure to Thrive (FTT)

Study	*n*	Intervention and control groups description	Weight outcome	Psychosocial and socioemotional outcome
Black, Dubowitz, Hutcheson, Berenson-Howard, & Starr (1995)	130	African American infants with nonorganic FTT (mean age at enrollment = 12. 7 months; *SD* 6. 4). Inner city, low income. Two interventions: (1) clinic + home intervention (*n* = 64) and (2) clinic only (*n* = 66). Clinic = "multidisciplinary growth and nutrition clinic." Home = weekly home visits by lay home visitors for 1 year to provide support, education on child nutrition and development, use of community resources, advocacy.	• Improved irrespective of treatment group	• Home intervention = slightly better receptive language • Cognitive development slightly better in home intervention (but only for children who were younger at enrollment) • No intervention effect on quality of parent–child interaction
Casey et al. (1994)	166	166 infants developed FTT in a cohort of 985 premature infants with low birthweights: 67 (20%) of 330 cohort infants who were randomized to an intensive intervention and 113 (22%) of 512 infants who were randomized to regular care. Intensive intervention included medical care, social services referral, support, infant stimulation. Weekly home visits during first year began at hospital discharge, then biweekly until age 3. Also, early intervention 5 days/week at child development center from 12 to 36 months. Control = pediatric care.	• Incidence of FTT not influenced by intervention • Greater amount of intervention related to better nutritional outcome	• No intervention effect on 3-year IQ, behavior problems, child health, and nutritional status • Children from families who were most compliant with home intervention had better intellectual and behavioral outcomes
Drotar & Sturm (1988)	59	36-month-old infants with nonorganic FTT diagnosed at ~5 months old. Low SES. Three interventions began shortly after diagnosis of FTT: (1) family therapy (*n* = 22), (2) parent support and education (*n* = 17), and (3) advocacy (*n* = 20). First two groups had weekly home visits for 12 months. Advocacy group had an average of six home visits (over ~2 months), followed by phone contacts.	n/a	• Decline in cognitive functioning or intelligence (Stanford–Binet) regardless of intervention

Note. FTT, failure to thrive; SES, socioeconomic status.

tritional status in the short term but have virtually no impact on socioemotional outcome and only inconsistent effects on development (ranging from minor to none).

INFANT OBESITY

Definition, Classification, and Etiology

Although obesity generally refers to the proportion of body fat to lean tissue, there are no established definitions for infants (Keller & Stevens, 1996; Whitaker et al., 1997). A growing number of studies use body mass index (defined as the weight in kilograms divided by the square of the height in meters) to assess the presence and degree of obesity (Harlan, 1993; Lissau & Sorensen, 1994; Whitaker et al., 1997).

Associated Features and Outcome

Few studies of obesity during childhood have examined infancy separately from other age groups. The examination of children under age 3 and older children and adolescents as separate groups is important because findings from recent studies that have done so have challenged common assumptions about the significance and outcome of obesity during infancy.

Inherited susceptibility has long been described as interacting with environmental factors to create risk for obesity (Moll, Burns, & Lauer, 1991; Stunkard, Harris, Pedersen, & McClearn, 1990). Environmental factors identified as increasing risk for adult obesity include parental neglect (independent of age, body mass index in childhood, gender, and social background; Lissau & Sorensen, 1994), high fat diet, limited physical activity, low maternal education (Moussa, Skaik, Selwanes, Yaghy, & Bin-Othman, 1994), and use of food for reward, punishment, or comfort measures (Keller & Stevens, 1996). However, studies that have documented these risk factors were conducted with older (school-age) children and not with infants. Other environmental factors that have been identified as risk factors for obesity include early introduction of solids and misinterpretation of infant cries as a sign of hunger (Keller & Stevens, 1996) and cultural beliefs that fat babies are healthy babies and that rapid weight gain in infancy is a measure of good health (Sherman, Alexander, Clark, Dean, & Welter, 1992). Unfortunately, many of the stud-

ies that have examined environmental contributors to childhood obesity are fraught with problems, the most significant of which may be the lack of examination of infancy separately from other age groups. A notable exception is a retrospective cohort study of 854 individuals (and both their parents) studied from infancy to young adulthood (Whitaker et al., 1997).

Whitaker et al. (1997) demonstrated that obesity at 1 or 2 years of age does not increase the risk for adult obesity for males and females (infant obesity was defined as body mass index at or above the 85th percentile for age and gender). However, compared with 1- and 2-year-olds who do not have an obese parent, obese and nonobese 1- and 2-year-olds have a greater chance of being obese as adults if at least one parent is obese (28% vs. 10%). The risk to become obese adults is even greater if both parents are obese. Very obese infants (i.e., body mass index at or above the 95th percentile for age and gender) with at least one obese parent are at the highest risk for obesity in adulthood (40% vs. 14% of very obese infant without an obese parent). Whitaker et al. (1997) demonstrated that neither the age of onset nor the duration of obesity during infancy increase the risk for adult obesity after adjusting for parental obesity and for whether or not the infant is very obese.

Management and Treatment

Whitaker et al. (1997) indicated that based on their findings, children under age 3 who do not have at least one obese parent should not be treated for obesity and should not be labeled as being at risk for later obesity as so few of them become obese as adults. Although 1- and 2-year-olds who have one or two obese parent(s) might benefit from some intervention to prevent obesity (Whitaker et al., 1997), there is no empirical evidence documenting the effectiveness of any intervention during infancy in preventing obesity during childhood and adulthood. Future prospective studies are needed to confirm Whitaker et al.'s findings and identify targets for intervention during infancy aimed at the prevention of later obesity for those infants who have at least one obese parent.

CONCLUSION

FDs and FTT continue to be viewed as complex, multifactorial problems and are associated with varying degrees of poor health, growth, emotional, behavioral, and developmental outcomes. The quality of the caregiver–infant relationship remains a focus of paramount importance when examining feeding context and factors contributing to or protecting against the development and perpetuation of FDs and FTT. On the other hand, infant obesity may have been overestimated as a serious problem, given that so few obese infants grow up to become obese children and adults, especially if they do not have an obese parent. Research on FDs, FTT, and obesity is limited by inconsistent definitions and methodologies. However, several randomized clinical trials have examined the effectiveness of interventions that clinicians always had believed to be effective in FTT. Although most studies on FTT convincingly have shown that increased caloric intake is associated with improved nutritional status (in the short term), results from randomized controlled trials have been less conclusive. Indeed, randomized clinical trials of interventions in FTT have included broad-based, intensive, and lengthy, multidisciplinary interventions traditionally used in FTT and have shown that these interventions have inconsistent and generally insignificant effects on the developmental, nutritional, and socioemotional outcomes of infants with FTT. The two randomized clinical trials of interventions in FD show a brighter picture as they confirm what many single case reports and small case series had reported in the past; that is, that various forms of behavior therapy may be helpful in eliminating problem feeding behaviors and getting infants to eat and drink. However, behavior therapy as treatment of FDs is not a panacea, as evidenced by the substantial proportion of infants with a FD who are not helped by current behavioral treatments. Future research should examine the criteria clinicians can use to determine what specific treatment methods most efficiently treat specific FDs, the limitations of each treatment method, and factors that mediate treatment success and failure. Future research also should explore new methods of prevention of obesity in infants at risk and new methods of treatment. Finally, much work is still needed to develop universally accepted and validated definitions and classifications for both FD and FTT.

REFERENCES

Arts-Rodas, D., & Benoit, D. (1998). Feeding problems in infancy and early childhood: Identification and management. *Paediatrics and Child Health, 3,* 21–27.

Babbitt, R. L., Hoch, T. A., Coe, D. A., Cataldo, M. F., Kelly, K. J., Stackhouse, C., & Perman, J. A. (1994). Behavioral assessment and treatment of pediatric feeding disorders. *Journal of Developmental and Behavioral Pediatrics, 15,* 278–291.

Bazyk, S. (1990). Factors associated with the transition to oral feeding in infants fed by nasogastric tubes. *American Journal of Occupational Therapy, 44,* 1070–1078.

Benoit, D. (in press). Regulation and its disorders. In C. Violato, M. Genuis, & E. Paolucci (Eds.), *The changing family and child development.* Aldershot, England: Ashgate.

Benoit, D., & Coolbear, J. (1998). Post-traumatic feeding disorders in infancy: Behaviors predicting treatment outcome. *Infant Mental Health Journal, 19,* 409–421.

Benoit, D., & Green, D. (1995). The Infant Feeding Behaviors—Rater checklist: Preliminary data. Scientific proceedings of the 42nd Annual Meeting of the American Academy of Child and Adolescent Psychiatry. New Orleans.

Benoit, D., Green, D., & Art-Rodas, D. (1997). Post-traumatic feeding disorder. *Journal of the American Academy of Child and Adolescent Psychiatry, 36,* 577–578.

Benoit, D., Zeanah, C. H., & Barton, M. L. (1989). Maternal attachment disturbances in failure to thrive. *Infant Mental Health Journal, 10,* 185–202.

Benoit, D., Zeanah, C. H., Parker, K. C. H., Nicholson, E., & Coolbear, J. (1997). "Working Model of the Child Interview": Infant clinical status related to maternal perceptions. *Infant Mental Health Journal, 18,* 107–121.

Benoit, D., Zlotkin, S. H., & Wang, E. E. L. (1999). Behavioral treatment of feeding disorders in infancy: A randomized clinical trial. Manuscript submitted for publication.

Berkowitz, C. D., & Senter, S. A. (1987). Characteristics of mother–infant interactions in nonorganic failure to thrive. *Journal of Family Practices, 25,* 377–381.

Bithoney, W. G., McJunkin, J., Michalek, J., Snyder, J., Egan, H., & Epstein, D. (1991). The effect of a multidisciplinary team approach on weight gain in nonorganic failure to thrive children. *Developmental and Behavioral Pediatrics, 12,* 254–258.

Black, M. M., Dubowitz, H., Hutcheson, J., Berenson-Howard, J., & Starr, R. H. (1995). A randomized clinical trial of home intervention for children with failure to thrive. *Pediatrics, 95,* 807–814.

Boddy, J. M., & Skuse, D. H. (1994). Annotation: The process of parenting in failure to thrive. *Journal of Child Psychology, 35,* 301–424.

Brinich, E., Drotar, D., & Brinich, P. (1989). Security of attachment and outcome of preschoolers with histories of nonorganic failure to thrive. *Journal of Clinical Child Psychology, 18,* 142–152.

Budd, K. S., McGraw, T. E., Farbisz, R., Murphy, T. B., Hawkins, D., Heilman, N., Werle, M., & Hochstadt, N. J. (1992). Psychosocial concomitants of children's feeding disorders. *Journal of Pediatric Psychology, 17,* 81–94.

Casey, P. H., Kelleher, K. J., Bradley, R. H., Kellogg, K. W., Kirby, R. S., & Whiteside, L. (1994). A multifaceted intervention for infants with failure to thrive—A prospective study. *Archives of Pediatrics and Adolescent Medicine, 148*, 1071–1077.

Chatoor, I. (1989). Infantile anorexia nervosa: A developmental disorder of separation and individuation [Special issue]. *Journal of the American Academy of Psychoanalysis, 17*, 43–64.

Chatoor, I., Conley, C., & Dickson, L. (1988). Food refusal after an incident of choking: A posttraumatic eating disorder. *Journal of the American Academy of Child and Adolescent Psychiatry, 27*, 105–110.

Chatoor, I., Egan, J., Getson, P., Menvielle, E., & O'-Donnell, R. (1987). Mother–infant interactions in infantile anorexia nervosa. *Journal of the American Academy of Child and Adolescent Psychiatry, 26*, 535–540.

Chatoor, I., Getson, P., Menvielle, E., Brasseaux, C., O'Donnell, R., Rivera, Y., & Mrazek, D. A. (1997). A feeding scale for research and clinical practice to assess mother–infant interactions in the first three years of life. *Infant Mental Health Journal, 18*, 76–91.

Chatoor, I., Kerzner, B., Zorc, L., Persinger, M., Simenson, R., & Mzarek, D. (1992). Clinical Round Table. Two-year-old twins refuse to eat: A multidisciplinary approach to diagnosis and treatment. *Infant Mental Health Journal, 13*, 252–268.

Coolbear, J., & Benoit, D. (1999). Failure to thrive: Risk for clinical disturbance of attachment? *Infant Mental Health Journal, 20*, 87–104.

Crittenden, P. M. (1987). Non-organic failure to thrive: deprivation or distortion. *Infant Mental Health Journal, 8*, 51–64.

Dahl, M. (1987). Early feeding problems in an affluent society: III. Follow-up at two years: Natural course, health, behaviour, and development. *Acta Paediatrica Scandinavia, 76*, 872–880.

Dahl, M., & Sundelin, C. (1992). Feeding problems in an affluent society. Follow-up at four years of age in children with early food refusal. *Acta Paediatrica, 81*, 575–579.

Dellert, S. F., Hyams, J. S., Treem, W. R., & Geertsma, M. A. (1993). Feeding resistance and gastroesophageal reflux in infancy. *Journal of Pediatric Gastroenterology and Nutrition, 17*, 66–71.

DiScipio, W. J., Kaslon, K., & Ruben, R. J. (1978). Traumatically acquired conditioned dysphagia in children. *Annals of Otolaryngology, 87*, 509–514.

Dowdney, L., Skuse, D., Heptinstall, E., Puckering, C., & Zur-Szpiro, S. (1987). Growth retardation and development delay amongst inner-city children. *Journal of Child Psychology and Psychiatry, 4*, 529–541.

Drotar, D. (1990). Sampling issues in research with non-organic failure to thrive. *Journal of Pediatric Psychology, 15*, 255–272.

Drotar, D., & Eckerle, D. (1989). The family environment in nonorganic failure to thrive: A controlled study. *Journal of Pediatric Psychology, 14*, 245–257.

Drotar, D., Eckerle, D., Satola, J., Pallotta, J., & Wyatt, B. (1990). Maternal interactional behavior with nonorganic failure to thrive infants: A case comparison study. *Child Abuse and Neglect, 14*, 41–51.

Drotar, D., & Sturm, L. (1988). Prediction of intellectual development in young children with early histories of nonorganic failure to thrive. *Journal of Pediatric Psychology, 13*, 281–296.

Frank, D. A., & Zeisel, S. H. (1988). Failure to thrive. *Pediatric Clinics of North America, 35*, 1187–1206.

Fryer, G. E. (1988). The efficacy of hospitalization of nonorganic failure to thrive children: A meta-analysis. *Child Abuse and Neglect, 12*, 375–381.

Gorman, J., Leifer, M., & Grossman, G. (1993). Nonorganic failure to thrive: Maternal history and current maternal functioning. *Journal of Clinical Child Psychology, 22*, 327–336.

Grantham-McGregor, S. M., Schonfield, W., & Powell, C. (1987). The development of severely malnourished children who receive psychosocial stimulation: Six year follow-up. *Pediatrics, 79*, 247–254.

Griffin, K. M. (1979). Swallowing training for dysphagic patients. *Archives of Physical Medicine and Rehabilitation, 55*, 467–470.

Harlan, W. R. (1993). Epidemiology of childhood obesity. *Annals of the New York Academy of Sciences, 699*, 1–5.

Heptinstall, E., Pickering, C., Skuse, D., Start, K., Zur-Szpiro, S., & Dowdney, L. (1987). Nutrition and mealtime behaviour in families of growth retarded children. *Human Nutrition: Applied Nutrition, 41A*, 390–402.

Hobbs, C., & Hanks, H. G. (1996), A multidisciplinary approach for the treatment of children with failure to thrive. *Child: Care, Health & Development, 22*, 273–284.

Hutcheson, J. J., Black, M. M., & Starr, R. H. (1993). Developmental differences in interactional characteristics of mothers and their children with failure to thrive. *Journal of Pediatric Psychology, 18*, 453–466.

Hyman, P. E. (1994), Gastroesophageal reflux: One reason why baby won't eat. *Journal of Pediatrics, 125*, 103–109.

Jolley, S. G., McClelland, K. K., & Mosesso-Rousseau, M. (1995). Pharyngeal and swallowing disorders in infants. *Seminars in Pediatric Surgery, 4*, 157–165.

Keller, C., & Stevens, K. R. (1996). Childhood obesity: Measurement and risk assessment. *Pediatric Nursing, 22*, 494–499.

Kerwin, M. E., & Berkowitz, R. I. (1996). Feeding and eating disorders: Ingestive problems of infancy, childhood, and adolescence. *School Psychology Review, 25*, 316–328.

Kristiansson, B., & Fallstrom, S. (1987). Growth at the age of four subsequent to early failure to thrive. *Child Abuse and Neglect, 11*, 35–40.

Larson, K. L., Ayllon, T., & Barrett, D. H. (1987). A behavioral feeding program for failure to thrive infants. *Behavior Research and Therapy, 25*, 39–47.

Lindberg, L., Bohlin, G., & Hagekull, B. (1991). Early feeding problems in a normal population. *International Journal of Eating Disorders, 10*, 395–405.

Lindberg, L., Bohlin, G., Hagekull, B., & Palmerus, K. (1996). Interactions between mothers and infants showing food refusal. *Infant Mental Health Journal, 17*, 334–347.

Lindberg, L., Bohlin, G., Hagekull, B., & Thunstrom, M. (1994). Early food refusal: Infant and family characteristics. *Infant Mental Health Journal, 15*, 262–277.

Linscheid, T. R. (1992). Eating problems in children. In C. E. Walker & M. C. Roberts (Eds.), *Handbook of clinical psychology* (pp. 616–639). New York: Wiley.

Linscheid, T. R., Tarnowski, K. J., Rasnake, L. K., & Brams, J. S. (1987). Behavioral treatment of food refusal in a child with short-gut syndrome. *Journal of Pediatric Psychology, 12*, 451–459.

Lissau, I., & Sorensen, T. I. (1994). Parental neglect during childhood and increased risk for obesity in young adulthood. *Lancet, 343*, 324–327.

Luiselli, J. K. (1994). Oral feeding treatment of children with chronic food refusal and multiple developmental disabilities. *American Journal of Mental Retardation, 98*, 646–655.

Marchi, M., & Cohen, P. (1990). Early childhood eating behaviors and adolescent eating disorder. *Journal of the American Academy of Child and Adolescent Psychiatry, 29*, 112–117.

Mathisen, B., Skuse, D., Wolke, D., & Reilly, S. (1989). Oral–motor dysfunction and failure to thrive among inner-city children. *Developmental Medicine and Child Neurology, 31*, 293–302.

Moll, P. P., Burns, T. L., & Lauer, R. M. (1991). The genetic and environmental sources of body mass index variability: The Muscatine Ponderosity Family Study. *American Journal of Human Genetics, 49*, 1243–1255.

Moussa, M. A., Skaik, M. B., Selwanes, S. B., Yaghy, O. Y., & Bin-Othman, S. A. (1994). Factors associated with obesity in school children. *International Journal of Obesity, 18*, 513–515.

Polan, H. J., Kaplan, M. D., Kessler, D. B., Shindledecker, M. N., Stern, D. N., & Ward, M. J. (1991). Psychopathology in mothers of children with failure to thrive. *Infant Mental Health Journal, 12*, 55–64.

Polan, H. J., Leon, A., Kaplan, M. D., Kessler, D. B., Stern, D. N., & Ward, M. J. (1991). Disturbances of affect expression in failure to thrive. *Journal of the American Academy of Child and Adolescent Psychiatry, 30*, 897–903.

Polan, H. J., & Ward, M. J. (1994). Role of the mother's touch in failure to thrive: a preliminary investigation. *Journal of the American Academy of Child and Adolescent Psychiatry, 33*, 1098–1105.

Pollitt, E. (1987). A critical review of three decades of research on the effects of chronic energy undernutrition on behavioral development. In B. Schurch & N. S. Scrimshaw (Eds.), *Chronic energy deficiency: Consequences and related issues* (pp. 77–93). Lausanne, Switzerland: International Dietary Energy Consultative Group.

Pollitt, E., Golub, M., Gorman, K., Grantham-McGregor, S., Levitsky, D., Schurch, B., Strupp, B., & Wachs, T. (1996). A reconceptualization of the effects of undernutrition on children's biological, psychosocial, and behavioral development. *Social Policy Report (Society for Research in Child Development), 10*, 1–22.

Powell, G. F., Low, J. F., & Speers, M. A. (1987). Behavior as a diagnostic aid in failure to thrive. *Journal of Developmental and Behavioral Pediatrics, 8*, 18–24.

Puckering, C., Pickles, A., Skuse, D., Heptinstall, E., Dowdney, L., & Zur-Szpiro, S. (1995). Mother–child

interaction and the cognitive and behavioural development of four-year-old children with poor growth. *Journal of Child Psychology and Psychiatry and Allied Disciplines, 36*, 573–595.

Raynor, P., & Rudolf, M. C. J. (1996). What do we know about children who fail to thrive? *Child: Care Health and Development, 22*, 241–250.

Rydell, A. M., Dahl, M., & Sundelin, C. (1995), Characteristics of school children who are choosy eaters. *Journal of Genetic Psychology, 156*, 217–229.

Sanders, M. R., Patel, R. K., Le Grice, B., & Shepherd, R. W. (1993). Children with persistent feeding difficulties: an observational analysis of the feeding interactions of problem and non-problem eaters. *Health Psychology, 12*, 64–73.

Sherman, J. B., Alexander, M. A., Clark, L., Dean, A., & Welter, L. (1992). Instruments measuring maternal factors in obese preschool children. *Western Journal of Nursing, 14*, 555–569.

Singer, L. (1987). Long term hospitalization of nonorganic failure to thrive infants: patient characteristics and hospital course. *Journal of Developmental and Behavioral Pediatrics, 8*, 25–31.

Skuse, D. (1993). Identification and management of problem eaters. *Archives of Diseases of Childhood, 69*, 604–608.

Skuse, D. H., Gill, D., Reilly, S., Wolke, D., & Lynch, M. A. (1995). Failure to thrive and the risk of child abuse: A prospective population survey. *Journal of Medical Screening, 2*, 145–149.

Skuse, D., & Wolke, D. (1992). The nature and consequences of feeding problems in infancy. In P. J. Cooper & A. Stein (Eds.), *Feeding problems and eating disorders in children and adolescents* (pp. 1–25). Chur, Switzerland: Harwood.

Skuse, D., Wolke, D., & Reilly, S. (1992). Failure to thrive: Clinical and developmental aspects. In H. Remschmidt & M. H. & Schmidt (Eds), *Developmental psychopathology* (pp. 46–71). Lewiston, NY: Hogrefe & Huber.

Stunkard, A. J., Harris, J. R., Pedersen, N. L., & McClearn, G. E. (1990). The body-mass index of twins who have been reared apart. *New England Journal of Medicine, 322*, 1483–1487.

Sturm, L., & Drotar, D. (1989). Prediction of weight for height following intervention in three year old children with early histories of nonorganic failure to thrive. *Child Abuse and Neglect, 13*, 19 28.

Super, C. M., Herrera, M. G., & Mora, J. O. (1990). Long term effects of food supplementation and psychosocial intervention on the physical growth of Colombian infants at risk of malnutrition. *Child Development, 61*, 29–49.

Turner, K. M. T, Sanders, M. R., & Wall, C. R. (1994). Behavioural parent training versus dietary education in the treatment of children with persistent feeding difficulties. *Behaviour Change, 11*, 242–258.

Valenzuela, M. (1990). Attachment in chronically underweight young children. *Child Development, 61*, 1984–1996.

Wachs, T. D., Sigman, M., Bishry, Z., Moussa, W., Jerome, N., Neumann, C., Bwibo, N., & McDonald, M. A. (1992). Caregiver–child interaction patterns in two cultures in relation to nutritional intake. *Interna-

tional Journal of Behavior and Development, 15, 1–18.

Ward, M. J., Kessler, D. B. & Altman, S. C. (1993). Infant–mother attachment in children with failure to thrive. *Infant Mental Health Journal, 14,* 208–220.

Werle, M. A., Murphy, T. B., & Budd, K. S. (1993). Treating chronic food refusal in young children: home-based parent training. *Journal of Applied Behavior Analysis, 26,* 421–433.

Weston, J. A., Colloton, M., Halsey, S., Covington, S., Gilbert, J., Sorrentino-Kelly, L., & Renoud, S. S. (1993). A legacy of violence in nonorganic failure to thrive. *Child Abuse and Neglect, 17,* 709–714.

Whitaker, R. C., Wright, J. A., Pepe, M. S., Seidel, K. D., & Dietz, W. H. (1997). Predicting obesity in young adulthood from childhood and parental obesity. *New England Journal of Medicine, 337,* 869–873.

Wilensky, D. S., Ginsberg, G., Altman, M., Tulchinsky, T. H., Yishay, B. & Auerbach, J. (1996). A community based study of failure to thrive. *Archives of Disease in Childhood, 75,* 145–148.

Wolke, D. (1996). Failure to thrive: The myth of maternal deprivation syndrome. *The Signal, 4,* 1–6.

Wolke, D., Meyer, R., Ohrt, B, & Riegel, K. (1995). Comorbidity of crying and feeding problems with sleeping prolems in infancy: Concurrent ad predictive associations. *Early Development and Parenting, 4,* 1–17.

Wolke, D., & Skuse, D. (1992), Management of infant feeding problems. In P. J. Cooper & A. Stein (Eds), *Feeding problems and eating disorders in children and adolescents* (pp. 27–59). Chur, Switzerland: Harwood.

Wolke, D., Skuse, D., & Mathisen, B. (1990). Behavioral style in failure-to-thrive: A preliminary investigation. *Journal of Pediatric Psychology, 15,* 237–253.

Wright, C. M., Waterston, A., & Aynsley-Green, A. (1994). Effect of deprivation on weight gain in infancy. *Acta Paediatrica, 83,* 357–359.

22

Disturbances and Disorders of Attachment in Early Childhood

❖

CHARLES H. ZEANAH, JR.
NEIL W. BORIS

It would be no occasion for surprise, I think, if it turned out ultimately that prototypes are the highest level of precision to which we can reasonably aspire in the field of psychopathologic taxonomy.

—CARSON (1991, p. 303)

Attempts to describe psychiatric syndromes can be traced back for centuries, though it was not until 1952 that the first *Diagnostic and Statistical Manual of Mental Disorders* of the American Psychiatric Association (DSM-I) was published (American Psychiatric Association, 1952). The DSM was created by committee and spelled out descriptions of categorical disorders that were based on the cumulative clinical judgment of members of the American Psychiatric Association (Widiger, Frances, Pincus, Davis, & First, 1991). As reviews of the history leading up to DSM-IV (American Psychiatric Association, 1994) have suggested, subsequent attempts to classify psychopathology have taken advantage of more sophisticated empirical studies using advanced psychometric analysis (Widiger et al., 1991; Clark, Watson, & Reynolds, 1995). Yet Carson's quote reflects the reality that creating valid categories that reliably delineate disease states in psychiatry may be an unreachable goal. Carson (1991) argues further, as others have (see Millon, 1991), that "to anticipate that the outcomes of . . . multiple, complexly interwoven and, one must assume, often highly idiosyncratic antecedent processes

. . . will fall out naturally into neat, digital packages of the kind envisaged by a monothetic diagnostic system is to strain the limits of credibility" (p. 303). On the other hand, the DSM diagnostic system in particular, and medical classification systems in general, is created to provide clinical usefulness, facilitate research, and ultimately improve scientific understanding (Clark et al., 1995). These are worthy goals and suggest the need to press forward with attempts to classify psychopathology, keeping the pitfalls of these attempts clearly in mind.

Unfortunately, clinicians and researchers working with infants and young children face pitfalls unique to infancy; defining psychopathology in infancy is particularly problematic for several reasons (Zeanah, Boris, & Scheeringa, 1997). First, infants are constantly developing and changing. Second, because they cannot report on their own experience, we are forced to rely on inferences about their experiences. Observers who report on infants' behaviors may not know them well, may know them only in some contexts but not others, or may have a variety of subjective biases that influence their reports of observed behavior. Infants also are less well differentiated than are older children, and their repertoire of behaviors may be limited as a result.

A specific problem with attempting to diagnose attachment disorders is that attachment is a central and almost ubiquitous developmental process. Although Bowlby's (1969/1982) attachment theory suggests that the biobehavioral attachment system is evident across the lifespan, it is clear from observational data that this system transforms remarkably in infancy (Boris, Aoki, & Zeanah, 1999). On the one hand, even young children with severe relatedness abnormalities, such as pervasive developmental disorders, demonstrate attachment behaviors in standardized laboratory paradigms (Capps, Sigman, & Mundy, 1994). This suggests the robustness of the attachment system, which may be evident even when other forms of social behavior are markedly disturbed. On the other hand, the organization and developmental trajectory of attachment behaviors are dependent partly on experience (Ainsworth, Blehar, Waters, & Wall, 1978). It follows that sustained deviations from expectable environmental variations may affect the infant's developing attachment system. The difficulty is deciding when symptoms are most appropriately considered to represent an attachment disorder rather than some other syndrome.

In the first edition of the *Handbook of Infant Mental Health*, Zeanah, Mammen, and Lieberman (1993) considered existing sets of criteria for reactive attachment disorder (RAD) of infancy and early childhood in light of findings from developmental research on attachment. The authors then proposed an alternate set of criteria for a number of subtypes of attachment disorders. These revised criteria were derived from clinical experience and more explicitly linked to developmental attachment research than were DSM or ICD criteria. The authors concluded: "We look forward to attempts to validate disorders of attachment through critical evaluation of these and other criteria" (Zeanah et al., 1993, p. 347).

Since the first edition of this volume was published, validation of attachment disorders using any set of criteria has been limited. In many ways, the limited progress on validation is not surprising. Validating any psychiatric disorder requires a sophisticated stepwise multistage process, beginning with description of the clinical phenomenology (Cantwell, 1996). The rapid developmental changes of infancy and the

central role of the caregiving relationship in modifying the infant's behavior make this process even more difficult for disorders of infancy (Zeanah, Boris, & Scheeringa, 1997). In effect, the clinical context in infancy is inherently unstable. Furthermore, defining attachment disorders has been a challenge for reasons that are considered throughout this chapter (see also Zeanah, 1996).

There are two reasons why we consider it important to continue to attempt to define the clinical phenomenon of attachment disorders. First, our clinical experiences, like those reported by others, leave us little doubt that serious disturbances, if not disorders, of attachment do exist (cf. Richters & Volkmar, 1994; Hinshaw-Fuselier, Boris, & Zeanah, 1999). Second, we believe that research on the interaction between experience and brain development suggests that the identification of infants who are clinically compromised, or even at significant risk for disorder, is an important goal.

As Nelson and Bousquet (Chapter 3, this volume) noted, though research on early brain development is rapidly evolving, we still have limited information on the degree to which and under what conditions adverse experiences exert lasting influence on a given infant. On the other hand, there appears to be a "natural advantage" to intervening during periods in whch the brain develops most rapidly, making attempts to define disorders in infancy particularly useful.

We begin this chapter by defining and summarizing the various ways that the term "attachment" has been used in the literature. This section focuses particularly on attachment as a relationship construct. Following that, we consider attempts to define attachment disorders, beginning with the history of RAD in the nosology, and ending with a detailed discussion and revision of the alternative criteria for attachment disorders originally proposed by Lieberman and Pawl (1988). Throughout the chapter, we consider many controversies about how best to conceptualize attachment disorders in early childhood. These controversies, and the questions they raise, make it apparent why progress on validation of attachment disorders has been slow.

MEANINGS OF ATTACHMENT

Some of the confusion in the literature concerning attachment disorders derives from the varied ways in which the term "attachment" is used. As noted by Zeanah et al. (1993), there are at least four different meanings of the term in contemporary usage: attachment bonds, attachment behaviors, attachment as a behavior control system, and attachment as a relationship construct.

Attachment Bonds

"Attachment bonds" refer to emotional connections between people in intimate relationships with others. Although attachments may occur in many different types of relationships, in this chapter we are restricting the terms "attachment" and "attachment disorders" to their application in parent–child relationships.

Attachment Behaviors

Bowlby (1969/1982) defined attachment behaviors as infant behaviors designed to promote proximity to the caregiver. Examples include smiling, crying, crawling to approach, and clinging to the caregiver. Most behaviors are neither inevitably nor exclusively attachment behaviors. What matters are how and for what purpose the behaviors are organized. When they are organized for purpose of promoting proximity to the caregiver, they function as attachment behaviors.

Attachment as a System

The "attachment behavioral system" describes one of four major motivational systems (see Lamb, Thompson, Gardner, & Charnov, 1985; Marvin & O'Connor, 1999, for discussion) in young children that Bowlby (1969/1982) suggested were on par with hunger in terms of their effects as motivators of young human infants.

Attachment System

The "attachment system" has an external goal of physical closeness with the caregiver. This goal is context dependent in the sense that the infant monitors its surroundings, interprets cues, and seeks proximity when frightened or distressed. Bowlby (1969/1982) inferred from this tendency that the internal goal of the system is to motivate the child to behave in ways that will make him or her feel more secure.

Human infants are not born attached to any particular adult caregivers, but through regular interactions they develop a hierarchy of a small number of preferred attachment figures by the latter part of the first year of life (Bowlby, 1969/1982). The normal developmental progression of attachment, captured in the organization of attachment behaviors, reflects ongoing developments in cognitive, social, emotional, and motor domains (Zeanah, Boris, & Scheeringa, 1996) and has been described in detail elsewhere (Zeanah, Boris, Bakshi, & Lieberman, in press).

The attachment system undergoes several developmental transformations during the first few years of life, but it is fully functional in non-developmentally delayed infants by 7 to 9 months of age. At this age, infants turn preferentially to their discriminated attachment figures for nurturance, comfort, support, and protection. The period of preferred attachment is manifest in part by the appearance of stranger wariness, as infants no longer readily accept interactions with unfamiliar adults. Infants also begin to protest separation from their attachment figures as another manifestation of preferred attachment.

Exploratory System

The exploratory system is linked to curiosity and mastery motivation. This system motivates the human infant to explore the physical environment. Although it follows a developmental trajectory, the early efforts at exploration are evident within the first few weeks of life. The attachment and exploratory systems activate and deactivate in response to opposite cues. For instance, when the child is feeling secure because of the caregiver's presence and availability, he or she is more motivated to explore the physical environment. On the other hand, if the child is frightened or tired or distressed, all of which activate the attachment system, the child's motivation to explore the physical environment diminishes, and the child's motivation to seek proximity intensifies. This balance between motivation to explore and to seek proximity when distressed is what the Strange Situation procedure (Ainsworth et al., 1978) is designed to capture in a laboratory paradigm.

Affiliative System

The affiliative system is tied to the construct of sociability and describes the young child's motivation to engage socially with others. This system is evident even in the newborn period, although it becomes functionally much more meaningful after the first qualitative biobehavioral advance that occurs at about 2 months of age (Zeanah et al., 1996). At this point, the human infant is highly motivated to engage socially with others, interacting reciprocally and comfortably with a range of familiar and unfamiliar caregivers.

Fear/Wariness System

The fear/wariness system describes the human infant's monitoring of and responses to social and nonsocial fearful cues. This system is closely linked to the attachment system through shared activators, as fear is a major activator of the attachment system. The evolutionary purpose of the attachment system, in fact, was to protect the vulnerable infant from possible predators (Bowlby, 1969/1982). In any case, the fear/wariness system appears in the latter half of the first year of life (Sroufe, 1995) and motivates the child to monitor and respond to perceived danger.

Attachment as a Relationship Construct

In parent–child relationships, few dispute the importance of attachment as a fundamental feature. On the other hand, there is clearly more to parent–child relationships than attachment. Research in attachment has been criticized for emphasizing a simplistic model linking early caregiving with a limited set of patterns of infant attachment and relating these patterns to a host of later social and emotional domains of functioning (see Kagan, 1992). Despite this criticism, research on the development of the attachment system has helped focus research and theory on how relationships regulate behavior in early childhood (Hofer, 1995). Though we have much to learn about how relationships affect the developing attachment system, there are some helpful ways to conceptualize this process.

As clinicians, we often consider what features of relationships appear to be related to infant attachment. Emde's (1989) description of the functional domains of the parent–child relationship provides a model for considering what features of relationships impact the development of attachment. We have modified Emde's model in

a number of areas since his original description (see Zeanah, Boris, Heller, et al., 1997; Zeanah, Larrieu, Heller, & Valliere, Chapter 13, this volume). In this model, emotional availability, nurturance and warmth, protection, and provision of comfort are the most salient caregiver behaviors for the attachment relationship, corresponding to security and trust, balanced emotion regulation, vigilance, and seeking comfort for distress in the young child. Parental behaviors less salient for attachment are play, teaching, instrumental care and routines, and discipline/limit setting. The corresponding behaviors in the young child that are less indicative of attachment include play, learning and curiosity, self-regulation, and self-control.

For purposes of understanding what disordered attachment comprises, we suggest that these functional domains of the parent–child relationship are most salient. This approach emphasizes that the behavior of the caregiver is an important consideration, although in considering disordered attachment we are discussing the relationship as perceived and experienced by the young child.

But how does the infant's perception of the relationship form? How do caregiving experiences translate to patterns of infant behavior, including those linked to psychopathology in the form of RAD? There are many possible models for this process, though it is only recently that a significant body of cross-species research has focused on early relationships and how experiences affect behavior (Nelson & Bousquet, Chapter 3, this volume). Contemporary research differs from that conducted in Bowlby's time in its increasingly sophisticated neuroscientific approach (Hofer, 1987). The field has begun to focus on the relationships between neuronal development and processing, experience, and behavior (Kraemer, 1992; Insel, 1997; Schore, 1997). Although we have known for some time that gross deprivation in infancy may lead to poor brain growth and persistent behavioral anomalies (see Nelson & Bousquet, Chapter 3, this volume, for a review), it is only recently that potential neuronal mechanisms for these processes have been identified.

In a series of carefully planned sequential experiments in the rat, Hofer and colleagues have documented that environmental perturbations (such as separation of infant rats from their mothers) set off a highly specific set of behaviors and predictable patterns of physiological responses in rat pups (Hofer, 1987, 1995). These physiological responses include metabolic changes, autonomic dysregulation, neurotransmitter shifts, and neuroendocrine and immunological responses (Hofer, 1987). Even if the argument is made that rat pups and human infants are phylogenetically unrelated, the multisystem impact of changing the rat's expectable experience (by removing or anesthetizing the caregiver) suggests the potential for similar biological responses in primates and humans. In fact, replication of this work with nonhuman primates has led to the presentation of a psychobiological theory of attachment applicable to humans (Kraemer, 1992).

It is indeed a long way from separation of rat pups and infant monkeys from their mothers to consideration of clinical disorders of attachment in human infants. Nevertheless, clinically relevant findings have emerged. First, there is evidence that "social experience plays a central role in determining what cognitive structures will form [in the brain]" (Kraemer, 1992, p. 530). In other words, there is evidence that experience "selects" and molds brain pathways in the developing organism or that maturation of these brain pathways is either experience expectant or experience dependent (Nelson & Bousquet, Chapter 3, this volume). Of course, this is likely an oversimplification, given that there is an expectable ontogenetic unfolding of development not just in the brain but in the entire organism (Schore, 1997). Experiential influence on brain pathways cannot be understood to occur through a single window; in fact, it seems likely that somatic autonomic systems organize together with neural pathways in the brain. The effects of environmental perturbations such as trauma, prolonged separation, or interaction with a depressed caregiver may have an impact on "lower" autonomic systems, which in turn moderate the impact on central nervous system neural pathways (Schore, 1997). What is undeniable, however, is that the genetically mediated unfolding we call development proceeds at a rapid pace in the first 3 years of life and is regulated by the caregiver–infant relationship through many thousands of interactions, each of which has biological potential (Zeanah et. al., 1996).

Our knowledge of how early relationships influence the development of attachment has unfortunately not led to a simple way to define pathological disturbances of the attachment process. We turn to a consideration of how attachment disorders might be conceptualized, beginning with the history of classification of RAD.

DEFINING ATTACHMENT DISORDERS

There is perhaps no more important factor limiting progress in our understanding of childhood disorders than problems with definition. Many questions about defining attachment disorders have plagued the field and limited progress from research (Boris & Zeanah, 1999). What is the line between normal and abnormal attachment? Are attachment abnormalities correlates of clinical disorders or disorders in their own right? At what point does an infant's attachment disturbances constitute a clinical disorder rather than merely a risk for subsequent disorder? Should attachment disorders include socially disturbed behaviors in general or attachment behaviors in particular? Should attachment disorders be considered categorically or dimensionally?

The History of Classification

Although clinical descriptions of putatively disordered attachments have been available for more than 50 years (Bowlby, 1944; Spitz, 1945; 1946), the formal nosological criteria for clinical disorders of attachment have a rather brief history. The diagnosis of RAD was first introduced in modern nosologies in 1980 with the publication of DSM-III (American Psychiatric Association, 1980). This early version of the disorder included growth failure and lack of social responsivity as central features, and it included the requirement that the disorder should be apparent prior to 8 months of age. This was problematic in that an attachment disorder had to be apparent prior to focused attachment in human infancy.

DSM-III-R (American Psychiatric Association, 1987) eliminated the link between failure to thrive and RAD and specified only that the age of onset be within the first 5 years. Two types of the disorder, "inhibited" and "disinhibited," also were introduced with DSM-III-R (American Psychiatric Association, 1987), and these persisted in both DSM-IV (American Psychiatric Association, 1994) and ICD-10 (World Health Organization, 1992) with only minor modifications. In the DSM-III-R (American Psychiatric Association, 1987), the disorder was centered around abnormal social relatedness across a range of social contexts.

ICD-10 (World Health Organization, 1992) and DSM-IV (American Psychiatric Association, 1994) maintained the focus on diffuse abnormalities of social relatedness across contexts, although ICD-10 allowed for relationship variability and the "capacity for normal social relatedness with 'non-deviant' adult caregivers." The two subtypes first introduced in DSM-III-R—inhibited and disinhibited—also were maintained. Further, the etiological link to adverse caregiving experiences remained explicit in DSM-IV and implicit in ICD-10. Similarly, those children who meet criteria for pervasive development disorder are explicitly excluded from consideration for RAD in DSM-IV and implicitly excluded by ICD-10 criteria. DSM-IV went further by also suggesting that mental retardation cannot explain the social abnormalities included in the criteria.

All these criteria were developed and refined without the benefit of data, as there were no published studies evaluating or even using the criteria for attachment disorders between 1980 and 1994. In fact, the criteria in DSM-IV received virtually no attention until Richters and Volkmar (1994) published a series of case studies illustrating clinical examples of RAD, and Zeanah et al. (1993) criticized the criteria as inadequate to describe children who had seriously disturbed attachment relationships rather than no attachment relationships.

ALTERNATIVE CRITERIA FOR DISORDERS OF ATTACHMENT

Because all these approaches to classifying disorders of attachment in early childhood seemed curiously removed from the hundreds of studies conducted on developmental research on attachment (Zeanah, 1996), our group proposed an alternative set of criteria describing disorders of attachment drawn from developmental attachment research. Building on Lieberman's (Lieberman & Pawl, 1988, 1990) descriptions of clinical disturbances of the secure base phenomenon, we proposed an alternative set of criteria to describe a broader range of attachment disorders than any of the previous approaches (Zeanah et al., 1993). These descriptions were substantially modified in a subsequent revision (Lieberman & Zeanah, 1995).

This alternative approach involves three broad types of attachment disorders: disorders of nonattachment, which are similar to the DSM-IV and ICD-10 disorders, secure-base distortions, in which the child has a seriously unhealthy attachment relationship with a particular caregiver, and disrupted attachment disorder, in which the child reacts to the loss of an attachment relationship.

We demonstrated that these alternative criteria were more reliable than the DSM-IV criteria in a clinically referred sample of infants and toddlers (Boris, Zeanah, Larrieu, Scheeringa, & Heller, 1998). Furthermore, this study generated preliminary convergent validity of the alternative criteria, based on the fact that overall ratings of infant–parent relationship adaptation were significantly lower in children who had attachment disorders compared to children with all other disorders.

Following this study, and additional clinical experience with the criteria, we recently suggested modifications in the alternative criteria (Zeanah, Boris, & Lieberman, in press; Zeanah, Boris, Bakshi, & Lieberman, in press). Still, the criteria remain at odds with the limited data currently available. Next, we review and critique the most recent conceptualization of the alternative criteria.

Disorders of Nonattachment

In keeping with the DSM-IV and ICD-10 criteria, the alternative approach maintains two types of disorders in which there is no preferred attachment figure: (1) nonattachment with emotional withdrawal, a pattern in which the child is emotionally withdrawn, inhibited, and unattached, and (2) nonattachment with indiscriminate sociability, a pattern in which the child seeks comfort and social interaction with relative strangers without the developmentally appropriate discrimination and reticence. There is no expectation of relationship variability in disorders of nonattachment. That is, disturbed attachment behaviors should be similar across different relationships because children with either of these patterns have no discriminated attachment figure. These alternative criteria introduce a requirement that affected children have a mental age of at least 10 months, in order that the failure to demonstrate a preferred attachment figure is not due to cognitive limitations. Furthermore, the link to pathogenic parental care is not a part of the criteria because reliable histories of caregiving are often unavailable or contradictory (see Hinshaw-Fuselier et al., 1999; Zeanah et al., 1993, for examples).

Nonattachment with Emotional Withdrawal

In this pattern, important such attachment behaviors as comfort seeking, showing affection, reliance for help, and cooperation are remarkably restricted. This syndrome also is associated with disturbances of exploration (Boris et al., 1999). Affected children not only demonstrate absence of a preferred attachment figure but also are emotionally blunted, avoid or fail to respond to social overtures, and demonstrate serious problems in emotional self-regulation. This symptom picture has been described in samples of institutionalized children (Tizard & Rees, 1974) and neglected children (Hinshaw-Fuselier et al., 1999; Zeanah et al., 1993; Zeanah, Boris, Bakshi, & Lieberman, in press).

Comments. There is general consensus about the features of this disorder, with similar definitions apparent in DSM-IV, ICD-10, and the alternative criteria. Still, a few controversies are apparent.

First, differentiating whether certain behavioral disturbances are related specifically to a disturbed attachment system as opposed to being general consequences of physical and psychological deprivation has been recognized as a major problem for some time (cf. Kovach, 1992). Physical and psychological neglect involves both lack of stimulation and little opportunity to form selective attachments. It is likely that some symptoms of nonattachment with emotional withdrawal, such as stereotypies, are due more to lack of stimulation than to disturbed attachment. For the clinician, this means that the core feature of the disorder (e.g. nonattachment) may be related to different environmental perturbations than associated features such as stereotypies. Whether all features need to be evident for the diagnosis is unclear.

Another area of controversy is how to distinguish nonattachment with emotional withdrawal from a depressive disorder (see Luby, Chapter 24, this volume). Spitz (1945) used the term "anaclitic depression" to describe the state of infants separated from their attachment figures. In related research, Robertson and Robertson (1989) documented three phases in the separation reaction of toddlers. Each of these three phases, dubbed "protest, despair, and detachment," is associated with signs suggesting mood disturbance, though controlled research across species suggests that each phase is qualitatively different from the others (Kraemer, 1992). On the other hand, toddlers may exhibit these same signs of mood disturbance and still maintain a preferred attachment. Thus, in early childhood, depressive symptomatology always accompanies nonattachment with emotional withdrawal, but nonattachment does not always accompany depressive symptomatology.

Nonattachment with Indiscriminate Sociability

In this pattern, children also fail to exhibit a preferred attachment figure, but instead of failing to seek proximity or comfort, they seek it indiscriminately, even from strangers. In addition, these children lack the expected social reticence around unfamiliar adults that is typical of children in the second through fourth years of life.

Factors that limit the opportunity for young children to develop selective attachments, such as frequent changes in foster care or institutionalization, are linked to this form of nonattachment (Tizard & Rees, 1974; Zeanah et al., 1993; Zeanah, Boris, Bakshi, & Lieberman, in press). Infants and toddlers who meet criteria for this disorder also may demonstrate serious problems with the ability to protect themselves.

Comments. This pattern has been referred to variously as indiscriminate sociability, indiscriminate friendliness, and disinhibited attachment. The disorder has been described and defined categorically and has been included in all contemporary conceptualizations of disordered attachment in the past 20 years. Nevertheless, some available data raise questions about whether the attachment behavior of the children is really indiscriminate or not, and whether this disorder may be a disorder of social behavior rather than an attachment disorder.

For example, in the Tizard study of children raised in institutions in London, some children were adopted out of the institution, some were returned to their biological families who had placed them in the institution originally, and some remained in the institution. Across all three of these groups, persistence of indiscriminate sociability occurred in some of the children. In contrast, none of the inner-city London comparison children (who had not been raised in an institution) exhibited this pattern of behavior (Hodges & Tizard, 1989; Tizard & Rees, 1975). Such a finding suggests that indiscriminate sociability may be a long-term complication of early institutionalization.

This association was studied further using a sample of Romanian babies adopted from orphanages into Canada. In this sample, "indiscriminate friendliness" was noted both at 11 months and 39 months postadoption, consistent with Tizard's results (Chisholm, Carter, Ames, & Morison, 1995; Chisholm, 1998). More important, indiscriminate friendliness measured concurrently was inversely related to attachment security at 11 months postadoption but unrelated to concurrently measured attachment security at 39 months postadoption. Further, although attachment security significantly increased from 11 to 39 months, there were no differences in the levels of indiscriminate friendliness from 11 to 39 months postadoption, adding further evidence of the persistence of this unusual behavior pattern even after attachment develops. In fact, ICD-10 explicitly noted the persistence of this pattern of behavior as characteristic of the syndrome.

All these findings are compatible with the idea that attachment disturbances (defined as problems in the child's use of a discriminated caregiver for comfort, support, protection, and nurturance) are distinct from the social behavior disturbance known as indiscriminate sociability. That is, indiscriminate sociability may be caused by some of the same factors that cause attachment disturbances but may be less likely to recover than attachment behavior once adequate caregiving environments are available.

Bowlby (1969/1982) argued that the attachment behavioral system was molded by natural selection; in other words, human infants are preprogrammed to seek out a discriminated attachment figure for survival needs. Though there is certainly controversy about this claim (cf. Kovach, 1992), the biological tendency for the species to "right itself" is evident in data that suggest that infants who appear nonattached may rapidly show attachment behavior with replacement caregivers after a sustained relationship is formed (O'Connor, Brendenkamp, & Rutter, 1999). If the central nervous system is organized in a way that facilitates development of preferred attachments even in maladaptive caregiving environments, it

becomes easier to understand infants in institutions who, despite limited opportunities, manage to develop focused attachments (e.g., see Skeels, 1966; Tizard & Rees, 1974; Zeanah et al., 1993). This same principle would account for the apparent capacity for recovery noted in postinstitutionalized children who become attached to their adoptive parents (Chisholm et al., 1995; Chisholm, 1998; O'Connor, et al., 1999). As noted, the data suggest that indiscriminate sociability is more persistent and less likely to disappear even after the child becomes attached to a new caregiver (Chisholm, 1998).

Questions also remain about the whether all the children with indiscriminate sociability are really overly "friendly" or "sociable" or, instead, whether some of the children have deficits in their capacities to read and interpret social cues. The disinhibited behavior they demonstrate may not be merely developmentally inappropriate but also may reflect abnormal social relatedness. In some case descriptions (Zeanah, Boris, Bakshi, & Lieberman, in press) but not others (Albus & Dozier, 1999), the indiscriminate behavior is qualitatively inappropriate rather than merely excessively friendly. Animal data suggest that persistent abnormal social behavior frequently follows early disruptions in attachment, even when the separated animal returns to long-term social interaction (Kraemer, 1992).

Finally, it may be that indiscriminate sociability should be considered dimensionally rather than categorically. The study by O'Connor et al. (1999) assessed this core feature dimensionally. As it stands, it is unclear how pervasive indiscriminate sociability needs to be to meet diagnostic criteria. It is also unclear as to how reliably caregivers report indiscriminate sociability, though some caregivers in this study reported the symptom (albeit mostly at low levels) in adoptees who had never been institutionalized and were adopted prior to 6 months of age.

Secure-Base Distortions

A second general type of disordered attachment, grouped under the heading of secure-base distortions, arose from observing patterns of clinically disturbed attachment relationships between young children and their caregivers. What distinguishes these disorders from the disorders of nonattachment is that the child with a secure-base distortion does have a preferred attachment figure, but the relationship with this caregiver is seriously disturbed. The disturbed attachment behaviors that characterize these disorders are relationship specific, in keeping with the important finding from developmental attachment research that infants may construct different types of relationships with different caregivers (Lyons-Ruth, Zeanah, & Benoit, 1996; Zeanah, 1996).

Four different types of secure-base distortions have been described: attachment disorder with self-endangerment, attachment disorder with clinging/inhibited exploration, attachment disorder with vigilance/hypercompliance, and attachment disorder with role reversal. In each of these disorders, the observed disturbances in the child's behavior are anticipated to be relationship specific rather than general characteristics of how the child interacts socially.

Attachment Disorder with Self-Endangerment

The primary function of the attachment behavioral system is to maintain proximity to the caregiver. This function is closely tied to safety and survival as the infant's capacities for mobility increase dramatically in the second year, and the infant must balance the motivation to explore with the motivation to maintain proximity to the attachment figure.

The self-endangering pattern of attachment disorder is characterized by expected ventures away from the attachment figure for purposes of exploration; however, the exploration is unchecked by the opposing tendency to maintain proximity or to return to the putative safe haven of the attachment figure. In addition, the child may engage in a variety of exceedingly dangerous and provocative behaviors in the presence of the attachment figure, such as running out into traffic, deliberately running away in crowded public places, climbing up on ledges, and so on. Accompanying behaviors include aggression that may be self-directed or directed at the caregiver, especially if the aggressive behaviors are displayed in the place of comfort-seeking behaviors.

Case reports have suggested that family violence, either physical abuse, partner violence, or both, often are associated with self-endangering attachment disorder (Lieberman & Zeanah, 1995; Zeanah et al., 1993). It appears as if the young child were attempting to attract the attention and protection of an unavailable or undependable caregiver, although what combination of intrinsic and environmental features might predispose to self-endangering behaviors and the mechanisms responsible for their production remain unknown.

Comments. Self-endangering behavior is a well-known concern in young children; it is typically associated with impulsivity and/or aggression. The question for self-endangerment as an attachment disorder is the degree to which the behavior is relationship specific. Bold, active, or uninhibited children may exercise poor judgment at times, but their provocative and self-endangering behaviors constitute signs of an attachment disorder only if they are severe, persistent, and relationship specific. Although this disorder has been described in case reports (Zeanah et al., 1993; Lieberman & Zeanah, 1995; Zeanah, Boris, Bakshi, & Lieberman, in press) and reliably diagnosed in a retrospective study of case records (Boris et al., 1998), it needs further validation. The presence of attention-deficit/hyperactivity disorder (ADHD) should probably be considered an exclusionary criterion for this disorder, though ADHD itself is a difficult diagnosis to make in children less than 3 years old.

Attachment Disorder with Clinging/Inhibited Exploration

At the other end of the clinical spectrum, some young children do not venture away from the attachment figure to engage in age-expected exploration. Here, the secure-base function of the attachment figure appears to be deficient, and the child's willingness to venture away and explore the object world is impaired. Curiously, this inhibition is not pervasive but rather situation specific. The inhibited behaviors and high levels of accompanying anxiety are observed when the child is in the presence of the attachment figure in an unfamiliar setting, or especially in the presence of the attachment figure *and* an unfamiliar adult.

Comments. Conceptually, it is easy to imagine proximity seeking out of balance with exploration. However, delineating a clinical disturbance or disorder from normal variations is difficult. How do we operationalize the line over which clinging behavior is deemed to represent a disorder? It is clear from observing Strange Situation behavior, for example, that wide ranges of clinging behavior may be demonstrated, even in low-risk samples (Ainsworth et al., 1978). Assuming that a reasonable cut point for distinguishing disorder from no disorder can be established, there is also the question of how this putative disorder differs from a temperamental attribute, such as behavioral inhibition. This is especially true in light of the fact that data gathered with a longitudinal sample suggest that maternal narratives that include either negative affect or overinvolvement are a factor in the persistence of behavioral inhibition (Hirschfeld, Biederman, Brody, Faraone, & Rosenbaum, 1997). Zeanah, Boris, Bakshi, & Lieberman, (in press) have suggested that this type of attachment disorder is relationship specific, whereas behavioral inhibition is generalized. That is, the disorder has been defined as clinging/inhibition in the presence of the attachment figure and a relatively unfamiliar adult.

Still, it remains unclear whether a relationship-specific inhibition is the most useful way to conceptualize this form of disordered attachment behavior. This disorder has been described in only a small number of reported cases, and the consistency of the clinical picture is not yet clear. Albus and Dozier (1999) described a case of a young maltreated child who exhibited "terror of strangers." This child was markedly fearful in the presence of strangers but less fearful when alone and separated from mother. This presentation was distinguished from behavioral inhibition primarily by the extreme nature of the child's fearful reaction and by its relationship variability.

The lack of smooth regulation of close proximity to the caregiver, exploration, and social engagement with those less familiar may reflect an attachment disturbance; however, an important questions is when this dysregulation is severe enough to be considered a disorder.

Attachment Disorder with Vigilance/Hypercompliance

Another form of disordered attachment behavior associated with strong inhibition of exploration occurs in attachment disorder with vigilance/hypercompliance. In this pattern, however, there is no clinging. Instead, the child is emotionally constricted, vigilant of the caregiver, and hypercompliant with caregiver requests and commands. Instead of fearing to leave the caregiver as in the clinging/inhibited pattern,

the child instead gives the impression of fearing to displease the caregiver. Virtually all spontaneity is gone in the service of vigilance, creating the impression of a child who is terrified of the caregiver. Although the behavioral pattern is specific to interactions with the attachment figure, it is not necessarily always evident. It is likely that certain cues trigger the response in young children, such as displays of intense or prolonged anger and frustration by the caregiver.

In the child abuse literature, this pattern has been described as "frozen watchfulness" (Steele, 1983), and it is believed to be an effort by the child to minimize the chances of harsh, punitive, or frankly abusive responses by the caregiver. Crittenden and DiLalla (1988) demonstrated that a closely related pattern of compulsive compliance was indeed relationship specific and related to intrusive caregiving. The disorder is distinguished both by the intensity of the fearful reactions in the child and by their relationship specificity.

Comments. This pattern has been recognized in child abuse literature for years, and "frozen watchfulness" is mentioned in the DSM-IV criteria for RAD as one example of the failure to initiate or to respond to social interactions. Although distinctive and apparently readily recognized, it is rare in our clinical experience, especially in its extreme form. Important questions remaining are whether to view the disorder as continuous or categorical, and to determine how to distinguish normal variations in inhibition from the extreme form this disorder characterizes and how much variability in the vigilant/hypercompliant behavior to allow.

Attachment Disorder with Role Reversal

A final distortion of the secure base occurs when the attachment relationship is inverted (Bowlby, 1980). Instead of the caregiver providing emotional support, nurturance, and protection to the child, the emotional well-being of the caregiver is a preoccupation and even responsibility of the child. To a developmentally inappropriate degree, the child assumes the emotional burden of the relationship. This may be associated with the child's efforts to control the caregiver's behavior, either punitively, oversolicitously, or in some other role-inappropriate manner (Main & Cassidy, 1988; Solomon, George & DeJong, 1995). In fact, "controlling behavior" is the hallmark of a pattern of attachment behavior identified using the Strange Situation procedure in children 20–60 months of age (Cassidy, Marvin, & MacArthur working Group, 1992). There is a link between disorganized attachment in infancy and controlling attachment in later childhood (Main & Cassidy, 1988).

Comments. Although widely recognized clinically (Zeanah & Klitzke, 1991), role reversal has proven elusive in empirical research. Boris et al. (1998) had unacceptably low levels of interrater agreement about the diagnosis of role reversal in their study of clinic-referred cases. Furthermore, in a pilot study of homeless infants and their mothers, three out of six infants diagnosed with role-reversed attachment disorder were classified securely attached to their mothers in the Strange Situation procedure (Boris, 1996).

Our clinical experience suggests that identifying potential cases of clinically significant role reversal is difficult. It is only when the child is old enough to show a pattern of overly empathic behavior toward the caregiver coupled with significant anxiety about the caregiver's well-being that the diagnosis is obvious. Typically, the child's behavior is not seen by the caregiver as inappropriate and observing role-reversed behavior in the clinical setting is difficult. An added criterion, that the child show functional impairment outside the relationship (e.g. delayed or disturbed peer or sibling relationships), might improve the reliability of the diagnosis.

Disrupted Attachment Disorder

A third general type of attachment disorder also is included, namely, disrupted attachment disorder. These criteria are applied in cases in which the child experiences the sudden loss of the attachment figure. Criteria for the disorder are consistent with the descriptions by Robertson and Robertson (1989) of young children separated from their caregivers for days to weeks, many of whom would be expected to develop the well-known sequence of protest, despair, and detachment.

Comments

The rationale for this disorder is that loss of the attachment figure for an infant or toddler is so devastating that it is qualitatively different from loss at another point in the life cycle. This disorder has not been well studied, although it has been described in children who have lost their only attachment figure through death or through changes in foster placement (Lieberman & Zeanah, 1995; Gaensbauer, Chatoor, Drell, Siegel, & Zeanah, 1995; Zeanah, Boris, Bakshi, & Lieberman, in press). Clinical experience suggests that the presence of other attachment figures may buffer the loss of the primary attachment figure. Under what circumstances disrupted attachment disorder develops following loss is an important consideration for further research. One compelling question is whether young children with healthy attachments may be more vulnerable to disruptions than children with more disturbed attachments (cf. Gaensbauer et al., 1995). Also, having more than one attachment figure may buffer the loss of the primary attachment figure.

Clinicians may encounter children in foster care who have histories of maltreatment (especially neglect), no demonstrable attachments to adult caregivers, and emotional blunting and social detachment. Determining whether this represents nonattachment with emotional withdrawal or disrupted attachment disorder may be quite difficult.

REVISIONS IN THE ALTERNATIVE CRITERIA

As indicated in Table 22.1, the first major change that we have made is in focusing what

TABLE 22.1. Alternative Criteria for Disorders of Attachment

Disorders of nonattachment

Nonattachment with emotional withdrawal
Nonattachment with indiscriminate sociability

Secure base distortions

Disordered Attachment with Self-Endangerment
Disordered Attachment with Inhibition
Disordered Attachment with
    Vigilance/Hypercompliance
Disordered Attachment with Role Reversal

Disrupted attachment disorder

Criteria for these types are described in Lieberman & Zeanah (1995) and Zeanah, Boris, Bakshi, & Lieberman (in press).

was formerly nonattachment disorder on the absence of a discriminated attachment figure. Such a focus addresses recent findings indicating that children who clearly have discriminated attachment figures to whom they turn for comfort, support, and nurturance still may exhibit the pattern of indiscriminate sociability with strangers (Chisholm, 1998; Marvin & O'-Connor, 1999). Indiscriminate sociability with relative strangers has become an associated feature in the revised version of the criteria (Table 22.2).

The second major change that we are proposing for the alternative criteria is to make the criteria dimensional, at least to the degree that the two different levels of disturbance and disorder are defined. If the behavioral signs are somewhat or sometimes evident, then an *attachment disturbance* is present; if the behavioral signs are usually or often present, an *attachment disorder* is defined. With regard to secure-base distortions, the dimensional approach is a way of attempting to capture different levels of relationship disturbances. What may be less clear is how this applies to the "no discriminated attachment figure" type of attachment disorder. Although it may seem that the presence or absence of an attachment figure is an either–or category, in our clinical experience, this distinction is not always easy to make—especially for those children who are reared in unusual circumstances. If young children do not have discriminated attachment figures, they may be in the process of developing preferred attachments after they are placed in more favorable environments. The dimensional approach may be a more reliable way of identifying attachment in these situations. In studies of Romanian orphans later adopted, both Chisholm (1998) and O'Connor et al. (1999) used dimensional measures of indiscriminate sociability, although the particular measures used in the two studies differed somewhat.

The third change in the revised alternative

TABLE 22.2. An Update on Alternative Criteria for Attachment Disorders

Attachment disorder: No discriminated attachment figure

1. Lack of evidence of a preferred caregiver as evidenced by:
   a. Lack of differentiation among adults *or*
   b. Seeking comfort preferentially from unfamiliar adults rather than from familiar caregivers *or*
   c. Failure to seek or to respond to comfort from caregivers when hurt, frightened, or distressed *or*
   d. Lack of emotional responsiveness to and reciprocity with familiar caregivers
2. Child has a mental age of at least 10 months.
3. Does not meet criteria for a pervasive developmental disorder

Associated features may include:
1. Poorly regulated emotions with dampened positive affect, irritability, or sadness
2. Failure to check back with caregiver after venturing away, especially in unfamiliar settings
3. Absence of usual social reticence with unfamiliar adults
4. Willingness to go off readily with relative strangers

Note: Disturbed attachment should be indicated if signs are only somewhat or sometimes evident in one or more of the preceding criteria. Disordered attachment should be noted if signs are usually or often present.

Attachment disorder: Secure base distortions

The child has a discriminated attachment figure, but the relationship is disturbed or disordered as indicated by a pattern of one or more of the following:

1. Self-endangering, risk taking, and/or aggressive behavior that is clearly worse in the presence of the attachment figure rather than other caregivers.
2. Inhibition of exploration and excessive clinging that occurs in the combined presence of the attachment figure and less familiar adults.
3. Excessive vigilance and anxious hypercompliance directed towards the attachment figure and an associated absence of spontaneous exploratory behavior. The child behaves as if he or she is afraid *of* the caregiver.
4. Inverted caregiving in which the child is preoccupied by and seems to feel responsible for the attachment figure's emotional well-being. The child behaves as if he or she is afraid *for* the caregiver.

Note: Disturbed attachment should be indicated if signs are somewhat or sometimes evident in one or more of the preceding. Disordered attachment should be noted if signs are usually or often present.

criteria is related to the idea of making the disorders dimensional rather than categorical. That is, it is possible in the proposed revision for different patterns of secure-base distortions to co-occur in the same relationship. This recognizes that mixed patterns of secure-base distortions in the same child have been described in case reports (see Zeanah et al., 1993) as well as in a small case series (Boris, 1996).

ASSESSMENT

As we have noted before, the first point is that what is being assessed is the child's relationships with attachment figures rather than any characteristic of the individual child (Boris et al., 1999; Zeanah, Boris, Bakshi, & Lieberman, in press). The domains of the parent–child relationship that should be assessed are those most salient for attachment. As noted, these include caregiver emotional availability and child emotion regulation, caregiver nurturance–warmth–sensitivity and child trust–security, caregiver protection and child vigilance–self-protection, and caregiver provision of comfort and child comfort seeking.

Second, the focus should be on attachment specifically, rather than on social relatedness in general (Boris, Fueyo, & Zeanah, 1997; Zeanah & Emde, 1994; Zeanah et al., 1993). Thus, it is necessary to determine whether attachment behaviors are present and how they are organized in each of the child's important caregiving relationships because of the potential relationship specificity of symptomatic behavior.

We also have suggested that the relevant infant behaviors for assessment of an infant's attachment to a caregiver include showing affection, comfort seeking, reliance for help, cooperation, exploratory behavior, controlling behavior, and reunion responses (Boris et al., 1999; Zeanah et al., 1993). Using a broad range of behaviors and thinking about their organization in the service of attachment-related goals is likely to be far more useful than relying on reunion behaviors alone. Reunion behaviors, in our view, always should be one of several components of the assessment.

Development is another important consideration in assessing attachment. In the first half of the first year of life, preattachment behaviors and patterns of infant–caregiver interaction may be observed. Once a child is old enough to have developed focused, preferred attachments,

that is, by about 9 or 10 months of age, it becomes possible to observe the balance between the child's proximity/comfort-seeking behavior, on the one hand, and exploratory behavior, on the other. The constructs of secure base and safe haven are readily observable in naturalistic settings and may be used as guides to obtain relevant history, as well as for organizing observations. With older toddlers, the balance between attachment and exploration occurs in the integration of the child's autonomous functioning and simultaneous reliance on the attachment figure for help when needed.

Several structured research methods of assessing attachment exist, but they are neither specific nor sensitive enough to be used diagnostically by the clinician. Use of the Strange Situation procedure diagnostically, in particular, is problematic (Boris et al., 1999; Rutter, 1995; Zeanah & Emde, 1994). The Attachment Q-set (Waters & Deane, 1985) is not well validated, especially in clinical populations.

As we have noted, an ideal approach to assessing attachment would include history and perceptions provided by caregivers, as well as observations of the child and caregiver in naturalistic and clinic settings (Zeanah, Boris, Bakshi, & Lieberman, in press). Given that multiple observations in multiple contexts are rarely possible and often inefficient, we are exploring efforts to develop valid methods for clinic-based assessment of attachment (Boris, 1996).

INTERVENTIONS

There have been no formal efforts to evaluate interventions for clinical disturbances or disorders of attachment to date. The definitional obstacles we have described in this chapter have meant that diagnosis of attachment disorder has been problematic. Thus, studies of intervention after diagnosis of attachment disorder do not yet exist. What has been studied is the effect of various preventive interventions on security of attachment as a dependent measure. Results from these studies have been mixed (see Lieberman & Zeanah, 1999, for review), and the need is great for carefully designed, implemented, and evaluated interventions.

Specific interventions proposed for clinical disturbances or disorders of attachment have included individual psychotherapy for child and/or caregiver, parent training with emphasis on developmental expectations and sensitive responsiveness, family therapy, or caregiver–child dyadic therapy (reviewed in Lieberman & Zeanah, 1999). As described by Lieberman (Lieberman, 1991; Lieberman & Pawl, 1993; Lieberman, Silverman, & Pawl, Chapter 30, this volume), infant–parent psychotherapy integrates crisis intervention, developmental guidance, including attention to instrumental issues (e.g., poor housing, inadequate medical care), and psychotherapy in which the baby is present. This treatment is most specifically tailored for disturbances of attachment and, in many instances, may be the treatment of choice for affected dyads. Nevertheless, evaluation of this method has been limited to a study of promoting secure attachments in at-risk dyads (Lieberman, Weston, & Pawl, 1991).

For children who have no preferred attachment figure, the first and most important component of the intervention is to make available to them a caregiving relationship context in which attachment can develop. Presumably, promoting parental behaviors known to facilitate secure attachments, namely, emotional availability and sensitive responsiveness, seems most likely to be helpful. At times this may be facilitated by instruction and information and at other times through intensive psychotherapy. As always, specifics of the intervention must be designed to address the particular case in question (see Zeanah, Boris, Bakshi, & Lieberman, in press, for an elaboration of treatment principles).

SUMMARY AND CONCLUSION

The complexity and the excitement of clinical disturbances of attachment are difficult to convey in words alone. Often, they are most palpable when we present case examples to clinicians, especially videotaped clinical vignettes. These cases remind us that the difficulties with classification of attachment disorders are outweighed by the usefulness of having a common description of the types of presenting symptoms to which all clinicians can refer.

We began this chapter with a discussion of the limitations of psychiatric classification systems in general and an overview of how these limitations are amplified when considering infants. This discussion led us to why the validation of attachment disorders remains an elusive goal and to a review of how to define and un-

derstand attachment as a clinical phenomenon. We then considered the complex issues surrounding the definition of attachment disorders, and we proposed an updated set of alternative criteria for disorders of attachment. We hope that the comments on each proposed disorder will engender further discussion about the most useful way to capture the varying clinical phenomena we have described. We anticipate that testing these criteria in clinical populations will lead to improved assessment protocols and eventually suggest more specific approaches to treatment.

As we unravel the secrets of how experience impacts brain development in infancy, we hope also to uncover clues as to how disturbed relationships beget the kind of behavioral problems that come to clinical attention. Attachment disorders have yet to be validated, but we see great promise in the relevant clinical and basic research that is already under way.

REFERENCES

Ainsworth, M. D. S., Blehar, M. C., Waters, E., Wall, S. (1978). *Patterns of attachment: A psychological study of the strange situation*. Hillsdale, NJ: Erlbaum.

Albus, K. E., & Dozier, M. (1999). Indiscriminate friendliness and terror of strangers: Contributions from the study of infants in foster care. *Infant Mental Health Journal, 20*, 30–41.

American Psychiatric Association. (1952). *Diagnostic and statistical manual of mental disorders* (1st ed.). Washington, DC: Author.

American Psychiatric Association. (1980). *Diagnostic and statistical manual of mental disorders* (3rd ed.). Washington, DC: Author.

American Psychiatric Association. (1987). *Diagnostic and statistical manual of mental disorders* (3rd ed., rev.). Washington, DC: Author.

American Psychiatric Association (1994). *Diagnostic and statistical manual of mental disorders* (4th ed.). Washington, DC: Author.

Boris, N. W. (1996, May). *Validating attachment disorders of infancy*. Paper presented to the K–12 Scientific Review Committee Meeting, American Academy of Child and Adolescent Psychiatry, Block Island, RI.

Boris, N. W., Aoki, Y., & Zeanah, C. H. (1999). The development of infant–parent attachment: Considerations for assessment. *Infants and Young Children, 11*, 1–10.

Boris, N. W., Fueyo, M. A., & Zeanah, C. H. (1997). The clinical assessment of attachment in children less than five. *Journal of the American Academy of Child Adolescent Psychiatry, 36*, 291–293.

Boris, N., & Zeanah, C. H. (1999). Reactive attachment disorder. In H. I. Kaplan & B. J. Sadock (Eds.), *Comprehensive textbook of psychiatry*. Philadelphia: Williams & Wilkins.

Boris, N., Zeanah, C. H., Larrieu, J., Scheeringa, M., & Heller, S. (1998). Attachment disorders in infancy and early childhood: A preliminary study of diagnostic criteria. *American Journal of Psychiatry, 155*, 295–297.

Bowlby, J. (1944). Forty-four juvenile thieves. *International Journal of Psycho-Analysis, 25*, 19–53.

Bowlby, J. (1980). *Attachment and loss: Vol. 2. Loss.* Basic Books: New York.

Bowlby, J. (1982). *Attachment and loss: Vol. 1. Attachment.* Basic Books: New York. (Original work published 1969)

Cantwell, D. (1996). Classification of child and adolescent psychopathology. *Journal of Child Psychology and Psychiatry, 37* (1), 3–12.

Capps, L., Sigman, M., & Mundy, P. (1994). Attachment security in children with autism. *Development and Psychopathology, 6*, 249–262.

Carson, R. (1991). Dilemmas in the pathway of the DSM-IV. *Journal of Abnormal Psychology, 100*, 302–307.

Cassidy, J., Marvin, R., & MacArthur Working Group. (1992, June). *Attachment organization in preschool children: Procedures and working manual.* Unpublished manual.

Chisholm, K. (1998). A three year follow-up of attachment and indiscriminate friendliness in children adopted from Romanian orphanages. *Child Development, 69*, 1092–1106.

Chisolm, K., Carter, M. C., Ames, E. W., & Morison, S. J. (1995). Attachment security and indiscriminantly friendly behavior in children adopted from Romanian orphanages. *Development and Psychopathology, 7*, 283–294.

Clark, L. A., Watson, D., & Reynolds, S. (1995). Diagnosis and classification of psychopathology: Challenges to the current system and future directions. *Annual Review of Psychology, 46*, 121–153.

Crittenden, P., & DiLalla, D. L. (1988). Compulsive compliance: The development of an inhibitory coping strategy in infancy. *Journal of Abnormal Child Psychology, 16*, 585–599.

Emde, R. N. (1989). The infant's relationship experience: Development and affective aspects. In A. J. Sameroff & R. N. Emde (Eds.), *Relationship disturbances in early childhood* (pp. 33–51). New York: Basic Books.

Gaensbauer, T., Chatoor, I., Drell, M., Siegel, D., & Zeanah, C. H. (1995). Traumatic loss in a one-year-old girl. *Journal of the American Academy of Child and Adolescent Psychiatry, 34*, 94–102.

Hinshaw-Fuselier, S., Boris, N. W., & Zeanah, C. H. (1999). Reactive attachment disorder in maltreated twins. *Infant Mental Health Journal, 20*, 42–59.

Hirschfeld, D. R., Biederman, J., Brody, L., Faraone, S V., & Rosenbaum, J. F. (1997). Associations between expressed emotion and child behavioral inhibition and psychopathology: A pilot study. *Journal of the American Academy of Child and Adolescent Psychiatry, 36*, 205–213.

Hodges, J. & Tizard, B. (1989). Social and family relationships of ex-institutional adolescents. *Journal of Child Psychology, Psychiatry, and Allied Disciplines, 30*, 77–97.

Hofer, M. A. (1987). Early social relationships: A psychobiologist's view. *Child Development, 58*, 633–647.

Hofer, M. A. (1995). Hidden regulators: Implications for a new understanding of attachment, separation and loss. In S. Goldberg, R. Muir, & J. Kerr (Eds.), *Attachment theory: Social, developmental and clinical perspectives* (pp. 203–230). Hillsdale, NJ: Analytic Press.

Insel, T. (1997). A neurobiological basis of social attachment. *American Journal of Psychiatry, 154*, 726–735.

Kagan, J. (1992). The meanings of attachment. *Behavioral and Brain Sciences, 15*, 517–518.

Kovach, J. K. (1992). Attachment and the sources of behavioral pathology. *Behavioral and Brain Sciences, 15*, 518–519.

Kraemer, G. (1992). A psychobiological theory of attachment. *Behavioral and Brain Sciences, 15*, 493–511.

Lamb, M., Thompson, R. A., Gardner, W., & Charnov, E. L. (1985). *Infant–mother attachment: The origins and developmental significance of individual differences in strange situation behavior.* Hillsdale, NJ: Erlbaum.

Lieberman, A. F. (1991). Attachment theory and infant–parent psychotherapy: Some conceptual, clinical and research issues. In D. Cicchetti & S. Toth (Eds.), *Rochester symposium on developmental psychopathology: Vol. 3. Models and integration* (pp. 261–268). Hillsdale, NJ: Erlbaum.

Lieberman, A. F., & Pawl, J. H. (1988). Clinical applications of attachment theory. In J. Belsky & T. Nezworski (Eds.), *Clinical implications of attachment* (pp. 327–351). Hillsdale, NJ: Erlbaum.

Lieberman, A. F., & Pawl, J. H. (1990), Disorders of attachment and secure base behavior in the second year of life: conceptual issues and clinical intervention. In M. T. Greenburg, D. Cicchetti, & E. M. Cummings (Eds.), *Attachment in the preschool years* (pp. 375–398). Chicago: University of Chicago Press.

Lieberman, A. F., & Pawl, J. H. (1993). Infant–parent psychotherapy. In C. H. Zeanah, Jr. (Ed.), *Handbook of infant mental health* (pp. 427–442). New York: Guilford Press.

Lieberman, A. F., Weston, D., & Pawl, J. (1991). Preventive intervention and outcome with anxiously attached dyads. *Child Development, 62*, 199–209.

Lieberman, A. F., & Zeanah, C. H. (1995). Disorders of attachment in infancy. In K. Minde (Ed.), *Child psychiatric clinics of North America: Infant psychiatry* (pp. 571–588). Philadelphia: Saunders.

Lieberman, A. F., & Zeanah, C. H. (1999). Contributions of attachment theory to infant–parent psychotherapy and other interventions with infants and young children. In J. Cassidy & P. R. Shaver (Eds.), *Handbook of attachment* (pp. 555–574). New York, Guilford Press.

Lyons-Ruth, K., Zeanah, C. H., & Benoit, D. (1996). Disorder and risk for disorder during infancy and toddlerhood. In E. J. Mash & R. A. Barkley (Eds.), *Child psychopathology* (pp. 457–491). New York: Guilford Press.

Main, M., & Cassidy, J. (1988). Categories of response to reunion with the parent at age 6: Predictable from infant attachment classifications and stable over a 1-month period. *Developmental Psychology, 24*, 1–12.

Marvin, R., & O'Connor, T. (1999, April). *The formation of parent–child attachment following privation.* Paper presented at the biennial meeting of the Society for Research in Child Development, Albuquerque, NM.

Millon, T. (1991). Classification in psychopathology: Rationale, alternatives, and standards. *Journal of Abnormal Psychology, 100*(3), 245–261.

O'Connor, T., Brendenkamp, D., & Rutter, M. (1999). Attachment disturbances and disorders in children exposed to early severe deprivation. *Infant Mental Health Journal, 20*, 10–29.

Richters, M. M., & Volkmar, F. (1994). Reactive attachment disorder of infancy or early childhood. *Journal of the American Academy of Child and Adolescent Psychiatry, 33*, 328–332.

Robertson, J., & Robertson, J. (1989). *Separations and the very young.* London: Free Association Books.

Rutter, M. (1995). Clinical implications of attachment concepts: Retrospect and prospect. *Journal of Child Psychology, Psychiatry, and Allied Disciplines, 36*, 549–571.

Schore, A. (1997). Early organization of the nonlinear right brain and development of a predisposition to psychiatric disorders. *Development and Psychopathology, 9*, 595–631.

Skeels, H. M. (1966). *Adult status of children with contrasting early life experiences. Monographs of the Society for Research in Child Development, 31*(Serial no. 105).

Solomon, J., George, C., & DeJong, A. (1995). Children classified as controlling at age six: Evidence of disorganized representational strategies and aggression at home and at school. *Development and Psychopathology, 7*, 447–464.

Spitz, R. (1945). Hospitalism: An inquiry into the genesis of psychiatric conditions in early childhood. *Psychoanalytic Study of the Child, 1*, 53–74.

Spitz, R. (1946). Anaclitic depression: An inquiry into the genesis of psychiatric conditions in early childhood II. *Psychoanalytic Study of the Child, 2*, 313–342.

Sroufe, L. A. (1995). *Emotional development.* Cambridge: Cambridge University Press.

Steele, B. (1983). Psychological effects of child abuse and neglect. In J. D. Call, E. Galenson, & R. E. Tyson (Eds.), *Frontiers of infant psychiatry* (pp. 235–244). New York: Basic Books.

Tizard, B., & Rees, J. (1974). A comparison of the effects of adoption, restoration of the natural mother, and continued institutionalization on the cognitive development of four-year-old children. *Child Development, 45*, 92–99.

Tizard, B., & Rees, J. (1975). The effect of early institutional rearing on the behavior problems and affectional relationships of four-year-old children. *Journal of Child Psychology and Psychiatry, 27*, 61–73.

Waters, E., & Deane, K. (1985), Defining and assessing individual differences in attachment relationships: Q-methodology and the organization of behavior in infancy and early childhood. In I. Bretherton & E. Waters (Eds.), Growing points of attachment theory and research. *Monographs of the Society for Research in Child Development, 50*(Serial No. 209), 41–65.

Widiger, T. A., Frances, A. J., Pincus, H. A., Davis, W. W., First, M. B. (1991). Toward an empirical classification for the DSM-IV. *Journal of Abnormal Psychology, 100*, 280–288.

World Health Organization. (1992). *The ICD-10 classification of mental and behavioral disorders: Clinical descriptions and diagnostic guidelines.* Geneva, Switzerland: Author.

Zeanah, C. H. (1996). Beyond insecurity: A reconceptualization of clinical disorders of attachment. *Journal of Consulting and Clinical Psychology, 64*, 42–52.

Zeanah, C. H., Boris, N. W., Bakshi, S., & Lieberman, A. (in press). Disorders of attachment. In J. Ososfsky & H. Fitzgerald (Eds.), *WAIMH handbook of infant mental health.* New York: Wiley.

Zeanah, C. H., Boris, N. W., Heller, S. S., Hinshaw-Fuselier, S., Larrieu, J., Lewis, M., Palomino, R., Rovaris, M., & Valliere, J. (1997). Relationship assessment in infant mental health. *Infant Mental Health Journal, 18*, 182–197.

Zeanah, C. H., Boris, N. W., & Lieberman, A. (in press). Attachment disorders of infancy. In M. Lewis & A. Sameroff (Eds.), *Handbook of developmental psychopathology.* New York: Basic Books.

Zeanah, C. H., Boris, N., & Scheeringa, M. S. (1996). Infant development: The first three years of life. In A. Tasman, J. Kay, & J. Lieberman (Eds.). *Psychiatry* (pp. 75–100). Philadelphia: W. B. Saunders.

Zeanah, C. H., Boris, N., & Scheeringa, M. (1997). Psychopathology in infancy. *Journal of Child Psychology, Psychiatry and Allied Disciplines, 38*, 81–99.

Zeanah, C. H., & Emde, R. N. (1994). Attachment disorders in infancy. In M. Rutter, L. Hersov, & E. Taylor (Eds.), *Child and adolescent psychiatry: Modern approaches* (pp. 490–504). Oxford: Blackwell.

Zeanah, C. H., & Klitzke, M. (1991). Role reversal and the self-effacing solution: Observations from infant–parent psychotherapy. *Psychiatry, 54*, 346–357.

Zeanah, C. H., Jr., Mammen, O. K., & Lieberman, A. F. (1993). Disorders of attachment. In C. H. Zeanah, Jr. (Ed.), *Handbook of infant mental health* (pp. 332–349). New York: Guilford Press.

23

Posttraumatic Stress Disorder

❖

MICHAEL S. SCHEERINGA
THEODORE J. GAENSBAUER

Posttraumatic stress disorder (PTSD) is a multidimensional syndrome through which many fields of research and clinical interest intersect. Exciting areas of study, such as memory, neurobiology, etiology of psychiatric disturbance, and relationship factors, are all critical issues in the study of trauma in infancy, arguably the most important time of development of a person's life. Adult trauma cases have been described clinically at least since the 19th century (reviewed in van der Kolk, Weisaeth, & van der Hart, 1996), but the first detailed, published case of a child who suffered a truly life-threatening experience and was evaluated prior to 48 months of age appeared relatively recently (MacLean, 1977). This chapter presents the current state of knowledge regarding PTSD in infancy and early childhood which has been accumulating during the last 20 years.

PTSD is a syndrome of symptomatic behaviors produced by an event that is life-threatening, or so overwhelming and out of the ordinary compared to one's usual experience that one's ability to cope with it is overwhelmed. Following such an event, three types of symptoms appear: reexperiencing symptoms, avoidance and numbing of responsiveness symptoms, and increased arousal symptoms (American Psychiatric Association, 1994). Other sequelae may be associated with the disorder, such as chronic personality changes (Terr, 1991), physiological changes (reviewed in Southwick, Bremner, Krystal, & Charney, 1994), and parental/family dysfunction (Scheeringa, Zeanah, & Peebles, 1997).

EPIDEMIOLOGY

No epidemiological studies using community samples have been completed on younger children, although several studies have measured the prevalence of PTSD in adult community samples. Rates were 2.6% (Shore, Tatum, & Vollmer, 1986), 1% (Helzer, Robins, & McEvoy, 1987), and 1.3% (Davidson, Hughes, Blazer, & George, 1991). A somewhat higher rate, 9.2%, was found in a survey of young urban adults enrolled in a health maintenance organization (Breslau, Davis, Andreski, & Peterson, 1991). Although the increase was not explained by the authors, their sample differed from previous studies by comprising exclusively urban subjects. A study of 18-year-old urban teens found a prevalence of 6.3% (Giaconia et al., 1995). Prevalence rates of PTSD within traumatized samples vary widely depending on the type of the traumatic event (McNally, 1993).

Determining the total number of young children exposed to traumas, regardless of symptom development, is difficult due to inexact records. The main routes of exposure include abuse, witnessing domestic violence, witnessing community violence, accidents, natural disasters, and painful medical procedures.

THE STRESSOR CRITERION

By definition, two characteristics of an event must be present to cause PTSD or to be "traumatogenic." First, the event must involve "actual or threatened death or serious injury, or a threat to the physical integrity of self or others" (American Psychiatric Association, 1994). This characteristic can be objectively determined for the most part. Second, the event must be perceived by the person as sufficiently threatening. This perception is difficult to determine after the fact with young children because of their limited verbal skills. Furthermore, whether an event is sufficiently "overwhelming" might depend on the individual and on developmental capacities. Not only will no two people experience the same event exactly the same way, but infants and toddlers may perceive some events as life-threatening, whereas most adults would not, or vice versa. For example, Drell, Siegel, and Gaensbauer (1993) described a 10-month-old boy who became phobic of the outdoors after a lawnmower was started beside him and startled him.

It is not yet clear if some types of traumatic events are more potent than others for producing PTSD. The variety of traumatic events that have been reported to cause symptomatic reactions in children under 48 months of age include animal attacks (e.g., MacLean, 1977), accidents (e.g., Gaensbauer, 1995), witnessing a parent murdered (e.g., Pruett, 1979), physical abuse (e.g., Gaensbauer, 1982), sexual abuse (e.g., Terr, 1988), natural disaster (Azarian, Lipsitt, & Skripchenko, 1996), combinations of domestic and community violence (Osofsky & Scheeringa, 1997), and, possibly, medical procedures (e.g., Wallick, 1979). Because most of these were case reports, there is an obvious selection bias confounding a determination of the likelihood of an event leading to PTSD.

DIAGNOSTIC CRITERIA

The criteria for PTSD according to the *Diagnostic and Statistical Manual of Mental Disorders* (DSM-IV; American Psychiatric Association, 1994) have shortcomings when applied to very young children. Scheeringa, Zeanah, Drell, and Larrieu (1995) formally tested the DSM-IV criteria on young children. In phase one of their study, 20 published cases of severely traumatized children under 48 months old

were rated on the DSM-IV criteria. None of the cases met the full criteria for PTSD despite the children exhibiting numerous symptoms. The most common problems with the criteria were that in only 2 of the 20 cases could it be determined that the children manifest the symptom of showing "fear, helplessness, or horror" at the time of the trauma, and only 3 of the cases had enough symptoms in the cluster of avoidance and numbing of responsiveness (cluster C) symptoms. However, 19 of the 20 cases showed sufficient reexperiencing symptoms (cluster B), which is the only cluster containing trauma-specific symptoms.

Two main limitations of content validity of the DSM-IV criteria were found. First, many of the criteria (8 out of 17) relied on verbalizations from patients to report subjective internal experiences, which is impossible in preverbal or barely verbal children. Second, the criteria were not sensitive to developmental differences of young children compared to older children and adults. Some of the DSM-IV criteria were not applicable to infants and toddlers because of cognitive immaturity (e.g., sense of a foreshortened future and lapses in memory). The wording of some existing criteria needed modification to suit the abilities and activities of infants and toddlers. Furthermore, some commonly observed symptoms in traumatized infants and toddlers (e.g., new separation anxiety, new aggression, fear of going into the bathroom alone, and loss of previously acquired developmental skills) were not part of the DSM-IV.

As a result, phase two of the Scheeringa et al. (1995) study proposed an alternative set of criteria. The following changes were incorporated: Some symptoms were reworded to be behaviorally anchored and not dependent on verbalizations; new items were added to reflect symptoms seen uniquely in this age group; a new symptom cluster was added involving new fears and aggression; and the diagnostic algorithm was altered. In phase three of the study, this alternative set was then compared to the DSM-IV criteria on 12 new cases of traumatized children under 48 months of age. The alternative criteria were considered more useful than the DSM-IV criteria for infants and toddlers because the alternative criteria led to diagnosis of PTSD in 69% of severely traumatized young children, whereas the DSM-IV criteria led to diagnosis of PTSD in only 13% of the children. This set of alternative criteria was used as a basis for the criteria that define "traumatic stress disorder" in the *Diagnostic Classi-fication: 0–3* (Zero to Three, 1994).

Investigations of diagnostic criteria also must take into account the diagnostic algorithm. The DSM-IV diagnosis of PTSD is based on an algorithm with three symptom clusters: One symptom is required from the reexperiencing cluster, three symptoms are required from the avoidance and numbing of responsiveness cluster, and two symptoms are required from the increased arousal cluster. The alternative criteria required only one symptom from each cluster plus one symptom from the proposed new fears and aggression cluster. Overall, the DSM-IV criteria require six symptoms, and the alternative criteria require four symptoms (as does the *DC: 0–3* criteria). Determining the optimal criteria set and algorithm for infants and toddlers must await more sophisticated studies involving convergent validity and longitudinal studies of predictive validity.

INDIVIDUAL DIFFERENCES

Only one study has examined a group of traumatized, clinic-referred children less than 4 years of age to explore individual differences in the children or the events that might moderate the expression of PTSD. Scheeringa and Zeanah (1995) analyzed the severity of PTSD symptoms in 41 cases in relation to six variables of the children or the traumatic event. Two of the variables were characteristics of the children: gender and age at the time of the trauma (younger than or older than 18 months). Four of the variables were characteristics of the traumatic event: whether the events were acute versus repeated, involved physical injury or not, were directly experienced by the children or witnessed occurring to someone else, and involved a threat to the childrens' caregiver or not. The most potent variable that predicted the development of PTSD in infants and toddlers was not an event that happened directly to their own bodies but whether they had witnessed their caregiver being threatened. None of the six variables significantly predicted the overall severity of symptoms (determined as the total number of PTSD symptoms); however, several of the variables predicted a differential expression of symptoms in certain PTSD symptom clusters. Specifically, children who were older than 18 months of age at the time of the trauma

developed more reexperiencing symptoms (cluster B) than did children who were younger than 18 months; children who suffered acute traumas also developed more reexperiencing symptoms compared to children who suffered repeated traumas; children who witnessed traumatic events happen to someone else manifested more hyperarousal symptoms (cluster D) than did children who directly experienced traumas to themselves; and children who witnessed a threat to their caregivers manifested fewer avoidance and numbing symptoms (cluster C), more hyperarousal symptoms, and more new fears and aggression symptoms than did those who did not witness a threat to their caregivers.

Future areas of study that may prove fruitful in examining individual differences in symptom severity include neurophysiological parameters, family characteristics, temperament, and deviations in developmental levels of cognitive, communicative, and socioemiotional capacities.

DEVELOPMENTAL CAPACITIES AND PTSD

We know little about the lower limits of age at which a young child can develop PTSD. What developmental abilities must have emerged in order to experience an event as traumatic and develop the necessary symptom picture? On review of 40 known published cases for this chapter, only one case showed sufficient symptoms to meet the diagnosis by DSM-IV criteria, a 34-month-old boy described by Gaensbauer (1997). However, when the alternative criteria (Scheeringa et al., 1995) were applied, the youngest published case with sufficient symptoms for the diagnosis was 3 months old (Gaensbauer, 1982). The next youngest cases were 16 months old at the time of evaluation (traumatized at 7 months) (Terr, 1988) and 22 months old (traumatized at 9 months) (Drell et al., 1993; Gaensbauer, 1995). To address the question of which developmental capacities are pertinent to PTSD and the earliest ages these capacities emerge, we next review six capacities that seem to be relevant to produce PTSD symptomatology.

Perceptual abilities of infants, which are necessary for awareness of traumatic events, have been reviewed by Haith (1986). Tactile and auditory senses are functionally equivalent to those of adults at birth, although hearing acuity in the first year is slightly less than that for adults. Vision is near-sighted at birth, about 20/300 or 20/800, which means vision is clear a foot or so away. Visual acuity improves steadily until it reaches 20/20 by about 6 months of age. Binocular vision, or stereopsis, which allows depth perception, has been estimated to emerge around 3 months of age. By 5 months of age, infants seem capable of differentiating faces as a distinct class of stimuli and then become increasingly able to discriminate one person's face from another (reviewed in Cohen, DeLoache, & Strauss, 1979). Thus, traumatic events can be visualized with varying degrees of clarity and depth perception depending on the visual abilities that have developed during the first 6 months and how far away the events occur.

Memory, of some sort, is needed for storing information about the traumatic event. A consensus exists among memory scholars for the existence of at least two major memory systems. The earliest developed type of memory, nondeclarative or implicit memory (Schacter, 1987), is essentially unconscious to the person. One example of implicit memory is that involved in conditioning, which has been accomplished experimentally with fetuses (DeCasper & Spence, 1986) and newborns (Papousek, 1967). The rate of conditioning dramatically increases during the first 5 months of life. The other major type of memory to develop, declarative or explicit memory (Schacter, 1987), is conscious to the person and can be expressed behaviorally or verbally. Studies on normal development have shown that the earliest evidence for the expression of recalled, conscious memory is around 9 months of age, when infants can reproduce behaviorally events from the day before (reviewed in Mandler, 1990).

Verbal recall, which is rare before 18 months, and spotty for events between 18 and 36 months, is generally present in a coherent narrative after 36 months. Between 18 and 36 months, children produce more recall when stimulated by a context that reminds them of the past event or when prompted by an adult (Fivush, Pipe, Murachver, & Reese, 1997). From clinical work with traumatized children, Terr (1988) reached a similar conclusion: that the cutoff point for the emergence of full verbal recollection, not just spotty memories, of a trauma was usually present if the trauma occurred around 28–36 months of age, but not

earlier, and some type of verbal recollection may be present at earlier ages, particularly if the children have advanced cognitive or verbal abilities (see Sugar, 1988). Two systematic group studies of memory in young children in real-life stressful situations produced similar findings (Howe, Courage, & Peterson, 1994; Peterson & Bell, 1996).

Affective expression is needed to manifest many of the DSM-IV symptoms of PTSD. The different affects that are needed include distress, wariness, fear, irritation, anger, sadness, and startle (or surprise). The ability to express distress is present from birth. Irritability is difficult if not impossible to differentiate from general distress by observation in infancy. Sadness emerges by 3 months of age. Anger and surprise can be discerned reliably by observers in children by 6 months of age (Lewis, 1993). The observable emotion of fear emerges around 9 months of age, although the probable precursor emotion, wariness, is present by 4 months of age (Sroufe, 1979). In summary, some of the affects that are components of the diagnostic criteria are present at birth, and the full complement needed for all symptoms is usually present by 9 months of age.

Furthermore, by at least 5 months of age, infants can discriminate fear from other affects *in others* (Schwartz, Izard, & Ansul, 1985), and this can influence their reflexive behavior (Balaban, 1995; Mumme, Fernald, & Herrera, 1996; Sorce, Emde, Campos, & Klinnert, 1985). These findings suggest that infants typically recognize fear in others before they can express fear themselves, much as they can comprehend language more than they can produce it in the second year of life.

Behavioral expression is not required solely for any of the DSM-IV symptoms of PTSD. However, symptoms such as flashbacks (and the concomitant physical reactions to flashback imagery) and avoidance of reminders depend on motor movement. Many symptoms in the alternative criteria, including reenactment play, constriction of play, regression in developmental skills (such as toilet training), and aggression involve behavioral expression. The basic motor components needed to manifest these behaviors include purposeful arm movements (evident at birth), multistep coordinated means–end behavior (evident around 7 to 9 months) (reviewed in Gratch & Schatz, 1987), walking (evident by 12 months), and imaginative play (evident around 18 months).

Verbal expression is required for many symptoms of PTSD (especially the DSM-IV criteria) in order to express subjective internal experiences, such as feelings and thoughts. The minimum language competence that is helpful in the assessment of symptoms is probably two-word sentences, which typically emerges around 18–20 months of age. However, there is great variability in the pace at which normal children develop language skills. As noted previously, the lower age limit for producing coherent narratives of trauma has been suggested by Terr (1988) as 28–36 months.

Socioemotional relationships are affected by the expression of several of the symptoms of PTSD. Such DSM-IV symptoms include feeling of detachment or estrangement from others, restricted range of affect, and irritability or outbursts of anger (the latter two usually shown in the context of relationships). Such alternative symptoms include separation anxiety and aggression. The sequence of social interaction developmental milestones has been reviewed by Zeanah, Boris, and Scheeringa (1997). The abilities for social interaction emerge over the period of 2–7 months of age, beginning with the social smile, enhanced eye contact, and longer periods of engagement with a partner. At the 7- to 9-month biobehavioral shift, two important developments emerge. A cognitive development is intersubjectivity, which means that infants now understand that their own inner experiences can be appreciated by and shared with others. A social development is the focused blossoming of attachment. By this time infants have developed unique relations with their caregivers, and the familiar reactions of separation protest and stranger anxiety appear.

Summary

This section has attempted to describe the developmental capacities pertinent to the development or expression of PTSD symptoms and the earliest ages these capacities emerge. Which of these capacities is needed in individual cases depends on the characteristics of each traumatic event and the developmental pace of each child. In short, each case must be assessed individually, and definitive statements cannot be made at this point about a lower age limit at which it is possible to express PTSD. Nevertheless, on average, the developmental components needed to express full-blown PTSD

symptomatology do not emerge until around 9 months of age. Extraordinary events or precociously developed individuals may produce some symptoms at earlier ages (see Gaensbauer, 1982). Abnormal behavioral reactions that occur as a result of repetitive events prior to 9 months of age might be better conceptualized as conditioning rather than the PTSD experienced by older children and adults.

ASSESSMENT

PTSD is one of the few psychiatric disorders for which an etiological event is required. Therefore, a traumatic event must be known in order to make the diagnosis, and the assessment must include a thorough characterization of the trauma. Applying the diagnosis indiscriminately, without a careful review of the actual event and demonstrating its temporal relation to any symptoms, runs the risk of trivializing the disorder.

PTSD, like other psychiatric disorders, may be approached usefully as a categorical disorder or as a continuous construct, depending on the goal of the assessment. For either approach, the clinical assessment of symptoms should be approached with care. Each symptom should be characterized for time of onset, frequency, duration, intensity, and level of functional impairment. The only known instrument for assessing children under 48 months of age is a semistructured parent interview that can be supplemented by observations (Scheeringa & Zeanah, 1994).

The method of gathering diagnostic information is as important as the content gathered. The variety and quality of sources of information available are distinctly less than for older children and adults. The majority of information must be gathered from mothers or other caregivers. Self-reports from barely verbal children obviously are limited. Teacher reports are usually not available for children less than 2 years of age. Symptoms are not easily observable by watching children in an office because most symptoms occur at home or in the community in specific situations. Young children have shown a remarkable ability to reenact traumatic events accurately with dolls and props either spontaneously (e.g., MacLean, 1977) or when guided by a clinician (e.g., Gaensbauer, 1995), but it is not clear how reliable this is as a method to elicit diagnostic symptoms. "Procedural validity," a term used by Spitzer and Williams (1980) to address how well a new diagnostic procedure produces a result similar to the result of an established diagnostic procedure, may be used to capture these concerns, although the field of infant psychiatry has poorly established diagnostic procedures for comparison. Nonetheless, "procedural validity" may be a useful term to use to describe these areas of study that are particularly important when evaluating young, pre- or barely verbal children due to the concerns described earlier.

No investigations have been published that evaluated procedural validity in young children; however, an unpublished study has provided data on a small sample on which types of observations or interactions elicit useful diagnostic information and whether clinician–raters can agree on the presence of diagnostic criteria when viewing the same evaluation (Scheeringa, Peebles, Cook, Zeanah, 1999). Scheeringa and colleagues performed videotaped, standardized evaluations on 15 severely traumatized young children, using a semistructured interview and five playroom sequences of observation or interaction with the child. The five sequences were (1) observation of the child while the caregiver was being interviewed about the child, (2) free play with the caregiver, (3) free play with the examiner, (4) examiner-guided reenactment of the trauma with dolls and props, and (5) observation of the child while the caregiver was being interviewed about his or her own symptoms. Two blinded raters, both experienced clinicians, rated the presence of PTSD criteria from the caregivers' reports or from directly observing the children. Interrater reliability was acceptable for rating the presence of symptoms, 87%, and for rating the presence of the diagnosis, 87%.

Fourteen percent of the childrens' PTSD criteria could be observed from the observational sequences, meaning that raters were dependent on caregiver reports alone for 86% of the diagnostic symptoms. The sequences that were most useful for eliciting diagnostic information were free play with the caregivers and the examiner-guided trauma reenactments. Free play with the examiner and observation of the children while the caregivers were being interviewed about their own symptoms were the least useful because fewer signs were observed and no signs were observed exclusively during those sequences. All the signs observed were within the reexperiencing and the avoidance/numbing of responsiveness clusters, meaning that no signs from the hyperarousal cluster were observed. Debriefing with the raters revealed the qualitative finding that, in some instances, they felt that their impression of the presence or absence of a criterion was more accurate than the caregivers' reports based on the raters' direct observation of the children on the videotape. This discrepancy occurred for seven of the criteria, and it is noteworthy that five of these criteria belong to the avoidance/numbing of responsiveness cluster, which are typically more internalizing, rather than externalizing, types of criteria. Finally, debriefing with the raters underscored the importance of the examiner's following up questions thoroughly to obtain specifics of symptom onset, duration, frequency, and intensity. In 4% of all possible signs and symptoms asked about, the interview did not or could not elicit enough information for the raters to feel certain about a rating, and it may prove to be remarkable that this problem was evident only with the nonspecific criteria (avoidance/numbing of responsiveness and hyperarousal clusters) but not with the trauma-specific criteria (the reexperiencing cluster). Overall, the findings from this study, although limited in validity due to the small sample, is an important first step in determining the optimal procedures for diagnosing young children.

Given that parent reports of infant behavior are an essential if problematic method, clinicians must carefully assess a parent's report of symptomatology, corroborating the report as much as possible by observed behavior and from other sources. Factors to consider in one's assessment method include the truthfulness of the informant, any bias of the informant to over- or underendorse symptoms, and the variety of sources of information. A significant complication in this area is the effect of the child's traumatic experience on the parent, and the effect of that experience on the parent's report of the child's symptomatology.

Neurophysiological Variables

Within the rather extensive studies on adults with PTSD, one of the most robust findings is the positive correlation between physiological differences and the presence of the diagnosis. Findings include overreactivity of heart rate, dysregulation of the hypothalamic–pituitary–adrenal axis, increased activity of the opioid pain relief system, and suggestions of diminished immune functioning (reviewed in Southwick et al., 1994). The leading theory to explain these changes is that the experience of an overwhelming trauma results in a chronic tendency to overreact physiologically to perceived threats in the future. Sympathetic overreactivity has been demonstrated preliminarily in older children (DeBellis et al., 1994; Ornitz & Pynoos, 1989; Perry, 1994), but no studies of physiological parameters have been conducted on children less than 8 years old.

Parent and Family Factors

The positive correlation between the parent's ability to function and children's severity of symptoms following trauma is one of the most robust and consistent findings in the field. This phenomenon was first recorded for the children and mothers in London who suffered aerial bombing during World War II (Freud & Burlingham, 1943; Carey-Trefzer, 1949). Since then, more than 15 studies of traumatized children and their families have supported a similar conclusion (e.g., Green et al., 1991; Silber, Perry, & Bloch, 1956). The parental factors that positively correlated with greater severity of children's symptoms were more symptoms of PTSD in the mothers and fathers, greater severity of general psychopathology in mothers, parents' denial of children's symptoms, and changed family functioning (reviewed in Scheeringa et al., 1997). Several of these studies included children less than 3 years of age in their samples, but analyses by age were not reported.

What is the mechanism that connects adverse family functioning to more severe children's symptoms following trauma? Several explanations are plausible: (1) Trauma that is overwhelming enough to produce symptoms in children may simply be so powerful as to affect other family members also—a "shotgun effect"; (2) parents who are symptomatic may be unable to provide the therapeutic support that is needed for children to recover from the effects of trauma—a "lack of protective shield effect"; or (3) parents who are symptomatic may have an active and direct relational effect which actually promotes or maintains symptoms in their children—a "toxic family effect."

This co-occurrence of symptoms in parents and children was noted by Drell et al. (1993), who called it "PTSD à deux." Scheeringa et al. (1997) termed this phenomenon "relational PTSD" and described two possible qualitative patterns derived from clinical experience, although more patterns are possible. One pattern is of *withdrawn* mothers who not only avoid any reminders of the traumas but essentially avoid their children. They have become emotionally unavailable to their children, similar to the description of depressed mothers. The second pattern is of mothers who are *preoccupied* with the trauma and reexpose their children to reminders. Each pattern, although polar opposite in the outward appearance of the mothers, has the effect of hindering children's recovery or may even promote development of symptoms.

DIFFERENTIAL DIAGNOSIS

Phobic reactions may occur to threatening stimuli without developing the full PTSD syndrome. This may have been the case of the boy startled by a lawn mower in Drell et al.'s (1993) vignette. The lack of the full algorithm of PTSD signs and symptoms differentiates phobias from PTSD. *Attachment disturbances* are likely to be common when traumas involved the caregivers. No study has been published yet which concurrently assessed for PTSD and attachment symptoms. However, Bowlby's anecdotal descriptions of many of the symptoms of young children who suffered maternal deprivation sound remarkably similar to PTSD symptoms (Bowlby, 1973). Theoretically, this overlap makes sense. What event would be more life-threatening to young children than the perceived loss of their protectors? Attachment disturbances may be distinguished from PTSD by the lack of a close attachment to a caregiver, the presence of indiscriminate sociability, or the presence of relationship-specific abnormalities in attachment behaviors. Similar to attachment, *complicated grief reactions* to the death of a parent may also resemble many of the PTSD symptoms, including intrusive thoughts of the deceased, avoidance of reminders, restricted range of affect, loss of interest in activities, difficulty concentrating, and sleep difficulties. Children suffering from grief may look predominantly sad whereas children with PTSD would appear more fearful, vigilant, and anxious. *Depressive disorders* also have symptoms in common with PTSD, including restricted range of affect, sleep difficulties, concentration difficulties, and decreased interest in significant activities; however, the presence of sadness and vegetative depressive symptoms ought to distinguish this condition. Symptoms consistent with *attention-deficit/hyperactivity disorder* (ADHD), such as restlessness and difficulty focusing attention, are often apparent following trauma, although there is no overlap in diagnostic criteria with PTSD. ADHD types of symptoms following trauma are probably more likely in cases of repeated and chronic exposure to dysregulating experiences, as in the complicated case reported by Thomas (1995). In clinical practice, cases of "pure ADHD" are more likely to show happy affects and a lack of defiance and irritability.

Not only may these other disorders have some symptoms in common with PTSD, but they may be associated features of posttraumatic reactions that are not reflected in the PTSD criteria.

TREATMENT

There are no systematic studies examining the efficacy of specific modalities in the treatment of PTSD in infants and toddlers. A growing clinical literature, however, is available. A variety of violent and terrifying experiences have been the subject of treatment reports, including animal bites (MacLean, 1977), the witnessing of parental death (Gaensbauer, 1996), sexual abuse (Cohen & Mannarino, 1993), medical trauma (Wallick, 1979), multiple physical traumas and abuse (Thomas, 1995), and accidental injury (Gaensbauer, 1995). This considerable literature provides extensive illustrative detail regarding effective treatment techniques and serves as a resource for the identification of generally applicable treatment approaches.

Not surprisingly, therapeutic tenets that emerge from the literature on infants and toddlers correspond closely to the essential elements of treatment that have been described for older children (Pynoos, 1990) and adults (van der Kolk, McFarlane, & van der Hart, 1996), highlighting the commonality of traumatic reactions across the lifespan. These principles include (1) *establishing a sense of safety*, both in real life and within the therapeutic setting; (2) *reducing the intensity of the overwhelming affects* associated with the traumatic experience; (3) *helping the patient to develop a coherent narrative* from the often fragmented memories elicited by the traumatic event; (4) *helping the patient to integrate the traumatic events psychologically* and to obtain a sense of mastery over them; (5) *addressing the numerous ripple effects* emanating from the traumatic experience, including, in children, behavioral problems and/or developmental disturbances; and (6) *providing support and guidance to the patient's family* so that they can both help the patient and deal with their own reactions to the trauma. Ideally, treatment planning for a traumatized infant or toddler will incorporate all of these elements into an organized whole, having as a goal the reestablishment of functioning as close to the previous level of functioning as possible. An example of a treatment approach that incorporates these various elements into a useful and replicable intervention methodology is the structured, time-limited therapeutic program for sexually abused preschoolers described by Cohen and Mannarino (1993).

A necessary precondition for the carrying out of any therapeutic work in the area of trauma is the establishment of a condition of safety. This need for safety refers both to physical safety in the child's real world and a sense of safety within the therapeutic setting. It is difficult, if not impossible, to carry out therapeutic work involving a previous trauma if the child is at risk for ongoing trauma in the present. Thus, a child living in a chaotic, abusive home or one who is exposed to ongoing community and/or domestic violence will not likely benefit from therapeutic efforts directed toward past traumas unless current stresses are reduced or eliminated.

Similarly, the therapeutic setting itself must provide sufficient structure and protection to contain and support the child in the midst of the therapeutic work. The therapist must be realistic in regard to goals and take care that the support available both during and outside sessions is sufficient to deal with the severity of the trauma that he or she is attempting to help the child assimilate. Patients need adequate emotional distance from the traumatic situation to be able to work productively. Such concerns are particularly relevant in working with children who have been physically and/or sexually abused or who have been victims of repeated trauma. These children may have difficulty distinguishing therapist from perpetrator and will have strong tendencies to become disorganized and overwhelmed as they are reminded of traumatic events. When children cannot achieve the necessary sense of safety and distance, decreased focus on trauma issues in the therapeutic work and increased focus on issues of trust and bonding, self-esteem and competence, and pleasurable activities may be required. The internalization of positive experience is a necessary counterbalance for children constantly confronted with traumatic memories that threaten to overwhelm them.

Beyond the issue of safety, the most immediate task in the face of a traumatic experience is to alleviate overwhelming distress and emotional dysregulation brought about by traumatic reminders or more generalized disturbances in arousal. Therapists can work closely with caregivers to identify effective interventions to reduce autonomic arousal and facilitate calm. With younger children especially, these will involve time-honored soothing techniques such as holding, rocking, nursing, gentle talking, and various forms of physical touch. Given the traumatized child's emotional fragility, the identification of effective soothing mechanisms may require ingenuity and specialized techniques, such as those developed in working with hypersensitive or poorly regulated infants (Greenspan & Weider, 1993). Such basic soothing techniques will be applicable throughout childhood, but with maturation, a broader range of soothing activities may be anticipated. These include verbal empathy and support, physical proximity, involvement in constructive play, and various activities that lighten the child's mood.

Effective calming techniques are also a necessary element in the ongoing process of desensitizing the intensity of the child's affective response to traumatic reminders. With younger children, soothing in the context of exposure and desensitization likely will occur in the immediate, day-to-day situations that trigger distress, particularly if the child's emotions are interfering with vital activities such as feeding, sleeping, social interaction, or exploration. Such desensitization will involve gradual exposure to distress-evoking activities, while paying close attention to the child's readiness to handle each increase in exposure. The stepwise desensitization program developed to reduce anxiety in feeding situations following a posttraumatic feeding disorder (Chatoor, 1991) and the desensitization protocol used by Wallick (1979) in the treatment of a medically traumatized toddler provide models for this type of gradual exposure. Opportunities for desensitization also will occur spontaneously. In this regard, each

instance of emotional reliving in the course of the child's daily life can be considered an opportunity for therapeutic desensitization, to the extent that caregivers can recognize the source of the child's distress and provide reassurance.

As children become older, desensitization can take place not only in the actual situation but also through more representational modalities. In the simplest sense, such desensitization might involve exposure to play materials representing some aspect of the traumatic situation, such as a toy car or animal or a doctor kit, depending on the circumstances. With further elaboration in the capacity for symbolic play, abreaction of pent-up affect associated with a traumatic event can be elicited using structured play situations such as those originally described by David Levy (1939). As Levy documented, with minor trauma, abreaction alone is often sufficient to relieve ongoing distress. With more severe traumas, reductions in affective intensity will require repeated psychological reworking over time. Because infants and toddlers rarely express their traumatic memories spontaneously, opportunities for repeated reworking must often be provided for them. Such opportunities can be encouraged both in therapy sessions and at home through the provision of toys and other props that facilitate expressive play, through direct verbal discussions (to the degree the child is able), and through other expressive techniques such as storytelling or drawing.

Evolving naturally from efforts to desensitize and encourage abreaction are approaches designed to facilitate integration of traumatic experience. In the preverbal period, integration is likely to be accomplished through the sensory–motor and affective relearning that takes place during desensitizing exposure to the specific situations eliciting distress. Yet, even at preverbal stages there is emerging evidence that children have deeply imprinted, internalized representations of salient aspects of their traumas which will require some form of cognitive assimilation (Gaensbauer, 1995; Terr, 1988). Young children are unlikely to be able to make sense of these recurring images, except to experience them as happening in the present (Gaensbauer, 1996; Pynoos, Steinberg, & Wraith, 1995). The therapeutic task is to help the child recognize that the emotionally charged imagery of the present belongs to the traumatic experience of the past. In addition, the child will need to develop an adequate narrative about what has occurred and to correct any misconceptions and distortions. Following Levy, fashioning play scenarios that recreate the traumatic situation in some manner and then allow the child to play out "what happens next" can be most useful for young children to express their own understanding of a trauma. Observing and participating in such play can allow therapists to identify important themes and affects and to take the child through the various elements of the experience in ways that facilitate narrative understanding. In this process, the child's perspective can also be expanded to include an understanding of the parent's feelings, addressing frequently held misperceptions that parents were indifferent or punitive in allowing the trauma to happen.

Within the framework of such therapeutic recreations, the therapist has a variety of traditional play therapy techniques through which he or she can provide support, guidance, and interpretation. These include direct anticipation in the play through action or through verbal observations, identification of important affects and motives, provision of narrative commentary regarding sequences and meanings, corrections of distortions and misunderstandings, promotion of mastery through compensatory play scenarios, facilitation of the expression of anger, and the teaching of strategies for self-protection in the future. At ages at which receptive language is in advance of expressive language, storytelling can be a particularly useful vehicle for articulating the child's experience.

While therapeutic reworking will play an important role in alleviating posttraumatic symptoms, front-line responsibility for helping the child to correct disturbed and/or regressed behavior will largely fall to parents in the home setting. Educating parents about PTSD can help them to recognize the child's disturbed behavior as originating in posttraumatic reactions rather than defects of character and to respond empathically rather than reflexively. Guidance around soothing techniques and communication strategies that parents can use in the home environment can be enormously helpful in allowing parents to play effective roles in their child's recovery, facilitating the reestablishment of trust and parental confidence. In most cases, some form of behavioral structuring is also required. Therapists can help in the development of behavioral management strategies and the identification of effective contingent reinforce-

ments for adaptive behavior. Ideally, parents will be able to provide such disciplinary guidance patiently and in a nonpunitive manner, in order to avoid escalating and destructive cycles of misbehavior and punishment that can lead to a consolidation of the child's maladaptive behavior and negative self-image.

To the extent that it is appropriate and they are able, parents' participation in sessions with the child can be very productive. Parents can provide crucial background information, can directly observe continuing effects of the trauma on the child, and can work together with the therapist to develop effective ways of addressing the child's emotional needs. Parents' confidence in their ability to help their child is often significantly shaken by a traumatic experience, as is the child's trust in the parents' protective role. The more that parents and children are able to work through posttraumatic reactions together, the more likely that mutual confidence will be restored.

Close involvement with parents also enables the therapist to monitor the parents' emotional reactions. Parents have a particularly difficult role, as they must deal not only with their child's needs but with their own reactions. There is probably no stronger elicitor of painful affect than actual or threatened harm to one's child. Given such strong emotion, support for parents separate from work with the child is frequently necessary. This is particularly true when the child's trauma reawakens traumas from a parent's own past, as is frequently the case in instances of physical and/or sexual abuse. In most cases such support can be provided within the framework of the child's therapy, through shared communication during parent–child sessions, or through separate parent counseling sessions. At times, separate therapeutic arrangements to deal with parents' emotional reactions are required.

The establishment of open dialogue between parents and child around the traumatic experience is particularly important in regard to the long-term effects of trauma. As has been discussed, trauma can produce developmental distortions that may not be evident at the time of initial treatment. In addition, children may be too young to assimilate fully what has happened to them or to understand how a traumatic experience in the past is influencing their behavior in the present. For these reasons, parental awareness of the possibility for delayed effects and the maintenance of open communication between parents and child around the traumatic experience are necessary preconditions for continued integration to take place. Therapeutic work subsequent to the initial treatment is frequently indicated when developmental distortions become evident or when persisting symptoms are not likely to be alleviated until the child reaches a certain level of cognitive and emotional understanding.

Clinicians working with traumatized children frequently will be confronted with situations in which the posttraumatic affects are so intense and disruptive as to threaten the child's and family's well-being, and in which psychosocial interventions are inadequate to bring relief. Although fraught with risks and uncertainties, medications are being used increasingly in this population. Harmon and Riggs (1996) recently reported on the effective use of clonidine in seven chronically traumatized preschool children attending a day treatment center. Anecdotal reports have also appeared describing the beneficial use of antidepressant medications (Gaensbauer & Siegel, 1995; Thomas, 1995). Although there is reason to believe that medications that have been helpful in older children and adults may be useful in preschool children as well, there are too many unanswered questions to be able to make specific recommendations, except that medications are likely to be adjunctive rather than first line treatments for young children.

CONCLUSION

The empirical study of PTSD in infants and toddlers has advanced further than for some other Axis I disorders in early childhood, although our understanding of key issues is still at an early stage. Systematic research has focused to date on diagnostic validity, and case report studies have focused on assessment and treatment. Important advances have been made in being able to make the diagnosis accurately, and to know which psychotherapy techniques appear to help reduce the suffering of children and families. In other words, contrary to the state of knowledge 20 years ago, it is recognized that infants and toddlers can become functionally impaired due to life-threatening trauma, and that clinicians have a useful role in helping them get better.

Little is known, however, about epidemiology, etiology, neurobiology, prognosis, course, or effectiveness of specific therapies. Advances in these areas require systematic studies in the future.

REFERENCES

American Psychiatric Association. (1994). *Diagnostic and statistical manual of mental disorders* (4th ed.). Washington, DC: Author.

Azarian, A., Lipsitt, L. P., & Skripchenko, V. (1996, April). *Behavioral psychopathology in infants of disaster.* Paper presented at the 10th biennial International Conference on Infant Studies. Providence, RI.

Balaban, M. T. (1995). Affective influences on startle in five-month-old infants: Reactions to facial expressions of emotion. *Child Development, 66,* 28–36.

Bowlby, J. (1973). *Attachment and loss. Separation* (Vol. 2, pp. 3–24). New York: Basic Books.

Breslau, N., Davis, G. C., Andreski, P., & Peterson, E. (1991). Traumatic events and posttraumatic stress disorder in an urban population of young adults. *Archives of General Psychiatry, 48,* 216–222.

Carey-Trefzer, C. J. (1949). The results of a clinical study of war-damaged children who attended the child guidance clinic, The Hospital for Sick Children, Great Ormond Street, London. *Journal of Mental Science, 95,* 535–559.

Chatoor, I. (1991). Eating and nutritional disorders of infancy and early childhood. In J. Wiener (Ed.), *Textbook of child and adolescent psychiatry* (pp. 351–361). Washington, DC: Academy of Child and Adolescent Psychiatry Press.

Cohen, J. A., & Mannarino, A. P. (1993). A treatment model for sexually abused preschoolers. *Journal of Interpersonal Violence, 8,* 115–131.

Cohen, L. B., DeLoache, J. S., & Strauss, M. S. (1979). Infant visual perception. In J. D. Osofsky (Ed.), *Handbook of infant development* (pp. 393–438). New York: Wiley.

Davidson, J. R. T., Hughes, D., Blazer, D. G., & George, L. K. (1991). Post-traumatic stress disorder in the community: an epidemiological study. *Psychological Medicine, 21,* 713–721.

DeBellis, M. D., Chrousos, G. P., Dorn, L. D., Burke, L., Helmers, K., Kling, M. A., Trickett, P. K., & Putnam, F. W. (1994). Hypothalamic-pituitary–adrenal axis dysregulation in sexually abused girls. *Journal of Clinical Endocrinology and Metabolism, 78,* 249–255.

DeCasper, A., & Spence, M. J. (1986). Prenatal maternal speech influences newborns' perceptions of speech sounds. *Infant Behavior and Development, 9,* 133–150.

Drell, M. J., Siegel, C. H., & Gaensbauer, T. J. (1993). Post-traumatic stress disorder. In C. H. Zeanah, Jr. (Ed.), *Handbook of infant mental health* (pp. 291–304). New York: Guilford Press.

Fivush, R., Pipe, M., Murachver, T., & Reese, E. (1997). Events spoken and unspoken: Implications of language and memory development for the recovered memory debate. In M. Conway (Ed.), *Recovered memories and false memories. Debates in psychology* (pp. 34–62). Oxford, UK: Oxford University Press.

Freud, A., & Burlingham, D. T. (1943). *War and children.* New York: Medical War Books.

Gaensbauer, T. J. (1982). The differentiation of discrete affects: A case report. *Psychoanalytic Study of the Child, 37,* 29–66.

Gaensbauer, T. J. (1995). Trauma in the preverbal period: Symptoms, memories, and developmental impact. *Psychoanalytic Study of the Child, 50,* 122–149.

Gaensbauer, T. J. (1996). Developmental and therapeutic aspects of treating infants and toddlers who have witnessed violence. *Bulletin of Zero to Three, 16,* 15–20.

Gaensbauer, T. J. (1997). Traumatic stress disorder. In A. Lieberman, S. Wieder, & E. Fenichel (Eds.), *DC: 0–3 casebook* (pp. 31–46). Washington, DC: Zero to Three.

Gaensbauer, T. J., & Siegel, C. H. (1995). Therapeutic approaches to posttraumatic stress disorder in infants and toddlers. *Infant Mental Health Journal, 16,* 292–305.

Giaconia, R. M., Reinherz, H. Z., Silverman, A. B., Pakiz, B., Frost, A. K., & Cohen, E. (1995). Traumas and posttraumatic stress disorder in a community population of older adolescents. *Journal of the American Academy of Child & Adolescent Psychiatry, 34,* 1369–1380.

Gratch, G., & Schatz, J. A. (1987). Cognitive development: the relevance of Piaget's infancy books. In J. D. Osofsky (Ed.), *Handbook of infant development* (2nd ed., pp. 204–237). New York: Wiley.

Green, B. L., Korol, M., Grace, M. D., Vary, M. G., Leonard, A. C., Gleser, G. C., & Smitson-Cohen, S. (1991). Children and disaster: Age, gender, and parental effects on PTSD symptoms. *Journal of the American Academy of Child and Adolescent Psychiatry, 30,* 945–951.

Greenspan, S. I., & Wieder, S. (1993). Regulatory disorders. In C. H. Zeanah, Jr. (Ed.), *Handbook of infant mental health* (pp. 280–290). New York: Guilford Press.

Haith, M. M. (1986). Sensory and perceptual processes in early infancy. *Journal of Pediatrics, 109,* 158–171.

Harmon, R. J., & Riggs, P. D. (1996). Clonidine for posttraumatic stress disorder in preschool children. *Journal of the American Academy of Child and Adolescent Psychiatry, 35,* 1247–1249.

Helzer, J. E., Robins, L. N., & McEvoy, L. (1987). Posttraumatic stress disorder in the general population: Findings of the Epidemiologic Catchment Area survey. *New England Journal of Medicine, 317,* 1630–1634.

Howe, M. L., Courage, M. L., & Peterson, C. (1994). How can I remember when "I" wasn't there? Long-term retention of traumatic memories and emergence of the cognitive self. *Consciousness and Cognition, 3,* 327–355.

Levy, D. (1939). Release therapy. *American Journal of Orthopsychiatry, 9,* 713–736.

Lewis, M. (1993). The emergence of human emotions. In M. Lewis & J. M. Haviland (Eds.), *Handbook of emotions* (pp. 223–235). New York: Guilford Press.

MacLean, G. (1977). Psychic trauma and traumatic neurosis: Play therapy with a four-year-old boy. *Canadian Psychiatric Association Journal, 22,* 71–75.

Mandler, J. M. (1990). Recall and its verbal expression. In R. Fivush & J. A. Hudson (Eds.), *Knowing and remembering in young children* (pp. 317–330). Cambridge: Cambridge University Press.

McNally, R. J. (1993). Stressors that produce posttraumatic stress disorder in children. In J. R. T. Davidson, & E. B. Foa (Eds.), *Posttraumatic stress disorder: DSM-IV and beyond* (pp. 57–74). Washington, DC: American Psychiatric Press.

Mumme, D. L., Fernald, A., & Herrera, C. (1996). Infants' responses to facial and vocal emotional signals in a social referencing paradigm. *Child Development, 67,* 3219–3237.

Ornitz, E. M., & Pynoos, R. S. (1989). Startle modulation in children with posttraumatic stress disorder. *American Journal of Psychiatry, 147,* 866–870.

Osofsky, J. D., & Scheeringa, M. S. (1997). Community and domestic violence exposure: Effects on development and psychopathology. In D. Cicchetti & S. L. Toth (Eds.), *Rochester symposium on developmental psychopathology, Vol. 8. Developmental perspectives on trauma: Theory, research, and intervention* (pp. 155–180). Rochester, NY: University of Rochester Press.

Papousek, H. (1967). Conditioning during early postnatal development. In Y. Brackbill & G. G. Thompson (Eds.), *Behavior in infancy and early childhood* (pp. 259–274). New York: Free Press.

Perry, B. D. (1994). Neurobiological sequelae of childhood trauma: Post-traumatic stress disorders in children. In M. Murberg (Ed.), *Catecholamines in posttraumatic stress disorder: Emerging concepts* (pp. 253–276). Washington, DC: American Psychiatric Press.

Peterson, C., & Bell, M. (1996). Children's memory for traumatic injury. *Child Development, 67,* 3045–3070.

Pruett, K. D. (1979). Home treatment for two infants who witnessed their mother's murder. *Journal of the American Academy of Child and Adolescent Psychiatry, 18,* 647–657.

Pynoos, R. S. (1990). Posttraumatic stress disorder in children and adolescents. In B. D. Garfinkel, G. A. Carlson, & E. B. Weller (Eds.), *Psychiatric disorders in children and adolescents* (pp. 48–93). Philadelphia: Saunders.

Pynoos, R. S., Steinberg, A. M., & Wraith, R. (1995). A developmental model of childhood traumatic stress. In D. Cicchetti & D. Cohen (Eds.), *Developmental psychopathology: Risk, disorder, and adaptation* (Vol. 2, pp. 72–95). New York: Wiley.

Schacter, D. L. (1987). Implicit memory: History and current status. *Journal of Experimental Psychology: Learning, Memory, and Cognition, 13,* 501–518.

Scheeringa, M. S., & Zeanah, C. H. (1994). *Semi-Structured interview and observational record for the diagnosis of PTSD in infants and young children (0–48 months).* New Orleans: Tulane University School of Medicine.

Scheeringa, M. S., & Zeanah, C. H. (1995). Symptom

expression and trauma variables in children under 48 months of age. *Infant Mental Health Journal, 16,* 259–270.

Scheeringa, M. S., Zeanah, C. H., Drell, M. J., & Larrieu, J. A. (1995). Two approaches to the diagnosis of posttraumatic stress disorder in infancy and early childhood. *Journal of the American Academy of Child and Adolescent Psychiatry, 34,* 191–200.

Scheeringa, M. S., Zeanah, C. H., & Peebles, C. D. (1997, October). *Relational posttraumatic stress disorder: A new disorder?* Paper presented at the 44th Annual meeting of the American Academy of Child and Adolescent Psychiatry, Toronto.

Schwartz, G. M., Izard, C. E., & Ansul, S. E. (1985). The 5-month-old's ability to discriminate facial expressions of emotion. *Infant Behavior and Development, 8,* 65–77.

Shore, J. H., Tatum, E., & Vollmer, W. M. (1986). Psychiatric reactions to disaster: The Mt. St. Helen's experience. *American Journal of Psychiatry, 143,* 590–595.

Silber, E., Perry, S. E., & Bloch, D. A. (1956). Patterns of parent-child interaction in a disaster. *American Journal of Psychiatry, 113,* 416–422.

Sorce, J. F., Emde, R. N., Campos, J., & Klinnert, M. D. (1985). Maternal emotional signaling: Its effect on the visual cliff behavior of 1-year-olds. *Developmental Psychology, 21,* 195–200.

Southwick, S. M., Bremner, J. D., Krystal, J. H., & Charney D. S. (1994). Psychobiologic research in post-traumatic stress disorder. *Psychiatric Clinics of North America, 17,* 251–264.

Spitzer, R., & Williams J. B. W. (1980). Classification in psychiatry. In H. I. Kaplan, A. M. Freeman, & B. J. Sadock (Eds.), *Comprehensive textbook of psychiatry* (3rd ed., pp. 1035–1072). Baltimore: Williams & Wilkins.

Sroufe, L. A. (1979). Socioemotional development. In J.

D. Osofsky (Ed.), *Handbook of infant development* (pp. 462–516). New York: Wiley.

Sugar, M. (1988). Toddlers' traumatic memories. *Infant Mental Health Journal, 13,* 245–251.

Terr, L. C. (1988). What happens to early memories of trauma? A study of twenty children under age five at the time of documented traumatic events. *Journal of the American Academy of Child and Adolescent Psychiatry, 27,* 96–104.

Terr, L. C. (1991). Childhood traumas: An outline and overview. *American Journal of Psychiatry, 148,* 10–20.

Thomas J. M. (1995). Traumatic stress disorder presents as hyperactivity and disruptive behavior: Case presentation, diagnoses, and treatment. *Infant Mental Health Journal, 16,* 306–317.

van der Kolk, B. A., McFarlane, A. C., & van der Hart, O. (1996). A general approach to treatment of posttraumatic stress disorder. In B. A. van der Kolk, A. C. McFarlane, & L. Weisaeth (Eds.), *Traumatic stress* (pp. 417–440). New York: Guilford Press.

van der Kolk, B. A., Weisaeth, L., & van der Hart, O. (1996). History of trauma in psychiatry. In B. A. van der Kolk, A. C. McFarlane, & L. Weisaeth (Eds.), *Traumatic stress* (pp. 47–74). New York: Guilford Press.

Wallick, M. M. (1979). Desensitization therapy with a fearful two-year-old. *American Journal of Psychiatry, 136,* 1325–1326.

Zeanah, C. H., Boris, N. W., & Scheeringa, M. S. (1997). Infant development: The first 3 years of life. In A. Tasman, J. Kay, & J. A. Lieberman (Eds.), *Psychiatry* (pp. 75–100). Philadelphia: Saunders.

Zero to Three, National Center for Clinical Infant Programs. (1994). *Diagnostic classification: 0–3. Diagnostic classification of mental health and developmental disorders of infancy and early childhood.* Washington, DC: Author.

24

Depression

❖

JOAN L. LUBY

The idea that clinical depression could occur during infancy and early childhood, a time of life we expect to be characterized by joyful exploration and growth, is difficult to accept. Whether very young children can experience clinically significant symptoms of depression or only transient adverse developmental effects of being reared by a depressed parent remains the key question in this area. Increasing evidence that depressive-like signs and symptoms do occur in high-risk infants and toddlers, combined with an appreciation of the importance of early mental health intervention, has increased public health attention to this area. This chapter reviews the history of our understanding of childhood depression and the early observations suggesting the presence of such syndromes in very young children. The recent proliferation of work on infant emotions in child development and developmental psychopathology and the application of these findings to our understanding of early clinical depression are explored. In addition, the usefulness of more recently described theoretical and empirical work on normative emotional development also is discussed. Although a specific nosology for infant/preschool depression is not yet clearly articulated, a number of clinical models have been proposed. Further, potentially related and very early clinical syndromes that involve impairments in mood and affect have been commonly observed for decades. The uses and limitations of these models and the importance of related clinical

syndromes encompassing impairment in mood and affect on our understanding of depression in early childhood are discussed.

HISTORY

Historically, the notion that children could experience clinical depression has been met with significant skepticism and resistance from both the lay public and the mental health community. In the 1960s and 1970s, the idea that depression could occur in school-age children was deemed inconsistent with developmental theory. That is, it was believed that prepubertal children did not have a sufficiently well-developed sense of self, and the concomitant expectations of self, to experience the core sense of self-deprecation believed to be associated with this disorder (Rie, 1966). Subsequently, clinical observations and numerous empirical investigations (Puig-Antich, Blau, Marx, Greenhill, & Chambers, 1978; Kovacs & Paulauskas, 1984; Ryan, Puig-Antich, Ambrosini, & Rabinovich, 1987) refuted these misconceptions. However, before the construct of childhood "depression" was accepted, some argued that depression in children was expressed as "depressive equivalents" (e.g., somatization), or so-called masked depression, rather than as overt depressive symptoms (Cytryn & McKnew, 1974). Subsequently, evidence that typical symptoms of depression could be identified in depressed children and classified using the adult *Diagnostic and Statis-*

382

tical *Manual of Mental Disorders* (DSM) taxonomy (Carlson & Cantwell, 1980) became available.

This extension of the adult nosology for major depression to apply to children as young as age 6 provided clinicians with the necessary tools to identify and treat depressive disorders earlier in life. As a result, the field of child mental health has been enhanced by a growing body of empirical research on the characteristics, course, and treatment of childhood depression. Although depression appears to occur at a lower prevalence in children than in adults, the public health importance of this advance is underscored by the outcome literature showing that the childhood onset disorder is serious, causing significant impairment and demonstrating a chronic and relapsing long-term course (Kovacs et al., 1984a, 1984b; Lewinsohn, Clarke, Seeley, & Rohde, 1994; for review, see Luby, Todd, & Geller, 1996). Therefore, in addition to the need to treat the acute manifestations of depression when it occurs early in childhood, it also became clear that this disorder was not a transient and spontaneously resolving phenomenon that children simply outgrew. On the contrary, childhood depressive disorders appear to be chronic illnesses responsible for significant morbidity during childhood and early adulthood (Luby et al., 1996).

Despite these advances for prepubertal children, whether clinically significant depressive disorders exist in infants and preschoolers remains an empirically understudied issue.

The landmark observations of Rene Spitz were the first to capture the possible manifestations of depression during infancy (Spitz, 1946). Spitz observed infants in long-term hospital settings who were separated from their caregivers and experiencing psychosocial deprivation. Spitz noted that these infants demonstrated depressed and withdrawn affects, and that they appeared apathetic and unresponsive when approached by alternative caregivers. Strikingly, he observed that these infants demonstrated signs of developmental delay and failure to thrive, despite the fact that their physical needs for growth and nourishment were met. Spitz also noted that when these infants were placed in more nurturing environments with greater opportunity for a primary caregiving relationship, these mental status changes appeared reversible. Spitz postulated that these psychosocially neglected infants were manifesting a form of depression secondary to separation from their primary caregivers, so-called anaclitic depression. These remarkable observations, made over half a century ago, strongly suggest the importance of early (and primarily relational) psychosocial phenomena on physiological development in infancy. Specifically, the observations also suggest that developing affective systems are vulnerable to early psychosocial deprivation. Although etiological conclusions about the psychosocial and biological antecedents of depression in early childhood cannot be drawn from these observations, the findings may provide important clues about physiological plasticity, affective vulnerability, and the very early manifestations of depressive disorders. Spitz's observations, although a landmark in infant mental health theory, have yet to be replicated in systematic and controlled empirical investigations.

DEVELOPMENTAL RESEARCH

Despite the dearth of direct studies on the clinical manifestations of very early depression, there have been numerous studies in the area of early emotional development that may have pertinence to our understanding of early depressive syndromes.

Development of Emotions and Emotional Competence in Infancy

Research Measuring Infant Emotions

Charles Darwin was the first to hypothesize that a limited number of discrete emotional states were biologically innate and present from birth in humans. Since this time, investigators have provided empirical data to validate this notion and to begin to outline the trajectory of the development of emotional milestones during infancy (Emde, Gaensbauer, & Harmon, 1976). The identification of specific affects and emotional states in infants is complicated, however, by the inherent difficulty in making inferences about an infant's feeling states from behavior alone without the benefit of subjective verbal confirmation (i.e., infants cannot describe their feeling states). Over the last decade, new tools to measure early affect expression based on objective observations of facial expressions have been developed (e.g., The Maximally Discriminative Facial Movement Coding System [MAX]; Izard, 1983). The notion that facial expression and feeling states are concordant has been demonstrated by several investigations in adults in which it has been possible to also obtain subjective verbal confirmation of emotional states. Subsequently, several investigations looking at the relationship between infant emotional expression and environmental stimuli have provided data that support a high level of specificity and, thus, the validity, of facial expression as an index of emotional state in infancy (Weinberg & Tronick, 1994; Izard, Haynes, Fantauzzo, Slomine, & Castle, 1994). These studies have shown that certain infant facial expressions are elicited by specific environmental events in a predictable and meaningful fashion (i.e., expressions of interest and joy in response to positive conditions and expressions of sadness and anger in response to negative conditions). As a result of these novel methods, significant progress has now been made in the understanding of the development of early emotional expression and emotional regulation (Emde et al., 1976; Izard, Huebner, Risser, McGinness, & Dougherty, 1980; Emde, 1980; Thompson, 1994). For example, it is now known that three discrete emotional states are evident in the human infant as early as 2 months of age (interest, contentment, and distress) and that the emotional repertoire differentiates into eight discrete emotions (joy, contentment, anger, disgust, surprise, interest, sadness) by 7 months of age (Izard et al., 1980).

Evidence of Emotional Competence in Infancy

While the infant's innate capability to express and (by inference) to experience multiple discrete emotions has been established, whether infants perceive and react to the emotional expressions of others is also key to understanding emotional development and the risk for early depressive disorders. This might be important, for example, when considering the effects on an infant of exposure to a caregiver suffering from major depressive disorder. Cohn and Tronick (1983) designed an experimental paradigm to test healthy infants' responses to their mother's expression of negative and flat or unresponsive affect. To investigate the infant's reactions to the emotional expression of others, infants and mothers were placed in a face-to-face interaction, while the mother was instructed to refrain

from responding to the infant's bids for interaction and to remain instead with a still-face expression. These investigators then rated the reactions (based on facial expression and body postures) of 3-month-old infants to their mother's simulated still and nonreactive faces thought to be a facsimile of a depressive affect. Cohn and Tronick (1983) found that these 3-month-old infants reacted with protest, appeared wary, and averted their mother's gaze during this time. These exciting findings suggested that even at this very early point in development, these infants displayed specific reactions to their caregiver's expression of negative or flat affect. These infant reactions were suggestive of their disappointment and anger in reaction to mother's expression of negative or flat affect (Cohn & Tronick 1989). This landmark study was the first to suggest that infants 3 months of age were sensitive and reactive to the expression of negative affect in their caregivers.

In addition to the young child's experience of and ability to perceive emotional states, the study of patterns of emotional reactivity and the ability to regulate emotional responses is also an important component of emotional development (for review, see Fox, 1994). There has been much recent interest in the pertinence of emotional regulation and reactivity to understanding psychopathology in early childhood (Thompson, 1994; Cole, Michel, & Teti, 1994). Emotional dysregulation can be described as impairments in the control of affective experiences and expression. Based on this definition, emotional dysregulation has obvious pertinence to externalizing or disruptive disorders in children. However, adaptive emotional regulation is also conceived of as the ability to experience a broad range of emotions and to modulate the intensity and duration of specific emotions. Along these lines, it may also be pertinent to early-onset depressive disorders in that the greater tendency to experience depressive affect states, and the inability to recover from these states, may be related to impairments in emotional regulation. For example, the high proportion of amplified or sustained experiences of sadness or anhedonia seen in depressive disorders could be understood as a problem in the modulation of negative affective states. In the infancy and toddler period, when the primary caregiver plays a relatively more important role in shaping and aiding the child's emotional regulatory capacities, these impairments might result from problems in caregiving relationships (e.g., poor fit between child and caregiver), constitutional problems in the child, or a combination of these factors.

Emotional Development during the Preschool Period

As might be expected, the capacity to understand and experience emotional states becomes significantly more sophisticated during the preschool period. Preschool children are able to provide accurate identification and verbally label a number of their own discrete emotional states as early as age 3 (Denham, 1986; Stifter & Fox, 1986). Also at this early age, they have the capability to accurately identify emotional states from drawings of facial expressions in addition to linking emotions with appropriate social situations (Dunn, Brown, Slomkowski, Tesla, & Youngblade, 1991). By ages 5–6, children are able to provide reasonable determinants of emotions (Strayer, 1986). Emotional regulation in the preschool period is also enhanced by the child's greater ability to think about and talk about emotions, as described earlier. By about the age of 5, children begin to more often verbalize their feelings instead of acting upon them. They are also better able to strategize independently about methods of self-regulation. Investigations have now demonstrated that children as young as preschool age can understand the experience of more than one emotion at one time, including understanding concurrent conflicting emotions (Stein & Trabasso, 1989).

Importantly, a number of studies have also demonstrated marked individual differences in these emotional competencies during the preschool period (Denham, 1986; Dunn et al., 1991, Howe & Ross, 1990). Evidence for a hierarchical progression of this emotional developmental trajectory has been suggested by studies showing that the emotional abilities of children at age 3 were predictive of their later ability to understand more complex emotions (e.g., ability to explain conflicting emotions) at age 6 (Brown & Dunn, 1996). These findings suggest that early emotional competence, demonstrated by the ability to accurately label emotions from pictures and to match emotions to their correlate contexts, is a predictor of higher-level emotional competencies later in childhood. These individual differences and the process by which higher-level skills are built on the earlier acquisition of skills could be important to an understanding of risk/protective factors for developing affective disorders. Nevertheless, data from studies investigating these early emotional developmental milestones and their possible relationship to the risk or protection from mood disorders are not yet available.

DEVELOPMENTAL PSYCHOPATHOLOGY

Infants of Depressed Mothers

Pertinent to our understanding of the developmental psychopathology of mood disorders, high-risk studies have focused on emotional development in the infant offspring of mothers experiencing mood disturbances, compared to the infant offspring of mothers without these symptoms (i.e., control mothers). Family studies have shown that the child offspring of parents with affective disorders have higher rates of these disorders than do children in the general population (Weissman et al., 1987). Based on this finding, investigations of the infant offspring of mothers with depression could be key to our understanding of the early developmental psychopathology of depressive disorders. In addition to genetic risk factors, psychosocial factors also may be salient, given the fact that the primary caregiver plays a key role in the early affective development of the infant. A number of studies have suggested that caregivers with mood disturbances may be more impaired than controls in their ability to act effectively in this role (Gelfand & Teti, 1990; Radke-Yarrow, Zahn-Wexler, Richardson, Susman, & Martinez, 1994).

High-risk studies have demonstrated a number of impairments in emotional expression in the offspring of mothers with varying degrees of depressed mood states and clinical depression. Several independent investigations have documented evidence of significantly higher levels of negative emotional expression and lower levels of positive emotional expression (measured by facial expression) in the infants of depressed mothers, compared to controls (Field, 1984; Field et al., 1985; Pickens & Field, 1993; Cohn, Matias, Tronick, Connell, &

Lyons-Ruth, 1986; Cohn, Campbell, Matias, & Hopkins, 1990; Murray, 1992). Several groups also have shown that the infants of depressed mothers demonstrated more difficult temperamental features. In particular, they are rated as having greater difficulty in self-soothing, displaying more irritability and lower levels of activity (Cummings & Davies, 1994; Field, 1992). Preschool offspring of depressed mothers evidence more complex depressive symptoms, such as excessive guilt (measured using story completion tasks) and empathic overinvolvement in the problems of others, than do controls (Zahn-Waxler, Iannotti, Cummings, & Denham, 1990; Zahn-Waxler & Kochanska, 1990). Preschool children of depressed parents also have been observed to demonstrate increased inhibition to unfamiliar situations (Kochanska, 1991). These findings suggest that impairments in mood and affect occur naturalistically and can be quantified in young children of depressed mothers early in development.

Using the still-face experimental paradigm described previously, Field and colleagues compared 3-month-old infants of control mothers to the infants of mothers experiencing postpartum depression (Field, 1984). Consistent with the original findings of Cohn and Tronick (1983), the infants of control mothers demonstrated anger and protestation in response to the still-face expressions of their mothers. However, in notable contrast to these findings, the infants of the mothers with depressed mood demonstrated an absence of these responses. The authors hypothesized that these high-risk infants did not respond with the typical show of protest because they had acclimated to the expression of flat or negative emotions in their primary caregivers. Thus, there may be more enduring effects of exposure to caregivers with depression that extend beyond the immediate interactions with the infant. Indeed, alterations in the infant's expectation of a depressed caregiver's behavior may be different.

Biological Correlates in Infants of Depressed Mothers

In addition to changes in the facial and bodily expression of emotions, a number of psychophysiological alterations have been identified in infants of depressed mothers (presumed to be high-risk infants). In particular, there has been much attention to the measurement of

heart rate variability or vagal tone as a measure of emotional reactivity and regulation. Vagal tone has been studied in a wide variety of child and adult populations and is believed to be a key psychophysiological marker. The measurement of vagal tone may be important to the understanding of emotions and emotional regulation, given the role of the vagal circuit in the modulation of cardiac response to stress.

Vagal tone can be measured by assessing heart rate variability, a measure of the parasympathetic nervous system's modulation of physiologic reactivity to stress. High vagal tone is associated with low environmental challenges and relatively greater autonomic nervous system tone, which, in general, facilitates innervation to the internal viscera. Decreased vagal tone, or heart rate variability, has been found in the infants of depressed mothers compared to controls (Field, Pickens, Fox, Nawrocki, & Gonzalez, 1995; Pickens & Field, 1995).

High vagal tone can be conceptualized as the ability to modulate the physiological response to stress. Therefore, the finding of decreased vagal tone in high-risk infants during face-to-face interactions with their mother is consistent with the hypothesis that these infants are relatively more physiologically stressed during interactions with their caregivers than are infants of nondepressed mothers. Similar findings of low vagal tone have been found in infants at high risk for anxiety disorders. In follow-up studies of these children, low vagal tone appeared to be a risk factor for the development of anxiety disorders later in childhood (Biederman, Rosenbaum, Chaloff, & Kagan, 1995). Therefore, although these findings may not be specific to depressive syndromes, they may be informative to longer-term risk for psychiatric disorders related to affective reactivity and regulation.

Right frontal electroencephalogram (EEG) asymmetry in the infant offspring of depressed mothers also has been demonstrated (Field, Fox, Pickens, & Nawrocki, 1995; Dawson, Grofer Klinger, Panagiotides, Hill, & Spieker, 1992). Field, Fox, et al. (1995) identified right frontal asymmetry in the infant offspring of mothers with symptoms of depression at both 3 and at 6 months of age. Dawson, Grofer Klinger, Panagiotides, Hill, (1992) studied the frontal and parietal activity of the infant offspring of mothers with depressive symptoms, compared to a control group. EEGs were recorded at rest and during emotionally evocative situations. High-risk infants demonstrated reduced left frontal activation both at rest and during dyadic play with mother, compared to controls. In addition, control infants demonstrated greater right frontal activation upon a distress-inducing separation from their mothers, but this pattern was not observed in the infants of symptomatic mothers.

The potential clinical importance of these changes is suggested by similar EEG findings in depressed adults during episodes of depression (Henriques & Davidson, 1991). EEG studies of healthy adult subjects have identified that hemispheric asymmetry characterized by relatively less left frontal activation and relatively greater right frontal activation (so-called right frontal asymmetry) is associated with normal or routine negative emotional states. The reverse pattern of asymmetry has been associated with positive emotional states (left frontal asymmetry). An equivalent pattern of asymmetry also has been observed in 10-month-old infants in response to happy and sad videotapes (Davidson & Fox, 1982). Further, this right frontal EEG asymmetry has also been found to be associated with expressions of negative affect in infants. This finding emerged in an experiment in which 10-month-old infants who demonstrated right frontal activation patterns were also shown to demonstrate more crying in response to maternal separations. Related to these findings, Calkins, Fox, and Marshal (1996) also found right frontal asymmetry in 9-month-old infants who were later identified as behaviorally inhibited during the preschool period. These compelling findings suggest that right frontal asymmetry may be associated with the proclivity to experience negative affect states and further that central nervous system changes may occur in advance of overt behavioral manifestation of depressive symptoms in very young children.

Relational versus Cross-Contextual Symptoms of Depression

Data derived from face-to-face studies of the infant offspring of depressed mothers, such as those discussed earlier, raise the question of whether depressive symptoms during infancy arise out of problems in specific relationships or whether they can be characterized as individual qualities of the child. This issue is confounded by the fact that much of the evidence for affective impairments in infants and toddlers has occurred in the context of dyadic interactions between the child and the primary caregiver. This raises a broader and more complicated question of whether it will be useful to define some disorders of early childhood as relationship disorders, as opposed to disorders inherent in the individual, similar to those coded on Axis I in the current DSM system. Nevertheless, this question may be particularly important to considerations of early affective disturbances, because affective development is known to be at least partially linked to an early caregiving relationship, as suggested by the numerous high-risk studies described above. As described previously, the findings of greater spontaneous negative emotional expressions and matching of more negative versus positive emotions arise in the context of interactions with the affectively disturbed primary caregiver. However, this finding may be an artifact of the methodology in which the primary caregiver is the feasible and effective elicitor of representative emotional states in the infant.

Other evidence more suggestive of specificity to the relationship with the affectively disturbed parent has now been reported. Field and her colleagues (Pelaez-Nogueras, Field, Cigales, Gonzalez, & Clasky, 1994; Hossain et al., 1994) found that that infants of depressed mothers interacted more positively with other important attachment figures, including their nondepressed day-care providers and their nondepressed fathers. Nevertheless, there does appear to be generalization of depressed infant behavior to interactions with unfamiliar adults. The question is whether biological changes in infants of depressed mothers are "trait" or state related. To the degree that brain changes are apparent independent of the relationship with the caregiver (Dawson, Grofer Klinger, Panagiotides, Spieker, & Frey, 1992; Field, Healy, Goldstein, Perry, & Bendell, 1988, Abrams, Field, Scafidi, & Prodromidis, 1995), they may be trait-like. If they vary with different interactive partners, then they may be state-like and indicate remarkable relationship specificity. In either case, depressive emotions seem to depend on the nature and quality of their caregiving relationships. Findings from these studies could suggest differing developmental pathways of early onset depressive disorders. Also, they underscore the possible importance of relationships with non-depressed caregivers as protective factors.

CLINICAL MODELS

Clinical Models That Include Depressive Symptoms

Reactive Attachment Disorder

Many of the signs and symptoms originally observed by Spitz in institutionalized infants as early as the 1940s have been observed subsequently by other investigators (Emde, Polak, & Spitz, 1965; Harmon, Wagonfeld, & Emde, 1982) and have been incorporated into the DSM (American Psychiatric Association, 1994) under the category of reactive attachment disorder (RAD). The RAD category, therefore, stands as the only category in the current DSM system that describes impairments in mood and affect as they are hypothesized to specifically manifest in infancy. RAD was originally described in DSM-III (American Psychiatric Association, 1980) and then more recently modified in the DSM-IV (American Psychiatric Association, 1994) to encompass two subtypes of the disorder: inhibited and uninhibited. This diagnosis remains a somewhat controversial one among clinicians and investigators in infant mental health (see Zeanah & Boris, Chapter 22, this volume). Although RAD is not a mood disorder, impairments in emotional expression are a central component of the disorder. Issues about whether RAD represents a primary developmental disorder or a disorder of attachment per se have been raised. In addition, the inclusion of necessary environmental preconditions has been criticized as a feature of the diagnostic criteria (Richters & Volkmar, 1994). Even in its modified form, RAD remains a descriptive category that applies to a small subpopulation of severely disturbed children, and as such, it may have limited clinical utility (Zeanah, 1996).

The signs and symptoms of mood and affect disturbance originally identified by Spitz have not been applied to the formal classification of mood disorders in infancy. Further, other symptoms have been identified that may be more common manifestations of depressive disorders seen in infants and preschoolers. These symptoms, such as persistent preoccupation with sad or pessimistic themes in play, extreme emotional withdrawal and expression of apathy, or the more nonspecific symptom of regression in development, are not currently captured in the DSM-IV mood disorder category, despite the observations and growing consensus of their importance among a body of infant/preschool clinicians (Luby & Morgan, 1997; Harmon, 1995).

Nonorganic Failure to Thrive

Depressive symptoms similar to those described earlier also have been noted in infants manifesting varying degrees of failure to thrive (FTT) and nonorganic FTT. Chatoor and others have suggested that the distinction between nonorganic and organic forms of FTT may be spurious because, in most cases, both organic and nonorganic factors appear to be at play (Benoit, Chapter 21, this volume; Chatoor, Egan, Getson, Menvielle, & O'Donnell, 1987). Children with FTT observed in clinical settings have been described as appearing withdrawn, depressed, apathetic, or wary (Benoit, Chapter 21, this volume; Chatoor et al., 1987; Drotar, Malone, & Negray, 1980). In more severe cases, these children have been observed to be disinterested in physical contact and interpersonal interactions, as well as engaging in self-stimulatory behaviors, symptoms more akin to those seen in the pervasive developmental disorders (Rosenn, Stein Loeb, & Bates, 1980, Powell & Low, 1983). Similar behavioral and emotional problems also have been observed in infants experiencing various forms of organically based malnutrition, such as kwashiorkor (Goodall, 1979). Although these children do not appear to suffer from primary disturbances of mood and affect, it appears that in disorders characterized by early physical and emotional deprivation, the developing affective system may also be vulnerable.

Posttraumatic Stress Disorder

The finding of depressive symptoms in infants who have undergone early and traumatic separations from their primary caregivers, physical or emotional neglect, and/or malnutrition suggest that depressive mood states can and do arise naturalistically as early as infancy, at least under conditions of severe stress. However, the findings of these depressive symptoms in infants and preschoolers who have undergone such trauma do not alone imply that these children are manifesting an early form of a major depressive disorder (MDD). It seems more likely, given the salient psychosocial stressors that appear to be precipitants of the symptoms, that they occur secondary to these traumas and might, therefore, be more appropriately classified as post-traumatic symptoms (see Scheeringa & Gaensbauer, Chapter 23, this volume).

It is now well-known that MDD is an illness characterized by familial inheritance (shown to be partially related to genetic transmission), environmental precipitants, and biological correlates. Potentially distinct from depressive symptoms arising secondary to traumatic disorders, MDD is characterized by a chronic and relapsing course in older children and adults. Therefore, it would seem more likely that infant and preschool children demonstrating depressive symptoms that represent early manifestations of MDD would arise spontaneously in the population under a variety of psychosocial conditions that include both stressful and nonstressful family and social environments. Based on this, studies that ascertain samples of infant and preschool children with depressive symptoms from community populations and mental health treatment programs are needed to determine the characteristics, prevalence, course, and correlates of very early-onset MDD.

Toward Defining a Clinical Depressive Disorder in Infancy

There has been much interest in the behaviors of high-risk infants and preschoolers as possible predictors or prodromes of later mental health problems, as described earlier. In contrast, there has been less consideration and little investigation of the possibility that some of these behaviors may represent active symptoms of early-onset depressive syndromes requiring clinical attention. This trend is reflective of the traditionally greater interest from the developmental research community in the behaviors of young children as markers of risk and protective factors for later competencies and/or impairments, as opposed to consideration of their significance for current functioning and adaptation. In part, this may be due to the inherent skepticism and difficulty with the conceptualization of mental disorders in children at such an early age. However, an unfortunate result of this limited focus is that attention to the behavioral and emotional status of very young children becomes restricted to its importance for later life transitions and loses sight of the potentially immediate mental health needs of the child. Related to this, clinicians who focus on the treatment of infant and preschool patients

are in need of guidelines to determine the clinical significance of signs and symptoms of depression in these very young children who present for mental health treatment. For these reasons, it is important to begin the scientific process of investigating the clinical significance of symptoms of depression as they manifest in very young children. This effort would serve as an exploration of the validity of a more developmentally specific nosology for depression during the infant/preschool period.

Identification of Syndrome, Disorder, and Disease

The sequential scientific process for defining clinical syndromes, disorders, and diseases has been well described in medicine and psychiatry (Robins & Guze, 1970; Feighner et al., 1972; Kendell, 1982). This process revolutionized adult psychiatry and led to the development of the DSM and *International Classification of Disease* (ICD; World Health Organization, 1990), systems that have provided categorical descriptions and operational criteria to define mental disorders that are now in use worldwide. Although this categorical model of mental disorders is far from ideal, there is little doubt that it has catalyzed advances in our knowledge of the etiology and treatment of a number of mental disorders. In this categorical model, increasingly restrictive criteria are required to move from the description of a clinical syndrome to that of a discrete clinical disorder, and from there, to a pathophysiological (i.e., disease) entity (see Table 24.1).

Assuming a categorical approach to infant and preschool mood disorders is useful, we must consider the several steps that have been used to establish valid categorical diagnoses of mental disorders in adults. At face value, it seems reasonable that to consider an affective disturbance in an infant or preschool child to be clinically significant, the affective disturbance should be associated with functional impairment; that is, the child's level of adaptive functioning would suffer as a result of the affective disturbance. Stability of impairment is another consideration that has been applied to validating mental disorders. Although this issue is significantly more complicated in early childhood, the presence of enduring symptoms is one factor that identifies a disturbance that is likely to require intervention (as opposed to one that is spontaneously resolving). One consideration

TABLE 24.1. Levels in the Validation of a Disease

Levels of disease concept	Criteria for validation
Clinical syndrome	1. Characteristics are distinguishable from other syndromes 2. Intercorrelated group of symptoms 3. Consistent clinical picture (stable and homogeneous correlational structure of symptoms)
Discrete clinical disorder	4. Explicit inclusion and exclusion rules 5. Predictable progression of interrelated syndromes as a unit 6. Rarity of intermediate or combined cases (discrete boundaries from other disorders)
Pathophysiological entity: Disease	7. Identification of biosocial risk factors 8. Pathophysiological explanation of symptoms, syndromes, and course 9. Specific pathway from risk factors to disturbed pathophysiology

Note. Adapted from Cloninger, Martin, Guze, and Clayton (1985). Copyright 1985 by the American Medical Association. Adapted by permission.

regarding stability for very young children is that shorter periods of time must be considered, given the proportionately greater importance of impairments over shorter periods in the lifespan of the very young child. Genetic family history also has been considered a useful factor in attempts to validate mental disorders. Although there are a number of mental disorders that are not known to be genetic in etiology, the finding of a family history of a disorder is of obvious importance in establishing generational continuity. Once clear criteria for clinical depressive syndromes in infants and preschoolers can be established, investigations of biological correlates may be more fruitful.

Special Issues in Defining Disorders in Young Children

Clinical Syndromes versus Transient Difficulties of Development. An issue central to establishing criteria for any mental disorder in infant and preschool populations is the distinction between clinically significant symptoms from those behaviors that are normative and more transient in nature. During this period of rapid development, it is well-known that behavioral difficulties arise as a part of normative, age-specific challenges (e.g., oppositional behavior during the "terrible twos"). Therefore, so that treatment may be directed toward those children most in need, it is important to establish when problematic behaviors reach a clinically significant threshold. There are currently no data to help distinguish which depressive symptoms in infant and preschool children are

normative and which are symptoms of clinical syndromes; however, data collection efforts directly pertinent to this question are under way.

Data are published, however, regarding this distinction with respect to disruptive behaviors in preschool children. Campbell and colleagues studied a sample of preschool children identified by their caregivers at age 3 years as having disruptive behavioral problems (Campbell, Breaux, Ewing, & Szumowski, 1984). Follow-up of this sample into the school-age period suggests that some disruptive problems evident in the preschool period are not "normative" and do not spontaneously resolve (Campbell & Ewing, 1990). Campbell (1995) concluded, based on these longitudinal data, that disruptive symptoms occurring in the preschool period are more likely to be persistent and, therefore, representative of clinical syndromes when (1) a pattern or constellation of symptoms, as opposed to a single symptom, is present; (2) a pattern of symptoms with at least short-term stability is present; (3) symptoms are evident in more than one setting and with multiple caregivers; (4) high levels of severity are present; and (5) symptoms are associated with developmental impairment. In addition, these investigators have identified that family contextual factors, specifically, a negative mother–child relationship, was a significant mediator of the persistence of symptoms at follow-up (Campbell, Breaux, Ewing, & Szumowski, 1986; Campbell, 1995). This cogent model may also be useful in our attempts to distinguish clinically significant symptoms of affective disturbance from those that are likely to be more transient and spontaneously resolving. It is precisely because of the potential dangers of early stigmatization that validated and developmentally specific clinical criteria for mental disorders in infants and preschool children are needed.

Relational versus within the Individual Disorders. Whether mental disorders during early childhood occur in the context of specific relationships or whether they can be attributable to the individual child has been a central debate in the field of infant mental health in general. Given the young child's fundamental dependence upon the primary caregiver and the notion that the child–caregiver dyad is the representative unit of the child's emotional functioning early in life, the clinical technique of assessing the young child in the context of the caregiving relationship has been emphasized (Zeanah, Larrieu, Heller, & Valliere, Chapter 13, this volume; Thomas et al., 1997). In theory, the child's early emotional experiences of the dyad become internalized characteristics of the child as he or she becomes a more autonomously functioning individual during the preschool period. Consistent with this, relationship specificity of mental health symptoms are more apparent in younger children, as opposed to older children and adults. Based on these considerations, it seems possible that some affective disturbances (those with origins in the early caregiving relationship such as hypothesized in the infants of depressed parents) might be relationship specific in the first years of life. Subsequently, if the young child experiences sustained negative affective interactions during this period (without sufficient protective factors present), it seems possible that these internalized experiences (and correlate neurobiological changes) could then become a disorder of the individual that occurs independent of the primary relationship.

Clinical Depressive Disorder in Infancy

It is well-known that there are basic substantive developmental differences in the areas of emotions, social behavior, and cognition between preschool and school-age children. Therefore, on this basis, the application of the specific clinical criteria that are currently used for school-age and adolescent children are not likely a priori to be appropriately descriptive for children younger than 6 years of age. The rapid developmental transformations known to occur during this period are an important consideration for diagnostic studies because it is likely that these developmental changes are associated with rapid changes in neurobiology as well. Therefore, it seems likely the neurobiological processes, similar to the behavioral manifestations, that are related to affective disorders might be different earlier, compared to later, in brain development. The pharmacological treatment literature for childhood depression to date is suggestive of such differences in the neurobiology of prepubertal versus adolescent depression. This is based on the finding that only a subgroup of pharmacological agents (in particular those targeting the serotonin systems) has demonstrated efficacy for the treatment of prepubertal depression, whereas a broader scope of pharmacological agents (targeting both noradrenergic and serotonergic systems) has demonstrated efficacy for adolescent depression (Emslie et al., 1997). Although there are numerous possible interpretations of these findings, they may suggest that serotonergic systems are more central in prepubertal depression, whereas the noradrenergic and serotonergic systems are both salient in depression occurring later in development during adolescence.

This issue of fundamental developmental discontinuities is a particularly important one for studies that aim to investigate the continuity of affective symptoms across early development. Based on the previous principle, one cannot necessarily assume phenotypic similarity between earlier and later manifestations of affective disorders even when we hypothesize that these disorders demonstrate longitudinal continuity. At the same time, core impairments specific to the affective system across the age span must be established so that the classification of symptoms into an affective disorder category will have heuristic value.

A related developmental issue that is key in conceptualizing any mental disorder early in development is whether sufficient normative developmental differentiation has taken place. Although this concern was the basis for early and misguided skepticism about mood disorders in childhood, it remains a valid concern when applied to the more advanced body of empirical data on emotional development. For example, it would be foolish to expect attachment disorders in infancy prior to the development of preferred attachment relationships at 7 to 9 months of age. A similar question can be applied to infant and preschool affective disorders. At what point has sufficient normative affective developmental differentiation taken place to warrant the possibility of a deviation significant enough to constitute a clinical affective disorder? In this area, the developmental literature has now shown that affective development is surprisingly differentiated at very early points in development (during the first year of life).

Naturalistic observations of affective disturbances in infants and preschoolers who present for mental health services and/or those in high-risk environments known to be associated with these symptoms must be systematically studied to address some of the developmental questions raised previously. Clinicians specializing in the treatment of infants and preschoolers have provided anecdotal accounts of a number of symptoms and behaviors in children who appear to have impairments in affect and mood. These young children have been observed to be preoccupied with pessimistic or negative play themes, to express negative self evaluations, and to lack confidence in interactions with peers. Social withdrawal and anxiety appear to be common concomitants of early-onset depressive symptoms, and these children are also noted to be excessively irritable or sensitive to criticism. As in a number of early-onset mental disorders, regression in development may also occur as well.

Although these specific symptoms are not currently included in the DSM system, some of these age-adjusted symptoms are described in the diagnostic manual designed for children younger than 5 years of age, *Diagnostic Classification of Mental Health and Developmental Disorders of Infancy and Early Childhood* (DC: 0–3; Zero to Three, 1994). For example, "Depression of Infancy and Early Childhood" describes a constellation of symptoms including "irritable mood, diminished interest or pleasure in developmentally appropriate activities, diminished capacity to protest, excessive whining, and a diminished repertoire of social interactions and initiative." Similar to the DSM, a duration of symptoms for at least 2 weeks is required. This category in the DC: 0–3 seems to be clinically useful in that it is more developmentally appropriate. In this way, this category offers the clinician more age-appropriate guidelines for identification of the disorder. However, it is important to keep in mind that currently, the category lacks more specific operational criteria to establish caseness (symptoms that reach a clinical threshold) and, related to this, the necessary empirical testing to validate the utility and appropriateness of the described symptoms.

Empirical Studies of Depressive Phenomenology in the Preschool Period

Poznanski and Zrull (1970) provided the first case report of a DSM-III depression occurring in a preschool child. Kashani and Carlson (1985) have also provided compelling case studies, theoretical papers (Kashani, 1982), and reports of a small number of preschoolers meeting DSM-III criteria for MDD, identified within a heterogeneous clinical sample (Kashani, Ray, & Carlson, 1984). Based on the identification of these few preschool children who met formal DSM-III criteria for MDD, these investigators concluded that typical DSM depression could occur in preschool children. In community samples, however, using multiple informants and an observational screening measure, Kashani and colleagues found few preschool children meeting formal DSM-III criteria for MDD, although a substantial number of children had "concerning symptoms" (Kashani & Ray, 1983; Kashani, Holcomb, & Oravaschel, 1986). Based on these findings, the investigators suggested that modifications in the DSM criteria for preschool children were warranted (Kashani & Ray, 1983).

Dimensional versus Categorical Approaches to Depressive Syndromes

Whether dimensional or categorical approaches will be most informative to our understanding of depressive syndromes in the infancy and preschool period remains unresolved. The exclusive choice of one of these models of psychopathology has important implications for diagnostic definitions (Richters & Cicchetti, 1993). Such definitions would affect estimates of prevalence, as well as our understanding and estimates of comorbidity (Caron & Rutter, 1991). Several principles would apply to either categorical or dimensional conceptualizations of depressive syndromes in the infancy and preschool period. Using a developmental model, it seems clear that there is a continuum between adaptive/normative affective development and maladaptive/pathological affect states. In addition, it is also clear that individuals may have psychopathological features or traits without meeting definitions for syndromes or disorders. Both of these principles, which are applicable to all populations, but perhaps most salient in young child populations, are compatible with either dimensional or categorical models. Because of the relevance of both approaches for research and clinical practice, and given the relative limited knowledge base in this area in general, it would seem that both dimensional and categorical models may be useful to conceptualizations of affective disorders in the infancy and preschool period.

PREVENTION AND TREATMENT

The severity, chronicity, and treatment resistance of childhood depressive disorders underscores the need for attention to this public health problem. Several factors point to the importance of targeting depressive symptoms for intervention at the earliest possible developmental period. First, it is now known that depression identified after school entry has a chronic and relapsing course. In addition, it is also known that school entry is a period of higher risk for both internalizing and externalizing mental health problems, given the greater social and academic demands (Pianta & Castaldi, 1989). Given these issues and the fact that there is evidence of biological changes, such as decreased vagal tone and right frontal EEG asymmetry associated with affective symptoms in high-risk infants and preschoolers, occurring prior to the manifestation of overt depressive symptoms (Field, Fox, et al., 1995; Field, Pickens, et al., 1995; Dawson, Grofer Klinger, Panagiotides, Hill, et al., 1992), the identification of depressive symptoms in the infancy and preschool period appears to be both feasible and worthwhile.

Potentially related to the poor long-term outcomes, the data also suggest that depressive syndromes identified after school entry are relatively resistant to standard pharmacological treatments that have proven efficacious in adult populations (Geller, Luby, Todd, & Botteron, 1996). The possibility of treatment resistance in the disorder after age 6 makes the potential for clinical intervention or prevention at an earlier stage of central nervous system and emotional development an important area of exploration. Preventive efforts focused on the impact of maternal depression on child development have proven efficacious in older children (Beardslee, Salt, et al., 1997; Beardslee, Versage, et al.,

1997). In addition, there are promising and unexplored opportunities for prevention that could be focused more directly on specific features of early emotional development, such as programs to enhance the child's ability to identify and label emotions, which could result in improved emotional coping skills. Such preventive efforts should now be applied and tested in very young children who demonstrate symptoms of depression. The potential for such early "windows of opportunity" to influence brain development are suggested by a multitude of related findings from the basic developmental neuroscience literature.

REFERENCES

Abrams, S. M., Field, T., Scafidi, F., & Prodromidis, M. (1995). Newborns of depressed mothers. *Infant Mental Health Journal, 16*, 233–239.

American Psychiatric Association. (1980). *Diagnostic and statistical manual of mental disorders* (3rd ed.). Washington, DC: Author.

American Psychiatric Association. (1994). *Diagnostic and statistical manual of mental disorders* (4th ed.). Washington, DC: Author.

Beardslee, W. R., Salt, P., Versage, E. M., Gladstone, T. R., Wright, E. J., & Rothberg, P. C. (1997b) Sustained change in parents receiving preventive interventions for families with depression. *American Journal of Psychiatry, 154*(4), 510–515.

Beardslee, W. R., Versage, E. M., Wright, E. J., Salt, P., Rothberg, P. C., Drezner, K. & Gladstone, T. R. (1997). Examination of preventive interventions for families with depression: evidence of change. *Development and Psychopathology, 9*(1), 109–130.

Biederman, J., Rosenbaum, J. F., Chaloff, J., & Kagan, J. (1995). Behavioral inhibition as a risk factor for anxiety disorders. In J. S. March (Ed.), *Anxiety disorders in children and adolescents* (pp.61–81). New York: Guilford Press.

Brown, J. R., & Dunn, J. (1996). Continuities in emotion understanding from three to six years. *Child Development, 67*, 789–802.

Calkins, S. D., Fox, N., & Marshal, T. R. (1996). Behavioral and physiological antecedents of inhibited and uninhibited behavior. *Child Development, 67*, 523–540.

Campbell, S. B. (1995). Behavior problems in preschool children: A review of recent research. *Journal of Child Psychology and Psychiatry, 36*, 113–149.

Campbell, S. B., Breaux, A. M., Ewing, L. J., & Szumowski, E. K. (1984). A one-year follow-up study of parent-referred hyperactive preschool children. *Journal of the American Academy of Child Psychiatry, 23*, 243–249.

Campbell, S. B., Breaux, A. M., Ewing, L. J., & Szumowski, E. K. (1986). Correlates and predictors of hyperactivity and aggression: A longitudinal study of parent-referred problem preschoolers. *Journal of Abnormal Child Psychology, 14,* 217–234.

Campbell, S. B., & Ewing, L. J. (1990). Follow-up of hard-to manage preschoolers: Adjustment at age 9 and predictors of continuing symptoms. *Journal of Child Psychology and Psychiatry, 31,* 871–889.

Carlson, G. A., & Cantwell, D. P. (1980). Unmasking masked depression in children and adolescents. *American Journal of Psychiatry, 137,* 445–449.

Caron, C., & Rutter, M. (1991). Comorbidity in child psychopathology: Concepts, issues and research strategies. *Journal of Child Psychology and Psychiatry, 32,* 1063–1080.

Chatoor, I., Egan, J., Getson, P., Menvielle, E., & O'-Donnell, R. (1987). Mother–infant interaction in infantile anorexia nervosa. *Journal of the Academy of Child Psychiatry, 22,* 294–301.

Cloninger, C. R., Martin, R. L., Guze, S. B., & Clayton, P. J. (1985). Diagnosis and prognosis in schizophrenia. *Archives of General Psychiatry, 42,* 15–25.

Cohn, J. F., Campbell, S. B., Matias, R., & Hopkins, J. (1990). Face-to-face interactions of postpartum depressed and nondepressed mother–infant pairs at 2 months. *Developmental Psychology, 26,* 15–23.

Cohn, J. F., Matias, R., Tronick, E. Z., Connell, D., & Lyons-Ruth, K. (1986). Face-to-face interactions of depressed mothers and their infants. In E. Z. Tronick & T. Field (Eds.), *Maternal depression and infant disturbance* (pp. 31–45). San Francisco: Jossey-Bass.

Cohn, J. F., & Tronick, E. Z. (1983). Three month old infants' reaction to simulated maternal depression. *Child Development, 54,* 334–335.

Cohn, J. F., & Tronick, E. Z. (1989). Specificity of infants' response to mothers' affective behavior. *Journal of the American Academy Child Adolescent Psychiatry, 28,* 242–248.

Cole, P. M., Michel, M. K., & Teti, L. O. (1994). The development of emotion regulation and dysregulation: A clinical perspective. *Monographs of the Society for Research in Child Development, 240*(59, Serial Nos. 2–3), 73–100.

Cummings, E. M., & Davies, P. T. (1994). Maternal depression and child development. *Journal of Child Psychology and Psychiatry, 1,* 73–111.

Cytryn, L., & McKnew, D. H. (1974). Factors influencing the changing clinical expression of the depressive process in children. *American Journal of Psychiatry, 131,* 879–881.

Davidson, R., & Fox, N. (1982). Asymmetrical brain activity discriminates between positive versus negative affective stimuli in human infants. *Science, 218,* 1235–1237.

Dawson, G., Grofer Klinger, L., Panagiotides, H., Hill, D., & Spieker, S. (1992). Frontal lobe activity and affective behavior of infants of mothers with depressive symptoms. *Child Development, 63,* 725–737.

Dawson, G., Grofer Klinger, L., Panagiotides, H., Spieker, S., & Frey, K. (1992). Infants of mothers with depressive symptoms: Electroencephalographic and behavioral findings related to attachment status. *Development and Psychopathology, 4,* 67–80.

Denham, S. A. (1986). Social cognition, pro-social behavior, and emotion in preschoolers: Contextual validation. *Child Development, 57,* 194–201.

Drotar, D., Malone, C. A., & Negray, J. (1980). Intellectual assessment of young children with environmentally based failure to thrive. *Child Abuse and Neglect, 4,* 23–31.

Dunn, J., Brown, J., Slomkowski, C., Tesla, C., & Youngblade, L. (1991). Young children's understanding of other people's feelings and beliefs: Individual differences and their antecedents. *Child Development, 62,* 448–455.

Emde, R. N. (1980). Emotional availability. In P. M. Taylor (Ed.), *Parent–infant relationships.* New York: Grune & Stratton.

Emde, R. N., Gaensbauer, T., & Harmon, R. (1976). *Emotional expression in infancy: A biobehavioral study.* New York: International Universities Press.

Emde, R. N., Polak, P. R., & Spitz, R. A. (1965). Anaclitic depression in an infant raised in an institution. *Journal of the American Academy of Child Psychiatry, 4,* 545–553.

Emslie, G. J., Rush, A. J., Weinberg, W. A., Kowatch, R. A., Hughes, C. W., Carmody, T., & Rintelman, J. (1997). A double-blind, randomized, placebo-controlled trial of fluoxetine in children and adolescents with depression. *Archives of General Psychiatry, 54*(11), 1031–37.

Feighner, J. P., Robins, E., Guze, S. B., Woodruff, R. A., Winokur, G., & Munoz, R. (1972). Diagnostic criteria for use in psychiatric research. *Archives of General Psychiatry, 26,* 57–63.

Field, T. (1984). Early interactions between infants and their post-partum depressed mothers. *Infant Behavior and Development, 7,* 537–532.

Field, T. M. (1992). Infants of depressed mothers. *Development and Psychopathology, 4,* 49–66.

Field, T., Fox, N., Pickens, J., & Nawrocki, T. (1995). Relative right frontal EEG activation in 3–6 month old infants of depressed mothers. *Developmental Psychology, 31,* 358–363.

Field, T., Healy, B., Goldstein, S., Perry, S., & Bendell, D. (1988). Infants of depressed mothers show "depressed" behavior even with non-depressed adults. *Child Development, 59,* 1569–1579.

Field, T., Pickens, J., Fox, N. A., Nawrocki, T., & Gonzalez, J. (1995). Vagal tone in infants of depressed mothers. *Developmental Psychopathology, 7,* 227–231.

Field, T., Sandberg, D., Garcia, R., Vega-Lahr, N., Goldstein, S., & Guy, L. (1985). Pregnancy problems, postpartum depression, and early mother–infant interactions. *Developmental Psychology, 21,* 1152–1156.

Fox, N. A. (1994). The development of emotion regulation: biological and behavioral considerations. *Monographs of the Society for Research in Child Development, 240*(59, Serial Nos. 2–3), 103–107.

Gelfand, D. M., & Teti, D. M. (1990). The effects of maternal depression on children. *Clinical Psychology Review, 20,* 329–353.

Geller, B., Luby, J. L., Todd, R. D., & Botteron, K. (1996). Treatment resistant depression in childhood. *Psychiatry Clinics of North America, 19,* 253–267.

Goodall, J. (1979). A social score for Kwashiorkor. *Developmental Medicine and Child Neurology, 21,* 374–384.

Harmon, R. J. (1995). Diagnostic thinking about mental health and developmental disorders in infancy and early childhood: A core skill for infant/family professionals. *Zero To Three, 15*(3), 11–15.

Harmon, R. J., Wagonfeld, S., & Emde, R. N. (1982). Anaclitic depression: A follow-up from infancy to puberty. *Psychoanalytic Study of the Child, 37*, 67–94.

Henriques, J., & Davidson, R. (1991). Left frontal hypoactivation in depression. *Journal of Abnormal Psychology, 100*, 535–545.

Hossain, Z., Field, T., Gonzalez, J., Malphurs, J., Del Valle, C., & Pickens, J. (1994). Infants of depressed mothers interact better with their nondepressed fathers. *Infant Mental Health Journal, 15*, 348–357.

Howe, N., & Ross, H. (1990). Socialization, perspective-taking, and the sibling relationship. *Developmental Psychology, 26*, 160–165.

Izard, C. E. (1983). *The Maximally Discriminative Facial Movement Coding System.* Newark, DE: Instructional Resources Center, University of Delaware.

Izard, C. E., Haynes, O. M., Fantauzzo, C. A., Slomine, B. S., & Castle, J. M. (1994). The morphological stability and social validity of infants' facial expressions in the first nine months of life. *Psychological Bulletin, 115*(2), 288–299.

Izard, C. E., Huebner, R. R., Risser, D., McGinness, G., & Dougherty, L. (1980). The young infant's ability to produce discrete emotional expressions. *Developmental Psychology, 16*, 132–140.

Kashani, J. H. (1982). Depression in the preschool child. *Journal of Children in Contemporary Society, 15*, 11–17.

Kashani, J. H., & Carlson, G. A. (1985). Major depressive disorder in a preschooler. *Journal of the American Academy of Child Psychiatry, 24*, 490–494.

Kashani, J. H., Holcomb, W. R., & Oravaschel, H. (1986). Depression and depressive symptoms in preschool children from the general population. *American Journal of Psychiatry, 143*, 1138–1143.

Kashani, J. H., & Ray, J. S. (1983). Depressive related symptoms among preschool-age children. *Child Psychiatry and Human Development, 13*, 233–238.

Kashani, J. H., Ray, J. S., & Carlson, G. A. (1984). Depression and depressive-like states in preschool-age children in a child development unit. *American Journal of Psychiatry, 141*, 1397–1402.

Kendall, R. E. (1982). The choice of diagnostic criteria for biological research. *Archives of General Psychiatry, 39*, 1334–1339.

Kochanska, G. (1991). Patterns of inhibition to the unfamiliar in children of normal and affectively ill mothers. *Child Development, 62*, 250–263.

Kovacs, M., Feinberg, T., Crouse-Novak, M., Paulauskas, S., Pollock, M., & Finkelstein, R. (1984a). Depressive disorders in childhood: I. A longitudinal prospective study of characteristics and recovery. *Archives of General Psychiatry, 41*, 229–237.

Kovacs, M., Feinberg, T., Crouse-Novak, M., Paulauskas, S., Pollock, M., & Finkelstein, R. (1984b). Depressive disorders in childhood: II. A longitudinal study of the risk for a subsequent major depression. *Archives of General Psychiatry, 41*, 643–649.

Kovacs, M., & Paulauskas, S. (1984). Developmental stage and the expression of depressive disorders in children: An empirical analysis. In D. Cicchetti & K. Schneider-Rosen (Eds.), *Developmental perspectives on affective disorders in childhood.* San Francisco: Jossey-Bass.

Lewinsohn, P., Clarke, G., Seeley, J., & Rohde, P. (1994). Major depression in community adolescents: Age at onset, episode duration, and time to recurrence. *Journal of the American Academy of Child and Adolescent Psychiatry, 33*, 809–818.

Luby, J. L., & Morgan, K. (1997). Characteristics of an infant/preschool psychiatric clinic sample: Implications for clinical assessment and nosology. *Infant Mental Health Journal, 8*(2), 209–220.

Luby, J. L., Todd, R.D., & Geller, B. (1996). Outcome of depressive syndromes: Infancy to adolescence. In K. I. Shulman, M. Tohen & S. P. Kutcher (Eds.), *Mood disorders throughout the life span* (pp. 83–101). New York: Wiley-Liss.

Murray, L. (1992). The impact of postnatal depression on infant development. *Journal of Child Psychology and Psychiatry, 33*, 543–561.

Pelaez-Nogueras, M., Field, T., Cigales, M., Gonzalez, A., & Clasky, S. (1994). Infants of depressed mothers show less "depressed" behavior with a familiar caregiver. *Infant Mental Health Journal, 15*, 358–367.

Pianta, R. C., & Castaldi, J. (1989). Stability of internalzing symptoms from kindergarten to first grade and factors related to instability. *Development and Psychopathology, 1*, 305–316.

Pickens, J., & Field, T. (1993). Facial expressivity in infants of depressed mothers. *Developmental Psychology, 29*, 986–988.

Pickens, J., & Field, T. (1995). Facial expressions and vagal tone in infants of depressed and nondepressed mothers. *Early Development and Parenting, 4*, 83–89.

Powell, G. F., & Low, J. (1983). Behavior in nonorganic failure to thrive. *Developmental and Behavioral Pediatrics, 4*, 26–33.

Poznanski, E. O., & Zrull, J. P. (1970). Childhood depression. *Archives of General Psychiatry, 23*, 8–15.

Puig-Antich, J., Blau, S., Marx, N., Greenhill, L. L., & Chambers, W. J. (1978). Prepubertal major depressive disorder: A pilot study. *Journal of the American Academy of Child Psychiatry, 17*, 695–707.

Radke-Yarrow, M., Zahn-Waxler, C., Richardson, D., Susman A., & Martinez, P. (1994). Caring behavior in children of clinically depressed and well mothers. *Child Development, 65*, 1405–1414.

Richters, J. E., & Cicchetti, D. (1993). Mark Twain meets DSM-III-R: Conduct disorder, development, and the concept of harmful dysfunction. *Development and Psychopathology, 5*, 5–29.

Richters, M. M., & Volkmar, F. R. (1994). Reactive attachment disorder of infancy and early childhood. *Journal of the American Academy of Child and Adolescent Psychiatry, 33*(3), 328–332.

Rie, H. (1966). Depression in childhood: A survey of some pertinent contributions. *Journal of the American Academy of Child Psychiatry, 5*, 653–685.

Robins, E., & Guze, S. B. (1970). Establishment of diagnostic validity in psychiatric illness: Its application to schizophrenia. *American Journal of Psychiatry*, *126*, 983–987.

Rosenn, D. W., Stein Loeb, L., & Bates, M. (1980). Differentiation of organic from nonorganic failure to thrive syndrome in infancy. *Pediatrics*, *66*, 698–704.

Ryan, N. D., Puig-Antich, J., Ambrosini, P., & Rabinovich, H. (1987). The clinical picture of major depression in children and adolescents. *Archives of General Psychiatry*, *40*, 1228–1231.

Spitz, R. (1946). Anaclitic depression: An inquiry into the genesis of psychiatric conditions in early childhood. *The Psychoanalytic Study of the Child*, *1*, 47–53.

Stein, N. L., & Trabasso, T. (1989). Children's understanding of changing emotional states. In C. Saarni & P. L. Harris (Eds.), *Children's understanding of emotion* (pp. 50–77). Cambridge: Cambridge University Press.

Stifter, C. A., & Fox, N. A. (1986). Preschool children's ability to identify and label emotions. *Journal of Nonverbal Behavior*, *10*, 255–266.

Strayer, J. (1986). Children's attributions regarding the situational determinants of emotions in self and others. *Developmental Psychology*, *22*, 649–654.

Thomas, J.M., Benham A. L., Gean M., Luby, J., Minde, K., Turner, S., & Wright, H. (1997). Practice parameters for the psychiatric assessment of infants and toddlers (0–36 months). *Journal of the American Academy of Child and Adolescent Psychiatry, 36* (10 suppl.).

Thompson, R. A. (1994). Emotion regulation: A theme in search of definition. *Monograph of the Society of Research on Child Development*, *240*(59, Serial Nos. 2–3), 25–52.

Weinberg, M. K., & Tronick, E. Z. (1994). Organization and specificity in infant affect, behavior and affective configurations. *Child Development, 65*(5), 1503–1515.

Weissman, M., Gammon, G., John, K., Merikangas, K., Warner, V., Prusoff, B., & Sholmskas, D. (1987). Children of depressed parents. *Archives of General Psychiatry*, *44*, 847–853.

World Health Organization. (1990). *International Classification of Disease* (10th ed.). Geneva: World Health Organization.

Zahn-Waxler, C., Iannotti, R., Cummings, E. M., & Denham, S. (1990). Antecedents of problem behaviors in children of depressed mothers. *Development and Psychopathology*, *2*, 271–291.

Zahn-Waxler, C., & Kochanska, G. (1990). The origins of guilt. In R. Thompson (Ed.), *Nebraska symposium on motivation: Vol 36. Socio-emotional development* (pp. 183–258). Lincoln: University of Nebraska Press.

Zeanah, C. H. (1996). Beyond insecurity: A reconceptualization of attachment disorders of infancy. *Journal of Consulting and Clinical Psychology, 64,* 42–52.

Zero to Three, National Center for Clinical Infant Programs. (1994). *Diagnostic classification: 0–3. Diagnostic classification of mental health and developmental disorders of infancy and early childhood: 0–3.* Arlington, VA: Author.

25

Aggressive Behavior Disorders

❖

DANIEL S. SHAW
MILES GILLIOM
JOYCE GIOVANNELLI

The very title of this chapter raises concerns. At issue is whether it is appropriate to use the term "disorder" to describe children with significant levels of aggression between the ages of 1 and 3.

Those who have doubts about establishing an aggressive disorder of infancy point to the following concerns.

- Intentionality, an important component of aggression, is difficult to infer among infants.
- Most children do not have the cognitive capacity to comprehend aggression *fully* until their third or fourth year (Maccoby, 1980).
- For most children who show aggressive behavior prior to age 3, it is likely to be transient.
- Age 2 represents the peak incidence rate of aggressive behavior during the life course (Tremblay, 1998), which means that the false-positive rate for predicting future aggression is likely to be high.

Alternatively, the following points support establishing a disorder of aggressive behavior during infancy.

- Children who are not aggressive during infancy are unlikely to develop clinically elevated levels of aggressive behavior in later childhood or adulthood—the false-negative rate is likely to be low.

- Infants have the capacity to inflict serious harm on siblings, parents, pets, and objects.
- Predictors of conduct problems during infancy are similar to those that are related to conduct problems in later childhood and adolescence (Shaw, Keenan, & Vondra, 1994; Tremblay, 1998).
- Basic and applied research on conduct problems in young children has increased recently (Fagot & Leve, 1998; Calkins, 1994; Webster-Stratton & Herbert, 1994), as interventions targeted at younger children have been shown to be more efficacious (Reid, 1993).

This chapter explores issues surrounding aggressive behavior problems during infancy. To understand fully the complexities of this topic, we review how the term "aggression" has been defined, its development and stability during early childhood, factors that influence its onset and maintenance, and current treatment approaches. Finally, a clinical case is presented to demonstrate the techniques and challenges involved in implementing treatment.

DEFINING AGGRESSION

Intentionality lies at the heart of more recent definitions of aggression. It is perhaps the primary reason for not using the term "aggression" to describe aggressive-like behavior during infancy. Earlier definitions of aggression varied. Some investigators focused solely on outcome (Buss, 1961); others established intent to injure another person as the primary criterion (Dollard, Doob, Miller, Mowrer, & Sears, 1939). More recent interpretations assume at least an intent to threaten another and a consensus that the behavior be viewed as aggressive by the aggressor, the victim, and society (Bandura, 1979). For purposes of the present discussion, aggressive behavior is defined as an act directed toward a specific other person or object with the intent to hurt or frighten, for which there is a consensus about the aggressive intent of the act (Grusec & Lytton, 1988; Maccoby, 1980).

Aggressive acts toward others are typically subdivided into two categories: hostile and instrumental aggression. Hostile aggression refers to instances in which the major goal is inflicting injury, whereas instrumental aggression involves using force or threat of force to achieve a nonaggressive end (e.g., obtaining an object or gaining territory) (Grusec & Lytton, 1988). Note that in both kinds of aggression, intentionality is considered to be salient in determining if a behavior is aggressive. This presents a challenge in judging whether an infant has acted aggressively because of his or her limited cognitive ability and an observer's inability to interpret the meaning of the behavior.

At issue in inferring aggressive intent is the child's developmental status. According to Maccoby (1980), a child must understand the following principles to carry out an intentionally hurtful act:

1. That the intended victim can help or hinder the child's goals, knows what the child wants the victim to do, and knows that the victim can experience distress.
2. That the child's actions can generate distress.
3. That specific actions can cause distress in specific individuals.
4. That the child can execute distress-producing actions.
5. That distress can cause the victim to act in ways the child desires.
6. That the victim's actions can serve the child's needs.

Maccoby stresses that the child need not be conscious of these principles to act aggressively but must have some rudimentary understanding of each to act in a fully aggressive manner. At a broader cognitive level, the young child must be able to understand the nature of the other, including the other's goals and plans (Bowlby, 1969). Typically, a child develops the capacities to understand fully the point of view of another person at the beginning of the preschool years (Piaget, 1952); however, Dunn and Kendrick (1982) have found that some children under the age of 3 are capable of demonstrating these capacities when interacting with younger siblings. Given that it would be unusual for a 2-year-old to understand the theoretical underpinnings of aggressive behavior, conservatism is warranted in interpreting the meaning of aggressive-like behavior, particularly from ages 1–2 years. Just as 10–11-year olds who commit murder with firearms are treated as children because of their limited ability to understand the long-term consequences of their actions, infants who cause injury to siblings, parents, or pets need to be viewed in light of their own cognitive limitations.

Despite and because of these cognitive limitations, the age span between 1 and 2 represents a watershed period in the development of aggressive-like behavior. For infants less than a year, physical immobility limits the frequency of aggressive-like behavior. Although children less than 8 months old are clearly capable of using physical force to obtain an object (see Piaget, 1952), their accessibility is constrained by their inability to walk and, in most cases, crawl. With the onset of walking at 12 months and gradual increase in coordination during the second year, the accessibility issue becomes moot. The increase in physical mobility is of great concern to parents, as the infant now has the capacity to explore unchartered territory without the requisite knowledge base. In some ways, it is comparable to parent's predicament in handling the behavior of adolescents. In both instances, the child has the necessary "equipment" to engage in behavior that may cause harm to self or others without sufficient decision-making skills.

Two examples discussed by Maccoby (1980) capture the developmental transition children and parents undergo between ages 1 and 2. The first is from a study of 1- to 2-year-olds by Bronson (1975), who observed groups of three to four children in a free-play activity. Both 1 and 2-year-olds showed a comparable number of disagreements over toys; however, children's emotional intensity surrounding reactions to conflicts increased with age. Two-year-olds were more distressed and angry when a toy was taken from them. The loss of the toy affected the quality of the child's play after the incident, but also it appeared to offend the child's very sense of self. This study points out how the child comes to understand the term "mine." As Maccoby writes, "between the ages of one and two years, is an increase in the intensity of involvement with objects, a staking out of claims, and an increasingly intense emotional reaction to encounters over possession" (p. 119). As Goodenough (1931) documented over 50 years ago, angry outbursts peak in the middle of the second year for both boys and girls. Tremblay (1998) recently has corroborated these findings with respect to aggressive behavior, reporting that by 17 months of age, 70% of children take toys away from other children, 46% push others to obtain what they want, and 21–27% engage in one or more of the following behaviors with peers: biting, kicking, fighting, or physically attacking. Tremblay also reports that aggression occurs more frequently for infants with siblings, especially for girls (e.g., hitting, kicking, and biting), providing daily opportunities for conflicts over possessions.

A second example points to the challenge parents must face in responding to a more physically mobile and potentially destructive child beginning in the second year. Ausubel (1958) characterizes the process by which parents set rules as an ego devaluation crisis for infants. This type of parenting differs markedly from the first year, when most parents serve the infant's wishes unconditionally. In the second year, parents are also more likely to interpret the infant's misbehavior as more intentional and, as such, meriting discipline. Ego devaluation is the shock an infant must contend with in responding to a formerly servant-like parent. Children begin to realize that parents are satisfying their needs because the parents want to, not because they have to. The implication is that children come to accept their role in the family as relatively powerless beings who ultimately must yield to parental authority. Thus, it is not surprising that the second and third years are marked by increasing negativity on the part of the infant as he or she tests the limits of adult authority in response to parents' attempts to expedite socialization. Of course, the infant's day of reckoning is not a foregone conclusion. It is quite possible that in cases in which children develop early conduct problems, a different lesson is learned; namely, if I persist long and hard enough, I can continue to get my way. Empirical support for such a coercive process is discussed later in the chapter.

STABILITY OF EARLY AGGRESSION

Children's limited ability to understand the impact of their aggressive behavior, coupled with the developmental transitions taking place during the second and third years, make it important to examine its stability. As children are trained to desist from using aggressive conflict resolution strategies, rates of aggressive behavior gradually decrease from age 2 to 5. The decrease in aggression is supported by data from our longitudinal study of 300 low-income boys. Using the same five items of aggressive behavior common to the age 2–3 and 4–16 versions of the Achenbach's Child Behavior Checklist (CBCL; Achenbach, 1992), maternal reports of boy's aggressive behavior (means) decrease from 2.6 to 2.5 to 1.6 and to 1.3 at 24, 42, 60, and 72 months, respectively. Statistically significant differences in rates of aggression were found between 24 and 42 months and 60 and 72 months (for all four comparisons, $p < .001$).

Unfortunately, there are relatively few studies of the stability of aggressive and other types of disruptive behavior beginning in infancy. Studies of slightly older children suggest that continuity is moderate from the preschool to school-age period. In one of the first studies of the latter type, Jersild and Markey (1935) found that among 2- to 4-year-olds, peer aggression showed a stability of 0.7 over a 9-month period. More recently, Richman, Stevenson, and Graham (1982) identified the top 14% of 3-year-olds from a parental questionnaire of behavioral problems and followed them in comparison to a control group of children from similar backgrounds. Problems persisted in 63% of these children at age 4 compared to 11% of the control group, and 62% at age 8 compared to 22% of the controls. Similarly, Campbell and colleagues have followed two cohorts of hard-to-manage children from preschool through school age (Campbell, 1990). In the first cohort, children identified at age 3 showed moderate continuity of behavioral problems at ages 6, 9, and 13. Fifty and 48% of those with problems at age 3 showed clinically significant problems at ages 6 and 9, respectively. Campbell (1994) followed a second cohort of overactive and inattentive boys and found comparable rates of continuity from preschool to school age.

The few longitudinal studies initiated prior to age 3 largely corroborate these results. Rose, Rose, and Feldman (1989) found a correlation of .73 on the CBCL Externalizing factor between the ages 2 and 5. In a study specifically focused on aggressive behavior conducted by Cummings, Iannotti, and Zahn-Wexler (1989), the stability of physical aggression from age 2 to 5 was as high as $r = .76$ for males among a sample of 43 subjects (22 boys). This study is notable because it is one of the few in which observational data were obtained at both assessment points to evaluate aggression, and because the stability was obtained while having children interact with same-age peers. In our own work, which relied on both observational measures and parental report, Keenan and Shaw (1994) found correlations ranging from .23 to .45 between 1½ and 2 years for object- and person-related aggressions among 89 toddlers. For boys only, observed aggression was also related to maternal report of CBCL Externalizing factor at age 3 ($r = .34$) (Shaw et al., 1994), and symptoms of disruptive behavior disorders according to the *Diagnostic and Statistical Manual of Mental Disorders* (DSM-IV; American Psychiatric Association, 1994) at age 5 using the Kaufman Schedule for Affective Disorders and Schizophrenia (K-SADS; Kaufman et al., 1997) ($r = .30$) (Keenan, Shaw, Delliquadri, Giovannelli, & Walsh, 1998).

Finally, in analyzing data from our more recent cohort of low-income boys, we found among boys identified at or above the 90th percentile on the CBCL Externalizing factor at age 2, 63% remained above the 90th percentile at age 5, and 97% remained above the median. At age 6, 62% remained in the clinical range and 100% (all 18) remained above the median. False-negative rates are relatively low for the same factors. Only 13 and 16% of boys below the 50th percentile on the Externalizing factor at age 2 moved into the clinical range at ages 5 and 6, respectively. When clinically elevated groups were formed at age 2 based solely on CBCL items involving aggressive behavior, and the outcome variable was the narrow-band CBCL Aggression factor (comprised of aggressive, destructive, and oppositional symptoms) at age 5, prediction to clinical outcome was fur-

ther improved. Approximately 88% of boys identified as aggressive at age 2 continued to show clinically elevated symptomatology at age 5 (false-negative rate 22%). At age 6, 58% remained in the clinical range on Aggression and 92% remained above the median (false-negative rate 27%). These data are comparable to those reported by Patterson (1982) concerning the stability of antisocial behavior from school age to late adolescence. Of those identified in the top 5%, Patterson found 38.5% stayed at or above the 95th percentile and 100% stayed above the sample mean 10 years later. Similar to Patterson's data with older children, the stability findings of early childhood also suggest that there are relatively few "late-starters" who begin to show clinically elevated rates of disruptive behavior after infancy.

Taken together, the results suggest that aggression shows moderate to strong continuity beginning in early childhood. The data from our own sample indicate comparable stability of clinically elevated scores as reported for older children. That 63–88% of those identified with clinically elevated scores at age 2 continued to maintain clinical status 3 to 4 years later is a strong endorsement of the need for early intervention programs. It should be noted that these stability levels may be limited to other high-risk samples. Still, the results suggest that aggressive behavior is relatively stable for the most aggressive children during a period of great developmental transition. Finally, as Rutter (1997) notes, despite the high stability of aggressive behavior problems from infancy, it remains to be established whether these very early starters will go on to demonstrate severe antisocial behavior during school age and adolescence.

CORRELATES OF AGGRESSION DURING INFANCY

Several factors have been theorized to influence the course of aggression in young children. Unfortunately, relatively few studies have been undertaken to validate these hypotheses with infants. In the next sections we review areas that have been postulated to affect early disruptive behavior and research studies that have addressed these issues. The domains include infant temperament, parental attributes and support, parenting, and cumulative family adversity.

Infant Temperament

Several investigators have examined the relation between early temperamental attributes and conduct problems. Most studies have focused on infant negative emotionality (Bates, Maslin, & Frankel, 1985), although recent research has begun to explore individual differences in attention-seeking behavior and the expression of anger (Rothbart, Ahadi, & Hershey, 1994; Shaw et al., 1994). Negative emotionality is thought to be directly related to later oppositional and aggressive behavior and indirectly through its effects on parenting (Bates et al., 1985). Studies examining the former pathway have shown modest to moderate predictive validity (Maziade, Cote, Bernier, Boutin, & Thivierge, 1989; Sanson, Oberklaid, Pedlow, & Prior, 1991). However, interpretation of these findings must be tempered by the use of maternal report to assess infant difficulty *and* later behavioral problems. In the few studies using multiple informants, relations between maternal report of infant difficulty and later externalizing problems have been modest or nonsignificant (Bates et al., 1985; Belsky, Hsieh, & Crnic, 1998). This indicates that the direct association between infant temperament and later externalizing problems may be at least partially due to the parent's stable perception of the child rather than the child's behavior. However, such a bias may still have a significant, albeit indirect, effect on child antisocial outcome. Mothers who perceive their infants as high on negative emotionality may be less responsive to their requests for attention and use more harsh discipline strategies in response to their behavior.

In our own work, we have sought to understand the relation between infant attention seeking, maternal unresponsiveness, and early conduct problems using an interactive measure of attention seeking. Employing an observational measure developed by Martin (1981), infants are placed in a high chair with nothing to do, while mothers are instructed to complete a questionnaire and attend to the infant's needs. Persistent attention seeking is assessed by coding infant bids for behavior following initial bids that are unresponded to by the caregiver. Viewed from an interactional context, persistent attention seeking is likely to be aversive to the caregiver who is initially unresponsive to the infant. Thus, attention seeking may be a direct precursor of disruptive problems but also indirectly lead to disruptive behavior by influencing caregiver's perception and parenting of the child. Attention seeking assessed observationally between 10 and 12 months has been directly related to conduct problems in between the ages of 2 and 3½ years in three studies, including observed and maternal report of aggression at age 2 (Martin, 1981; Shaw et al., 1994; Shaw, Winslow, Owens, Vondra, et al., 1998).

A related interest has grown in exploring individual differences in infant's expression of anger, stemming from work on the affective bases of aggression. It has been hypothesized that infants who respond to goal frustration with intense and prolonged anger may be at elevated risk for aggressive behavior problems (Calkins, 1994; Cole, Michel, & Teti, 1994).

Longitudinal studies from infancy to early childhood provide preliminary support for this premise. Zahn-Waxler, Iannotti, Cummings, and Denham (1990) examined relations between aggression at age 2 and subsequent behavior problems in the offspring of well and depressed mothers. Both normative (object struggles, rough play) and dysregulated (hostility toward adults, out-of-control behavior) forms of infant aggression were identified. Only dysregulated aggression predicted externalizing problems reported by mothers at age 5 and children's reports of problem behavior at age 6. Similarly, Kuczynski and Kochanska (1990) identified several noncompliance strategies used by 2-year-olds, including passive noncompliance, simple refusal, direct defiance, and negotiation. Of these subtypes, only direct defiance, that is, noncompliance accompanied by poorly controlled anger, predicted externalizing problems at age 5. These studies indicate that the long-term consequences of aggressive, noncompliant behavior may depend on concomitant patterns of emotion regulation.

Parental Attributes and Support

Parental characteristics and support have been hypothesized to influence infant aggressivity in multiple ways. At an environmental level, parental maladjustment and low social support may compromise parenting. Parents who are impaired by psychopathology are also more likely to model maladaptive problem-resolution strategies for children to observe, including higher rates of interparental conflict and the use of physical force to resolve disagreements.

From a genetic perspective, maladaptive characteristics may be passed on to children, including such traits as impulsivity and low frustration tolerance (Raine, 1997). Among older children, conduct disorder and delinquency are associated with antisocial personality characteristics in both mothers and fathers (Robins, West, & Herjanic, 1975). This relationship has since been corroborated in three samples of infants. Keenan and Shaw (1994) found that familial criminality was related to boys' aggression at age 2, after controlling for aggression at 18 months and maternal age, a result we have replicated in our larger cohort of low-income boys (Shaw, Winslow, Owens, & Hood, 1998). In a large sample of 17-month-olds, Tremblay (1998) also found that a father's antisocial behavior prior to the birth of the child to be related to infant aggression. The relations between criminality and infant aggression tend to be modest (r's range from .15 to .25) but statistically significant.

Parental mood disorders have also been examined as risk factors for early conduct problems. However, the majority of these studies have ascertained child disruptive behavior during preschool age or thereafter. When young children with disruptive behavior problems are compared to normal controls, mothers of children with externalizing problems report more depressive symptomatology (Mash & Johnston, 1983), and these differences persist at follow-up (Campbell, 1994; Webster-Stratton, 1990). In our own work, depressive symptoms at 18, 24, and 42 months have been related to both concurrent and subsequent conduct problems from 18 to 72 months of age according to both parent and teacher report (Owens, 1998).

In addition to examining parental personality and adjustment, investigators have identified sources of stress and support within and outside the family system that are related to the occurrence of child behavioral problems. Again, the majority of these studies begin at preschool age. Among preschoolers and school-age children, marital conflict has been found to be associated consistently with externalizing problems, particularly when conflicts involve disagreements over child-rearing practices (Dadds & Powell, 1991; Jouriles, Murphy, & O'Leary, 1989). This finding has been corroborated repeatedly with infants (Gable, Belsky, & Crnic, 1992; Shaw, Winslow, Owens, & Hood, 1998) beginning with assessments of marital satisfaction/conflict at ages 1–2 years. In addition, quality of maternal social support outside the family has been positively related to responsive parenting and negatively related to maternal depressive symptoms and child disruptive behavior in the first 2 years (Burchinal, Follmer, & Bryant, 1996; Shaw, Winslow, Owens, & Hood, 1998).

Parenting

During infancy, maternal responsiveness has been the focus of research on parenting factors associated with externalizing behavioral problems. According to attachment theory, contingent responsiveness is critical to the development of self-regulation skills, the resultant bond between parent and infant, and later patterns of the child's behavior (Bowlby, 1969; Sroufe, 1983). An infant who receives less contingent caregiving may engage in disruptive behavior to obtain parental attention (Greenberg & Speltz, 1988) and also have less at stake to lose by being noncompliant and aggressive (i.e., loss of love) (Shaw & Bell, 1993). Thus, maternal unresponsiveness could trigger the initiation of coercive interaction patterns and the development of more serious conduct problems at school age.

Research examining infant attachment security and direct observations of maternal responsiveness during infancy have found support for their relation with later externalizing problems (Erickson, Sroufe, & Egeland, 1985; Renken, Egeland, Marvinney, Mangelsdorf, & Sroufe, 1989). Regarding infant attachment security, a consistent association has emerged between the insecure disorganized (type "D") category and later externalizing problems, particularly problems of aggression for boys (Lyons-Ruth, 1996; Shaw, Owens, Vondra, Keenan, & Winslow, 1996). The D category is yet to be associated with constitutional or genetic attributes (e.g., negative emotionality) but has been related to specific behavioral and psychological problems in caregivers. These include the caregiver's own maltreatment, unresolved loss or trauma, depression, and interparental conflict—all of which may impair the quality of parenting (van IJzendoorn, Schuengel, & Bakermans-Kranenburg, 1999). A recent meta-analysis found a combined effect size of $r = .29$ in 12 studies (total $n = 734$) examining the relation between disorganized attachment status and conduct problems. It should be noted that the meta-analysis included studies of attachment security that occurred at preschool age; however, effect sizes are similar across age periods (van IJzendoorn et al., 1999).

Direct observations of maternal responsiveness have also been related to concurrent and later externalizing problems, particularly for boys (Gardner, 1987). Using the same high chair task described above, three studies have found low maternal responsiveness between 10 and 12 months to be associated with boys' disruptive behavior at ages 2 to 3½ years (Martin, 1981; Shaw et al., 1994; Shaw, Winslow, Owens, Vondra, et al., 1998). In all three studies, the interaction of low maternal responsiveness and infant attention-seeking behavior added unique variance to the prediction of later disruptive behavior above and beyond the individual parent and child factors.

As it follows from developmental theory that maternal responsiveness should be studied as a correlate of early disruptive behavior in the first year, discipline practices should play a more salient role in the development of disruptive behavior in the second and third years. While maintaining a positive relationship, parents also begin exerting their will to protect the infant and other family members' physical well-being. In addition, parents begin to expect greater self-regulatory control insofar as the child can perform developmentally appropriate tasks that require greater social and cognitive competence. Parents, in fact, do report the second year to be a time of increased stress, during which patience and coping mechanisms are tested (Fagot & Kavanaugh, 1993). From a social learning perspective, rejecting parents might unintentionally reinforce children's disruptive behavior by attending only to negative behavior. The child may learn that the most successful way to terminate a parent's noncontingent rejecting behavior is to act in a highly aversive manner. The parent, in response, may withdraw from the confrontation, thereby increasing the likelihood of future coercive interaction (Patterson, 1982). In addition, rejected children may fail to internalize moral values pertaining to concern for the rights and well-being of others (Shaw, Winslow, Owens, Vondra, 1998). Parental warmth has been considered an important component of children's willingness to accept messages from parents regarding moral behavior (Grusec & Goodnow, 1994). Yet, there is a dearth of studies on the effects of parental rejection on child behavior prior to preschool age despite consistent associa-

tions between rejection and antisocial behavior among older children (Loeber & Stouthamer-Loeber, 1986). Recently we found observed parental rejection at age 2 to be moderately related to parental report of externalizing problems at age 3½ (Shaw, Winslow, Owens, Vondra, 1998). Interestingly, maternal rejection added unique variance after accounting for concurrent child problem behavior and earlier maternal unresponsiveness. Maternal rejection was also one of the few predictors of conduct problems for both boys and girls.

Chronic Family Adversity

A number of investigators have noted that the accumulation of risk factors is related to several types of child problem behavior, including disruptive behavior problems (Sameroff, Seifer, Barocas, Zax, & Greenspan, 1987; Zeanah, Boris, & Scheeringa, 1997). Rutter, Cox, Tupling, Berger, and Yule (1975) were perhaps the first to suggest that the presence of multiple familial stressors may be a better predictor of child behavioral problems than any specific factor alone. Consistent with this hypothesis, several investigators have found that the likelihood of behavioral problems increases with the number of stressors present (Sameroff et al., 1987). In the past decade this hypothesis has been corroborated with infants (Sanson et al., 1991; Shaw, Winslow, Owens, & Hood, 1998). In two studies of chronic family adversity assessed when infants were between 1 and 2 years of age, consistent relations were found with later disruptive behavior problems between ages 2 and 3½. Relations were more robust for externalizing verus internalizing problems. In addition, when groups were dichotomized based on clinical symptomatology, families with stressors present from four different domains had a 15 times greater probability of having clinically elevated scores than those with no stressors present. Stressor domains included maternal adjustment, family climate, parental aggressivity, and sociodemographic risk. The findings on chronic family adversity raise issues about the need to intervene with families at levels beyond the door of the therapist's office. It is also a reason the stability data are likely to be "inflated" in samples from impoverished backgrounds because of the number and type of stressors facing such families. Preventionists and interventionists need to consider these nonpsychological factors that affect parenting ability, including social support with-in and outside the family, overcrowding in the home, neighborhood dangerousness, and family income.

TREATMENT

While knowledge of the course and correlates of infant aggression is growing, psychosocial interventions that target this problem have yet to be evaluated empirically. In the absence of such data, the treatment recommendations provided here are guided by two principles that emerge from the preceding review.

First, early aggressive behavior must be considered within the interpersonal context in which it occurs. The research discussed previously suggests that infant aggression originates in and is maintained by multiple, interacting factors in the caregiving milieu, including characteristics of the infant and his or her parents as well as environmental pressures that impinge on the parent–infant relationship. We assume that the reduction of infant aggression requires identifying and addressing major etiological influences that are cooperating in a particular case. Hence, the focus of treatment must be broadened beyond the infant to include factors such as the emotional quality of parent–infant interactions, the ways in which parents respond to their infant's misbehavior, and stressors that impair parents' ability to provide adequate care.

Second, aggression should be viewed from a developmental perspective. A developmental framework dictates that clinicians approach aggressive behavior in light of the salient issues of a given age period (Sroufe & Rutter, 1984). For example, the establishment of an effective attachment relationship is a central goal of the first year of life. Aggressive behavior may be a result of an attachment relationship that is characterized by anger and frustration (Zeanah & Boris, Chapter 22, this volume). Similarly, the development of autonomy is a primary task in year 2, while the establishment of flexible self-regulation is a critical issue in the third year and beyond. Aggression may occur when factors within the child or family prevent the realization of these age-specific goals. It is critical that the timing and content of treatment be attuned to the developmental status of the child.

This section describes clinical approaches to aggression in the first 3 years of life. In keeping with relevant research findings and theoretical models, the strategies presented here are oriented toward relational and developmental processes that are thought to contribute to aggressive behavior in infancy. Each approach is covered in greater detail elsewhere, but usually in reference to other problems or to older children. Our goal is to illustrate how these interventions may be applied to infant aggression in an integrated fashion.

Parental Responsiveness

According to attachment theory, the emotional bond formed between an infant and his or her parents has far-reaching consequences for adjustment (Bowlby, 1969). Parental responsiveness is thought to be a primary determinant of the quality of the attachment relationship and, therefore, the behavioral tendencies of the developing child. Infants with unresponsive parents may resort to aggression to gain attention and are less likely to fear losing their parents' love by acting out. As an initial intervention, the clinician must attempt to optimize parental responsiveness to an infant who may already pose considerable challenges to even the most patient caregiver.

Several approaches have been developed to modify the ways in which parents relate to their infant. Infant–parent psychotherapy (Lieberman, Silverman, & Pawl, Chapter 30, this volume) is based on the psychoanalytical hypothesis that parents reenact with their children unresolved conflicts from important relationships in their own childhood. For instance, conflicts of parents with an aggressive infant may involve themes of aggression (e.g., abuse or domestic violence), resulting in feelings of anger or rejection toward their child. From this perspective, behavioral disturbance is codetermined by the mother's projections and the infant's reactions to them (Robert-Tissot et al., 1996). Treatment involves helping parents to understand the relationship between childhood experiences and current behavior as caregivers. In addition, the unconditional support of the therapeutic relationship affords a corrective attachment experience for the parent. These changes permit parents to respond more effectively to the needs and emotions of their infant.

Interaction guidance (McDonough, Chapter 31, this volume) also focuses on parents' perceptions of and responses to their infants; however, the emphasis is on observed interactional sequences rather than unconscious representations arising from past experience. The clinician assists parents in interpreting accurately the infant's signals (e.g., differentiating between anger and distress) and determining appropriate reactions to these cues. By providing an environment that is optimal for the formation of secure attachment, the parents and clinician maximize the child's ability to form a harmonious, reciprocal emotional bond, not only with the parent but with siblings, peers, and other adults.

Approaches that target parental responsiveness provide a cornerstone for the treatment of aggression in the first year. However, the clinician should remain sensitive to attachment issues beyond the first birthday and may choose to implement the foregoing strategies in combination with treatments that are appropriate for older infants. The work of Greenberg and Speltz (1988) illustrates how learning theory and attachment conceptualizations may be integrated in the treatment of early conduct problems.

Discipline Practices

Discipline practices become increasingly important in shaping infants' behavior in the second and third years. Support is accumulating for a hypothesis that states that the manner in which parents impose and enforce limits has important implications for the development of aggression (Patterson, 1982; Webster-Stratton & Herbert, 1994). Parent management training seeks to change discipline practices that may inadvertently foster and maintain young children's use of aggression (Webster-Stratton & Herbert, 1994). Because treatment targets specific patterns of reinforcement that occur within a family, it is important to make a detailed assessment of parent–child interactions, preferably in the home environment. A central focus in parent management training is helping caregivers to avoid the development of coercive interactions, wherein parent and child each employs increasingly aversive behaviors in an attempt to control the outcome of discipline encounters. In service of this goal, parents learn to observe their infant's behavior in an objective, unemotional manner and to implement appropriate consequences in response to aggression.

Time out is a useful discipline technique because it curtails negative parent–child interchanges while ensuring that aggressive behavior goes unrewarded. Time out may be used with infants as young as 18 months and can be implemented in the same fashion as with older children, but for shorter durations (a minute per year of the child). Parents should warn infants in advance about the unacceptability and consequences of aggressive behavior. When aggression occurs, the infant is removed immediately to an area in which alternative stimulation is not available. Time out should be used judiciously. Less extreme misbehavior may desist in the absence of parental attention. The clinician can discuss with parents which behaviors merit time out and which may be ignored and should emphasize the importance of applying these criteria consistently. Finally, parents should learn to identify behaviors that indicate that the infant may soon become aggressive (e.g., physical signs of anger or frustration) and events that serve as triggers. It may be possible to intervene before aggression occurs.

Just as parent management training shows caregivers how to make aggressive behavior less worthwhile for their infant, parents also learn to increase the frequency of prosocial behavior through the use of positive reinforcement (Webster-Stratton & Herbert, 1994). The clinician can aid parents in identifying and monitoring desired behaviors, choosing appropriate reinforcers (e.g., praise and treats) and providing rewards in a consistent fashion. Social modeling affords a second method for increasing prosocial behavior. Parents and siblings should be encouraged to use appropriate problem-solving strategies in dealing with one another.

Family Adversity

The clinician may find that parents are unable to comply with treatment recommendations. If this occurs, it is possible that the family's social resources are too overwhelmed by the challenges of daily life to permit significant change. For instance, there may be too many family members and too little privacy for parents to provide one-on-one attention for the infant. A parent's depression may prevent him or her from instituting time-out procedures in a consistent manner. Or the neighborhood may be so dangerous that parents are unwilling to become less restrictive with their children. Factors that may interfere with treatment should be examined carefully during the assessment period. Home visits are particularly useful in making an accurate evaluation of family adversity and offer the clinician a chance to observe the circumstances in which aggression occurs.

Multisystemic therapy (MST), a treatment approach developed by Henggeler and Bourdin (1990), provides a useful framework for addressing contextual processes that adversely affect parent and child functioning. Originally used with conduct-disordered adolescents, preliminary efforts are under way to apply MST to infants and their families (Pickrel, 1997). Rather than applying a single therapeutic technique, MST draws from a variety of treatment modalities. For example, a multisystemic treatment plan may include family-based interventions (e.g., structural family therapy) to increase family cohesion and decrease hostility, as well as more concrete assistance with problems of living, such as helping the family find adequate housing, in addition to the infant–parent approaches described previously.

Depending on the type and severity of challenges the family faces, the clinician can provide needed services and/or put the family in contact with appropriate agencies. The clinician should evaluate the effects of the services on parental functioning throughout the course of treatment and introduce appropriate adjustments as needed.

Interventions Outside Therapy

Infants in their second or third year may be aggressive in a variety of settings, such as day care or play groups. Individuals in contact with an aggressive infant in these contexts can augment the efforts of the clinician and the child's family by becoming active participants in the ongoing treatment of aggression. The clinician should consult with and instruct these individuals on how to develop and maintain appropriate interventions to reduce the infant's aggressive behavior. The clinician can also provide those involved with the support to continue during difficult times.

As noted in the section on parent management training, the young child may have learned to use aggression to gain control over the environment. Thus, one way adults in the infant's life can help to reduce aggressive behavior is by being consistent in when and how they afford the control the infant seeks. Praise and rewards should be given for periods in which no aggression occurs. Equally important are others' responses to aggression by the in-

fant. Adults should carefully avoid giving in to demands accompanied by aggression or threats of force and should be prepared to respond to aggressive behavior using consequences agreed on in advance by members of the treatment group. The clinician and members of the treatment network should review periodically the consequences of both prosocial and aggressive behavior so that they are understood by all parties and can be modified according to the infant's progress.

CASE ILLUSTRATION

The following example is based on a composite of several clinical cases. It is presented to illustrate the challenges inherent in meeting the needs of aggressive infants and their families.

Mrs. Amy Williams called the mental health clinic complaining about the destructive behavior of her 2-year-old son, Tommy. Mr. and Mrs. Williams lived in a two-bedroom apartment with their three children: Melissa, age 6; Tommy; and Joan, 7 months old. Mrs. Williams sounded very worried over the phone about Tommy's interactions with herself, Melissa, and Joan. She reported that Tommy had always been a child who became angry easily and took out his frustrations on others physically. This had not been a problem until the past year when he became more physically mobile. Tommy's aggressive behavior reportedly increased following the arrival of Joan, which resulted in less attention from both parents. In the past few months, Tommy had broken several family valuables and toys and had scratched the dining room table and wood floor. On several occasions he had been found pulling forcefully on Joan's legs and arms. Mrs. Williams no longer felt safe leaving Tommy with Joan in the same room unattended. In addition, Tommy responded to his parents' requests to stop destructive or noncompliant behavior with verbal obstinance and physical force. Mrs. Williams reported that her "patience had been growing thin" with Tommy, and believed it had adversely affected her caregiving with the other children and the quality of her marriage. According to Mrs. Williams, Mr. Williams had been helpful when he was home but often arrived from work after dinner around the children's bedtime. When asked about other sources of support, Mrs. Williams stated that she "used to" have two or three close friends, but had had relatively little contact with them since the births of Tommy and Joan. Mr. Williams's parents lived in the area, but Mrs. Williams expressed reluctance about using them for emotional support or child care. Mrs. Williams worked part-time until the arrival of Tommy. Since then, she had been a full-time mother.

An intake session was arranged to gain a better sense of Tommy's problematic behavior, the quality of Tommy's relationships with family members, and the family's coping resources. Mr. Williams was able to attend an early-evening session but expressed concern about being able to attend meetings on a regular basis. With encouragement from the therapist, Mrs. Williams was able to recruit Mr. Williams's mother to babysit Joan during the visit. It is notable that even setting up the initial appointment had tested the family's coping resources (e.g., flexibility from Mr. Williams's employer and making use of extended family for child care).

During the initial part of the interview, Tommy and Melissa were allowed to play with a set of toys in the same room to observe Tommy's behavior with his elder sibling. In addition to evaluating the quality of the sibling relationship, the free-play procedure provided an opportunity to observe how the parents responded to the children's conflict, should it arise. Based on Mrs. Williams's report, the therapist was confident that Tommy would act aggressively toward Melissa during the session. After 10 minutes, during which time the children had become involved in pretend play with action figures, Tommy became upset about a statement made by Melissa acting as "Batgirl." In response, Tommy forcefully removed Batgirl from Melissa's hand, threw the toy against the wall, and hit Melissa on the arm. Both parents simultaneously looked at each other, then at the therapist for assistance, following which Mr. Williams forcefully picked up Tommy while yelling and moved him to the couch beside his parents. Tommy responded by calling Mr. Williams several unflattering names and only allowed his father to pick him up after continued physical and verbal resistance. After a few minutes, Tommy was allowed to return to play with the action figures. However, after this sequence of events repeated itself two more times during the next 20 minutes, he was instructed to play in a different part of the room from his sister.

When not dealing with Tommy's disruptive behavior, the parents discussed their troubles in dealing with Tommy. A pattern was described in which Tommy "got inside" each parent emotionally, eliciting a punitive response. Mr. Williams confirmed having felt this way earlier in the session. The pattern was similar to Patterson's (1982) coercive cycle, in which parents and child reinforced the aversive behavior of the other, leading to an escalation of the problem behavior.

The therapist also examined the history of Tommy's attachment to the parents, particularly prior to the arrival of Joan. In comparison to Melissa, Mrs. Williams described Tommy as more difficult to "connect with" as a young infant, a pattern that persisted during his first year. Since he was approximately 15 months old, she had found herself spending most of her time reprimanding Tommy for dangerous or aggressive behavior. Mrs. Williams stated that she still had positive interactions with Tommy, but these had become more fleeting in the past 6 months. She also reported feeling guilty about not being able to provide Tommy with enough attention since the arrival of Joan. Mr. Williams also expressed remorse about his inability to assist more with child care but felt he had no other choice given his job demands. When the therapist inquired about working different hours or slightly shorter days, he expressed doubts about his employer's willingness to reduce his hours and concern about the possible financial consequences for the family. However, he said he would consider the option given the situation. The Williamses also agreed that dealing with Tommy had affected their own relationship adversely, particularly their ability to support one another.

Assessment Findings

The Williams family faced several issues typical of infants with aggressive behavior problems. These included an aggressive child who had previously shown a tendency to become angry easily, parenting discipline strategies that had unintentionally exacerbated the child's aggressive behavior and further compromised the quality of the relationship between parents and child, a marital relationship that was "on edge," and limited use of support from friends and relatives. In addition, the family was facing a normative developmental transition with the arrival of Joan. Older siblings often regressed to behavior typical of younger children in response to the depletion of parental attention necessitated by the newborn's birth.

Treatment Selection

A multifaceted treatment package was designed which incorporated elements from several modalities. Treatment included components from Webster-Stratton's and Patterson's parent-training approaches, Lieberman and Pawl's (1993) infant–parent psychotherapy, and Minuchin's (1974) structural family therapy. Before the therapist sought to implement change, a concerted effort was made to place the family's issues in a normative developmental context. Without minimizing the seriousness of Tommy's problems and the parents' distress, the family was informed of how typical behavior problem issues were for older siblings of newborns. Then, before addressing discipline techniques, an effort was made to improve the quality of the relationship between Tommy and his parents. Patterson (personal communication, January 15, 1993) has suggested that by encouraging parents to be more warm and reinforcing, it increases their "bank account" with the child. There are various reasons for parents to resist being warm with their infants. In some instances, parents may be inexperienced in reading and/or responding effectively to infant cues. In cases such as this one, in which the child has come to be seen as unmanageable, parents may become "blocked" from interacting in a warm manner because of "battle scars" from their experience with the child. Thus, it was necessary for the therapist to play an active role in modeling warm and responsive behavior to show the parents that Tommy was still capable of reciprocating in a positive manner. Once over their initial hesitation, both parents approached Tommy in a friendly, engaging manner. The second session was facilitated by having Mr. Williams's mother watch both Melissa and Joan, providing an hour of undivided attention for Tommy with his parents.

Discipline issues also were addressed in the latter half of the second session. Following guidelines recommended by Webster-Stratton and Herbert (1994), the parents were instructed to intervene with Tommy in a more objective, unemotional manner and to use discipline techniques that decreased the emotional valence of their interactions. Consistency and firmness were emphasized, but given the Williams's admitted reactivity to Tommy, significance was

placed on the emotional tenor of their delivery; the parents must simultaneously demonstrate that aggressive behavior would not be tolerated or modeled in administering punishment. At the end of the session, Tommy was recruited to help the parents in practicing a 2-minute time-out procedure, agreeing to engage in a pretend fight with the therapist to elicit a calm parental response. The therapist and parents also brainstormed about behaviors Tommy displayed when he was about to act aggressively so they might intervene prior to more explosive outbursts.

Both relational and discipline issues were revisited each week. At the same time, the therapist explored how intra- and extrafamilial resources could be better used. These included interventions designed to improve the quality of relations between Mr. and Mrs. Williams, provide child-care assistance for Mrs. Williams, and use extrafamilial sources of support for both Mrs. and Mr. Williams. To improve the Williams's relationship, couple sessions were held every fourth week to discuss parenting and marital issues. Mr. Williams's mother continued to provide child care during therapy sessions and also during weekend evenings so the Williamses could spend time alone. Mr. Williams arranged his schedule to make three out of four monthly sessions. Mr. Williams's mother also attended two sessions to improve consistency in the administration of discipline practices. After initial resistance, the elder Mrs. Williams agreed to use time outs with Tommy when she cared for him in her son's house (but not necessarily in her own house). Mr. Williams also negotiated more family-friendly work hours at a slight financial cost to the family. As a result, Mr. Williams arrived home at 5:00 P.M. two days a week, prior to the witching hours of parental care before bedtime. Finally, both Mr. and Mrs. Williams were encouraged to spend time with adult friends individually on occasion (once every 3 weeks) to provide external support.

Treatment progressed in a two-steps-forward-one-step-back manner. After responding initially to the increased positive attention and more consistent and less emotionally laden discipline, Tommy's behavior improved. However, after 2 weeks, Tommy's behavior deteriorated. The parents were encouraged to stay with the regimen, particularly continuing to approach Tommy proactively in a warm manner and maintaining a calm demeanor when administering discipline. During subsequent weeks, Tommy's behavior showed gradual improvement with fewer and less extreme bouts of aggressive behavior. After 14 weeks of therapy, his behavior had improved sufficiently to reduce meetings to monthly check-ups. Treatment was successfully concluded 6 months after the initial intake.

SUMMARY

This chapter has described the current state of knowledge on aggressive behavior problems during infancy. Despite cognitive limitations in fully understanding aggression and the high frequency of the behavior, aggression during infancy shows comparable stability and similar correlates to aggressive behavior at older age periods during childhood. The implications of these findings are that prevention and intervention efforts need to be directed at similar targets as they are for older children, with special attention to parent–child relationships. Given infant's greater dependence on relationships in the home, approaches that reinforce responsive caregiving and consistent, even-tempered discipline practices and address factors that affect parental functioning appear the most logical. A case example illustrated how successful intervention might be implemented. It is recommended that an ecologically based treatment package be employed to deal with the multiple challenges facing families with aggressive infants.

ACKNOWLEDGMENTS

The research reported in this chapter was supported by Grant Nos. MH 46925 and MH 50907 to Daniel Shaw from the National Institute of Mental Health.

REFERENCES

Achenbach, T. M. (1992). *Manual for the Child Behavior Checklist 2/3 and 1992 profile.* Burlington, VT: University of Vermont Department of Psychiatry.

American Psychiatric Association. (1994). *Diagnostic and statistical manual of mental disorders.* (4th ed.). Washington DC: Author.

Ausubel, D. P. (1958). *Theory and problems of child development.* New York: Grune & Stratton.

Bandura, A. (1979). Psychological mechanisms of aggression. In M. von Cranach, K. Foppa, W. Lepenies, & D. Ploog (Eds.), *Human ethology: Claims and limits of a new discipline* (pp. 316–356). Cambridge: Cambridge University Press.

Bates, J. E., Maslin, C. A., & Frankel, K. A. (1985). Attachment security, mother-child interaction, and temperament as predictors of behavior-problem ratings at age three years. In I. Bretherton & E. Waters (Eds.), Growing points of attachment theory and research. *Monographs of the Society for Research in Child Development, 50*(1–2), 167–193.

Belsky, J. Hsich, K., & Crnic, K. (1998). Mothering, fathering, and infant negativity as antecedents of boys' externalizing problems and inhibition at age 3 years: Differential susceptibility to rearing experience? *Development and Psychopathology, 10,* 301–320.

Bronson, W. C. (1975). Developments in behavior with age mates during the second year of life. In M. Lewis & L. A. Rosenblum (Eds.), *The origins of behavior: Friendship and peer relations* (pp. 131–153). New York: Wiley.

Bowlby, J. (1969). *Attachment and loss: Vol. 1. Attachment.* New York: Basic Books.

Burchinal, M. R., Follmer, A., & Bryant, D. M. (1996). The relations of maternal support and family structure with maternal responsiveness and child outcomes among African American families. *Developmental Psychology, 32,* 1073–1083.

Buss, A. H. (1961). *The psychology of aggression.* New York: Wiley.

Calkins, S. (1994). Origins and outcomes of individual differences in emotion regulation. In N. A. Fox (Ed.), The development of emotion regulation: Biological and behavioral considerations. *Monographs of the Society for Research in Child Development, 59*(2–3, Serial No. 231), 53–72.

Campbell, S. B. (1990). *Behavior problems in preschool children: Clinical and developmental issues.* New York: Guilford Press.

Campbell, S. B. (1994). Hard-to-manage preschool boys: Externalizing behavior, social competence, and family context at two-year-follow-up. *Journal of Abnormal Child Psychology, 22,* 147–166.

Cole, P. M., Michel, M. K., & Teti, L. (1994). The development of emotional regulation and dysregulation. In N. A. Fox (Ed.), The development of emotion regulation: Biological and behavioral considerations. *Monographs of the Society for Research in Child Development, 59*(Serial No. 240), 73–100.

Cummings, E. M., Iannotti, R. J., & Zahn-Waxler, C., (1989). Aggression between peers in early childhood: Individual continuity and developmental change. *Child Development, 72,* 887–895.

Dadds, M. R., & Powell, M. B. (1991). The relationship of interparental conflict and global marital adjustment to aggression and immaturity in aggressive and nonclinic children. *Journal of Abnormal Child Psychology, 19,* 553–567.

Dollard, J., Doob, L. W., Miller, N. E., Mowrer, O. H., & Sears, R. R. (1939). *Frustration and aggression.* New Haven: Yale University Press.

Dunn, J., & Kendrick,, C. (1982). *Siblings: Love, envy, and understanding.* Cambridge, MA: Harvard University Press.

Erickson, M. F., Sroufe, L. A., & Egeland, B. (1985). The relationship between quality of attachment and behavior problems in preschool in a high-risk sample. In I. Bretherton & E. Waters (Eds.), Growing points of attachment theory and research. *Monographs of the Society for Research in Child Development, 50*(1–2, Serial No. 209), 147–167.

Fagot, B., & Kavanaugh, K. (1993). Parenting during the second year: Effects of children's age, sex, and attachment classification. *Child Development, 64,* 258–271.

Fagot, B., & Leve, L. D. (1998). Teacher ratings of externalizing behaivor at school entry for boys and girls: Similar early predictors and different correlates. *Journal of Child Psychology and Psychiatry, 39,* 555–566.

Gable, S., Belsky, J., & Crnic, K. (1992). Marriage, parenting, and child development: Progress and prospects. *Journal of Family Psychology, 5,* 276–294.

Gardner, F. E. (1987). Positive interaction between mothers and conduct-problem children: Is there training for harmony as well as fighting? *Journal of Abnormal Child Psychology, 15,* 283–293.

Goodenough, F. L. (1931). *Anger in young children.* Minneapolis: University of Minnesota Press.

Greenberg, M. T., & Speltz, M. L. (1988). Contributions of attachment theory to the understanding of conduct problems during the preschool years. J. Belsky & T. Negworski (Eds.), *Clinical implications of attachment* (pp. 177–218). Hillsdale, NJ: Erlbaum.

Grusec, J., & Goodnow, J. (1994). Impact of parental discipline methods on the child's internalization of values: A reconceptualization of current points of view. *Developmental Psychology, 30,* 4–19.

Grusec, J. E., & Lytton, H. (1988). *Social development.* New York: Springer-Verlag.

Henggeler, S. W., & Bourdin, C. M. (1990). *Family therapy and beyond: A multisystemic approach to treating the behavior problems of children and adolescents.* Pacific Grove, CA: Brooks/Cole.

Jersild, A. T., & Markey, F. V. (1935). Conflicts between preschool children. *Child Development, 21,* 170–181.

Jouriles, E., Murphy, C., & O'Leary, K. D. (1989). Interspousal aggression, marital discord, and child problems. *Journal of Consulting and Clinical Psychology, 57,* 453–455.

Kaufman, J., Birmaher, B., Brent, D., Rao, U., Ryan, N., Flynn, C., & Moreci, P. (1997). The Schedule for Affective Disorders and Schizophrenia for School-Aged Children: Present and lifetime version—Initial reliability and validity data. *Journal of the American Academy of Child and Adolescent Psychiatry, 36,* 980–988.

Keenan, K., & Shaw, D. S. (1994). The development of aggression in toddlers: A study of low-income families. *Journal of Abnormal Child Psychology, 22,* 53–77.

Keenan, K., Shaw, D. S., Delliquadri, E., Giovannelli, J., & Walsh, B. (1998). Evidence for the continuity of early problem behaviors: Application of a developmental model. *Journal of Abnormal Child Psychology, 26,* 441–454.

Kuczynski, L., & Kochanska, G. (1990). Development of children's noncompliance strategies from toddlerhood to age 5. *Developmental Psychology, 26*(3), 398–408.

Lieberman, A. F., & Pawl, J. H. (1993). Infant–parent psychotherapy. In C. H. Zeanah, Jr. (Ed.), *Handbook of infant mental health* (pp. 427–442). New York: Guilford Press.

Loeber, R., & Stouthamer-Loeber, M. (1986). Family factors as correlates and predictors of juvenile conduct problems and delinquency. In M. Tonry & N. Morris (Eds.), *Crime and justice: An annual review of research* (Vol. 7). Chicago: University of Chicago Press.

Lyons-Ruth, K. (1996). Attachment relationships among children with aggressive behavior problems: The role of disorganized early attachment patterns. *Journal of Consulting and Clinical Psychology, 64,* 572–585.

Maccoby, E. E. (1980). *Social development.* New York: Harcourt Brace.

Martin, J. (1981). A longitudinal study of the consequences of early mother–infant interaction: A microanalytic approach. *Monographs of the Society for Research in Child Development, 46,* (Serial No. 190).

Mash, E., & Johnston, C. (1983). Parental perceptions of child behavior problems, parenting self-esteem, and mothers' reported stress in younger and older hyperactive and normal children. *Journal of Consulting and Clinical Psychology, 51,* 86–99.

Maziade, M., Cote, R., Bernier, H., Boutin, P., & Thivierge, J. (1989). Significance of extreme temperament in infancy for clinical status in preschool years. *British Journal of Psychiatry, 154,* 544–551.

Minuchin, S. (1974). *Families and family therapy.* Cambridge, MA: Harvard University Press

Owens, E. B. (1998). *Resilience to chronic psychosocial stressors: A longitudinal study of preschool-aged boys at risk for developing externalizing behavior problems.* Unpublished doctoral dissertation, University of Pittsburgh.

Patterson, G. (1982). *Coercive family processes* (Vol. 3). Eugene, OR: Castalia.

Piaget, J. (1952). *The origins of intelligence in children.* New York: International Universities Press.

Pickrel, S. (1997). *Multisystemic therapy for infant, toddlers, and their families.* Presentation at Zero to Three 12th National Training Institute, Nashville, TN.

Raine, A. (1997). Antisocial behavior and psychophysiology: A biosocial perspective and a prefrontal dysfunctio hypothesis. In D. Stoff, J. Breiling, & J. D. Maser (Eds.), *Handbook of antisocial behavior* (pp. 289–304). New York: Wiley.

Reid, J. B. (1993). Prevention of conduct disorder before and after school entry: Relating interventions to developmental findings. Toward a developmental perspective on conduct disorder [Special issue]. *Development and Psychopathology, 5,* 243–262.

Renken, B., Egeland, B., Marvinney, D., Mangelsdorf, S., & Sroufe, A. (1989). Early childhood antecedents of aggression and passive withdrawal in early elementary school. *Journal of Personality, 57,* 257–281.

Richman, M., Stevenson, J., & Graham, P. J. (1982).

Preschool to school: A behavioral study. London: Academic Press.

Robert-Tissot, C., Cramer, B., Stern, D. N., Serpa, S. A., Bachmann, J., Palacio-Espasa, F., Knauer, D., De Muralt, M., Berney, C., & Mendiguren, G. (1996). Outcome evaluation in brief mother–infant psychotherapies: Report on 75 cases. *Infant Mental Health Journal, 17,* 97–114.

Robins, L. N., West, P., & Herjanic, B., (1975). Arrests and delinquency in two generations: A study of black urban families and their children. *Journal of Child Psychology and Psychiatry, 16,* 125–140.

Rose, S. L., Rose, S. A., & Feldman, J. F. (1989). Stability of behavior problems in very young children. *Development and Psychopathology, 1,* 5–19.

Rothbart, M. K., Ahadi, S. A., & Hershey, K. L. (1994). Temperament and social behavior in childhood. *Merrill–Palmer Quarterly, 40,* 21–39.

Rutter, M. (1997). Antisocial behavior: Developmental psychopathology perspectives. In D. Stoff, J. Breiling, & J. D. Maser, (Eds.), *Handbook of antisocial behavior* (pp. 115–124). New York: Wiley.

Rutter, M., Cox, A., Tupling, C., Berger, M., & Yule, W. (1975). Attainment and adjustment in two geographical areas: 1. The prevalence of psychiatric disorder. *British Journal of Psychiatry, 126,* 493–509.

Sameroff, A. J., Seifer, R., Barocas, R., Zax, M., & Greenspan, S. (1987). IQ scores of 4-year-old children: Social–environmental risk factors. *Pediatrics, 79,* 343–350.

Sanson, A., Oberklaid, F., Pedlow, R., & Prior, M. (1991). Risk indicators: Assessment of infancy predictors of pre-school behavioural maladjustment. *Journal of Child Psychology and Psychiatry, 32,* 609–626.

Shaw, D. S., & Bell, R. Q. (1993). Developmental theories of parental contributors to antisocial behavior. *Journal of Abnormal Child Psychology, 21,* 493–518.

Shaw, D. S., Keenan, K., & Vondra, J. I. (1994). Developmental precursors of externalizing behavior: Ages 1 to 3. *Developmental Psychology, 30,* 355–364.

Shaw, D. S., Owens, E. B., Vondra, J. I., Keenan, K. & Winslow, E. B. (1996). Early risk factors and pathways in the development of early disruptive behavior problems. *Development and Psychopathology, 8,* 679–699.

Shaw, D. S., Winslow, E. B., Owens, E. B., & Hood, N. (1998). Young children's adjustment to chronic family adversity: A longitudinal study of low-income families. *Journal of the American Academy of Child and Adolescent Psychiatry, 37,* 545–553.

Shaw, D. S., Winslow, E. B., Owens, E. B., Vondra, J. I., Cohn, J. F., & Bell, R. Q. (1998). The development of early externalizing problems among children from low-income families: A transformational perspective. *Journal of Abnormal Child Psychology, 26,* 95–107.

Sroufe, L. A. (1983). Infant–caregiver attachment and patterns of adaptation in preschool: The roots of maladaption and competence. In M. Perlmutter (Ed.), *Minnesota symposium in child psychology* (Vol. 16, pp. 41–81). Hillsdale, NJ: Erlbaum.

Sroufe, L. A., & Rutter, M. (1984). The domain of developmental psychopathology. *Child Development, 55,* 17–29.

Tremblay, R. (1998). *On the origins of physical aggression.* Paper presented at the meeting of the Life History Society, Seattle, WA.

van IJzendoorn, M. H., Schuengel, C., & Bakermans-Kranenburg, M. J. (1999). Disorganized attachment in early childhood: Meta-analysis of precursors, concomitant, and sequelae. *Development and Psychopathology, 11,* 225–250.

Webster-Stratton, C. (1990). Long-term follow-up of families with young conduct problem children: From preschool to grade school. *Journal of Clinical Child Psychology, 19,* 144–149.

Webster-Stratton, C., & Herbert, M. (1994). *Troubled families, problem children: Working with parents: A collaborative process.* Chichester, UK: Wiley.

Zahn-Waxler, C., Iannotti, R. J., Cummings, E. M., & Denham, S. (1990). Antecedents of problem behaviors in children of depressed mothers. *Development and Psychopathology, 2,* 271–292.

Zeanah, C. H., Boris, N. W., & Scheeringa, M. S. (1997). Psychopathology in infancy. *Journal of Child and Adolescent Psychology, 38,* 81–99.

26

Gender Identity Disorder

❖

KENNETH J. ZUCKER
SUSAN J. BRADLEY

As a point of departure, it might be worth asking why a chapter on gender identity disorder (GID) is included in a volume concerned with infant mental health? Two rationales may suffice. First, there is now little doubt that gender is a rather substantive, perhaps paramount, part of the emerging self (Stoller, 1968); thus, to ignore gender during late infancy and early toddlerhood misses out on something important. Second, normative studies show that aspects of the phenotypical expression of gender identity typically emerge between the ages of 2 and 3 years (Ruble & Martin, 1998), if not earlier in intellectually precocious toddlers. As noted later, the behavioral signs of GID often emerge during this same chronological time frame, thus implicating late infancy and early toddlerhood as crucial for understanding its genesis. It is probably for this reason that GID was included as a primary diagnosis in the recently published *Diagnostic Classification of Mental Health and Developmental Disorders of Infancy and Early Childhood* (Zero to Three, 1994), the criteria for which were borrowed from the fourth edition of the *Diagnostic and Statistical Manual of Mental Disorders* (DSM-IV; American Psychiatric Association, 1994).

PHENOMENOLOGY

Boys and girls diagnosed with GID show both a strong preference for sex-typed behaviors more characteristic of the opposite sex and a rejec-

tion or avoidance of sex-typed behaviors more characteristic of their own sex. In addition, such youngsters also express a strong desire to be of the opposite sex and often verbalize their unhappiness about being boys or girls. The behaviors that characterize GID occur in concert, not in isolation. It is this behavioral patterning that is of clinical significance, and recognizing it is extremely important in conducting a diagnostic assessment. Table 26.1 shows the DSM-IV diagnostic criteria for GID. For a discussion of the reliability and validity of the DSM criteria and consideration of extant assessment procedures, both of which have been reviewed in detail elsewhere, see Zucker (1992), Zucker and Bradley (1995), and Zucker et al. (1998).

At the time of assessment, parents sometimes remark that their child had behaved in a cross-gendered manner "since day one." Upon questioning, what parents usually mean is that their child first displayed cross-gender behaviors once they were old enough to engage in particular sex-dimorphic activities (e.g., toy play and dress-up play). Most typically, this is during the toddler and preschool years (2 to 4 years).

Identity statements and cross-dressing are two of the more commonly first-noticed behaviors reported by parents. For example, some parents recall that when their child was between 2 and 3 years old, gender self-labeling was of the opposite sex or that there seemed to be a period of prolonged gender identity confusion; for example, one mother of a 4-year-old boy

TABLE 26.1. DSM-IV Diagnostic Criteria for Gender Identity Disorder

A. A strong and persistent cross-gender identification (not merely a desire for any perceived cultural advantages of being the other sex).

In children, the disturbance is manifested by at least four (or more) of the following:

(1) repeatedly stated desire to be, or insistence that he or she is, the other sex
(2) in boys, preference for cross-dressing or simulating female attire; in girls, insistence on wearing only stereotypical masculine clothing
(3) strong and persistent preferences for cross-sex roles in make-believe play or persistent fantasies of being the other sex
(4) intense desire to participate in the stereotypical games and pastimes of the other sex
(5) strong preference for playmates of the other sex

B. Persistent discomfort with his or her sex or sense of inappropriateness in the gender role of that sex

In children, the disturbance is manifested by any of the following: in boys, assertion that his penis or testes are disgusting or will disappear or assertion that it would be better not to have a penis, or aversion toward rough-and-tumble play and rejection of male stereotypical toys, games, and activities; in girls, rejection of urinating in a sitting position, assertion that she has or will grow a penis, or assertion that she does not want to grow breasts or menstruate, or marked aversion toward normative female clothing.

C. The disturbance is not concurrent with a physical intersex condition.

D. The disturbance causes clinically significant distress or impairment in social, occupational, or other important areas of functioning.

Note. From American Psychiatric Association (1994). Copyright 1994 by the American Psychiatric Association. Reprinted by permission. Only criteria for children are listed.

(IQ = 103) recalled that "he would say things like 'I'm a girl' . . . [it] took a lot to convince him [that] he was a boy . . . [he] didn't want to believe that he would grow up to be a man." Other parents report that, although they could not remember a period of errors in self-labeling, their child was "always" expressing the desire to be of the opposite sex.

Several years ago, we developed a 12-item structured gender identity interview for children (Zucker, Bradley, Lowry Sullivan, et al., 1993). Factor analysis identified two factors, which were labeled "Cognitive Gender Confusion" and "Affective Gender Confusion," respectively. Portions of an interview with a 5-year-old boy (IQ = 95) illustrate:

Interviewer (I): Are you a boy or a girl?

Child (C): Girl.

I: Are you a boy?

C: No.

I: When you grow up, will you be a mommy or a daddy?

C: A mom.

I: Could you ever grow up to be a daddy?

C: Sometimes.

I: Are there any good things about being a boy?

C: No.

I: Are there any things that you don't like about being a boy?

C: Yes.

I: Tell me some of the things that you don't like about being a boy.

C: I don't like being a boy Power Ranger and I don't like being a boy pig or something, like an animal. I like being a girl, girls are better. . . .

I: In your mind, do you ever think that you would like to be a girl?

C: Yes.

I: Can you tell me why?

C: 'Cause it's funner [*sic*] and you can fling your hair around and do it in ponytails and pigtails. . . .

The interview contains two additional questions, in which the child is asked about parents' prenatal gender preference:

I: When you were in your mom's tummy, do you think she wanted you to be a boy or a girl?

C: Girl.

I: When you were in your mom's tummy, do you think your dad wanted you to be a boy or a girl?

C: Girl.

I: What do you think about that?

C: Maybe 'cause girls are good and boys are bad . . . all these boys are bad . . . you get the point of mine?

Cross-dressing is probably the most common early sign of GID *in statu nascendi*. In toddlerhood, the use of the mother's clothes by boys is very common, including high-heeled shoes, wigs, dresses, jewelry, and makeup. In Green's (1987) study, the modal time of onset of cross-dressing was between ages 2 and 3. Although these boys invariably wear conventional masculine clothing in social settings, typically they spend hours in the dress-up center at day care or nursery school wearing feminine apparel. Indeed, some teachers report that it is difficult to convince the boy to engage in alternative activities, even if they are gender neutral.

In girls, it is common for parents to report that during the toddlerhood or preschool years their daughters began to reject wearing stereotypical feminine clothing. In some cases, this coincides with the girl's gender self-labeling as a boy or the expression of the wish to be a boy. In other cases, particularly in girls who are less verbally expressive, the marked aversion toward normative feminine clothing, at least in retrospect, was the first behavioral sign of gender identity conflict. The preference of these girls for a masculine style of dress does not simply result from a desire for more comfortable clothing (e.g., slacks or sweatpants, which many girls wear in social settings for this reason) but appears to be associated with the marked distress about being a girl. Some parents report that asking their daughters to wear stereotypical feminine clothing on special occasions gives rise to intense, catastrophic temper tantrums. Many of the girls also demand that their hair be cut extremely short, which results in the phenotypical social appearance of a boy; indeed, it is common for girls with GID to be perceived by others as boys because of their hairstyle and clothing style (for a more extended discussion of the physical appearance of both boys and girls with GID, see Fridell, Zucker, Bradley, & Maing, 1996; McDermid, Zucker, Bradley, & Maing, 1998; Zucker, Wild, Bradley, & Lowry, 1993).

Apart from the GID itself, these children also show other behavioral problems; for example, on measures such as the Child Behavior Checklist (CBCL) and the Teacher's Report Form, clinic-referred boys and girls with GID have significantly more general behavioral problems than their siblings and normal children. Compared to demographically matched clinical controls, they have similar levels of behavioral problems. On the CBCL, boys with GID show a predominance of internalizing behavioral difficulties, whereas girls with GID do not (Zucker & Bradley, 1995). Boys with GID have also been found to show high rates of separation anxiety traits (Coates & Person, 1985; Zucker, Bradley, & Lowry Sullivan, 1996).

DEVELOPMENTAL COURSE

After late infancy and toddlerhood, what is known about the developmental course of GID? From a cross-sectional standpoint, it is clear that GID can be diagnosed at any point during childhood, adolescence, and adulthood. Indeed, among children, the mean age of referral is around 6 or 7 years—this may reflect the fact that, by school age, children with extreme cross-gender behavior are beginning to experience more social ostracism within the peer group, which may be an added impetus for parents to seek out a clinical assessment (Zucker, Bradley, & Sanikhani, 1997). Almost all youngsters who are seen for the first time during middle or late childhood will have had an onset of cross-gender behaviors and feelings during late infancy or toddlerhood.

The same early-onset developmental pattern also holds among adolescents, who often present with the request for both hormonal and surgical sex reassignment, and with whom it is even more apparent that the cross-gender behaviors and feelings have not remitted over time (Cohen-Kettenis & van Goozen, 1997; Zucker & Bradley, 1995). It should, however, be noted that such adolescents represent an extreme subgroup, because follow-up studies of children suggest a more variable outcome:

1. Like those youngsters assessed for the first time in adolescence, a small minority of youngsters who were assessed in childhood and then followed over time remain gender dysphoric and eventually seek out physical sex transformation procedures during adolescence

or young adulthood. Such youngsters invariably report an attraction to members of their own biological sex but characterize their sexual identity as "heterosexual," not "homosexual," because of their cross-gender identification.

2. Some youngsters, probably the majority, show a partial diminution of cross-gender behaviors during childhood, but the gender dysphoric feelings remit entirely. Many of the youngsters that constitute this subgroup report a homosexual sexual orientation by late adolescence (Green, 1987).

3. Other youngsters, also a minority, show an almost complete diminution of cross-gender behaviors in childhood, and the gender-dysphoric feelings remit entirely. Many of the youngsters in this group report a heterosexual sexual orientation by late adolescence.

RISK FACTORS

Risk factors are variables that predispose an individual to psychiatric disorder (and, more broadly, to behavioral problems and maladaptation). Regarding GID, the study of putative risk factors has been rather piecemeal, with various investigators examining selected variables of interest. Proposed integrative models have been largely descriptive (e.g., Coates & Wolfe, 1995; Green, 1987; Stoller, 1968; Zucker & Bradley, 1995), rather than based on formal statistical approaches, as in experimental epidemiology or path analysis. In this section, we discuss some of the factors identified in the literature believed to be associated with an increased "risk" for the development of GID. Following O'Connor and Rutter (1996), we attempt also to characterize the putative risk mechanism.

Risk Factors in the Child

A Sensitive Period for Gender Identity Formation?

Over four decades ago, Money, Hampson, and Hampson (1957), influenced by the emerging discipline of ethology and the phenomenon of imprinting, suggested that there was a process analogous to a critical period in the formation of gender identity, beginning some time after birth and up to around the age of 18–24 months. Since then, the critical period construct has been the subject of a great deal of empirical scrutiny, and the concept of a "sensitive" or an "optimal" period was introduced to expand the window of time in which certain environmental experiences might exert their greatest impact, but without the irreversibility that was believed to characterize critical periods (e.g., Bornstein, 1989; Hess, 1973).

The claim that there is a sensitive period for gender identity formation suggests a certain malleability or plasticity in which gender identity differentiation can move in one direction or another, but after some imprecisely defined window of time, this becomes more difficult. Such malleability would suggest that all children are at risk for developing a gender identity discordant with their biological sex.

Along similar lines, Coates, Friedman, and Wolfe (1991) have argued that there is an inherent vulnerability to gender identity confusion because children need to acquire a stable cognitive representation and understanding of gender invariance, which typically does not occur until the preschool years or older (Kohlberg, 1966). Because this developmental task is required of all children, it lacks specificity in explaining why only a very small number of children develop GID; thus, such cognitive vulnerability may be a necessary but not sufficient condition for GID to occur. Nonetheless, cross-sectional data suggest that children with GID may well have a "developmental lag" in gender constancy acquisition compared to demographically matched controls (Zucker, Bradley, Kuksis, et al., in press).

The concepts of a sensitive period and a co-occurring cognitive vulnerability are intriguing because we know that GID almost invariably develops at a time when the cognitive understanding of gender is in its most rudimentary form. Although the sensitive period construct has not been subjected to adequate empirical scrutiny vis-à-vis gender identity formation (Meyer-Bahlburg, 1998), it is helpful heuristically in thinking about the genesis of GID.

Sex

Although formal prevalence studies are not available, there is reasonable evidence that boys are referred for gender identity concerns at a much higher rate than are girls—6.6:1 in one study (Zucker, Bradley, & Sanikhani, 1997). If one assumes, for the sake of argument, that this sex disparity in referral rates partially reflects true prevalence rates, what are possible explanations?

Boys and girls with GID invariably do not show any gross evidence for somatic intersexuality; for example, their genitalia are normal in appearance and configuration at birth, which would rule out a marked prenatal hormonal anomaly. Of course, this does not rule out more subtle prenatal hormone variations, particularly with regard to the masculinizing class of androgenic steroids that might influence sex-dimorphic brain differentiation (but not genital differentiation) and then subsequent postnatal sex-dimorphic behavior. One line of experimental research on nonhuman female primates has suggested that such a behavior–genital dissociation can occur (Goy, Bercovitch, & McBrair, 1988), but the applicability of this model to humans is unknown.

Another biological explanation of the possible sex difference in prevalence pertains to maternal immune reactions during pregnancy. The male fetus is experienced by the mother as more "foreign" (antigenic) than the female fetus. Based on studies with lower animals, it has been suggested that one consequence of this antigenicity is that the mother produces antibodies that have the consequence of demasculinizing or feminizing the male fetus, but no corresponding masculinizing or defeminizing of the female fetus (Blanchard & Klassen, 1997). This model would predict that males born later in a sibline might be more affected, because the mother's antigenicity increases with each successive male pregnancy. Thus, it is of interest that boys with GID are, on average, later born, and that this appears to occur largely in relation to the number of older brothers, not older sisters (Blanchard, Zucker, Bradley, & Hume, 1995; Zucker, Green, et al., 1997). At present, however, this proposed mechanism has not been formally tested in humans.

It is, of course, quite tenable that social factors also contribute to the putative sex difference in prevalence. Both classical and neo-Freudian accounts of normative psychosexual differentiation emphasize the importance of same-sex identification. Given the mother's particularly important role in the first few years of life, it has been argued that boys may be at more risk than girls, because they need to "deidentify" from their mothers as part of the process of consolidating a masculine gender identity (Greenson, 1968; Stoller, 1968). Because girls are not in the same position, it is possible that normative gender identity development is more likely to be derailed in boys than in girls.

Temperament

Activity Level and Rough-and-Tumble Play. Activity level (AL) is a commonly accepted dimension of temperament. Regarding children with GID, AL as a risk factor is a promising possibility, because it shows a rather strong sex difference, with boys having a higher AL than girls (Eaton & Enns, 1986). Rough-and-tumble (RT) play bears some similarity to AL in that it is often characterized by high energy expenditure; however, a distinguishing feature of RT play is that it is a social–interactive behavior involving such sequences as "play fighting" and "chasing." Several studies have shown RT play to be more common in boys than in girls, particularly in same-sex groups (Ruble & Martin, 1998).

Using parent-report measures of AL, two studies found that boys with GID had a lower AL than did control boys (Bates, Bentler, & Thompson, 1979; Zucker & Bradley, 1995). Zucker and Bradley (1995) also found that girls with GID had a higher AL than did control girls; indeed, the girls with GID had a higher AL than did the boys with GID, whereas for the controls, the typical sex difference was observed. It is conceivable, therefore, that a sex-atypical AL is a risk factor that predisposes to the development of GID. For example, a low-active boy with GID may find the typical play behavior of other boys to be incompatible with his own behavioral style (cf. Ruble & Martin, 1998), which might make it difficult for him to integrate successfully into a male peer group.

Marked avoidance of RT play is also characteristic of boys with GID (Green, 1974); indeed, aversion toward RT play is part of the Point B criteria for GID in boys (see Table 26.1). Thus, the risk factor would not be aversion of RT play per se, but the factors that predispose to such aversion, such as general behavioral inhibition (Coates, Wolfe, & Hahn-Burke, 1994) or parental traits that might make a boy anxious about engaging in such activity.

Sensory and Interpersonal Sensitivities. Stoller (1968) reported that young boys with GID have a heightened sensitivity to sensory stimuli and apparent artistic (creative) ability. Coates, Hahn-Burke, Wolfe, Shindledecker, and Nierenberg (1994) administered a 19-item sensory reactivity questionnaire (with unknown psychometric properties) to the mothers of 36 boys with GID ages 4 to 6 years and 16 mothers of normal control boys who were comparable in age and social class. Coates et al. (1994) found that the GID boys were judged to be more sensory reactive than the controls boys. For example, more of the GID boys were reactive to both "pretty" and "ugly" colors and to "good" and "bad" odors. Coates, Hahn-Burke, et al. (1994) suggested that such reactivity might be associated with the heightened empathy that they believe is characteristic of boys with GID (Coates et al., 1991). It has been noted, for example, that boys with GID are often quite attuned to their mother's emotional state and well-being. Unfortunately, we do not yet have available an empirical study on empathy in boys with GID, so this intriguing hypothesis remains to be tested.

Risk Factors in the Family

Prenatal Gender Preference

It is common for parents to express a prenatal gender preference. Other things being equal, parents will have a child of the nonpreferred sex about 50% of the time. Are parents of children with GID more likely than control parents to report having had a desire for a child of the opposite sex? The simple answer appears to be no, at least with regard to the mothers of boys with GID (Zucker et al., 1994). We did find, however, that the maternal wish for a girl was significantly associated with the sex composition and birth order of the sibship. Among the GID boys with only older brothers, the percentage of mothers who recalled a desire for a daughter was significantly higher than among the probands with other sibship combinations (e.g., those who had at least one older sister); however, the same pattern was observed in a control group (Zucker et al., 1994).

Although the wish for a daughter per se is not a risk factor, maternal reactions to bearing a child of the nonpreferred sex may be. In our clinical experience, we have observed several quite striking examples of maternal disappointment, which appears to influence the mother's ongoing relationship with her son—it is this factor that may well be the risk mechanism. We have tentatively labeled these reactions examples of maternal *pathological gender mourning*.

Among mothers of boys with GID, Zucker (1996) identified at least 10 possible signs of pathological gender mourning, including severe postpartum depression related to the birth of a son, recurrent nightdreams about being pregnant with a girl, and active cross-dressing of the boy (for further details, see Zucker & Bradley, 1995; Zucker, Bradley, & Ipp, 1993).

A particularly illuminating example of pathological gender mourning was reflected in diary notes of a mother, who, during her pregnancy with her third-born son, recorded on a regular basis her desire for a girl. The first entry in the diary was:

"I'm not sure how I feel but I think I'm pregnant again.... My nerves are less with the boys [her two other sons]. I yell more and if I'm not preg [*sic*] then I better find out the problem. We prayed directly at the retreat for a girl and I so wish this— if it's not I'll be [accepting] another boy with love."

Many subsequent entries pertained to the mother's strong wish for a daughter. The last entry prior to delivery was:

"[My friend] bought a pair of pink booties . . . she said they were 'in hope.'"

The next entry occurred two weeks after delivery:

"Well little tiny [name of boy], I'm home and feeling somewhat settled.... I'm worn out yelling at the other two boys.... All the neighbours and people that see you say you are an exceptionally beautiful baby boy.... [The doctor] did your circumcision and didn't do a good job, it was like it was half done. You don't look anything like your brothers...."

Three years later, similar entries occurred during the pregnancy with a fourth-born son. Just prior to the delivery, the mother wrote:

"Last week you [the third-born son] and I were shopping and you picked up a little blue denim dress and a bright pink belt . . . you held on to it and said it was for baby Mary [the hoped for daughter].... I bought it. You were so taken by it. I thought it would be nice to give it to the new baby *if* it was a girl."

A few months later, the mother wrote:

"I'm a little afraid of the future. I've noticed you [the third-born son] play what I feel is too much of house where you *always* are the lady figure. It got to the point you'd take a towel to make believe it was hair . . . your teacher . . . is concerned that there is too much female role playing. . . . I think it may have been you alone with me for four years, you play my role. . . ."

In a review of our clinical cases to document such reactions, we found that they occurred almost exclusively when the mother had desired a daughter and had had only older sons. In our clinical experience, the most common psychological trait associated with the strong wish for a daughter is the need to nurture and be nurtured by a female child, which often reflects compensatory needs originating in childhood (cf. Gibson, 1998).

Social Reinforcement

Clinical experience with GID from diverse quarters suggests that the parental response to early cross-gender behavior is typically neutrality (tolerance) or positive encouragement (for review, see Zucker & Bradley, 1995). Regarding boys with GID, Green (1974) assessed parental recall of such responses taken from clinical and structured interviews at the time of assessment and concluded that "what comes closest so far to being a *necessary* variable is that, as any feminine behavior begins to emerge, there is *no* discouragement of that behavior by the child's principal caretaker" (p. 238, emphasis in original) (see also Green, 1987; Roberts, Green, Williams, & Goodman, 1987). In our clinic, Mitchell (1991), in a structured interview study, found that mothers of GID boys were more likely to tolerate/encourage feminine behaviors and less likely to encourage masculine behaviors than were the mothers of both clinical and normal control boys.

These empirical studies are consistent with the clinical case report literature regarding maternal responses to feminine and masculine behaviors in boys with GID. However, the limitations of both studies, including reliance on interview data, should be recognized. From the standpoint of demand characteristics, one aspect of these data deserves special comment. As noted previously, clinicians of diverse theoretical persuasions have observed the apparent tolerance, or even encouragement, of feminine behavior shown by parents of boys with GID. However, the fact that these parents have sought out a clinical assessment usually means that they are now concerned about their child's gender identity development (Zucker, in press). From the standpoint of attribution theory (Weiner, 1993), one might predict that parents would minimize their encouragement or tolerance of cross-gender behavior, because it has such an obvious bearing on "causality." Yet a majority of the parents whom we have assessed do not recall systematic efforts to limit their child's cross-gender behavior.

Maternal Emotional Functioning

The role of maternal psychopathology in the genesis and perpetuation of GID has received a great deal of clinical and theoretical attention but, unfortunately, only limited empirical evaluation. At the outset, it should be noted that the available empirical studies have been delimited to the mothers of boys with GID—comparable studies are not available regarding the mothers of girls with GID (for descriptive data, however, see Zucker & Bradley, 1995).

Marantz and Coates (1991) found that the mothers of boys with GID showed more signs of psychopathology than did the mothers of demographically matched normal boys, including more pathological ratings on the Diagnostic Interview for Borderlines and more symptoms of depression on the Beck Depression Inventory.

Over the past several years, our group has collected systematic data on maternal psychopathology and marital discord, some of which was reported by Mitchell (1991) and Zucker and Bradley (1995). To date, our data show that, on average, mothers of boys with GID have levels of emotional distress and psychiatric impairment comparable to that of clinical control mothers but higher than that of normal control mothers. We did not, however, detect between-group differences on a measure of marital discord.

On one measure, the Symptom Checklist 90—Revised, mothers of GID boys had higher scores on most of the subscales and the composites than did the mothers of the normal control boys, whereas the scores of the clinical control mothers fell in between the two other groups. The GID mothers had peak scores on the Obsessive–Compulsive, Depression, and Hostility subscales.

On another measure, the Diagnostic Interview Schedule (DIS), 30% of the mothers of GID boys (total $n = 140$) had two DIS diagnoses, and 24% had three or more DIS diagnoses. The most common diagnoses were major depressive episode (39.6%) and recurrent major depression (32.1%). Overall, the rate of psychiatric impairment appears to be higher than our available data on mothers of both the clinical control and normal boys. Because more control group mother data are required, these results should, of course, be viewed cautiously. Nonetheless, it is apparent by reference to epidemiological data that, on average, mothers of GID boys have a history of psychiatric disorder that is elevated.

The emerging data on emotional distress and psychiatric impairment in the mothers of boys with GID indicate that it is more common than in the mothers of normal control boys and at least comparable to the mothers of clinical control boys. Still, we are left with the problem of specificity (Garber & Hollon, 1991) in that these maternal characteristics are not unique to the mothers of GID boys but common to the mothers of clinic-referred boys in general. Accordingly, maternal emotional distress/impairment functions, at best, only as a nonspecific risk factor in the development of GID. If the mother's emotional state truly is involved in the genesis of GID, there should be evidence of psychiatric impairment prior to and during the emergence of the child's symptoms. The data are suggestive that this is the case, and that the presence of emotional difficulties in the mothers is not simply a reaction to having a child with GID (Zucker & Bradley, 1995).

Coates and her colleagues have argued that the presence of psychopathology renders the mothers emotionally unavailable, which results in anxiety and insecurity in the son, and that it is this state of affairs that is partly responsible for symptom onset. Indeed, Coates and Person (1985) advanced a specific hypothesis, namely, that the erratic and uneven emotional availability of the mothers activated separation anxiety in the boys, which, in turn, activated the symptoms of GID: "In imitating 'Mommy' [the boy] confuse[s] 'being Mommy' with 'having Mommy.' [Cross-gender behavior] appears to allay, in part, the anxiety generated by the loss of the mother" (p. 708). Indeed, boys with GID appear to have high rates of separation anxiety traits, as judged by maternal report on a structured interview schedule (Zucker, Bradley, & Lowry Sullivan, 1996) and their own responses on the Separation Anxiety Test (Birkenfeld-Adams, Zucker, & Bradley, 1998a).

The possible role of separation anxiety in the genesis of GID raises more general questions about the quality of the mother–son relationship. Over the past few years, our group has examined the quality of attachment to the mother among young boys and girls with GID (ages 3 to 6). Among a sample of 22 boys, Birkenfeld-Adams, Zucker, and Bradley (1998b) found that the majority (73%) were classified as insecurely attached, a rate comparable to that of an internal clinical control group and of other studies of clinical populations (e.g., Greenberg, Speltz, DeKlyen, & Endriga, 1991).

Because insecure attachments and separation anxiety are likely nonspecific risk factors (i.e., many boys who have these qualities do not have GID), the crucial question that remains is why only a small minority of boys develop the "fantasy solution" of wanting to be a girl. Various predisposing factors have been implicated, including temperamental characteristics of the child, the premorbid relationship with the mother, the position of the father in the family system, that the family psychopathology must occur during the sensitive period for gender identity formation, and so on. At present, however, the question of specificity remains unanswered in any satisfactory manner.

One possible mediating variable might be the importance of the child's gender to the mother or her attitudes toward men and masculinity in general. In this regard, pathological gender mourning, as discussed earlier, may be a potential prototype. As noted elsewhere (Zucker, 1996), however, pathological gender mourning appears to be part of the family history in only a small minority of cases, and thus other pathways are required to account for the role of maternal impairment in the genesis of GID. The following vignette illustrates one such alternative pathway:

Fred was a 7-year-old boy with an IQ of 102. He lived with his parents, who were of a lower-middle-class background. At the time of referral, the parents were primarily concerned about

Fred's general behavior, which included lying, stealing, defiance, and being "hyper." This was manifested mainly in parent–child interactions, and less so in the school setting, where he was judged to be more withdrawn and aloof. The parents were extremely frustrated with Fred, finding him needy, attention seeking, and "always in [your] face." He had been previously diagnosed by a child psychiatrist with attention-deficit/hyperactivity disorder and was on Ritalin (methylphenidate).

Fred's mother reported that she never had a desire to become a parent, but did so to please her husband. When asked about a prenatal gender preference, Fred's mother stated that she wanted a boy because "it's easier for a man, it's a man's world . . . men dictate, men get paid more . . . I wish I was a man." In contrast, she stated that her husband wanted a girl, to which she laughed and said somewhat dismissively, "Now he has both."

From infancy on, the mother felt little connection to Fred and returned to work when he was 1 month old. Care was deferred to babysitters and Fred's father. At present, the mother reported that she would do anything to avoid having to interact with Fred and would often drink to the point of blackouts to distance herself from him.

Fred's mother had a psychiatric history consistent with a diagnosis of borderline personality disorder. On the DIS, she met criteria for four diagnoses: major depressive episode; major depression, recurrent; alcohol abuse; and alcohol dependence. Fred's mother also reported a history of sexual assault, in which she was raped in her late adolescence by a friend. She also believed that she had sexual intercourse with a friend when her husband was at work but was too drunk to remember it. The episode of rape appeared to be associated with symptoms of posttraumatic stress disorder. In general, Fred's mother reported highly ambivalent feelings about men and sexuality. She recalled that her maternal aunt told her that she should "watch out for men because all they want to do is get their dicks wet . . . it's sad, but true . . . I wished I listened to her." After the rape, Fred's mother moved to a large city and was promiscuous for several years: "[I] was hell-bent on getting revenge . . . I'd pick men up, use them, and lose them . . . sex was a weapon. . . ." The marital relationship was stable, in part because she viewed her husband as being very tolerant and accepting of her deficits; however, the parents no longer had sex as Fred's mother had developed a strong aversion toward it.

Fred showed all the behavioral signs of GID, including a preoccupation with long hair. He was constantly trying to stroke his mother's hair and professed an interest in her occupation, which, interestingly enough, had something to do with hair. From the time Fred first began to manifest cross-gender behavior, the parents reported virtually no concern about it. They thought the behavior was funny and amusing and reported no concern if Fred wanted to change his sex when he was older. Fred provided several reasons for his desire to be a girl—one reason was that if he were a girl, then he would not be "bad," and his parents would like him better.

In this case, one sees no evidence of a mother who was overinvolved or enmeshed with her son or who showed signs of pathological gender mourning. Indeed, the most striking aspects of the mother's history included the extent of her psychiatric impairment and her marked underinvolvement in the parenting role, which included rather transparent displays of rejection. Mother's underinvolvement appeared to be buffered somewhat by father's parenting role, but the father reported that he too was often frustrated with Fred, and yelled at him frequently. Indeed, father reported difficulty in regulating his angry feelings in general and struggled with homicidal urges toward strangers who irritated him. Regarding gender issues, father did not seem to support Fred's identity as a boy. One way of understanding Fred's GID is that it evolved in the context of equating being a boy with being bad. His effort to be close to his mother only worked when she would allow him to stroke her hair, but even this she often found aversive and smothering and thus would push him away. Because the parents often laughed at Fred in a positive way when he acted like a girl, this may well have reinforced the behavior and functioned as a perpetuating factor.

It is, of course, not clear whether the cross-gender behavior would have accelerated over time if the parents had reacted to it negatively, and thus Fred would have had to develop a different "solution" to dealing with his mother's detachment from him. In addition, one might speculate that the mother's angry feelings toward men (although not her husband), secondarily to the date rape, colored her relationship with her son in a way that made it difficult for her to connote positively his masculinity.

It appears that there are diverse pathways that lead to how parents respond to the child's early cross-gender behavior (either by encouraging or tolerating it). Thus, from a clinical and therapeutic point of view, it is important to identify the putative motivations with regard to the selective reinforcement of sex-typed behaviors. This is consistent with the principle of *equifinality* (Cicchetti & Rogosch, 1991), in which a similar outcome (in this case, tolerance/encouragement of cross-gender behavior) begins from different starting points and through different processes.

Paternal Emotional Functioning

The role of paternal influences in the genesis and perpetuation of GID has also received a great deal of clinical and theoretical attention but, again, only limited empirical evaluation, which has been delimited to the fathers of boys with GID.

One account implicates the father's role by virtue of his absence from the family matrix. Across 10 samples of boys with GID, the rate of father absence (e.g., due to separation or divorce) was 34.5% (summarized in Zucker & Bradley, 1995). It is unlikely, however, that this rate would differ significantly from the rate found in clinical populations in general, if not the general population. Green (1987) found that paternal separations occurred earlier in the families of GID boys than in normal control boys, so it is possible that timing is an additional variable to consider. Green (1987) also found that the fathers of GID boys (both father-present and father-absent) recalled spending less time with their sons than did the fathers of control boys during the second year of life, years 3 to 5, and at the time of assessment. The inclusion of a clinical control group would be helpful in gauging the specificity of this finding.

Unfortunately, there is little in the way of systematic research on paternal psychopathology. Wolfe (1990) conducted a small but detailed study of 12 fathers, predominantly of an upper-middle-class background, of boys with GID. On the Structured Clinical Interview for DSM-III, all the fathers received an Axis I diagnosis for either a current or past disorder (most frequently substance abuse and depression), and eight also received at least one Axis II diagnosis. Unpublished DIS data from our own clinic on 90 fathers indicate that alcohol abuse (22.2%) has been the most common diagnosis. This percentage may underestimate the prevalence of alcohol abuse in fathers of GID boys, as we were not able to interview a substantial number of fathers who were no longer part of the family matrix. On the other hand, it should be noted that about half the fathers who were interviewed did not meet criteria for any DIS diagnosis. Whatever the exact patterning of paternal emotional functioning proves to be, the same issues of interpretation discussed earlier regarding mothers apply.

THERAPEUTICS

Therapeutic interventions for GID per se are entirely psychosocial in nature, taking into account temperamental and psychological factors in the child and family dynamics.

Several therapeutic approaches have been employed, including behavior therapy, psychotherapy, family therapy, parental counseling, group therapy, and eclectic combinations. As reviewed elsewhere (Zucker & Bradley, 1995), all these strategies appear to have some clinical utility; unfortunately, formal comparative studies have not been conducted, so the most efficacious types of treatment remain unclear.

Three general comments about treatment of GID can be made. First, clinical experience suggests that intervention can more readily reduce gender identity conflict during early childhood than during late childhood and adolescence. Perhaps for this reason more than any other, it is important to give careful clinical consideration to the earliest signs of GID in late infancy and early toddlerhood. The prognosis for reducing severe gender dysphoria after puberty is rather poor. Second, the importance of working with the parents of children with GID has been much discussed in the literature. When there is a great deal of marital discord and parental psychopathology, treatment of these problems will greatly facilitate more specific work on gender identity issues. Management of the child's gender behavior in his or her daily environment requires that the parents have clear goals and a forum in which to discuss difficulties. Because parental dynamics and parental ambivalence about treatment may contribute to the perpetuation of GID (Newman, 1976), it is important for the therapist to have an appropriate relationship with the parents in order to address and work through these issues. Finally, the therapist needs to consider closely the goals of treatment (Zucker & Bradley, 1995). In part, this issue will be conceptualized within the therapist's theoretical framework, but it will also be a function of the parents' concern and, to some extent, of the child's concerns. Two short-term goals have been discussed in the clinical literature: the reduction or elimination of social ostracism and conflict and the alleviation of underlying or associated psychopathology. Longer-term goals have focused on the prevention of postpubertal gender dysphoria and homosexuality. Little disagreement about the advisability of preventing gender dysphoria in adolescence or adulthood has been expressed in the clinical literature. Contemporary and secular-minded clinicians are, however, sensitive to the importance of helping people integrate a homosexual sexual orientation into their sense of identity (Green, 1987). Not surprisingly, however, the development of a heterosexual orientation is probably preferred by most parents of children with GID. It is, therefore, important that clinicians point out to such parents that, as of yet, there is no strong evidence that treatment affects later sexual orientation. Both authors, as well as other experienced clinicians in the field, have preferred to emphasize the merit of reducing childhood gender identity conflict per se and, when it is present, associated behavioral problems and to orient the parents of children with GID to the short-term goals of intervention.

SUMMARY

In this chapter, we have reviewed aspects of the core phenomenology, some of the associated features, and selected (putative) risk factors pertaining to GID in children. Like other psychiatric disorders of childhood, it is apparent that complexity, not simplicity, is the guiding rule of thumb in an effort to make sense of the origins of GID. From an etiological standpoint, perhaps the most vexing issue is to make progress in solving the problem of specificity. It is likely that both biological and psychosocial factors will be implicated, and a model of cumulative risk (partly sex-specific) will be required to understand this relatively uncommon psychiatric disorder of childhood.

REFERENCES

American Psychiatric Association. (1994). *Diagnostic and statistical manual of mental disorders* (4th ed.). Washington, DC: Author.

Bates, J. E., Bentler, P. M., & Thompson, S. K. (1979). Gender-deviant boys compared with normal and clinical control boys. *Journal of Abnormal Child Psychology, 7*, 243–259.

Birkenfeld-Adams, A., Zucker, K. J., & Bradley, S. J. (1998a, October). *Boys with gender identity disorder: Signs of separation anxiety and distress.* Poster presented at the Second International Conference on Attachment and Psychopathology, Toronto, Ontario.

Birkenfeld-Adams, A., Zucker, K. J., & Bradley, S. J. (1998b, October). *Quality of attachment in young boys with gender identity disorder.* Poster presented at the Second International Conference on Attachment and Psychopathology, Toronto, Ontario.

Blanchard, R., & Klassen, P. (1997). H-Y antigen and homosexuality in men. *Journal of Theoretical Biology, 185*, 373–378.

Blanchard, R., Zucker, K. J., Bradley, S. J., & Hume, C. S. (1995). Birth order and sibling sex ratio in homosexual male adolescents and probably prehomosexual feminine boys. *Developmental Psychology, 31*, 22–30.

Bornstein, M. H. (1989). Sensitive periods in development: Structural characteristics and causal interpretations. *Psychological Bulletin, 105*, 179–197.

Cicchetti, D., & Rogosch, F. A. (1996). Equifinality and multifinality in developmental psychopathology. *Development and Psychopathology, 8*, 597–600.

Coates, S., Friedman, R. C., & Wolfe, S. (1991). The etiology of boyhood gender identity disorder: A model for integrating temperament, development, and psychodynamics. *Psychoanalytic Dialogues, 1*, 481–523.

Coates, S., Hahn-Burke, S., Wolfe, S., Shindledecker, R., & Nierenberg, O. (1994, June). *Sensory reactivity in boys with gender identity disorder: A comparison with matched controls.* Poster presented at the meeting of the International Academy of Sex Research, Edinburgh, Scotland.

Coates, S., & Person, E. S. (1985). Extreme boyhood femininity: Isolated behavior or pervasive disorder? *Journal of the American Academy of Child Psychiatry, 24*, 702–709.

Coates, S., & Wolfe, S. (1995). Gender identity disorder in boys: The interface of constitution and early experience. *Psychoanalytic Inquiry, 15*, 6–38.

Coates, S., Wolfe, S., & Hahn-Burke, S. (1994, June). *Do boys with gender identity disorder have a shy, inhibited temperament?* Poster presented at the meeting of the International Academy of Sex Research, Edinburgh, Scotland.

Cohen-Kettenis, P. T., & van Goozen, S. H. M. (1997). Sex reassignment of adolescent transsexuals: A follow-up study. *Journal of the American Academy of Child and Adolescent Psychiatry, 36*, 263–271.

Eaton, W. O., & Enns, L. R. (1986). Sex differences in human motor activity level. *Psychological Bulletin, 100*, 19–28.

Fridell, S. R., Zucker, K. J., Bradley, S. J., & Maing, D. M. (1996). Physical attractiveness of girls with gender identity disorder. *Archives of Sexual Behavior, 25*, 17–31.

Garber, J., & Hollon, S. D. (1991). What can specificity designs say about causality in psychopathology research? *Psychological Bulletin, 110*, 129–136.

Gibson, L. A. (1998). *Adult attachment and maternal representations of gender during pregnancy: Their impact on the child's subsequent gender-role development*. Unpublished doctoral dissertation, City University of New York.

Goy, R. W., Bercovitch, F. B., & McBrair, M. C. (1988). Behavioral masculinization is independent of genital masculinization in prenatally androgenized female rhesus macaques. *Hormones and Behavior, 22,* 552–571.

Green, R. (1974). *Sexual identity conflict in children and adults*. New York: Basic Books.

Green, R. (1987). *The "sissy boy syndrome" and the development of homosexuality*. New Haven, CT: Yale University Press.

Greenberg, M. T., Speltz, M. L., DeKlyen, M., & Endriga, M. C. (1991). Attachment security in preschoolers with and without externalizing behavior problems: A replication. *Development and Psychopathology, 3,* 413–430.

Greenson, R. R. (1968). Dis-identifying from mother. *International Journal of Psychoanalysis, 49,* 370–374.

Hess, E. H. (1973). *Imprinting*. New York: Van Nostrand.

Kohlberg, L. (1966). A cognitive-developmental analysis of children's sex-role concepts and attitudes. In E. E. Maccoby (Ed.), *The development of sex differences* (pp. 82–173). Stanford, CA: Stanford University Press.

Marantz, S., & Coates, S. (1991). Mothers of boys with gender identity disorder: A comparison of matched controls. *Journal of the American Academy of Child and Adolescent Psychiatry, 30,* 310–315.

McDermid, S. A., Zucker, K. J., Bradley, S. J., & Maing, D. M. (1998). Effects of physical appearance on masculine trait ratings of boys and girls with gender identity disorder. *Archives of Sexual Behavior, 27,* 253–267.

Meyer-Bahlburg, H. F. L. (1998). Gender assignment in intersexuality. *Journal of Psychology and Human Sexuality, 10*(2), 1–21.

Mitchell, J. N. (1991). *Maternal influences on gender identity disorder in boys: Searching for specificity*. Unpublished doctoral dissertation, York University, Downsview, Ontario.

Money, J., Hampson, J. G., & Hampson, J. L. (1957). Imprinting and the establishment of gender role. *Archives of Neurology and Psychiatry, 77,* 333–336.

Newman, L. E. (1976). Treatment for the parents of feminine boys. *American Journal of Psychiatry, 133,* 683–687.

O'Connor, T., & Rutter, M. (1996). Risk mechanisms in development: Some conceptual and methodological considerations. *Developmental Psychology, 32,* 787–795.

Roberts, C. W., Green, R., Williams, K., & Goodman, M. (1987). Boyhood gender identity development: A statistical contrast of two family groups. *Developmental Psychology, 23,* 544–557.

Ruble, D. N., & Martin, C. L. (1998). Gender development. In W. Damon (Series Ed.) & N. Eisenberg (Vol. Ed.), *The handbook of child psychology* (5th ed.): *Vol. 3. Social, emotional, and personality development* (pp. 933–1016). New York: Wiley.

Stoller, R. J. (1968). *Sex and gender: Vol. I. The development of masculinity and femininity*. New York: Jason Aronson.

Weiner, B. (1993). On sin versus sickness: A theory of perceived responsibility and social motivation. *American Psychologist, 48,* 957–965.

Wolfe, S. M. (1990). *Psychopathology and psychodynamics of parents of boys with a gender identity disorder of childhood*. Unpublished doctoral dissertation, City University of New York.

Zero to Three, National Center for Clinical Infant Programs. (1994). *Diagnostic classification: 0–3. Diagnostic classification of mental health and developmental disorders of infancy and early childhood*. Washington, DC: Author.

Zucker, K. J. (1992). Gender identity disorder. In S. R. Hooper, G. W. Hynd, & R. E. Mattison (Eds.), *Child psychopathology: Diagnostic criteria and clinical assessment* (pp. 305–342). Hillsdale, NJ: Erlbaum.

Zucker, K. J. (1996, March). *Pathological gender mourning in mothers of boys with gender identity disorder: Clinical evidence and some psychocultural hypotheses*. Paper presented at the meeting of the Society for Sex Therapy and Research, Miami Beach, FL.

Zucker, K. J. (in press). Gender identity disorder. In M. Lewis & A. J. Sameroff (Eds.), *Handbook of developmental psychopathology* (2nd ed.). New York: Plenum.

Zucker, K. J., & Bradley, S. J. (1995). *Gender identity disorder and psychosexual problems in children and adolescents*. New York: Guilford Press.

Zucker, K. J., Bradley, S. J., & Ipp, M. (1993). Delayed naming of a newborn boy: Relationship to the mother's wish for a girl and subsequent cross-gender identity in the child by the age of two. *Journal of Psychology & Human Sexuality, 6,* 57–68.

Zucker, K. J., Bradley, S. J., Kuksis, M., Pecore, K., Birkenfeld-Adams, A., Doering, R. W., Mitchell, J. N., & Wild, J. (in press). Gender constancy judgements in children with gender identity disorder: Evidence for a developmental lag. *Archives of Sexual Behavior.*

Zucker, K. J., Bradley, S. J., & Lowry Sullivan, C. B. (1996). Traits of separation anxiety in boys with gender identity disorder. *Journal of the American Academy of Child and Adolescent Psychiatry, 35,* 791–798.

Zucker, K. J., Bradley, S. J., Lowry Sullivan, C. B., Kuksis, M., Birkenfeld-Adams, A., & Mitchell, J. N. (1993). A gender identity interview for children. *Journal of Personality Assessment, 61,* 443–456.

Zucker, K. J., Bradley, S. J., & Sanikhani, M. (1997). Sex differences in referral rates of children with gender identity disorder: Some hypotheses. *Journal of Abnormal Child Psychology, 25,* 217–227.

Zucker, K. J., Green, R., Bradley, S. J., Williams, K., Rebach, H. M., & Hood, J. E. (1998). Gender identity disorder of childhood: Diagnostic issues. In T. A. Widiger, A. J. Frances, H. A. Pincus, R. Ross, M. B. First, W. Davis, & M. Kline (Eds.), *DSM-IV sourcebook* (Vol. 4, pp. 503–512). Washington, DC: American Psychiatric Association.

Zucker, K. J., Green, R., Coates, S., Zuger, B., Cohen-Kettenis, P. T., Zecca, G. M., Lertora, V., Money, J.,

Hahn-Burke, S., Bradley, S. J., & Blanchard, R. (1997). Sibling sex ratio of boys with gender identity disorder. *Journal of Child Psychology and Psychiatry, 38,* 543–551.

Zucker, K. J., Green, R., Garofano, C., Bradley, S. J., Williams, K., Rebach, H. M., & Lowry Sullivan, C. B. (1994). Prenatal gender preference of mothers of feminine and masculine boys: Relation to sibling sex composition and birth order. *Journal of Abnormal Child Psychology, 22,* 1–13.

Zucker, K. J., Wild, J., Bradley, S. J., & Lowry, C. B. (1993). Physical attractiveness of boys with gender identity disorder. *Archives of Sexual Behavior, 22,* 23–34.

27

Somatic Expression of Disease

❖

DAVID A. MRAZEK

Interactions between "mind" and "body" can be vividly demonstrated by very young children who often respond physically to their early emotional experiences. Developmental theorists have responded to their inability to probe the inner world of the nonverbal child by first hypothesizing and then trying to demonstrate direct links between early emotional experiences, physiological processes, somatic symptoms, and illnesses. Clinical observations of the psychotherapy of adults with "psychosomatic" illnesses led to theories that linked "preverbal memories" to symptoms that did not emerge until much later in life. These ephemeral "somatic" memories of the first years of life could be detected only through their expression in adult behaviors which were triggered by parallel interpersonal experiences. Theories emerged hypothesizing that temperamental limitations interacting with pathogenic early experiences were associated with problems in the verbal expression of emotions in children with psychosomatic diseases. Patients who lacked the verbal capacity to express what were essentially preverbal experiences were described as alexithymic because they struggled to find words (i.e., alexi) for feelings (i.e., thymia).

During the conduct of psychotherapy with older children who had both physical illnesses and psychiatric symptoms, similar difficulties in their ability to express feeling states were documented. For these older verbal children, it was hypothesized that the somatic processes as-sociated with these illnesses were the product of internal emotional conflicts that were expressed as bodily symptoms, because they had no alternative available mode of expression. Subsequent "confirmatory" clinical observations were presented as evidence to support these theories. Although these speculations have captured the imagination of clinicians over the years, currently there is little empirical research being conducted to clarify or define these processes.

This chapter reviews empirical evidence that provides support for an alternative, albeit still speculative, model of psychosomatic interactions (Mrazek, 1998). The first central principle in this model is that genes control key proteins and these proteins control physiological processes. Abnormal gene expression is a core vulnerability that precedes physiological dysfunction. What is needed to understand these processes more fully is a comprehensive theory of developmental psychosomatic psychopathology that links the experience of the child with the child's unfolding biological potential. After a brief historical review, the chapter focuses on current understandings of three illustrative somatic problems that begin in the first year. These three clinical conditions—infantile onset obesity, early-onset asthma, and atopic dermatitis—are discussed as each illness reflects an interaction between genetic vulnerability and early environmental stressors. In addition, all three diseases are candidates for early intervention strategies.

HISTORICAL CONSIDERATIONS

The Chicago school of psychoanalysis provided the original conceptualization of psychoanalytic psychosomatic processes (Alexander, 1950). While fascinating individual clinical phenomena were described, these psychoanalytical formulations were difficult to test empirically. Furthermore, historical misconceptions regarding normal physiology led to the suggestion of relatively implausible mechanisms for the explanation of quite complex pathophysiological processes. However, two major contributions of these investigations continue to influence current practice. First, the importance of focussing clinical attention on the earliest responses of infants to distress was established with full recognition that these responses occurred at a point in the cognition development when children had no language. Second, the theoretical perspective that early traumatic emotional experiences in the first year of life could result in life-long changes in psychophysiological regulation was articulated. However, the mechanisms by which these permanent changes in function emerge have remained essentially unknown.

Piaget committed his career to understanding cognitive structure and how the minds of infants and children actually emerge. His work led to a new level of appreciation for the links between cognitive "schema" and physical processes. The work of Piaget was strongly influenced by the empirical studies of Pavlov who experientially manipulated discrete physiological processes in what have become classic conditioning experiments. Piaget (1952) appreciated the possibility that physiological processes could become linked to environmental signals. He conceptually expanded Pavlov's simple reflex theory of relationships to reflect a more complex and fascinating set of early associational patterns or schemas that he demonstrated inevitably to evolve in normal children over the first months and years of life. Through precise observations, he catalogued evidence that vividly demonstrated how an infant gradually creates cognitive connections between emotions, ideas, and sensations. As these schemas evolve, they create a network of cognitive templates that are ultimately the basis by which a child defines reality. To the degree that Piaget considered these learned associational relationships to be incorporated as somatic components during the sensorimotor phase of development, this work provided a phenomenonological de-

scription of how a physiological experience (e.g., hunger) actually becomes the signal sensation that can drive a set of behaviors (e.g., crying) designed to achieve a discrete homeostatic state (e.g., satiety). Within this framework, a number of both sensory stimuli (e.g., sight of mother) and motor responses (e.g., sucking on thumb) can become linked to the original signal and to each other. The physiological processes involved in such a process can be measured with increasing sophistication. The behaviors elicited are readily observable. What has been more elusive has been the demonstration of the neural processes and the elaboration of biochemical control systems that include both the translation of central nervous system processes and the expression of genetic information.

With the advent of an increasingly sophisticated understanding of operant conditioning, a new theory to explain the origin of psychosomatic illness became available and was used to formulate the process by which physical symptoms become "reinforced" in childhood. The work by Creer (1976) in respiratory diseases provided a greater clarification of the mechanisms by which physiological processes could be manipulated behaviorally. However, virtually no behavioral strategies have focused on the evolution of physical symptoms in infancy.

The evolution of attachment theory has provided a context in which to evaluate the role that primary attachment figures play in mediating the emotional experience of children. The specific protective factor provided by the attachment figure resides in her ability to help her child maintain homeostatic control in the presence of intense physiological distress. Incorporating the early psychodynamic observations of Spitz (1965), Emde's developmental studies further charted the early landmarks of normal early development (Emde, Gaensbauer, & Harmon, 1982). Within this context, Parmelee (1989) explicitly elaborated the importance of early supportive relationships during periods of physical illness. He hypothesized that successful adaption to the illness stressors led to the development of well-modulated emotional regulation, whereas failure to adapt could lead to deviant patterns of development.

Sameroff expanded a transactional model of environmental influence to specifically address how the interactions of multiple risk factors affect physically ill children (Sameroff & Chandler, 1975; Sameroff, 1986). Physically ill children were shown to be able to cope reasonably well with one or two environmental stressors, but when a critical threshold is exceeded, the likelihood of a major perturbation is enhanced. How infants can be helped to gain control of their own emotional homeostasis during periods of internal distress remains a compelling question for those interested in preventive interventions (Sameroff & Emde, 1989).

THE IMPORTANCE OF NATURE IN THE NATURE–NURTURE EQUATION

A complex interaction exists between the genetic potential of the infant and the environmental experiences provided by the parents. However, the contributions of these environmental factors has rarely been a target of early interventions that could be designed to minimize the likelihood of the expression of an anticipated phenotype. This is particularly intriguing given that models have existed which describe successful early behavioral preventive efforts for more than a generation. An illustrative example is phenylketonuria (PKU). PKU is an autosomal recessive metabolic disorder that, if untreated, results in a dramatic decrease in intelligence of an affected child. A deficiency of phenylalanine hydroxylase was identified as a cause of this disorder. As a consequence of this single genetic error, a patient cannot appropriately metabolize phenylalanine, resulting in its subsequent accumulation, which in turn causes subnormal intelligence.

Based on this discovery, infants were identified as having PKU based on early elevations in serum phenylalanine, through a universal screening procedure. Subsequently, these infants were placed on a diet that contained very low quantities of this amino acid. Instituting this restrictive diet within the first week of life effectively preserves the cognitive abilities of these infants.

One striking lesson to learn from the successful treatment of PKU is that parents are able to follow even complex diets in a dramatically compliant fashion. The most probable reason that these parents can restrict the diet of their children is that the consequences of noncompliance are so ominous and inevitable. It is noteworthy to remember that parents have virtually complete control of their infant's eating behavior unless a feeding disorder develops.

Given the dramatic success of a low phenylalanine diet, it is surprising that little extension of this effective intervention has occurred with other illnesses where diet is presumed to be a critical factor.

Why is it that parents often ignore medical advice despite concrete evidence that the prescribed course of action is in the best interest of their own child? No single answer has emerged, but the phenomenon has resulted in many physicians being excessively cautious when considering early interventions based on their beliefs that parents have a limited ability to change their behaviors. For example, allergists who identify that a child is allergic to the family cat are regularly told by the child's parents that they have decided to keep the cat because they felt that the cat was a "part of the family." Similarly, physicians must deal with situations that arise when family members are in conflict regarding their priorities. What is the correct response when an infant of an asthmatic father begins to wheeze, and the nonasthmatic mother of the child decides to continue to smoke because she does not want to gain weight? Yet another example is the behavior of obese parents who are told by their pediatrician that their toddler son is already in the 99th percentile for weight while only in the 50th percentile for height. Clearly, their child needs to lose weight and a correct clinic prescription is to place the child on a restrictive diet (Epstein, McCurley, Voloski, & Wing, 1990). All too often, it is impossible for these parents to restrict their child's eating successfully because they believe that a normal diet would leave their child with a sense of deprivation.

This dread of inflicting a state of deprivation is often more disturbing than facing the reality that their child will almost certainly become obese in a family in which most members are overweight. One of the core differences between these examples of noncompliance and the faithful adherence of parents who provide phenylalanine-free diets for their children with PKU is almost inevitably their understanding of the certainty and nature of the negative consequence. For most psychosomatic problems that may arise in infancy, parents can "play the odds" that their child will not suffer if they persist in their preferred behaviors. Because the parents of children with PKU have strong evidence that they will cause immediate permanent damage to their child's intelligence if they do not alter their behavior, they do make the change.

The genome of a child is fixed at conception. At this time, every allele has been selected and the sequence is immutable. Therefore, change in the environment of the child must be the focus of early intervention until more effective methods of providing alternative DNA are developed. To modify a young child's environment, it is essentially necessary to help the family alter either the physical or the emotional experience of a child. What has only recently been appreciated is that whereas gene structure does not change in accordance with environmental events, the function of the genes does change. Gene expression can be controlled by a range of factors including genetically coded information that regulates gene action and environmental signals that affect the genes themselves. The realization that genetic control is possible through environmental manipulation has led to the development of a new focus of intervention. These treatment strategies can be described as MERGER (management of environmental regulation of gene expression and reactivation) interventions. In short, genes can be turned off and on. The exact mechanism by which this happens is only beginning to be understood. Nevertheless, the clinical implications of the management of these processes may be far reaching.

EARLY-ONSET OBESITY

In reviewing psychosomatic processes, there is no more basic consideration than the structure and shape of the body. Of public health significance, obesity in the United States has increased dramatically over the past 20 years (Schonfeld-Warden & Warden, 1997). Although there is a strong focus on environmental factors, a series of new studies has focused on the genetic control of obesity that promise to identify infants at risk. Using large twin samples where one of the twins has been raised by nonbiological parents, the importance of the role of genetics in the development of obesity in children becomes more vivid (Stunkard et al., 1986; Price & Gottesman, 1991). Some studies suggest that heritability may be as high as 80%; in other samples, a heritability estimate of closer to 50% has been suggested. Some substantial portion of this heritability, perhaps 25%, may be the result of genetic control of metabolic rate and energy expenditure (Bouchard, Depres, & Tremblay, 1991;

Bouchard & Perusse, 1993). What appears to be true is that there is a strong genetically controlled tendency for excessive calorie consumption and excessive body weight. Although no conclusive set of genes has been identified, localization of candidate genes is progressing (Clement et al., 1998; Montague et al., 1997).

Nevertheless, it is equally critical to consider the role that environmental factors play in the development of obesity in children who are genetically at risk. Environmental risk factors such as low socioeconomic status are known to be strong predictors of subsequent obesity. Perhaps the most straightforward and undeniable demonstration of the influence of environmental factors on the expression of obesity can be found in those identical twin pairs in which one individual is strikingly obese and the other twin has maintained his weight within normal limits. Their genetic endowment is identical, but their phenotypical expression is dramatically different. Shields (1962) supported this clinical observation in his classic monograph on monozygotic twins. Here, he reported that two pairs of twins who were reared apart varied in weight by more than three stone (e.g., 42 pounds).

Many obese parents have had a particularly difficult struggle with controlling their own weight. Ironically, this may be one factor that contributes to their "overfeeding" of their children. This paradoxical behavior is an appropriate area of focus for the infant mental health clinician. Certainly, the risk factors involved with the development of obesity are clear and straightforward. Children should be carefully weighed throughout the first year of life. A growing discrepancy between the percentile of weight versus the percentile of height is an indication of a need to become proactive in monitoring the diet of a child. Because these children do not have problems with consuming food and do not hesitate in becoming active participants in the feeding process, they contrast sharply with children who fail to thrive, and a different proactive approach is warranted. How a child becomes obese is not a total mystery. The two primary issues are consumption of calories and expenditure of energy. In the first years of life, parents have virtually total control of the diet of their child and a substantial influence on their child's level of activity. The range of possibilities for problems in overfeeding are again straightforward. In terms of quantity of food consumed, parents need to be motivated to take active control. Both gradually decreasing the quantities of food consumed at mealtime and restricting food between meals are reasonable strategies. Yet, another key factor in calorie consumption is the choice of foods. The current wisdom is to avoid foods with either high fat or high sugar content, because there is some evidence that these choices tend to lead quickly to the development of strong food preferences that can contribute to problems in long-term weight management. It is important for parents to ensure that young children consume adequate protein in order to maintain appropriate growth. Other risk factors for obesity have been more difficult to define. Interestingly, less sleep at 5 years of age has recently been linked to an increased risk (Locard et al., 1992). In addition, a child's diet must contain the basic vitamins and minerals necessary to maintain good health. With proper precautions, dietary interventions during the preschool years have been reported to demonstrate some promise (Davis & Christoffel, 1994).

Prevention of obesity promises to be a far more effective strategy for eventual weight control than are attempts to change the eating pattern of children who have already become obese. Critical periods for the onset of obesity have been reported to occur during early childhood (Dietz, 1994). Of children at the 95th percentile of weight at birth, 58% are likely to be obese at 7 years of age. Although this is already a strong predictive factor, it provides optimistic evidence that many children, even in uncontrolled environments, will adopt appropriate eating behaviors and develop a normal body size. However, this plasticity diminishes rather quickly. Specifically, the future of those children who are obese at 4 years of age is far more problematic. Virtually all (98%) these children will still be obese 3 years later, when they are 7. (Fisch, Bilek, & Ulstrom, 1975).

Despite the importance of early intervention, many parents are resistant to dealing with the problem of early-onset obesity. In part, this may reflect the psychological meaning of eating for these parents. An obese mother who uses food as a primary method for modulating her own distress will almost certainly find it difficult to restrict the food intake of her daughter when the daughter signals that she wants to consume more.

Some parents fear that by restricting the intake of their child, they may in some way do harm. Currently, the American Academy of Pediatrics advocates restricting the consumption of high levels of fat. Still, until recently, a baby's "chubbiness" was a sign of "good health." Fortunately, there is now good evidence that appropriate early dieting does not lead to negative outcomes and, particularly, does not lead to a permanent effect on the ultimate height of a child (Epstein et al., 1990). Yet another parental anxiety is that focusing too soon on weight control may lead a child to develop an unhealthy preoccupation with eating. The ultimate fear in this regard is that early food restriction might lead to the later development of anorexia nervosa. Although there has been some suggestion that intense preoccupation with thinness, particularly involving a mother and her daughter during the preadolescent years, can sensitize some girls to developing anorexia, there is no evidence to link early conservative weight control to increased risk of eating disorders.

In summary, the problem of obesity in the first 3 years of life illustrates how the emotional needs of parents can interact with a strong hunger drive in an infant to lead the family to ignore warning signs of excessive weight gain. Establishing patterns of overeating early in life can lead to chronic obesity and a wide range of negative medical outcomes including hypertension, cardiac disease, and diabetes.

The infant mental health clinician has a major opportunity to assess the complexity of the psychological context in which children begin overeating and to intervene in the process at an early stage in their development. A collaboration with pediatric practitioners provides practical opportunity to identify children at risk for developing obesity. If pediatric counseling targeted at straightforward methods to maintain the weight of children at appropriate levels fails, referral to an infant mental health clinician is strongly indicated. The focus of this intervention requires a strong educational component but must also take into account how the emotional needs of parents influence a child's eating behavior. It is ultimately a child's eating pattern and activity level that will result in the expression of obesity in those children who are genetically vulnerable.

EARLY-ONSET ASTHMA

Asthma is a "psychosomatic" illness that illustrates many of the clinical issues relevant to the care of young children who have medical problems. All psychosomatic illnesses are "real" diseases that present with tangible signs and symptoms. These illnesses do not reside in the "child's head," as punitive caregivers have historically asserted with pathological consequences. The evidence demonstrates that the onset and course of these illnesses are influenced by the emotional, immunological, and endocrinological homeostasis of the child. Some of the most fascinating questions in medicine focus on specific disruptions in this homeostasis and how they are linked to the expression of physical illnesses. These essential questions are focused on defining the "root cause" of both the physical and emotional symptoms. Progress in understanding etiology will be based on defining the bidirectional processes involved in symptom expression. One direction is defined by how the early difficult emotional experiences lead to the expression of physical symptoms and, ultimately, illness in genetically vulnerable children. The reciprocal direction is regulated by illness-specific stressors that are associated with physical disease and play a central role in the development of early psychopathological symptoms and, ultimately, psychiatric illness. Regardless of whether a child's first symptom is one of emotional distress or physical dysfunction, the eventual process becomes what is classically described as a "vicious cycle." With increasing emotional disturbance, the somatic symptoms of the infant become acute. Reciprocally, with increasing physical symptoms, the emotional state of the child becomes increasingly compromised, and a wide range of problems in adaptation begin to emerge.

Asthma is one of the most common pediatric illnesses. It affects approximately 7% of all children in the United States (Smith, 1988). Conservatively, more than 4,000,000 U.S. children are coping with asthma. Given that nearly three quarters of these children develop their first respiratory symptoms in the first 3 years of life, the public health implications are staggering.

Asthma is normally an illness that is characterized by sudden reversible bronchoconstriction and concomitant inflammation. It usually is accompanied by high-pitched expiratory wheezing and acute difficulty in breathing. Asthma has both a strong genetic (Daniels et al., 1996) and a prominent environmental component (Mrazek & Klinnert, 1991; Peat, 1996).

Furthermore, there is wide variability in the nature of symptoms in young asthmatic children. These symptoms range from mild chest tightness that occurs in a seasonal pattern at one extreme to life-threatening bronchoconstriction that can close down the airways of the child at the other end of the continuum. Some children have an allergic form of the illness that is triggered by exposure to antigens that may be derived from pets, dust, foods, or more exotic allergens. The asthmatic attacks of young children may be triggered by respiratory infections, exercise, or exposure to intense emotional stress and may often involve an allergic component.

Psychiatric disturbances occur in asthmatic children at a somewhat increased incidence when compared to healthy children (Mrazek, 1992). However, the occurrence of psychiatric symptoms is linked to the severity of the asthma. More than half of the children with serious illness have been reported to demonstrate psychiatric symptoms. Children with mild illness have rates of psychiatric disturbance that only slightly exceed those found in carefully geographically selected epidemiological populations. The severity of illness varies greatly in young infants and has considerable implications for their long-term prognosis. Children with severe early asthma are unlikely to "grow out of it" and have a higher risk for serious episodes later in life (Blair, 1977). In contrast, infants and toddlers who have mild asthma may be symptom-free after their third or fourth year of life, when the diameter of their airways has reached a critical threshold.

In a classic study conducted in Montreal, key parameters characterizing the interactions between mothers and their infants with mild asthma were examined (Gauthier et al., 1977, 1978). Though subtle differences in the interactions of mothers and their young asthmatic children were noted, these asthmatic children were adapting well overall. Furthermore, this study demonstrated that there was minimal evidence that serious problems existed in the parenting of infants with mild asthma.

In contrast, a sample of 75 preschool children with severe asthma who had experienced multiple hospitalizations and required multiple medications to control their symptoms were shown to be at high risk for psychiatric disturbance (Mrazek, Anderson, & Strunk, 1983; Mrazek, 1994). More than half of this sample had developed a behavioral disturbance when they were systematically assessed using a semi-structured maternal report interview methodology. These quite severely asthmatic children had more problems with sleep and depressed mood than did a healthy comparison group. In addition, their mothers had difficulty establishing compliance in completing a standardized task when their interactions were assessed using a microanalytical interactional coding technique.

If severity of illness were not considered, these two studies of young children with asthma would appear to yield contradictory findings. Instead, they provide empirical support for what has become an increasingly central component of our understanding of developmental psychopathology. Risk factors may interact in an additive or synergistic manner, and as the number of risk factors increase, there is an escalation in the probability that there will be a breakdown in the adaptation of the child.

Illness-specific risk factors associated with mild asthma are actually quite limited. Although the symptoms associated with mild asthma may provide intermittent limitations on a preschooler's activity and contribute to "a sense of being different," the stressors associated with mild disease rarely become an organizing principle in the identity of the child. In contrast, a child with severe asthma must cope with a number of major stressors. Often, respiratory symptoms limit the child's capacity to attend nursery school and develop normal peer relationships. Changes in body image can be dramatic, particularly if there is a need to maintain the child on steroid medication. Growth retardation, obesity, and changes in facial appearance can all be disturbing and serve as a constant reminder to these children that they are different. Eventually, many children with severe asthma become sensitized to their symptoms and develop a sense of vulnerability that becomes linked to a growing fearfulness of a severe life-threatening attack.

Given that the nature of the emotional difficulties of children usually reflects the specific aspects of the stressors they experience, it is not surprising that severely asthmatic children often develop symptoms of anxiety and depression. Furthermore, they are more likely to develop sleep disturbances in part because they are more likely to experience severe attacks during the night. The primary interactional difficulties noted in the preschool study reflects the inability of some of the parents to set limits successfully. Given that asthmatic attacks can occur as a consequence of emotional conflicts or when children become agitated and distressed, parents sometimes chose to avoid such confrontations even at the cost of "giving in" to the child. A recent study confirmed the occurrence of the same pattern of behavioral problems in children of a second cohort. Sleeping difficulties, depression, and fearfulness were again associated with early-onset asthma (Mrazek, Schuman, & Klinnert, 1998).

The role that emotional stressors play in the initial expression of symptoms in genetically at-risk asthmatic children has been a controversial area of study. The W. T. Grant Study conducted in Denver focused on a group of 150 infants of asthmatic mothers and a comparison sample. Sixty of the index children also had paternal relatives with asthma. An estimate of the risk for the development of asthma is about 20% if one parent has asthma and 50% if both parents are affected. A prospective and longitudinal design was used in the Denver study, with all children being identified during their mother's pregnancy. Families were recruited into the study during the second or third trimester. Both biological and environmental risk factors were carefully monitored from before the birth of the child. These included biological risk factors such as the occurrence of atopic dermatitis in infancy, frequent respiratory infections (Frick, German, & Mills, 1979; Dodge, Martinez, Cline, Lebowitz, & Burrows, 1996), or high levels of serum IgE (immunoglobulin E) (Mrazek, Klinnert, & Brower, & Harbeck, 1990). IgE levels from cord blood samples had been shown statistically to predict both the onset of asthma and atopic dermatitis in large samples of infants (Michel, Bousquet, Greillier, Robinet-Levy, & Coulomb, 1980). However, from a psychiatric perspective, the most interesting hypothesis tested in this study was that early problems in parenting would act as an emotional stressor and further increase the risk for these children to develop asthma. All the risk factors were prospectively measured. Only three of these risk factors, when considered together, contributed to the ability to predict onset: frequent infections, parenting difficulties, and elevated IgE. When considered together, these risk factors were able to predict the onset of asthma with a 70% probability (Mrazek et al., 1999).

These findings lead to new questions regarding the mechanism by which these factors were able to predict disease expression. Focusing on the parenting assessment, a systematic range of diverse parenting problems were assessed, but all were judged clinically as being capable of causing the emotional dysregulation of the child. These parenting problems included maternal depression, overt parental marital unhappiness, and observed insensitivity regarding the emotional needs of the child. These judgments of parenting difficulties were noted after an hour-long semistructured interview with the mother and an opportunity to observe the mother interacting with the child in the family home (Mrazek, Mrazek, & Klinnert, 1995; Mrazek, Klinnert, Mrazek, & Macey, 1991). Of major methodological significance, these judgments were made before the onset of any respiratory symptoms. Therefore, these early disruptions in the emotional experience of the child, as mediated through specific caretaking parental practices, may have led to increased environmental dysregulation for the child, thereby increasing the likelihood of the genetic expression of underlying respiratory symptoms (Klinnert, Mrazek, & Mrazek, 1994). Other studies have also demonstrated that the onset of asthmatic symptoms can be associated with increasing dysfunction within families (Gustafsson, Bjorksten, & Kjellman, 1994). This finding supports the testing of programs designed to modulate the expression of genes associated with asthma through environmental manipulation.

ECZEMA

Eczema or atopic dermatitis is an illness that is closely related to asthma. It has a substantial allergic component, but like asthma, a complex genetic environment interaction is required to actually result in clinical symptoms (Bos, Kapsenberg, & Smitt, 1994). Most important, it is not at all clear what the salient environment triggers are that initiate gene expression. Once expressed, IgE mediated reactions in the skin appear to play a prominent role in the aggravation of the atopic form of the illness.

Eczema is a common skin disorder that usually begins in the first year of life. Some reports suggest that the prevalence of the full range of expression of the disorder reaches 20% in children less than 12 years of age (Kay, Gawkrodger, Mortimer, & Jaron, 1994). It is characterized by an intense puritis or itching, which leads to extensive scratching and ultimately a scaly rash. With persistent scratching, the rash will bleed and form scabs. Eczema is the older name. Atopic dermatitis is a more recent label, which has been referred to as one form of eczema that is particularly linked to food sensitivity (Sampson, 1997). Given that this illness has a complex etiological basis, I use the more generic and shorter name to discuss this problem.

Considerable controversy has surrounded the links between stress and the onset of eczema. Perhaps most striking is that if the child does not scratch, the disease does not emerge. The dilemma is that it is extremely difficult to prevent an infant or toddler from responding to the intense puritis that suddenly develops. To further compound the problem, the excessive use of restraints can be quite disturbing to young children even in the absence of physical discomfort. When restraint is imposed to frustrate an intense need to seek some relief from compelling but incomprehensible physical discomfort, the infant and toddler does not have the cognitive capacity to become a partner in his or her own care.

Prospective studies that examine the risk factors associated with gene expression have become increasingly available. Unfortunately, it is difficult to develop a comprehensive strategy to be able to identify the interaction of a full range of risk factors. The result has been that few consistent risk factors have been determined. However, a positive family history of eczema is usually noted and consistently supports the genetic diathesis that has been largely accepted as a necessary condition for the development of the disease (Arshad, Stevens, & Hide, 1993). Further evidence of the genetic nature of the illness is supported by twin studies that report a concordance rate of 0.73 in monozygotic twins and 0.23 in dyzygotic twin pairs (Larsen, 1993).

Though the problems of caring for these acutely uncomfortable infants have been the focus of discussions for many years (Cohen, 1975; Lourie, 1955), empirical data regarding psychiatric outcome have been difficult to establish. A primary factor that has contributed to the dilemma is the wide range of severity of the illness and the reality that strong associations between emotional and behavioral difficulties occur only in those children with more severe forms of eczema. A study that included only preschool children with 10% or more of their skin surface being affected revealed a number of interesting differences in their adaptation when compared to normal controls. Specifically, greater problems with dependency, fearfulness, and sleep patterns were noted. Mothers of these children with eczema were also more likely to feel unsupported and be distressed (Daud, Garralda, & David, 1993).

MERGER INTERVENTIONS

The management of the environmental regulation of gene expression is a reorganizing clinical concept. Until recently, clinicians viewed the expression of genes as inevitable. Consequently, there was little clinical interest in developing psychosocial interventions for any disease that was believed to be "genetically" controlled.

Converging lines of evidence have made it clear that genes are expressed at specific points in development. A gene may remain dormant throughout life and never be expressed. To the degree that a particular genetic trait has variable "penetrance," it can be understood as having a variable probability of expression. Both medical and environmental interventions can be tested to determine their influence on the timing of expression of a target gene. A simple example of variability in timing of the expression of a gene is male baldness. During the first 20 years of a boy's life, there is no physical sign to identify whether he carries a gene that will result in premature hair loss. For more than 20 years, his baldness genes remain silent. Then, during early adulthood, a genetic "switch" is suddenly "flipped."

The data related to the differential expression of genetically controlled traits in monozygotic twins are of particular interest. Some genes have very powerful penetrance. Currently, we have little expectation of being able to influence the expression of powerfully penetrant genes. For example, it is extremely rare that identical twin pairs are discordant for eye color. Also, if one identical twin develops cystic fibrosis, it is still virtually inevitable that the second twin will eventually develop this disease. However, as we come to understand the precise variability of the different alleles that result in the development of cystic fibrosis, it may be possible to develop a "gene therapy" that can prevent its expression. However, it does suggest that environmental interventions are less likely to be successful.

In contrast, early-onset obesity, early-onset asthma, and eczema present attractive models for MERGER interventions. The first necessary strategy is to identify the children at risk. One straightforward method is to use a pedigree analysis. Those children with a high incidence of first- and second-degree relatives who have expressed the phenotype are quantitatively at greater risk. This is equally true for excessive weight, asthma, or atopic dermatitis.

To be able to mount an effective intervention for a specific child, it is helpful to know if the child in fact is carrying a vulnerable gene, or genes, for the disorder. It is highly probable that within a decade, more of the gene sites that control obesity and asthma will be identified. Furthermore, the sequence of specific alleles should be fully explicated. At that point, only children who actually have a known genetic vulnerability would be appropriate candidates for a MERGER intervention. However, at this time, any child who has a high probability of having an affected gene or genes, based on pedigree analysis, is an appropriate candidate for such a therapeutic strategy. This implies that some children who are at no actual genetic risk for the biological expression inevitably will be treated. Given this circumstance, MERGER interventions currently have few, if any, major negative sequellae or side effects.

In the case of obesity, a disproportionate weight-to-height ratio should signal the need for early intervention. For asthma, wheezing during the course of an infectious illness in the first years of life is a good indicator of bronchial hyperactivity and an increased risk for the development of the disease. For eczema, the unwelcome appearance of a scaly rash with intense puritis, often with the introduction of a new food, is a clear signal.

A MERGER intervention has recently been developed for the prevention of asthma, and its effectiveness is currently being assessed. This comprehensive intervention includes three specific treatment components that were each hypothesized to be effective. None of these interventions had potential negative sequellae. The intervention included an educational module designed to sensitize parents to the known risk factors associated with asthma onset, a hypoallergic diet module designed to minimize the exposure of the infant to foods known to have high antigenic properties, and a home-visiting module designed to help mothers to respond to their infants more sensitively and to make decisions related to child care and family management that would minimize the exposure of these children to increased emotional distress. Some 140 families were enrolled in the study, and ongoing data are available for the entire sample. Only preliminary findings are available, but what is striking is the low incidence of wheezing and the even lower frequency of diagnosis of asthma in this sample. Although these results may represent only a temporary delay in the onset of wheezing symptoms in these genetically at risk young children, the overall good health of this cohort is encouraging already.

A parallel MERGER intervention has been conceptualized for obesity that involves an educational, a dietary, and a parental support component. This obesity program is designed to support families in which obese parents identify an infant who has begun to gain weight excessively.

Infant mental health clinicians will play an increasingly prominent role in the implementation of such interventions. Effecting change in young families requires sensitivity to the developmental needs of infants and toddlers as well as to the emotional needs of these children and their parents. A multidisciplinary team is usually in the best position to mount such interventions. For such teams to be effective, they must include a clinician who can communicate the key intervention concepts to the parents and, most important, be able to effect a behavioral change in how these parents relate to their infants. The field of infant mental health will play an instrumental role in providing insights into effective methodologies for effective behavioral changes. However, until recently, the range of families with children who could benefit from such interventions has actually been quite narrow. As the number of illnesses with well-demonstrated genetic bases becomes better documented, the role of the environment in the regulation of gene function will become more defined. As more effective strategies to prevent the onset of psychosomatic illnesses are developed and are put into place, the public health implications of such efforts should be substantial.

REFERENCES

Alexander, F. (1950). *Psychosomatic medicine.* New York: Norton.

Arshad, S. H., Stevens, M., & Hide, D. W. (1993). The effect of genetic and environmental factors on the prevalence of allergic disorders at the age of two years. *Clinical Experimental Allergy, 23*(6), 504–511.

Blair, H. (1977). Natural history of childhood asthma. *Archives of Diseases of Children, 52,* 613–619.

Bos, J. D., Kapsenberg, M. L., & Smitt, J. H. (1994). Pathogenesis of atopic eczema. *Lancet, 343*(8909), 1338–1341.

Bouchard, C., Depres, J., & Tremblay, A. (1991). Genetics of obesity and human energy metabolism. *Proceedings of the Nutrition Society, 50,* 139–147.

Bouchard, C., & Perusse, L. (1993). Genetic Aspects of obesity. *Annals of the New York Academy of Science, 699,* 26–35.

Clement, K., Vaisse, C., Lahlou, N., Cabrol, S., Pelloux, V., & Cassuto, D. (1998). A mutation in the human leptin receptor gene causes obesity and pituitary dysfunction. *Nature, 392*(6674), 398–401.

Cohen, D. J. (1975). Psychosomatic models of development. In E. J. Anthony (Ed.), *Explorations in child psychiatry* (pp. 197–212). New York: Plenum.

Creer, T. L. (1976). Behavioral contributions to rehabilitation and childhood asthma. *Rehabilitation Literature, 37,* 226.

Daniels, S. E., Bhattacharrya, S., James, A., Leaves, N. I., Young, A., & Hill, M. R. (1996). A genome-wide search for quantitative trait loci underlying asthma. *Nature, 383*(6597), 247–250.

Daud, L. R., Garralda, M. E., & David, T. J. (1993). Psychosocial adjustment in preschool children with atopic eczema. *Archives of Disease in Childhood, 69*(6), 670–676.

Davis, K., & Christoffel, K. K. (1994). Obesity in preschool and school-age children: Treatment early and often may be best. *Archives of Pediatric and Adolescent Medicine, 148,* 12.

Dietz, W. H. (1994). Critical periods in childhood for the development of obesity. *American Journal of Clinical Nutrition, 59*(5), 955–959.

Dodge, R., Martinez, F. D., Cline, M. G., Lebowitz, M. D., & Burrows, B. (1996). Early childhood respiratory symptoms and the subsequent diagnosis of asthma. *Journal of Allergy and Clinical Immunology, 98*(1), 48–54.

Emde, R. N., Gaensbauer, T. J., & Harmon, R. J. (1982). Using our emotions: Some principles for appraising emotional development intervention. In M. Lewis & L. Taft (Eds.), *Developmental disabilities: Theory assessment and intervention* (pp. 409–424). New York: Spectrum.

Epstein, L. H., McCurley, J., Voloski, A., & Wing, R. R.

(1990). Growth in obese children treated for obesity. *American Journal of Diseases of Children, 144,* 1360–1364.

Fisch, R. O., Bilek, M. K., & Ulstrom, R. (1975). Obesity and leanness at birth and their relationship to body habitus in later childhood. *Pediatrics, 56*(4), 521–528.

Frick, O. L., German, D. F., & Mills, J. (1979). Development of allergy in children. I: Association with virus infections. *Journal of Allergy and Clinical Immunology, 63,* 228–241.

Gauthier, Y., Fortin, C., Drapeau, P., Breton, J. J., Gosselin, J., Quintal, L., Weisnagel, J., Tetreault, L., & Pinard, G. (1977). The mother–child relationship and the development of autonomy and self-assertion in young (14–30 months) asthmatic children. *Journal of the American Academy of Child Psychiatry, 16,* 109–131.

Gauthier, Y., Fortin, C., Drapeau, P., Breton, J. J., Gosselin, J., Quintal, L., Weisnagel, J., Tetreault, L., & Pinard, G. (1978). Follow-up study of 35 asthmatic preschool children. *Journal of the American Academy of Child Psychiatry, 17,* 679–694.

Gustafsson, P. A., Bjorksten, B., & Kjellman, N-I. M.(1994). Family dysfunction in asthma: A prospective study of illness development. *Journal of Pediatrics, 125*(3), 493–498.

Kay, J., Gawkrodger, D. J., Mortimer, M. J., & Jaron, A. G. (1994). The prevalence of childhood atopic eczema in a general population. *Journal of the American Academy of Dermatology, 30*(1), 35–39.

Klinnert M., Mrazek D. A., & Mrazek P. (1994). Early asthma onset: The interaction between family stressors and adaptive parenting. *Psychiatry, 57*(1), 51–61.

Kumanyika, S. (1993). Ethnicity and obesity development in children. *Annals of the New York Academy of Science, 699,* 81–92.

Larsen, F. S. (1993). Atopic dermatitis: A genetic–epidemiologic study in a population-based twin sample. *Journal of the American Academy of Dermatology, 28*(5 pt. 1), 719–723.

Locard, E., Mamelle, N., Billette, A., Miginiac, C., Munoz, F., & Rey, S. (1992). Risk Factors of Obesity in a Five year Old Population. Parental versus environmental factors. *International Journal of Obesity Related Metabolic Disorders, 16*(10), 721–729.

Lourie, R. S. (1955). Experience with therapy of psychosomatic problems in infants. In P. H. Hoch & J. Rubin (Eds.), *Psychopathology of childhood* (pp. 254–266). New York: Grune & Stratton.

Michel, F. B., Bousquet, J., Greillier, P., Robinet-Levy, M., & Coulomb, Y. (1980). Comparison of cord blood immunoglobulin E concentrations and maternal allergy for the prediction of atopic diseases in infancy. *Journal of Allergy and Clinical Immunology, 65,* 422–430.

Montague, C. T., Farooqi, S., Whitehead, J. P., Soos, M. A., Reau, H., & Wareham, N. J. (1997). Congenital leptin deficiency is associated with severe early-onset obesity in humans. *Nature, 387*(6636), 903–908.

Mrazek, D. A. (1992). Psychiatric complications of pediatric asthma. *Annals of Allergy, 69*(4), 285–290.

Mrazek, D. A. (1994). Disturbed emotional develop-

ment of severely asthmatic children. In A. West & M. J. Christie (Eds.), *Quality of life in childhood asthma* (pp. 71–80). Chichester, UK: Carden.

Mrazek, D. A. (1998). The new genetic paradigm in child psychiatry. *Current Opinion in Psychiatry, 11*(4), 371–372.

Mrazek, D. A., Anderson, I., & Strunk, R. (1983). Disturbed emotional development of severely asthmatic preschool children. In J. Stevenson (Ed.), *Recent research in developmental psychopathology, Journal of Child Psychology and Psychiatry book supplement no. 4* (pp. 81–93). Oxford, UK: Pergamon Press.

Mrazek, D. A., & Klinnert, M. (1991). Asthma: Psychoneuroimmunologic considerations. In R. Ader, E. L. Felton, & N. Cohen (Eds.), *Psychoneuroimmunology II* (2nd ed., pp. 1013–1035). Orlando, FL: Academic Press.

Mrazek, D. A., Klinnert, M., Brower, A., & Harbeck, R. J. (1990). Predictive capacity of elevated serum IgE for early asthma onset. *Journal of Allergy and Clinical Immunology, 85,* 194.

Mrazek, D. A., Klinnert, M., Mrazek, P., Brower, A., McCormick, D., Rubin, B., Ikle, D., Kastner, W., Larsen, G., Harbeck, R., & Jones, J. (1999). Prediction of early onset asthma in genetically at risk children. *Journal of Pediatric Pulmonology, 27,* 89–94.

Mrazek, D. A., Klinnert, M., Mrazek, P., & Macey, T. (1991). Early asthma onset: Consideration of parenting issues. *Journal of the American Academy of Child and Adolescent Psychiatry, 30,* 277–282.

Mrazek, D. A., Mrazek, P. B., & Klinnert, M. (1995). The clinical assessment of parenting. *Journal of the American Academy of Child and Adolescent Psychiatry, 34*(3), 272–282.

Mrazek, D. A., Schuman, W. B., & Klinnert, M. (1998). Early asthma onset: Risk of emotional and behavioral difficulties. *Journal of Child Psychology and Psychiatry, 39*(2), 247–254.

Parmelee, A. H. (1989). The child's physical health and the development of relationships. In A. J. Sameroff & R. N. Emde (Eds.), *Relationship disturbance in early childhood: A developmental approach* (pp. 145–162). New York: Basic Books.

Peat, J. K. (1996). The epidemiology of asthma. *Current Opinion in Pulmonary Medicine, 2,* 7–15.

Piaget, J. (1952). *The origins of intelligence in children.* New York: International Universities Press.

Price, R. A., & Gottesman, I. I. (1991). Body fat in identical twins reared apart: Roles of genes and environment. *Behavioral Genetics, 21*(1), 1–7.

Sameroff, A. J. (1986). Environmental context of child development. *Journal of Pediatrics, 109,* 192–200.

Sameroff, A. J., & Chandler, M. J. (1975). Reproductive risk and the continuum of caretaking causality. In F. D. Horowitz, M. Heatherington, S. Scan-Salapatek, & G. Siegel (Eds.), *Review of child development research* (Vol. 4, pp. 187–244). Chicago: University of Chicago.

Sameroff, A. J., & Emde, R. N. (Eds.). (1989). *Relationship disturbances in early childhood: A developmental approach.* New York: Basic Books.

Sampson, H. A. (1997). Food sensitivity and the pathogenesis of atopic dermatitis. *Journal of the Royal Society of Medicine, 90*(S30), 2–8.

Schonfeld-Warden, N., & Warden, C. H. (1997). Pediatric obesity: An overview of etiology and treatment. *Pediatric Clinics of North America, 44*(2), 339–361.

Shields, J. (1962). *Monozygotic twins brought up apart and together.* London: Oxford University Press.

Smith, J. M. (1988). Epidemiology and natural history of asthma, allergic rhinitis, and atopic dermatitis (eczema). In E. Middleton, C. E. Reed, & E. F. Ellis (Eds.), *Allergy: Principles and practice* (3rd ed., pp. 891–929). St. Louis: Mosby.

Spitz, R. (1965). *The first year of life.* New York: International Universities Press.

Stunkard, A. J., Sorensen, T. I., Hanis, C., Teasdale, T. W., Chakraborty, R., Schull, W. J., & Schulsinger, F. (1986). An adoption study of human obesity. *New England Journal of Medicine, 314*(4), 193–198.

V

INTERVENTION

❖

Concerned as it must be with development, infant mental health is inherently involved with the process of change. Intervention efforts are designed to effect change, more rapidly and more effectively than might occur otherwise. Some interventions target infants' developmental trajectories, attempting to enhance the subsequent development of infants who are deviating from early adaptive pathways. Other interventions are designed to provide treatment to infants who are not merely at risk for symptoms or disorders but who are disturbed or disordered already. Across diverse approaches is an emphasis on relationships between infant and caregiver and between clinician and family. In fact, it may well be that the nature of the therapeutic relationship is one of the best predictors of the success of intervention efforts.

A key feature of therapeutic relationships is the working alliance, that shared sense between clinician and parent of working together in the best interest of the infant. For this reason, virtually all successful interventions make establishing and maintaining a therapeutic alliance between parents and therapists vital steps. For infant mental health clinicians, how the baby is incorporated into the alliance is a central question.

In Chapter 28, Beckwith reviews what is known about preventive intervention efforts in the United States. This review clearly indicates that prevention programs are more effective when they are based on prior knowledge of the risk behaviors, as well as the risk conditions, of the target population. Providing interventions indiscriminately, without regard to a detailed knowledge of specific needs of the participants, is unlikely to be effective. In keeping with the other chapters in Part V, Beckwith also notes the centrality of the relationship between intervenor and family as crucial to successful outcomes.

In Chapter 29, Gilkerson and Stott provide an important overview of the historical roots and philosophical framework of early intervention. This approach to infants and toddlers with disabilities has grown out of the tradition of education rather than health care. As mandated by U.S. government guidelines, early intervention emphasizes values and principles of family-centered services and a belief in natural environments—that is, settings that are natural for the child's age peers—as the primary resource for child development. Gilkerson and Stott consider in detail the philosophical similarities and differences in the approaches of early intervention and infant mental health. They point out that although these two orientations have come together through a more relational focus on infancy in the past few years, it is clear that considerable misunderstandings and some real differences between the two approaches remain. They conclude that exploring similarities and differences in frameworks may enhance our capacity to respond to infants and families in need.

In Chapter 30, Lieberman, Silverman, and Pawl describe infant–parent psychotherapy, perhaps the best known and most widely practiced intervention in infant mental health. Described originally by Selma Fraiberg and her colleagues in Michigan, infant–parent psychotherapy is a multimodal method of intervention that uses joint work with parents, infants, toddlers, and, more recently, preschoolers. The ultimate goal is improving parent–child relationships and children's socioemotional functioning. In this chapter, they describe both core concepts and recent innovations in this therapeutic approach that always has emphasized the therapeutic relationship as a basic catalyst for change.

McDonough, in Chapter 31, describes interaction guidance, another form of intervention that is widely practiced in infant mental health settings around the world. Developed originally for use with difficult-to-engage families, this approach has applicability at all levels of social class and psychological resources. At its core are principles of a focus on strengths and on self-observation as a vehicle for change.

Finally, Field describes infant massage as a therapeutic intervention in Chapter 32. She points to its worldwide popularity and to a small but growing body of literature suggesting its efficacy. Although this clearly is an infant-directed intervention, her review makes clear that it provides ample opportunities for infant–caregiver change. This approach may be a primary intervention in some settings and a useful adjunct in others.

28

Prevention Science and Prevention Programs

❖

LEILA BECKWITH

PRINCIPLES OF PREVENTION SCIENCE

Preventive intervention, as discussed in this chapter, is a process between child development professionals and families whereby family conditions, parenting behavior, and/ or children's behavior are altered. The purpose is to increase the probability of normal developmental trajectories in childhood and adolescence and to decrease potential later disorders. Prevention programs aim to prevent a condition that has not yet occurred and, generally, are conducted with children who do not show diagnosable disorders or disabilities. The premise is that prevention is easier and results in less serious consequences for the family, the child, and the community than does treatment of a disorder. The interventions discussed in this chapter were geared to infants and young children who were at an increased statistical risk for later developmental problems. The prevention efforts were based on a model of human development in which risk and protective factors, arising from both biological and social influences, shape the paths by which individuals become vulnerable or resistant to developmental deviance.

Risk factors are those characteristics or hazards that increase the possibility of the occurrence, severity, duration, or frequency of later psychological disorders (Coie et al., 1993). Risks arise in multiple spheres: within the child

as in physiological, attentional, or temperamental vulnerabilities or impairments within the parent–child relationship resulting in deficits in involvement, nurturance, and protection (Bowlby, 1982), as well as ineffective or punitive discipline. Risks also arise from the individual characteristics of the parents, as in their model of attachment derived from the adverse caregiving they received within their family of origin (Main, Kaplan, & Cassidy, 1985), psychological disorders, or alcohol and drug abuse. Risks may also originate in the structure and functioning of the family unit or in the marital interaction in discord, divorce, or single parenting. Intensely stressful life events within the family ecology, such as unemployment or extreme poverty, are another possible source.

Risk factors often co-occur. For example, mothers subjected to adverse experiences in the family of origin, who dismiss the formative influence of parent–child relationships, or are preoccupied with them, are less likely to form stable marital relationships and more likely to experience marital discord and/or divorce (Greenberg, Speltz, & DeKlyen, 1993). Marital discord and divorce increase the likelihood of financial strain and parent–child conflict (O'Connor & Rutter, 1996).

Risk factors also are additive, and with respect to some later disorders, each exposure to a new risk may increase the vulnerability exponentially (Sameroff, Seifer, Baldwin, & Baldwin, 1993). Because they tend to affect a number of developing adaptive functions, most risk conditions, dependent on the biological and social context of development, can potentiate a variety of later disorders (Coie, et al., 1993). Similarly, multiple paths that include different combinations of risk factors can lead to the same outcome. Still, risks do not fully determine outcome, because some children in a risk group will develop the anticipated adverse consequences but some will not.

The balance between risk and protective factors is most potent in affecting development (Lester et al., 1995). *Protective factors* are those conditions that increase resilience under conditions of adversity and increase resistance to later disturbances (Masten & Coatsworth, 1998). Protective factors, akin to risks, also exist in multiple domains. They may exist within the child, as with intelligence or skills in self-regulation; or within the parent, as commitment and sensitivity to the needs of the child and appropriate discipline, monitoring, and supervision. A close attachment with an effective parent or parent figure has been found to be a universal protective factor for children growing up under adversity (Werner & Smith, 1982). Similarly, a powerful protective factor for parents is their close relationships to other adults. Social support, social transactions through which needed emotional, informational, and concrete resources are exchanged, buffers the effects of life stresses. Mothers who have more satisfactory social relationships with other adults, particularly stable, supportive marital relationships, manifest better parent–child interaction (Crockenberg, 1981) and feel more competent as parents and less stressed by their parenting responsibilities (Crnic, Greenberg, Ragozin, Robinson, & Basham, 1983). Therefore, the relationship with the intervenor to provide social support is a widely used intervention strategy (Thompson, 1995).

Developing and implementing effective prevention programs is extremely challenging. The difficulties are conceptual as well as methodological (O'Connor & Rutter, 1996). The developmental tasks that young children confront with the help of their families—physiological regulation, attachment (Ainsworth, Blehar, Waters, & Wall, 1978), exploration/learning (White, 1959), emotional self-regulation (Robinson, Emde, & Korfmacher, 1997), sense of self, and autonomy (Emde & Buchsbaum, 1990), and internalization of rules (Kochanska, 1997)—are vastly different from those to be

faced later, including school achievement, work, friendships, resistance to substance use, and avoidance of delinquency. What are the developmental pathways? How can more normative trajectories be effected? An organizational perspective of development suggests that positive adaptation to one developmental task increases the likelihood of adaptively resolving subsequent tasks (Cicchetti & Toth, 1998; Sroufe, 1988). But what factors within the family and/or the child should be addressed, knowing that development also will be influenced by forces that have yet to occur, such as peers, schoolteachers, and changes in the family's structure and functioning?

Prevention programs are a promising route for understanding normative and pathological developmental processes. Prevention is embedded in epidemiological, child development, and clinical research and, in turn, contributes to and can be used as experimental tests of theoretical models of development. The classic, brilliant work by Skeels (1966) during the 1930s is an example. Out of concern for the lack of emotional care received by infants and young children in orphanages, he placed individual infants in wards of mentally retarded adolescents and adults, who showered the infants with loving, social interactions. Those fortunate infants became socially and cognitively competent young children, were attractive enough to be adopted, and went on to live normal, useful lives, in marked contrast to those who received ordinary orphanage care. The brilliant intervention contributed immeasurably to the understanding of the powerful effects for children's development of early parent–child attachments and led to a social policy promoting adoption rather than orphanages.

In this chapter, we describe and evaluate examples of prevention efforts addressed to illustrative protective factors, maternal sensitivity and child's security of attachment, and a range of risk conditions that are relevant to the lives of young children and their families. The risk conditions chosen, coercive parental discipline, child prematurity, family marital discord/divorce, and family poverty, are not exhaustive but represent a span from those in which there is extensive knowledge of developmental paths, many efforts at prevention, and long-term follow-up to conditions with much less information. Whenever possible, we select from prevention studies that occurred post-birth-hospitalization, that endured for more than the first month of life, and that evaluated effectiveness in changing children's development by comparing randomly assigned intervention groups to control groups. Some exceptions are made to illustrate a risk condition for which prevention efforts are only beginning.

The multiple nature of risks, often overlapping, provides multiple foci for prevention. Prevention efforts can target the child directly, parenting and the parent–child relationship, the parent's individual strengths and vulnerabilities, and/or the family's ecology and functioning (see Figure 28.1 for a model of prevention paths). The programs described and evaluated in this chapter illustrate one or more of the paths and have used multiple means of intervention: home visits, parent groups, couple groups, and/or early education daycare/preschool. Universal interventions that are addressed to the general population are not reviewed.

SELECTED PREVENTION PROGRAMS

Protective Factors in Parenting: Sensitive Responsiveness and Security of Attachment

Maternal sensitivity to child signals has been shown to influence a range of developing cogni-

tive and social/emotional competencies. Moreover, sensitive, responsive caregiving moderates the effects of high-risk environments and promotes resilience and positive change for children who have experienced poverty, family stress, and maltreatment (Egeland, Carlson, & Sroufe, 1993). Further, sensitive caregiving during infancy is a significant causal factor in attachment security concurrently (Ainsworth et al., 1978) and, in the context of benign life experiences, endures to early adulthood as a representational model of attachment relationships (Beckwith, Cohen, & Hamilton, 1999). Secure attachments are a general protective factor that buffer both parents and their children against risk conditions and diminish the likelihood of later disorders in the children (Egeland et al., 1993).

One of the most effective interventions aimed at enhancing maternal sensitivity and infant security is that of van den Boom (1994, 1995). She instituted a short-term, behaviorally focused, skill-based training program to enhance maternal sensitivity of lower-class Dutch mothers with first-born irritable babies. The temperamental quality of negative emotionality was chosen as a risk condition because it has been linked to increased insecure attachments (Miyake, Chen, & Campos, 1985) and more internalizing and externalizing behavior problems (Lyons-Ruth, Easterbrooks, & Cibelli,

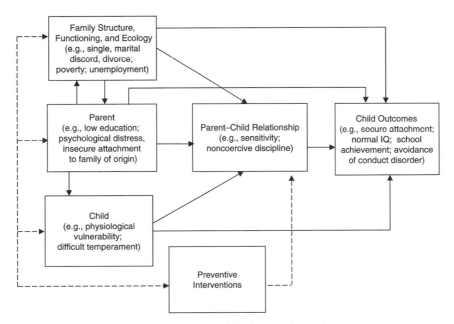

FIGURE 28.1. Model of prevention paths.

1997). Infants were identified at birth by high irritability scores on two separate Brazelton examinations. When the infants were 6 months and continuing to 9 months, the intervenor made three home visits, promoting maternal skills in responding to negative and positive infant cues during everyday interactions. The 6- to 9-month period was chosen because it is a point at which mothers may lose confidence in their mothering of more difficult babies, and when mothers would be very motivated to learn adequate behavioral responses. At the conclusion of intervention, mothers in the intervention group were significantly more responsive to their infants than were the control mothers. At 12 months, 68% of the infants in the intervention group (the proportion found in middle-class normative samples) were securely attached to their mothers, whereas only 28% of the infants in the control group were. The infants and their mothers were further evaluated at 18 and 24 months and at 3½ years, in naturalistic and structured situations at home and in the laboratory with the mother and with unfamiliar peers (van den Boom, 1995). Intervention continued to be associated with secure attachment: 72% at 18 months in the intervention group were secure as compared to 26% in the comparison group. Almost 3 years after the end of intervention, mothers in the intervention group remained significantly more sensitive and responsive to their children; their children were more cooperative with them and with unfamiliar peers and were more likely to be chosen by unfamiliar peers for play.

van IJzendoorn, Juffer, and Duyvesteyn (1995) conducted a meta-analysis of 12 studies that aimed to enhance parental sensitivity and thereby increase children's attachment security. Whereas both parental sensitivity and child attachment security were significantly enhanced in the van den Boom (1994) study, van IJzendoorn et al. (1995) found that some efforts increased parental sensitivity without increasing infant security. Some studies found no differences in the proportion of security between their intervention and control groups (Barnard et al., 1988, with poor, single, socially isolated mothers; Beckwith, 1988, with poor, low-educated mothers of preterms with respiratory distress; Brinich, Drotar, & Brinich, 1989, with children diagnosed as nonorganically failure to thrive). One study (Lieberman, Weston, & Pawl, 1991) provided intervention to Latina mothers and their insecurely attached toddlers

and increased proximity-seeking behavior and decreased avoidant behaviors of the children to their mothers, but did not increase the overall secure attachment. Some studies even found decreased, rather than increased, proportions of secure attachments associated with intervention (Barnett, Blignault, Holmes, Payne, & Parker, 1987; Erickson, Korfmacher, & Egeland, 1992).

van IJzendoorn et al. (1995) concluded that (1) more focused programs—that is, those programs that addressed directly the desired changes in behavior—tended to be more effective than those that addressed more general qualities of the parent such as social support or mental representation of attachment; (2) more focused programs tended to be given to more well-functioning families, whereas the more comprehensive programs were directed to more multiproblem families. Thus, comprehensiveness was confounded with the degree of vulnerability within the populations. Because security of attachment is more likely to occur in families with more psychological resources, rather than less, the likelihood of intervention effectiveness is markedly decreased in multiproblem families, regardless of the nature of the intervention. Nonetheless, there are exceptions, with at least one study reporting success with intensive interventions with high-risk families (Lyons-Ruth, Connell, Grunebaum, & Botein, 1990).

As of now, the evidence suggests that short, behaviorally focused interventions do work to enhance security of attachment of infants in relatively well-functioning families. Longer, more intense interventions with multiproblem families work sometimes, but under what conditions is not yet clear.

Risk Factor in Parenting: Coercive Discipline

Parents who regulate their children's behavior through criticism, lack of praise, physical coercion, and inconsistent monitoring are more likely to have children who develop externalizing behavior problems (Shaw, Gilliom, & Giovannelli, Chapter 25, this volume). In contrast, parents who promote autonomy, engage in more shared positive affect, and are more cooperative with their child are more likely to have children who internalize the parent's rules and values (Kochanska, 1997). Theory-based parent training, in which parents learn to reinforce prosocial child behavior and to reduce negative child behavior, is one of the more well-examined, effective intervention techniques for children and adolescents with externalizing behavioral problems. Webster-Stratton (1990, 1998; Webster-Stratton & Hammond, 1997), in a series of studies, has formed parent groups for families with young, conduct-disordered children and used videotaped materials with a discussion leader to train parents in noncoercive behavioral management and ways to engage in more positive interactions with their child. An individually administered videotape-modeling parent training program has been used as well (Webster-Stratton, Kolpacoff, & Hollinsworth, 1988). At short-term follow-up, children's aggressiveness and noncompliance in the family were reduced, as were parental use of criticism and physical discipline, possibly changing the trajectory of the children's development (Webster-Stratton, 1990).

Risk Conditions within the Child: Prematurity

Children born prematurely, particularly those of very low birthweight, and those with perinatal complications of respiratory distress and intracranial hemorrhages of severe degree are at increased risk for later cognitive limitations, attentional problems, difficulties in school achievement, and behavioral disturbances (Minde, Chapter 10, this volume). The Infant Health and Development Project (IHDP), in 10 sites across the country, provided intervention to 985 families and their preterm children, from the early months of life to age 3 years (Brooks-Gunn et al., 1994; Brooks-Gunn, Gross, Kraemer, Spiker, & Shapiro, 1992; IHDP, 1990; McCarton, Brooks-Gunn, Wallace, & Bauer, 1997; Ramey et al., 1992). Home visits were used to guide parenting behavior, and a full-day, center-based, educational day-care program was provided in order to directly change the child. Children in both intervention and control groups received medical, developmental, and social assessments, with referral for further care as indicated. The home visitor met weekly for the first year and then biweekly for the next 2 years with the mother and used a prescribed curriculum to encourage specific, developmentally appropriate games between parent and child. The center-based, educational day-care program began at 12 months of age and continued for the next 2 years. There were scheduled parent group meetings as well.

At the end of intervention, at age 3, children in the intervention group achieved significantly higher cognitive test scores, significantly so across all birthweights, but with larger effects for the infants with higher birthweights. They also had higher receptive vocabulary test scores and lower scores on maternal reports of behavior problems (Ramey et al., 1992). At 5 and 8 years of age, significant differences in IQ were no longer apparent for the intervention group, although the heavier birthweight children still had significantly higher IQ scores and higher math achievement scores than the comparison group (McCarton et al., 1997). At age 8, the last published follow-up, there were no differences in rates of grade repetition or special education or in behavioral problems (McCarton et al., 1997).

During the intervention, the intervention mothers interacted more positively with their children at age 2 1/2 years and were more likely to be employed and for more months (Brooks-Gunn, Klebanov, & Liaw, 1995; Spiker, Ferguson, & Brooks-Gunn, 1993). There were no differences in rates of subsequent pregnancy, welfare use, or months in schooling.

Risks from Maternal Psychological Distress: Depressive Symptoms and Anxiety

Children whose mothers experience severe, chronic depressive symptoms during pregnancy and postbirth are vulnerable to later poorer achievement and increased rates of diagnosable psychopathology, particularly depression, but also including conduct disorder, attention-deficit disorder, and substance abuse (Zahn-Waxler, Cummings, Iannotti, & Radke-Yarrow, 1984). The causes are found in multiple risks arising from genetic influences, altered parenting behavior, and associated disrupted family functioning (Dickstein et al., 1998).

There are, as yet, few preventive intervention studies that have specifically addressed depressed mothers and their children (Field, 1997). Lyons-Ruth et al. (1990) offered weekly home visits for 13 months to 31 depressed mothers, living in poverty, whose caretaking of their infants was considered inadequate. The intervenor aimed to increase maternal competence in obtaining basic needs, model and reinforce more positive and developmentally appropriate parenting, and decrease social isolation. When the infants were 18 months of age, infants of mothers who had received home visits were cognitively more competent than were infants of unserved mothers and were more likely to be classified as securely attached in their relationship with their mothers, 57% as compared to 20% secure in the comparison group. Intervention did not alter maternal depressive symptoms. Infants of unserved, depressed mothers showed not only poorer cognitive functioning but also high rates of angry, rejecting behaviors and an increased proportion of the disorganized pattern of attachment, linked to later behavioral problems in school.

High levels of anxiety often co-occur with depressive symptoms. Children of parents with anxiety disorders, with or without depression, are more likely themselves to suffer behavioral inhibition, social avoidance, and anxiety disorders than are children of nonanxious parents (Manassis, Bradley, Goldberg, Hood, & Swinson, 1995; Rosenbaum et al., 1988; Silverman, Cerny, Nelles, & Burke, 1988). Barnett et al. (1987), in a nonclinical sample, screened 134 mothers after delivery as to level of anxiety and randomly assigned them to professional intervention with a social worker, nonprofessional support from an experienced mother, or a control group. Although maternal anxiety was reduced in the professional intervention group as compared to the other two groups, attachment security was reduced for their children; 59% secure as compared to 74% secure in the control group.

These studies underscore a principle of prevention science: Preventive interventions depend on and contribute to the understanding of developmental pathways from risk conditions to later disorders. In one study, children's behavioral functioning improved even when maternal symptoms did not; in the other, children's adaptive functioning decreased when maternal well-being increased. Although the evidence thus far is sparse, it does suggest that even though maternal psychological distress is a risk condition, it does not mediate children's adaptation directly. If so, prevention needs to address parenting behavior and the parent–child relationship, rather than, or in addition to, parental psychological symptoms.

Risks and Family Functioning: Single Parent, Marital Discord, Divorce

Single parenting, marital conflict, and divorce are associated with increased likelihood of a wide range of deleterious effects in children, including more behavioral problems, poorer academic performance, depression, conduct disorders, and, as young adults, more difficulty in attaining intimate relationships (Hetherington, Bridges, & Isabella, 1998). Moreover, marital satisfaction may act as a protective factor against cross-generational transmission of negative parenting (Belsky, Youngblade, & Pensky, 1989). Prevention programs to increase marital satisfaction and constructive handling of conflictual issues have used a strategy of weekly couples' groups, meetings with a professional intervenor, and focusing on marital roles and communication. Using a brief five-session program to teach effective communication and conflict management skills, Markman, Renick, Floyd, Stanley, and Clements (1993) found that intervention was associated with half as many divorces, fewer marital problems, and greater satisfaction through 4 to 5 years after intervention. Cowan and Cowan (1987, 1997) instituted a prevention program for nonclinical couples who were becoming parents to work out troubling marital issues and parental roles. Program couples, in comparison to the controls, reported more marital satisfaction and intact marriages throughout the second year of parenthood.

Risks in the Family Ecology: Poverty and Associated Factors

Poverty is a complex phenomenon associated with alterations in community stresses and supports, family structure, maternal psychological resources, and parenting attitudes and behaviors (Aber, Jones, & Cohen, Chapter 6, this volume). The Prenatal/Early Infancy Project (the Elmira project) provided home visits by public health nurses trained in parent education, methods of involving family and friends in assisting the mother, and linkage of the family with other health and human services, to 400 first-time mothers and their children, 85% of whom had at least one of the following risk factors: less than age 19 at intake, single, and low socioeconomic status; nearly 25% of the women had all three risk factors. Two intervention groups were randomly constituted: home visiting only during pregnancy, home visits beginning in pregnancy and continuing through the first 2 years of life; and two control groups, one receiving free transportation to prenatal and well-child visits and one receiving only health and developmental screening and follow-up referrals at 1 and 2 years of age (Olds, Henderson, Tatelbaum, & Chamberlin, 1986a, 1986b; Olds et al., 1997; Olds et al., 1998; Olds & Korfmacher, 1998). The home visits, on average 9 during pregnancy and 23 from birth to age 2, focused on health-related behaviors during pregnancy and infancy; maternal life-course development as to family planning, education, and employment; and parenting behavior.

Significant effects of the intervention were seen immediately during pregnancy in less cigarette use and more social support (Olds et al., 1986a, 1986b). In the two intervention groups, mothers who smoked had significantly fewer preterm infants than did control mothers who smoked, and birthweights were higher for intervention teenage mothers than for their comparison peers. However, only for the intervention group that received both prenatal and postnatal home visits were later changes in parenting behavior and maternal life course evident. For that group, during the intervention there were decreased reports of child abuse and neglect among the higher-risk families, as well as fewer safety hazards in their homes. Two years after the end of intervention, their children were seen less frequently in the hospital emergency department. Through age 4 and continuing until the final published follow-up at age 15, there were no significant differences in children's IQ, completed years of education for the mother, or home environment. The follow-up at age 15 years found fewer reported acts of child abuse and neglect for the full intervention sample and the higher-risk subsample (Olds et al., 1997). The most at-risk mothers in the prenatal–postnatal intervention group had fewer subsequent pregnancies and births, had a longer birth interval between the first and second child, spent fewer months receiving Aid for Dependent Children (AFDC), and had lower levels of criminal activity. Children in the prenatal–postnatal intervention group also had fewer arrests than children in the other groups.

Project CARE randomly assigned 66 children to a control group or either of two intervention groups to compare two intervention strategies: (1) home visits in which the intervenor promoted parent problem solving and demonstrated to the mother developmentally appropriate activities and (2) home visits plus an educational day-care program for the child (Ramey & Ramey, 1992; Wasik, Ramey, Bryant, & Sparling, 1990). Interventions began during the first few months after birth and continued throughout the child's preschool years. Children's IQ scores, beginning at 12 months and continuing until the last assessment at 54 months, were significantly higher for children in the group receiving educational day-care and home visits, as compared to those whose parents received only the home visits or no intervention at all, groups that did not differ from each other. Neither intervention influenced the home environment or maternal attitudes about parenting.

The Carolina Abecedarian Project (Campbell & Ramey, 1994; Ramey & Campbell, 1991) provided first-born infants of mostly single, poor mothers with a full-day, year-round, quality early education day care, beginning in early infancy and continuing until kindergarten. Medical services also were provided. Early intervention was associated with significantly higher IQ scores from the end of intervention through age 12. Although IQ differences were no longer significant by age 15, children from the preschool program continued to show higher scores on achievement tests, as well as a decreased likelihood of being retained in grade and fewer special educational placements (Ramey & Campbell, 1991). Further, mothers in the program achieved significantly more years of education and were less likely to be unemployed. There were no changes in the cognitive stimulation in the home environment or in maternal parenting attitudes.

The Syracuse University Family Development Research Program (Honig, Lally, & Mathieson, 1982; Lally, Mangione, & Honig, 1988) provided prenatal and postnatal weekly home visits by paraprofessionals, as well as quality early education day care beginning when the children were 6 months of age, to 108 poor, mostly single mothers with less than a high school education. At 3 years, intervention children had significantly higher IQ scores, but by 5 years of age, there were no differences between the groups. On follow-up at adolescence, 10 years after the end of intervention, the intervention and comparison groups differed in the rate of delinquent behavior, with 22% of the control group as compared with 6% in the intervention group having been processed in the legal system.

The Yale Child Welfare Project (Provence & Naylor, 1983) began home visits at birth to 17 families and continued with quality day care, pediatric care, developmental examinations, and home visits through 30 months postpartum. When the children were 12 years old, 10 years after intervention had ended, there were no differences in IQ, but those in the intervention group had better school attendance and adjustment and had required fewer remedial services than did the children in the comparison families (Seitz, Rosenbaum, & Apfel, 1985). Further, mothers who had received intervention, in contrast to the comparison women, had had fewer children, with births spaced more widely and had obtained more education. Moreover, 19 years after completion of intervention, benefits of the intervention had been diffused to later-born children, who also had better school attendance, required less remedial services, and were more likely to be making normal school progress than were the younger siblings in the comparison families (Seitz & Apfel, 1994).

The High/Scope Perry Preschool Project provided weekly home visits and a 2-year, daily, center-based preschool education program to 3- to 4-year-old low IQ children of single, low-educated, poor mothers (Berrueta-Clement, Schweinhart, Barnett, Epstein, & Weikart, 1984; Schweinhart & Weikart, 1997; Weikart & Schweinhart, 1992). There were short-term effects in raising children's IQ at ages 4 to 7 years, followed by decreased years in special education, higher achievement scores during high school, more students graduating high school and attending postsecondary education, and, by age 28 years, more young adults who were employed for longer periods, earning higher wages, and less involved in delinquency, crime, and teenage pregnancy. At age 28, one third of the intervention group as compared to 14% of the comparison group had never been identified as handicapped, never arrested, did not drop out of high school, and were never on welfare.

EFFECTIVENESS OF PREVENTION PROGRAMS

Short-Term Effects

Table 28.1 summarizes changes in children's functioning, maternal life course, and parenting behavior associated with the interventions in each of the 11 studies described in some detail (omitting studies that did not assess children's outcomes). Any integration of these efforts is

biased by the selection of the studies and the limited nature of the assessments used in some studies, particularly of parenting behavior and parental lives. However, 9 of the 11 studies enhanced children's functioning, at least in the short term. The five studies that provided an early education program directly to the children aimed to enhance cognitive functioning (as denoted by increases in IQ) were successful in almost every case (80%). The six studies that provided preventive interventions only to the parents were less successful in raising IQ (16%), but most targeted social–emotional functioning, rather than cognitive, and succeeded in decreasing behavioral problems, improving peer relations, increasing school achievement, and increasing rates of secure attachment. Adequate research has not yet been conducted as to the long-term effects of many of these social–emotional changes. Of the effective studies that enhanced children's functioning, five of them also affected parenting behavior and four changed maternal lives. On the basis of the limited information, it appears that effective prevention for young children at risk occurs with and without direct interventions with the child, often when parenting behavior is changed and often accompanied by changes in mothers' lives.

Long-Term Effects

Information about the sequelae in adolescence or adulthood of preventive interventions exists for only some studies—those that began at least 15–20 years ago and showed large early effects. Thus, the data are incomplete and may be misleading. Still, some trends are apparent. Impressive long-lasting effects, despite fadeout effects in some domains, have been demonstrated both in those interventions that affected the children directly with an educational day-care or preschool program and those that worked only with the mother.

Cognitive gains, as in IQ scores, eroded over time but enhanced school and work achievement, and less involvement in delinquency and crime followed in adolescence and adulthood. Less involvement in crime as an adult was evident even in the absence of IQ gain during intervention (Olds et al., 1997), contrary to the assertion that only those who derived short-term large cognitive benefits will show later effects (Yoshikawa, 1994). Still, sleeper effects and later enduring effects probably do not occur

TABLE 28.1. Prevention Programs and Their Effects

Program	Effects		
	Child	Maternal life course	Parent–child relationship
Abecedarian (Campbell & Ramey, 1994)	↑ IQ; ↑ achievement ↓ Retention in grade ↓ Special education	↑ Education ↑ Employment	n.s. HOME, positive child-rearing attitudes
Barnett, Blignault, Holmes, Payne, & Parker (1987)	n.s. Security of attachment	↓ Anxiety	Not measured
High/Scope Perry Preschool (Weikart & Schweinhart, 1992)	↑ IQ; ↑ achievement	n.s. Employment	n.s. Child-rearing attitudes
IHDP (Ramey et al., 1992; McCarton, Brooks-Gunn, Wallace, & Bauer, 1997)	↑ IQ; ↑ achievement ↓ Behavior problems n.s. Special education	↑ Employment n.s. Education, welfare, subsequent pregnancies	↑ Sensitive responsiveness
Lyons-Ruth, Connell, Grunebaum, & Botein (1990)	↑ Security ↑ IQ ↓ Behavior problems	n.s. Depression	n.s. Responsiveness
Prenatal/Early Infancy (Olds et al., 1997)	↑ Achievement ↓ Delinquency	↓ Welfare ↓ Crime ↓ Subsequent pregnancies ↑ Family and partner support	↓ Child abuse ↑ Positive child-rearing attitudes ↓ Restrictive and punishing discipline
Project CARE (Wasik, Ramey, Bryant, & Sparling, 1990)	n.s. IQ (parent component)	Not reported	n.s. HOME
Syracuse University Family Development Research (Lally, Mangione, & Honig, 1988)	↑ IQ ↓ Delinquency	Not reported	Not reported
van den Boom (1995)	↑ Security ↑ Peer relations	Not reported	↑ Sensitive responsiveness ↑ Fostering autonomy
Webster-Stratton (1998)	↓ Negative behavior ↑ Cooperation ↑ Positive affect	Not reported	↓ Criticism ↓ Physical punishment ↑ Praise
Yale Child Welfare (Provence & Naylor, 1983)	n.s. IQ ↑ School attendance ↑ Peer relations ↓ Special education	↑ Education ↑ Delay in subsequent pregnancies	↑ Sensitive responsiveness ↑ Fostering autonomy

Note. n.s. refers to nonsignificant statistical differences between intervention on and comparison group.

in the absence of large and significant changes in the child, in cognition and/or social–emotional functioning, and in parenting behavior (Yoshikawa, 1994).

The findings underscore the fact that in prevention science, developmental tasks change over time. Continuity in specific behaviors is not the goal of prevention but, rather, successful resolution of developmental tasks as they emerge. Whereas cognitive effects fade, effects of increased mastery motivation and enhanced emotional and behavioral regulation continue, as evident in increased involvement in achievement and good citizenship.

Limits of Prevention Programs

In general, even the most effective prevention programs did not achieve the goal of enabling a group of children whose families had multiple risks to be indistinguishable from their nonrisk peers. Although children who had been members of high-quality successful prevention projects, as a group, were significantly less compromised in achievement and social–emotional competence than were their high-risk peers who had not received intervention, outcomes remained more problematic when compared to those of nonrisk children. Results from the High/Scope Project (Weikart & Schweinhart, 1992) illustrate. By age 19, there were 68 teen pregnancies per 100 females in the intervention group. At age 27, many children, 34%, in the experimental group had not graduated high school. A high percentage of individuals, 57%, in the experimental group had been arrested; the average number of arrests for the group was 2.3. On one hand, the percentages in these indices of life problems were significantly reduced for the intervention group as compared to the controls; on the other hand, intervention did not prevent serious difficulties for many individuals.

However, programs targeted to families with fewer risks do achieve higher levels of children's functioning, as in security of attachment (van den Boom, 1995), comparable to the nonrisk, normative population. Not surprisingly, the nature of the sample, particularly the balance between protective and risk conditions, affects the degree to which the group will be helped.

STRUCTURE OF PREVENTION

Timing

There is some evidence that, when feasible, pregnancy, as a time of transition to parenting, is a particularly effective time to begin intervention (Olds et al., 1998). The Elmira project began during pregnancy with women who expected to deliver their first-born child, in order to capitalize on their openness to learning and their increased motivation for guidance as they began their transition to parenting, as well as to address behaviors during pregnancy, (e.g., smoking) that compromise fetal development. Other projects, although they did not start during pregnancy, did begin at times of family transitions—for example, marriage (Cowan & Cowan, 1987) or parenting, and/or did include only first-born children and their families in order to maximize motivation for help and flexibility to change (van den Boom, 1995).

For those conditions that have not yet occurred during pregnancy (e.g. prematurity, infant irritability, infant insecurity of attachment, and child low IQ) initiating an intervention during pregnancy is not possible. Moreover, some strategies of intervention would also not be possible (e.g., an early educational program for the child or guided parent–child interaction as to responsiveness or discipline). The onset of intervention, therefore, must be shaped by the parental or child behaviors being targeted, as well as by the life stages of the family.

Duration

Other than timing of onset, duration of the intervention also contributes to effectiveness. In the Elmira project, the maximum benefits in maternal life changes and children's development were found for the group that received prenatal and postnatal home visits. Intervention only during pregnancy was much less effective. The Abecedarian intervention plus a follow-on program during elementary school was more effective than the Abecedarian alone but when not combined with the Abecedarian intervention contributed little to children's functioning (Campbell & Ramey, 1994). As expected, these studies suggest that longer duration is more effective than shorter duration.

Components

Congruent with the finding that longer duration increases effectiveness is the assumption that more components, directed both to the parent and the child, are more effective than single components. For example, Webster-Stratton and Hammond (1997) compared a parent training intervention, a child training group, and a combined child and parent training group for parents of children with early-onset conduct problems. Comparison of the three intervention conditions indicated that the combined child training and parent training condition produced the most significant improvements in child behavior at 1-year follow-up.

Despite the reasonableness of the position that more is better, there is some startling evidence to the contrary. As discussed previously, the more focused, shorter, less comprehensive interventions were more effective in promoting parental sensitivity and children's attachment security (van IJzendoorn et al., 1995). Intensity, duration, and the number and kinds of components in prevention programs need to match the participants, their needs, their motivation, and their abilities and the developmental pathways being addressed.

WHO BENEFITS FROM PREVENTION PROGRAMS?

Not all participants in an intervention benefit, in part because of the heterogeneity of children and parents within a risk group. They differ in many initial characteristics, both as to resources and vulnerabilities, that are not part of the risk designation. Initial characteristics within the individual families and their children decrease or increase the benefits from the intervention, as well as the degree and quality of participation in the intervention. Often it is not the best-functioning parents and children who benefit the most—or even benefit at all—from specific interventions.

For example, Olds et al. (1986a), in the Elmira study, found that during the first 2 years after birth, the combination of prenatal and postnatal intervention reduced the instances of child abuse and neglect to 4% in the highest-risk group, those who were young and single and poor, as compared to 19% in the comparable group without intervention. There were no differences associated with intervention for the lower-risk individuals. Similarly, there were fewer injuries and ingestions for nurse-visited children during the first 2 years of life, with the greatest effects for children born to women with fewer psychological resources, those who had a lower IQ, mental health symptoms, and an external locus of control (Olds et al., 1998). In the IHDP, intervention was associated with lower behavioral problem scores at ages 2 and 3 years, with the most marked benefits for those children with high initial scores (Brooks-Gunn, Klebanov, Liaw, & Spiker, 1993). In the Abecedarian program, children who showed the greatest relative IQ gains compared to controls were those whose mothers had the lowest IQ scores, below 70 (Ramey & Ramey, 1992).

Prevention can be effective only if it addresses behaviors with a high rate of occurrence in the selected sample. When problem behavior

has a low base rate, intervention may be irrelevant. Targeting a group on the basis of one risk condition probably overidentifies the number of children at risk and results in families and children in intervention who will do well regardless of the presence or absence of intervention. Interventions with those parents who do "good enough" parenting or those children who are developing well are either unnecessary or show diminishing returns.

On the other hand, the association between more risks and greater effectiveness of intervention holds within limits; too many risk factors may impede prevention. In the IHDP, the lighter babies, those below 2,000 grams, benefited less from the program than heavier-birthweight children. Ramey and Ramey (1992) suggested that the lower-birthweight children may have suffered more central nervous system effects so that their behavior was less malleable to the educational program than that of their less biologically affected peers. Similarly, in the IHDP, intervention acted to increase HOME (Home Observation of the Environment Scale) scores for those mothers who were subject to more adverse conditions (as measured by ethnicity, unemployment, low education, poor verbal ability, teenage mother, single parent, psychological distress)—but who were not poor (Brooks-Gunn et al., 1995). Presumably, there was already a ceiling effect for low-risk mothers, and high-risk mothers who were poor found it too difficult to change their home conditions. Moreover, among poor families, the size of the effects of the IHDP program varied with the number of risks: larger effects for those with none to four risks but no effects for those with six or more risks (Liaw, Meisels, & Brooks-Gunn, 1995). The Memphis study affected maternal life course by a reduction in second pregnancies and subsequent live births but only for women with high levels of psychological resources (Olds et al., 1998). Webster-Stratton (1998) reported that poor, single-parent women tended to derive the least benefit from a 9-week behaviorally oriented parent training program.

There appears to be an inverted-U-shaped association between number of risks and efficacy of prevention. "Too few" risk factors and the behavior to be prevented, such as child abuse, is too infrequent in either the control group or the intervention group for intervention effects to be evident. Too many risk factors, and either the child or the mother cannot change her behavior sufficiently for the program to be effective. Thus, there must be a match between the program goals and the needs, abilities, and malleability of behavior in the parent and the child.

Participant Involvement in the Prevention Program

Simply providing an opportunity to partake of an intervention does not necessarily bring about changes in children and their parents, in part because individuals do not participate equally. Participants differ in their needs and resources, in the degree of their involvement in the project, and in the quality of their relationship to the intervenor. Thus, the "dosage" of an intervention, the number of contacts actually made, differs among participants and differs from the number of contacts planned by the program. For example, average attendance in the Perry Preschool Program was 69% in the center-based program (Weikart & Schweinhart, 1992), many parents did not attend even once a year the parent support groups in IHDP (Liaw et al., 1995), and mothers received only approximately half the number of home visits as expected by protocol in the Memphis study, a replication of the Elmira project (Korfmacher, Kitzman, & Olds, 1998).

An examination of how women's psychological characteristics influenced their use of nurse home visitation services in the Elmira and in the Memphis projects (Olds & Korfmacher, 1998) indicated that the number of home visits decreased, and the number of phone contacts increased, as the maternal sense of control over life circumstances increased, or as the level of psychological resources increased. Thus, although it would seem that more face-to-face contacts should be associated with greater benefits for the child and family, the number of face-to-face contacts in this study, and probably in other studies as well, was confounded with poorer maternal functioning.

However, when the measure of "dose" depends on a more active involvement of the participant, quantity becomes linked to more competent maternal functioning and does relate to enhanced children's development. Thus, Osofsky, Culp, and Ware (1988), in an intervention program for teenage mothers, found that those mothers who established a working relationship with the intervenor and followed through on activities—"takers"—had higher HOME scores and better interaction with their infants during play and feeding, and their children had higher Bayley Mental Scale scores as compared to "nontakers."

Whereas quantity is a necessary measure to determine the degree to which families actually participated in an intervention, the quality of their participation may be more key to whether or not they will benefit. The IHDP measure of attendance, combining the number of home visits received with days attended at child centers and number of parent meetings attended, was compared to a quality of involvement measure, "Active Experience," in which intervenors rated the interest of parents in the intervention and the children's mastery of the curriculum. "Active Experience" explained more of the variance in children's IQ than did the quantity measure (Liaw et al., 1995). Lieberman et al. (1991), in their intervention with Latina mothers of avoidantly attached children, found that the development of a trusting and working relationship by the mother with the intervenor was directly associated with the children's increased proximity seeking-behaviors and decreased avoidance of the mother.

The Memphis study assessed the quality of the contact between intervenor and mother by measuring both the intervenor's perception of the mother's emotional engagement in the sessions and the mother's perception of her nurse's empathy with her. In addition, the interest of the mother in parenting issues was assessed by the percentage of each visit spent covering parenting concerns as contrasted to concerns about subsistence or relationships to friends, spouse, partner, and so on (Korfmacher et al., 1998). All three elements of the quality of the intervention process were associated with enhanced parenting but moderated by initial characteristics. Among mothers with low levels of psychological resources, a more concentrated focus on parenting issues was associated with higher HOME scores, that is, more cognitively stimulating homes. In contrast, among mothers with high levels of psychological resources (most of whom already provided stimulating homes), those who were more focused on parenting concerns and who felt that their nurses were empathic to them reported the highest level of empathy toward their children.

Who benefits in the intervention group depends in part on who participates, in how many contacts, and to what degree of involvement, trust, and interest. The degree and quality of involvement influence how much help the prevention program can provide.

REPLICATION OF PREVENTION PROGRAMS

Both scientific rigor and social policy require that successful programs be replicated. Multisite projects, such as the IHDP, are simultaneous replications, and the IHDP has impressively demonstrated that the model worked in all but one of the sites in different locations, with different staff. However, it must be remembered that the outstanding quality of the programs was maintained with great effort. All were directed by experienced, highly motivated university researchers; they selected, trained, and funded their intervention staff and set up the preschool centers; they collaborated with each other as well as with a central group of sophisticated researchers who monitored recruitment, evaluation, and intervention.

Other examples serve to illustrate some of the relevant issues when an intervention model is used with a different population, moved to a different community, or conducted by different staff and/or the nature of the relationship between the participant and the intervenor changes. Olds moved the Elmira, New York, project to Memphis, Tennessee (Olds et al., 1998) and, in so doing, changed the ethnic group but not the social class of the target sample. Trained nurses continued to administer the intervention, but there were more changes in nursing staff than had occurred in Elmira. The results were essentially the same, and the changes did not endanger the effectiveness of the prevention model. A more drastic change is now under way in which not only has the site and community been changed but paraprofessionals, rather than nurses, conduct the intervention. However, findings are not available as of now (Robinson et al., 1997).

Two replications of van den Boom's model for increasing security of attachment used samples with different kinds of risk conditions. The results were mixed. Juffer (van IJzendoorn et al., 1995) implemented maternal skills training with middle-class adoptive parents. The intervention did enhance maternal sensitivity and did result in a significant increase of securely attached infants, but the results were not as dramatic as in van den Boom's study (1994), as the control group on its own achieved 70% securi-

ty, as compared to 90% in intervention. Meij (van IJzendoorn et al., 1995) did not target parents of irritable infants but simply implemented the intervention with lower-class families and found no effects either for maternal sensitivity or for security of attachment, with both groups showing high rates of security: 88% in the intervention group and 77% in the control group. Thus, duplicating a parental skills training developed for mothers of irritable infants, for middle-class adoptive families with nonirritable infants, and for lower-class families with nonirritable infants altered the effectiveness of the intervention, presumably as a result of differences in salient issues across families (van den Boom, 1995).

To a more extreme degree, replications of the Mother/Child HOME program (Levenstein, 1992) did erode intervention effectiveness by changing the mode of group assignment and by using different communities, populations, and staff. The program made twice-weekly home visits for 2 years to low-income, single mothers and their 2- to 3-year-old children. "Toy demonstrators" brought gifts of books and toys and guided verbal interaction and sequenced play activities between the mother and child. When Levenstein changed the procedure of group assignment, resulting in a higher maternal education level than in previous years, the effects of intervention were not as apparent. A similar deterioration in efficacy occurred when the program model was implemented in Bermuda (Scarr & McCartney, 1988). Parents tended not to be single mothers of low education, and the program was not effective. The model also was tried unsuccessfully in a community setting in which clinical staff, not being researchers, referred the most needy families to the intervention group and the least needy to the comparison group. The initial differences in the groups obscured any possible effects of the intervention.

Weikart and Schweinhart (1992) compared three "replications" of their High/Scope quality early educational program for low-IQ children of poor, low-educated parents. One was High/Scope and used a language-enhancing curriculum in which children initiated their own learning activities with teacher support. One used the same curriculum and equally well-trained staff but provided direct instruction in which the teacher initiated and the children responded. The other was a quality nursery school, without curriculum, in which the teacher encouraged children to engage in free play. All groups showed impressive rises in IQ during the first year, dropping during the second year, with no differences in IQ after kindergarten. There also were no differences in academic performance. However, by age 15, the direct instruction group had engaged in twice as many delinquent acts and twice as many acts of drug abuse as had the other two groups. Nearly all the High/Scope group members participated in sports, but fewer than half of those in the direct instruction group did so. Only half of the direct instruction group expected to get postsecondary education, whereas two thirds and three fourths of the other groups did. One third of the members of the direct instruction group reported that their families thought they were doing poorly, as compared to one thirty-sixth in the other groups.

The Weikart and Schweinhart (1992) example demonstrates that the nature of the interaction between the intervenor and the child, as well as that between intervenor and parent, is a crucial aspect of the prevention program. The experience of being encouraged and supported in self-initiated learning activities may be an important mediator of later prosocial behavior.

Successful replication of a prevention program cannot occur without careful attention to the new sample, the balance of risk and protective factors among the participants, and the participants' interest in the program. The stability, commitment, and training of staff must continue to be of high quality. The emotional nuances of trust and empathy in the intervenor–participant relationship must be guarded.

INEFFECTIVE PROGRAMS

A recent evaluation of the effectiveness of 21 of the 24 sites of the Comprehensive Child Development Programs (CCDP) (St. Pierre, Layzer, Goodson, & Bernstein, 1997), whose aim was to provide comprehensive services to enhance child development and help low-income families achieve economic self-sufficiency, found that participation in CCDP did not produce any important positive effects on participating families: not on economic self-sufficiency of mothers, not on their parenting skills, and not on the cognitive or social–emotional development of their children. Also, there were no differential effects on subgroups of participants, nor was the length of time that a family was enrolled in

the program associated with any substantive change in family or child functioning. The problem did not appear to be in implementation, as the programs were closely monitored: There were detailed programmatic regulations and guidance, data collection staff were well-trained, there were more than 100 different outcome measures, and there were high response rates. Moreover, the problem was not in duration, as the program was provided from birth until entry to kindergarten.

Rather, St. Pierre et al. (1997) conclude that the model of CCDP relied too heavily on a case management approach in which the intervenor tried to promote the delivery of comprehensive social services to everyone in the entire family, and to do so either directly or by referral to agencies in the community. The authors further conclude that the CCDP, as well as other high-quality studies, provide no evidence that the case-management approach is effective in promoting positive outcomes for parents or children.

Moreover, the approach may rely too heavily on indirect effects in influencing children's outcomes. While case-management services have been included in several successful intervention projects with multiple-risk families, those services were supplementary and not the major focus. In addition, the CCDP may have failed because they depended on the indirect provision of basic services to enhance parents' and children's behavior rather than using the intervention as a collaboration in which participants gain a sense of control over themselves and their environments and initiate their own activities.

Other programs have failed because they, too, tried to affect children's development indirectly, by addressing too many problems simultaneously in families with many risk conditions. Focus (Howard, 1995), designed to provide comprehensive health, drug treatment, parent education services to mothers who were poor, single, low-education, and chronic heavy polydrug users with comorbid mental health problems, did not provide a direct intensive educational program to the children, and the mothers did not participate sufficiently in any part of the program.

The failure of CCDP and Focus does not mean that social support and social work services do not need to be included with multiple-risk families (Guralnick, 1998). Nor does it mean that community services are not essential to the well-being of families and children. Rather, it does indicate that case management, albeit, integrated, does not succeed on its own, and that social support and its effects are more complex than is usually assumed (Thompson, 1995).

CONCLUSIONS

Prevention programs are more effective when they are based on prior knowledge of the risk behaviors, as well as the risk conditions, of the participants. For example, the Prenatal/Postnatal Project (Olds et al., 1986b) was very effective in reducing smoking during pregnancy of young, single women and thereby decreasing the number of preterm infants and increasing birthweights in the offspring. Replicating that effort with a group of women who are known to be at increased likelihood of having preterm infants and infants of lower birthweights would seem worthwhile. However, when Olds et al. (1998) replicated the Prenatal/Postnatal program with black women in Memphis, they had to select other behavioral targets because the rate of smoking in the new sample was already low. Designing programs to target risk behaviors that occur with some frequency and that are amenable to change is central to prevention science.

To the extent that hypothesized, developmental pathways can be specified, both the participants of prevention programs and child development science benefit. Thus, maternal depressive symptoms and anxiety are risk factors for their offspring's development, but reducing maternal distress appears not to be the causal influence for the children. More normative developmental trajectories will occur for them when there is more precise specification of the family interactions and parental behaviors, associated with maternal distress, that mediate adverse functioning for the children. Several domains of parenting behavior, not restricted to cognitive stimulation or the teaching context, will have to be considered, including sensitive responsiveness, fostering autonomy, and appropriate monitoring, and these likely will vary with the age of the child.

Similarly, whereas social support is a protective factor, enhancing physical health and psychological well-being for parents, providing social support indiscriminately in prevention programs, without regard as to whether it meets specific needs of the participants, is unlikely to be effective (Thompson, 1995). Support that reinforces competent role functioning and is directed at the isolated or those undergoing difficult role transitions may be most useful (Heller, 1990; Olds & Kitzman, 1993). Programs that have a clear behavioral focus in which behaviors to be changed and behavioral skills to be acquired are specified for either the parent (Olds et al., 1997; Webster-Stratton, 1990; van den Boom, 1995) or the child (Brooks-Gunn et al., 1994; Weikart & Schweinhart, 1992) appear to be most successful.

Finally, most prevention programs embed prevention efforts in a personal relationship between the intervenor and the parent and/or child. The degree of participant engagement and the efficacy of the intervention will depend on the nature of the relationship (Greenspan & Wieder, 1987). Several investigators (Robinson et al., 1997; Webster-Stratton, 1998) have stressed the need for a collaborative relationship that is nonblaming and actively solicits ideas, feelings, and experiences of the participants. Concepts and skills are adapted cooperatively to fit the particular circumstances of the parents' or children's lives. The intervenor conveys empathic understanding as well as expectations of personal efficacy for the participants.

REFERENCES

Ainsworth, M. D. S., Blehar, M. C., Waters, E., & Wall, S. (1978). *Patterns of attachment. A psychological study of the strange situation.* Hillsdale, NJ: Erlbaum.

Barnard, K. E., Magyary, D., Sumner, G., Booth, C. L, Mitchell, S. K. & Spieker, S. (1988). Prevention of parenting alterations for women with low social support. *Psychiatry, 51,* 248–253.

Barnett, B., Blignault, I., Holmes, S., Payne, A., & Parker, G. (1987). Quality of attachment in a sample of 1-year-old Australian children. *Journal of the American Academy of Child and Adolescent Psychiatry, 26,* 303–307.

Beckwith, L. (1988). Intervention with disadvantaged parents of sick preterm infants. *Psychiatry, 51,* 242–247.

Beckwith, L., Cohen, S. E., & Hamilton, C. E. (1999). Maternal sensitivity during infancy and subsequent life events relate to attachment representation at early adulthood. *Developmental Psychology, 35,* 693–700.

Belsky, J., Youngblade, L., & Pensky, E. (1989). Childrearing history, marital quality, and maternal affect: Intergenerational transmission in a low-risk sample. *Development and Psychopathology, 1,* 291–304.

Berrueta-Clement, J. R., Schweinhart, L. J., Barnett, W.

S., Epstein, A. S., & Weikart, D. P. (1984). *Changed lives: The effects of the Perry Preschool Program on youths through age 19* (Monographs of the High/Scope Educational Research Foundation, No. 8). Ypsilanti, MI: High/Scope Program.

Bowlby, J. (1982). *Attachment and loss: Vol. 1. Attachment* (2nd ed.). New York: Basic Books.

Brinich, E., Drotar, D., & Brinich, P. (1989). Security of attachment and outcome of preschoolers with histories of nonorganic failure to thrive. *Journal of Clinical Child Psychology, 18,* 142–152.

Brooks-Gunn, J., Gross, R. T., Kraemer, H. C., Spiker, D., & Shapiro, S. (1992). Enhancing the cognitive outcomes of low birthweight, premature infants: For whom is the intervention most effective? *Pediatrics, 89,* 1209–1215.

Brooks-Gunn, J., Klebanov, P. K., & Liaw, F. (1995). The learning, physical, and emotional environment of the home in the context of poverty: The Infant Health and Development Program. *Children and Youth Services Review, 17*(1–2), 251–276.

Brooks-Gunn, J., Klebanov, P. K., Liaw, F., & Spiker, D. (1993). Enhancing the development of low-birth-weight, premature infants: Changes in cognition and behavior over the first three years. *Child Development, 64,*736–753.

Brooks-Gunn, J., McCarton, C. M., Casey, P. H., McCormick, M. C., Bauer, C. R., Bernbaum, J. C., Tyson, J., Swanson, M., Bennett, F. C., Scott, D. T., Tonascia, J., & Meinert, C. L. (1994). Early intervention in low-birth-weight premature infants. *Journal of the American Medical Association, 272,* 1257–1262.

Campbell, F. A., & Ramey, C. T. (1994). Effects of early intervention on intellectual and academic achievement: A follow-up study of children from low-income families. *Child Development, 65,* 684–698.

Cicchetti, D., & Toth, S. L. (1998). The development of depression in children and adolescents. *American Psychologist, 53*(2), 221–241.

Coie, J. D., Watt, N. F., West, S. G., Hawkins, J. D., Asawnow, J. R., Markman, H. J., Ramey, S. L., Shure, M. B., & Long, B. (1993). The science of prevention: A conceptual framework and some directions for a national research program. *American Psychologist, 48*(10), 1013–1022.

Cowan, C. P., & Cowan, P. A. (1987). A preventive intervention for couples becoming parents. In C. F. Z. Boukydis (Ed.), *Research on support for parents and infants in the postnatal period* (pp. 225–251). Norwood, NJ: Ablex.

Cowan, C. P., & Cowan, P. A. (1997). Working with couples during stressful transitions. In S. Dreman (Ed.), *The family on the threshold of the 21st century: Trends and implications* (pp. 17–47). Mahwah, NJ: Erlbaum.

Crnic, K. A., Greenberg, M. T., Ragozin, A. S., Robinson, N. M., & Basham, R. B. (1983). The effects of stress and social support on mothers of premature and full-term infants. *Child Development, 45,* 209–217.

Crockenberg, S. (1981). Infant irritability, mother responsiveness, and social influences on the security of infant-mother attachment. *Child Development, 51,* 209–217.

Dickstein, S., Seifer, R., Hayden, L. C., Schiller, M., Sameroff, A. J., Keitner, G., Miller, V., Rasmussen, S., Matzko, M., & Magee, K. D. (1998). Levels of family assessment. II. Impact of maternal psychopathology on family functioning. *Journal of Family Psychology, 12,* 23–40.

Egeland, B. R., Carlson, E., & Sroufe, L. A. (1993). Resilience as process. Milestones in the development of resilience [Special issue]. *Development and Psychopathology, 5,* 517–528.

Emde, R. N., & Buchsbaum, H. K. (1990). "Didn't you hear my mommy?": Autonomy with connectedness in moral self-emergence. In D. Cicchetti & M. Beeghly (Eds.), *The self in transition* (pp. 35–60). Chicago: University of Chicago Press.

Erickson, M. F., Korfmacher, J., & Egeland, B. (1992). Attachments past and present. Implications for therapeutic intervention with mother–infant dyads. *Development and Psychopathology, 4,* 495–507.

Field, T. (1997). The treatment of depressed mothers and their infants. In L. Murray & P. J. Cooper (Eds.), *Postpartum depression and child development* (pp. 221–236). New York: Guilford Press.

Greenberg, M. T., Speltz, M. L., & DeKlyen, M. (1993). The role of attachment in the early development of disruptive behavior problems. *Development and Psychopathology, 5,* 191–213.

Greenspan, S. I., & Wieder, S. (1987). Dimensions and levels of the therapeutic process. Infants in multirisk families: Case studies in prevention intervention [Special issue]. *Clinical Infant Reports, 3,* 391–430.

Guralnick, M. J. (1998). Effectiveness of early intervention for vulnerable children: A developmental perspective. *American Journal on Mental Retardation, 102*(4), 319–345.

Heller, K. (1990). Social and community intervention. *Annual Review of Psychology, 41,* 141–168.

Hetherington, E. M., Bridges, M., & Isabella, G. M. (1998). What matters? What does not? Five perspectives on the association between marital transitions and children's adjustment. *American Psychologist, 53*(2), 167–184.

Honig, A. S., Lally, J. R., & Mathieson, P. H. (1982). Personal and social adjustment of schoolchildren after five years in the Family Development Research Program. *Child Care Quarterly, 11,* 136–146.

Howard, J. (1995). *Final report: FOCUS project.* Prepared for the National Institute on Drug Abuse, National Institutes of Health, Bethesda, MD.

Infant Health and Development Program. (1990). Enhancing the outcomes of low birthweight, premature infants: A multisite randomized trial. *Journal of the American Medical Association, 263,* 3035–3042.

Kochanska, G. (1997). Mutually responsive orientation between mothers and their young children: Implications for early socialization. *Child Development, 68*(1), 94–112.

Korfmacher, J., Kitzman, H., & Olds, D. (1998). Intervention processes as predictors of outcomes in a preventive home-visitation program. *Journal of Community Psychology, 26,* (1), 49–64.

Lally, J. R., Mangione, P. L, & Honig, A. S. (1988). The Syracuse University Family Development Research Program: Long-range impact of an early intervention with low-income children and their families. In D. R. Powell (Ed.), *Advances in applied developmental psychology: Vol. 3. Parent education as early childhood intervention: Emerging directions in theory, research, and practice* (pp. 79–104). Norwood, NJ: Ablex.

Lester, B. M., McGrath, M. M., Garcia-Coll, C., Brem, F. S., Sullivan, M. C., & Mattis, S. G. (1995). In H. E. Fitzgerald, B. M. Lester, & B. Zuckerman (Eds.), *Children of poverty. Research, health, and policy issues* (pp. 197–227). New York: Garland.

Levenstein, P. (1992). The mother–child home program: Research methodology and the real world. In J. McCord & R. E. Tremblay (Eds.), *Preventing antisocial behavior: Interventions from birth through adolescence* (pp. 43–66). New York: Guilford Press.

Liaw, F. Meisels, S. J., & Brooks-Gunn, J. (1995). The effects of experience of early intervention on low birth weight, premature children: The Infant Health and Development Program. *Early Childhood Research Quarterly, 10*, 405–431.

Lieberman, A. F., Weston, D. R., & Pawl, J. H. (1991). Preventive intervention and outcome with anxiously attached dyads. *Child Development, 62*, 199–209.

Lyons-Ruth, K., Connell, D. B., Grunebaum, H. U., & Botein, S. (1990). Infants at social risk: Maternal depression and family support services as mediators of infant development and security of attachment. *Child Development, 61*, 85–98.

Lyons-Ruth, K., Easterbrooks, M. A., & Cibelli, C. D. (1997). Infant attachment strategies, infant mental lag, and maternal depressive symptoms: Predictors of internalizing and externalizing problems at age 7. *Developmental Psychology, 33*(5), 681–692.

Main, M., Kaplan, N., & Cassidy, J. (1985). Security in infancy, childhood and adulthood. A move to the level of representation. In I. Bretherton & E. Waters (Eds.), Growing points of attachment theory and research. *Monographs of the Society for Research in Child Development, 50*(2, Serial No. 209), 66–104.

Manassis, K., Bradley, S., Goldberg, S., Hood, J., & Swinson, R. P. (1995). Behavioral inhibition, attachment and anxiety in children of mothers with anxiety disorders. *Canadian Journal of Psychiatry, 40*(2), 87–92.

Markman, H. J., Renick, M. J., Floyd, F. J., Stanley, S. M., & Clements, M. (1993). Preventing marital distress through communication and conflict management training: A 4- and 5-year follow-up [Special section: Couples and couple therapy]. *Journal of Consulting and Clinical Psychology, 61*, 70–77.

Masten, A. S., & Coatsworth, J. D. (1998). The development of competence in favorable and unfavorable environments. *American Psychologist, 53*(2), 205–220.

McCarton, C. M., Brooks-Gunn, J., Wallace, I. F., & Bauer, C. R. (1997). Results at age 8 years of early intervention for low-birth-weight premature infants: The Infant Health and Development Program. *Journal of the American Medical Association, 277*(2), 126–132.

Miyake, K., Chen, S., & Campos, J. J. (1985). Infant temperament, mother's mode of interaction, and attachment in Japan: An interim report. In I. Bretherton & E. Waters (Eds.), Growing points of attachment

theory and research. *Monographs of the Society for Research in Child Development, 50*(2, Serial No. 209), 276–297.

O'Connor, T. G., & Rutter, M. (1996). Risk mechanisms in development: Some conceptual and methodological considerations. *Developmental Psychology, 32*, 787–795.

Olds, D. L., Eckenrode, J., Henderson, C. R., Kitzman, H., Powers, J., Cole, R., Sidora, K., Morris, P., Pettitt, L. M., & Luckey, D. (1997). Long-term effects of home visitation on maternal life course and child abuse and neglect. Fifteen-year follow-up of a randomized trial. *Journal of the American Medical Associations, 278*(8), 637–643.

Olds, D., Henderson, C. R. Jr., Kitzman, H., Eckenrode, J., Cole, R., & Tatelbaum, R. (1998). The promise of home visitation: Results of two randomized trials. *Journal of Community Psychology, 26*(1), 5–21.

Olds, D. L., Henderson, C. R., Tatelbaum, R., & Chamberlin, R. (1986a). Preventing child abuse and neglect: A randomized trial of nurse home visitation. *Pediatrics, 78*, 16–28.

Olds, D. L., Henderson, C. R., Tatelbaum, R., & Chamberlin, R. (1986b). Improving the delivery of prenatal care and outcomes of pregnancy: A randomized trial of nurse home visitation. *Pediatrics, 78*, 16–28.

Olds, D. L., & Kitzman, H. (1993). Review of research on home visiting for pregnant women and parents of young children. *The Future of Children, 3*(3), 53–92.

Olds, D. L., & Korfmacher, J. (1998). Maternal psychological characteristics as influences on home visitation contact. *Journal of Community Psychology, 26*(1), 23–36.

Osofsky, J. D., Culp, A. M., & Ware, L. M. (1988). Intervention challenges with adolescent mothers and their infants. *Psychiatry, 51*, 236–241.

Provence, S., & Naylor, A. (1983). *Working with disadvantaged children and parents: Scientific issues and practice.* New Haven, CT: Yale University Press.

Ramey, C. T., Bryant, D. M., Wasik, B. H., Sparling, J. J., Fendt, K. H., & LaVange, L. M. (1992). Infant Health and Development Program for low birthweight, premature infants: Program elements, family participation, and child intelligence. *Pediatrics, 89*, 454–465.

Ramey, C. T., & Campbell, F. A. (1991). Poverty, early childhood education, and academic competence: The Abecedarian experiment. In A. Huston (Ed.), *Children reared in poverty* (pp. 190–221). New York: Cambridge University Press.

Ramey, C. T., & Ramey, S. L. (1992). Effective early intervention. *Mental Retardation, 30*(6), 337–345.

Robinson, J. L., Emde, R. N., & Korfmacher, J. (1997). Integrating an emotional regulation perspective in a program of prenatal and early childhood home visitation. *Journal of Community Psychology, 25*(1), 59–75.

Rosenbaum, J. F., Biederman, J., Gersten, M., Hirschfield, D. R., Meminger, S. R., Herman, J. B., Kagan, J., Reznick, S., & Snidman, N. (1988). Behavioral inhibition in children of parents with panic disorder and agorophobia. *Archives of General Psychiatry, 45*, 463–470.

Sameroff, A. J., Seifer, R., Baldwin, A., & Baldwin, C. P. (1993). Stability of intelligence from preschool to adolescence: The influence of social and family risk factors. *Child Development, 64,* 80–97.

Scarr, S. & McCartney, K. (1988). Far from home: An experimental evaluation of the mother–child home program in Bermuda. *Child Development, 59,* 531–543.

Schweinhart, L. J., & Weikart, D. P. (1997). The High/Scope Preschool Curriculum Comparison study through age 23. *Early Childhood Research Quarterly, 12*(2), 117–143.

Seitz, V., & Apfel, N. H. (1994). Parent-focused intervention: Diffusion effects on siblings. *Child Development, 65,* 677–683.

Seitz, V., Rosenbaum, L. K., & Apfel, N. H. (1985). Effects of family support intervention: A ten year follow-up. *Child Development, 56,* 376–391.

Silverman, W. K., Cerny, J. A., Nelles, W. B., & Burke, A. E. (1988). Behavior problems in children of parents with anxiety disorders. *Journal of the American Academy of Child and Adolescent Psychiatry, 27,* 779–784.

Skeels, H. M. (1966). Adult status of children with contrasting early life experiences: A follow-up study. *Monographs of the Society for Research in Child Development, 31*(3, Serial No. 105), 1–65.

Spiker, D., Ferguson, J., & Brooks-Gunn, J. (1993). Enhancing maternal interactive behavior and child social competence in low birthweight, premature infants. *Child Development, 64,* 754–768.

Sroufe, L. A. (1988). The role of infant–caregiver attachment in development. In J. Belsky & T. Nezworski (Eds.), *Clinical implications of attachment* (pp. 18–40). Hillsdale, NJ: Erlbaum.

St. Pierre, R. G., Layzer, J. I., Goodson, B. D., & Bernstein, L. S. (1997). *The effectiveness of comprehensive case management interventions: Findings from the national evaluation of the comprehensive Child Development Program.* Cambridge, MA: Abt.

Thompson, R. A. (1995). *Preventing child maltreatment through social support: A critical analysis.* Thousand Oaks, CA: Sage.

van den Boom, D. (1994). The influence of temperament and mothering on attachment and exploration: An experimental manipulation of sensitive responsiveness among lower-class mothers with irritable infants. *Child Development, 65,* 1449–1469.

van den Boom, D. (1995). Do first-year intervention effects endure? Follow-up during toddlerhood of a sample of Dutch irritable infants. *Child Development, 66,* 1798–1816.

van IJzendoorn, M. H., Juffer, F., & Duyvesteyn, M. G.

(1995). Breaking the intergenerational cycle of insecure attachment: A review of the effects of attachment-based interventions on maternal sensitivity and infant security. *Journal of Child Psychology and Psychiatry, 36*(2), 225–248.

Wasik, B. H., Ramey, C. T., Bryant, D. M., & Sparling, J. J. (1990). A longitudinal study of two early intervention strategies: Project CARE. *Child Development, 61,* 1681–1696.

Webster-Stratton, C. (1990). Long-term follow-up of families with young conduct problem children: From preschool to grade school. *Journal of Clinical Child Psychology, 19*(2), 144–149.

Webster-Stratton, C. (1998). Parent training with low-income families. Promoting parental engagement through a collaborative approach. In J. R. Lutzker (Ed.), *Handbook of child abuse research and treatment* (pp. 183–210). New York: Plenum.

Webster-Stratton, C., & Hammond, M. (1997). Treating children with early-onset conduct problems: A comparison of child and parent training interventions. *Journal of Consulting and Clinical Psychology, 65,* 93–109.

Webster-Stratton, C., Kolpacoff, M., & Hollinsworth, T. (1988). Self-administered videotape therapy for families with conduct-problem children: Comparison with two cost-effective treatments and a control group. *Journal of Consulting and Clinical Psychology, 56*(4), 558–566.

Weikart, D. P., & Schweinhart, L. J. (1992). High/Scope Preschool program outcomes. In J. McCord & R. E. Tremblay (Eds.), *Preventing antisocial behavior. Interventions from birth through adolescence* (pp. 67–86). New York: Guilford Press.

Werner, E. E., & Smith, R. S. (1982). *Vulnerable but invincible: A longitudinal study of resilient children and youth.* New York: McGraw-Hill.

White, R. W. (1959). Motivation reconsidered: The concept of competence. *Psychological Review, 66,* 297–333.

Yoshikawa, H. (1994). Prevention as cumulative protection: Effects of early family support and education on chronic delinquency and its risks. *Psychological Bulletin, 115*(1), 28–54.

Zahn-Waxler, C., Cummings, E. M., Iannotti, R. M., & Radke-Yarrow, M. (1984). Young offspring of depressed parents: A population at-risk for affective problems. In D. Cicchetti & K. Schneider-Rosen (Eds.), *New directions for child development: No. 26. Childhood depression* (pp. 81–105). San Francisco: Jossey-Bass.

29

Parent–Child Relationships in Early Intervention with Infants and Toddlers with Disabilities and Their Families

❖

LINDA GILKERSON
FRANCES STOTT

Since 1987, the U.S. Department of Education, through what is now referred to as Part C of the Individuals with Disabilities Education Act (IDEA; Public Law 101-476), assists states in developing and maintaining statewide, comprehensive, coordinated, mutlidisciplinary, interagency systems that offer early intervention services to all eligible infants and toddlers and their families. IDEA does not require states to participate in Part C and, thus, to serve children less than 3 years old, but the legislation provides financial assistance to states that choose to do so. Currently, all 50 states and 5 territories provide early intervention services through Part C. The legislation permits each state to define its eligible population from three targeted groups of infants and toddlers: (1) children who are experiencing a developmental delay, (2) children who have a diagnosed physical or mental condition that has a high probability of developmental delay, or (3) at the state's discretion, children at risk. Only 10 states serve at-risk infants and toddlers. Although each state has the authority to define eligibility, the law serves as an entitlement requiring participating states in their fifth year of Part C funding (and thereafter) to provide appropriate services for

every child who meets the eligibility requirements.

Each state system must provide, at a minimum, 14 required services (see Table 29.1). The Governor of each state must appoint (1) a lead agency to administer, supervise, and monitor the statewide program and (2) a state interagency council to advise and assist the lead agency. The federal legislation is under the U.S. Department of Education, but in only 18 states is education the lead or co-lead agency. Each state is to have a comprehensive child-find program, a public awareness program, a central directory of services, a comprehensive system of personnel development, and a system of procedural safeguards.

The most striking aspect of Part C, however, is the philosophical orientation of the law: its emphasis on the values and principles of family-centered services and the belief in natural environments—that is, settings that are natural for the child's age peers—as the primary resource for child development. Evaluation includes a timely, multidisciplinary evaluation and a family-directed assessment of the resources, priorities, and concerns of the family related to enhancing the child's development.

TABLE 29.1. Early Intervention Program for Infants and Toddlers with Disabilities: Part C of the Individuals with Disabilities Education Act (IDEA), Public Law 105-17 as Amended in 1997

Required services

1. Family Training, Counseling, and Home Visits
2. Special Instruction
3. Speech–Language Pathology and Audiology Services
4. Occupational Therapy
5. Physical Therapy
6. Psychological Services
7. Service Coordination Services
8. Medical Services Only for Diagnostic or Evaluation Purposes
9. Early Identification, Screening, and Assessment Services
10. Health Services Necessary to Enable the Infant or Toddler to Benefit from the Other Early Intervention Services
11. Social Work Services
12. Vision Services
13. Assistive Technology Devices and Assistive Technology Services
14. Transportation and Related Costs

These assessments provide the basis for an Individualized Family Service Plan (IFSP).

One of the current dilemmas in implementing Part C is the degree to which early intervention services should focus on parent–child relationships as a tool for child change. On the one hand, this focus is compatible with accepted theories of infant development and years of developmental research. Yet there are concerns about overburdening families with the role of interventionist and interfering with the naturally occurring interactions between parent and child. Further, there is concern about the compatibility of a parent–child relationship approach with the cultural practices of families and with a family-centered philosophy. Finally, there is concern regarding the capacities, training, and supervision needed for the interventionist.

The purpose of this chapter is to explore the issues related to supporting parent–child relationships within the context of Part C services. We begin by considering the influence of the changing perceptions of disability in the larger social environment on parent–child relationships and, ultimately, on the child's development of self. Next, we describe the prevailing philosophy of early intervention—family-cen-

tered services—as the framework within which all early intervention efforts are embedded. Then, we explore different intervention approaches developed to support parent–child relationships with infants and toddlers with disabilities. We consider not only the opportunities that each of these approaches offer but also the cautions and concerns relevant to their implementation within Part C. A theme throughout the chapter is the interface between infant mental health and early intervention: the contributions each has to make to the development of infants and toddlers with disabilities, and the tensions inherent when two frameworks with different theoretical and historical roots come together.

A FULLY HUMAN LIFE

> Parents compose for their baby an ongoing biography, which they constantly consult. Thus, this biography serves as framework and dictionary for both how they see their baby and how she sees herself—and, hence, for her life.
> —STERN (1990, p. 3)

> Disability, from the inside out, is different from . . . the outside looking in . . . we must always be receptive and respectful of that difference.
> —ROUSSO (1985, p. 30)

Parents imagine an inner life for their baby: what their baby likes or dislikes; who their baby resembles, what their baby wants next. Parenting depends on these very interpretations (Stern, 1985). For parents of babies born with disabilities, the early chapters of these biographies are full of unexpected and emotionally powerful experiences, shaped in part by the nature of the responses of others. Insensitive, hurtful comments are seared into memory; moments of genuine human caring and connection are safely stored away, to be returned to again and again. For some parents, learning about disability or developmental delay is a longer, slower process, one that involves holding on to the child whom they know and the family they have created, simultaneously coming to terms with a whole new dimension of human experience. All the while, another world view is being shaped and molded—that of the child: how he experiences his world, what she is coming to know about herself, and how she is perceived by others.

Examining the meaning of disability is a crucial yet often unrecognized aspect of the context for early development and, thus, for early intervention. The central question for individuals, families, and society is as follows: Is being disabled an acceptable way for a person to be? (Hauerwas, 1986). As noted, current theories of infant development see the child's emerging self as a social creation; that is, as defined, maintained, and transformed in reference to others (Stern, 1985). Zola (1993), a sociologist and founder of the Society for Disability Studies, proposed that in addition to a social construction of self, there is also a social construction of disability. These two phenomena interact and have a powerful influence on how a child comes to see him- or herself.

In our society, attitudes toward persons with disabilities have been predominately negative: disability viewed as tragedy. Positive views have tended to stereotype in the opposite direction; persons with disabilities are seen as exceptionally courageous or saintly (Wright, 1960). The roots of disability as tragedy are illustrated in Olshansky's (1962) classic article on chronic sorrow. He asserted that the birth of a child with a disability was a tragedy that gave parents little to look forward to; parents always would be burdened by unrelenting demands and unabated dependency until either their own or their child's death. Olshansky suggested that the deep symbolism of giving birth to a child with a disability further contributed to the parents' chronic sorrow. In his view, chronic sorrow was a natural response to tragedy. Olshansky believed that framing parental responses in this way was a step forward from the previous portrayal of parental responses as pathological.

These negative views of disability and of the family, including the family as the cause of autism, have been associated with psychoanalytic theory and thus with mental health. As a result, some families and professionals in the disability field feel that there is an incompatibility between the needs of families of children with disabilities and the perspectives of mental health. We mention this lingering tension not to single out mental health, for education and health also have operated from inadequate frameworks, but because understanding the past provides a context for understanding current paradigms that place families in primary decision-making roles and that focus on strengths, resiliency, and coping.

In fact, many parents do experience and reexperience pain and sadness. In one father's

words: "It hurts, and it comes in waves." Without recognizing the potential for hardship—for emotional pain, isolation, fatigue—we convey a limited view of the experience of disability and family life. Yet, using the concept of "tragedy" as *the* standard for disability, particularly in mainstream Western society, which places a premium on beauty and performance, may reflect external projections and evaluations more than the actual experience of disability for the individual or the family (Asch & Rousso, 1985; Vohs, 1993) and, therefore, may be inaccurate and limiting. Further, part of the stress and pain that have been associated with disability may arise out of struggles with the very systems that have been established to help.

Although there is no one standard for disability and no one way in which it affects individuals or their families and friends, Zola (1993) believed that we must reach for perspectives that "allow for the full development of the individual" and simultaneously recognize the "reality of our conditions." Saxton, in Gilkerson (1983), proposed that disability involves a loss, that there are objective hardships, and that disability is a fully human lifestyle. Asch (personal communication, January 15, 1999) stressed that loss may not be a part of the experience for all persons with disability, and that the impact of disability changes given the context. When there are ramps available and easy access to public transportation, a physical disability may have minimal or no effect. When the opposite is the case, the same disability may absorb almost all of one's attention and energy.

There is an extensive body of literature in the health field which indicates that the perceptions of health providers regarding the quality of life of persons with disabilities are more negative than the perspectives of the persons themselves (Gething, 1992). National studies of adults with disabilities indicate that the majority of persons consider their lives somewhat to very satisfying (National Organization on Disability, 1994). Turnbull and Turnbull (1986) noted that we too often assume that children without disabilities are easy to raise whereas children with disabilities inevitably will be a burden. As a result, the research on children and families is biased toward stress.

Investigation of positive contributions reveals that persons with disabilities can be a source of joy to the family; a source of learning life's lessons, such as patience or the dignity of all individuals; a source of love, blessing, and fulfillment; and a source of pride and strengthening of the family (Turnbull, Blue-Banning, Behr, & Kerns, 1986). Asch (1998) pointed out that there is a tendency to view such positive statements from persons with disabilities or their families as "defense mechanisms" or as exceptions. Yet, she also warned that although there is evidence that many disabled persons do find life rewarding, this may not tell us anything about the next child or family that we meet. As with any kind of major life event, the outcome of disability is not predetermined. Rather, it is mediated by a range of individual, familial, cultural, and social factors (McCubbin & McCubbin, 1987; Turnbull et al., 1993).

For adults, it is well established that the meaning an individual gives to the disability is more predictive of eventual functioning than is the degree or type of the disability itself (Wright, 1960). The key to framing the experience of disability is to differentiate what is inherent in the disability from what is held within the social and cultural environment. The facts of disability may not change (although they may with advances in research and new technology), but the meanings attributed to disability can. The challenge for the parents is to figure disability into their knowledge of their child in the same way that parents know their child's personality, temperament, likes, and dislikes (Ferguson & Asch, 1989) and to realize that this child will bring another experience of the world to the family, part of which will be shared and part of which will not, unique to the child's life as a person with a disability (Gill, 1994).

Rousso (1985), a psychotherapist and an adult with a disability, has explained that children who have a congenital disability may experience disability as an inherent part of their body and self. Like other aspects of the child, the disability contributes to a sense of identity and is in need of acceptance, appreciation, and affirmation. She has pointed to the response of the social environment and the ways that the child is helped to develop strategies to address the responses of others as a key to the child's development of self. She suggested that infants initially develop unimpeded by an awareness of their disability. However, the moment with the most potential for emotional trauma comes not when the child realizes he or she is different but when the child discovers that the differences are perceived by society as inferior (Rousso, 1985).

The child's discovery of disability is "not a one-time thing with a single meaning"; rather, it "occurs at different developmental stages with different developmental meanings" (Rousso, 1985, p. 25). As Zola (1993) points out, these meanings do not occur within a vacuum. Turnbull and Turnbull (1986) describe the toll that a unidimensional, fix-it model of disability can take on a child's development of self. The child is viewed as broken rather than whole, the child is differentially valued according to the degree of progress he or she makes, the mode for relationships is instruction rather that interaction, and normality is the only avenue to full humanness. For children with disabilities to hold the dual notion of being intact and being disabled at the same time, Rousso (1985) emphasized the importance of parental acceptance, appreciation, and love. Thus, the nature of parent–child relationships is central to the child's development of an integrated self.

How parents come to view themselves as parents, their child, and their circumstances will depend, in part, on the attitudes of those who work with them and on the approaches taken to the intervention process. The professional's own cultural values, biases, training, and experience will play a part in how they view families and how they view their roles in relationship to families. A potential danger is that the professional may use theory to work deductively from general principles to the details of a particular child, adult, or family (Stott, 1997). If the parent's own subjective experience is not included in the formulation, the individual will not feel understood. Thus, it seems important for professionals to be open to all possibilities—to accept the legitimacy of parents' personal and cultural thinking and feeling and to validate them in their own community while still honoring the full humanness and potential of the child.

To understand another's subjective reality, how you are may be more important than what you see or do (Pawl, 1995; Tronick, 1998). Years later, parents of children with disabilities can describe with chilling anger or with warmth and appreciation, the tone of voice, facial expression, and manner of the persons who first spoke with them about their child's disability. Parents seek information delivered with emotional sensitivity (Summers et al., 1990). Authentic human connection is highly valued and registered by parents of children with disabilities. This same authenticity has been noted recently in the infant mental health literature as a key to the change process in psychotherapy:

"Early in our discussions, our attention was drawn to the observation that most patients remember 'special moments' of authentic person-to-person connection with their therapists. We believe that these moments of intersubjective meeting constitute a pivotal part of the change process" (Lyons-Ruth, 1998, p. 284).

Bruschweiler-Stern (1998), a pediatrician, has asserted that these "moments of meeting" occur not just in a psychotherapeutic relationship but in other therapeutic or helping relationships, and that these authentic moments have as much impact on the professional as on the individual or family. The essential characteristic of these moments is that there is a specific recognition of the other's subjective reality (Sander, 1995).

The professional, regardless of discipline, must be open to the full range of human emotions and experiences—both positive and negative. Although a focus on either end of the continuum can be a violation of a parent's experience, the beginning assumption, by definition, is that strengths already exist and can be drawn on. This requires participating in an authentic person-to-person connection with the parents—perhaps one in which the professional can both hold the feelings of the parents and depart from past perceptions of disability. If the professional truly believes in the full development of each child and family and is aware of his or her own responses to disability, he or she can help co-construct the meaning of disability with the parents, helping the family to create in those early chapters of their child's biography the rich, sustaining relationships that are at the heart of a fully human life.

FAMILY-CENTERED SERVICES IN EARLY INTERVENTION

Family-centered is one of those terms that probably means something different to everybody. But for our family, it meant services delivered in a way that helped us feel glued together, instead of pulled apart. You hope that as a family you will keep that togetherness because when you don't, there are ripple effects into the rest of your life.

—Sue Walter, parent and past vice chair, Illinois Interagency Council on Early Intervention (personal communication to L. Gilkerson, January 12, 1999)

Early intervention for infants and toddlers with disabilities and their families had its roots in models and approaches developed for preschool-age children. These approaches focused on the amelioration of developmental deficits through child-focused, stimulation models using primarily developmentally prescriptive, Piagetian, or behavioral approaches to develop training programs or recommendations for families that would enable them to teach their children at home (Garland, 1993).

The prevailing philosophy of early intervention today is family-centered. Baird and Peterson (1997) summarized the major tenets of the family-centered philosophy as a recognition of and respect for the following:

(1) the family as the expert on the child
(2) the family as the ultimate decision maker for the child and the family
(3) the family as the constant in the child's life and professional service provided as temporary
(4) the family's priorities and goals for services
(5) the family's choices regarding their level of participation
(6) the need for a collaborative, trusting relationship between parents and professionals
(7) the need to respect differences in cultural identify, beliefs, values, and coping styles (p. 140)

Klein and Gilkerson (2000) cited two major influences on the shift to a family-centered approach: (1) the introduction of a family systems perspective to the field of special education (Barber, Turnbull, Behr, & Kerns, 1988) and (2) the articulation of a family empowerment philosophy (Dunst, Trivette, & Deal, 1988). The family systems perspective challenged child-oriented professionals to understand that the family functions as a whole and that gains from child-oriented interventions needed to be considered in relation to each subsystem of the family. Interventionists were encouraged to consider the preexisting family style—the way the family communicates, solves problems, facilitates child growth, and relates to the community—as a window into how a family might organize itself around intervention goals. Family systems theory focused attention on family meanings and family coping styles and, eventually, on family diversity, which led to a major focus on cross-cultural understanding and competence (Lynch & Hanson, 1998). The grief and loss model was challenged as the only framework for understanding disability.

With a systems perspective came an aware-ness of the family life cycle. Turnbull (1987) urged that early interventionists adopt a longer time frame to help families develop "marathon skills"—skills such as knowledge of yourself and your family, building relationships, loving the child unconditionally, experiencing and benefiting from emotions, anticipating the fu-ture, and seeking a balance: The field of early intervention needs to seek a balance in its goals and methods, because balance is what families seek. Bernheimer, Gallimore, and Weisner (1990) proposed that interventions should be meaningful in terms of family beliefs and val-ues, congruent with child characteristics, and sustainable over time, given family strengths and opportunities.

A core assumption of the empowerment ap-proach is that strengths and competencies al-ready exist within the family and the child (Dunst et al., 1988). Within this framework, families operate from a needs hierarchy; goals must be relevant for action. Resistance or lack of follow-through result from a lack of consen-sus about what is important. Nearly a decade later, Able-Boone (1996) found that different parent–professional priorities are the leading source of conflict in the delivery of early inter-vention and proposed that parent–professional interaction should have as a goal communica-tion which achieves "uncoerced consensus and non-manipulated understanding and agree-ment" (p. 19).

The expectations for the family-centered practitioner for communication and for rela-tionships is extremely high, implying the need for a high degree of intrapersonal and interper-sonal awareness, knowledge, and effectiveness. The capacity to listen and to understand the family's point of view is at the heart of family-centered practice (Seligman & Darling, 1989). While families differ and needs change over time, families of children with disabilities place a high value on informality in parent–profes-sionals relationships. Summers et al. (1990) found that parents of children with disabilities preferred relationships characterized by an un-hurried atmosphere, with an informal conversa-tional style including some degree of mutual self-disclosure. Families viewed their relation-ships with early intervention providers as per-sonal relationships, people who over time come to know one another in a way that is meaningful to each. It appears that families blend informal and formal support systems and, as noted, value

authentic relationships with the providers who work closely with them and with their child.

The implementation of family-centered ser-vices has presented significant challenges to the field. Brinker (1994) cautioned that the no-tion of family-centered intervention may be based on a "dominant prototype of families as autonomous, self-enhancing centers of deci-sion-making" (p. 313). In a complex, multicul-tural society, this prototype may conflict with the cultural practices and wishes of some fami-lies. Turbiville, Turnbull, Garland, and Lee (1996) proposed that placing one member in the "power position" is not the goal of family-centered collaboration. Rather, the goal is "col-lective empowerment"—a perspective that stresses the family's role as ultimate decision maker *and* the need for flexible leadership pat-terns that take advantage of everyone's skills and resources. Although this view stresses flex-ibility in roles, "when it comes to the final deci-sion, that decision must be one that works for the family" (Turbiville et al., 1996, p. 82).

Slentz and Bricker (1992) challenged the ca-pacity of early intervention programs to encom-pass a broad family support mission and pro-posed that programs adopt a child-focused, family-guided approach. McWilliams, Tocci, and Harbin (1995) suggested that early inter-vention services are child-centered and that families expect them to be so. Wehman (1998) found that families differed in the degree of in-volvement that they wanted in early interven-tion practices: Families wanted a higher degree of involvement in areas that directly concerned families, such as family assessment and service coordination, and were more reliant on profes-sionals to lead in areas such as child assess-ment. Beckman (1996) pointed out that child-centered may be an inappropriate contrast with family-centered, for the child provides the cata-lyst and the reason for the dialogue between providers and families. Rather, Beckman sug-gested that a more appropriate contrast is be-tween family-centered and program-centered frameworks.

Recognizing the centrality of families is key in understanding the ethos of early interven-tion. Through the requirements of Part C and the leadership of families and professionals, families are viewed as stakeholders and deci-sion makers for more than their individual child (Vincent & McLean, 1996). Their perspectives are sought in program evaluation, on policy councils, and in personnel efforts. Part C requires that 20% of the members of state interagency councils on early intervention are parents. Early intervention has built a tradition of parent–professional collaboration in preservice and in-service education of professionals (McBride, Sharp, Hains, & Whitehead, 1995), including models that involve family members as co-instructors, adjunct faculty, field supervisors, and mentors.

As defined by Part C, the purpose of family–professional engagement is to promote the development of the child with special needs. Mahoney and Wheeden (1997) assert that family-centered practices are not an end in and of themselves but a means to engage parents as active participants in the early intervention process, a process that will enhance their effectiveness as caregivers and primary influences on their children's development. How does a family-centered approach address the needs of the child? Longitudinal research on early intervention provides possible directions.

Whereas Shonkoff, Hauser-Cram, Krauss, and Upshur (1992) found that the severity of disability was the best predictor of developmental outcome at 1 year of age, later follow-up at ages 3 and 5 revealed that relationship variables, such as family cohesion and mother–child interaction, supersceded child characteristics or family demographic variables as the best predictors of communication, social skills, and adaptive behavior (Hauser-Cram et al., 1999). As with typically developing children, the development of children with biologically based disabilities is significantly enhanced in families in which the members feel more connected to each other, and in which mothers are emotionally supportive and engage in contingently responsive and cognitive-growth-promoting interactions. These findings support the premise of family-centered practices and the centrality of the family in the child's life and point the way to considering relationships—within the family and between parent and child—as central to early intervention.

RELATIONSHIP APPROACHES TO EARLY INTERVENTION: THEME AND VARIATIONS

Before her diagnosis, we had a hard time bonding. I felt frustration and fear; then came the initial sadness, but it was also the starting point of really getting to know my daughter, this new little baby. I wasn't doing the exercises with her until the

therapist started thinking of intervention in terms of games and fun times she and I could have together. It was these times of just being relaxed with each other that gave us the opportunity to fall in love. Those are times you hold onto when your child or you are having a rough day.
—SUE WALTER, parent and past Vice-Chair, Illinois Interagency Council on Early Intervention

As suggested, it has long been recognized that the parent–child relationship is both a context and a mediator of child development. Now, new research expands accepted child development theory to document the power of the family environment, especially relational processes, in promoting the development of children with disabilities (Hauser-Cram et al., 1999). This view suggests that improvement of child outcome depends on working with some aspects of the parent–child–family relationship. In fact, the most potent, lasting outcomes of early intervention—the "marathon skills" that Turnbull and Turnbull (1986) identified—may be in the relational domain: family cohesion, emotional attunement, responsive caregiving, and parental satisfaction with the child. These are the same qualities that underlie the parental acceptance, nurturance, and approval so vital to the child's development of self (Rousso, 1985).

Presently, leaders from varying perspectives have argued for a relationship perspective within early intervention. In fact, Mahoney, Boyce, Fewell, Spiker, and Wheeden (1998) assert that the omission of a focus on parent–child interaction may be a factor in the limited results obtained in early intervention research. However, it is not clear that there is agreement on the elements of a relationship approach or on the exact fit for this focus within a family-centered framework.

One way to look at differing approaches to intervention is to use Stern's (1995) conceptualization of the parent–child relationship as four interdependent elements: the parent's and the infant's overt behaviors and the parent's and the infant's mental representations of the interaction and of each other. Approaches differ in which elements they target (e.g., overt interactive behaviors or subjective representations) and in terms of the modalities used (e.g., modeling, education, and support). In this section, we explore relationship approaches developed for young children with disabilities from two perspectives. First, we consider those that work *through* the relationship, focusing on parent–child interactive behaviors to achieve child outcome. Second, we consider approaches that work *with* the relationship by attending to the subjective experience of infants, parents, and providers, as well as with their interactive behaviors.

Working through the Relationship: Supporting Parent–Child Interactions

Parent–Child Interactions

Beginning with this view of the centrality of the parent–child relationship to all aspects of development, Bromwich (1981, 1997) developed one of the first parent–child interaction models of early intervention for infants at medical or environmental risk or for infants with disabilities. Avoiding infant curriculum models, on one hand, and parent education models, on the other, Bromwich (1981) built on psychodynamic, attachment and cognitive theories and research on parent–child interactions and aimed directly at altering or enhancing the interactive behaviors of both partners in the relationship. While Bromwich (1997) begins with the primary objective of helping mothers and infants develop a mutually satisfying social relationship, her ultimate aim for early intervention "is to offer the best possible opportunity for each infant and young child to achieve his/her optimal potential in development and physical and mental health" (pp. 40–41).

Bromwich begins with the assumption that parents of children who are medically vulnerable or disabled experience stress and need support and assistance with coping. Home visits are tailored to the needs and interests of parents and not guided by a written curriculum. Staff use a variety of approaches, including videotapes, to help parents learn to observe their children, enjoy interacting with them, and eventually become able to provide stimulating activities appropriate to their level of development. If it is difficult for a parent to interact in a positive way with the child, the interventionist works directly with the infant until the parent can see the child in a new light. When modeling is used, it is in the interest of experimenting or trying out a new behavior with a child that may or may not be successful.

Although Bromwich has a strong behavioral focus on the interaction, she nevertheless relies on a therapeutic alliance between a parent and an interventionist and hopes to have an impact on parents' perceptions of their infants. Thus,

although the focus is on working through the relationship to enhance child outcome, the relationship is also often changed. In evaluating her program, Bromwich argued for a perspective that recognizes the inherent transactional process of change in parent and infant and that sustained changes in the infant cannot be achieved without concomitant changes in caregiving responses of adults.

Triadic Strategies

A decade later, basing their work less on theory and more on developmental research primarily within the context of language and cognitive learning, special educators McCollum and Yates (1994) focused on parent–child interactions as both a means of ensuring family participation and enhancing child outcome. Believing, like Bromwich, that the parent must change in order to support changes in the infant, McCollum and Yates advocated supporting and enhancing the roles of parents as competent and confident caregivers of their young children. They enabled parents to establish developmentally supportive interactions by providing information about the child's developmental agenda in the context of parent–child play.

McCollum and Yates (1994) framed the interaction unit as a triad: child, parent, and interventionist. Thus, this approach makes the traditionally child-oriented professional explicitly aware of the other partners in the dance. "Triadic strategies" serve as a means to build on and expand the strengths of the parent–child interaction by providing contextual and interpersonal support. The strategies include (1) establishing a supportive context to increase the probability of playful interaction, (2) acknowledging parent competence by recognizing and expanding developmentally facilitative behaviors, (3) focusing attention on particular competencies or actions in the interaction, (4) providing child development information in context, (5) modeling by momentarily taking on dyadic interaction roles, and (6) suggesting options for dealing with the child. Most significantly, the interventionist must be consciously aware of the strategies and strive to match them to the dyad—focusing on the individual strengths and interests of the parent—*moment by moment*.

Like Bromwich, the triadic strategies influence the parent–child relationship through a focus on parent and child *behaviors* rather than through the parent's representation of the child. McCollum and Yates acknowledged parents' perceptions but focused primarily on supporting parents' self-efficacy and perceptions of themselves as competent in their parenting role. They conceived supervision as a parallel process in which the supervisor has a respectful, supportive relationship with the interventionist and supports her knowledge, competence, and self-efficacy. The supervisor also assists each interventionist in focusing on her own perspectives and recognizing how these perspectives color her relationships with families and children.

Parents Taking the Lead

Like McCollum and Yates (1994), Baird and Peterson (1997) subscribe to the major tenets of family-centered philosophy including a collaborative relationship wherein professionals "do things with, not to, families" (p. 140). Yet, they also subscribe to the notion that a child's developmental course may be altered by changing the nature of the interactions between infants and caregivers. Being respectful of the cultural relativity of child-rearing goals and practices creates a dilemma. On one hand, the basic tenets of family-centered practice and law involve parental choice and decision making—not a contract for changing parents' behavior. On the other hand, there is evidence that interactions in infancy mold and integrate the child's development.

Thus, Baird and Peterson (1997) proposed a model for incorporating infant–parent interaction into family-centered intervention by explicit family choice. The model involves four strategies for assisting families, rather than professionals, to make subjective decisions about the appropriateness of infant–parent interactions relative to their values and goals for their child and to be active decision makers about addressing infant–parent interaction within the early intervention process. These strategies include (1) identification of the family's vision for the future, (2) discussions with the family about interaction implications, (3) family decisions about intervention, and (4) family evaluation of outcomes.

Baird and Peterson (1997) demystify parent–infant interaction by explaining the child's role and the parent's role in understandable terms and in intervention topics or choices. In-

terventionists discuss infant parameters such as (1) clarity of infant signals, (2) infant patterns of social interaction, and (3) infant temperament. Caregiver interaction variables such as (1) identification and interpretation of infant signals, (2) style of caregiving, (3) acoustic properties of interactive behavior compatible with "motherese," (4) pacing of interactive behaviors, (5) perceptions of self-efficacy, and (6) feelings of enjoyment.

With a virtual map of parent–infant interactive behaviors, the model assists parents in making decisions about the desirability of parent–infant interactions within the early intervention process. Using this map, parents can help monitor progress, assess the degree to which their goals are respected, and report satisfaction with the intervention. Parent–child interaction may be identified as a prioritized outcome, incorporated into strategies for obtaining child development outcomes, or may not be formally addressed at all. The authors acknowledge that for a variety of reasons—emotional, social, environmental—families may not want to focus in this area, and professionals must respect this wish and support families in other ways. However, they also note that professionals maintain a responsibility to provide families with recommendations as part of the evaluation process, and professionals "must be aware of their ethical obligation when interactions are clearly detrimental to the child's development" (p. 159) including mandatory reporting.

Reflections on Supporting Parent–Child Interactions

Thus, one emerging theme in the field of early intervention is a focus on parent–child interaction to facilitate parental competence and child outcome. For educators and therapists who have trained in a hands-on, child-focused approach, these strategies offer a broader view of the relationship as the context for learning and an indirect route to child outcome. They may be most helpful with families for whom one-to-one interaction is comfortable and/or who share the assumption that a high degree of reciprocity will enhance their child's development. Because the child may be difficult to engage, it may be easier for adults to change their overt interactive behavior first. Thus, adapting parental behavior is a potent entry point to change the infant's behaviors. None of these models explicitly discusses how specific disabilities influence the approach to parent–child interaction. The implicit assumption is that the interventionist begins with knowledge about disability and that general principles of interaction apply. Mahoney and Wheeden (1997) suggest that the goal is to help parents become *more effective* at teaching the developmental and social behaviors they desire for their children. This goal involves high levels of maternal responsiveness and moderate to low levels of directiveness in parents' interactions with their infants. These approaches may increase the effectiveness of early intervention, in part because they serve as a proxy for child engagement, encouraging children to be active agents in constructive learning efforts. Facilitating attachment is not explicitly mentioned in the early intervention literature, but supporting responsivity presumably facilitates it.

Nonetheless, concerns and cautions have also been expressed about a focus on parent–child interactions within early intervention by some of the same persons who have advocated for such an approach. As noted, one of the major concerns is the extent to which addressing infant–parent interaction is compatible with the tenets of family-centered philosophy; that is, with parental choice regarding intervention goals. There is also a growing awareness about cultural differences and the possibility that subjective intervention methods based on ethnocentric values may compromise family-centered practice (Baird & Peterson, 1997; McCollum & McBride, 1997). Are the same interactive characteristics meaningful and important across cultures? What is "adequate" or appropriate caregiving? How much "responsivity" or "sensitivity" is enough? How much "intrusiveness" is too much? To what extent are intervention methods compatible with the parents' own child-rearing goals (Gilkerson & Stott, 1997), daily routines, and family-identified IFSP goals?

Questions also arise regarding the validity and appropriateness of parent–infant assessment tools. Because of these concerns, Mahoney, Spiker, and Boyce (1996) proposed that intervention can focus on interactions without formal assessment. They cautioned that assessment and intervention with parent–infant relationships are emotionally charged issues and, if approached insensitively, have the potential to undermine the trusting relationship essential for effective early intervention.

Another major concern is with the level of preparedness of the professional team members to address the observed interaction. In addition, these models are directed toward overt parent–child behaviors, but they also have the potential to both influence parental representations and to be influenced by parental representations. These approaches do not explicitly address the possibilities for pain or problems in the relationship, nor do they require the kind of clinical supervision that would help the interventionist deal with those issues. Mahoney et al. (1996) raised ethical questions about interventionists addressing parent–child interactions without a full understanding of the complexity of this endeavor. In training professionals, Baird (personal communication, February 12, 1999) stressed the seriousness of the work, the potential for harm, the wisdom for restraint given uncertainty, and the process of referral when relationship issues go beyond the preparation of the worker. Opportunities to experience reflective supervision as part of training or ongoing practice would enhance the effectiveness of the worker in understanding and respecting the boundaries inherent in these approaches (Gilkerson & Shamoon-Shanok, in press).

In sum, informed by the cautions and concerns, these models offer promising approaches for early intervention specialists to move from child-oriented, hands-on interventions to promoting parent and child interactive behaviors which have the potential to enhance parental effectiveness and promote child development.

Working with the Relationship: An Infant Mental Health Perspective

In the context of Part C, the need for intervention originates in the child in the form of a developmental delay or specific disability. Yet, this infant is embedded in a relationship that is influenced by a rich history on the parents' part and a quickly accumulating "biography" on the infant's part. Another approach to facilitating relationships within early intervention posits that these subjective experiences of the parents and the child are central to understanding motive and meaning of overt behavior. These approaches are process oriented and draw from the perspectives of infant mental health. In recent years, there have been several attempts to bring the fields of early intervention and infant mental health together in a variety of ways. At one end of the continuum is the suggestion that the two fields be completely integrated; at the other end are more modest suggestions that aspects of each inform the other. We describe three approaches that appear to represent different points on the continuum, beginning with the most integrated.

A Holistic Relationship Perspective

Weston, Ivins, Heffron, and Sweet (1997) proposed a new organizing construct for the field of early intervention which involves the integration of relationship-based concepts at all service levels. Weston et al. (1997) suggested that the changes related to focusing on family relationships in early intervention have been largely additive rather than integrative because the organizing principles have not changed. In their view, the construct of "centrality of relationships" exemplifies a fundamental reconceptualization of early intervention services by (1) recognizing relationships as both organizers of development and as the basis of all interventions and (2) focusing on the process of intervention as well as the content. This means that the focus is not just on child progress but on the complexity of the child's social–emotional experience and the quality of the parent–child relationship. Thus, the model focuses on "how behaviors feel from the inside, not just how they look from the outside" (Lieberman, 1998). In this model, interventionists are prepared to help parents find ways to understand and identify with their child's inner experience and thus become more accepting and helpful.

Weston et al. (1997) proposed that the relationship perspective needs to permeate the whole organization, serving as the organizing construct at the direct service, program, and agency level. This model assumes that the organization's mission, structures, and process also are shaped by a recognition of the power of relationships. The model suggests that infant mental health and early intervention should be seen as aspects of a single field of inquiry and integrated practice. This parallel process model is required so that the organizational structure and process reflect the same philosophy as that of the service provider. Others who are interested in bringing the fields together focus less on integration and more on complementarity, perhaps in recognition of the inevitable limits of any single practitioner's knowledge, skill, and professional passion (Fenichel, 1997–1998) or any agency's capacity.

Focusing on Emotional Development

Moss and Gotts (1997–1998) proposed a relationship approach that (1) focuses on provider–parent relationships in specific families, using a case study approach, and (2) uses an affective curriculum (Partners in Parenting Education [PIPE]; Butterfield, 1996) as a resource, adapting selected activities to fit the early intervention system. Staff volunteers were asked to select families who had parenting needs (in part determined by referral) or those whose IFSPs included child objectives that implied a desire on the part of the parents to change some aspect of their relationship with their child.

This new emphasis on relationships resulted in a range of strategies. Some parents were helped at the behavioral level (e.g., to read their infant's cues better). Other parents demonstrated change at the representational level (e.g., understanding both the meaning of the child's behaviors and feelings as well as their own feelings and perceptions). In still other families, the impact seemed to be more on the provider, who developed insights and a deeper understanding of the range of outside resources that were needed. The model includes regular reflective supervision as a critical element.

Infant Mental Health Consultation

A third possible model of bringing infant mental health to early intervention—outside consultation—is elaborated by Hirshberg (1998). First, he strove to incorporate an infant mental health point of view into the functioning of all the early intervention professionals through a monthly case consultation process. Second, he provided specific guidance when more traditional mental health issues, such as parental psychopathology, were identified. The approach to consultation emphasized careful and thorough reflection and had several important outcomes: early intervention professionals recognized infant mental health issues in their work; many of the professionals were able to integrate the perspective into their professional work, and it helped the staff see that the perspective is not a "good fit" for everyone. Hirshberg had hoped to include a mental health evaluation as part of every early intervention assessment and notes that he failed to achieve this goal. Perhaps the reason is that this aspect of mental health seems to be the most antithetical to the family-centered focus of early intervention.

Reflections on Infant Mental Health

The infusion of infant mental health principles has allowed programs to look at external behavior as an expression of inner, subjective experience and to frame their interventions in a way that respects motive and meaning from both participants' and professionals' points of view. There are at least three reasons for including infant mental health principles into early intervention. One is that the early intervention system seems to be well-organized to respond to the stressors that families may face (Guralnick, 1997); another is that relationships are central to development *and* intervention; finally, the expectations for interpersonal effectiveness and intrapersonal self-knowledge of the family-centered practitioner are high. The emphasis on motive and psychological meaning and the ability to deal with intense emotion, including conflict and pain, that is a part of infant mental health lends itself to each of these rationales. Paradoxically, it is this strength that also can be perceived as a limitation. As noted, infant mental health has roots in psychodynamic theories that have been associated primarily with negative views of disability and of the families involved. While infant mental health has moved beyond these views, the cloud of pathologizing families hangs over and runs counter to the philosophy and practice of family-centered services.

The tensions involved in bringing the two systems together exist at two levels. First, there may be aspects of each framework that are not compatible. For example, within a family-centered model, the case consultation process (Hirshberg, 1998) might need to be renamed and restructured to include informed parent consent and opportunities for families to participate. Likewise, whenever one becomes involved in a family's coping strategies or relationships, there is potential for misapplication of theory and principles. Thus, reflective supervision is essential to the thoughtful implementation of these approaches. Another major concern is that attending to parents' subjective experiences can be like opening "Pandora's box"—for the parent and for the provider. Identified problems create considerable anxiety about role definitions and how to proceed within the framework of Part C, even when appropriate training and supervision are in place.

Yet, the blending of a strength-based, family-centered approach which also draws from infant mental health principles offers great potential to both validate the family's experience—whatever it may be—while holding a view of the full potential of the infant. The Family Administered Neonatal Activities (Cardone & Gilkerson, 1992) is an example of a brief postnatal intervention (over three contacts) adapted for families of infants born with Down syndrome, which is informed by principles of classic psychotherapeutic interviewing, an awareness of the role of behavior and representations in shaping parenting, and a belief in the power of the assumption of parental competence. The role of the facilitator is to hold the process: to hear the parental observations, to acknowledge the feelings associated with them, and to support their very beginning efforts at getting to know *this* baby. McDonough's (1995 and Chapter 31, this volume) work on interaction guidance provides another example of an integrated model that has rich potential for adaptation for infants and toddlers with disabilities and their families. As the field of early intervention continues to develop, we hope there will be more efforts to integrate multiple perspectives, thus providing the field with more viable options for enhancing the development of very young children with disabilities and their families.

CONCLUSION

Infants and toddlers can grow and develop with a disability, but they cannot thrive without the love and care of their families. Greenspan (1992) has asserted that perhaps the primary goal for children who have significant delays is to enable them to form a sense of their own personhood—a sense of themselves as intentional, interactive individuals. This sense of self is developed and shaped within the circle of primary relationships. Thus, supporting and enhancing primary relationships is a part of any birth to 3 intervention effort. This work can be done in different ways: through focusing on parent–child interactions directly or through understanding representations and meaning or both. A focus on parent–child relationships may be a large part or a small part of the work with an individual family. Like all other aspects of early intervention, the decision to work in this area will be mutual, that is, one negotiated with the family. In either approach, it is crucial to remember that early relationships are also held within the larger social environment. The prevailing views of disability are shifting toward perspectives that redefine wholeness and, thus, allow for the full development of the child and family. While the broader context of disability is changing toward more positive and empowering paradigms, each family and each child's experience is uniquely their own. To be truly family-centered, early intervention providers must be open to the full range of emotions—positive and negative, providing information *with* emotional sensitivity.

Early intervention and the disabilities field have led us to an understanding of the social construction of the meaning of disability, the values and practices of family-centered services, and promising models for facilitating parent–child interactions which promote parental competence and child outcome. Infant mental health helps us focus on how people understand, respond to, and make meaning of their own experiences. It offers the possibility for holding the pain as well as the hope. The crux of early intervention rests on how individual practitioners respond to individual children and families. By exploring differences in position and values, we are more likely to recognize other ways of knowing and to deepen our capacity to respond to the richness and complexity of lives of very young children with disabilities and their families.

ACKNOWLEDGMENTS

We thank Adrienne Asch, Carol Gill, Harilyn Rousso, and Jeanette McCollum for sharing their work with us; Sue Walter for sharing her family's experience; and Bridget Scott and David Wilson for their help in preparing the manuscript.

REFERENCES:

Able-Boone, H. (1996). Ethics and early intervention: Toward more relationship-focused interventions. *Infants and Young Children, 9*(2), 13–21.

Asch, A. (1998). Distracted by disability. *Cambridge Quarterly of Healthcare Ethics, 7*, 77–87.

Asch, A., & Rousso, H. (1985). Therapists with disabilities: Theoretical and clinical issues. *Psychiatry, 48*(1), 1–12.

Baird, S., & Peterson, J. (1997). Seeking a comfortable fit between family-centered philosophy and infant–parent interaction in early intervention: Time for a paradigm shift? *Topics in Early Childhood Special Education, 17*(2), 139–164.

Barber, P. A., Turnbull, A. P., Behr, S. K., & Kerns, G. M. (1988). A family systems perspective on early childhood special education. In S. L. Odom & M. B. Karnes (Eds.), *Early intervention for infants and children with handicaps: An empirical base* (pp. 179–198). Baltimore: Brookes.

Beckman, P. J. (Ed.). (1996). *Strategies for working with families of young children with disabilities.* Baltimore: Brookes.

Bernheimer, L. P., Gallimore, R., & Weisner, T. S. (1990). Eco-cultural theory as context for the individual service plan. *Journal of Early Intervention, 14*, 219–233.

Brinker, R. P. (1994). Family involvement in early intervention: Accepting the unchangeable, changing the changeable, and knowing the difference. *Topics in Early Childhood Special Education, 12*(3), 307–332.

Bromwich, R. (1981). *Working with families and their infants at risk.* Austin, TX: Pro-Ed.

Bromwich, R. (1997). *Working with families and their infants at risk* (2nd ed.). Austin, TX: Pro-Ed.

Bruschweiler-Stern, N. (1998). Reflections on the process of psychotherapeutic change as applied to medical situations. *Infant Mental Health Journal, 19*(3), 320–323.

Butterfield, P. M. (1996). The Partners in Parenting Education Program: A new option in parent education. *Zero to Three, 17*(1), 3–10.

Cardone, I. A., & Gilkerson, L. (1992). Family administered neonatal activities: An adaptation for infants born with down syndrome. *Infants and Young Children, 5*(1), 40–48.

Dunst, C. L., Trivette, C. M., & Deal, A. G. (1988). *Enabling and empowering families: Principles and guidelines.* Cambridge, MA: Brookline Books.

Fenichel, E. (1997–1998). Introduction. *Zero to Three, 18*(3), 1–3.

Ferguson, P. M., & Asch, A. (1989). Lessons from life: Personal and parental perspectives on school, childhood, and disability. In D. Biklen, D. Ferguson, & A. Ford (Eds.), *Schooling and disability: Eighty-eighth yearbook of the National Society for the Study of Education* (pp. 108–140). Chicago: University of Chicago Press.

Garland, C. W. (1993). Beyond chronic sorrow: A new understanding of family adaptation. In A. P. Tunbull, J. M. Patterson, S. K. Behr, D. L. Murphy, J. G. Marquis, & M. J. Blue-Banning (Eds.), *Cognitive coping, families and disability* (pp. 67–80). Baltimore: Brookes.

Gething, L. (1992). Judgements by health professionals of personal characteristics of people with a visible physical disability. *Social Science and Medicine, 34*, 809–815.

Gilkerson, L. (1983). A fully human life. *Family Resource Coalition Report, 2*, 3.

Gilkerson, L., & Shahmoon-Shanok, R. (in press). Relationships for growth: Cultivating reflective practice in infant, toddler, and preschool programs. In J.D. Osofsky & H. E. Fitzgerald (Eds), *WAIMH handbook of infant mental health* (Vol. 2). New York: Wiley.

Gilkerson, L., & Stott, F. (1997). Listening to the voices of families: Learning through caregiving consensus groups. *Zero to Three, 18*(2), 9–16.

Gill, C. J. (1994). A bicultural framework for understanding disability and the family. *Family Psychologist, 10*(4), 13–16.

Greenspan, S. I. (1992). *Infancy and early childhood: The practice of clinical assessment and intervention with emotional and developmental challenges.* Madison, CT: International University Press.

Guralnick, M. J. (1997). *The effectiveness of early intervention.* Baltimore: Brookes.

Hauerwas, S. (1986). Suffering the retarded: Should we prevent retardation? In P. R. Dokecki & R. M. Zaner (Eds.), *Ethics of dealing with persons with severe handicaps: Toward a research agenda* (pp. 53–70). Baltimore: Brookes.

Hauser-Cram, P., Warfield, M. E., Shonkoff, J. P., Krauss, M, Upshur, C. C., & Sayer, A. (1999). Family influences on adaptive development in young children with Down syndrome. *Child Development, 70,* 979–989.

Hirshberg, L. M. (1998). Infant mental health consultation to early intervention programs. *Zero to Three, 18*(3), 19–23.

Klein, N. K., & Gilkerson, L. (2000). Personnel preparation for ealy childhood intervention. In J. P. Shonkoff & S. J. Meisels (Eds.), *Handbook of early childhood intervention* (2nd ed.). New York: Cambridge University Press.

Lieberman, A. F. (1998). An infant mental health perspective. *Zero to Three, 18*(3), 3–5.

Lynch, E. W., & Hanson, M. J. (1998). *Developing cross-cultural competence: A guide for working with children and their families* (2nd ed.). Baltimore: Brookes.

Lyons-Ruth, K. (1998). Implicit relational knowing: Its role in development and psychoanalytic treatment. *Infant Mental Health Journal, 19*(3), 282–289.

Mahoney, G., Boyce, G., Fewell, R., Spiker, D., & Wheeden, C.A. (1998). The relationship of parent–child interaction to the effectiveness of early intervention services for at-risk children and children with disabilities. *Topics in Early Childhood Special Education, 1*(1), 5–17.

Mahoney, G., Spiker, D., & Boyce, G. (1996). Clinical assessments of parent–infant interaction: Are professionals ready to implement this practice? *Topics in Early Childhood Special Education, 16,* 26–50.

Mahoney, G., & Wheeden, C. (1997). Parent–child interaction—The foundation for family-centered early intervention practice: A response to Baird and Peterson. *Topics in Early Childhood Special Education, 17*(2), 165–184.

McBride, S., Sharp, L., Hains, A., & Whitehead, A. (1995). Parents as co-instructors in pre-service: A pathway to family-centered practice. *Journal of Early Intervention, 19,* 377–389.

McCollum, J. A., & McBride, S. L. (1997). Ratings of parent–infant interaction: Raising questions of cultural validity. *Topics in Early Childhood Special Education, 17,* 494–519.

McCollum, J. A., & Yates, T. J. (1994). Dyad as focus, triad as means: A family-centered approach to supporting parent–child interactions. *Infants and Young Children, 6*(4), 54–63.

McCubbin, H. I., & McCubbin, M. A. (1987). Family stress theory and assessment: The T-double ABCX model of family adjustment and adaptration. In H. I. McCubbin & A. Thompson (Eds.), *Family assessment for research and practice* (pp. 3–32). Madison: University of Wisconsin–Madison.

McDonough, S. C. (1995). Promoting positive early parent–infant relationships through interaction guidance. *Child and Adolescent Psychiatric Clinics of North America, 4,* 661–672.

McWilliams, R. A., Tocci, L., & Harbin, G. (1995). *Services are child-oriented and families like it that way—but why?* Chapel Hill: Carolina Policy Studies Program, Frank Porter Graham Child Development Center, University of North Carolina.

Moss, B., & Gotts, E. (1997–1998). Relationship-based early childhood intervention. *Zero to Three, 18*(3), 24–32.

National Organization on Disability (1994). *NOD/Harris survey of disabled Americans.* New York: Author.

Olshansky, S. (1962). Chronic sorrow: A response to heaving a mentally defective child. *Social Casework, 43,* 190–193.

Pawl, J. (1995). The therapeutic relationship as human connectedness: Being held in another's mind. *Zero to Three, 15,* 2–5.

Rousso, H. (1985). Fostering health self esteem. In M. J. Schleifer & S. D. Klein (Eds.), *The disabled child and the family: An exceptional reader* (pp. 24–30). Boston: Exceptional Parent Press.

Sander, L. (1995). *Thinking about developmental process: Wholeness, specificity, and the organization of conscious experiencing.* Paper presented at the annual meeting of the division of psychoanalysis, Santa Monica, CA.

Seligman, M., & Darling, R. (1989). *Ordinary families, special children: A systems approach to childhood disability.* New York: Guilford Press.

Shonkoff, J.P., Hauser-Cram, P., Krauss, M.W., & Upshur, C.C. (1992). Development of infants with disabilities and their families: Implications for theory and service delivery. *Monographs of the Society for Research in Child Development, 7*(6, Serial No. 230).

Slentz, K., & Bricker, D. (1992). Family-guided assessment for the IFSP development: Jumping off the family assessment bandwagon. *Journal of Early Intervention, 16,* 11–19.

Stern, D. N. (1985). *The interpersonal world of the infant: A view from psychoanalysis and developmental psychology.* New York: Basic Books.

Stern, D. N. (1990). *Diary of a baby.* New York: Basic Books.

Stern, D. (1995). *The motherhood constellation.* New York: Basic Books.

Stern, D. N. (1998). The process of therapeutic change involving implicit knowledge: Some implications of developmental observations for adult psychotherapy. *Infant Mental Health Journal, 19*(3), 300–308.

Stott, F. (1997, July–September). A view from the classroom: Changing minds. *The Signal,* pp. 6–9.

Summers, J. A., Dell'Oliver, C., Turnbull, A. P., Benson, H. A., Santelli, E., Campbell, M., & Siegel-Causey,

E. (1990). Examining the individual family service plan process: What are family and practitioner preferences? *Topics in Early Childhood Special Education, 10,* 78–99.

Tronick, E.Z. (1998). Dyadically expanded states of consciousness and the process of therapeutic change. *Infant Mental Health Journal, 19*(3), 290–299.

Turbiville, V. P., Turnbull, A. P., Garland, C. W., & Lee, I. M. (1996). Development and implementation of IFSPs and IEPs: Opportunities for empowerment. In S. L. Odom & M. E. McLean (Eds.), *Early intervention/early childhood special education* (pp. 77–100). Austin, TX: Pro-Ed.

Turnbull, A. P. (1987). *Accepting the challenge of providing comprehensive support to families.* Paper presented at the Early Childhood Developmental Association of Washington, Seattle, WA.

Turnbull, A. P., Blue-Banning, M., Behr, S., & Kerns, G. (1986). Family research and intervention: A value and ethical examination. In P. R. Dokecki & R. M. Zaner (Eds.), *Ethics of dealing with persons with severe handicaps: Toward a research agenda* (pp. 119–140). Baltimore: Brookes.

Turnbull, A. P., Patterson, J. M., Behr, S. K., Murphy, D. L., Marquis, J. G., & Blue-Banning, M. J. (1993). *Cognitive coping, families, and disability.* Baltimore: Brookes.

Turnbull, A. P., & Turnbull, H. R. (1986). Stepping back from early intervention: An ethical perspective. *Journal of the Division of Early Childhood, 10,* 106–117

Vincent, L. J., & McLean, M. E. (1996). Family participation. In S. L. Odom & M. E. McLean (Eds.), *Early intervention/early childhood special education* (pp. 59–76). Austin, TX: Pro-Ed.

Vohs, J. (1993). On belonging: A place to stand, a gift to give. In A. Turnbull, J. M. Patterson, S. K. Behr, D. L. Murphy, J. G. Marquis, & M. J. Blue-Banning (Eds.), *Cognitive coping, families and disability* (pp. 51–66). Baltimore: Brookes.

Wehman, T. (1998). *Parental perceptions of current and ideal levels of family participation in early intervention program practices in Illinois.* Unpublished doctoral dissertation, Loyola University, Chicago.

Weston, D. R., Ivins, B., Heffron, M. C., & Sweet, N. (1997). Formulating the centrality of relationships in early intervention: An organizational perspective. *Infants and Young Children, 9*(3), 1–12.

Wright, B. (1960). *Physical disability: A psychological approach.* New York: Harper & Row.

Zola, I. K. (1993). Self, Identity, and the naming question: Reflections on the language of disability. *Social Science and Medicine, 36*(2), 167–173.

30

Infant–Parent Psychotherapy: Core Concepts and Current Approaches

❖

ALICIA F. LIEBERMAN
ROBIN SILVERMAN
JEREE H. PAWL

A father names his son Lucifer and then boasts that his now severely disturbed 2-year-old "fits his title." A mother is convinced that her 3-month-old infant is kicking her "on purpose" when she changes the child's diaper. Absorbed in her thoughts, another mother consistently fails to notice the crying of her 1-month old. Home alone with his 8-month-old baby, a father believes that the child's naptime presents the ideal opportunity to go jogging. A toddler's mother refuses his entreaties to play for fear of "spoiling" him. In each of these situations we bear witness to an infant who holds no parental focus as an individual in his or her own right but, rather, becomes the unwitting participant in a deeply conflictual aspect of the parent's experience that impedes an empathic awareness of the baby's own developmental and emotional needs.

Certain themes predominate, although their psychological origins and behavioral manifestations are as varied and unique as the individuals who enact them.

In these examples, the "evil" infant, the "destructive" infant, the "invisible" infant, the "independent infant," and the "insatiable" infant represent recurrent parental constructions of what Stern (1985) called the clinical infant.

Each of these constructions, expressed in the resulting set of caregiving behaviors, stands for an important but unconscious aspect of the parent's sense of self and other that interferes with an emotionally satisfying relationship with the child and has a negative effect on the baby's development.

Infant–parent psychotherapy aims at protecting infant–toddler mental health by aligning the parents' perceptions and resulting caregiving behaviors more closely with the baby's developmental and individual needs within the cultural, socioeconomic, and interpersonal context of the family. The therapeutic process may take a variety of forms, but the core component involves the therapist's effort to understand how the parent's current and past experiences are shaping perceptions, feelings, and behaviors toward the infant (Fraiberg, 1980). The baby's contribution to the interactional difficulties, for example, through physical or temperamental characteristics that hold particular meaning for the parents, has become an increasingly recognized aspect of infant–parent psychotherapy as well. The intervention focuses on what transpires between the baby and the parent, regardless of its constitutional, psychological or historical origins. The "identified patient" is the child–parent relationship, and the therapy painstakingly examines and addresses the transactions between the partners (Lieberman & Pawl, 1993; Pawl & Lieberman, 1997).

In many cases, only one of the parents experiences conscious conflict toward the baby and is motivated to seek change through therapeutic intervention. Other times, only one parent—usually the mother—is actually present in the child's life. In these situations, infant–parent psychotherapy focuses on the dyad, although the absent parent may be actively represented in the clinical work. When both parents are physically present and willing to participate, and/or when siblings are an intrinsic part of the clinical picture involving the baby, the dyadic format is expanded to include whatever family configuration is appropriate. In these circumstances, what distinguishes infant–parent psychotherapy from family therapy is that the clinical focus remains on the baby, with the goal of achieving improvement in the baby's emotional health by enhancing the emotional quality of the relationship network in which she is embedded.

It is important to point out that this clinical focus on the baby may be not always be explicitly articulated to the parents. The infant–parent psychotherapist may judge that in some circumstances the best way of helping the baby is to first help those who take care of the baby. However, infant–parent psychotherapy always involves at least a tacit expression of the baby's relevance to the treatment. This is the case even when the clinical picture of the parents prevents the therapist from pursuing an ongoing articulated focus on the baby. In this sense, the final outcome of infant–parent psychotherapy is always evaluated in terms of improvement in the *baby's* social-emotional well-being as the result of treatment.

CORE CONCEPTS

Perhaps the most succinct and enduring description of infant–parent psychotherapy was made by its originator, Selma Fraiberg (1980), when she wrote that this form of treatment is used in situations in which the baby has become

> the representative of figures within the parental past, or a representative of an aspect of the parental self that is repudiated or negated. In some

cases the baby himself seems engulfed in the parental neurosis and is showing the early signs of emotional disturbance. In treatment, we examine with the parents the past and the present in order to free them and their baby from old "ghosts" who have invaded the nursery, and then we must make meaningful links between the past and the present through interpretations that lead to insight. At the same time . . . we maintain the focus on the baby through the provision of developmental information and discussion. We move back and forth, between present and past, parent and baby, but we always return to the baby. (p. 61)

This passage highlights the meaning of the baby as a transference object to the parents. The transferential component obscures the baby's selfhood for the parents, so that their perceptions of the baby's personality and behavior are colored and distorted by their own experiences. Because of such perceptions, the baby's presence during the therapeutic session is a central ingredient of infant–parent psychotherapy. Parental report cannot be a substitute for direct observation of the baby and of the parent–baby interaction. The therapist's observational skills allow her to identify themes, detect defensive distortions, capture emotional nuances, and monitor infant development in ways that would not be possible in the baby's absence. Moreover, the baby's real contributions allow for therapeutic intervention in the immediacy of the moment, while affect is being keenly experienced and can be addressed most directly.

Neurotic Conflict or Character Structure?

The baby's function as a transference object for the parents stems from a particular theoretical perspective: the classical psychoanalytical concept of neurotic conflict as the interplay between an id impulse seeking discharge and an ego defense warding off or diverting the impulse's direct discharge or access to consciousness (Greenson, 1967). The metaphor of "ghosts in the nursery" illustrates the psychoanalytical concept of the struggle between an impoverished ego and forbidden, unconscious impulses that find partial expression in parental anger and ambivalence toward the baby.

In its original formulations, infant–parent psychotherapy saw its goal as uncovering and making conscious the childhood sources of these unconscious impulses so that the baby would no longer serve as their representative.

However, since the inception of infant–parent psychotherapy in the mid-1970s, this theoretical core has evolved in response to three major influences: recent developments in psychoanalytical theory, the emergence of attachment theory as a clinically relevant conceptual frame, and research findings about the early affective, cognitive, and interpersonal capacities of infants (Lieberman, 1991, 1997, Lieberman & Zeanah, 1999; Pawl & St. John, 1998; Pawl & Lieberman, 1997; Seligman, 1994, 1999).

It is certainly still the case that enormous improvement in the parents' feelings toward the baby, in the infant–parent relationship and in the baby's well-being, can be accomplished when the parents are able to link their negative feelings toward the baby with their childhood experiences, gradually creating a tapestry of new meaning from initially fragmented and isolated early memories. At the same time, it is also true that retrieving the past is not necessarily or invariably the avenue to healing in the present. This is often the case, for example, when the parent does not rely on language as the primary form of self-expression, when he or she is not psychologically minded, when childhood trauma is of such magnitude that the parent's capacity for symbolization is substantially damaged, or when the parent's psychological functioning is too fragile or constricted to tolerate delving into painful early memories. In addition, some parents state forthrightly that they do not want to speak about their past. Working within these clinical constraints, it is helpful to remember that the present exists in its own right and not solely as a mirror of the past, and that childhood is not the only developmental stage when formative emotional experiences can take place. Speaking in depth about recent experiences can bring about transformative change. Moreover, in some situations the most effective interventions are not verbal but rather enacted through the therapist's empathic attitude and behavior (Lieberman & Pawl, 1993).

Infant–parent psychotherapy, as originally practiced in Ann Arbor and currently in San Francisco, is a socially minded psychological intervervention. It does not require a prerequisite level of parental psychological sophistication, motivation, knowledge, or ability to pay. It does assume that all parents have the right to receive respectful, skillful, and culturally appropriate interventions to help them overcome the obstacles they face toward adequate parenting. Selma Fraiberg's training as both a social worker and a psychoanalyst made her keenly aware of the important role of real life events and circumstances in molding psychological experience, and she appreciated the need for clinical flexibility and versatility in working with families that would not ordinarily choose to undergo psychotherapy. Infant–parent psychotherapists are trained to think carefully about therapeutic boundaries but not to be reflexively obedient to the traditional guidelines that define them. One example is the routine use of home visiting as the medium for intervention in situations in which families have difficulty with transportation, firsthand observation can provide an understanding of the conditions endured by the family and the baby, or the therapist's willingness to enter into the family's neighborhood and home can serve as an affirmation of the parent's dignity that strengthens the motivation to participate in treatment.

Mutative Factors

There is a long clinical tradition of searching for the discrete factors that promote enduring change in clinical treatment. Is it insight into the childhood origins of the patient's conflicts? Is it the novel ways of relating that are experienced in the course of a genuine, supportive relationship with an empathic therapist? Is it learning and rehearsing new ways of thinking and behaving in stressful situations? These questions apply to the mutative factors in infant–parent psychotherapy as well.

Initially, the parent's insight into the childhood conflicts that fueled the present ambivalence toward the baby was considered the pivotal factor in clinical improvement (Fraiberg, 1980). Current approaches to infant–parent psychotherapy give less primacy to conflict analysis and to clarifying links between the past and the present. Rather, similar importance as a mutative factor is attributed to the corrective attachment experiences provided by the therapeutic relationship, which becomes a vehicle for change in rigidly constricted or disorganized internal representations of the self in relation to attachment and other intimate relationships (Lieberman, 1991). Much importance is also attributed to the transformational power of learning and practicing reciprocal, mutually satisfying forms of interaction that give a positive emotional valence to the network of meanings being constructed between parent and child (Pawl & St. John, 1998). As noted in the previous section, these developments in infant–parent psychotherapy have been spearheaded by advances in psychoanalysis, infant research, and attachment theory.

Recent Developments in Psychoanalysis

A review of this literature is beyond the scope of this chapter, but it is worthwhile to highlight Wallerstein's (1986) Psychotherapy Research Project, a seminal effort to explore the mutative effects of different therapeutic factors by comparing and contrasting the techniques of classical psychoanalysis (four to five sessions a week on the couch, with the analyst restricted to primarily interpretive interventions) with the techniques of expressive–supportive psychotherapy (involving less frequent, face-to-face sessions and a more active stance on the therapist's part). The interpretive, insight-oriented techniques were defined as those analyzing the defenses, including resistances and transference reactions, as an essential step toward the integration of id impulses and subsequent symptom reduction. In contrast, supportive techniques were described as ego supportive or ego building and included, but were not limited to, a reality-oriented position, the use of encouragement and praise, recognition of and respect for basic defenses, and occasional reeducation. All these interventions, together with allowing for a positive transference and the suspension of judgment with regard to the patient's inner life, are presumed to facilitate new emotional and relational experiences which, with repetition, can serve as the vehicle for profound and lasting change.

The Psychotherapy Research Project found greater than expected success for supportive psychotherapy approaches and lesser than expected success for psychoanalytical approaches. Furthermore, the theoretical distinctions between these two groups did not hold up in practice because psychoanalysis carried more supportive elements than originally appreciated. Moreover, changes in personality structure that occurred via insight-oriented, interpretive techniques were virtually indistinguishable from those structural changes that occurred via supportive techniques.

The timing of these findings coincided with Kohut's (1966; Kohut & Wolf, 1978) writings, which emphasized the importance of explicit responsiveness, emotional attunement, attention, and respect in the treatment of narcissistic disorders. Kohut suggested that narcissistic imbalances reflected deficits in the formation of the self brought about by failures in the caregiving environment. In this paradigm, incapacity to modulate rage resulted from the infant's repeated failures in his or her efforts to have needs met and was not an expression of constitutional drive endowment, as proposed in classical psychoanalysis.

In response to Kohut's theory and its implications for treatment, proponents of classical psychoanalysis argued that an empathic and supportive stance on the therapist's part might represent little more for the patient than an experience of idealized reparenting. In their view, such a stance would inevitably fail while fostering a problematic dependence on the therapist and on the therapeutic process. The theoretical debate that ensued was characterized by an unfortunate and inaccurate binarism: the cure by empathy as opposed to the cure by interpretation, with which many practitioners are still struggling today.

Infant–parent psychotherapy relies on both interpretive and supportive techniques. It has been influenced by relational theories, such as attachment theory, American intersubjective theory, British object relations theory, self psychology, and current trends in Freudian theory. A primary characteristic of relational theories is the notion of the human subject as an open system, "always in interaction with others, always responsive to the nature of the relationship with the other . . ." (Aron, 1990, p. 481). This idea, which has been both supported and elaborated by infant research, has implications for the nature of psychopathology, transference, and change—in short, all of what constitutes psychotherapy. Aron writes: "In the relational or two-person model, the analytic relationship and the transference are always contributed to by both participants in the interaction. One can no longer think of associations as solely emerging from within the patient; all associations are responsive to the analytic interaction . . . psychological events are never just a function of inner structures and forces, but are always derivative of interaction with others" (p. 481). This construction is eminently applicable to infant–parent psychotherapy. In fact, infant research has made a significant contribution to furthering the progress of intersubjective theory, as elucidated in the section below.

The Influence of Infancy Research

In the 1970s there was a major transformation in the theoretical orientation of infant research, which evolved from a unidirectional examination of the parent's influence on the child to a bidirectional model of reciprocal influences (see Lewis & Rosemblum, 1974; Sameroff & Chandler, 1975). The cumulative effect of countless studies of the sensory, perceptual, cognitive, and interpersonal capacities of infants led to the emergence of a "theoretical baby" that is not a passive recipient of the parent's ministrations but rather communicative, participatory, oriented both to relationships and to reality, and able to make various distinctions and to express preferences from the first weeks of life (for comprehensive reviews, see Stern, 1985; Beebe, Lachmann, & Jaffe, 1997; Crockenberg & Leerkes, Chapter 4, this volume). Given this early capacity for mutuality and reciprocal relationships, the baby's behavior is best understood in the context of the dyad. In this paradigm, the organizing themes for infant behavior become interpersonal rather than individual—for example, arousal and affect regulation through transactional processes, matching and mismatching of affect through facial mirroring, sequences of disruption and repair in affective matches, and the centrality of interpersonal timing in all these processes (Beebe et al., 1997). This paradigmatic change has implications not only for infant–parent psychotherapy but for adult psychotherapy as well because the central themes of treatment, such as motivation, repetition, historical significance, fantasy, perceptual processes, regulation of affect, and information processing, are viewed through a relational lens. The form of treatment most compatible with this theoretical model gives equally close attention to infant and caregiver affect, thought, and action and to the intricate interactions between them in a relational context.

Contributions from Attachment Theory

The emphasis of attachment theory (Bowlby, 1969/1982) on the importance of real-life events in shaping internal experience, on the impact of maternal sensitivity in influencing quality of attachment, and on the use of behavior as an avenue for understanding and analyzing psychological processes were incorporated into the core of infant–parent psychotherapy, although this influence was not explicitly ac-

knowledged in Fraiberg's writings (Lieberman, 1991; Lieberman & Zeanah, 1999). In addition, the construct of internal working models of attachment is compatible with the practice of infant–parent psychotherapy because it complements the emphasis on behavior with an emphasis on symbolic representation as the vehicle for the intergenerational transmission of relationship patterns (Bowlby, 1969/1982; Main, Kaplan, & Cassidy, 1985; Main & Hesse, 1990). Changes in maladaptive internal representations of the self in relation to attachment are hypothesized to occur both in the parent and in the baby through the transformational power of the therapeutic relationship, insight-oriented interpretation, and the acquisition of new interactive and caregiving behavioral patterns (Lieberman, Weston, & Pawl, 1991). Such changes go beyond circumscribed processes of conflict resolution to posit changes at the level of the person's relationship to the self and to intimate others.

Infant–parent psychotherapy has not to date made formal use of infant or adult attachment categories in devising treatment strategies. This is because attachment categories are considered useful ways of organizing information for research purposes rather than road maps for treatment, which need to be constructed jointly by the participants and the therapist and specifically tailored to the unique characteristics of the infant and the parents. However, the behavioral patterns and representational themes discovered and described in attachment theory and research (Ainsworth, Blehar, Waters, & Wall, 1978a; Main & Solomon, 1990; Main & Hesse, 1990; Main & Goldwyn, in press) enrich the vocabulary and clinical repertoire of infant–parent psychotherapy.

"Theoretical Targets" and "Ports of Entry"

In his illuminating discussion of how different clinical approaches conceptualize what needs to be changed in what he calls "the parent–infant clinical system," Stern (1995) speaks of two aspects that characterize these approaches. The "theoretical aim or target" is the basic element of the parent–infant system that the therapist ultimately wants to change. The "port of entry" is the basic element of the system that is the immediate object of clinical attention—the avenue through which the therapist enters into the clinical system.

The theoretical target of infant–parent psychotherapy is the web of mutually constructed meanings in the infant–parent relationship (Pawl & St. John, 1998). The focus here is on mutuality. Does the baby have parental permission to participate in this construction of meaning? Are her signals and behaviors accepted with an effort to incorporate them into the ongoing flow of the interaction? Or is meaning arbitrarily imposed from the outside, as the parent mandates what happens and when without using the baby's signals as a guide? Or, alternatively, is the parent so afraid of imposing meaning on a supposedly hapless infant that every signal is anxiously responded to and every initiative allowed to unfold for fear that saying "no" will bring lasting harm to the child?

Mutually constructed meanings have many components. The list of ingredients includes the most concrete daily caregiving procedures as well as the baby's emerging understanding of what is happening and his incipient theories about why an event is taking place (i.e., infantile theories of causality and the role of the self in making things happen); the parents' sometimes rigidly entrenched general ideas of who babies are and what they need; the parents' specific representations of this particular baby and his or her place in the parents' life at this point in time; and the contribution of the family's cultural, social, and economic circumstances. These individual ingredients gradually come together to form an intricate, multifaceted, and multilayered intersubjective space that for parent and baby represents the reality of their being, both individually and in relation to each other.

The infant–parent psychotherapist surveys the meanings constructed by parent and child in search of the most parsimonious or timely port of entry. The presence, appropriateness, and modulation of affect or its absence when expected are time-tested guideposts in this search. The specific port of entry selected may vary from family to family or, within a family, from session to session or from one time frame to another within a session. Commonly used ports of entry are the *child's behavior*, the *parent–child interaction*, the *child's representations of the self and of the parent*, the *parent's representations of the self and of the baby*, and the *parent–therapist relationship*. In the second year of life, toddlers' greater mastery of language and locomotion generates a more differentiated sense of personal autonomy and assertiveness vis-à-vis the parents, at the same time heightening concerns about separation, parental disapproval, and the danger of losing the parent's love (Mahler, Pine, & Bergman, 1975; Lieberman & Pawl, 1993). The resulting increased complexity of toddlers' inner life means that they become more active participants in giving shape and content to the web of meanings between themselves and their parents. Projective identification processes take place where parental attributions are internalized by the child and become an integral part of the child's sense of self (Lieberman, 1997; Silverman & Lieberman, 1999; Seligman, 1999). When the parental attributions are negative and critical, the child finds himself in a psychological quandary because he feels compelled to accept and comply with the negative parental image while at the same time experiencing anger and fear toward the parent and anxiety about the integrity of the self. The *intertwined parent–child representations* can become a useful port of entry for therapeutic intervention as well. Clinical vignettes illustrating each of these clinical possibilities are presented below.

Child's Behavior as Port of Entry

The baby's behavior is a powerful vehicle for therapeutic intervention, whether this behavior is developmentally expected or a particular expression of the baby's individuality. The meaning attributed by the parent to the baby's behavior may be quite different than the meaning the therapist finds in it. The construction of a meaning that takes benevolent account of the baby's experience then becomes a goal of the therapeutic endeavor, as in the situation described next.

When the therapist arrived, Jason, 2 months old, was lying on his back on the mother's bed, crying hard. His 17-year-old single mother picked him up and handed him over to the therapist, saying, "Here. You take him." Without taking him, the therapist came close to mother and child and said, "Hi, Jason. Are you having a hard morning?" The mother replied, "He has a hard everything. He hollers and hollers when he's hungry. Nursing babies get hungry every 2 hours." The therapist nodded in agreement and said sympathetically, "So that makes for a lot of hollering. Not all babies are so regular either. Does he cry every two hours?" The mother answered, "Sometimes more, sometimes less." Jason was calmer now and oriented to his mother's voice. The therapist commented, "He knows your voice and he likes listening to you." The mother smiled and fixed the blanket so that it covered the baby's toes. She said, "They told me in the breastfeeding class that it would be every 2 hours. Anyway, that class was a waste. He doesn't like nursing, so I'm gonna stop and just give him a bottle. But I could nurse him. I used to drink, but I stopped 'cause they said it was bad for him." The therapist said, "You wanted to make sure he was healthy and strong." The mother nodded in agreement. The therapist asked, "What makes you think he doesn't like nursing?" The mother rolled her eyes as if to say it was obvious, and said, "'Cuz he turns away and cries harder and harder, gets all worked up and then when he finally drinks he gets so worn out that he falls asleep at the breast." Jason was crying again and flailing in his mother's arms. The mother lifted her shirt and said, "See, I try to feed him, but he turns away." Indeed, the baby was wiggling around, keeping his head oriented toward the breast but kicking his legs and twisting. The mother tightened her hold on Jason, holding him belly to belly as Jason struggled to turn away. The therapist asked how she had decided to hold him belly to belly, and the mother replied that she was taught to do that in her nursing class. The therapist said, "You know, Jason seems to have a different idea about how he'd like to be held. Maybe we could see what position might work for the two of you." The mother loosened her hold on the baby, and as the therapist watched and made encouraging noises, she followed Jason's lead until they found a rather unique position that the baby seemed to find comfortable, "over his shoulder," as the mother came to call it. From this position, Jason nursed absorbedly. The mother was surprised and excited by this discovery, which over time proved to be the position from which Jason nursed most successfully.

In this example, the baby's fretfulness over his inability to nurse became a guideline to look for a mutually comfortable nursing position that satisfied the baby and made the mother feel confident about her competence in feeding him. Most important, the baby's emotional expressions were the guide to this accommodation. He had been heard.

Parent–Child Interaction as Port of Entry

Because harsh, punitive, or otherwise developmentally inappropriate interactions are often the trigger for a referral to an infant mental health program, miscommunications and angry exchanges between parent and child are common during the sessions and can provide a ripe opportunity for exploring the sources of conflict and for helping in the mutual construction of meaning, as in the example that follows.

Linda, 18 months old, was eagerly trying to get a sip of orange juice from her mother's glass. The mother lifted her glass high in the air so Linda couldn't reach it, and said harshly, "You have your own glass. Go drink from it yourself." Linda cried as she reached way up in the air. She then gave up and tried to take a piece of cheese from her mother's plate. The mother took the plate away and yelled, "Stop trying to take things away from me!" She looked at the therapist and said, in exasperation, "She just started this. She won't let me eat in peace. Everything I have, she wants." The therapist asked, "Is it only food, or other things as well?" The mother says, in an angry voice, "Everything! She almost tore off my ear trying to get my earring. I found her putting my best sunglasses on—lucky I caught her before she broke them. She is always trying to take what I have for herself." The therapist said, with much feeling in her voice, "You know, I think I recognize what you are describing. She just became a toddler and toddlers are trying really hard to be like their moms and dads. She wants to be you—like you, as close as she can. She thinks you are the greatest and she copies everything you do. It can be a real pain in the neck! Can you believe that you are so important that she wants to be just like you in every way she can?" The mother's mood changed abruptly. She looked serious and surprised. There was a silence where she seemed to be trying to come to grips with the therapist's explanation. The therapist used this time to talk to Linda, saying, "You want to be just like your mom, eat just like her, look just like her." Linda had plopped herself on the floor, chewing on a piece of cheese. The mother asked, "What am I supposed to do? I hate it when my things are messed with." The therapist said, "Well, of course you have a right to keep your things safe, and she needs to learn what is OK and what is not OK for you. I wonder if there are things that you don't mind so much sharing with her, because it will make her feel so good that she has a little piece of you." The mother turned to Linda and said, "Hey, kid, what about a grape?" as she handed her one. Mother and daughter ate a few grapes looking intently at each other.

In this exchange, the therapist's tactfully phrased developmental guidance may have begun a process that could prevent the emergence of a negative maternal attribution of greediness or selfishness to her child. The therapist chose this course of action in spite of knowing that there were direct links between the mother's past experiences and her present anger at her daughter. This mother had been embroiled in a bitter and losing battle with her older sister, who constantly took things from her and interfered with her activities. She remembered her own mother as indifferent to her plight and as always taking her sister's side by telling her that she needed to learn how to share. This knowledge influenced the therapist's careful phrasing, which emphasized the mother's right to her own things and to her own experience. However, the therapist chose not to make a direct link between past and present because she believed that such an interpretation would be experienced by the mother as a repetition of earlier situations, when her frustration as a child had been belittled by her mother. Instead, the therapist anchored her approach in this mother's unfulfilled childhood wish to be recognized as important and worthy of love and admiration, and appealed to her potential to empathize with similar longings in her little girl. The coaching of the therapist's intervention in a general description of toddler development was intended to normalize Linda's behavior by making her comparable to other children her age.

Child's Representations as Port of Entry

Children's internal representations can serve as a useful therapeutic tool. Paying attention to how they feel about themselves and how they interpret the behavior of those closest to them legitimizes their experience and serves as a basis for further exploration. It can also expand the parent's appreciation for what the child thinks and feels.

Mario, 3 years, 8 months old, was a child who witnessed a lot of domestic violence between his mother and father before his parents divorced. This included an incident when his mother threatened his father with a knife. In this session, Mario was playing with a kitchen set. He took a toy carving knife and excitedly said to the therapist, "This is like the knife in my dream." The mother commented that a few days earlier Mario had had a terrifying dream and could not be awakened—he

kept crying and screaming and holding on to his mother for a long time, until she finally had to lay down and sleep with him. The therapist asked Mario about his dream, and he said, with much emotion, "There was this mommy . . . no, this monster, who came up to me with a knife and cut out my heart!" The mother asked if she was in the dream, and Mario replied, "No, I wanted you to be there to help me, but you weren't." The mother turned to the therapist and said she felt guilty for making Mario feel so scared. The therapist encouraged her to speak directly to her son. The mother said to Mario, "Mario, listen to me. I know I threatened your daddy with a knife because I was very mad at him, but I am very sorry that I scared you so much and I will never do it again." Mario looked at her very seriously, came close to her, and said, "Sometimes you get very mad at me, Mommy." The mother looked helplessly at the therapist, who said, "Mario, I think you are trying to tell your mom that you are scared of what she can do to you when she gets mad." Suddenly understanding, the mother said, "Mario, I love you very much, and no matter how angry I get I will never, ever, do anything to hurt you like taking a knife at you." Mario relaxed visibly and turned to the doctor's kit. For the rest of the session he proceeded to put bandages on his mother, his baby brother, and the therapist. When his mother tried to broach the issue of the knife again, he said, "Mommy, we're done with the knife for today. Put it in the bag."

The aspect of Mario's complex representation of his mother that portrayed her as a dangerous murderer was heard and understood by his mother, who became appropriately distraught by her contribution to the child's experience. The mother's empathic response and promise to protect him from her anger were an important counterweight to Mario's fear, and enabled him to begin re-forming a more coherent representation of his mother in such a way that her protective and benign aspects began to outweigh her frightening side.

It is useful to point out that Mario's mother was not a woman who started treatment with any explicit interest in becoming more aware of her child's or her own psychological processes. When she started child–parent treatment 7 months before this session, she was an angry disciplinarian who relied on rigid standards of right and wrong to raise her child, and her stated desire for treatment was to "make Mario behave." Her ability to make use of treatment to become more aware of psychological complexity illustrates the transformational potential of infant–parent psychotherapy when offered to parents who would not ordinarily seek conventional psychotherapy.

Parental Representations as Port of Entry

This is the best known avenue for therapeutic intervention in infant–parent psychotherapy because some of the most dramatic examples of distorted meanings in the parent–infant relationship involve parental representations of the child as willfully malevolent or as harboring adult-like motives (Fraiberg, 1980; Lieberman, 1997). In many cases, the parents' negative attributions are triggered by their subjective experience of the child's behavior, but the experience is so congruent, self-evident, and ego-syntonic and the negative attribution is so self-evident to the parent that a therapeutic effort to clarify the meaning of the behavior from the child's perspective is most often futile. Instead, the therapist tries to explore the associations to the parent's sense of being tricked, overlooked, disrespected, abused, or whatever affective experience the parent holds the child responsible for. This is sometimes done while simultaneously providing a context that suggests another meaning to the child's behavior, a meaning that is more consistent with the child's developmental stage. Pathological parental representations of a baby can occur even during pregnancy, as illustrated in the example that follows.

Eva and Sean, about 40 years old and expecting their first baby, had just found out that the baby was in a breach position and that a C-section might be necessary. Both parents were recovering drug users and had a long history of lawless and violent behavior which they were struggling to overcome. They were both quite shaken by the possibility of a C-section. Eva was trying hard to keep a positive attitude, but Sean was furious with the baby. "Who the hell does that little bastard think he is?" he bellowed, his face red with anger. "I'm gonna beat the hell out of him to teach him a lesson." Clearly embarrassed by this display, his wife tried to soothe him by assuring him that she would go for massages to turn the baby around. He calmed down a little. There was an uncomfortable silence. Looking for a way to introduce the baby's experience without sounding confrontational, the therapist said lightly, "If I were the

baby and saw how upset you were, I'd be scared stiff and wouldn't be able to turn around." Mother and father laughed. The therapist added, "Sean, I know how much you love Eva and how upset you are that she might get hurt. I think that the idea of her being cut and your not being able to protect her takes you back to the times when you were a violent man and could not control your anger." Sean said, with a muffled sob, "It took me so long to find her, and it is so hard to make a new life. I can't stand the idea of anything happening to her." The therapist pointed out that when that when people feel helpless they often try to figure out who is to blame and asked Sean whether perhaps he was blaming the baby as if the child were in breach position out of stubborness, just to spite the parents. The remainder of the session involved Sean's recollection of his father's physical abuse, how it was often triggered by behaviors Sean had not intended to be naughty, and how Sean turned fear into aggression as a form of self protection.

Intertwined Parent–Child Representations as Port of Entry

Negative parental attributions are coercive in the sense that they are expressed through behaviors that impel the child to identify with the parent's perceptions and to internalize these attributions into the child's sense of self (Lieberman, 1997; Silverman & Lieberman, 1999). Such intertwined representations can be a starting point for therapeutic intervention, as in the example that follows.

Brian, 3 years old, sat on the floor near his mother as she listed her complaints about him. She said, in a harsh voice, "People don't want to be around him. He hit another kid in school today. He gets everyone mad at him, so they don't like him. He's just like his father, and I worry that he'll grow up to hit women just like his father hit me." Without looking up or acknowledging in any direct way that he heard what his mother was saying, Brian began twisting the heads and mangling the limbs on the human figures he was playing with. The therapist said, "You have a lot of complaints for someone as little as Brian." The mother continued, "He doesn't listen; he has tantrums if he doesn't get his way. I don't know what to do with him anymore." Brian stood up, walked across the room and yanked a toy from his 12-month old sister's hands. The mother yelled at him, saying, "Give it back to her! I will kill you before I let you terrorize my family!" Brian went back to the doll he had been playing with and stomped on it repeatedly. The mother yelled at him not to break the therapist's toys. The therapist said, "The toys are not breakable. Brian, what is happening with the doll?" Brian answered, "It's a bad, bad baby and I'm gonna kill it." The mother looked at the therapist and said, "I just said that about Brian, didn't I?" The therapist answered, "That is what Brian heard and what I heard." Brian stopped stomping on the doll and looked at his mother, who began to cry and said, "I'm so mean to him, I get convinced that he's my enemy and I have to protect myself from him. In my mind I know that he's just a little boy and that this is crazy." This was the beginning of a long therapeutic process where the mother's attributions of badness and dangerousness to Brian and Brian's internalization and enactment of this attribution were examined and corrected again and again.

Parent–Therapist Relationship as a Port of Entry

Transference phenomena are as ubiquitous in infant–parent psychotherapy as in other forms of clinical intervention. The same emotional impediments that parents face in forming solid relationships with their children are also at work as impediments to the formation of a working alliance. This is even more apparent when the client belongs to a disadvantaged social group in which powerlessness and discrimination are rampant, creating a perceptual filter that makes it difficult for the parent to trust the therapist's competence and good intentions (Fraiberg, 1980; Seligman & Pawl, 1984). As a result, the parent's motivation to participate in infant–parent psychotherapy often needs to be patiently fostered. This process involves the therapist's ability to engage in a genuinely felt human connection with the parents, which often involves surmounting biases and preconceptions. The following vignette illustrates how the therapist's ability to repair an empathic break in nondefensive ways can provide the basis for a parallel process where the therapist's acknowledgement of his or her mistakes can soften the parent's angry stance toward the child.

The therapist arrived to meet with this 22-year-old mother and her daughter, Isabella. It was their seventh meeting, and the therapist was surprised to find that the mother, who had been resentful of the child protective services (CPS) referral to the infant mental health program, was waiting eagerly to see her. The mother ran out to meet the therapist while holding the child in her arms. The therapist commented that it was nice to see them. The mother sighed heavily and said that it had been a hard day because a child protective services worker had come to see her. She was interrupted by Isabella, who jumped into the therapist's arms. As they walked into the house, Isabella chattered away with the therapist, who answered her playfully. The mother started speaking again, "CPS did a surprise visit today. My ex called them. . . ." Isabella took the therapist's hand smilingly and said, "Go." For the next 10 minutes, therapist and child played together while the mother looked at them from a distance. Suddenly, while Isabella was jumping on the bed, the mother yelled, "Stop jumping! This house is a mess! All I do is clean all day long, and it is never clean! Get off the bed right now, Isabella!" As the mother started cleaning up, she spoke harshly to the child, telling her to move out of the way. It took the therapist several moments of feeling confused and rejected to realize her series of errors. She gently said to the mother, "Jenny, you met me at the door and told me that this had been a hard day, and I'm afraid I made it even worse. I think you wanted to talk to me about the CPS visit and I ignored you. I only paid attention to Isabella. I treated Isabella like her feelings were really important and I treated you like your feelings weren't important at all." The mother continued cleaning while ignoring the therapist. After a few minutes she yelled, "Isabella, you better start cleaning up. We have to go and I don't want this house to be a mess when we come back." The therapist took the dust pan and said casually, "Is it okay if I help?" The mother nodded unenthusiastically. The therapist took the dustpan and held it on the floor for the mother to sweep into it. After a few minutes of silence, the therapist added, "I am afraid I made you hurt and angry, but it's hard for you to tell me. I mean, you know, I was insensitive from the start today, and I think it might be easier for you to get mad at Isabella than to get mad at me, especially on a day when a CPS worker dropped in unexpectedly." The mother nodded, then she said with some embarrassment, "Both Isabella and I were a little sick, and the house was such a mess." The therapist said, "It is a small place, just a few things lying around can make it feel that way." The mother shook her head and said, in a resigned voice, "No, it was a mess. I have been sick and tired lately and just don't feel like keeping up with things." Isabella pulled on her mother's leg and asked for some juice. Her mother put down the broom and in a nice voice said, "I have to make some, Isabella, it will take a minute." The therapist followed mother and child into the kitchen and sat at the table while the mother made juice. "So," she asked, "why did CPS drop by today?" Jenny gave the child her juice, pulled Isabella on her lap, and explained that her ex-husband had reported a diaper rash on Isabella that did not exist. She added that the CPS worker had asked a few questions, checked Isabella, and left. The therapist said sympathetically, "It's very stressful even if nothing came of it." Jenny nodded vigorously and answered, "And it's not like I don't have enough to worry about already, like how I'm gonna get me and my kid out of this hellhole." Once her relationship to the mother was back on track, the therapist was able to move her attention back to a consideration of the stresses that interfered with this young mother's ability to be emotionally responsive to her child. The therapist's willingness to speak openly about her mistakes and to apologize for the distress she caused were a turning point in this mother's attitude toward herself, her child, and the therapeutic endeavor. The therapist was, in effect, showing the mother a new way to be, quite different from the critical and dismissive responses the mother had encountered from her parents.

These examples, taken together, illustrate the readiness of the infant–parent psychotherapist to make use of whatever promising entry he or she encounters to change the infant–parent relationship for the better, moving seamlessly (or trying to) between behavior and internal representation, between individual, dyadic, and family issues, and between the past and the present to construct a rich joint narrative between parent and child.

This variety of therapeutic approaches and modalities can be bewildering to a therapist used to working within a different clinical tradition. Therapists who were trained in an individual psychotherapy model can find it difficult to attend to the partners in a dyadic or triadic therapeutic format. Therapists who work with adults and rely on words as the carriers of meaning may not attend to the nonverbal signals of a baby or to the unspoken exchanges between parent and child. These difficulties can lead to serious therapeutic mistakes. Among the most common of these mistakes are the following: The therapist becomes so involved in the parental experience that he or she does not include the baby in the evolving understanding of

the situation; the therapist is too timid or unsure of his or her knowledge about babies and does not introduce the baby's experience into the therapeutic process; the therapist colludes with the parent in the maltreatment of the child; or, alternatively, the therapist is so identified with the infant that he or she cannot be empathically attuned to the parent's experience (Lieberman & Pawl, 1993). The ability to be evenly attuned to the individual needs of the partners while remaining keenly devoted to their interpersonal experience with each other is a hallmark of the seasoned and skillful infant–parent psychotherapist.

THE EFFECTIVENESS OF INFANT–PARENT PSYCHOTHERAPY: RESEARCH EVIDENCE

The conceptual compatibility of infant–parent psychotherapy with attachment theory (Lieberman, 1991) was used for measure selection. Difficulties in the infant–mother relationship was assessed using the Strange Situation procedure (Ainsworth, Blehar, Waters, & Wall, 1978b). Anxiously attached infants were randomly assigned to an intervention or a control group. Securely attached dyads comprised a second control group.

At outcome, the intervention group performed significantly better than anxious controls in measures of goal-corrected partnership, child avoidance, resistance and anger at mother, and maternal empathic responsiveness to the child. The intervention group did not differ from the securely attached comparison group at outcome.

Within the intervention group, mothers who formed a strong positive relationship with the intervenor tended to be more empathic to their infants and to have less avoidant babies at outcome. However, the mother's ability to use infant–parent psychotherapy to explore her feelings about herself and her child had the most positive outcomes. This measure was significantly correlated in the expected directions with maternal empathy, child anger and avoidance, security of attachment, and goal-corrected partnership in the negotiation of conflict. These findings indicate that the human quality of the therapeutic relationship has significant repercussions on both mother and child behavior, but that the most powerful results emerged from the mother's capacity to make use of the therapeutic relationship as a "secure base" to increase her self-knowledge and understanding of her child.

Many of the paremeters of infant–parent psychotherapy are currently being applied with preschoolers who witnessed severe domestic violence (Lieberman, Van Horn, Grandison, & Pekarsky, 1997; Lieberman & Van Horn, 1998). The basic format of intervention in the child–parent relationship is being employed in family situations in which the abuser (most commonly the child's father) has left the home, and in which the child and the mother are reenacting with each other the patterns of abuse and victimization that previously were played out between the adult partners. Outcome evaluation does not yet incorporate a randomized control design, but preliminary analyses of maternal and child behavior before and after intervention using standardized measures show significant statistical differences pointing to improvement in quality of the child–mother interaction as well as in child cognitive performance, decreases in child behavioral problems, and decreases in and maternal posttraumatic stress disorder symptomatology. Although preliminary, these findings echo the more systematic research findings that intervening in the child–parent relationship can lead to beneficial individual effects in both partners.

CONCLUSION

Infant–parent psychotherapy is a multimodal method of intervention that uses joint work with parents, infants, toddlers, and, more recently, preschoolers with the ultimate goal of improving the parent–child relationship and the children's socioemotional functioning. The therapist strives to create a therapeutic relationship characterized by flexibility and receptiveness to the parents' and the child's needs. This therapeutic relationship is a basic catalyst for change, and it becomes the vehicle for utilizing a combination of intervention modalities that include insight-oriented psychotherapy, unstructured developmental guidance, emotional support, and concrete assistance as well as crisis intervention when needed. The underlying assumption is that the corrective experience of the therapeutic relationship (a "corrective attachment relationship"), generated through the therapist's supportive and empathic stance, coa-

lesces with the new knowledge, self-understanding, and behaviors fostered and practiced through the different therapeutic modalities. It is these processes, created jointly by parent, child, and therapist, that can lead to enduring changes in the parent's and child's experiences of each other, the meanings they construct together, and their sense of themselves both individually and in relation to each other.

REFERENCES

Ainsworth, M. D. S., Blehar, M., Waters, E., & Wall, S. (1978a). *Patterns of attachment.* Hillsdale, NJ: Erlbaum.

Ainsworth, M. D. S., Blehar, M. C., Waters, E., & Wall, S. (1978b). *Patterns of attachment: Assessed in the Strange Situation and at home.* Hillsdale, NJ: Erlbaum.

Aron, L. (1990). One person and two person psychologies and the method of psychoanalysis. *Psychoanalytic Psychology, 7*(4), 475–485.

Beebe, B., Lachmann, F., & Jaffe, J. (1997). Mother–infant interaction structures and presymbolic self and object representations. *Psychoanalytic Dialogues, 7*(2), 133–182.

Bowlby, J. (1982). *Attachment and loss: Vol. 1. Attachment* (2nd ed.). New York: Basic Books. (Original work published 1969)

Fraiberg, S. (1980). *Clinical studies in infant mental health.* New York: Basic Books.

Greenson, R. (1967). *The technique and practice of psychoanalysis.* New York: International Universities Press.

Kohut, H. (1966). Forms and transformations of narcissism. *Journal of the American Psychoanalytic Association, 14,* 243–272.

Kohut, H., & Wolf, E. S. (1978). The disorders of the self and their treatment: An outline. Reprinted in Andrew Morrison (Ed.), *Essential papers on narcissism* (pp. 175–196). New York: New York University Press.

Lewis, M., & Rosenblum, L. (Eds.). (1974). *The effect of the infant on its caregiver.* New York: Wiley-Interscience.

Lieberman, A. F. (1991). Attachment theory and infant–parent psychotherapy: Some conceptual, clinical and research considerations. In D. Cicchetti (Ed.), *Rochester symposium on developmental psychopathology* (Vol. 3, pp. 261–287). Rochester, NY: University of Rochester Press.

Lieberman, A. F. (1997). Toddlers' internalization of maternal attributions as a factor in quality of attachment. In L. Atkinson (Ed.), *Attachment and psychopathology* (pp. 277–291). New York: Guilford Press.

Lieberman, A. F., & Pawl, J. H. (1993). Infant–parent psychotherapy. In C. H. Zeanah, Jr. (Ed.), *Handbook of infant mental health* (pp. 427–442). New York: Guilford Press.

Lieberman, A. F., & Van Horn, P. (1998). Attachment, trauma, and domestic violence. *Child Custody, 7,* 423–443.

Lieberman, A. F., Van Horn, P., Grandison, C. M., & Pekarsky, J. H. (1997). Mental health assessment of infants, toddlers and preschoolers in a service program and a treatment outcome research program. *Infant Mental Health Journal, 18*(2), pp. 158–170.

Lieberman, A. F., Weston, D. R., & Pawl, J. H. (1991). Preventive intervention and outcome with anxiously attached dyads. *Child Development, 62,* 199–209.

Lieberman, A. F., & Zeanah C. H. (1999). Contributions of attachment theory to infant–parent psychotherapy and other interventions with infants and young children. In J. Cassidy & P. R. Shaver (Eds.), *Handbook of attachment: Theory, research, and clinical applications* (pp. 555–574). New York: Guilford Press.

Mahler, M. S., Pine, F., & Bergman, A. (1975). *The psychological birth of the human infant.* New York: Basic Books.

Main, M., & Goldwyn, R. (in press). *Adult attachment classification system.* Unpublished manuscript, University of California, Berkeley.

Main, M., & Hesse, E. (1990). Parents' unresolved traumatic experiences are related to infant disorganized attachment status: Is frightened and/or frightening parental behavior the linking mechanism? In M. Greenberg, D. Cicchetti, & E. M. Cummings (Eds.), *Attachment in the preschool years: Theory, research and intervention* (pp. 161–184). Chicago: University of Chicago Press.

Main, M., Kaplan, N., & Cassidy, J. (1985). Security in infancy, childhood and adulthood: A move to the level of representation. *Monographs of the Society for Research in Child Development, 50*(1–2, Serial No. 209), 66–104.

Main, M., & Solomon, J. (1990). Procedures for identifying infants as disorganized/disoriented during the Ainsworth Strange Situation. In M. Greenberg, D. Cicchetti, & E. M. Cummings (Eds.), *Attachment in the*

preschool years: Theory, research, and intervention* (pp. 121–60). Chicago: University of Chicago Press.

Pawl, J. H., & Lieberman, A. F. (1997). Infant–parent psychotherapy. In S. Greenspan, S. Wieder, & J. Osofsky (Eds.), *Handbook of child and adolescent psychiatry* (pp. 339–351). New York: Wiley.

Pawl. J. H., & St. John, M. (1998). *How you are is as important as what you do.* Washington, DC: Zero-to-Three, National Center for Clinical Infant Programs.

Sameroff, A. J., & Chandler, M. J. (1975). Reproductive risk and the continuum of caretaking casualty. In F. D. Horowitz (Ed.), *Review of child development research* (Vol. 4, pp. 187–244). Chicago: University of Chicago Press.

Seligman, S. (1994). Applying psychoanalysis in an unconventional context: Adapting infant–parent psychotherapy to a changing population. *Psychoanalytic Study of the Child, 49,* 481–500.

Seligman, S. (1999). Integrating Kleinian theory and intersubjective infant research: Observing projective identification. *Psychoanalytic dialogues* (Vol. 9, pp. 129–160). Hillsdale, NJ: Analytic Press.

Seligman, S., & Pawl, J. H. (1984). Impediments to the formation of the working alliance in infant–parent psychotherapy. In J. D. Call, E. Galenson, & R. Tyson (Eds.), *Frontiers of infant psychiatry* (Vol. 2, pp. 232–237). New York: Basic Books.

Silverman R. C., & Lieberman, A. F. (1999). Negative maternal attributions, projective identification and the intrgenerational transmission of violent relational patterns. *Psychoanalytic diagogues* (Vol. 9, pp. 161–186). Hillsdale, NJ: Analytic Press.

Stern, D. (1985). *The interpersonal world of the infant: A view from psychoanalysis and developmental psychology.* New York: Basic Books.

Stern, D. (1995). *The motherhood constellation.* New York: Basic Books.

Wallerstein, R. (1986). *Forty-two lives in treatment: A study of psychoanalysis and psychotherapy.* New York: Guilford Press.

31

Interaction Guidance: An Approach for Difficult-to-Engage Families

❖

SUSAN C. McDONOUGH

Despite our various professional backgrounds, theoretical orientations, and disciplinary practices, the field of infant mental health seems to coalesce around several common assumptions. Infant behavior cannot be viewed separately from the young child's relationships. During infancy, the most important relationships are with primary caregivers. In turn, infants' caregivers have relationships with their social context. These assumptions provide a nesting of the infant within multiple contexts: the baby's caregivers and extended family members and the broader social and cultural networks in which these families live.

The transactional model of the baby affecting and being affected by the caregiver, who in turn is influencing and being influenced by the broader social and cultural contexts, is considered more thoroughly in Sameroff Chapter 1, this volume. Because the baby's development and emotional well-being seem to be simultaneously influencing and being influenced by others, we are offered opportunities for both nurturing and supporting early caregiving relationships. My goal in this chapter is to illustrate how a relationship-focused orientation can illuminate and guide our interventions with the most challenging families.

To meet this goal, I describe interaction guidance, a therapeutic model that incorporates prin-

ciples of a family system theory into a multigenerational transactional intervention. The resulting approach focuses therapeutic treatment on the infant–caregiver relationship rather than on either the *infant* or the caregiver alone. Caregiver *interactions* with the infant are understood both as reflection of family structure and caregiving nurturance and as a reflection of the caregiver's and baby's representational world. Because many overburdened families are preoccupied with everyday life challenges, observable interactions between baby and caregiver serves as the therapeutic intervention focus.

DEVELOPMENT OF THE INTERACTION GUIDANCE TREATMENT APPROACH

The interaction guidance treatment approach was created specifically to meet the needs of infants and their families that previously were not successfully engaged in mental health treatment or that refused treatment referral. Many of these families could be described as being "overburdened" by risk factors such as poverty, poor education, family mental illness, substance abuse, inadequate housing, large family size, lack of a parenting partner, or inadequate social support.

In an effort to reach overburdened families, we sought to create a treatment approach that would invite families to take an active role in the creation and evaluation of their family's treatment. Our goal was to develop a therapeutic approach that was sensitive to each family's strengths and vulnerabilities. We reviewed the intervention and treatment literature for components of successful clinical interventions with the aim of using these elements to create a unique treatment approach.

Successful clinical interventions have both structural and process elements. Structural elements are the specific content of the intervention—for example, addressing the unique needs of each family, involving extended family or household members in the treatment plan when appropriate or necessary, offering supplemental assistance when such help is asked or deemed critical to treatment success, providing the option of follow-up services at the conclusion of treatment, and including the family in the evaluation of treatment progress (McDonough, 1995).

The process elements of successful clinical interventions address how the clinician offers the therapeutic assistance. The key process features of interaction guidance are (1) encouraging the family to define the problem or issue of concern as they see it, (2) emphasizing a family's strengths while recognizing their vulnerabilities and limitations, (3) embracing a nonjudgmental stance in work with families while conveying societal norms for the family's caregiving behavior, (4) using an egalitarian and cooperative approach in the engagement and treatment of families, and (5) offering alternative perspectives to the family about their child caregiving through individually designed treatment (McDonough, 1995).

The interaction guidance treatment approach for parent–child relationship disturbances is designed to assist the family in gaining enjoyment from their child and in developing an understanding of their child's behavior and development through interactive play experience. The approach also seeks to foster the development of adult family members in their role as their child's parents or primary caregivers. Interventions to modify problematic behavior or to promote healthy patterns of interactional behavior are provided by a therapist who provides guidance but does not undermine the parents' role as primary caregivers.

This egalitarian treatment method has proven successful for families caring for infants with growth failure, pediatric regulation disorders (sleeping, feeding, or excessive crying), biological vulnerabilities (substance-exposed), and genetic disorders (Robert-Tissot et al., 1996; McDonough, 1995, 1996a; Stern, 1995). Parents who are resistant to participating in other forms of psychotherapy, who are young or inexperienced, or who are cognitively limited often respond positively to this treatment approach (McDonough, 1995, 1996b).

INFLUENCE OF FAMILY SYSTEM THINKING

The interaction guidance approach seeks to nurture the development of adult family members in their role as the child's parents or caregivers. Implicit in that goal is the importance of structural balance as it affects generational boundaries among grandparents, parents, children and siblings; parental coalitions such as scapegoating and triangulation; family roles and relationships; and the experience of childhood to the parent. The interaction guidance approach shares these and other common elements with other family system therapy treatments (e.g., emphasizing the separation of self from other within the family system). Structural family therapy (Minuchin, 1974), solution-focused therapy (Berg, 1994; Miller, Duncan, & Hubble, 1996), and strategic family therapy (Haley, 1976) communicate a similar model of individuation of self as an important aspect of successful family development.

Each approach addresses the importance of generational "boundaries," although the language among the approaches differs. For example, Bowenian therapy highlights the necessity of adults separating successfully (differentiating) from their family of origin but still remaining in emotional contact with them (Bowen, 1971). In the structural family framework, on the other hand, the importance of individual, spousal, parental, and sibling boundaries is clearly delineated. The structural family approach further addresses how power is executed in relation to whom and for what purposes as a focal point of treatment (Aponte & Van Deusen, 1981). The attention paid to the importance of the parent–child relationship makes the interaction guidance approach more narrowly focused on the importance of the early child–caregiver relationship than other forms of family treatment.

The conceptual underpinnings of narrative therapy (Freedman & Combs, 1996) are quite similar to the approach embraced by the interaction guidance therapist. While narrative therapists may capture a family story through the translation of oral to visual words, the interaction guidance therapist focuses on captured video images as the window into the family's thinking about themselves and their child. In each therapeutic approach, the clinician embraces the role of listener and recorder, checking with the family to ascertain whether the story that they are recording is correct. In many instances the therapist helps the family reflect on or to restory a particular incident. In so doing, the therapist presents alternative perspectives for the family to consider. Both treatment methods embrace an egalitarian approach in working with families. In each method, family and therapist share in identifying the sources of concern, are actively involved in treatment formulation and implementation, and measure treatment success using family identified treatment goals.

PRINCIPAL GOALS OF THE INTERACTION GUIDANCE APPROACH

The principal goals of the interaction guidance approach are to assist the family in gaining enjoyment from their child and in developing an understanding of their child's behavior and development through interactive family play experiences. These observable family interactions are understood as a reflection of infant–caregiver relationship and family functioning in the present and a representation of the parent's own caregiving experience. The approach also seeks to foster the development of adult family members in their role as their child's parents or primary caregivers. Efforts to intervene with parent–child problems take place within the context of the parent–child relationship rather than focusing singularly on problems in the child or in the parent.

When observing parent–infant interactions, both the content and style of the interaction can provide important clinical information to the therapist. Content refers to what the dyad or family is doing. Are they playing, talking, negotiating, or fighting? Style addresses how the family goes about interacting. For example, when the parent plays with his or her infant,

does the parent follow the infant's lead or does the parent try to have the baby do what he or she wants? If the child does not comply, does the parent permit the child to continue playing, make an effort to redirect the activity, or attempt to force or coerce the child to do what the parent wants?

The interaction guidance approach attempts to engage families in the therapeutic process by highlighting existing family strengths and competence before attempting to intervene in areas of family concern. One way to begin this process is to focus on preexisting aspects of quality caregiver–infant interaction. Field (1982) is one of the original investigators to identify elements of interaction style. She presented five stylistic characteristics of quality interactions. They include both interactive partners speaking at the same level, relating to the same thing, taking turns in communicative exchanges, observing each other's signals, and responding contingently. These characteristics are not only essential for good communication but also are easily observable in any family play. By observing family members together, the interaction guidance therapist can both draw attention to the pleasurable feelings derived from family interactions and nurture and coach these behaviors from reluctant or insensitive interactive partners.

THE STRUCTURE OF INTERACTION GUIDANCE

Families generally are seen weekly for hourly treatment sessions. Although the total number of sessions varies from family to family, it is often in the range of 10–12. Treatment lasts generally from 2 to 6 months, with later sessions often occurring less frequently.

The treatment structure of interaction guidance includes assessing the family situation; arranging who comes to treatment, and delivering the treatment. Each treatment session involves three phases: videotaping the family play session, viewing the videotape, and concluding the session.

Assessing the Family Situation (Caregiving Environment)

In an effort to understand as vividly as possible the family's experience, the therapeutic process begins with meeting of family household members at the referral source, that is, at the hospital or human service agency or in the family home. The child's primary caregiver (often the mother) is asked to invite all family members who assist in the care of the infant to an initial family meeting. The purpose of this household gathering is to gain a clear understanding of how the family views their situation, to describe the interaction guidance program, and to offer the family an opportunity to participate.

During the initial family meeting and/or on subsequent visits to the family home, the therapist encourages the family to tell their own "family story," that is, the history of their relationship with the infant (Zeanah & McDonough, 1989). The family meeting also permits the therapist to gain an understanding of the family's perspective of their own child, their belief system, family rituals, rules, and mores. Because treatment interventions that are sensitive to family and cultural beliefs and practices seem to offer the greatest likelihood of success (McGoldrick, Pearce, & Giordano, 1982), the interaction guidance therapist places emphasis on acquiring a clear understanding of the family's view of the problem or situation. The therapist completes a clinical assessment of family functioning, social support, and interaction style.

The meetings conclude with the development of family treatment goals that are generated by family members and discussed with the therapist. In contrast to some family interventions that hold the family responsible for treatment success, (Aponte, 1992; Aponte & Van Deusen, 1981; Bowen, 1971; Minuchin, 1974, Minuchin & Nichols, 1993), the interaction guidance therapist invites the family to monitor treatment progress on a weekly basis and to suggest changes in their treatment goals as necessary. The treatment plan is modified according to input from both the family and the therapist. Joint responsibility between the family and the therapist for treatment goal setting and monitoring treatment progress reflects the more equitable stance assumed by the interaction guidance approach regarding the relationship between client and therapist.

Throughout the intake period the therapist works to involve all family members in the treatment planning process. Even if other family members choose not to participate in the treatment sessions, their cooperation and support of the child's parents or primary caregivers is necessary to implement and maintain any therapeutic change in family functioning.

Who Comes to Treatment?

A common aspect among many relationship-based treatments is the focus on working with at least two family generations. In interaction guidance treatment, the infant's caregiver is encouraged to invite a parenting partner into the treatment sessions. Treatment "families" can be the child's biological parents and siblings, a single parent and friend, or an adolescent mother and her own mother. The treatment session always includes at least two family generations: caregiver and child. Although families often bring siblings to the sessions, in some cases it is advisable to work initially with the caregiver(s) and a single child. For example, in the case of a fragile infant who easily becomes overstimulated, it may be more advantageous to work with the parent and child alone until the caregiver is confident of being able to soothe and calm the infant. Gradually other family members can join the treatment session.

Implementing Interaction Guidance

The treatment sessions usually are held in a specially designed playroom equipped with developmentally appropriate toys, a playmat, comfortable chairs or sofa, and a bassinet. A video camera is available to record the play session for viewing by the family and therapist. The room is arranged to be comfortable for the needs of both adults and very young children. Although the therapist usually sits on the floor to encourage more interactive play between the infant and the caregivers, some adults initially choose to sit on a seat and join in the floor play sometime later in the session. Prior to the family's arrival, the therapist selects a variety of toys that the caregivers and infant can use during play. Toys and play materials (e.g., mirror, book, and music box) are chosen because they invite use by more than one person. Some of these toys create an unusual display when moved or make a musical sound. For caregivers that seem initially uncomfortable playing with their infant, the toys seem to provide a helpful aid.

While the family interacts, the therapist videotapes approximately six minutes of the play sequence. The family and therapist following family–infant play will view this 6-minute "movie." In situations in which an assistant mans the camera, the therapist remains in the treatment room but sits apart from the family and tries not to interact with family members. Whether videotaping or observing the family in the treatment room, the therapist makes particular note of existing positive caregiving behavior and parental sensitivity. The therapist also makes note of behaviors that need to be modified or altered because of their critical importance, for example, caregivers failing to provide adequately for infant's safety.

The sequence of activities during each family session remains fairly consistent throughout treatment. Families whose own lives are disorganized and chaotic seem to find this predictable routine comforting. Once the family is welcomed into the playroom, the therapist inquires about what has occurred in the family's life since the last visit. This is an opportunity to learn about the issues and topics with which the family has dealt and how comfortable family members are with what has transpired. Early in the treatment process, this is a time of information solicitation and exchange. The family members share their story, offer opinions, and ask questions of the therapist. As the family displays more trust in the therapeutic relationship, often members display spontaneously a wider range of emotions with the therapist. Families speak of the frustration and disappointment they encounter in their efforts to make changes in their lives, or, conversely, they express the increased enjoyment and satisfaction they receive from their interactions with one another. Consequently, as treatment evolves, the therapist spends more time initially listening to and speaking with the family. In each session, once the therapist judges that family members appear satisfied that their concerns were heard or addressed, the therapist invites the family to play with their infant the way they would if they were home.

Reviewing the Videotape

To facilitate the parents' understanding of growth and development of their own child, the caregivers are actively involved in observing both the behavior of their infant and their own style of interaction and play with their child. The use of videotape in treatment allows for immediate feedback to the parent(s) or family regarding their own behavior and its effect on the infant's behavior. Through viewing samples of parent–child play interaction, family members become more aware of important interactive behaviors that are positive and need to be

reinforced, elaborated, and extended and those interactions that were less enjoyable or inappropriate and require redirection, alteration, or elimination. The use of videotape also provides the parents with the opportunity to listen more carefully to what they say to their child and the manner in which they say it.

After taping the play interaction session, the family and the therapist view the videotape. Initially, the clinician attempts to solicit comments from the parent(s) concerning their perception of the session and their thoughts and feelings regarding their infant and their role as parents. A series of systematic probes are posed to the family, such as, "Was this play session typical of what happens at home?" Or, "Were you surprised by anything that happened during the session?" These questions often stimulate discussion among family members and the therapist about what the family saw on the screen, what it meant to them, how they felt about what they saw, how they thought their children felt, and how they felt about themselves as parents.

Following the caregivers' comments, the therapist then highlights specific examples of positive parenting behavior and parental sensitivity in reading and interpreting their infant's behavior. Focusing on what family and therapist agree is mutually satisfying and enjoyable to all interactive partners seems to convey a sincere sense of caring and concern on the part of the therapist. During these repeated occasions, most families begin to realize that the focus of treatment is positive in nature and that the therapist will address family identified problems through the use of family competence and strength.

The videotape viewing and feedback aspect of the sessions seem especially meaningful to the family at the beginning of treatment. As families become more comfortable verbalizing their thoughts and concerns spontaneously with the therapist, they seem to view the videotape feedback as an opportunity to reflect on what the televised event represents to them in a broader context. For example, some families use the videotape viewing as a stimulus to discuss events of the past week, whereas others reflect on experiences from years past and the feelings that accompany these memories.

Another advantage of videotaping is the opportunity it affords both the family and therapist to review the changes that occur across sessions. In situations in which change is subtle and progress is slow, a retrospective viewing of progress over time can often encourage a family's effort at continuing treatment.

Concluding the Play Session

After the videotape is shown and discussed, the therapist continues talking with family members while they play with their infant. Sometimes issues raised by family members during the video replay are discussed for the remainder of the session. Other times the conversation expands into other aspects of family life beyond the caregiver's parenting role. The therapist attempts to follow the client's lead in exploring areas of concern and conflict but also raises issues the therapist believes are interfering with the growth and development of family members, particularly the infant.

The session concludes with a therapist-led discussion regarding treatment progress or lack of progress. The family is encouraged to comment candidly on the treatment process. The family is asked if they would like to schedule a visit for the coming week. The purpose of offering another appointment to the family rather than assuming a standing meeting is to convey the importance of active family decision making concerning their own treatment participation and progress.

Therapeutic Considerations for Video Use

At the end of treatment, the clinician prepares an edited videotape that documents the changes that occur in parent–child interactions and family transactions over the course of the treatment. This videotape is given to the family as a record and an example of their sensitive and positive parenting. There are several situations in which offering a copy of the videotape to the family before the completion of treatment may assist in treatment progress. Sometimes a spouse or co-parent (friend, relative, household member) is unable or refuses to participate in the treatment sessions. Sharing a "movie" of what happens during a play session often alleviates unspoken concerns or fears by the resistant party about what actually occurs during the treatment hour. Also, having other household members view and hear what is done and said by the therapist often provides a source of validation for clients in their attempt to restructure or to change previous ways of thinking or behaving. Finally, viewing the videotape is a con-

crete way for the family to share the experience with other persons interested and concerned about the infant's well-being and happiness.

THE PROCESS OF INTERACTION GUIDANCE

The interaction guidance approach rests on certain basic assumptions about working with families. These beliefs are helpful both in understanding the important role of family members in the infant's life and in working with family members to broaden their thinking and to change their behavior.

1. Embrace the position that parents and caregivers are doing the best they know how to do. Although this sounds simple, it can be challenging to implement consistently. By emphasizing the phrase "the best they know how to do," one is able to keep open the possibility that the parents can acquire new ways of thinking, coping, behaving, and feeling. This approach also conveys acceptance and respect of where parents are now without assuming that it is all they are capable of. Use existing positive parental behavior and attitudes to assist in building feelings of self-confidence in the caregivers.

2. Address what parents believe to be the problem or issue of concern. As professionals working with multiproblem families, it is frustrating and often heartbreaking to see parents worry excessively about things that they can not change or fail to take some direct action that could minimize or alleviate some difficulty. Sometimes what appears to be a critical family need is not identified as an area of concern by the family. The family may chose to use their resources differently. Acknowledge and accept the family's negative feelings and attributions of child behavior without feeling either as if you need to change them immediately or that you concur with their assessment. To maintain your relationship with the family, it is necessary only to make clear that you understand their perspective. Often caregivers are seeking to be heard.

3. Ask the family directly what you can do to be helpful. At the simplest level, the helping process involves two components: (1) a person offers some assistance or aid and (2) another person accepts what is offered. Professionals working with families can increase the likeli-

hood that the offered help will be accepted by encouraging the family to decide what, if any, assistance they desire or need rather than assuming that a clinician identified problem is the family's source of concern. Reinforce the role of the parents as decision makers in the family and protectors of the child by deferring to their expertise as the individuals who know their child "best." Consider the ramifications of "doing for" (including handling the baby) without being asked to do so *before* initiating an intervention. Sometimes our "assistance" may be interpreted as the clinician knowing better, taking over, criticizing, or correcting.

4. Answer questions posed by the family directly; provide information when asked. Many families begin treatment with questions they hope to have answered by the therapist. Occasionally the information requested by the family may be unknown or unanswerable, or the material requested may be too technical for the family to use. Often families need to have things repeated many times, in many different ways, and sometimes by more than one person before they grasp the meaning of what is being said to them. Even then the family's understanding of the long-term implications of particular circumstances or conditions may change as the family acquires additional information or experiences new insights. Families report that what a professional tells them is not always as important as the manner in which the information is shared. Consequently, minimize the role as "the authority"; rather, convey expertise in a nonjudgmental way by providing perspective on caregivers' beliefs and feelings.

5. Jointly decide with the parents the definition of treatment success—make it explicit. Families that are having difficulties in raising their children or have experienced a parenting failure already need some reassurance that things are capable of changing. Short-term, problem-focused therapy is one way to begin addressing this concern. Involving the family in an active negotiation of treatment success affords the therapist another opportunity to learn how the family attempts to solve problems and to prioritize their goals. For example, is treatment success dependent on whether the symptoms go away? Do they reflect both on internal changes (feelings, thoughts, beliefs) and behavioral manifestations (child sleeps through the night)? Or do they reflect only on one? Are these indices of treatment success child focused, parent focused, or relational? Responses

to questions such as these provide the therapist with insight into how to establish the therapeutic alliance with the family. Maintaining and strengthening that alliance often occur when caregivers feel respected and accepted. Therapists should make note of behavior they wish to alter or modify but address only that which they believe to be of critical importance.

6. Monitor treatment progress weekly with the family. Involving families in monitoring their own treatment progress assists the therapist in observing areas of growth and development within the family, as well as issues of resistance and relapse from the family's point of view. If treatment is proceeding positively, the family can share feelings of achievement and accomplishment. If one party is dissatisfied, those feelings can be explored openly and the therapist can suggest changes or a redirection in treatment focus. This weekly monitoring appears to be especially helpful in dealing with resistant clients whose anger often can be addressed and worked through by providing a regular opportunity for them to express their thoughts and feelings about the treatment process. Because one of the principal partners in the relationship may not be able to speak on his or her own behalf, the therapist should use his or her own voice to gain the family's attention and interest by articulating the baby's needs and desires.

PROCESS CHARACTERISTICS OF INTERACTION GUIDANCE

A few specific process characteristics of the interaction guidance approach are included here to further illustrate treatment implementation. The first concerns the importance of establishing and maintaining a working alliance, and the second concerns the nonauthoritarian role of the therapist.

Working Alliance

The therapist should work hard and quickly to establish a positive working alliance. When working with families that have a history of unproductive contacts with social service professionals, it is useful to acknowledge where the "system" and those working within it have failed the family in the past. Clearly, many overburdened families have spent years struggling mightily to resolve complex life problems. What needs to be conveyed during an initial family session is that the therapist is asking to join in an alliance with the family rather than assuming that family members will join with the therapist. Because disappointment and failure often characterized past dealing with professionals, it seems particularly important to offer concrete assistance that produces some tangible result for the family during the initial family meeting. This may involve arranging a scheduled appointment at the family's convenience. The message to be conveyed is that *the therapist* intends to work hard toward making this experience a productive one for the family.

Nonauthoritarian Role

The therapist should play down or minimize the role of authority; rather he or she must convey expertise in a nonjudgmental way. Every family wants to play a meaningful role in their child's life. Often the strategies that overburdened families use are not fulfilling this family desire. Asking the family what they have discovered about what works best and not so well for them invites an egalitarian discussion between the therapist and the family. It also offers the possibility for therapists to share what other families have shared with them about the family's own successful efforts to adapt and cope. Using other families' life lessons can be a less threatening way for family members to entertain new ideas or to broaden their perspectives about different ways to think and to behave.

The therapist should make note of behavior he or she wishes to alter or modify but should address only those that he or she believes to be of critical importance. For therapists learning the technique, this is often the most unsettling and unusual aspect of the approach. We are drawn naturally to a problem-focused approach by babies in distress, by our interest in psychopathology, and/or by our mission as change agents. Nevertheless, forcing ourselves to ask, "What is going well?," allows us to attempt to establish links between the present and the future and possible parent–infant relationship that is the focus of treatment.

Related to the third principle is using existing positive parental behavior and attitudes to help build feelings of self-confidence in the parents. Sooner or later the interaction guidance therapist will be asking the caregiver to find value in the baby—even in situations of serious conflict with the baby or when characteristics of the baby are especially burdensome. As a way of demonstrating how to find strengths, it is useful for the therapist to identify and reinforce what is positive in the parent, and to use that as a basis for building a more satisfying relationship with the baby. The implicit message to the parents is as follows: Having seen your relationship with your baby at close hand and having learned about the problems you described to me, I believe we already have a foundation for improving things because you are able to be a good/loving/sensitive/etc. parent in this moment that I am pointing out to you. For parents burdened by guilt and disappointment, this can be a powerful message.

SUMMARY

The interaction guidance treatment approach for parent–infant relationship problems was developed primarily to reach families that have been difficult to engage and help using more traditional psychotherapeutic approaches. It is informed by a transactional and contextual model of development in which infant–caregiver relationships are nested within larger contextual systems. Similar to other family therapy methods and approaches, it is both here and now and multigenerationally focused on interactional sequences and the meanings they convey to family members. Perceived family needs and family treatment goals are developed within the therapeutic relationship rather than imposed from the outside. Interaction guidance is explicitly strengths based and emphasizes the working alliance between therapist and family as partners in the process of change.

The basic assumption of this approach is that infants can be helped through strengthening their relationships with their primary caregivers. Preliminary data support that this treatment can be effective in enhancing the development of both infants and caregivers through careful attention to the process and content of therapist–family transactions.

REFERENCES

Aponte, H. J. (1992). Training the person of the therapist in structural family therapy. *Journal of Marital and Family Therapy, 18,* 269–281.

Aponte, H. J., & Van Deusen, J. M. (1981). Structural family therapy. In A. S. Gurman & D. P. Kniskern

(Eds.), *Handbook of family therapy* (pp. 196–216). New York: Brunner/Mazel.

Berg, I. K. (1994). *Family based services: A solution-focused approach*. New York: Norton.

Bowen, M. (1971). Family therapy and family group therapy. In H. Kaplan & B. Sadock (Eds.), *Comprehensive group psychotherapy* (pp. 345–362). Baltimore: Williams & Wilkins.

Field, T. (1982). Interaction coaching for high-risk infants and their parents. In H.A. Moss, R. Hess, & C. Swift (Eds.), *Prevention in human services: Vol. 1. Early intervention programs for infants* (pp. 5–24). New York: Haworth Press.

Freedman, J., & Combs, G. (1996). *Narrative therapy*. New York: Norton.

Haley, J. (1976). *Problem-solving therapy*. San Francisco: Jossey-Bass.

McDonough, S. C. (1995). Promoting positive early parent–infant relationships through interaction guidance. *Child and Adolescent Clinics of North America, 4*, 661–672.

McDonough, S. C. (1996a). Models of interaction for parents and children. In J. Gomes-Pedro & M. Folque Patricio (Eds.), *Bebe XXI: Infants and families in the next century* (pp. 221–233). Lisbon: Fundacao Calouste Gulbenkian.

McDonough, S. C. (1996b). *Using video replay to change adolescent mothers' interactions with their infants*. Paper presented at the meetings of the International Society for the Study of Behavioral Development, Quebec, Canada.

McGoldrick, M., Pearce, J. K., & Giordano, J. (Eds.). (1982). *Ethnicity and family therapy*. New York: Guilford Press.

Miller, S. D., Duncan, B. L., & Hubble, M. A. (1996). *Escape from Babel: Toward a unifying language for psychotherapy practice*. New York: Norton.

Minuchin, S. (1974). *Families and family therapy*. Cambridge, MA: Harvard University Press.

Minuchin, S., & Nichols, M. P. (1993). *Family healing: Tales of hope and renewal from family therapy*. New York: Free Press.

Robert-Tissot, C., Cramer, B., Stern, D. N., Serpa, S., Bachman, J., Palacio-Espasa, F., Knauer, D., De Muralt, M., Berney, C., & Mendiguren, G. (1996). Outcome evaluation in brief mother–infant psychotherapies: Report on 75 cases. *Infant Mental Health Journal, 17*, 97–114.

Stern, D. N. (1995). *The motherhood constellation: A unified view of parent–infant psychotherapy*. New York: Basic Books.

Zeanah, C. H., & McDonough, S. C. (1989). Clinical approaches to families in early intervention. *Seminars in Perinatology, 13*, 513–522.

32

Infant Massage Therapy

❖

TIFFANY FIELD

Infant massage is practiced throughout much of the world, especially in Africa and Asia (Auckett, 1981; McClure, 1989). In many countries, including Nigeria, Uganda, India, Bali, Fiji, New Guinea, New Zealand (the Maiori), Venezuela, and the Soviet Union, infants are given a massage with oil after the daily bath and before sleep time for the first several months of their lives. Many of the techniques they are using have been introduced to the Western world and are beginning to be practiced by parents and clinicians.

In India, infant massage is a daily routine that begins in the first days of life. The infant is laid on his or her stomach on the mother's outstretched legs, and each body part is individually stretched. Warm water and soap are applied to the legs, then the arms, back, abdomen, neck, and face. The massage looks to an observer like scrubbing clothes on an old washboard because it is administered so vigorously. After infants are massaged and swaddled, typically they sleep for prolonged periods.

Although no data have been collected on infant massage as it is practiced in India, some infant massage therapists have attributed the precocious motor development of these infants to their daily massage. Infant massage therapists have made several claims based on anecdotal data. For example, benefits claimed include that the massage provides both stimulation and relaxation that helps respiration, circulation, digestion, and elimination (Grossman, 1985). Some have claimed that infants who are mas-

saged sleep more soundly and that the massage relieves gas and colic and helps the healing process during illness by easing congestion and pain (Eisenberg, 1985). Further, they have suggested that massage promotes parent–infant bonding and warm and positive relationships; reduces distress following painful procedures such as inoculations, pain from teething and constipation, and sleep problems; and makes parents "feel good" while they are massaging their infants. The infant massage therapy groups also have reported that infants with special needs (e.g., those who are blind and deaf or paralyzed, cerebral palsied, or premature) benefit from massage. Massage seems to help them become more aware of their bodies, among other benefits.

Infant massage has been discovered and researched much more recently in the Western world. In the United States there is a national organization of infant massage therapists with 4,000 members. There are also massage therapy schools in almost every major city in the United States, teaching parents how to massage their infants based primarily on the teachings of two massage therapists who trained in India (Amelia Auckett and Vimala Schneider McClure). The popularity of this form of intervention appears to derive in large part from the mutual enjoyment for infants and caregivers, although data are beginning to accumulate indicating that some significant effects are associated with therapeutic massage. Table 32.1 outlines the techniques used, which are repre-

TABLE 32.1. Infant Massage Instructions for Infants 3–24 Months Old

The massage procedure for older infants (3–24 months) provides more complexity and is a little more interesting than the young infant (0–3 months) procedure described in Table 32.2. Older infants like more variety, so this massage uses a greater variety of techniques. This massage lasts approximately 15 minutes and proceeds as follows:

A. Begin with the infant, face up.

1. *Face*—Strong stroking motions along both sides of the face.

2. *Legs*—Apply oil with gentle strokes from hip to foot. Long milking strokes toward ankle with hand wrapped around leg. Squeeze and twist hands as if you were wringing wet clothes from foot to hip. Massage foot using a thumb-over-thumb motion covering the entire bottom of the foot. Squeeze each toe gently and finish with a soothing pull. Use thumbs to press into bottom of baby's foot. Make small circles all over the top of the ankle and foot. Use long milking strokes with hands wrapped around leg toward the heart and back to the ankle. Roll baby's leg in between your hands from knee to ankle. Long gentle strokes toward ankle. Repeat above movements on other leg.

3. *Stomach*—Hand over hand in paddlewheel fashion, higher to lower on the stomach. Circular motion with fingers in a clockwise direction starting at appendix. Gently feel for gas bubbles and work them out in a clockwise direction.

4. *Chest*—Make strokes on both sides of the chest with the flats of fingers, going from middle to outward directions. Make cross strokes from center of chest and going over the shoulders. Then, make strokes on both sides of the chest simultaneously with flats of hands over chest to shoulders.

5. *Arms*—Apply oil with long gentle strokes from shoulders to hands. Use the same procedure as for legs.

6. *Face*—Apply strokes along both sides of the face using flats of fingers across the forehead. Make circular strokes over the temples and hinge of the jaw. Use flats of fingers over nose, cheeks, jaw, and chin. Lightly massage area behind ears and continue the circular movements to the rest of the scalp.

B. Turn *baby face down.*

1. Back—Gently apply oil in long downward strokes. Hands from side to side caress infant's back including infant's sides. Hand over hand from upper back to buttocks with flats of hands contoured to shape of back. Gentle strokes along length of back to the bottom of the feet. Circular motion with finger tips, from head to buttocks over the long muscles next to the spine. Do not rub over the spine. Lightly massage baby's neck and shoulders using soothing circular strokes.

---

sentative of most approaches in the United States.

In this chapter, I review preliminary research that suggests that massage is useful for facilitating infant development and, perhaps, promoting infant–parent relationships. Specifically, I review studies in low-risk infants and studies regarding infant regulatory problems (e.g., colic and sleep problems), preterm infants, drug-exposed infants, and HIV-exposed infants. Following that, I turn to preliminary data evaluating the effects of massage on the caregivers who administer it to infants. Many more questions than answers have been raised by what we have learned to date, but given that infant massage is being practiced as an adjunctive therapy by infant mental health clinicians (see Fava-Vizzielo, 1993), it seems that such emphasis is warranted while we await more clarity about the mechanisms through which the technique exerts its effects.

MASSAGING LOW-RISK INFANTS

In many parts of the world, as noted earlier, massage is considered a routine caregiving activity as opposed to an intervention for a particular problem. In these cultures, massage is practiced routinely because it is enjoyable and "good for babies," although often it is practiced without any explicit developmental goals in mind. Nevertheless, it seems reasonable to ask whether there are any demonstrable differences associated with massage when it is applied to low-risk populations of infants as opposed to those with specific problems. My group at the Touch Research Institutes, in a preliminary study, has studied massage in low-risk infants.

We randomly assigned 60 1-month-old low-risk infants to a massage group with oil and a massage group without oil. Massage had a soothing/calming influence on the infants, particularly when given with oil. The infants who received massage with oil were less active and showed fewer stress behaviors and head averting, and their saliva cortisol levels decreased more. In addition, vagal activity increased more following massage with oil versus massage without oil (Field, Schanberg, Davalos, & Malphurs, 1996). Still we know little about individual differences in responsiveness to massage in these infants.

MASSAGING HIGH-RISK INFANTS

The preliminary data regarding low-risk infants beg the question whether infant massage may be helpful with various groups of high-risk infants. We and others have conducted the following research evaluating potential benefits of massage as applied to several different groups of high-risk infants, including those with regulatory problems, those born preterm, those who were drug exposed, and those who were HIV exposed.

Massage and Regulatory Problems

Colic and sleep problems are the most frequently presenting problems to pediatricians by parents of infants in the United States. Although there are various approaches advocated for treatment of these problems, we were curious about the potential usefulness of massage as an intervention for infants with these common regulatory difficulties. In a recent study, we taught parents whose infants attended our university nursery school to massage their 3- to 6-month-old colicky infants for a 15-minute period prior to bedtime. The massaged infants became less irritable, fell asleep faster, experienced fewer night wakings, and spent more time in quiet, alert states during the daytime than did control (nonmassaged) infants (Field & Hernandez-Reif, 1999). Several parents who participated in this study and who encountered us years later, told us that we had "saved their marriages" by helping them to calm their infants and get them to sleep. Others expressed chagrin that as late as age 7 years, their child still needed a massage to go to sleep, as though it had become an addiction.

Massage and Preterm Infants

Most of the data on the effects of infant massage come from studies on preterm (premature) infants. During the last two decades, a number of studies have been conducted, most of them purporting to evaluate tactile/kinesthetic stimulation because of the negative connotations of the word "massage." A recent meta-analysis of data from 19 of these studies revealed that 72% of the massaged infants were positively affected (Ottenbacher et al., 1987). Most of them experienced greater weight gain and better performance on developmental assessments. Those studies that did not report significant weight gain had used a light stroking procedure. Their failure to demonstrate an effect may have been due to this technical difference. Our group has noted that babies do not like light touch, probably because it feels like tickling. The babies who gained weight had been given deeper pressure massage, thus stimulating both tactile and pressure receptors.

One of the studies used in this global analysis was conducted in our lab (Field et al., 1986). In that study, we gave massage therapy to preterm newborns for 45 minutes a day (in doses of three 15-minute periods) for 10 days. The infants averaged 9 weeks premature and 1,200 grams and were treated in intensive care for an average of 3 weeks before the study. The study began when they had graduated from the "Grower Nursery." At this time, their main agenda was to gain weight. Table 32.2 illustrates the massage therapy protocol we used.

The massaged infants in this study averaged

TABLE 32.2. Preterm Infant Massage

Massage therapy sessions are divided into three phases. For the first and last phase, the newborns are placed on their stomachs and gently stroked for 5, 1-minute periods (12 strokes at approximately 5 seconds per stroking motion) over each region in the following sequence:

1. From the top of the head to the neck.
2. From the neck across the shoulders.
3. From the upper back to the waist.
4. From the thigh to the foot to the thigh on both legs.
5. From the shoulder to the hand to the shoulder on both arms.

The Swedish-like massage was given because, as already noted, infants preferred some degree of pressure. During the middle phase the infants' arms and legs were moved back and forth much like bicycling motions while the infants lay on their backs.

47% greater weight gain (even though the groups consumed the same amount of formula). They were awake and active more of the time, even though we expected they would sleep more, and they were more alert and responsive to the examiner's face and voice, and showed more organized limb movements on the Brazelton Neonatal Behavioral Assessment Scale (BNBAS) (Brazelton, 1973). Finally, they were discharged from the hospital an average of 6 days sooner, saving approximately $3,000 per infant in hospital costs. The comparable cost savings today would be $10,000 per infant. If all 470,000 premature infants born each year in the United States were massaged, that figure potentially would translate into $4.7 billion in hospital costs savings per year. Further, it is possible that that figure could even double based on more recent data suggesting that the same weight gain can be achieved in 5 versus 10 days of massage therapy (Dieter & Field, 1999).

In another study on massage with premature infants, 33 mother–infant pairs were randomly assigned to one of three groups: control, talking, or interactive groups (White-Traut & Nelson, 1988). The interactive group received massage, talking, eye contact, and rocking. The treatments were given at specific times 24 hours after delivery. Before being discharged, the mothers and infants were observed during a feeding. The interactive group that received the massage was more responsive and easier to feed during their feeding interactions.

In still another study, preterm infants' biochemical and clinical responses to massage were assessed (Acolet et al., 1993). The 11 infants in the study were born 11 weeks prematurely, weighed approximately 2 pounds, and were hospitalized for 3 days. Blood samples were obtained for stress hormone (cortisol) levels 45 minutes before the start of massage and approximately 1 hour after the end of the massage. Cortisol levels decreased consistently after massage. There was also a slight decrease in skin temperature.

Replication studies have been conducted in Israel (Goldstein-Ferber, 1998) and the Philippines (Jinon, 1996). In the Philippines study (Jinon, 1996), which was an exact replication of the Field et al. (1986) methodology, the preterm infants who were massaged gained 45% more than the nonmassaged infants. In the Israeli study (Goldstein-Ferber, 1998), a 31 % greater weight gain was reported for the massaged versus control, preterm infants. In addition, the mothers who provided the massage

experienced a decrease in depression. The Philippine and the Israeli studies, respectively, approximated the weight gain data (47% and 31%) published a decade ago by Field et al. (1986) and Scafidi et al. (1990), respectively. Finally, a recent study by Deiter, Hernandez-Reif, and Field (1998) found that a 46% greater weight gain can be achieved in preterm infants following only 1 week of massage.

At the time we began our studies with preterm infants, colleagues at Duke University Medical Center were conducting similar studies on rat pups (Schanberg & Field, 1988). They removed rat pups from their mother to explore touch deprivation. Separation led to dramatic decreases in ornithine decarboxylase, an enzyme critical for protein synthesis. This decrease was noted in all body organs, including heart, liver, and all parts of the brain. Levels of ornithine decarboxylase returned to normal once mother rats were reunited with their pups and began to tongue lick them. The investigators were able to restore levels of the enzyme by simulating the tongue licking by stroking the rat pups with a paint brush dipped in water and briskly applied all over the body of the rat pup. The Duke team's more recent discovery of a growth gene that responds to touch suggests a strong genetic influence on the relationship between touch and growth, although the underlying mechanism remains unclear at this time (Schanberg, 1995).

This observation plus the results of a study in Sweden led us to some ideas about mechanisms that might explain the relationship between touch and weight gain (Uvnas-Moberg, Widston, Marchini, & Winberg, 1987). The Swedish study reported that stimulating the mouth of the human newborn (and the breast of the breastfeeding mother) led to an increase in food absorption hormones, such as gastrin and insulin. Therefore, it is plausible that massage therapy on several parts of the body might lead to an even greater increase in food absorption hormones, which in turn could explain the weight gain. Our later assays of insulin levels before, during, and after massage therapy suggested that they were significantly elevated in those preterm infants who received massage therapy versus those who did not (a 61% increase vs. a 4% decrease in insulin levels) (Field, Schanberg, Davalos, & Malphurs, 1997). Of course, future studies could assay the relative changes of several food absorption hormones and other vagally mediated changes, such as an increase in gastric motility.

Massage and Cocaine-Exposed Preterm Infants

Cocaine-exposed preterm infants also were included in the massage therapy protocol, initially merely because of their preterm status. We thought that they might benefit from the same type of massage three times a day for a 10-day period. Nevertheless, we did not know whether they would demonstrate the same kind of beneficial response as did non–drug-exposed preterm infants, and we decided to evaluate formally the efficacy of massage therapy for this group (Wheeden, Scafidi, Field, & Ironson, 1993). After treatment, the massaged, cocaine-exposed, preterm infants had fewer medical complications and less irritability; they had a 28% greater daily weight gain than infants not massaged, and they showed more mature motor activity.

Massage and HIV-Exposed Neonates

The worldwide epidemic of acquired immune deficiency syndrome (AIDS) has led to increasing numbers of babies being exposed to HIV prenatally. These infants are at risk for multiple reasons, and we decided to evaluate the efficacy of massage in improving the growth and development of HIV-exposed preterm newborns. Therefore, we taught the mothers how to massage their infants (Scafidi & Field, 1996). We predicted that this group of preterm infants would demonstrate improved weight gain as a result of the massage therapy, much as their non-HIV-exposed counterparts had benefited in our earlier study. Interestingly, we experienced an unusually high rate of compliance in this investigation (nearly 100%). This near-perfect compliance may have resulted from mothers feeling guilty about exposing their infants to HIV. In any case, after 2 weeks of massage therapy these infants showed greater weight gain, better performance on the social and motor items of the BNBAS, and fewer stress behaviors than control infants (Scafidi, Field, & Schanberg, 1993).

CONTEXTUAL CONSIDERATIONS: CAREGIVERS AS MASSAGE THERAPISTS

We are beginning to teach parents to provide massages to their infants routinely. Initially, we did this because it was advantageous to us for the infants to be massaged daily at no cost. Nevertheless, we began to notice what we believed to be beneficial effects on caregivers themselves of administering massage to their infants. Therefore, we have begun to examine effects of massage not only on infants but also on parents and other caregivers.

Depressed Mothers Massaging Their Infants

We have conducted a large number of investigations of infants of depressed mothers, and we were curious about the effects of massage on this group. In a study in which we taught depressed mothers to massage their infants, we found not only less distress behavior and disturbed sleep patterns in the infants but also improvements in mothers' moods and behaviors (Field, Grizzle, Scafidi, Abrams, & Richardson, 1996). In this study, we asked the depressed mothers to perform a 15-minute massage daily on their infants for 2 weeks. After the intervention, the infants were able to fall asleep faster, slept longer, and were less fussy.

During these interactions, the infants were positioned in an infant seat on a table face-to-face with their mothers. Video cameras, which were partially hidden, filmed the mother's face and torso and the infant's face and body. The videotapes were subsequently coded for the mother's and the infant's eye contact, facial expressions, and vocalizations. We found that mothers who had massaged their infants also interacted more favorably during the face-to-face interactions.

Fathers as Massage Therapists

Interest in fathers' involvement in massaging their infants appears to be growing. A film made for Australian television, in which U.S. fathers were shown giving their infants massage, was aired in Australia rather than in the United States because the producers wanted the fathers to be more involved in caregiving. Since the television broadcast, a study has been conducted on Australian fathers massaging their infants (Scholz & Samuels, 1992). In this study, Australian fathers with first-born babies were given a monthlong training program in a bathing massage technique to be used at bathtime. Based on data analyzed from a home observation conducted when the infants were 3 months old, the intervention fathers showed greater involvement with their infants. At this time, the intervention infants also greeted their fathers with more eye contact, smiling, vocalizing, and reaching responses and less avoidance behavior. This study did not explicitly consider effects of massaging their infants on fathers, but it is plausible that this instrumental task might be one that many fathers would find engaging.

Elderly Volunteers as Massage Therapists

Teaching elderly volunteers is another no-cost way to deliver massage therapy. In a recent study, elderly volunteers massaged infants and toddlers in a nursery school (Field, Hernandez-Reif, Quintino, Schanberg, & Kuhn, 1998). The study was designed to measure the massage therapy effects on the volunteer grandparents who were giving the massage. Elderly people themselves can experience failure to thrive because of touch deprivation (Campion, Berkman, & Fulmer, 1986). A survey indicates, for example, that failure to thrive and depression are fairly common among the elderly (Copeland et al., 1987). Depressive symptoms in the elderly are similar to those in younger persons (Gaylord & Zung, 1987). They can have negative mood states, poor concentration, feelings of hopelessness and worthlessness, and complaints of physical problems and memory impairments (Gaylord & Zung, 1987). In addition, they may experience frequent night wakings, increased stress hormone levels, and immune system problems (Post, 1982). Failure to thrive may develop, leading to decreased appetite and weight loss. Pet therapy (having and holding pets) has been shown to be effective with the elderly (Grossberg & Alf, 1985). The question is whether massage therapy also might be helpful, especially when the elderly are giving massages themselves.

In our elderly volunteer study, the "grandparent-aged" volunteers were randomly assigned to either give massages to infants (following the massage therapy protocol in Table 32.1) or to receive massage therapy themselves. At the end of the first month, the volunteers then received the opposite treatment to that received in the first month (either massaging the infants or being massaged themselves). These sessions were 15 minutes for the infant massage and 30 minutes for the elderly volunteer massage. The latter session was longer only because it takes longer to provide a full body table massage for

an adult. The infant and elderly massages occurred twice a week for 4 weeks.

After the baseline and end-of-study sessions the grandparent volunteers reported lower anxiety levels and fewer depression symptoms and an improved mood after both giving and receiving massage. Their stress hormone levels also decreased. After 1 month of giving or getting the therapy (the order of giving massages for 1 month was counterbalanced with getting massages for 1 month) their lifestyle improved, including having more social contacts, making fewer trips to the doctor's office, and drinking fewer cups of coffee. These changes may have helped to improve their sleep and their self-esteem. Somewhat surprising, these improvements were greater after 1 month of giving the infant massages than they were after 1 month of receiving their own massages. All this needs further exploration, but preliminary results are encouraging.

CONCLUSIONS

Infant massage has a long tradition in many parts of the world as a caregiving activity for young infants. Its popularity is beginning to spread to a greater number of Western countries. In these countries it is also beginning to be applied as a therapeutic technique for many high-risk infants. A preliminary but growing body of data support the efficacy of infant massage for enhancing the growth and development of infants with various high-risk conditions. Intriguing preliminary evidence suggests that beneficial effects for the caregivers who provide the massage also may accrue.

Several important questions remain to be determined by future research. First, is infant massage as effective at enhancing infants' primary caregiving relationships? Second, who responds more and who responds less to this approach? Third, how may this approach be usefully integrated into a comprehensive intervention approach? Answers to these questions will better enable infant mental health clinicians to determine when and for whom this technique is most appropriate.

ACKNOWLEDGMENT

Preparation of this chapter was supported in part by an NIMH Senior Research Scientist

Award (No. MH00331) and an NIMH Research Grant (No. MH46586) to Tiffany Field, and funds from Johnson and Johnson.

REFERENCES

Acolet, D., Giannakoulopoulos, X., Bond, C., Weg, W., Clow, A., & Glover, V. (1993). Changes in plasma cortisol and catecholamine concentrations in response to massage in preterm infants. *Archives of Disease in Childhood, 68,* 29–31.

Auckett, A. D. (1981). *Baby massage.* New York: Newmarket Press.

Brazelton, T. B. (1973). *Neonatal Behavior Assessment Scale.* London: Spastics International Medical Publications.

Campion, E., Berkman, B., & Fulmer, T. (1986). *Failure to thrive in the elderly.* Unpublished manuscript, Harvard Medical School.

Copeland, J. R. M., Dewey, M. E., Wood, N., Searle, R., Davidson, I. A., & McWilliams, C. (1987). Range of mental illness among the elderly in the community: Prevalence in Liverpool using the GMS–AGECAT package. *British Journal of Psychiatry, 150,* 815–823.

Dieter, J. & Field, T. (1999). *Preterm infants gain more weight after 5 days of massage therapy.* Manuscript under review.

Dieter, J., Hernandez–Reif, M., & Field, T. (1998, April). *Weight gain can increase in preterm infants following only one week of massage.* Paper presented to the International Conference on Infant Studies, Atlanta.

Eisenberg, D. (1985). *Encounters with Oi (exploring Chinese medicine).* New York: Norton.

Fava-Vizziello, G. (1993). Clinical use of infant massage in Italy. *The Signal, 1,* 5–8.

Field, T., Grizzle, N., Scafidi, F. Abrams, S., & Richardson, S. (1996). Massage therapy for infants of depressed mothers. *Infant Behavior and Development, 11,* 109–114.

Field, T., & Hernandez-Reif, M. (1999). *Sleep problems in infants decrease following massage therapy.* Manuscript under review.

Field, T., Hernandez-Reif, M., Quintino, O., Schanberg, S., & Kuhn, C. (1998). Elder retired volunteers benefit from giving massage therapy to infants. *Journal of Applied Gerontology, 17,* 229–239.

Field, T., Schanberg, S., Davalos, M., & Malphurs, J. E. (1996). Massage with oil has more positive effects on normal infants. *Pre- and Perinatal Psychology Journal, 11*(2), 75–80.

Field, T., Schanberg, S., Davalos, M., & Malphurs, J. E. (1997). Massage therapy effects on infants. *Pre- and Perinatal Psychology Journal, 12,* 73–78.

Field, T., Schanberg, S., Scafidi, F., Bower, C., Vega-Lahr, N., Garcia, R., Nystrom, J., & Kuhn, C. M. (1986). Tactile/kinesthetic stimulation effects on preterm neonates. *Pediatrics, 77,* 654–658.

Gaylord, S. A., & Zung, W. W. K. (1987). Affective disorders among the aging. In L. L. Carstensen & B. A. Edelstein (Eds.), *Handbook of clinical gerontology.* New York: Pergamon Books.

Goldstein–Ferber, S. (1998). *Massage in premature infants.* Paper presented at child development conference, Bar-Ilaon, Israel.

Grossberg, J. M., & Alf, E. F., Jr. (1985). Interaction with pet dogs: Effects on human cardiovascular response. *Journal of the Delta Society, 11,* 20–27.

Grossman, R. (1985). *The other medicine (an invitation to understanding and using them for health and healing).* Garden City, NJ: Doubleday.

Jinon, S. (1996). The effect of infant massage on growth of the preterm infant. In C. Yarbes-Almirante & M. De Luma (Eds.), *Increasing safe and successful pregnancy* (pp. 265–269). Netherlands: Elsevier Science.

McClure, V. (1989). *Infant massage: A handbook for loving parents.* New York: Bantam Books.

Ottenbacher, K. J., Muller, L., Brandt, D., Heintzelman, A., Hojem, P., & Sharpe, P. (1987). The effectiveness of tactile stimulation as a form of early intervention: A quantitative evaluation. *Journal of Developmental and Behavioral Pediatrics, 14,* 68–76.

Post, F. (1982). Functional disorder 11. Treatment and its relationship to causation. In R. Levy & F. Post (Eds.), *The psychiatry of late life* (pp. 28–39). London: Blackwell Scientific.

Scafidi, F., & Field, T. (1996). Massage therapy improves behavior in neonates born to HIV positive mothers. *Journal of Pediatric Psychology, 21,* 889–898.

Scafidi, F., Field, T., & Schanberg, S. M. (1993). Factors that predict which infants benefit most from massage therapy. *Journal of Developmental and Behavioral Pediatrics, 11,* 176–180.

Scafidi, F., Field, T., Schanberg, S., Bauer, C., Tucci, K., Roberts, J., Morrow, C., & Kuhn, C. M. (1990). Massage stimulates growth in preterm infants: A replication. *Infant Behavior and Development, 13,* 167–188.

Schanberg, S., (1995). The genetic basis for touch effects. In T. Field (Ed.), *Touch in early development* (pp. 67–79). Hillsdale, NJ: Erlbaum.

Schanberg, S., & Field, T. (1988). Maternal deprivation and supplemental stimulation. In T. Field, P. McCabe, & N. Schneiderman (Eds.), *Stress and coping across development* (pp. 3–25). Hillsdale, NJ: Erlbaum.

Scholz, K., & Samuels, C. (1992). Neonatal bathing and massage intervention with fathers, behavioral effects 12 weeks after birth of the first baby: The Sunraysia Australia Intervention Project. *International Journal of Behavioral Development, 15,* 67–81.

Uvnas-Moberg, K., Widston, A. M., Marchini, G., & Winberg, J. (1987). Release of GI hormones in mother and infant by sensory stimulation. *Acta Paediatrica Scandinavica, 76,* 851–860.

Wheeden, A., Scafidi, F., Field, T., & Ironson, G. (1993). Massage effects on cocaine-exposed preterm neonates. *Journal of developmental and Behavioral Pediatrics, 14,* 318–322.

White-Traut, R., & Nelson, M. (1988). Maternally administered tactile, auditory, visual and vestibular stimulation: Relationship to later interactions between mothers and premature infants. *Research in Nursing and Health, 11,* 31–39.

VI

APPLICATIONS OF INFANT MENTAL HEALTH

❖

Knowledge about infant development and psychopathology is vital to determining the kind of world we want for infants and their families. Nevertheless, this presents challenging dilemmas for the field of infant mental health about how to integrate facts and inferences in the service of important questions. Translating research findings into social policy pits the caution, skepticism, and circumspection of science against the urgency of pressing problems and the hyperbole of political arenas. This creates many opportunities for misunderstanding, confusion, or distortion.

Contemporary examples of conflicting perspectives of science and advocacy concern the developmental sequella of prenatal cocaine exposure (see Lester, Boukydis, and Twomey, Chapter 9, this volume) and the effects of early experience and brain development (Nelson & Bosquet, Chapter 3, this volume). In each case, the rush to embrace advocacy positions has led to the selection of specific facts that support a particular position rather than a painstaking scrutiny of the whole. On the one hand, research findings about these vitally important topics are of little use until we can translate them into the improved understanding of how to allocate our resources to improve the lives of infants and families. On the other hand, the space between facts and inferences provides fertile ground for unintended consequences. Thus, we are challenged simultaneously to learn as many of the facts about infant development as we can but also to exert care in deriving conclusions about their meaning.

In Chapter 33, Shonkoff, Lippitt, and Cavanaugh provide an overview of social policy issues in the United States that are relevant for infant mental health. They note the increasing attention that "the early years" are receiving in policy circles, and they underscore the importance of responsible advocacy. Along these lines, Shonkoff (in press) has distinguished recently among proven facts, reasonable inferences, and irresponsible assertions. The translation of scientific findings about development into policy arenas is delicate work that requires nothing short of our best efforts.

Chapter 34 illustrates this dilemma well by addressing the important social concern of child care and infant development. Hungerford, Brownell, and Campbell point out that child care varies enormously in quality and does not operate independently of family and child characteristics. They conclude by pointing to emerging areas of research on the effects of child care, and they emphasize the need for longitudinal and process-oriented research to understand how child-care experiences exert their influences on young children's' development.

Kaplan and Pruett consider the intricacies of divorce as a developmental context for young children in Chapter 35. They point out that decision makers such as judges are likely to turn to clinicians for advice regarding what is in young children's best interests in these situations. They caution about distinguishing between personal, intuitive opinions and those supported by research. The specificity of the questions asked sometimes renders what research is available less useful, further complicating the task of providing information to decision makers. They conclude by reminding us of diverse outcomes in young children whose parents divorce, and they reassert basic principles of child development as essential to the well-being of infants and toddlers in these situations.

In the concluding chapter of the volume, Zeanah, Larrieu, and Zeanah consider a variety of issues relevant for training in infant mental health. Although not a social policy issue per se, training is another example of the application of knowledge about infant mental health to other arenas. The authors suggest that the challenges of training in infant mental health derive from its multidisciplinary nature, developmental orientation, multigenerational focus, and emphasis on prevention. Infant mental health is a specialized body of knowledge relevant to trainees and others from a variety of different professions. As a result, the authors suggest that a core body of knowledge about infant mental health may be relevant to all disciplines but that many aspects of the field will be more or less relevant depending upon an individual's professional discipline and context. They conclude by noting an apparent increase in the number and types of programs available for training in infant mental health.

REFERENCE

Shonkoff, J. (in press). Science, policy and practice: Three cultures in search of a shared mission. *Child Development.*

33

Early Childhood Policy: Implications for Infant Mental Health

❖

JACK P. SHONKOFF
JOHN A. LIPPITT
DOREEN A. CAVANAUGH

Although there is no specific infant mental health policy in the United States, many social policies have an impact on the mental health of young children. Such policies include those that affect infant and toddler general health and well-being, as well as those that have a broader impact on families and the contexts in which they live, thereby influencing the care, protection, and nurturance that young children receive (Shonkoff & Meisels, 2000).

Infant mental health is inseparable from infant physical health and early childhood development. Each is shaped by biologically driven maturation, the influence of individual experience, and inextricably linked transactions between the two. At the most proximal level of analysis, the mental health and development of young children are influenced by the nature of their relationships with key caregivers, generally beginning with their mothers (Crockenberg & Leerkes, Chapter 4, this volume; Emde & Robinson, 2000; Lewis, Chapter 5, this volume; Osofsky & Thompson, 2000; Sameroff, Chapter 1, this volume). At more distal levels, child well-being is affected by a range of factors that have an impact on the family unit (including its social network, economic circumstances, and physical living conditions), as well as by broader contextual variables that characterize the community and the larger society (Bronfenbrenner, 1986; Bronfenbrenner & Ceci, 1994; Garbarino & Ganzel, 2000; Jacobs, 1994; Sameroff & Fiese, 2000; Schorr, 1997).

Public policy, as it addresses the needs of young children in the United States, is influenced by a host of cultural, political, economic, and historical forces. These forces include such complex issues as contrasting perspectives on the scope and scale of public responsibility for children, the appropriateness of nonparental care for infants, and the value of targeted versus universal service programs (Grubb & Lazerson, 1982; Jacobs, 1994; Meisels & Shonkoff, 2000). Furthermore, the growing racial and ethnic diversity of U.S. families and the multiplicity of cultural differences they bring to child rearing present increasing challenges for the policymaking process (Garcia Coll et al., 1996; Garcia Coll & Magnuson, 2000). This chapter provides a broad overview of these influences and challenges, examines selected policies and programs in the United States, and concludes with comments about future policy directions.

NATURE AND CONTEXT OF CHILD AND FAMILY POLICY

Many of the policies that have an impact on infant mental health are not focused solely on young children, let alone on their mental health. Public policies that affect the well-being of children and families are reflected in both formal governmental actions (such as laws) and strategies designed to affect their implementation (such as regulations and their enforcement by the public bureaucracy). Although this chapter focuses primarily on federal policies, there has been a recent trend toward "devolving" greater discretion and policymaking to the state and local levels—for example, in welfare reform and publicly funded health care (Gold, 1998). It is important to note that other domains (e.g., corporate policies) also have a significant impact. For example, individual workplace policies that affect the number, flexibility, and schedule of work hours, as well as the availability of parental leave for the birth or illness of a child, have important influences on parenting, family life, and child well-being. Employer subsidies for child care and health insurance premiums, including the availability of family medical coverage, have a similar impact.

Policies that affect child health and well-being can be grouped into three categories. The first, *explicit policies*, are those directed intentionally toward families and children. Examples include protective services for children who are abused and tax breaks for families with dependent children. The second, *implicit policies*, are those that affect families and children indirectly and/or unintentionally. These include minimum wage laws, the home mortgage interest deduction, and public transportation policy. The third, *policies of omission*, include those areas in which the absence of a decision or action leads to policy by default. The lack of federal child care standards and the failure to establish a national health care system that guarantees universal access are examples of this third category (Jacobs & Davies, 1994).

Despite the formalization of many public policies in the law, gaps often emerge between the legally mandated policy and the actual experience of those for whom it was developed. In the area of health care, for example, an estimated 4.7 million children under 19 years of age who are eligible for Medicaid remain uninsured (Selden, Banthin, & Cohen, 1998). In the area of child protective services, legislation originally passed to authorize the provision of increased support for "high risk" families in order to decrease out-of-home placements has been replaced by a law with broader treatment mandates but little increase in funding. Thus, spending levels and the management of service delivery are key factors that influence the actual implementation and ultimate impact of many public policies (Schorr, 1997).

Several aspects of society and the political decision-making process set the stage for the formulation of public policies. These factors focus selective attention on certain problems, limit the range of potential solutions that are considered, and channel the decision-making process itself (Grubb & Lazerson, 1982; Jacobs, 1994). Issues appear on the agenda when they gain policymakers' attention, which is typically (but not always) driven by the level of public interest. Solutions are developed with variable levels of input from "experts," and the politics of decision making is influenced by both the process of deliberation and the cultural and historical context that frames the decision options (Kingdon, 1995).

The fundamental problem-driven nature of policymaking means that it tends to be reactive (i.e., responsive to crises and dramatic public events). The political nature of decision making means that it involves negotiation and compromise and often leads to an end result that does not fully satisfy any of the parties involved (Kingdon, 1995). The values and attitudes that individuals and groups hold about each other and about their own and "other people's children," as well as their differential views of the role of government, all affect the development of child and family policy. Although there have been major changes in recent decades in the role and structure of the family, the evolution of social policies is generally a constrained process that proceeds slowly. The significant value conflicts and policy inconsistencies that characterize our approach to the work force participation of mothers and the care of very young children are striking examples of this reality (Davies, 1994; Grubb & Lazerson, 1982; Jacobs, 1994).

Although the family is still identified as the basic unit in our society, from both an economic and socialization perspective, it is no longer the self-sufficient, self-determining entity it was 150 years ago (Hernandez, 1997). In contrast, modern societies have been characterized by the growing impact of the corporate and public sectors on the nature of work and community life and, therefore, on family functioning, child rearing, and child health and well-being (Davies, 1994; Grubb & Lazerson, 1982). Notwithstanding these dramatic changes in public influences on family life, mainstream culture in the United States clings to the traditional belief that the family is (or should be) a private, self-sufficient entity. Consequently, child rearing is viewed by many as a personal affair anchored to a strong ethos of individual accountability. Public responsibility for the care and protection of children is deemed appropriate only in highly selected situations, thereby limiting the circumstances, scope, and scale of formal public intervention (Grubb & Lazerson, 1982; Jacobs, 1994).

Nonvoluntary public involvement in family life (whether by removing a child from the home or mandating specific social services) is seen as an "intrusion" and a last resort. It is viewed as appropriate only when a family is judged to have failed in its basic child-rearing responsibilities, a judgment that is often complicated by bias related to race, ethnicity, class, gender, and/or sexual orientation. Thus, intervention in the life of a family often carries a strong stigma of inadequacy. Notwithstanding the consistent popular support for services needed by "deserving" families (e.g., parents of children with developmental disabilities), parents who are labeled as "failures" (e.g., poor, teenage mothers) are increasingly likely to be viewed as "undeserving" of public benefits. In turn, their young children become indirect victims of public neglect, as they are relegated to the status of "other people's children" (Grubb & Lazerson, 1982).

This juxtaposition of "deserving" children and "undeserving" parent(s) presents a policy-making conundrum given the contemporary understanding of ecological theory as a model for human development and the importance of a family-centered approach to best serve the needs of children. Welfare reform in the late 1990s provides a compelling example of this paradox in its focus on changing the behavior of parents (mainly mothers) through work requirements, strict time limits, and other sanctions, with little consideration for the potential adverse impact of this fundamental policy change on the well-being of their children (Schorr, 1997). When complicated by discrimination based on race, ethnicity, culture, language, or family structure and composition, the challenges for policymaking and service delivery are intensified.

The typical disregard for a broad contextual approach to the needs of children leads to social policies that are limited in scope and that focus on specific concerns in targeted populations. The consequence for society is a tendency for policies to emphasize the treatment and/or remediation of problems rather than health promotion and the prevention of illness, disability, and maladaption. Perhaps most important, child policies rarely address the underlying structural inequalities (e.g., poverty, discrimination, and social exclusion) that have a significant adverse impact on families and serve as important risk factors for compromised infant mental health (Grubb & Lazerson, 1982).

This limited, treatment-oriented philosophy is based on an implicit assumption that all a child's needs can be met by his or her parents, and that most families can fulfill those needs without public support. In contrast to this myth of family self-sufficiency, middle- and upper-income families rely on a wide variety of supportive services, some of which they purchase and some of which they secure through informal networks. In the absence of public subsidies, poor families have limited access to comparable supports, despite their equal or greater needs (Grubb & Lazerson, 1982; Halpern, 1993).

Another serious impediment to unified child and family policies is that advocates often focus on narrow issues and frequently compete against each other for attention and resources (State Legislative Leaders Foundation, 1995). The consequence of such battles is a diffuse collection of policies and programs that are fragmented and underfunded. Competition for resources for child care, for example, often engages advocates representing the interests of a broad range of socioeconomic and age constituencies. Should subsidies be provided preferentially for those receiving or leaving welfare, for low-income working families, or for the middle class? Are subsidies needed most for infants and toddlers, for preschoolers, or for school-age children? These conflicting demands result in multiple funding streams for child care, serving different target populations, without a coherent, integrated policy.

Finally, power and political processes ultimately shape public programs in many ways. Generally speaking, parents with greater political capital (i.e., those who are white and of high socioeconomic status) are better able to influence public institutions to serve their needs. Consequently, policies designed (at least in part) to compensate for structural inequalities in opportunities for children frequently fail to achieve their goal (Grubb & Lazerson, 1982). The progressive income tax structure in the United States, for example, includes numerous provisions that primarily benefit middle- and upper-income families (e.g., the home mortgage interest deduction and the dependent care tax credit), thereby undermining its actual progressivity.

The absence of a broad-based policy agenda on behalf of all children and families comparable to that advanced by advocates for the elderly is a critical problem. In part, this is related to the broad scope of policies that potentially affect families and the value-driven nature of conflicting views on private and public responsibility for children. The increasing politicization of "family values," however, has further complicated this dilemma by producing a policymaking environment in which ideology often eclipses the influence of scientific knowledge and professional expertise.

POLICIES AND POPULATIONS

A wide variety of policies and programs affect the mental health of young children (Knitzer, 1996; Knitzer, 2000). The specific federal policies and programs discussed in this chapter are selected examples from among many others. Those that address universal needs are presented first, followed by policies that target progressively smaller subsets of the early childhood population. For each policy, we describe relevant mental health issues for young children, identify potential policy options, and outline the current U.S. policy response.

Universal Needs

All infants and toddlers need care, protection, and nurturance within an environment that is supportive of their physical, cognitive, social, and emotional development. To a considerable extent, these needs are viewed within "mainstream" U.S. culture as private family responsibilities. It is generally acknowledged, however, that even the most self-sufficient family requires health care and basic social support.

Health Care

Health care is a universal need that requires access to professional services. Payment or insurance for these services can be provided by the public sector, offered as a fringe benefit by employers, or left up to individuals. Thus, child health care in the United States is a shared responsibility of both the private and public sectors. Government policy affects health care delivery through publicly provided programs as well as through policies that affect the availability, affordability, and nature of both public and private insurance (Klerman, 1996).

The largest public investment in children's health care in the nation is Medicaid (Title XIX of the Social Security Act). In 1995, 17.5 million children under age 18 were covered by Medicaid, including one of every three infants in the United States. As a result of ongoing expansions, Medicaid has moved from covering only children of the poor and unemployed to providing health care for increasing numbers of children living in low-income working families, as well as those with developmental disabilities and other special health care needs (who qualify through the Supplemental Security Income [SSI] program) (Kaiser Commission on the Future of Medicaid, 1997). Nevertheless, Selden et al. (1998) estimate that despite their eligibility for Medicaid, 4.7 million children under 19 years of age were uninsured in 1996, representing approximately 40% of the uninsured children in the United States.

Since 1967, the Early and Periodic Screening, Diagnosis, and Treatment (EPSDT) Program has been the component of Medicaid with the greatest potential for prevention and early detection of infant and toddler problems. In fact, it represents the only attempt in the United States to provide a right to comprehensive child health services nationwide (Sardell & Johnson, 1998). EPSDT requires early and periodic medical, dental, vision, and developmental screening, diagnosis, and treatment of all Medicaid-covered children. However, despite credible research that has identified a range of preventable problems (Sardell & Johnson, 1998), implementation of the EPSDT benefit across the states has been, and remains, uneven. The Omnibus Budget Reconciliation Act of 1989 amended EPSDT to require that states provide reimbursement not only for screening, but also for diagnostic and treatment services determined (as the result of a screen) to be necessary to correct or ameliorate a physical or mental condition (Fox, McManus, Almeida, & Lesser, 1997; Kamis-Gould, Hadley, & Markel-Fox, 1994). In spite of its promise, however, the success of EPSDT remains limited, with participation rates of roughly 25–35% of eligible children nationally (Sardell & Johnson, 1998).

One of the newest pieces of child health legislation, the Children's Health Insurance Program (CHIP) (Title XXI of the Social Security Act), was enacted in 1997 to address further the problem of uninsured children. This legislation (Public Law No. 105–33) entitles states to federal allotments for health insurance targeted to low-income children who are ineligible for other coverage, including Medicaid (Rosenbaum, Johnson, Sonosky, Markus, & DeGraw, 1998). Additional requirements of the CHIP legislation include outreach and enrollment initiatives, public involvement in the design and implementation of the state plan, and both annual and long-term assessments of program operation and progress toward reducing the number of uninsured children (Reiss, 1998; Rosenbaum et al., 1998; Ullman, Bruen, & Holahan, 1998).

Regardless of funding source, one of the most sweeping changes in the financing and delivery of health care over the past decade has been the shift to a managed care model. To control escalating costs, managed care strategies were first introduced by private insurers. Their early success in cost containment prompted the introduction of managed care into the Medicaid program through demonstrations and waivers granted to individual states. Little research has been conducted on the impact of these changes on the health of infants and toddlers, but managed care constraints could result in either of two scenarios: reduced screening and less early treatment of developmental problems or expansion of prevention and early intervention services as a strategy designed to minimize the need for more costly services later. Further research clearly is needed on the effect of managed care on both the physical and mental health of infants and toddlers (Office of Inspector General, 1997; Rosenbach & Gavin, 1998).

Another important federal policy domain relates to publicly supported health care for children and families that goes beyond the financing of personal medical services. The longest-standing programs, administered by the Maternal and Child Health Bureau in the Health Resources and Services Administration of the U.S. Public Health Service, were enacted in 1935 as Title V of the Social Security Act. These federal programs direct funds to the states through block grants and support a vital framework within which each state has built and maintained its system of care for children and pregnant women. Early childhood goals and activities supported by the Maternal and Child Health Block Grant include ensuring access to health care for all mothers and children, comprehensive medical care for pregnancy and childbirth, and preventive and primary care services; meeting the nutritional and developmental needs of mothers, children, and families; and immunization programs, adolescent pregnancy prevention programs, injury and violence prevention programs, national standards for prenatal care, and healthy and safe child care. One-third of all pregnant women in 1997 received health services through this block grant, and preventive and primary care services were provided to nearly 8 million infants, children, and adolescents (Rani, 1997). The block grant language also requires that a minimum of 30% of the funds be used to support programs for children with special health care needs.

The Healthy Start program also is administered by the Maternal and Child Health Bureau. With roots in both prenatal nursing and public health research, its theoretical underpinning is derived from data that demonstrate the importance of successful mother–infant attachment for preventing future parenting disturbances. This initiative also funds the development of services and strategies to reduce infant mortality in targeted high-risk communities. Program components may include prenatal screening for medical and psychosocial risk, home visiting, spousal abuse services, respite and child care, substance abuse counseling, housing assistance, medical services, and child and family support services (Breakey & Pratt, 1991; Pecora, Whittaker, Maluccio, Barth, & Plotnick, 1992).

Family Support

Beyond the provision of health care by trained professionals, all young children need the basic care and nurturance that is provided by the family itself. However, few, if any, families meet the day-to-day demands of child rearing without the support of others. Most are able to rely on a wide range of informal social networks; a subset of the population requires public-sector services to meet their basic needs.

The Carnegie report (Carnegie Corporation of New York, 1994) charged that despite our extensive knowledge about the importance of the first 3 years of life and about the requirements for optimal development in this period, the care and nurturance of young children are deteriorating. The report called for integrated action in four areas: promoting responsible parenting, guaranteeing the availability of quality child care, ensuring basic health and safety, and mobilizing community support for families and their young children.

Although there is no single public policy that ensures the provision of family support, there has been a proliferation of community-based programs that address this critical need. The underlying concepts that have driven the growth of the family support movement include integrated service delivery, universal availability, voluntary participation, empowerment of parents in service planning and delivery, building on families' strengths, focusing on prevention, and ensuring that services are delivered in a culturally and linguistically appropriate manner (Adams & Krauth, 1994; Barnes, Goodson, & Layzer, 1995; Kagan, 1996; Venner et al., 1995; Weissbourd & Kagan, 1989).

Family support programs in the United States are not uniform in either their services or their delivery mode. They vary considerably in their auspices and funding sources, and generally are not comprehensive in their nature. Indeed, their focus typically has been on services for targeted, high-risk populations rather than on universal, voluntary support (Kamerman & Kahn, 1995).

In recent years, home visiting has received growing attention as an effective approach to providing family support. As a service delivery strategy rather than a uniformly defined, specific program, home-visiting services typically provide developmental and health screening, service referral, parenting education, and/or general social support (Powell, 1993; Schorr, 1997). Home visits typically target families of newborns or those who are expecting their first child and may be conducted by a professional (often a nurse) or a paraprofessional. Home visiting offers the opportunity to observe a parent and child in their natural environment, which facilitates both greater understanding of their needs and the capacity to better tailor individual services. It also avoids the requirement that a family come to the service provider, therefore reaching those who might otherwise fail to obtain assistance (Gomby, Larson, Lewit, &

Behrman, 1993). In 1991, the U.S. Advisory Board on Child Abuse and Neglect recommended a federal policy of universal home visiting (Krugman, 1993), and the Carnegie report called for home-visiting services on a voluntary basis for all first-time parents (Carnegie Corporation of New York, 1994).

The diversity among home visitation and family support programs and among the families they serve, makes these services difficult to evaluate. Nevertheless, several studies have demonstrated multiple benefits, including improved child development and health outcomes, reductions in preterm or low-birthweight births, increased use of preventive health services, reductions in reported child abuse and neglect, improved interaction between parents and children, reduced rates of subsequent pregnancy, and improved maternal education and employment (Beckwith, Chapter 28, this volume; Duggan et al., 1999; Olds et al., 1999; Wagner & Clayton, 1999). In general, benefits appear to be most significant for families and children with the greatest needs and when a broad range of child and family issues is addressed (Barnes et al., 1995; Barnett, 1993; Olds & Kitzman, 1993; Ramey & Ramey, 1993). However, a recent review of the results of evaluations of six home visiting models illustrated the overall modest level of program effects and underscored the need for realistic expectations regarding how much impact a limited intervention can have in the face of substantial social and economic vulnerability (Gomby, Culross, & Behrman, 1999).

Widespread Needs

Some service needs of young children and their families, although not universal, are relevant to a large proportion of the population. Nonparental child care is an example of such a need.

Child Care

The care of children in the infant and toddler years traditionally has been a family (and especially a maternal) responsibility. Over the past three decades, however, the work-force participation of mothers of children under age 3 in the United States has grown from 27% in 1970 to 42% in 1980 to over 50% in the 1990s. With this increase in maternal employment, more than one-quarter of children under 3 years of age now receive out-of-home care from nonrelatives. Of these, roughly one-third are in childcare centers and two-thirds are cared for in a home setting (i.e., family child care) (Kamerman & Kahn, 1995).

As the influence of early relationships on infant–toddler development has become better understood, the need for public policies to address the care of young children has received increased attention, particularly with respect to the impact of nonparental care on mental health and maternal attachment behaviors (Barnett, 1995; Crockenberg & Leerkes, Chapter 4, this volume; Kagan & Neuman, 2000; Zeanah & Boris, Chapter 22, this volume; Zeanah, Larrieu, Heller, & Valliere, Chapter 13, this volume; Zigler & Gilman, 1996). Nevertheless, the growing reliance on nonparental care for infants and toddlers has been accompanied by a slow recognition of the public responsibility to ensure the affordability, accessibility, and quality of that care (Kamerman & Kahn, 1995). For many families, the cost (which can be more than $12,000 annually for infant care in some metropolitan areas, Stoney & Greenberg, 1996) is prohibitive, and public subsidies do not approach the level necessary to make it affordable. Moreover, the quality of less expensive care for infants and toddlers may actually be harmful to their development and mental health (Frede, 1995; Helburn & Culkin, 1995; Hofferth, Brayfield, Deich, & Holcomb, 1991; Hungerford, Brownell, & Campbell, Chapter 34, this volume).

Greater attention has been focused on the child-care issue by changes in both state and federal welfare laws in the late 1990s, which were based on the premise that public assistance for low-income mothers (with limited exceptions) should be linked to mandated work and time-limited benefits. This premise represented a fundamental change in direct contradiction to the policies of the preceding 60 years (established under the provisions of the Social Security Act's Aid to Dependent Children and its successor, Aid to Families with Dependent Children [AFDC]), which were based on the belief that the health and well-being of young children were best served by being cared for at home by their mothers. Thus, the mandates for maternal employment under the new welfare laws have underscored the need for child care and highlighted the public responsibility to make quality care affordable through subsidies for low-income working parents.

Two policy options are available to address the child care needs of low-income families with young children. The public sector can subsidize nonparental care, or policies can make it more viable financially and acceptable socially for a parent to forego working and stay home to care for his or her children. The policy response in the United States, with respect to both options, has been dramatically weak in comparison to other industrialized countries. U.S. child care policies typically offer targeted, means-tested subsidies, in contrast to the universal financial supports commonly available in most European countries (Kamerman, 2000; Kamerman & Kahn, 1995). Furthermore, when child care is subsidized publicly in the United States, the goal is often to provide inexpensive care to maximize the number of parents who can work, rather than to provide high-quality care that enhances the health and development of children. Although standards do exist for some early childhood programs (e.g., Head Start), there are no universal federal standards for child care (Zigler, 1997). Where standards do exist at the state level, they vary markedly across the country (Hungerford, Brownell, & Campbell, Chapter 34, this volume).

In 1998, the federal government spent $8 billion on child care, allocated through 22 separate programs funded by multiple agencies (not including other programs in which child care was a minor component). Over three-quarters of these funds are distributed through three programs: the Dependent Care Tax Credit (which is of no value to low income families who do not owe taxes), the Child Care and Development Block Grant (which largely benefits those on or leaving welfare), and a portion of the Social Services Block Grant (which benefits low- and moderate-income working families) (Committee on Ways and Means, 1998; Kamerman & Kahn, 1995; Office of the Assistant Secretary for Planning and Evaluation, 1998). Taking into account the widely varying levels of support provided by state and local governments, it is estimated that parents pay 70–75% of the costs of preschool child care (Stoney & Greenberg, 1996).

Public policies that support parents who stay at home and care for their young children are even less extensive in the United States than are those that support nonparental child care. Although there is broad consensus that parenting time is critical to the mental health and development of infants and toddlers, conflict persists about whether the protection of parenting time is an individual, employer, or public responsibility. There is deep reluctance in the United States to enact laws requiring the type of paid, job-protected leave that is common in most European countries (Kamerman, 2000; Kamerman & Kahn, 1995; Zigler, 1997). This is reflected in the relatively weak provisions of the Family and Medical Leave Act (FMLA) of 1993, which provides for only 12 weeks of unpaid, job-protected leave for workers in companies with over 50 employees, after they have worked at that company for at least 1 year and for 1,250 hours in the previous 12 months (Frank & Zigler, 1996). Under these criteria, only 55% of the work force are eligible for this modest benefit. Moreover, the unpaid nature of the mandated leave effectively restricts its impact to those who can afford to give up 3 months of income. Consequently, early evaluations of the FMLA indicate that only 1.2% of all employees have taken an "FMLA leave," while 16.8% of all employees have taken some type of family or medical leave. Approximately 25% of leaves are taken by parents to care for a child at birth, adoption, or during a serious illness (Commission on Family and Medical Leave, 1995). Prior to 1993, federal parental leave policy was based on requiring short-term disability insurance, when available, to cover pregnant and postpartum women (Gomby et al., 1996).

Finally, greater attention has begun to focus on fathers and their impact on infant mental health and early childhood development (Lamb, 1997). The social and emotional development of boys who grow up without fathers has been a particular area of increased research interest (Pruett, 1997). Concurrently, incentives for establishing paternity and enhanced attention to collecting child support payments have been an area of growing concern to policymakers within the context of welfare reform (Garfinkel, McLanahan, Meyer, & Seltzer, 1998).

Specialized Needs

Certain subgroups of the general population of infants and toddlers have specialized needs. Three are discussed here as illustrative examples: (1) children experiencing significant economic hardship and social disorganization, (2) children with special health care needs, and (3) children who have been abused.

Children Experiencing Significant Economic Hardship and Social Disorganization

Extensive research has shown that a combination of risk factors better explains mental health problems and developmental disorders in young children than does any single variable (Halpern, 1993; Sameroff, Seifer, Barocas, Zax, & Greenspan, 1987; Upshur, 1990). The concurrence of significant economic hardship and social disorganization puts infants and toddlers at particular risk. Although the federal poverty line ($12,500 for a family of three in 1998) is the standard definition of poverty, this income level is well below what would be conducive to the healthy development and well-being of young children (Pearce & Brooks, 1998).

A family that lives in poverty generally is preoccupied with the basic subsistence challenges of day-to-day survival. Under such circumstances, parent–child interactions frequently are affected by a drain on parent time and energy that can have a significant adverse impact on a child's mental health. Excessive levels of family stress, an increased incidence of maternal depression and/or parental substance abuse, a higher likelihood of violence in the home and the community, and an elevated risk of child abuse and neglect all present an increased threat to the mental health of children living in poverty (Duncan & Brooks-Gunn, 1997; McLoyd, 1990). The likelihood of reduced access to basic health care and mental health services, as well as to quality child care, further underscores the vulnerability of such children (Aber, Jones, & Cohen, Chapter 6, this volume).

The increase in risk factors experienced by children living in poverty can be addressed through a variety of policies that provide both financial and social supports. U.S. public policies that provide financial support can be grouped into three categories: (1) direct financial benefits, (2) income tax code benefits, and (3) minimum wage laws.

Direct financial benefits consist of cash welfare payments and a variety of noncash benefits, including Medicaid (or other health care support) and a host of subsidies for food, housing, and child care. Food subsidies are provided primarily through two federal programs: the Food Stamp Program, which provides subsidies for low income households generally, and the Special Supplemental Nutrition Program for

Women, Infants, and Children (WIC), which provides nutritional screening and food assistance for pregnant and postpartum women and their children up to age 5 (Committee on Ways and Means, 1998).

In the late 1990s, changes in cash welfare policies occurred at both the federal and state levels. The major federal law, the Personal Responsibility and Work Opportunity Reconciliation Act of 1996 (PRWORA), represented a fundamental change in child and family policy, as it eliminated the open-ended entitlement to welfare payments for families with dependent children, dramatically restructured federal subsidies for child care, tightened eligibility criteria for child nutrition subsidies, increased the emphasis on child support by noncustodial parents, and restricted children's eligibility for SSI (Committee on Ways and Means, 1996).

As an alternative to AFDC, PRWORA created Temporary Assistance to Needy Families (TANF). TANF provided the states with block grants and greater decision-making flexibility, but it limited funds, mandated work requirements for all recipients after 2 years on welfare, and imposed a 5-year limit on the collection of benefits. TANF also encouraged reductions in births to teenagers and unwed mothers and provided incentives for the establishment of paternity. Although single parents of children under 1 year of age and those who cannot find child care for a child under age 6 cannot have their cash benefits reduced for failure to work, they are still bound by the overall time limit (Administration for Children and Families, 1998d; Office of the Assistant Secretary for Planning and Evaluation, 1998; Committee on Ways and Means, 1996). Most of the political motivation that led to these dramatic welfare changes was focused on the adult recipients, with little consideration given to the potential adverse effects on their children (Schorr, 1997). Although the full impact of the new law is not yet known, the economic effects on families as parents leave welfare for work are of great concern, given the likelihood of low wages and the potential loss of other public benefits (such as health care and child-care subsidies) that may not be replaced by employee benefits.

In addition to the direct financial benefits of welfare programs, three major income tax code benefits are available to help poor families: (1) the earned income tax credit (EITC), (2) the dependent care tax credit (DCTC), and (3) the dependent exemption.

The EITC is a refundable tax credit (i.e., a refund is sent if the credit is greater than the taxes owed) that is targeted at poor, working families with children. Although the amounts are modest and are phased out at income levels at which a family is still struggling financially, the $27 billion in benefits (in 1998) is significant. The DCTC and the dependent exemption provide additional support of a few hundred dollars per family annually, although the benefits accrue mainly to middle- and high-income families (Committee on Ways and Means, 1998).

The federal minimum wage ($5.15 per hour in 1998) is another source of support for poor, working families. Although the minimum wage establishes a floor for what a working parent earns, it is not sufficient to lift a single-parent family above the poverty line, even with full-time, year-round work. Furthermore, it does not put a two-working-parents family at an income level that is conducive to the healthy development and well-being of a young child, particularly in the absence of public or private subsidies for child care and health insurance (Pearce & Brooks, 1998).

Finally, the adverse effects of significant poverty and social disorganization on families and young children also can be attacked through the delivery of direct services (Halpern, 2000; Zigler & Styfco, 1996). Early Head Start, created in 1994 to serve children between birth and age 3 in low-income families, reflects many of the elements of the basic early childhood intervention and family support models (Lally & Keith, 1997; Mann 1997). In 1998, it served roughly 38,000 children (out of a total of 2.6 million eligible children between birth and age 3 in families below the poverty line) (Administration for Children and Families, 1998a; U.S. Bureau of the Census, 1998).

Children with Special Health Care Needs

Approximately 18% of children in the United States have special health care needs, most notably chronic health conditions and disabilities (Newacheck et al., 1998). Many of these children require specialized medical services, while their families require both financial and nonfinancial supports.

The federal response to the needs of children with chronic health conditions or disabilities includes both a cash subsidy and direct service provision. The former is provided through SSI, a means-tested program that provides monthly cash payments based on national eligibility standards. In 1996, PRWORA (the federal welfare reform law) significantly changed the SSI eligibility criteria for children by eliminating "maladaptive behavior" as a criterion and introducing a more restrictive definition of childhood disability, which terminated the individualized functional assessment process for qualification (Committee on Ways and Means, 1996). Among the children most likely to lose their SSI benefits under the new guidelines are those with emotional and behavioral problems, developmental disabilities, mental retardation, or multiple impairments (none of which alone may be severe enough to meet the more stringent disability criteria established under PRWORA). The Social Security Administration estimates that 95,180 children receiving benefits under the previous law will be denied SSI when their cases are reassessed (Grantmakers in Health, 1997).

Direct services for infants and toddlers with special health care needs are provided through two major federal programs. The first, Part C of the Individuals with Disabilities Education Act, is administered through the U.S. Department of Education. This federally mandated program requires states to provide services for infants and toddlers with disabilities and specifies inclusion of the emotional development of the child in the required comprehensive assessment. Part C also allows states to provide services for "at-risk" children up to 3 years of age, and it requires an Interagency Coordinating Council to ensure coordination among the systems that are involved in delivering services for this population (Harbin, McWilliams, & Gallagher, 2000).

The other major federal program, the Maternal and Child Health Block Grant, provides specialized health and family support services for children with chronic medical conditions or developmental disabilities. Funds may be used by the states to provide a broad array of services, including home visiting, coordination of care, genetic counseling, staff training, and research designed to improve service delivery. This program serves half of the nation's children with severe disabilities and approximately 20% of children with chronic conditions (Meisels & Shonkoff, 2000; Rani, 1997).

Children Who Have Been Abused

Children who have been maltreated require highly sophisticated and sensitive care, and their families need a variety of specialized services to address a host of complex mental health concerns. Beyond the immediate physical protection of the child, services must be provided to address both short- and long-term emotional needs, as well as to consider alternative custody arrangements including family reunification, foster-care placement, and adoption (Chalk & King, 1998; Kaufman & Zigler, 1996).

Although the federal government has been involved in child welfare since the early 1900s, there still is no coherent federal policy or continuum of services for children who have been abused. By 1994, incremental approaches to child protection had resulted in approximately 40 federal programs, administered by four different cabinet agencies, authorized to provide an array of services for this highly vulnerable population (Committee on Ways and Means, 1998; Robinson & Forman, 1994).

Primary responsibility for child welfare services rests with the states. Nevertheless, the federal government is an integral part of the child protection system, influencing it through both legislative language and budget appropriations. The largest federal programs addressing child abuse and neglect are Title IV-B and Title IV-E of the Social Security Act.

The Title IV-B Child Welfare Services Program provides funds to the states for screening, investigation, and treatment. In addition, it authorizes funds for direct federal grants to public and private agencies for child welfare staff training and for demonstration activities. One section of Title IV-B, the Family Preservation and Family Support Act, focuses solely on state grants to prevent out-of-home placements. In 1997, this act was amended by the Adoption and Safe Families Act (Public Law No. 105–89), which requires that the child's health and safety be of paramount concern and that termination of parental rights and adoption processes be made more efficient and timely (Committee on Ways and Means, 1998). Whereas the more recent legislation requires states to spend increased resources on adoption-related activities, limited appropriations have prompted concerns that monies for preventive family support programs may be diverted.

Foster Care and Adoption Assistance, Title IV-E of the Social Security Act, is administered by the Administration for Children and Families in the U.S. Department of Health and Human Services. This law provides open-ended federal matching funds to support foster care for income-eligible children and adoption for children who are difficult to place. Title IV-E addresses the long-standing concern of "foster-care drift" (i.e., inappropriately long stays in out-of-home care) by allowing states that control foster-care expenditures to reallocate these funds to programs for child welfare and family preservation (Administration for Children and Families, 1998b; Committee on Ways and Means, 1998).

The Child Abuse Prevention and Treatment Act provides funds and technical assistance to states for prevention and intervention in cases of child abuse and neglect through community-based family resource and support programs. Treatment and support services also are funded through the Social Services Block Grant, which was created in 1974 as Title XX of the Social Security Act. These funds are given to states to help them meet a wide range of social policy goals including prevention of child maltreatment and reunification of families (Administration for Children and Families, 1998c; Committee on Ways and Means, 1996).

Stated simply, after a century of experience in the broad domain of child welfare, the child protection dimension of child and family programs and policies continues to be overwhelmed. Despite substantial amounts of funding that have been allocated to address the crisis of child abuse and neglect, it has been estimated that between 40 and 60% of substantiated cases of maltreatment receive no follow-up services (McCurdy & Daro, 1993).

CONCLUSIONS AND FUTURE DIRECTIONS

To have a positive impact on the mental health of young children in the United States, public policy must be guided by an ecological and family-centered approach and be responsive to the cultural and structural diversity of contemporary family life in the United States. Within this framework, contentious political struggles over preferred "family values" often sabotage well-intentioned efforts, occasionally paralyze progress, and invariably compromise the effective provision of sustained assistance to infants and toddlers in need (Jacobs, 1994). Sound policy in this area must be both child-focused and family-centered. It must recognize the futility

of past attempts to support children as independent agents, in a manner that did not fully address the nature of their caregiving contexts. Further, effective policy on behalf of young children and their families must reflect the critical importance of both economic and social support, each of which can help reduce stress and, thereby, enhance parenting and child well-being.

Social policies and programs for young children must offer a range of interventions and supportive options that can respond to a broad diversity of needs. Those that address the normative requirements of all (or a large majority of) young children and their families should be universally available, accessible, and affordable. The use of targeting strategies to limit resource allocations for services that address widespread needs produces inevitable inequities and may create perverse incentives for those who are potential program beneficiaries. In addition, targeted programs create significant bureaucratic complexity and expense by requiring the definition, determination, and policing of eligibility. In contrast, targeting policies and programs to address the specialized needs of well-defined population subgroups can be efficient and make good sense.

Most European countries offer paid and job-protected leave to all mothers (and sometimes fathers) of new children, and provide free (or highly subsidized) child care for children between age 3 and primary school entry. In addition, 82 countries (not including the United States) provide income supplements through child or family allowances based on the number of children in a family. These allowances tend to be a flat amount (like our dependent exemption) distributed in the form of a refundable tax credit (like our EITC). In other words, families may either reduce their income tax liability or receive a refund that reflects a fixed amount per child (Kamerman, 2000; Kamerman & Kahn, 1995).

These differences in child and family policies between the United States and most industrialized countries appear to be related primarily to two key cultural distinctions. First, there is a greater focus on personal and family responsibility in the United States, in contrast to an attitude of shared responsibility for children that is found in other societies throughout both the industrialized and developing world. Second, the greater ethnic and racial diversity, immigrant status, and cultural heterogeneity of the population of the United States contributes to a more pervasive problem with intergroup conflict and a greater reluctance to use public resources to support "other people's children" (Grubb & Lazerson, 1982).

The mental health and physical well-being of infants and toddlers can be promoted by a wide variety of policies that promote economic security, reduce family stress, strengthen parenting skills, enhance the parent–child relationship, and reduce the social isolation of the nuclear family (Upshur, 1990). To address issues of both diversity and private/public responsibility, effective social policies must respect individual choice about *whether* to make use of available services (except in such circumstances as child abuse) and *which* specific services one wishes to use. Enlightened policies recognize the impact on children of underlying economic and social conditions and make realistic efforts to eliminate, or at least ameliorate, those factors that have an adverse impact on family functioning. To be affordable for all, universal preventive programs could include subsidies that vary with family income, thereby reflecting a recognition of unequal resources in the face of shared, normative needs (Grubb & Lazerson, 1982). Furthermore, such programs could counteract the fragmentation of services among multiple policies, funding streams, areas of professional expertise, and service delivery systems.

Child and family policy in the United States generally evolves slowly. Given the lack of a strong, unified voice for all children, and the weak voices of many of the families that need public support the most, it is imperative that a broad constituency speaks out on behalf of our youngest citizens. To this end, the recent devolution of policy and program initiatives from the federal to the state level may make the child and family policymaking process more accessible to advocates, service providers, and the general public. Although this shift in control creates the potential for significant disparities among the states, it provides new opportunities for broader participation in the creation of more integrated family and child policy. Fifty states with different policies (in welfare, child care, health care, etc.) in the absence of federal standards may produce a variety of creative responses or may engage in a "race to the bottom" in the delivery of health and human services. History suggests that children in some states will be the focus of sympathetic atten-

tion, whereas others will be the victims of serious apathy or frank neglect. In all cases, however, constraints on public expenditures indicate vulnerability for children in general, particular danger for those who are poor, and further disadvantage for children of color. Moreover, an adverse impact is likely to be felt most seriously during economic recessions, when the weakness of the public safety net will be particularly apparent.

In view of the trend toward greater state control over social policies, it is essential that the multiple federal agencies that administer the plethora of programs affecting young children make greater efforts to speak to the states with one voice. To this end, it would be immensely helpful if each federal agency were to take an inventory of its relevant policies, identify duplications and gaps in the overall policy infrastructure, focus on promising points of intersection with other agencies, and select priorities for action. Each federal agency could then reassess its charge and articulate its distinctive contribution to improved policy and practice. If the trend toward greater state control continues, the states could be supported further in their increased policymaking roles through efforts to integrate data collection systems and provide incentives for greater coordination (if not true integration) of services at the state and local levels.

The evaluation of new state policy initiatives is generally neither required nor funded by the federal government. This is especially true for policies affecting the population from birth to age 3. Thus, it is essential that a plan be developed and implemented to document the mental health needs of infants and toddlers, evaluate existing systems level responses, and demonstrate and evaluate new models for promoting emotional and behavioral competence (UNOC-CAP Oversight Board, 1998). Longitudinal studies that document changes in the organization, financing, and impact of infant and toddler services would be particularly instructive.

In conclusion, it is clear that the early childhood years are the subject of increasing public attention. This has generated a greater appreciation of the critical importance of both child development, in general, and mental health, specifically, in the period from birth to age 3 years. Public policies and their implementation can have a significant impact on the well-being of young children and their families. In the final analysis, the best hope for enlightened policies and programs in the future is a combination of carefully crafted advocacy, the knowledgeable application of the science of early childhood development, and a spirit of self-examination and continuous improvement in the delivery of services.

REFERENCES

Adams, P., & Krauth, K. (1994, Fall). Community-centered practice to strengthen families and neighborhoods: The patch approach. *The Prevention Report,* pp. 2–5.

Administration for Children and Families. (1998a, June 4). *Fact sheet: Head Start.* Retrieved from the World Wide Web: http://www.acf.dhhs.gov/programs/opa/facts/headst.htm.

Administration for Children and Families. (1998b, June 4). *Fact sheet: Protecting the well-being of children.* Retrieved from the World Wide Web: http://www.acf.dhhs.gov/programs/opa/facts/chilwelf.htm.

Administration for Children and Families. (1998c, June 8). *Fact sheet: Social Services Block Grant (SSBG).* Retrieved from the World Wide Web: http://www.acf.dhhs.gov/programs/opa/facts/ssbg.htm.

Administration for Children and Families. (1998d, June 4). *Fact sheet: Temporary assistance for needy families (TANF).* Retrieved from the World Wide Web: http://www.acf.dhhs.gov/programs/opa/facts/tanf.htm.

Barnes, H. V., Goodson, B. D., & Layzer, J. I. (1995). *National evaluation of family support programs: Review of research on supportive intervention for children and families.* Washington, DC: Administration on Children, Youth and Families, U.S. Department of Health and Human Services.

Barnett, W. S. (1993). Economic evaluation of home visiting programs. *The Future of Children, 3*(3), 93–112.

Barnett, W. S. (1995, Winter). Long-term effects of early childhood programs on cognitive and school outcomes. *The Future of Children, Long-Term Outcomes of Early Childhood Programs, 5*(3), 25–50.

Breakey, G., & Pratt, B. (1991, April). Healthy growth for Hawaii's "Healthy Start": Toward a systematic statewide approach to the prevention of child abuse and neglect. *Zero to Three, 11*(4), 16–22.

Bronfenbrenner, U. (1986). Ecology of the family as a context for human development: Research perspectives. *Developmental Psychology, 22*(6), 723–742.

Bronfenbrenner, U., & Ceci, S. J. (1994). Nature–nurture reconceptualized in developmental perspective: A bioecological model. *Psychological Review, 101*(4), 568–586.

Carnegie Corporation of New York. (1994, April). *Starting points: Meeting the needs of our youngest children* (Report of the Carnegie task force on meeting the needs of young children). New York: Author.

Chalk, R., & King, P. A. (Eds.). (1998). *Violence in families: Assessing prevention and treatment programs.* Washington, DC: National Academy Press.

Commission on Family and Medical Leave. (1995). *A workable balance: Report to Congress on family and medical leave policies* [Executive summary]. Washington, DC: U. S. Department of Labor, Employment Standards Administration, Wage and Hour Division.

Committee on Ways and Means, U.S. House of Representatives. (1996). *1996 green book: Background material and data on programs within the jurisdiction of the Committee on Ways and Means.* Washington, DC: U.S. Government Printing Office.

Committee on Ways and Means, U.S. House of Representatives. (1998). *1998 green book: Background material and data on programs within the jurisdiction of the Committee on Ways and Means.* Washington, DC: U.S. Government Printing Office.

Davies, M. W. (1994). Who's minding the baby? Reproductive work, productive work, and family policy in the United States. In F. H. Jacobs & M. W. Davies (Eds.), *More than kissing babies? Current child and family policy in the United States* (pp. 37–64). Westport, CT: Auburn House.

Duggan, A., McFarlane, E., Windham, A., Rohde, C., Salkever, D., Fuddy, L., Rosenberg, L., Buchbinder, S., & Sia, C. (1999). Evaluation of Hawaii's Healthy Start Program. *The Future of Children, 9*(1), 66–90.

Duncan, G. J., & Brooks-Gunn, J. (Eds.). (1997). *Consequences of growing up poor.* New York: Russell Sage.

Emde, R. N., & Robinson, J. A. (2000). Guiding principles for a theory of early intervention: A developmental–psychoanalytic perspective. In J. P. Shonkoff & S. J. Meisels (Eds.), *Handbook of early childhood intervention* (2nd ed.). New York: Cambridge University Press.

Fox, H. B., McManus, M. A., Almeida, R. A., & Lesser, C. (1997, Summer). Medicaid managed care policies affecting children with disabilities: 1995 and 1996. *Health Care Financing Review, 18*(4), 23–36.

Frank, M., & Zigler, E. F. (1996). Family leave: A developmental perspective. In E. F. Zigler, S. L. Kagan, & N. W. Hall (Eds.), *Children, families, and government: Preparing for the twenty-first century* (pp. 117–131). New York: Cambridge University Press.

Frede, E. C. (1995, Winter). The role of program quality in producing early childhood program benefits. *The Future of Children, Long-Term Outcomes of Early Childhood Programs, 5*(3), 115–132.

Garbarino, J., & Ganzel, B. (2000). The human ecology of early risk. In J. P. Shonkoff & S. J. Meisels (Eds.), *Handbook of early childhood intervention* (2nd ed.). New York: Cambridge University Press.

Garcia Coll, C., Lamberty, G., Jenkins, R., McAdoo, H., Crnic, K., Wasik, B., & Garcia, H. (1996). An integrative model for the study of developmental competencies in minority children. *Child Development, 67*(5), 1891–1914.

Garcia Coll, C., & Magnuson, K. (2000). Cultural differences as sources of developmental vulnerabilities and resources. In J. P. Shonkoff & S. J. Meisels (Eds.), *Handbook of early childhood intervention* (2nd ed.). New York: Cambridge University Press.

Garfinkel, I., McLanahan, S., Meyer, D., & Seltzer, J. (1998). Fathers under fire: The revolution in child support enforcement. *Focus, 19*(3), 24–28.

Gold, S. D. (1998, November 12). *Issues raised by the new federalism.* Washington, DC: The Urban Institute. Retrieved from the World Wide Web: http://newfederalism.urban.org/html/ntj.htm.

Gomby, D., Culross, P., & Behrman, R. (1999). Home visiting: Recent program evaluations—analysis and recommendations. *The Future of Children, 9*(1), 4–26.

Gomby, D. S., Krantzler, N., Larner, M. B., Stevenson, C. S., Terman, D. L., & Behrman, R. E. (1996, Summer/Fall). Financing child care: Analysis and recommendations. *The Future of Children, Financing Child Care, 6*(2), 5–25.

Gomby, D. S., Larson, C. S., Lewit, E. M., & Behrman, R. E. (1993, Winter). Home visiting: Analysis and recommendations. *The Future of Children, Home Visiting, 3*(3), 6–22.

Grantmakers in Health. (1997, September 15). Children with special health care needs: Challenges, opportunities, & models for improving their access to care. *Safety Net Focus.* Retrieved November 10, 1998, from the World Wide Web: http://www.gih.org/bulletin/safetynet.htm.

Grubb, W. N., & Lazerson, M. (1982). *Broken promises: How Americans fail their children.* New York: Basic Books.

Halpern, R. (1993, Winter). The societal context of home visiting and related services for families in poverty. *The Future of Children, Home Visiting, 3*(3), 158–171.

Halpern, R. (2000). Early intervention for low-income children and families. In J. P. Shonkoff & S. J. Meisels (Eds.), *Handbook of early childhood intervention* (2nd ed.). New York: Cambridge University Press.

Harbin, G., McWilliams, R. A., & Gallagher, J. J. (2000). Services for young children with disabilities and their families. In J. P. Shonkoff & S. J. Meisels (Eds.), *Handbook of early childhood intervention* (2nd ed.). New York: Cambridge University Press.

Helburn, S., & Culkin, M. L. (1995). *Cost, quality, and child outcomes in child care centers.* Denver: Economics Department, Center for Research in Economics and Social Policy, University of Colorado at Denver.

Hernandez, D. (1997). Child development and the social demography of childhood. *Child Development, 68*(1), 149–169.

Hofferth, S. L., Brayfield, A., Deich, S., & Holcomb, P. (1991). *National child care survey, 1990.* Washington, DC: Urban Institute Press.

Jacobs, F. H. (1994). Child and family policy: Framing the issues. In F. H. Jacobs & M. W. Davies (Eds.), *More than kissing babies? Current child and family policy in the United States* (pp. 9–35). Westport, CT: Auburn House.

Jacobs, F. H., & Davies, M. W. (1994). Introduction. In F. H. Jacobs & M. W. Davies (Eds.), *More than kissing babies? Current child and family policy in the United States* (pp. 1–8). Westport, CT: Auburn House.

Kagan, S. L. (1996). America's family support movement: A moment of change. In E. F. Zigler, S. L. Kagan, & N. W. Hall (Eds.), *Children, families, and government: Preparing for the twenty-first century* (pp. 156–170). New York: Cambridge University Press.

Kagan, S. L., & Neuman, M. J. (2000). Early childhood care and education. In J. P. Shonkoff & S. J. Meisels (Eds.), *Handbook of early childhood intervention* (2nd ed.). New York: Cambridge University Press.

Kaiser Commission on the Future of Medicaid. (1997, November). Medicaid's role for children. *Medicaid Facts.* Washington, DC: Henry J. Kaiser Family Foundation.

Kamerman, S. B. (2000). An international perspective on early childhood intervention. In S. J. Meisels & J. P. Shonkoff (Eds.), *Handbook of early childhood intervention* (2nd ed.). New York: Cambridge University Press.

Kamerman, S. B., & Kahn, A. J. (1995). *Starting right: How America neglects its youngest children and what we can do about it.* New York: Oxford University Press.

Kamis-Gould, E., Hadley, T., & Markel-Fox, S. (1994). *Mental health services offered through Early Periodic Screening, Diagnosis and Treatment (EPSDT).* Retrieved June 2, 1998, from the World Wide Web: http://www.med.upenn.edu/cmhpsr/epsdt.html.

Kaufman, J., & Zigler, E. F. (1996). Child abuse and social policy. In E. F. Zigler, S. L. Kagan, & N. W. Hall (Eds.), *Children, families, and government: Preparing for the twenty-first century* (pp. 233–255). New York: Cambridge University Press.

Kingdon, J. W. (1995). *Agendas, alternatives, and public policies* (2nd ed.). New York: HarperCollins.

Klerman, L. V. (1996). Child health: What public policies can improve it? In E. F. Zigler, S. L. Kagan, & N. W. Hall (Eds.), *Children, families, and government: Preparing for the twenty-first century* (pp. 188–206). New York: Cambridge University Press.

Knitzer, J. (1996). Children's mental health: Changing paradigms and policies. In E. F. Zigler, S. L. Kagan, & N. W. Hall (Eds.), *Children, families, and government: Preparing for the twenty-first century* (pp. 207–232). New York: Cambridge University Press.

Knitzer, J. (2000). Early childhood mental health programs. In J. P. Shonkoff & S. J. Meisels (Eds.), *Handbook of early childhood intervention* (2nd ed.). New York: Cambridge University Press.

Krugman, R. D. (1993, Winter). Universal home visiting: A recommendation from the U. S. Advisory Board on Child and Abuse Neglect. *The Future of Children, Home Visiting, 3*(3), 184–191.

Lally, J. R., & Keith, H. (1997, October/November). Early Head Start: The first two years. *Zero to Three, 18*(2), 3–8.

Lamb, M. E. (Ed.). (1997). *The role of the father in child development* (3rd ed.). New York: Wiley.

Mann, T. L. (1997, October/November). Promoting the mental health of infants and toddlers in Early Head Start: Responsibilities, partnerships, and supports. *Zero to Three, 18*(2), 37–40.

McCurdy, K., & Daro, D. (1993). *Current trends in child abuse reporting and fatalities: The results of the 1994 fifty state survey.* Chicago: National Center on Child Abuse Prevention Research, National Committee to Prevent Child Abuse.

McLoyd, V. C. (1990). The impact of economic hardship on black families and children: Psychological distress, parenting, and socio-emotional development. *Child Development, 61*(2), 311–346.

Meisels, S. J., & Shonkoff, J. P. (2000). Early childhood intervention: A continuing evolution. In J. P. Shonkoff & S. J. Meisels (Eds.), *Handbook of early childhood intervention* (2nd ed.). New York: Cambridge University Press.

Newacheck, P. W., Strickland, B., Shonkoff, J. P., Perrin, J. M., McPherson, M., McManus, M., Lauver, C., Fox, H., & Arango, P. (1998). An epidemiologic profile of children with special health care needs. *Pediatrics, 102*(1), 117–123.

Office of the Assistant Secretary for Planning and Evaluation, Department of Health and Human Services. (1998, June 4). *Comparison of prior law and the Personal Responsibility and Work Opportunity Reconciliation Act of 1996 (P.L. 104–193)*. Retrieved from the World Wide Web: http://aspe.os.dhhs.gov/hsp/isp/reform.htm.

Office of Inspector General, Office of Evaluation and Inspections. (1997). *Medicaid managed care and EPSDT* [WAIS document]. Washington, DC: Department of Health and Human Services.

Olds, D., Henderson, C., Kitzman, H., Eckenrode, J., Cole, R., & Tatelbaum, R. (1999). Prenatal and infancy home visitation by nurses: Recent findings. *The Future of Children, 9*(1), 44–65.

Olds, D. L., & Kitzman, H. (1993, Winter). Review of research on home visiting for pregnant women and parents of young children. *The Future of Children, Home Visiting, 3*(3), 53–92.

Osofsky, J., & Thompson, D. (2000). Adaptive and maladaptive parenting: Risk and resilience. In J. P. Shonkoff & S. J. Meisels (Eds.), *Handbook of early childhood intervention* (2nd ed.). New York: Cambridge University Press.

Pearce, D., & Brooks, J., with Russell, L. H. (1998). *The self-sufficiency standard for Massachusetts: Selected family types* (Report prepared for the Massachusetts Project for Family Economic Self-Sufficiency, convened by the Women's Educational and Industrial Union). Washington, DC: Wider Opportunities for Women.

Pecora, P. J., Whittaker, J. K., Maluccio, A. N., Barth, R. P., & Plotnick, R. D. (1992). *The child welfare challenge: Policy, practice, and research*. New York: Aldine de Gruyter.

Powell, D. R. (1993, Winter). Inside home visiting programs. *The Future of Children, Home Visiting, 3*(3), 23–38.

Pruett, K. D. (1997, August/September). How men and children affect each other's development. *Zero to Three, 18*(1), 3–11.

Ramey, C. T., & Ramey, S. L. (1993, Winter). Home visiting programs and the health and development of young children. *The Future of Children, Home Visiting, 3*(3), 129–139.

Rani, M. (1997). *Fact sheet: Maternal and Child Health Block Grant FY 1998 appropriations*. Washington, DC: American Public Health Association.

Reiss, J. (1998). *Does your state's Title XXI SCHIP plan promote the development and maintenance of quality systems of care for children with special needs? Issues and criteria for SCHIP plan review and analysis* [Policy brief]. Gainesville, FL: Institute for Child Health Policy.

Robinson, D., & Forman, M. R. (1994, November 8). *Comparison of selected federal child welfare and child abuse programs* (memorandum to the Committee on Ways and Means). Washington, DC: Congressional Research Service.

Rosenbach, M. L., & Gavin, N. I. (1998). Early and periodic screening, diagnosis, and treatment and managed care. *Annual Review of Public Health 19*, 507–525.

Rosenbaum, S., Johnson, K., Sonosky, C., Markus, A., & DeGraw, C. (1998). The children's hour: The state children's health insurance program. *Health Affairs 17*(1), 75–89.

Sameroff, A. J., & Fiese, B. H. (2000). Transactional regulation: The developmental ecology of early intervention. In J. P. Shonkoff & S. J. Meisels (Eds.), *Handbook of early childhood intervention* (2nd ed.). New York: Cambridge University Press.

Sameroff, A. J., Seifer, R., Barocas, R., Zax, M., & Greenspan, S. (1987, March). Intelligence quotient scores of 4-year-old children: Social-environmental risk factors. *Pediatrics 79*(3), 343–350.

Sardell, A., & Johnson, K. (1998). The politics of EPSDT policy in the 1990s: Policy entrepreneurs, political streams, and children's health benefits. *Milbank Quarterly, 76*(2), 175–205.

Schorr, L. B. (1997). *Common purpose: Strengthening families and neighborhoods to rebuild America*. New York: Doubleday.

Selden, T. M., Banthin, J. S., & Cohen, J. W. (1998). Medicaid's problem children: Eligible but not enrolled. *Health Affairs, 17*(3), 192–200.

Shonkoff, J. P., & Meisels, S. J. (Eds.). (2000). *Handbook of early childhood intervention* (2nd ed.). New York: Cambridge University Press.

State Legislative Leaders Foundation. (1995). *State legislative leaders: Keys to effective legislation for children and families*. Centerville, MA: Author.

Stoney, L., & Greenberg, M. H. (1996, Summer/Fall). The financing of child care: Current and emerging trends. *The Future of Children, Financing Child Care, 6*(2), 83–102.

Ullman, F., Bruen, B., & Holahan, J. (1998). *The State Children's Health Insurance Program: A look at the numbers*. Washington, DC: The Urban Institute.

U.S. Bureau of the Census. (1998, October 21). *March 1998 Current population survey*. Retrieved from the World Wide Web: http://www.census.gov/hhes/poverty/poverty97/pv97est1.html.

UNOCCAP Oversight Board. (1998, November 9). *Charting the mental health status and service needs of children: Recommendations from the UNOCCAP Oversight Board*. Retrieved from the World Wide Web: http://www.nimh.nih.gov./research/unoccap.htm.

Upshur, C. (1990). Early intervention as preventive intervention. In S. J. Meisels & J. P. Shonkoff (Eds.), *Handbook of early childhood intervention* (pp. 633–650). New York: Cambridge University Press.

Venner, S., Sullivan, B., Burns, V., Healey, G., Keaney, W., Miller, J., Mitchell, C., & Rathblott, R. (1995).

What's working in Massachusetts: Models of support and empowerment. Boston: Special Committee on Family Support and the Child Welfare System.

Wagner, M., & Clayton, S. (1999). The Parents as Teachers Program: Results from two demonstrations. *The Future of Children, 9*(1), 91–115.

Weissbourd, B., & Kagan, S. (1989). Family support programs: Catalysts for change. *American Journal of Orthopsychiatry, 59*(1), 20–31.

Zigler, E. (1997, June 5). *Testimony at Pre to 3: Policy implications of child brain development* (hearing before the Senate Subcommittee on Children and Families of the Committee on Labor and Human Re-

sources). Washington, DC: U. S. Government Printing Office.

Zigler, E. F., & Gilman, E. (1996). Not just any care: Shaping a coherent child care policy. In E. F. Zigler, S. L. Kagan, & N. W. Hall (Eds.), *Children, families, and government: Preparing for the twenty-first century* (pp. 94–116). New York: Cambridge University Press.

Zigler, E. F., & Styfco, S. (1996). Head Start and early intervention: The changing course of social science and social policy. In E. F. Zigler, S. L. Kagan, & N. W. Hall (Eds.), *Children, families, and government: Preparing for the twenty-first century* (pp. 132–155). New York: Cambridge University Press.

34

Child Care in Infancy: A Transactional Perspective

❖

ANNE HUNGERFORD
CELIA A. BROWNELL
SUSAN B. CAMPBELL

Recent reviews of child care research (Barton & Williams, 1993; Hayes, Palmer, & Zaslow, 1990; Lamb, 1998) have emphasized that asking whether child care in infancy is good or bad for children's development is too simple a question for our current state of understanding. Child care is embedded in a rich ecology that includes characteristics and needs of the child as well as of the family, culture, and sociohistorical era, and child-care arrangements themselves are diverse and multifaceted. Research in the last decade has increasingly recognized the complex interplay between child-care experiences and these other factors in predicting developmental outcome. The questions, therefore, have changed: Under what circumstances do children thrive or suffer in early child care, and how do different sources of influence mutually shape development? The answers, as suggested by more complex conceptual models, are neither straightforward nor well delineated. It is clear that child care does not inevitably harm children, nor is it inevitably beneficial. However, it is not yet known under which conditions child care adds risk or buffers children's development against risk, particularly when child care begins in infancy. The focus of this chapter is on research since 1990 that has contributed to our growing but still limited understanding of those conditions that, together with varia-

tions in child-care experience during infancy, influence individual differences in developmental outcome.

CHILD CARE IN THE 1990s

The debate still rages about the advisability of child care for infants, particularly in the popular press, largely because of vestiges of the strong early experience position inherent in the psychoanalytic tradition (Lamb, 1998). However, child care in the early years of life is now the norm for most children in the United States and other industrialized countries. In this country, over half the mothers of infants under 12 months old are employed (Scarr, 1998). The National Institute of Child Health and Human Development (NICHD) Study of Early Child Care, a multisite study of roughly 1,200 families from all major regions of the country, found that 58% of infants under 12 months were in child care for 30 or more hours a week and 74% were in care for at least 10 hours a week (NICHD Early Child Care Research Network [ECCRN], 1997a).

The term "child care" is meant to capture the wide variety of settings in which infants are cared for by someone other than their mothers. These include center-based care, child-care homes, care by relatives, and in-home care by nonrelatives. In general, studies find that most infants in child care are in home settings (their own or another's), with only about 12% of infants younger than 1 year in child-care centers. By toddlerhood more children are entering formal care, but the majority are still in home-based care arrangements rather than center-based care (Kisker, Hofferth, Phillips, & Farguhar, 1991; NICHD ECCRN, 1997a). These trends are important in evaluating the research on child care because the majority of research has focused on center-based care (Lamb, 1998; Scarr, 1998). Given that young infants are more likely to be cared for in home settings, the findings from center-based studies may not generalize to the experiences of most infants.

As more attention is paid to different types of care arrangements, it is important to note that the type of care parents select, as well as other parameters of care (i.e., age of entry, quality, and amount), are correlated with demographic, economic, and psychosocial variables. Although some studies have considered such correlates of care, most studies consider only a few. As Scarr (1998) notes, there are likely to be many factors that differentiate groups of infants with varying care experiences, and it is impossible to control for all of them. Thus, when significant differences emerge between groups, they are often difficult to interpret.

The most comprehensive study to date of child care and children's development is the NICHD Study of Early Child Care (NICHD ECCRN, 1997c). In this study, a wide variety of factors that frequently have been implicated in parents' decisions regarding care arrangements were controlled. The most consistent predictors of parameters of care were the importance of maternal income to the family's economic status, maternal attitudes about child rearing, and maternal beliefs about the effects of mothers' employment on children. Infants of more poorly educated mothers and of mothers who worked longer hours spent more time in child care. In general, the amount of child care infants received was related to families' reliance on maternal income. In addition, mothers who believed that the effect of maternal employment on their children was positive and who held less authoritarian child-rearing attitudes were more likely to enroll their infants in more hours of child care.

Economic factors also predicted the type of care parents chose for their infants. Higher family income was related to the use of in-home care by nonrelatives, whereas lower family income was associated with care by fathers and grandparents. In addition, mothers who were least concerned about risks of maternal employment for children's development were more likely to select center-based care, whereas those who were most concerned tended to have their children cared for by relatives.

The quality of care infants received was also related to economic variables. Infants of more affluent families generally were in child-care settings of higher quality. However, income did not predict the quality of care provided by fathers and grandparents. In child-care centers, infants from poor and affluent families were in better-quality care arrangements than were infants whose families were in the middle economically. This curvilinear relationship is consistent with past findings regarding center care for preschoolers and may be because economically disadvantaged families often receive federal subsidies for child care of higher quality (Hayes et al., 1990).

Maternal child-rearing attitudes were also associated with quality of care for infants in grandparent care, in-home care, and child-care homes; less authoritarian beliefs were related to higher-quality child care. The quality of infants' home environments also was related positively to the quality of care provided in child-care homes. Neither maternal child-rearing attitudes nor the quality of infants' home environments were related to the quality of center-based care. Because each of these correlates of care influences development in its own right, these patterns highlight the importance of considering the factors associated with child-care usage that may account for differences between children with varying care experiences.

A BRIEF HISTORY OF CHILD-CARE RESEARCH

Child-care research in the 1960s and 1970s focused predominantly on children whose experiences began after infancy and was limited to children in high-quality university-based child-care centers or to children who participated in child-care programs as part of early interventions designed to ameliorate the effects of poverty on school achievement. This "first wave" of child-care research was motivated by the simple question of whether child care was harmful for young children (Hayes et al., 1990; Lamb, 1998).

Research in the 1980s began to recognize the importance of the quality of children's experiences in child care. Thus, this "second wave" of child care research addressed the question of how child-care of varying quality affected children's development. During this decade, measurements of "quality" became increasingly complex and sophisticated. By the decade's close, researchers recognized two related aspects of child-care quality: (1) "structural" measures such as group size; adult-child ratio; caregiver education, training, and commitment; staff turnover; and the safety, cleanliness, and developmental appropriateness of the environment and (2) "process" measures, usually obtained by direct observation in the child-care setting, such as the amount and type of stimulation caregivers provided, the quality of their interactions with the children, and the nature of child–caregiver relationships. Many studies have now found systematic relations between various measures of child-care quality in infancy and a variety of developmental outcomes (Lamb, 1998).

As research began to accrue concerning the effects on development of variations in quality of child care, it became evident that quality of child care is not independent of the child's experiences in other contexts outside the child-care setting. In particular, as noted previously, family characteristics, including economic status, education, and attitudes toward child rearing often covary with the age that children enter child care, the type of care parents choose, and both the amount and the quality of care provided (Howes & Olenick, 1986; NICHD ECCRN, 1997c; Scarr, 1998). Thus, the infant's experiences in child care are not independent of experiences at home. The "third wave" of child care research is therefore focused on the multiple, interacting features of the child's experiences in shaping development. Much of the research conducted since 1990, but by no means all, is premised on this model.

TRANSACTIONAL AND ECOLOGICAL MODELS: THEIR RELEVANCE TO CHILD-CARE RESEARCH

It is clear from the preceding discussion that simple models that examine "main effects" of child care are inadequate. In general, whatever the outcome, "main effects" studies of child care in infancy have not provided a clear picture and results have been inconsistent. In addition, studies have varied widely in their attention to possible confounding variables and in how they operationalized aspects of child care. As a result, when child-care effects are discerned, it is difficult to know how to interpret them. Do the effects really reflect differences *solely* as a function of parameters of care? Or are they partly or wholly accounted for by the preexisting differences among families that are also associated with child care-choices? Or do they reflect something fundamental about family environments that may mediate or moderate child-care effects, such as the quality of the mother–infant relationship or family stability (e.g., Crockenberg & Litman, 1991; Egeland & Hiester, 1995)? What role do child characteristics such as sex and temperament play in moderating outcomes (e.g., Crockenberg & Litman, 1991; Volling & Feagans, 1995)? As our models of development become more complex and ecologically based, our questions about the impact of child care initiated during infancy on young children's development obviously need to be reformulated to take this complexity into account.

From this framework, then, questions should not be directed at the effects of child care per se on infants. Questions must focus instead on the combined influence of child characteristics, family relationships and contexts, and multiple aspects of the child care itself on specific developmental outcomes in toddlerhood and the preschool period (NICHD ECCRN, 1994). Potentially important child characteristics include sex, temperament, and intelligence. Family demographic factors such as educational and occupational level, maternal age, family income, family composition, and place of residence (e.g., urban–rural; poor inner-city neighborhood or stable community) may function as "selection effects," influencing the availability and choice of care, including type (e.g., relative care, family child care, center care) and quality. Selection variables may also influence when a new mother returns to work. For example, occupational level is likely to be associated with job stability, family finances, and length of paid maternity leave, if any.

Other aspects of the family environment beyond demographic characteristics may also mediate or moderate child-care effects. Important family-level variables to consider include aspects of the parent–child relationship, such as attachment security, parental warmth and sensitivity, cognitive stimulation and involvement, and, in toddlerhood, styles of limit setting and control; family climate, including the quality of the marital relationship and spousal support, both generally and in regard to child rearing; social support from spouse and other network members; and the emotional adjustment of the parents (Bates et al., 1994; NICHD ECCRN, 1994, 1997b). Finally, as already noted, aspects of child care itself also are important to consider. Studies have examined type of care, age of entry, stability, amount, and quality defined in terms of regulatable features of the child-care setting (e.g., child-caregiver ratio, group size, and caregiver education) and the quality of the caregiver–infant relationship.

The "dual risk" and "cumulative risk" models suggest that the combination of two or more risk factors will place young children at a disadvantage with respect to later cognitive and/or socioemotional outcomes, whereas the impact of just one risk factor may be less evident. For example, infants living in a dysfunctional family with a depressed and/or insensitive mother or infants who have developed an insecure attachment during the first year may fare especially poorly if they also attend low-quality child care (NICHD ECCRN, 1997b). That is, the impact of unresponsive or unstimulating care both at home and in child care may exacerbate each other.

Predictions may be made still more accurate by the addition of child characteristics to the model. For example, the combined effect of poor-quality care in both contexts may be stronger for boys, who are more vulnerable to negative outcomes than are girls (Campbell, 1995), or for children with fussy–difficult temperaments (who may become even fussier given low-quality care across contexts); or boys may become more aggressive and noncompliant, whereas girls may express their frustration and unhappiness via internalizing symptoms such as sleep disturbances, social withdrawal, or separation anxiety. Cumulative risk models have received much attention in the developmental psychopathology literature (e.g., Sameroff, Seifer, Baldwin, & Baldwin, 1993), and it seems logical that low-quality child care should function as an additional risk factor for infants and toddlers who are already at risk because of biological vulnerabilities and/or psychosocial factors.

A second possible model posits "compensatory" or "buffering" factors when high-quality child care helps young children at risk overcome some of the negative outcomes associated with being reared in a punitive, uninvolved, or disorganized family setting or in a family that fails to provide adequate cognitive stimulation (Burchinal, Roberts, Nabors, & Bryant, 1996; Caughy, DiPietro, & Strobino, 1994; Volling & Feagans, 1995). This is the model on which early intervention and prevention programs such as Head Start rest (Ramey & Ramey, 1998). In this model, high-quality child care helps the young child develop coping strategies and cognitive and social skills that support more adaptive early development, despite less sensitive and stimulating care at home.

Finally, the "lost resources" model hypothesizes that children in well-functioning and stimulating home environments may lose something by attending child care (Egeland & Hiester, 1995). This model proposes that children at home with more sensitive, involved, and stimulating mothers may do better than children from such homes who attend child care, especially low-quality child care (e.g., Caughy et al., 1994). Moreover, if child care serves as a risk for children in optimal home environments, as this model suggests, it is most likely to take its toll on young boys, who seem to be more vulnerable to the negative impact of child care, or on children who are already fussy and difficult and who may react more negatively to change and disruption in their daily schedule.

These models highlight the complexity of disentangling the effects of child care from factors internal to the child and factors in the child's family environment that are known to influence developmental outcomes. Although some recent studies have begun to examine child care using more complex models (e.g., Bates et al., 1994; Deater-Deckard, Pinkerton, & Scarr, 1996; Howes & Olenick, 1986), most extant studies of child care have not been comprehensive enough to examine multiple influences on young children's development simultaneously or have not included a large enough sample to permit analyses of multiple factors.

The NICHD Study of Early Child Care was designed from an ecological and transactional perspective to examine these very issues (NICHD ECCRN, 1994). This study has provided a description of child-care usage in infancy and toddlerhood with an emphasis on quality of care (NICHD ECCRN, 1997a, 1997c) while also examining multiple aspects of family functioning and parent–child interaction over time in relation to a range of child outcomes including attachment security (NICHD ECCRN, 1997b), compliance and self-control (NICHD ECCRN, in press-a), cognitive and language development (NICHD ECCRN, 1998b), and the early development of behavior problems (NICHD ECCRN, in press-a). In addition, peer competence and friendship skills are being explored (NICHD ECCRN, 1998a).

The data examined so far underscore the combined importance of child-care quality and family context in predicting developmental outcomes. In addition, they do not support the contention of Howes (1990) that the influence of family characteristics is lessened for children in full-time infant child care. In a series of analyses conducted on a subgroup of children with early and extensive care who were compared to a subgroup with only limited formal care, minimal differences were found in the predictors of cognitive, language, and socioemotional outcomes at 24 and 36 months (NICHD ECCRN, in press-b). Scarr (1998) recently concluded that family variables were much more robust predictors of children's functioning than parameters of child care. With this background, we turn now to a review of recent studies of child care in infancy.

CHILD CARE IN INFANCY AND ATTACHMENT SECURITY

One of the most controversial issues concerning the "effects" of child care is the association between child care in infancy and attachment security. Beginning in the 1980s, several studies noted elevated rates of insecure attachment as assessed with the Strange Situation (Ainsworth, Blehar, Waters, & Wall, 1978) among infants in child care as compared to home-reared infants (e.g., Barglow, Vaughn, & Molitor, 1987; Belsky & Rovine, 1988). However, findings across these earlier studies were somewhat conflicting, with some studies failing to find any relation between child care and infants' attachment security (e.g., Chase-Lansdale & Owen, 1987).

In attempts to clarify the association, several researchers aggregated independent samples in multistudy analyses (Belsky, 1988; Clarke-Stewart, 1989; Lamb, Sternberg, & Prodromidis, 1992). Although these analyses provided support for an association between child care and insecure attachment, the magnitude of differences between home-reared infants and infants in child care was small and the interpretation of the findings has remained controversial (Barton & Williams, 1993; Lamb, 1998). Thus, some researchers have argued that extensive child care in infancy is a risk factor for insecure infant–parent attachment, whereas others have argued against this interpretation on both methodological and conceptual grounds. First, it has been suggested that the Strange Situation, with its sequence of separations and reunions, may be experienced differently by infants in regular child care (Clarke-Stewart, 1989; Thompson, 1988). Because these infants have experience with daily separations and reunions with primary caregivers, the Strange Situation may not be sufficiently stressful to activate the attachment system. In particular, their avoidant behavior toward their mothers may simply reflect greater independence and less distress. However, this argument has not received much empirical support (NICHD ECCRN, 1997b).

Another important issue concerns the magnitude of the differences in attachment security and/or avoidant behavior found between infants with and without child-care experience (Barton & Williams, 1993; Clarke-Stewart, 1989; Thompson, 1988). With regard to avoidant behavior, Lamb et al. (1992) noted that although infants with child-care experience were significantly more avoidant than were home-reared infants in their analysis, the mean difference between the two groups was quite small. In addition, although the multistudy analyses demonstrate a slightly elevated rate of insecure attachment among infants in care relative to infants not in care, the overall distribution of attachment classifications for infants in care is not significantly different from the distribution typically found in middle-class samples. That is, the majority of infants in child care are securely attached to their mothers. Thus, there are statistically significant differences in average rates of security between home-reared infants and those in child care, but these differences may not be particularly meaningful when considered in the context of typical distribution patterns (Barton & Williams, 1993; Clarke-Stewart, 1989; Lamb, 1998).

This conclusion is bolstered by the fact that more recent studies generally have failed to find relations between child care and attachment security (e.g., Burchinal, Bryant, Lee, & Ramey, 1992; Stifter, Coulehan, & Fish, 1993). Roggman, Langlois, Hubbs-Tait, and Rieser-Danner (1994) conducted a recent replication of Belsky's (1988) multistudy analysis and found no consistent relations between child care and attachment security. These authors suggest that studies in which no differences are found are less likely to be published (the "file drawer problem"). Thus, they contend that reviews and meta-analyses of the published literature are likely to overestimate the relation between child care and insecure attachment.

Finally, in most studies of child care and attachment security, the quality of care is not measured, despite its importance for understanding child-care effects. Further, as noted earlier, because infants are not randomly assigned to child care or home care, it is quite possible that associations between child care and attachment security may be the product of preexisting differences between families that do or do not place their infants in child care. Although researchers are increasingly likely to consider such "selection effects" in their models, they have not been systematically or comprehensively included in the work on attachment security.

The NICHD Study of Early Child Care (NICHD ECCRN, 1997b) is the most comprehensive study to date on the relation between child care and developmental outcomes, including attachment security. The results indicated no main effects of child care on attachment security at 15 months, with or without selection effects controlled. However, maternal sensitivity observed at 6 and 15 months was related to attachment security. Several interactions consistent with both the "dual risk" and "compensatory" models also were significant. Specifically, low maternal sensitivity coupled with low-quality child care, more extensive child-care, or unstable child care arrangements predicted an elevated rate of insecure attachment, suggesting the dual risks of insensitive maternal behavior and less favorable conditions of child care. However, compensatory effects of child care also are suggested: When maternal sensitivity was low but quality of child care was high, children were more likely to be securely attached than when quality of care was low in both contexts. Taken together, the small effects found in earlier studies and the absence of effects found in more recent studies suggest that child care in infancy, in

and of itself, does not increase the risk of insecure infant–mother attachment.

COMPLIANCE, SELF-CONTROL, AND BEHAVIOR PROBLEMS

Compliance, self-control, and behavior problems are among the most common socioemotional outcomes studied in early childhood. Behaviors such as the ability to comply with adult requests and to inhibit inappropriate or prohibited responses are major developmental achievements during toddlerhood, and these behaviors set the stage for the continued development of autonomy, social engagement in group settings, and a sense of self. Moreover, high levels of noncompliance and poor self-regulation are among the early signs of behavior problems in toddlerhood and the preschool years (Campbell, 1995). However, only a few studies have actually examined these outcomes as a function of child care instituted in infancy.

Child Care and Family Predictors

Crockenberg and Litman (1991) examined child compliance and defiance as a function of maternal employment and consequent child-care usage, but their more complex model implicated maternal control strategies, aspects of employment status that may contribute to or ameliorate stress (role satisfaction and social support), and child sex as moderators of any relations between child behavior and maternal employment in their sample of toddlers. Consistent with transactional and ecological models, as well as research on the determinants of parenting (Belsky, 1984), employed mothers who felt more stressed because of lower role satisfaction and less social support used more negative control with their toddlers during a laboratory clean-up task than did less stressed employed mothers and nonemployed mothers.

Consistent with other data on the quality of parenting and children's adjustment (Maccoby & Martin, 1983), when employed mothers were more negative their toddlers were also more defiant. When employed mothers were observed at home at dinner time, however, a time of especially high stress, they were *less* negative and *more* responsive than were nonemployed mothers. Despite this, boys of employed mothers seemed somewhat more vulnerable to the effects of maternal employment; they were more defiant than girls of employed mothers, and they were especially likely to be defiant when they were in multiple child-care arrangements, suggesting the possible impact of several risk factors simultaneously.

Other studies also suggest interactions between child care and relationship quality in predicting problematic outcomes. Egeland and Hiester (1995) studied high-risk mothers and children longitudinally and reported that attachment security in infancy interacted with child-care experience to predict behavior at 42 months and in kindergarten. Secure children who had been in child care in infancy were more hostile when observed in a structured interaction with their mothers at 42 months, and they were rated by their teachers as more aggressive, with more externalizing problems in kindergarten, in comparison to secure children who had remained at home through 18 months. In contrast, insecure children who had attended early child care were less withdrawn and more agentic than were insecure children who remained at home. This suggests that child care may serve as a compensatory social experience for insecurely attached children but may represent a "lost resource" for children who are secure. In a similar vein, Volling and Feagans (1995) suggested that high-quality child care may serve a compensatory function for children who are temperamentally difficult in infancy.

Child Care Quality

Howes and colleagues (Howes, 1990; Howes & Olenick, 1986) also examined children's cooperative behavior with adults and their ability to resist temptation as a function of child-care usage and quality, defined in terms of child:adult ratio and caregiver training and stability. Parents of children in high-quality center-based care were more invested in gaining compliance than were parents of children in low-quality center care, and the children in high-quality care also were more compliant when observed in child care. Moreover, during a resistance-to-temptation task, children with child-care experience were more likely to resist touching the attractive toy than children who were home full time, and children in high-quality care were the most able to resist. There also was some suggestive evidence that boys might be more sensitive to the effects of low-quality child care than are girls.

Howes (1990) followed this sample longitu-

dinally and reported that low-quality care predicted poorer adjustment in kindergarten, as reflected in teacher ratings of hostility and poor peer relations. Children who entered low-quality child care in infancy were especially likely to be rated by their kindergarten teachers as distractible and as less task-oriented and considerate of others than were children who entered later. When the relative contributions of child, family, and child-care characteristics were examined for children who entered child care before 12 months, child-care quality was a stronger predictor of problem behavior in kindergarten than were family variables; conversely, family variables were more predictive of kindergarten behavior problems among children who had entered care after infancy.

Deater-Deckard et al. (1996) also examined behavior problems and adjustment as a function of child-care quality and family factors, using a larger sample and more rigorous statistical tests. In this sample, all the children entered care before their first birthday, the care was characterized as average to low quality, and most children (70%) were in center care. There were no relations between structural features of child care and maternal or teacher ratings of behavior problems or social withdrawal 4 years later. When child (sex, age, prior behavior problems) and family characteristics (socioeconomic status [SES], parenting stress, and use of physical discipline) were statistically controlled, child-care quality did not predict either teacher or mother reports of behavior problems. Maternal ratings of behavior problems were predicted by maternal stress and negative discipline; teacher ratings of social withdrawal were likewise predicted by maternal use of physical punishment but not by child-care quality. Thus, in contrast to the findings of Howes (1990), family variables were stronger predictors of behavior problem outcomes even in this sample of children who entered child care early.

Age of Entry

The data of Deater-Deckard et al. (1996) are consistent with Bates et al. (1994), who reported only minimal effects of age of entry into child care in a sample of over 500 children studied in kindergarten. Child-care histories were obtained retrospectively, so quality of care could not be assessed. Bates et al. (1994) proposed a complex model in which possible mediators and moderators of age of entry and amount of care were examined. These included family processes such as negative discipline and family stress that may account for child-care effects, potential child effects such as sex and temperament, and selection factors such as SES and family structure. Outcome measures were derived from multisource (parent, teacher, and peer) and multimethod (observations, questionnaires, peer nominations) assessments of children's prosocial behavior and negative, aggressive behavior.

When potential confounding variables were controlled, entry into child care during infancy or toddlerhood predicted less positive adjustment but never accounted for more than 1.7% of the variance in outcomes. SES and child sex were the strongest predictors, with boys showing less positive and more negative outcomes than girls and children from higher SES families showing better adjustment to school. These authors concluded that there was "slim support" for the "special significance" of early child care as a predictor of behavior problems at school entry. On the other hand, because quality of care was not measured in this study, it is possible that positive effects of high-quality care and negative effects of low-quality care canceled each other out, leading to the modest effects of age of entry found here.

This interpretation is plausible when the work of Andersson (1989, 1992) in Sweden is considered. Social policies in Sweden mandate not only generous maternity leave for mothers who wish to stay home with their babies but also government-operated high-quality child-care centers and family child-care homes. Therefore, studies of child care in Sweden are based on the assumption that all children are in child care of high quality. Andersson examined age of entry into child care and type of care as predictors of teacher ratings of social adjustment in a sample of 119 eight-year-olds. After controlling for maternal education, family occupational level, family structure, and child sex, earlier age of entry predicted greater persistence, lower anxiety, and an easier transition to school. Children who entered care in the first year were seen as more persistent, independent, and socially confident as well as less anxious than children who entered care later. When this same sample was followed at age 13, child-care effects were still in evidence, but they were mediated by adjustment at age 8. Field (1991) also has reported follow-up data on two small samples of children who attended high-quality

child care beginning in infancy in the United States and who were followed up in elementary school. More time in quality care was associated with better social adjustment and emotional well-being.

Complex Models: The NICHD Study

The NICHD Study of Early Child Care (NICHD ECCRN, in press-a) also examined the development of compliance and behavior problems among children in child care. Measures were obtained across contexts, methods, and sources and included rating scales completed by mothers and caregivers and observations of child compliance in the laboratory and in child care. When maternal sensitivity and responsiveness were controlled, only caregiver reports of problem behavior and observations of compliant behavior in child care were predicted by characteristics of the child-care experience. Moreover, family variables (selection effects and mother–child relationship quality) accounted for up to 18% of the variance in child outcomes; when child-care variables were entered after selection effects, but before mother–child relationship variables, they accounted for only 3% or less of the variance in child outcomes. Thus, even when child-care effects were statistically significant, they accounted for only a small proportion of the variance in children's social adjustment and behavioral control; once family variables were controlled, predictions were specific to the child-care setting and did not generalize to mother–child interaction or maternal reports.

Taken together, then, these studies suggest that child care, especially when it is low quality, may account for small variations in children's compliance and behavior problems. However, interaction effects between characteristics of child care and characteristics of children and/or families are also in evidence. Unfortunately, these effects are not totally consistent, and studies vary widely in the nature of the sample, sample size, child-care parameters, and outcome measures. Even so, there is some support for "compensatory," "lost resources," and "dual risk" models, and effects may be clearer as children enter school and their behavioral adjustment becomes easier to measure. In addition, in line with other research in developmental psychopathology, boys may have a more difficult time in unstable or low-quality child-care arrangements, and this may carry over to less adaptive behavior later on.

PEER RELATIONSHIPS

Children's peer relationships are recognized as major contexts for socialization, including aggression and conflict management, cooperation and other aspects of prosocial behavior, communication skills, moral reasoning, and normative social behavior such as sex-typed behavior (Berndt & Ladd, 1989; Hartup, 1996). Because individual differences in preschool and middle-childhood peer relationships predict a variety of other important outcomes, including behavior problems, delinquency, and school dropout, researchers have become interested in the origins of these individual differences in both family and peer contexts (Parke & Ladd, 1992).

Limitations of Past Research

Two recent studies have controlled for some family factors in predicting peer outcomes from infants' child-care experience (Bates et al., 1994; Vandell & Corasiniti, 1990). In both cases, extensive child-care experience during infancy predicted poorer peer relationships in childhood relative to children who had been reared exclusively by their mothers during infancy. However, in both studies information about infants' child-care experience was obtained retrospectively and the quality of child care in infancy was not measured. In fact, these authors speculated that the quality of care experienced by the children in their samples may have been relatively poor. Thus, whether it is child-care experience in infancy per se that predicts poorer peer relationships or only child care of substandard quality cannot be answered by this research. Likewise, it remains unknown whether the positive effects of early child care reported in other studies are accounted for by higher-quality care or by different sample characteristics. It should be evident that conclusions about the role of child care in children's developing peer relations are incomplete, perhaps even inaccurate, when they do not also take into account both family factors and features of the child's actual experiences in child care.

Quality of Child Care

A converging body of research now suggests that higher-quality child care relates to more competent peer relationships (Holloway & Reichart-Erickson, 1989; Howes, 1988, 1990; Howes, Matheson, & Hamilton, 1994; Phillips, McCartney, & Scarr, 1987; Vandell, Henderson, & Wilson, 1988). In an extensive study of the role of early child-care quality, Howes (1990) found that when infants and toddlers in center-based child care experienced greater teacher involvement and investment, they later engaged in more advanced social play with peers in kindergarten, exhibited more positive affect with peers, and were less likely to be hesitant or withdrawn with peers. When child-care quality is high, it appears that earlier enrollment and longer participation translate into greater peer social competence, even into adolescence (Andersson, 1992; Field, 1991). Further, high-quality child care may help temperamentally inhibited children overcome some of their fearfulness with peers, whereas low-quality child care appears to exacerbate it (Volling & Feagans, 1995). It should be noted that most of the research on child-care quality has been conducted in child-care centers and only sometimes controls for family characteristics that covary with the quality of child care.

The NICHD Study of Early Child Care (NICHD ECCRN, 1998a) also addressed which aspects of child-care experience, including quality, predict peer social competence at 24 and 36 months. Family and child factors were controlled to determine how child-care experiences relate to the growth of peer skill above and beyond family socialization effects. Peer competence was assessed by mother and caregiver report, as well as by observations in the child-care setting and in a semistructured dyadic play setting outside child care with a familiar peer. Child-care quality was assessed by on-site observations of children in their child-care environments at 6, 15, 24, and 36 months of age.

Although family and child factors contributed the most variance to peer outcomes at both 24 and 36 months, child-care experiences did play an additional role, particularly at 24 months. Two-year-olds who had spent more time in child care and who had experienced more sensitive, responsive caregiving in child care were more positive and prosocial with their peers and less aggressive. On the other hand, 2-year-olds whose child care had included more time in settings with other children were more negative and aggressive with peers. By age 3, however, children who had had more experience in child-care settings with other children were more positive and skilled with their peers. Thus, early child-care experiences with both adults and peers seem to play important roles in shaping the growth of peer skills in the first 3 years of life. At age 2, positive experiences with adult caregivers may translate into positive interactions with peers; at age 3, greater experience with other children predicts more positive, skilled interactions with peers.

Other Parameters of Care

Research addressed to the effects of other aspects of child-care experience on early social development is neither as plentiful nor as systematic as research concerning child-care quality. Results of studies examining age of entry and social competence are inconsistent, with some studies showing positive effects for earlier entry into high-quality child care (Andersson, 1989, 1992; Field, 1991) and other studies finding negative effects (Bates et al., 1994; Volling & Feagans, 1995) or no effects (Howes et al., 1994). It is noteworthy that in the studies that report negative effects of early child care on children's peer social competence, quality of care is typically not assessed. A handful of investigators have now reported no effects of child-care type, whether the comparisons are between child-care homes versus centers or relative versus nonrelative care (Holloway & Reichart-Erickson, 1989; Howes et al., 1994; Lamb et al., 1988). Howes also has reported that more caregiver changes for young children in child care are related to reduced peer sociability and greater aggression (Howes & Hamilton, 1993).

Future Directions

In nearly all the research on early child-care effects, the question of mechanism remains open, even when effects are found. Whether children themselves, via temperament, cognitive ability, verbal facility, sociability, gender, or some other quality, are likely to elicit different kinds of care from caregivers and at the same time to acquire different kinds of peer skills is unknown. And the relative role of experience with caregivers versus experience with other children also remains relatively unexplored, as does the influence of experiences with same-age versus mixed-age peer groups, or with larger or smaller peer groups, or with siblings versus peers. Finally, the fact that family factors continue to carry the most variance (Deater-Deckard et al., 1996; NICHD ECCRN, 1998a) suggests that

satisfactory models will have to integrate family influences with child-care influences. Child-care influences neither replace nor outweigh family influences; rather, child-care experiences act in concert with and/or complement family experiences in shaping children's social development, whether it is optimal or problematic.

COGNITIVE AND LANGUAGE DEVELOPMENT

As with other domains of developmental outcome, contemporary research on children's cognitive development as a function of early child-care experiences has progressed to more complex questions. These include which particular aspects of child care are most influential in cognitive development; whether there are different effects of child care at different ages; whether child care, especially low-quality care, poses unique risks for cognitive development at different ages, for boys more than for girls (because boys are more vulnerable to cognitive and attentional deficits in childhood), and for some cultures or ethnic groups more than others; which aspects of cognitive and language development are most influenced by variations in early care; and how child-care environments act together with family environments to facilitate or impede cognitive developmental achievements.

The largest and longest intervention study of child-care effects on IQ and school achievement among children from low-income families is the Abcedarian Project (Ramey & Ramey, 1998). Infants who were assigned to receive early, extensive, high-quality, center-based child care consistently scored higher on a variety of standardized measures of cognitive performance beginning in infancy and extending through second grade. They also had better school achievement and were less likely to be retained in grade or to be referred to special education services (Campbell & Ramey, 1994; Ramey & Campbell, 1992). Other similar but smaller-scale intervention studies have reported similar results (Burchinal, Campbell, Bryant, Wasik, & Ramey, 1997; Goelman & Pence, 1987). These findings suggest that child care can contribute to cognitive achievements even when family factors are taken into account. It must be noted, however, that intervention studies are geared to children who are likely to receive less optimal levels of cognitive stimulation and structure at home, and that the interventions are typically designed specifically to produce cognitive gains in children at risk. As a consequence, their results do not necessarily generalize either to children from families with more normative levels of stimulation and structure or to community-based child-care settings.

Research based on more diverse samples of children and a wider variety of child-care settings has produced mixed results. Although several researchers have recently reported no effects of child care on infant and later cognitive performance, particularly when family factors are taken into account statistically or controlled by sampling (Ackerman-Ross & Khanna, 1989; Burchinal, Ramey, Reid, & Jaccard, 1995), others have reported main effects for quality of care above and beyond family influences (Field, 1991; Galinsky, Howes, Kontos, & Shinn, 1994; Rosenthal, 1994), and still others have reported interactions between child-care experience and family socioeconomic status (Caughy et al., 1994). The latter finding can occur in two ways. First, children from economically disadvantaged environments may be buffered against the risks for cognitive development carried by these environments if they attend high-quality child care beginning in infancy ("buffering" hypothesis). Second, children from economically advantaged environments may perform less well cognitively if they attend child care that is less stimulating than the care they would receive at home ("lost resources" hypothesis). The intervention research reviewed earlier clearly supports the "buffering" hypothesis. The "lost resources" hypothesis has received suggestive support from several analyses of data from the National Longitudinal Study of Youth (Baydar & Brooks-Gunn, 1991; Caughy et al., 1994).

Based on findings from recent research that point to language stimulation in child-care settings as being especially important for early cognitive development as well as for early language development (McCartney, 1984; Melhuish, Lloyd, Martin, & Mooney, 1990), the NICHD Study of Early Child Care (NICHD ECCRN, 1998b) addressed the roles of child-care quality (as generally stimulating and responsive) and the specific feature of language stimulation in child care in predicting cognitive and language development in the first 3 years of life. Findings from this study indicated that child care during infancy and early childhood

did not, in and of itself, predict differences in cognitive or linguistic performance at 15, 24, or 36 months. Children reared exclusively by their mothers did not differ from children who experienced even extensive child care beginning in infancy, once family influences on cognitive development were taken into account. However, the quality of child care did predict differences in cognitive outcomes for those children who were enrolled in care, even after controlling for family factors. Although the general quality of caregiving was relevant, the amount of language stimulation was especially predictive of outcomes. More language stimulation in child-care settings predicted higher scores on standardized assessments of cognitive development, language comprehension, and language production at 15, 24, and 36 months. Sensitive, responsive caregiving also predicted both cognitive and language outcomes but less consistently across ages. Finally, there was no support for the "buffering" hypothesis in this sample and only limited support for the "lost resources" hypothesis. The larger conclusions from this study are that family and child variables continue to carry most of the weight in predicting cognitive and language development in early childhood, and that child care in and of itself does not alter the predictive significance of family influences. Importantly, however, child-care quality does play a role in shaping cognitive development for those children who are in child care.

CONCLUSIONS AND FUTURE DIRECTIONS

What can we say about child care experiences and children's development at this time? In general, there is evidence to support both the "dual risk" and "compensatory" models. Thus, child care of low quality, particularly when it is coupled with other risk factors, appears to be detrimental to a range of developmental outcomes. Conversely, child care of moderate to high quality, particularly for children at psychosocial or socioeconomic risk, appears to have beneficial effects, especially for cognitive outcomes. An interesting question for future research is whether high-quality child care might facilitate more positive socioemotional outcomes for children at risk due to psychosocial factors (e.g., parental mental illness).

As noted in the preceding discussion, child-care experiences may influence development differently for different children, depending on other family and child characteristics. Thus, high-quality child care appears to be particularly beneficial for children at socioeconomic or psychosocial risk, but it may have fewer or less obvious influences on the development of children from middle-class or higher-functioning families. Low-quality child care appears to negatively influence the development of children from many different backgrounds, although the proposed mechanisms are different. Children from more optimal home environments may lose potential benefits by attending low-quality care (the "lost resources" model), whereas children already at risk because of their home environments may be exposed to added risk as a function of low-quality child-care experience (the "dual risk" model), and their development more severely compromised.

Although much progress has been made in understanding the influence of varying care experiences on children's development, there is still much about the "effects" of child care that remains unknown. The "third wave" of child-care research has focused attention on how child care and its associated parameters, in concert with family and child characteristics, influence development. This research has shown us the complexity of the relations that exist between child-care characteristics and family and child factors. More recent studies have begun taking this complexity into account in predicting individual differences in development. This work has also highlighted important methodological and conceptual issues that must be addressed in future research. As has been emphasized throughout this chapter, child-care experiences are not independent of other features of children's lives. Whether and when children enter child care, as well as the type and amount of care they receive and its quality, are related to factors such as family income, child-rearing attitudes, and parental beliefs about maternal employment, to name just a few. More research integrating family, child, and child-care influences longitudinally is needed. Such integration must consider the mediating functions, as well as the moderating roles, of family environments and relationships as well as children's characteristics, including their developmental status.

Now that child-care experience is normative in early development, issues will emerge regarding long-term cumulative and "sleeper" ef-

fects, both positive and negative, in middle childhood. Moreover, there may be repercussions for normative development (Hoffman, 1981) of such a widespread change in children's early experiences. Only by expanding the range of outcomes studied will such effects, if they exist, be detected. For example, will children's age-related sex-role stereotypes and gender understanding shift? Moral and social reasoning? Understanding of authority? Peer group norms? Perhaps most important, we need to begin exploring the mechanisms underlying the observed effects of child-care experiences in interaction with family and child characteristics; to this end, process-oriented research must be emphasized.

REFERENCES

Ackerman-Ross, S., & Khanna, P. (1989). The relationship of high quality day care to middle-class 3-year-olds' language performance. *Early Childhood Research Quarterly, 4,* 97–116.

Ainsworth, M. D. S., Blehar, M. C., Waters, E., & Wall, S. (1978). *Patterns of attachment.* Hillsdale, NJ: Erlbaum.

Andersson, B.-E. (1989). Effects of public day care: A longitudinal study. *Child Development, 60,* 857–866.

Andersson, B.-E. (1992). Effects of day care on cognitive and socioemotional competence of thirteen-year-old Swedish school children. *Child Development, 63,* 20–36.

Barglow, P., Vaughn, B. E., & Molitor, N. (1987). Effects of maternal absence due to employment on the quality of infant–mother attachment in a low-risk sample. *Child Development, 53,* 53–61.

Barton, M., & Williams, M. (1993). Infant day care. In C. H. Zeanah, Jr. (Ed.), *Handbook of infant mental health* (pp. 445–461). New York: Guilford Press.

Bates, J. E., Marvinney, D., Kelly, T., Dodge, K. A., Bennett, D. S., & Pettit, G. S. (1994). Child-care history and kindergarten adjustment. *Developmental Psychology, 30,* 690–700.

Baydar, N., & Brooks-Gunn, J. (1991). Effects of maternal employment and child care arrangements on preschoolers' cognitive and behavioral outcomes: Evidence from the children of the National Longitudinal Survey of Youth. *Developmental Psychology, 27,* 932–945.

Belsky, J. (1984). The determinants of parenting: A process model. *Child Development, 55,* 83–96.

Belsky, J. (1988). The "effects" of infant daycare reconsidered. *Early Childhood Research Quarterly, 3,* 235–272.

Belsky, J., & Rovine, M. J. (1988). Nonmaternal care in the first year of life and the security of infant–parent attachment. *Child Development, 59,* 157–167.

Berndt, T., & Ladd, G. (1989). *Peer relationships in child development.* New York: Wiley.

Burchinal, M. R., Bryant, D. M., Lee, M. W., & Ramey, C. T. (1992). Early day care, infant–mother attachment, and maternal responsiveness in the infant's first year. *Early Childhood Research Quarterly, 7,* 383–396.

Burchinal, M. R., Campbell, F. A., Bryant, D. M., Wasik, B. H., & Ramey, C. T. (1997). Early intervention and mediating processes in cognitive performance of children of low-income African-American families. *Child Development, 68,* 935–954.

Burchinal, M. R., Ramey, S. L., Reid, M. K., & Jaccard, J. (1995). Early child care experiences and their association with family and child characteristics during middle childhood. *Early Childhood Research Quarterly, 10,* 33–61.

Burchinal, M. R., Roberts, J. E., Nabors, L. A., & Bryant, D. M. (1996). Quality of center child care and infant cognitive and language development. *Child Development, 67,* 606–620.

Campbell, F. A., & Ramey, C. T. (1994). Effects of early intervention on intellectual and academic achievement: A follow-up study of children from low-income families. *Child Development, 65,* 684–698.

Campbell, S. B. (1995). Behavior problems in preschool children: A review of recent research. *Journal of Child Psychology and Psychiatry and Allied Disciplines, 36,* 113–149.

Caughy, M. O'B., DiPietro, J. A., & Strobino, D. M. (1994). Day care participation as a protective factor in the cognitive development of low-income children. *Child Development, 65,* 457–471.

Chase-Lansdale, P. L., & Owen, M. T. (1987). Maternal employment in family context: Effects on infant–mother and infant–father attachments. *Child Development, 58,* 1505–1512.

Clarke-Stewart, K. A. (1989). Infant day care: Maligned or malignant? *American Psychologist, 44,* 266–273.

Crockenberg, S., & Litman, C. (1991). Effects of maternal employment on maternal and two-year-old child behavior. *Child Development, 62,* 930–953.

Deater-Deckard, K., Pinkerton, R., & Scarr, S. (1996). Child care quality and children's behavioral adjustment: A four-year longitudinal study. *Journal of Child Psychology and Psychiatry, 37*(8), 937–948.

Egeland, B., & Hiester, M. (1995). The long-term consequences of infant daycare and mother–infant attachment. *Child Development, 66,* 474–485.

Field, T. (1991). Quality infant daycare and grade school behavior and performance. *Child Development, 62,* 863–870.

Galinsky, E., Howes, C., Kontos, S., & Shinn, M. (1994). *The study of children in family child care and relative care.* New York: Families and Work Institute.

Goelman, H., & Pence, A. R. (1987). Effects of child care, family, and individual characteristics on children's language development: The Victorian day care research project. In D. A. Phillips (Ed.), *Quality in child care: What does research tell us?* (pp. 89–104). Washington, DC: National Association for the Education of Young Children.

Hartup, W. (1996). The company they keep: Friendships and their developmental significance. *Child Development, 67,* 1–13.

Hayes, C. D., Palmer, J. L., & Zaslow, M. J. (Eds.). (1990). *Who cares for America's children?: Child care policy for the 1990s* (pp. 67–81). Washington, DC: National Academy Press.

Hoffman, M. L. (1981). Perspectives on the difference between understanding people and understanding things: The role of affect. In J. H. Flavell & L. Ross, (Eds.), *Social cognitive development: Frontiers and possible futures.* New York: Cambridge University Press.

Holloway, S. D., & Reichhart-Erickson, M. (1989). Child care quality, family structure, and maternal expectation: Relationship to preschool children's peer relations. *Journal of Applied Developmental Psychology, 10,* 281–298.

Howes, C. (1988). The peer interactions of young children. *Monographs of the Society for Research in Child Development, 53*(1, Serial No. 217).

Howes, C. (1990). Can the age of entry into child care and the quality of child care predict adjustment in kindergarten? *Developmental Psychology, 26,* 292–303.

Howes, C., & Hamilton, C. E. (1993). The changing experience of child care: Changes in teachers and in teacher–child relationships and children's social competence with peers. *Early Childhood Research Quarterly, 8,* 15–32.

Howes, C., & Matheson, C. C., & Hamilton, C. (1994). Maternal, teacher, and child care correlates of children's relationships with peers. *Child Development, 65,* 253–263.

Howes, C., & Olenick, M. (1986). Family and child care influences on toddler compliance. *Child Development, 57,* 202–216.

Kisker, E., Hofferth, S., Phillips, D., & Farguhar, E. (1991). *A profile of child care settings: Early education and care in 1990.* Princeton, NJ: Mathematica Policy Research.

Lamb, M. E. (1998). Nonparental child care: Context, quality, correlates, and consequences. In W. Damon (Series Ed.) & I. E. Sigel & K. A. Renninger (Vol. Eds.), *Handbook of child psychology: Vol. 4. Child psychology in practice* (5th ed., pp. 73–133). New York: Wiley.

Lamb, M. E., Hwang, C. P., Bookstein, F. L., Broberg, A., Hult, G., & Frodi, M. (1988). Determinants of social competence in Swedish preschoolers. *Developmental Psychology, 24,* 58–70.

Lamb, M. E., Sternberg, K. J., & Prodromidis, M. (1992). Nonmaternal care and the security of infant–mother attachment: A reanalysis of the data. *Infant Behavior and Development, 15,* 71–83.

Maccoby, E. E., & Martin, J. (1983). Socialization in the context of the family: Parent–child interaction. In P. H. Mussen (Series Ed.) & E. M. Hetherington (Vol. Ed.), *Handbook of child psychology: Vol. 4. Socialization, personality, and social development* (4th ed., pp. 1–101). New York: Wiley.

McCartney, K. (1984). Effect of quality of day care environment on children's language development. *Developmental Psychology, 20,* 244–260.

Melhuish, E. C., Lloyd, E., Martin, S., & Mooney, A. (1990). Type of child care at 18 months—II. Relations with cognitive and language development. *Journal of Child Psychology and Psychiatry, 31*(6), 861–870.

National Institute of Child Health and Human Development Early Child Care Research Network. (1994). Child care and child development: The NICHD study of early child care. In S. L. Friedman & H. C. Haywood (Eds.), *Developmental follow-up: Concepts, domains and methods* (pp. 377–396). New York: Academic Press.

National Institute of Child Health and Human Development Early Child Care Research Network. (1997a). Child care experiences during the first year of life. *Merrill–Palmer Quarterly, 43,* 340–360.

National Institute of Child Health and Human Development Early Child Care Research Network. (1997b). The effects of infant child care on infant–mother attachment security: Results of the NICHD study of early child care. *Child Development, 68,* 860–879.

National Institute of Child Health and Human Development Early Child Care Research Network. (1997c). Familial factors associated with characteristics of nonmaternal care of infants. *Journal of Marriage and the Family, 59,* 389–408.

National Institute of Child Health and Human Development Early Child Care Research Network. (1998a). *Early child care and children's peer relationships at 24 and 36 months.* Manuscript submitted for publication.

National Institute of Child Health and Human Development Early Child Care Research Network. (1998b). *The relations of child care to cognitive and language development in the first three years of life: Results of the NICHD study of early child care.* Manuscript submitted for publication.

National Institute of Child Health and Human Development Early Child Care Research Network. (in press-a). Early child care and cooperation, compliance, defiance, and problem behavior at 24 and 36 months of age. *Child Development.*

National Institute of Child Health and Human Development Early Child Care Research Network. (in press-b). Relations between family predictors and child outcomes: Are they weaker for children in child care? *Developmental Psychology.*

Parke, R. D., & Ladd, G. W. (Eds.). (1992). *Family–peer relationships: Modes of linkage.* Hillsdale, NJ: Erlbaum.

Phillips, D. A., McCartney, K., & Scarr, S. (1987). Child-care quality and children's social development. *Developmental Psychology, 23,* 537–543.

Ramey, C. T., & Campbell, F. A. (1992). Poverty, early childhood education, and academic competence: The Abecedarian experiment. In A. C. Huston (Ed.), *Children in poverty: Child development and public policy* (pp. 190–221). New York: Cambridge University Press.

Ramey, C. T., & Ramey, S. L. (1998). Early intervention and early experience. *American Psychologist, 53,* 109–120.

Roggman, L. A., Langlois, J. H., Hubbs-Tait, L., & Rieser-Danner, L. A. (1994). Infant daycare, attachment, and the "file drawer problem." *Child Development, 65,* 1429–1443.

Rosenthal, M. K. (1994). *An ecological approach to the study of child care: Family day care in Israel.* Hillsdale, NJ: Erlbaum.

Sameroff, A. J., Seifer, R., Baldwin, A., & Baldwin, C. (1993). Stability of intelligence from preschool to adolescence: The influence of social and family risk factors. *Child Development, 64,* 80–97.

Scarr, S. (1998). American child care today. *American Psychologist, 53,* 95–108.

Stifter, C. A., Coulehan, C. M., & Fish, M. (1993). Linking employment to attachment: The mediating effects of maternal separation anxiety and interactive behavior. *Child Development, 64,* 1451–1460.

Thompson, R. A. (1988). The effects of infant day care through the prism of attachment theory: A critical appraisal. *Early Childhood Research Quarterly, 3,* 273–282.

Vandell, D. L., & Corasaniti, M. A. (1990). Variations in early child care: Do they predict subsequent social, emotional, and cognitive differences? *Early Childhood Research Quarterly, 5,* 555–572.

Vandell, D. L., Henderson, V. K., & Wilson, K. G. (1988). A longitudinal study of children with day care experiences of varying quality. *Child Development, 59,* 1286–1292.

Volling, B. L., & Feagans, L. V. (1995). Infant day care and children's social competence. *Infant Behavior and Development, 18,* 177–188.

35

Divorce and Custody: Developmental Implications

❖

MICHAEL D. KAPLAN
KYLE D. PRUETT

The normative family experience for many children in this country has been redefined over the course of one generation. Estimates suggest that divorce affects nearly 1 million children per year (American Academy of Child and Adolescent Psychiatry, 1997). Of those divorcing, nearly 10% involve custody litigation. Nearly half of all children in this country will spend time in a single-parent home (Glick & Lin, 1986). While the rate of divorce in this country has declined in the last decade, approximately half of all first marriages end in divorce (U.S. Bureau of the Census, 1992). An additional 17% separate but do not divorce. Postdivorce children usually live with a custodial mother who remains single for an average of 5 years (Castro-Martin & Bumpass, 1989). Many of these homes will include other family members or new male partners. Remarriage rates have been falling, suggesting that many children will remain with a single custodial parent until they leave home. The majority experience, however, is for two-thirds of divorced women and approximately three-quarters of divorced men to remarry (Bumpass, Sweet, & Castro-Martin, 1990). With divorce rates even higher among remarriages, many children find themselves in the position of adapting to ever-changing family constellations.

Divorce typically leads to multiple disruptions in the lives of children. The concrete effects include reconfigured living arrangements, potential change(s) in residence, and, with shared custody or visitation, increased number of transitions from home to home as well as home to school to home. Familial patterns realign. Stepparents and stepsiblings are often introduced. Children may be adopted by new parents. For the majority of children who live with their mother, their economic well-being is threatened.

Divorce is a unique disruption to the nurturing domain. Nurturance is an attitude, an instinct, and a set of observable behaviors. It encompasses a broad range of feelings and skills that can be innate or learned and enhanced with practice (Yogman, Cooley, & Kindlon, 1988). The nurturing domain surrounds and scaffolds the young child. Unlike the loss of a parent to death, neglect, illness, or separations due to employment-related travel, divorce places the child in a process and context of ongoing cognitive and emotional adjustment in their relationship with each parent. The nurturing domain, while important throughout childhood, is especially salient in the first years of life. The risk to the child in a divorcing family is that the nurturing domain will be set off its developmental trajectory, placing the child at risk for emotional, behavioral, and relational disturbances.

A developmental framework for conceptualizing issues in divorce and custody is essential. Although the literature on the impact of divorce on children's development has taken such a perspective, the needs of the youngest children have received less attention. The impact on children in the first years of life is not well understood, and few, if any, guidelines exist to shape policy and decisions regarding the best interests of infants and toddlers. Given the rapid advances in cognitive and emotional development in the first 2 to 3 years of life, divorce and custody will have different meanings depending on the age of the child. Even in amicable divorces with minimal custody deliberations, most proceedings require at least 12 months. For an infant, following this process to its legal conclusion could occupy (and for parents, preoccupy) 50–100% of their life.

The significance of the role of the expert witness in child custody cases cannot be underestimated. In one of the only large-scale reviews (282 disputed child custody cases) examining the relative influence on judges' decision-making processes, child preference, and the opinion of the expert witness emerged as the only significant factors (Kunin, Ebbesen, & Konecni, 1992). This study has particular relevance for those consulting to cases involving infants and young children. In such cases, the first factor is undiscernible, making the expert's recommendations paramount. Taking the significance of this role into account, this chapter addresses issues in divorce and custody from the infant mental health perspective. Given the paucity of data regarding this developmental grouping, however, general principles related to child custody are discussed and, when appropriate, perspectives on infancy are addressed. The constraints of an overview chapter prevent in-depth coverage or exploration of this topic. References are provided for those seeking more detailed examination. This chapter begins with an enumeration of the standards for custody and visitation decisions, proceeds with the literature on the impact of divorce on children, and then addresses the developmental issues in this population. An outline for conducting a child custody evaluation follows. The chapter then addresses the training experiences of family court judges and lawyers, and finally, recommendations to improve the system are offered.

STANDARDS FOR CUSTODY AND VISITATION DECISIONS

Social and legal approaches to custody have changed over the past century. Several paradigm shifts have occurred in response to broad social movements and alterations in family structure. Before the Victorian era, children were viewed as property, and fathers maintained absolute rights for their children. The Victorian image of the child placed new emphasis on the moral and spiritual needs of children and the unique ability of mothers to provide nurturance in these domains. Maternal custody replaced paternal preferences (Shear, 1998), culminating in the "tender years" doctrine, which held that mothers, who were better suited to meet the needs of young children, should be granted custody in divorce disputes. Some have argued that many judges cling to this doctrine, particularly for children under the age of 7 (American Academy of Child and Adolescent Psychiatry, 1997).

The current conceptual model driving custody decisions is "the best interests of the child" (*Finlay v. Finlay,* 1925). This legal test, which placed primary importance on the child's needs, assumed prominence in the 1970s. Many more women were working out of the home, and gender distinctions were becoming less rigidly defined. Fathers sought more intimate relationships with their children and the gender-neutral best interests standard emerged. Distinctions between "custody" and "visitation" diminished as courts and legislatures decided that children should have "frequent and continuing contact" with both parents. The "friendly parent" doctrine guided custody decisions toward the parent most likely to facilitate the child's relationship with the noncustodial parent (Shear, 1998).

Under the best interests standard, which gradually replaced the tender-years doctrine, judges were accorded broader, more discretionary, and more ambiguous latitude. Statutory provisions emphasize an array of factors while still encouraging courts to favor past parental participation in child rearing. Section 402(3) of the Uniform Marriage and Divorce Act (1968) describes one factor for consideration as the "interaction and interrelationship of the child with his parent or parents." On its face, the best interests standard does not require that more weight be given to past parental roles than to other factors. Yet, evidence that mothers still are favored in the majority of cases indicates that past participation in child care is accorded substantial weight (Emery, 1994).

The vulnerability of the best interests standard as a decision rule has been well documented. In brief, the rule seems to attenuate the link between custody and past parental care, laying open ambiguous decision-making rules that are more likely to result in prolonged adversarial conflicts (Pruett & Pruett, 1998a). Goldstein et al. (1973) proposed one solution to the indeterminacy of the best interests standard. They advocate for swift decisions that regard the child's sense of time and, with finality, to preserve caretaking continuity and a child's sense of security. They posit that the goal of custody is to preserve and protect the child's relationship with his or her psychological parent. The proposal has received wide support, but the main controversy surrounding the authors' ideas is the designation of a primary caretaker when parents cannot cooperate, leaving the survival and continuity of the relationship between the child and the noncustodial parent to the primary parent's discretion. Although the proposal makes intuitive and clinical sense, it does not account for situations in which the child has two psychological parents. With some high-conflict couples, supporting the child's continuity with one psychological parent requires supporting permanent discontinuity with the other psychological parent.

The strength of Goldstein et al.'s (1973) proposal regarding custody issues in early childhood lies in its conceptual structure. It follows a developmental framework that emphasizes the nature of time for children, highlights the concept of a psychological parent, and values continuity of caretaking. Swift decisions decrease the potential for protracted periods of stress and adversarial combat, although they create a risk for premature conclusions being drawn from incomplete data.

Concerns about the consequences of an ambiguous standard for father–child relationships have resulted in additional movements in decision making. Father advocates and other concerned individuals spurred the joint custody movement beginning in the 1980s. Joint legal custody literally and symbolically articulates a norm of shared parenting. Many states' custody statutes include a policy statement expressing legislative commitment to joint custody. Although the joint custody presumption corrects for the gender imbalance, it is still used far less than sole custody (Pruett & Pruett, 1998b).

IMPACT OF DIVORCE
ON CHILDREN

The past two decades have witnessed an increase in research on the effects of divorce on children. Most of the research has focused on school-age children and older, with few studies focusing on young children, preschoolers, and, even more rarely, children under 12 months of age. In fact, an exhaustive review of this literature produced only a small handful of studies that examined divorce and its impact on infants. Therefore, we present a review of the literature on divorce in families with older children, with the expectation that the conceptual framework produced by these findings has implications for young children and their families.

In the 1970s and 1980s, the literature on the effect of divorce on children took a narrow view, conceptualizing divorce in a simple cause–effect model. Divorce was conceived as a static concept, without relation to history or present functioning. It was also seen as a unitary concept, one that was equal to all (mothers, fathers, children) in all situations. Early research failed to place children and families in a developmental framework. The divorce itself was stripped of its own longitudinal force. The research seemed to ignore the common finding that divorce usually took longer than 12 months to complete. Using anecdotal, cross-sectional, uncontrolled studies, children from divorced families were found to have a whole range of emotional, behavioral and academic problems when compared to their peers from nondivorced families. Over time, the model has grown and now takes a more complex view of the multiple mediating factors involved. The leading view is that divorce does not invariably or inevitably lead to poor outcome but should be viewed as a family transition or disruption that usually places a child at risk for variable amounts of time (Hetherington & Stanley-Hagan, 1995).

In reviewing the literature on divorce and its effect on children, Kelly (1998) cites conflicting findings. Some studies have found that children are more at risk for disruptive behavior and conduct-related problems, lower academic achievement, and deficits in social relationships. Even in those studies that document differences between these two groups of children, for those from divorced families, the differences are rarely very large and, as a whole, fall in the normal range. Much has been made of the found differences rather than focusing on what is clinically relevant. Following children into adulthood also has documented statistically significant differences, but the effect sizes are generally modest. Gender and age differences also have been explored but, again, with conflicting results. In general, review of the literature does not yield consistent findings, as the studies have used very different methodological approaches: groups sampled, instruments used, definitions of terms, the length of time followed, and the age of children at the time of divorce.

When studying the effect of divorce, many factors play a role in child outcome. It is difficult to tease apart the relative impact of child variables, parent variables, and the quality of marital conflict. Longitudinal studies are required to understand the impact of predivorce variables on postdivorce functioning. Does divorce exacerbate or uncover underlying psychopathology, or do problems emerge de novo as a direct impact of the separation from married parents?

Two longitudinal studies that have examined child, parent, and family factors prior to divorce have led to similar conclusions. In the first, Cherlin et al. (1991) followed a group of children from age 7 to 11 and found that differences in child outcome between children from divorced versus intact families lie in three sources. First, growing up in a dysfunctional family may have a deleterious effect on child development. Second, severe and protracted marital conflict often accompanies the first and takes a toll on young children. A third difference between divorced and nondivorced families is the partner's emotional upset, diminished parenting capacities, and continued conflict that can continue after the separation.

Cherlin et al. (1991) looked at the effects of the marital separation and the conflictual nature of the couple's functioning before the couple considered divorce. Any impact of divorce was diminished once the investigators controlled for behavioral problems, achievement levels, and family difficulties that predated the separation. These effects were true for boys and girls.

The presence of prolonged marital conflict may play a greater role than divorce itself on child outcome. Studies have examined the nature of high-conflict marriages compared to children of divorced families. Psychological adjustment for school-age children was found to be lowest in those with intact, high-conflict marriages, best for those in low-conflict, intact families, whereas children from divorcing families fell in between the other two groups (Emery, 1982; Hetherington, Cox, & Cox, 1982). The literature on children raised in high-

conflict, intact marriages with frequent and chronic expression of high levels of anger are more likely to have difficulties with attention, depression, anxiety, and behavioral problems (Cummings & Davies, 1994). In addition, the children in these families with frequent conflict have been shown to respond with feelings of heightened vulnerability—sadness, distress, helplessness, and anger (Grych & Fincham, 1990). This suggests that the quality of the predivorce marriage plays an important role in child outcome.

Block, Block, and Gjerde (1986, 1988) also conducted a longitudinal study following children and families from early in life, when the child was 3 years old. They detected differences between children from intact versus divorced families beginning at age 3 and up through age 14. At age 3, boys whose families eventually divorced were rated as more inconsiderate and labile. At age 7, boys from predivorce families were rated as more impulsive, aggressive, and energetic. While boys from predivorcing families demonstrated difficulties in the domains of aggression and impulsivity, girls from these families were more likely to demonstrate difficulties with interpersonal relationships. Parent reports in the years prior to divorcing found fathers describing themselves as detached and uninvolved, whereas mothers described themselves as having poor self-esteem and feeling out of control of their lives. Thus, factors prior to the divorce—child measures and parent measures—showed differences between those whose marriages remained intact and those who divorced.

As mentioned previously, few studies have followed families from early in the family's life. Cowan and Cowan (1992) followed families who divorced by the time the children reached age 4. In this study, they found an increase in marital conflict in the first 18 months, with 20% divorcing by the time the children had finished kindergarten. Heinecke, Guthrie, and Ruth (1997) followed a cohort of families, weaving both child and parent variables into a model of postdivorce functioning. Their early reports found that marital adaptation was a powerful predictor of later functioning. Identifying families before the birth of their child, Heinecke et al. showed that the level of post-birth couple adaptation predicted both parents' responsiveness to their infant at 6 months of age. The infants of parents who demonstrated adaptive competence were more secure in their relationship to their parents (Heinicke & Guthrie, 1992). Heinecke concluded that marital adaptation along with the level of child functioning needs to be considered in postdivorce adaptation. Follow-up reports (Heinecke et al., 1997) continued to support their thesis that initial family status predicts the likelihood of divorce and its effects. They linked a "continuing negative marital pattern" to "a tendency for the preschool child to externalize control, and be uncontrolled and antisocial." Highlighting the powerful continuity between early disruptive behavior and later conduct problems, they noted this to be a critical time for intervention.

CASE EXAMPLE: TIME 1

Sole custody of Rebecca age 4 years, 7 months, and Sara aged 2 years, 4 months, was the object of caustic litigation between their parents. A controlling, bitter father and a narcissistic, somewhat paranoid mother, both professionals with sufficient family resources to fuel protracted motion filing and legal wrangling, had kept their fate in limbo from the time Sara had been born. Raucous screaming matches, police callings, and some pushing, shoving, and minor blood letting on both sides, all in regular and full view of the children, had filled both girls with more information about adult troubles than they could possibly manage. Although the parents had eventually separated their residences, access was so embittered that two-thirds of "visitations" somehow failed to happen with either parent as planned.

When the second author saw them for a custody evaluation at the request of the court, Rebecca was initially well related, with a sweet disposition and a slight speech initiation stutter, she poured out her heartache about her parents' fighting. "I try to stop them, but I'm too little, I can't." She broke off eye contact for the rest of the session as she talked about her parents' fighting. "Daddy doesn't poison me, but mommy thinks he does—why? . . . I try to tell mommy nice things about daddy but she yells at me." When she drew a family picture, she drew her father on the reverse side of the paper, after she had drawn herself so close to the mother that the stick figure looked like it had a shadow, not a companion. She told a poignant story about how her father had tried to help her clean her fish tank and lost one of the fish. She found it dried up on the carpet the next day.

Sara spoke well for her age and had good motor control. As she played house between two houses,

she crashed cars repeatedly head-on as they traveled back and forth, crammed full of food, small stuffed animals, and babies. As she repeatedly licked the face of the daddy doll, Rebecca explained, "Every time she goes to daddy's house, 'Saree' licks his face a long time and he giggles." Upon hearing this, Sara elaborated, "I want mommy to live at daddy's house and be nice . . . be nice . . . be nice," her affect draining away like water down a drain.

Research into the effects of divorce, although suggestive of potential risks for children, has produced equivocal findings. The National Child Development Study, a long-term follow-up into adulthood, found a minimal effect of divorce, especially for men (Chase-Lansdale, Cherlin, & Kiernan, 1995). In this study, 94% of men and 82% of women whose parents divorced fell below clinical cutoffs for adult emotional disorders. These findings, if replicated, suggest minimal impact, tremendous recovery, or discontinuity from childhood into adulthood. One study, however, does not answer the important question of long-term effects. Our research methodology, while effective in detecting threshold disorders, may miss more subtle intrapsychic or interpersonal phenomenon.

One area in which research results are not conflicted pertains to family violence. Multiple studies have documented the serious and pervasive problems that characterize children reared in such families (Hughes, 1988; Fantuzzo et al., 1991; Johnston & Campbell, 1993; Jouriles, Norwood, McDonald, Vincent, & Mahoney, 1996). They are more likely to be aggressive, be anxious, have behavioral problems and low self-esteem compared to children who have not witnessed violence, and to approve of violence as a way of resolving conflict (Davies & Cummings, 1994; Grych & Fincham, 1990). The younger the child, the more severe the symptoms. Compared to older children, preschool children have been found to exhibit more behavioral problems, higher levels of distress, and lower self-esteem than school-age children enduring similar circumstances (Fantuzzo et al., 1991; Hughes, 1988). Maltreatment of infants has been linked to disorganized attachment (reviewed in Cicchetti & Toth, 1995), but a recent study suggested that exposure to partner violence alone produces similar disturbances of attachment (Zeanah et al., in press). In addition, children who witness threats to a caregiver are more likely exhibit aggressive behavior, fear, and symptoms of hyperarousal than exposure to other types of trauma (Scheeringa & Zeanah, 1995).

CASE EXAMPLE: TIME 2

Sara, when she was about 22 months old, following yet another separation of her warring parents, began to grab her mother's small calico cat by the neck and squeeze as she gritted her teeth excitedly and growled. Sometimes she screamed "Stop it, stop it . . . no no!," until Rebecca intervened. The mother thought "it was cute," but Sara's intensity and behavior scared Rebecca, and she often cried or hit Sara afterward. Given Sara's age, it was hard to differentiate the developmentally expected inability to appreciate the cat as an animate object from a possible enactment of domestic violence.

When consulting on issues of violence to the courts, physical safety must be the top priority. In a finding reported by two separate investigators, the incidence of violence increases after separation. Separated battered women have been found to be battered 14 times as often than battered women who remain with their partners (Lieberman & Van Horn, 1998). In addition, 70% of the violence reported by battered women occurred after the separation (Lieberman & Van Horn, 1998).

Few studies have looked at the impact of divorce on infants or preschool children. The impact on toddlers was explored in one study that found that children reared in high-conflict families compared to those from low-conflict families are more likely to develop insecure attachments to their parents (Kelly, 1998). In reviewing the literature on divorce, Kelly (1998) concluded that in general, most children do not assume responsibility for causing the divorce. This is more likely to happen when parents provide adequate, age-appropriate explanations. Those at risk for taking the blame are preschool children, those with psychological vulnerability, and those in homes in which marital conflicts have centered on the children.

What about the effect of divorce on parents? On the one hand, the parent has potentially severed a relationship that was the cause of great distress, leading to relief and personal satisfaction at overcoming a challenging situation. Alternatively, the parent might feel spurned, jealous, and angry. A third possibility is a mixture of intense positive and negative feelings. Given the complexity of human nature, a "typical" portrait of the divorced parent is difficult to design. It is likely that the nature of the divorce, the level of pre- and postdivorce conflict, will be predictors of parental outcomes.

CASE EXAMPLE: TIME 3

One year after the final divorce decree, which occurred 2 months after the psychiatrist's report was submitted to the court, just before the case was scheduled for trial, both parents were interviewed separately as part of a research protocol. The diminished capacity to parent, so painfully obvious in both parents during the maelstrom of their litigation, had eased noticeably. The violence and nearly unbearable tension and suspiciousness had softened, and they tolerated weekly 15-minute phone calls in which they discussed the children's development, health, social needs, and so on. They had each fired their lawyers and were using a collaborator of one of the authors as a conflict resolution consultant. Both parents expressed guilt over the havoc they wrought in their children's lives, albeit with different levels of awareness and remorse. Their denial, however, urges them to minimize their appreciation for the ongoing risk in their children's lives regarding impulse control, trust, and developing empathy.

Divorce has been shown to have several short-term effects. Parents have been found to be more vulnerable to physical and psychological disorders in the year following divorce (Hetherington & Stanley-Hagen, 1995). Other early symptoms include problems with depression, anxiety, and behavioral control. These early effects are replaced by more optimistic later adjustments. In a fairly consistent finding, 2 years after divorce, 75% of women are happier than in their last year of marriage, and most find it easier, although stressful, to be rearing their children alone. However, feelings of anger and resentment continue, and 25% remain in conflicted parenting relationships (Hetherington, 1993). The main mediators of positive, postdivorce outcomes for women include financial security, job satisfaction, neutral or positive relationships with ex-spouses, and forming new, intimate relationships (Hetherington & Stanley-Hagen, 1995). Research on psychological effects of divorce on fathers lags significantly behind similar research with mothers.

To evaluate divorce as a risk factor, it needs to be placed in the context of prior and ongoing parental harmony/disharmony and functioning because these variables more reliably predict outcome. The parenting environment creates the frame for child development and the structure around which children thrive and adapt or succumb to the effects of parental strife. The stability in the parent's relationship before and after the divorce, the ability of parents to maintain cooperative and invested relationships with each other and their children, and the quality of children's relationship with stepparents all lead to normal adjustment (Hetherington & Stanley-Hagen, 1995). Divorce becomes less of a risk factor and more of a conduit for a complexity of risk factors. For some children, as well as for parents, divorce is a welcome relief to the storm that filled their lives. In fact, the literature demonstrates consistently that most children from divorced families do not display enduring behavioral problems.

DEVELOPMENTAL ISSUES

A recent review of the literature on infant development proposed three major biobehavioral shifts in the first 3 years of life (Zeanah, Boris, & Larrieu, 1997). These three periods of qualitative reorganization occur at ages 2–3 months, 7–9 months, and 18–20 months. Observable, qualitative changes occur in multiple domains—regulatory, cognitive, emotional, communicative, and social development. Contrasting with these qualitative shifts are quantitative developmental advances that occur in between these time frames. A familiarity with these periods of developmental activity and quiescence may aid custody evaluations with infants and young children.

The hallmark of development in the first 12 months of life is the establishment of a stable attachment relationship with significant caregivers in the child's life. Bowlby (1969/1982) theorized that the attachment system, which serves to promote proximity to the caregiver, is based on evolutionary needs to protect the infant from external dangers. In his view, the caregiver serves as a secure base from which the infant can explore the world and to which the infant retreats to maintain security from environmental threats. Attachment represents individual differences in how infants regulate emotions and behaviors vis-à-vis their primary caregivers (Cicchetti, Rogosch, & Toth, 1997). Attachment styles organize evolving affective states, cognition, and behavior (Sroufe, 1979), while the nurturing domain also shapes underlying patterns of physiological regulation (Gun-

nar & Nelson, 1994; Hofer, 1987). The pattern of attachment that evolves represents and reflects the quality of the relationship between primary caregiver and infant. The caregiver's physical and emotional availability, as well as his or her sensitivity and responsiveness, contribute to the individual differences in the ways infants negotiate attachment relationships.

The infant's capacity for memory, ability to hold another in mind, and development of the capacity to internalize representations, which then guide relational styles, are all in evolution in the first few years of life. Parents serve as regulators of these multiple levels of functioning (Lyons-Ruth & Zeanah, 1993). The stress of divorce contributes to a diminished capacity to parent (Wallerstein & Blakeslee, 1989). How divorce and custody proceedings influence these levels [1] of development is not fully understood. Several salient features of infant development, however, should be accounted for in a custody evaluation. First, infants have tremendous needs that change over time. Initially, feeding, protection from danger, state regulation, and relief from distress (hunger, pain, internal discomfort) predominate. These parenting functions persist, though in somewhat altered forms, as the parent accommodates to the growing infant. Social and cognitive stimulation begins at birth but assumes greater importance over the first year of life. Second, the need for caretaking continuity over time is paramount. While the capacity for resilience in the face of alternative caregivers has been demonstrated (National Institute of Child Health and Human Development [NICHD] Early Child Care Research Network, 1998), poor care coupled with insensitive mothering has been found to be predictive of poor outcome (NICHD Early Child Care Research Network, 1997). Third, an infant's sense of time differs from that of an adult. It is unusual for a coherent sense of time to develop before the end of preschool. The typical time frame to complete a custody proceeding exceeds the capacity of a young child's comprehension.

TESTIFYING AND ETHICAL ISSUES IN CHILD CUSTODY PROCEDURES

Serving as an expert witness raises many issues for the clinician. The ingredients that make for competent clinical practice are not always successful on the witness stand and vice versa. The careful, thoughtful deliberation, use of empathic responses, clinical curiosity, and shared mission to understand strength and vulnerability do not always serve one well when testifying. It is the unusual clinical situation that becomes adversarial. The ways in which the court process evolves—confrontational, requiring quick, terse responses, not having all the data, testifying in a vacuum, the process of direct and cross-examination (see Table 35.1)—is foreign to the general practitioner. The languages rarely overlap.

Four specific principles of providing expert testimony in custody cases have been described by the second author elsewhere and include (Pruett & Solnit, 1998): (1) maintain a distinction between professionally informed opinion and personally held value preference, (2) resist the temptation to exceed one's authority or competence on a given question, (3) avoid serving as both evaluator and therapist, and (4) understand the boundary between the clinically informed expert witness and arbiter of fact.

There is a critical distinction between the expert witness and the witness of fact. Witnesses providing fact testimony usually have a standing in the case. They may be subpoenaed because of information they might have acquired or generated in the course of routine practice. Very often, witnesses of fact need to have counsel themselves.

TABLE 35.1. Contrasting Roles For Clinicians and Expert Witnesses

Clinical situation	Custody hearing
Collaborative	Adversarial
Thoughtful responses valued	Rapid response to questioning
Complete data available to clinician	Limited data
Confidential atmosphere	Open system
Therapist as facilitator	Therapist as follower, responder
Focus on healing	Competitive focus
Limited variables	Unlimited variables (judge, lawyers, calendar)
Facilitating decisions	"Decision maker"
Understanding, knowledge valued	Presentation, persuasiveness valued

The expert witness, however, is selected because of a proven competence as a practitioner, researcher, or scientist. Unlike witnesses of fact, the expert witness is called on to address larger medical or scientific issues. Experts are chosen with an eye toward their knowledge base and skill, as well as an expectation that they do not have any standing in the case. Among groups of well-trained clinicians or researchers, attorneys are less likely to select witnesses based on accomplishments. Rather, they will choose "the most articulate, understandable, predictable, and persuasive expert ... whose presentation and interpretation of the data is most supportive to the attorney's case" (Sales & Shulman, 1993, p. 225). In selecting an expert witness, more value is often placed on performance in court, than on who is the better scientist.

When clinicians are brought in for fact testimony, they are fulfilling their role as advocates for the patient. This is best accomplished by giving factual accounts and avoiding the tendency to espouse opinions. The expert witness, on the other hand, does not represent the patient; rather, he or she is there to testify to fact, opinion, and truth. According to Schetky (1998), "the guiding ethical principals for a forensic evaluation are truthfulness, compassion, and respect for patients."

These differences highlight the danger involved in serving dual roles of clinician and evaluator, particularly in child custody matters. Multiple temptations wait for the witness: stretching the science to fit the problem, overstepping boundaries, blurring boundaries between clinician and evaluator, assuming an overly didactic style, failing to constrain empathy, and turning the relationship into a therapeutic encounter.

The legal process itself is often frustrating for the developmental clinician. The adversarial nature of the process, which attempts to polarize the witness's opinion, might influence and distort an expert's neutrality. The witness might find themselves identifying with one party over the other. Clinicians who are comfortable when placed in the position of child advocate must temper their reactions during the court proceedings. The witness may find that while they are interested in the child's developmental needs, the parents' competing needs will sway the court's decision. The clinician also needs to be conscious of potential biases toward different lifestyles, sexual orientation, paternal custody, and economic or racial issues. In addition, clinicians should be relatively free of personal boundary issues, such as being concurrently (especially if conflictually) involved in their own divorce or legal proceedings, as well as professional boundary issues, such as potential social or professional contact with the parties involved.

The clinical encounter in custody cases differs from therapeutic encounters in many ways. The purpose of a clinical examination in the child placement process is to answer questions posed by the court or counsel, not those generated from a clinical referral (Goldstein, Solnit, & Freud, 1979). The clinical interview is nonconfidential and is often not voluntary for the parties involved. The data are handled differently as well. Unlike the clinical situation in which the therapist weighs each piece of information on the scale of neutrality, the legal team's goal is to win the case. Subsequently, attorneys will maximize data supportive to their case and minimize data that conflict with their theory (Holden, 1989). All these factors construct a frame with few similarities to the standard clinical interview. Given the complexities outlined previously, for the clinical trainee or the clinician with limited experience as an expert witness, supervision becomes essential for developing competence and providing effective, informed, and ethical testimony (Pruett & Solnit, 1998). In addition, the American Academy of Child and Adolescent Psychiatry (1997) recently released a set of practice parameters for child custody evaluation. Highlights of these parameters are presented here, and they helped to inform one perspective in preparing this chapter.

Special Issues in Court Work

1. *Setting fees.* It is important to make clear to the attorney that payment is for time and expertise, not a partisan opinion. Most agree that contracting for the fee prior to initiating a custody consultation protects the objectivity (and integrity) of the expert (Melton, Petrilla, & Poythress, 1987; Pruett & Solnit, 1998). It is not that uncommon for a party to terminate services if the expert's conclusions do not support the attorney's case.

2. *Report writing.* The goal of the report is to answer directly and succinctly the specific questions posed by the legal process. To conduct a thorough evaluation and complete a written report, the expert must have access to all available relevant data. While experts use varying styles in report writing, we tailor our reports to the legal situation. The report is fact based, making clear the number and types of encounters, the sources of information, a summary of all assessment instruments used or observational techniques employed, an assessment of overall developmental and psychological functioning, and, most important, how the clinical material informed the decision-making process. Data must support the conclusions and recommendations. The style should be clear and nonjudgmental.

3. *Testifying.* The pitfalls of testifying in court have been well described by Haas (1993) and include arrogance, advocating, and ignorance regarding the judicial process. Pruett and Solnit (1998) added two important measures of competence for court work: "acknowledging the limits of knowledge and the awareness of strongly held value preferences" (p. 132).

Special Issues in Custody Evaluations with Infants and Young Children

1. While the measures for assessing parental competence and children's attachments are sparse, the measures for young children are even less objective.

2. In making custodial decisions, it is commonplace to ask the older child for his or her residential preference. This procedure is precluded by the cognitive capacities of infants and toddlers. The evaluator is forced to rely on observed patterns of attachment to assess how each parent meets his or her child's needs.

3. Fathers and mothers often serve very different functions for their children (Pruett, 1987). Experts need to be aware of their biases regarding appropriate parent–infant interaction when conducting evaluations. Fathers are more likely to engage in rough-and-tumble play with their young children, whereas mothers tend to assume caregiving roles. Maternal play is more often verbal, didactic, and toy mediated (Parke, 1995). This pattern holds for very young infants as well as for older preschoolers (MacDonald & Parke, 1986). Infants learn these patterns early. They elicit and seek out different behaviors; it has been shown that infants prefer to be picked up by fathers, most likely because fathers pick up children to engage in physical activity rather than for caretaking responsibilities (Parke, 1995). If the well-intentioned evaluator is look-

ing for the "nurturing" parent, he or she should know what is being nurtured and how the nurturing is taking place. Mothers and fathers nurture different components of development.

4. Developmental change is greatest in the period from birth to 3 years. Another factor that should be examined is whether the parent has expressed preferences for different-age children. Some parents prefer and are more competent with infants and toddlers, whereas others find comfort and confidence with school-age children. Interactions that appear rigid or less mutually enjoyable might soften and evolve as the child ages and vice versa. Though the evaluator should be aware of these developmental processes in parenting, the usual goal is to assess the current situation based on history and presentation.

5. Whether to conduct a developmental evaluation is an important question. Developmental evaluations are not mandatory during the custody evaluation. If there is any suspicion for even mild developmental delay, an evaluation is indicated. Regardless of the need for a developmental assessment, the process of conducting an evaluation, which requires parental presence, provides information beyond the child's developmental level. Because the stated focus of a developmental evaluation is on the child, the parent will experience less pressure than a traditional "parent–child interaction." Alternating the presence of each parent permits the consultant to assess the parent's conduct during a structured experience. The consultant may observe the way in which the child uses the parent's presence, the way in which the parent responds to the testing and their child's overtures, the way in which the parents understand their child, manage the information, and incorporate the results into their concept of their child's expectations and needs.

6. Observational data are essential. A key component of the early childhood custody evaluation is the nature of the attachment relationship. Infants form separate and distinct attachments to their mothers and fathers (Steele, Steele, & Fonagy, 1996). Attachments are bidirectional, and observing the relationship over one or two sessions will inform the evaluator as to the degree of attachment from parent to infant and infant to parent. A mixture of structured and unstructured observations is most effective for identifying the salient features of the relationship. Zeanah, Larrieu, Heller, and Valliere (Chapter 13, this volume) have formalized

a set of observational procedures for the evaluating child–caregiver relationships from ages 12 to 54 months. Unfortunately, in the name of assessing "attachment," some evaluators artificially induce a separation from the parents in order to "rate" the attachment. It is fairly clear that the classic attachment paradigm is not a useful clinical procedure, as it is intentionally artificial in structure and requires extensive training to draw conclusions from the observations (Crowell & Fleischmann, 1993).

Unstructured play sessions, observed through a one-way mirror if possible, provide the most direct information regarding attachment. The setting can be the evaluator's consultation room or in the home. The results often surprise; the evaluator must separate his or her reactions from the informational session and observe with neutrality. A parent who is highly verbal and describes a coherent portrait of his or her child's development and needs might not have a psychological or emotional connection with his or her infant. On the other hand, the less verbal parent who presents poorly in the information-gathering stage of the evaluation may be exquisitely attuned to their child's inner world, anticipating needs and meeting expectations.

CHALLENGES TO THE EXPERT WITNESS: TRAINING ISSUES IN THE LEGAL SYSTEM

To understand the context of the legal proceedings, a brief review of the background, training, and orientation of the professionals involved follows. The training of family law judicial officers and family court practitioners is variable. Few specialize in family law; most who practice family law are generalists. In general, the legal professionals who are involved in making decisions regarding custody and divorce have little or no family law experience. Even fewer have any training in child development (Shear, 1998).

Kass (1998) has provided a useful review of legal issues in custody cases. Her main points are summarized later. The traditional legal process is fault based, with investigations geared to assign responsibility, resulting in a polarized process. An underlying assumption in most judicial proceedings is that the parties have no shared future and may have no further contact. As Kass describes, these principles run counter to the goals of promoting healthy family development and serve to increase conflict, diminishing prospects for reasonable solutions. Another complicating factor is that family relationships are universal. Judges and lawyers have all been in families, and many will have been affected by divorce either as children or as spouses. Legal professionals involved in family law expose themselves to personal biases and place themselves at risk of emotional entanglements if they are unable to examine their own beliefs and attitudes regarding family life.

The ambiguity in the law regarding "best interests," as described previously, further facilitates judges relying on personal preferences rather than objective criteria and empirical data. Unlike most other areas of law, such as contract disputes, which require black-and-white, right-versus-wrong thinking, family law is nonlinear, uncertain, and subject to swings in social fashion. Judges may respond to this situation of uncertainty by adopting a set of rules that are applied regardless of the age of the child (e.g., always granting equal amounts of time to each parent). Finally, boundary issues are managed differently in the legal profession. Conflicts of interest, which are a central concern for mental health professionals, are not prohibited or discouraged. Lawyers may represent family members, colleagues, or people in their social world. Kass (1998) describes lawyers and judges who assume the role of rescuer and avengers, by "doing for someone what they can and should do for themselves and giving people what we think they deserve instead of what they need" (p. 252).

On the other hand, legal professionals involved in family law are often hungry for and appreciative of expert opinion. This has particular relevance for early childhood. Nonverbal, nonwalking infants are difficult for nonprofessionals to assess. Although the courts might have moved beyond the tender years doctrine, it has left the legal system without much structure to determine the best interests or the least detrimental alternative for young children. Lawyers and experts have relied on degrees of attachment to determine custody arrangements but the Ainsworth-attached child and the clinically attached child are not always reconcilable. Broader developmental concepts need to be infused into the custody process. Mental health consultants who provide coherent, jargon-free information regarding child development and its utility for a custody proceeding frequently find their opinions respected and followed. Adopting a nonpatronizing tone will enhance the educative nature of these consultations.

NEW DIRECTIONS: PARENTING PLANS

In recent years, advocates for change in family law practice have implemented several programs and paradigm shifts in their approach to custody decisions. Two of these approaches include the formation of parenting plans and mediation to solve disputes. With the acknowledgment that children's needs might be best served with continuity of contact with both parents, joint custody has become the preferred arrangement in many states. This reframing of custody decisions has not been without problems. The notion that both parents in postdivorce families should play active roles in child rearing, although appropriate, is often difficult to implement. The custody question has been changed from *who* will raise a child to *how* will both parents be involved (Shear, 1998).

The concept of a parenting plan has been replacing the term "joint custody." Shared parenting emphasizes parental roles and responsibilities over child ownership (Pruett & Hoganbruen, 1998). Detailed, court-ordered parenting plans serve as a template for complementary parenting arrangements. They are court ordered, signed by a judge and legally enforceable. Plans can formalize expectations, concretize understandings, and help decrease the need for continual renegotiation. Shared parenting plans should have the following features: (1) the language is understandable and unambiguous, (2) the terms balance flexibility with certainty, (3) the child's social and peer worlds are incorporated, (4) clear indications for modifications are included, (5) guidelines for how the parents will exchange information are established, (6) the authority for decision making is defined, and (7) mechanisms for review and adaptation are included (Shear, 1998). The research on parenting plans or joint legal custody has found some advantages, but the major findings indicate that moderating variables in the family play a greater role than any particular custody arrangement (Pruett & Hoganbruen, 1998).

RECOMMENDATIONS

There is great distress with the current way in which the legal system becomes involved with familial disputes. Situations of high conflict are usually fueled by the legal system, exacerbating tensions and decreasing parental functioning.

As mental health professionals, we can make a difference in setting the tone, establishing policy, and effecting change. Consultation to a range of society's institutions (schools, hospitals, residential treatment centers) is a significant area of expertise for our profession. Given the number of children affected by divorce and custody proceedings, active efforts are required to make an impact. Seven areas of change are recommended and include the following (Pruett & Pruett, 1998a):

1. A simpler, shorter, and less expensive legal process.
2. A process guided by a family focus, with emphasis on varying needs within families.
3. A more collaborative process that reduces the adversarial nature of divorce.
4. Involving the children in the process. Tell them who the people are who entered their lives during the divorce, explain what the divorce is within developmentally appropriate limits, and listen to what they are trying to tell the adults in their lives.
5. Connect parents' own language and goals to those used by legal personnel.
6. Families need information that helps them set realistic expectations, and makes the divorce understandable to parents and children.
7. Specialized training for judges and attorneys is an area in need of augmentation.

Future Research Agenda

The burning questions regarding child custody still hover around visitation and custody in the first years of life. The last two decades have seen a slow but steady increase in the quality of research on the impact of divorce on the young child as well as on the vital relationships to significant objects in their lives. Although methodological constraints still hobble some of the findings, several researchers have produced work of quality significant enough to draw the attention of policymakers and the judiciary. Judith Solomon's prospective studies of the effect of overnight visitation on toddlers' and preschoolers' attachment behaviors are examples of sophisticated clinical research with significant policy implications (Solomon & George, 1996; Solomon, in press).

The *Culture of Litigation Project,* directed by M. Kline Pruett and K. Pruett, has taken clinical findings from 20 families who had recently undergone divorce proceedings and investigated the perceptions of young children (2 years, nine months to 5 years), their mothers, and their fathers (and their lawyers) regarding the effect of divorce litigation and proceedings on their family and, possibly more significant, their relationships with each other (Pruett & Pruett, 1998a). The compelling findings led to an intervention to be tested on a large scale. The design proposes to reduce the morbidity of divorce on the capacity to parent appropriately and feel appropriately parented during and after divorce. Other reports by Howes and Markman (1989) and Hetherington (1989) also contribute increasing wisdom to the clinical realm of decision making regarding the early years.

Decision makers such as judges, magistrates, and special masters turn to clinicians repeatedly for advice regarding their custody decisions for young children. The following presents a preliminary list of clinical questions that require empirical attention:

1. How much contact should a noncustodial parent have with the 6-, 12-, 18-, or 24-month-old infant/toddler? With a previously involved parent? With a previously uninvolved parent?
2. Does such contact appreciably change the infant's attachment to either the custodial or noncustodial parent?
3. What constitutes a meaningful, if not necessarily "attachment," relationship under such circumstances, and what are the long- or short-term effects on the principals involved?
4. For children 3 years or younger whose parents have moved significant distances apart, who does the traveling, for how long, and how far, without paying too heavy a price?
5. What are the warning signs that a young child is not coping well, or at all, with what is so often a brokered agreement, and what are the least intrusive mediating steps to correct the problem?

Clinicians (including us), have their prejudices regarding the answers to such crucial and relevant questions, but the research base to support that advice remains worrisomely small. Nevertheless, thoughtful attempts at proposing developmentally appropriate guidelines have become available, such as the *Child Centered*

Residential Schedules, compiled by the Spokane County Bar Association (Hoffman, Etter, Thomar, Iverson, & Jorgensen, 1996).

CONCLUSIONS

Understanding the process of divorce as it relates to infants is complicated, on one hand, by the rapidity of development that occurs in the first years of life and, on the other, by the lack of communication skills. Infant reactions are inferred, perceived, observed, and, by definition, subjective. The tools one uses with older children are not applicable to the youngest children. Broad principles of child development—continuity, predictability, the importance of attachment, and psychological parents—suffice in the absence of empirical data. More research on the impact of divorce, marital conflict, and the effects of various custodial arrangements is needed. More education of and collaboration with our colleagues in the legal profession is indicated. If we extrapolate downward from school-age children, we would hypothesize that the combination of ongoing marital conflict, violence, and economic stress with divorce is a more powerful risk factor than divorce alone. In fact, the literature suggests that divorce is not always a negative experience for families. Divorce often decreases pressures and preoccupations, freeing up the nurturing domain in either or both parents. It is the nurturing domain that needs to be supported and protected, whether parents remain together or separate.

REFERENCES

American Academy of Child and Adolescent Psychiatry. (1997). Child custody evaluations. *Journal of the American Academy of Child and Adolescent Psychiatry, 36*, 57S–68S.

Block, J. H., Block, J., & Gjerde, P. F. (1986). The personality of children prior to divorce: A prospective study. *Child Development, 57*, 827–840.

Block, J., Block, J. H., & Gjerde, P. F. (1988). Parental functioning and the home environment in families of divorce: Prospective and concurrent analyses. *Journal of the American Academy of Child and Adolescent Psychiatry, 27*, 207–213.

Bowlby, J. (1982). *Attachment and loss. Vol. 1: Attachment.* New York: Basic Books. (Original work published 1969)

Bumpass, L. L., Sweet, J. A., & Castro-Martin, T. (1990). Changing patterns of remarriage. *Journal of Marriage and the Family, 52*, 747–756.

Castro-Martin, T., & Bumpass, L. (1989). Recent trends and differentials in marital disruption. *Demography, 26*, 37–51.

Chase-Lansdale, P. L., Cherlin, A. J., & Kiernan, K. E. (1995). The long-term effects of parental divorce on the mental health of young adults: A developmental perspective. *Child Development, 66*, 1614–1634.

Cherlin, A. J., Furstenburg, F. F., Chase-Lonsdale, P. L., Kiernan, K. E., Robins, P. K., Morrison, D. R., & Teitler, J. O. (1991). Longitudinal studies of effects of divorce in children in Great Britain and the United States. *Science, 252*, 1386–1389.

Cicchetti, D., Rogosch, F. A., & Toth, S. L. (1997). Ontogenesis, depressotypic organization, and the depressive spectrum. In S. S. Luthar, J. A. Burack, D. Cicchetti, & J. R. Weisz. (Eds.), *Developmental psychopathology* (pp. 273–313). Cambridge: Cambridge University Press.

Cicchetti, D., & Toth, S. L. (1995). A developmental psychopathology perspective on child abuse and neglect. *Journal of the American Academy of Child and Adolescent Psychiatry, 34*, 541–565.

Cowan, C. P. & Cowan, P. A. (1992). *When partners become parents.* New York: Basic Books.

Crowell, J. A. & Fleischmann, M. A. (1993). Use of structured research procedures in clinical assessments of infants. In C. H. Zeanah, Jr. (Ed.), *Handbook of infant mental health* (pp. 210–221). New York: Guilford Press.

Cummings, E. M., & Davies, P. T. (1994). *Children and marital conflict: The impact of family dispute and resolution.* New York: Guilford Press.

Davies, P. T., & Cummings, E. M. (1994). Marital conflict and child adjustment: An emotional security hypothesis. *Psychological Bulletin, 16*, 387–411.

Emery, R. E. (1982). Interparental conflict and the children of discord and divorce. *Psychological Bulletin, 92*, 310–325.

Emery, R. E. (1994). *Renegotiating family relationships: Divorce, child custody, and mediation.* New York: Guilford Press.

Fantuzzo, J. W., DePaoia, L. M., Lambert L., Martino, T., Anderson, G., & Sutton, S. (1991). Effects of interparental violence on the psychological adjustment and competencies of young children. *Journal of Consulting and Clinical Psychology, 59*, 258–265.

Finlay v. Finlay, 148 N.E. 624 (New York 1925).

Glick, P. C., & Lin, S. (1986). Recent changes in divorce and remarriage. *Journal of Marriage and the Family, 48*, 737–747.

Goldstein, J., Solnit, A. J., & Freud, A. (1973). *Beyond the best interests of the child.* New York: Free Press.

Goldstein, J., Solnit, A. J., & Freud, A. (1979). *Before the best interests of the child.* New York: Free Press.

Gunnar, M., & Nelson, C. A. (1994). Event-related potentials in year-old infants: Relations with emotionality and cortisol. *Child Development, 65*, 80–94.

Grych, J. H., & Fincham, F. D. (1990). Marital conflict and children's adjustment: A cognitive–contextual framework. *Psychological Bulletin, 108*, 267–290.

Haas, L. J. (1993). Competence and quality in the performance of forensic psychologists. *Ethics and Behavior, 3*, 251–266.

Heinecke, M. H., & Guthrie, D. G. (1992). Stability and change in husband–wife adaptation, and the development of the positive parent–child relationship. *Infant Behavior and Development*, *15*, 109–127.

Heinecke, M. H., Guthrie, D. G., & Ruth, G. (1997). Marital adaptation, divorce, and parent–infant development: a prospective study. *Infant Mental Health Journal*, *18*, 282–299.

Hetherington, E. M. (1989). Coping with family transitions: Winners, losers, and survivors. *Child Development, 60,* 1–14.

Hetherington, E. M. (1993). An overview of the Virginia longitudinal study of divorce and remarriage with a focus on early adolescence. *Journal of Family Psychology*, *7*, 1–18.

Hetherington, E. M., Cox, M. J., & Cox, R. (1982). Effects of divorce on parents and children. In E. M. Lamb (Ed.), *Non-traditional families* (pp. 233–288). Hillsdale, NJ: Erlbaum.

Hetherington, E. M., & Stanley-Hagan, M. M. (1995). Parenting in divorced and remarried families. In M. Bornstein (Ed.), *Handbook of parenting* (pp. 233–254). Hillsdale, NJ: Erlbaum.

Hofer, M. A. (1987). Early social relationships: A psychobiologist's view. *Child Development, 58,* 633–647.

Hoffman, K., Etter, P., Thomar, C., Iverson, M., & Jorgensen, C. (1996). *Child centered residential schedules.* Spokane, WA: Spokane County Bar Association.

Holden, C. (1989). Science in court. *Science, 243,* 1658–1659.

Howes, P., & Markman, H. (1989). Marital quality and child functioning: A longitudinal investigation. *Child Development, 60,* 1044–1055.

Hughes, H. M. (1988). Psychological and behavioral correlates of family violence in child witnesses and victims. *American Journal of Orthopsychiatry, 18,* 77–90.

Johnston, J., & Campbell, L. (1993). A clinical typology of interparental violence in disputed-custody divorces. *American Journal of Orthopsychiatry, 63,* 90–112.

Jouriles, E., Norwood, W., McDonald, R., Vincent, J. P., & Mahoney, A. (1996). Physical violence and other forms of marital aggression: Links with children's behavior problems. *Journal of Family Psychology, 10,* 223–237.

Kass, A. (1998). Clinical advice from the bench. *Child and Adolescent Psychiatric Clinics of North America, 7,* 247–257.

Kelly, J. B. (1998). Marital conflict, divorce, and children's adjustment. *Child and Adolescent Psychiatric Clinics of North America, 7,* 259–272.

Kunin, C. C., Ebbesen, E. B., & Konecni, V. J. (1992). An archival study of decision making in child custody disputes. *Journal of Clinical Psychology, 48,* 564–573.

Lieberman, A. F., & Van Horn, P. (1998). Attachment, trauma, and domestic violence: Implications for child custody. *Child and Adolescent Psychiatric Clinics of North America, 7,* 423–443.

Lyons-Ruth, K., & Zeanah, C. H., Jr. (1993). The family context of infant mental health: I. Affective development in the primary caregiving relationship. In C. H. Zeanah, Jr. (Ed.), *Handbook of infant mental health* (pp. 14–37). New York: Guilford Press.

MacDonald, K., & Parke, R. D. (1986). Parent–child physical play: The effects of sex and age of children and parents. *Sex Roles, 7–8,* 367–379.

Melton, G., Petrilla, J., & Poythress, N. G. (1987). Consultation, report writing and expert testimony. *Psychological evaluations for the court* (pp. 347–371). New York: Guilford Press.

National Institute of Child Health and Human Development Early Child Care Research Network. (1997). The effects of infant child care on infant–mother attachment security: Results of the NICHD Study of Early Child Care. *Child Development, 68,* 860–879.

National Institute of Child Health and Human Development Early Child Care Research Network. (1998). Early child care and self-control, compliance, and problem behavior at twenty-four and thirty-six months. *Child Development, 69,* 1145–1170.

Parke, R. D. (1995). Fathers and families. In M. Bornstein (Ed*.), Handbook of parenting (*pp. 27–63). Hillsdale, NJ: Erlbaum.

Pruett, K. D. (1987). *The nurturing father.* New York: Warner.

Pruett, K. D., & Solnit, A. J. (1998). Psychological and ethical considerations in the preparation of the mental health professional as expert witness. In S. J. Ceci & H. Hembrooke (Eds.), *Expert witnesses in child abuse cases* (pp. 123–135). Washington, DC: American Psychological Association.

Pruett, M. K., & Hoganbruen, K. (1998). Joint custody and shared parenting: Research and interventions. *Child and Adolescent Psychiatric Clinics of North America, 7,* 273–294.

Pruett, M. K., & Pruett, K. D. (1998a). *Divorce in legal context: outcomes for children.* Westport CT: Smith-Richardson Foundation.

Pruett, M. K., & Pruett, K. D. (1998b). Fathers, divorce and their children. *Child and Adolescent Psychiatric Clinics of North America, 7,* 389–407.

Sales, B. D., & Shulman, D. W. (1993). Reclaiming the integrity of science in expert witnessing. *Ethics and Behavior, 3–4,* 223–229.

Scheeringa, M. S., & Zeanah, C. H. (1995). Symptom expression and trauma variables in children under 48 months of age. *Infant Mental Health Journal, 16,* 259–271.

Schetky, D. H. (1998). Ethics and the clinician in custody disputes. *Child and Adolescent Psychiatric Clinics of North America, 7,* 455–463.

Shear, L. E. (1998). From competition to complementarity: legal issues and their clinical implications in custody. *Child and Adolescent Psychiatric Clinics of North America, 7,* 311–334.

Solomon, J. (in press). Parenting schedules for the very young child: Summary of a longitudinal study on the development of attachment in separated and divorced families. *Attachment and Human Development, 1*(1).

Solomon, J., & George, C. (1996, April). *The effects on attachment of overnight visitation in divorced and separated families.* Paper presented at the biennial meeting of the International Conference on Infant Studies, Providence, RI.

Sroufe, L. A. (1979). The coherence of individual development: Early care attachment and subsequent developmental issues. *American Psycholoigst, 34,* 834–841.

Steele, H., Steele, M., & Fonagy, P. (1996). Associations among attachment classifications in mothers, fathers and their infants. *Child Development, 67,* 541–555.

Uniform Marriage and Divorce Act, 9A U.L.A.561 (1968).

U. S. Bureau of the Census. (1992). *Studies in marriage and the family: Married couple families with children* (Current Population Reports, Series P–23, No. 162). Washington, DC: U. S. Government Printing Office.

Wallerstein, J. S., & Blakeslee, S. (1989). *Second chances.* New York: Ticknor & Fields.

Yogman, M. W., Cooley, J., & Kindlon, D. (1988). Fathers, infants and toddlers: A developing relationship. In P. Bronstein & C. Cowan (Eds.), *Fatherhood today: Men's changing role in the family.* New York: Wiley.

Zeanah, C. H., Boris, N. W., & Larrieu, J. A. (1997). Infant development and developmental risk: A review of the past 10 years. *Journal of the American Academy of Child and Adolescent Psychiatry, 36,* 165–178.

Zeanah, C. H., Danis, B., Hirshberg, L., et al. (in press). Disorganized attachment associated with partner violence: A brief report. *Infant Mental Health Journal.*

36

Training in Infant Mental Health

❖

PAULA DOYLE ZEANAH
JULIE A. LARRIEU
CHARLES H. ZEANAH, JR.

The knowledge base and clinical applications of infant mental health have expanded rapidly in the past two decades. The short- and long-term ramifications of ensuring or failing to ensure the physical, social, and emotional health and well-being of our youngest children are receiving the urgent attention of researchers and clinicians across diverse fields, as well as social policy planners around the world.

Still, little has been written about training in infant mental health. The field is young, and many of its senior practitioners are self-trained rather than graduates of any formal programs. On the other hand, Fraiberg's training program in Michigan began over 25 years ago, and Zero to Three, the National Center for Infants and Families (formerly the National Center for Clinical Infant Programs), has sponsored enrichment fellowships for professionals from different disciplines almost continually since 1981. In addition, there appears to us be an unprecedented interest in infant mental health across many disciplines. All this suggests that a consideration of training issues for the field of infant mental health is justified.

Many features of infant mental health pose relatively unique challenges to any consideration of training. Two overarching questions come to mind immediately: What is unique about infancy as a developmental epoch? And, what is distinct about the mental health perspective on infancy? Related to these overarch-

ing questions are more specific questions regarding the uniqueness of infant mental health. Should infant mental health practitioners be credentialed? What are the distinctive features of specific training programs? What are some of the problems and issues that are evolving as training becomes more systematic? In this chapter, we present an overview of training and begin to address some of these emerging issues and dilemmas.

INFANT MENTAL HEALTH: CHALLENGES

Emde, Bingham, and Harmon (1993), writing about diagnostic classification, asserted that the uniqueness of infant mental health derived from four basic characteristics: its multidisciplinary nature, developmental orientation, multigenerational focus, and emphasis on prevention. We believe that these same features are relevant for training, and we consider each of them briefly.

Multidisciplinary Nature

From its inception, infant mental health has required a multidisciplinary perspective. Thus, a large portion of the field is "shared" among a variety of clinical disciplines. On the other hand, infant mental health is becoming increasingly specialized in terms of knowledge base, assessment, and intervention techniques. The juxtaposition of the need for a broad-based perspective and the need for specialized knowledge and skills has implications for training and how one becomes an "infant mental health specialist." Is infant mental health uniquely a mental health subspecialty? Or, are non–mental health clinicians who work with infants and/or their caregivers considered infant mental health specialists? Which aspects of infant mental health are unique to specific clinical disciplines, and which aspects are generic to the knowledge base for all disciplines?

With the possible exception of a graduate certificate program in infant mental health at the Merrill–Palmer Institute Wayne State University in Michigan (Weatherston, in press), infant mental health is not a program of study that leads to a degree in universities in the United States. Instead, infant mental health is a field that currently is mastered after one already has completed training in a specific discipline. Grounding in education or psychology or pediatrics, for example, provides professionals with relevant theoretical and clinical underpinnings that may enhance their understanding of infant mental health. Nevertheless, this process of training raises another dilemma in that even professionals with extensive experience with children are likely to find a considerable amount of new material to master in infant mental health. The additional investment of time and money needed to master the unique perspective, skills, and knowledge of infant mental health may be a significant barrier to seeking the additional required training.

Developmental Orientation

The developmental orientation derives from the fact that changes in the first 3 years of life are unparalleled in the life cycle. This orientation has significant implications for training because it means that details about development across biological, cognitive, communicative, emotional, and social domains are fundamental to the knowledge base of infant mental health professionals. Clearly, there will be inevitable differences in the details about development among individuals from different disciplines, but there is no clinical field that requires a more detailed working knowledge of development than does infant mental health.

Multigenerational Perspective

The relational approach to infant mental health includes a multigenerational perspective that is not only quantitatively greater than other mental health or allied disciplines but also qualitatively different. That is, because infants are so embedded within and dependent on their caregiving contexts (see Sameroff, Chapter 1, this volume), and because of the remarkable amount of evidence for intergenerational transmission of patterns of relating in caregiving relationships (see Benoit & Parker, 1994), consideration of multiple generations is more central to infant mental health than to most other disciplines.

Prevention Emphasis

The emphasis on prevention in infant mental health, perfectly familiar for some disciplines, is likely to be unsettling for others. Infant mental health is concerned not only with instances in which development has gone awry but also about situations in which development is at increased risk for going awry in the future. This means that interventions are often applied even before problems are apparent.

DISCIPLINES

As Table 36.1 illustrates, professional disciplines that have made contributions to and have an active role in various aspects of infant mental health include child and adult mental health, pediatric and primary health care, education and early intervention, child welfare, and legislative and social policy planning. Each discipline has a unique perspective, although there may be overlapping interests and roles.

Mental Health Professionals

For mental health practitioners, the unique aspect of infant mental health is the infant. These professionals are trained to attend to the emotional and behavioral difficulties of individuals, as well as to the importance of the context of relationships: clinician–client, parent–child, and client–other. On the other hand, preverbal or barely verbal children who are developing rapidly and continually may be much less familiar.

TABLE 36.1. Infant Mental Health Involved Disciplines and Roles

Disciplines	Roles
Mental health	
Psychiatry	Assessment
Psychology	Secondary and tertiary
Psychiatric social work	interventions
Psychiatric nursing	Referral/collaboration
Licensed professional counselor	
Health care	
Pediatrics	Assessment
Family practice	Primary, secondary, and
Pediatric, obstetric, and public health nursing	tertiary interventions
	Referral/collaboration
Pediatric social work	
Nutritionists	
Early interventionists	
Child development specialists	Assessment
Speech and language	Secondary and tertiary interventions
Occupational therapists	Referral/collaboration
Physical therapists	
Education	
Early childhood educators	Assessment
Child-care providers	Primary, secondary, and
Special education teachers	tertiary interventions
	Referral/collaboration
Child welfare	
Child protection workers	Assessment
Attorneys	Secondary and tertiary
Judges	interventions
	Referral/collaboration
	Permanency planning

Understanding how relationships develop, the strengths and stressors inherent in close relationships, and how relationships affect and are affected by environmental influences as well as individual functioning are common areas of concern and exploration by the mental health professional. An important therapeutic aim is to develop a good "working alliance" between the caregiver and the clinician and to use this relationship to work collaboratively in the best interests of the infant. Mental health roles include assessment, diagnosis, and treatment, but because families of infants usually do not have contact with mental health clinicians until a problem has become apparent, mental health involvement generally occurs at the secondary and tertiary levels; primary prevention generally is not a major focus.

Primary Health Care

Pediatric and primary care clinicians, in contrast, are more likely to see problems as they begin to emerge. Because pediatric and primary care professionals are universally available and are not stigmatized, this group of professionals has access to large numbers of mothers and babies, and its members perform primary, secondary, and tertiary interventions. Pediatric health care professionals may not consider their work with young children to be "infant mental health." Nevertheless, for at least the past two decades, there has been increasing recognition of how family, social, and environmental factors contribute to the incidence and treatment of the "new morbidities" in child and adolescent health (e.g., learning, behavioral and emotional problems, accidents and injuries, and child abuse and neglect), which account for a substantial portion of the morbidity and mortality in children today (Haggerty, Roghmann, & Pless, 1975). Prevention and early recognition of such problems are viewed as within the scope of current pediatric practice (Green, 1994) and, thus, developing a good working relationship between parent and clinician, finding ways to help parents and babies develop or strengthen nurturing and protective family relationships, and supporting social and emotional development increasingly are recognized as important and fundamental functions of pediatric health care (Green, 1994). These activities clearly fall within the domain of infant mental health, yet the typical pediatric setting requires different approaches than those used by mental health professionals.

Pediatric professionals receive variable amounts of training in developmental issues and contextual influences on health and development, but it is widely recognized that the usual methods of delivering health care often do not address children's cognitive, social, and emotional development adequately (Fenichel, 1997). Numerous practical obstacles, such as lack of time, cost/reimbursement issues, lack of referral services, large caseloads, and the need to attend to urgent medical problems (Burnst & Burke, 1985) often prohibit adequate attention to psychosocial and developmental issues. In addition, pediatricians frequently report that they feel undertrained and are uncomfortable in addressing psychosocial concerns of their patients, are reluctant to attach perceived deleterious labels to their patients, and tend to underidentify problems even when parents bring them to the attention of the provider (Costello, 1986). A number of strategies and programs have been developed to address such issues (Fenichel, 1995, 1997).

Early Intervention/Education

Early interventionists are similar to mental health professionals in that they become involved with infants and their caregivers in order to clarify a concern about an infant or after problems have been identified. Formerly, some of the roles of early interventionists were quite specialized, but federal government mandates have broadened their roles (see Gilkerson & Stott, Chapter 29, this volume) and even increased their involvement with families considered "at risk." They have the opportunity to develop and to observe the effects of the clinician–caregiver relationship on their work as well as to observe the developing relationship between caregiver and infant. Although their initial involvement may be at the tertiary care level, they also are in a position to identify the emergence of parent–infant problems and to provide brief interventions aimed at enhancing the parent–infant relationship.

Child Welfare

Child welfare professionals range from child protective services workers to attorneys involved in child protection cases to judges who make decisions regarding permanency planning. This group of professionals often makes critical decisions that have substantial short- and long-term effects on young children, yet, in our experience, their knowledge base and degree of sophistication regarding how such issues should be understood and approached are quite variable.

Child protective services workers are not directly involved with clinical care of infants and young children, yet their decisions can result in preventing later developing problems, and enhancing and supporting current development. Foster care is a powerful intervention, and differences in the quality of care are likely to be even more important for infants and young children than for older children and adoles-

cents. In addition, it is crucial that protective services workers recognize signs of delayed or deviant development, because, in partnership with foster parents, they act as gatekeepers for young children with regard to access to services. Finally, if assessment and intervention methods are familiar to child protective services workers, then their expectations from referrals may be more realistic. Clearly, it is important that child protective services workers appreciate the importance of relationships and how to incorporate relationship considerations into their decisions.

Social Policy Planners

As the empirical base of infant mental health has grown and strengthened, legislators and policy planners are increasingly interested in examining programs and developing policies aimed at preventing problems and/or facilitating the social and emotional development of our youngest citizens. Federal guidelines that recognize the importance of addressing mental health needs of infants, children, and adolescents continue to be developed and refined (U.S. Department of Health and Human Services, 1997). Explicit attention is given to increasing the number of primary-care providers who are trained to screen, assess, and provide brief interventions (e.g., counseling, education, and appropriate referrals) for mental health problems in infants through adolescents and to improve access to and collaboration with mental health practitioners.

Although policy planners do not provide direct services, their understanding of infant development and the factors that enhance or impede development, as well as the long-term effects of early experiences, is critical. Further, they must be familiar with the importance of assessments and the efficacy of interventions as their decisions and directions will affect funding priorities at local, national, and international levels.

Others

In addition to those disciplines mentioned previously, other groups have a stake in the content of infant mental health. Specifically, developmental investigators and developmental psychopathologists may make important contributions to infant mental health through better characterization of risk groups, delineation of deviant and healthy developmental trajectories, and evaluation of the validity and usefulness of various types of assessments and by testing the efficacy of various interventions. On the other hand, infant mental health as practiced can often shape or focus important questions for investigators to address systematically.

Of course, parents of infants are clearly stakeholders and consumers of the content of infant mental health. From the original *The Common Sense Book of Baby and Child Care* (Spock, 1946), through more contemporary works, such as *The Earliest Relationship* (Brazelton & Cramer, 1991), *The Emotional Life of the Toddler* (Lieberman, 1993), and the American Academy of Child and Adolescent Psychiatry's *Your Child* (Pruitt, 1998), there have been many efforts to communicate to parents important aspects of infant mental health.

Conclusions

In sum, each of the many disciplines (including others we have not specifically mentioned) involved in and with infant mental health has different roles and, therefore, concerns; yet each shares a stake in the body of knowledge comprising this field. By recognizing the specific as well as the complementary roles, interests, and goals within each discipline, it becomes possible to determine the universal and unique training needs in infant mental health.

CONTENT OF TRAINING

Table 36.2 lists the topics we feel are important to be addressed in an infant mental health training program, regardless of the discipline involved. Clearly, however, although the general content areas may be similar across disciplines, there will be differences in emphasis and explicit content.

Development in Context

Understanding infant social and emotional development and the familial, social, and cultural influences on development is essential for any professionals working with parents and infants. Of course, these are vast topics. Appreciating development includes the neurobiological underpinnings of behavior, cognitive and communicative development, and social and emotional development and how they interrelate.

TABLE 36.2. Core Components of Clinical Infant Mental Health Training

Infant development in context (biological, relationship, family and culture)

Developmental psychopathology (developmental trajectories, risk and protective factors)

Disorders of infancy and diagnostic classification

Assessment

Interventions

Prevention

Professional–family relationships

Interdisciplinary collaboration

Legal and ethical issues

Further, because of the importance of context for infant development (see Part 1, Chapters 1–5, this volume), training should consider infant development in context. Contextual influences should include both aspects of development that seem to be neurobiologically "hardwired" and found across cultures and those aspects of development that are particularly sensitive to environmental influences. Therefore, social expectations regarding infant behavior and sex-role development and parenting roles and behavior; the effects of impaired caregiver functioning (e.g., maternal physical and mental illness, depression, and substance abuse); the effects of the parents' own relationship experiences (attachment relationships, early abuse, partner violence); the effects of major environmental risk factors, such as poverty and domestic and community violence; and other contemporary issues (e.g., day care, divorce, and teenage parents) are "basic" content.

Psychopathology

This foundation naturally leads to a discussion of the manifestations of psychopathology in infancy, including the topic of developmental psychopathology. Here, the emphases are on risk and protective factors that increase or decrease the probability of various outcomes and on understanding the process of development and how various maladaptive trajectories can be modified. This approach is closely linked to prevention efforts because it is possible to consider modifying risk factors for infants even before problems have become manifest.

Disorders of infancy are another way of considering psychopathology. Although the diagnoses of autism and pervasive developmental disorders, as well as feeding and sleeping problems, are widely recognized, the idea of infants having psychopathology or disorders is surprising to some and offputting to others (Zeanah, Boris, & Scheeringa, 1997). The topic often is of great interest, however, and can underscore powerfully the importance of attending to infant mental health issues. Although psychiatrists and psychologists are most likely oriented toward making psychiatric diagnoses and require the most extensive training in diagnoses, we believe that all professionals need to have a general understanding of how psychopathology in infancy is conceptualized, to be aware of the range of abnormal behaviors and interactions which may be observed, and to know when to make a referral for further assessment or treatment.

Assessment and Intervention

The content areas of assessment and intervention are likely to be the most discipline specific yet likely build on the basic foundations of social and emotional development, consider contextual influences, and have the general goal of identifying problems and preventing further problems. Despite a discipline-specific focus, however, there are aspects of infant mental health which are fundamental to all disciplines. For example, developing good interviewing skills and systematic approaches to assessing parent–infant interactions are important, whether in an extended (e.g., in a permanency planning) or a brief (e.g., pediatric well-child exam) context. Similarly, there are interventions that can be used by a variety of clinicians: speaking in the baby's voice and from the baby's perspective (Carter, Osofsky, & Hann, 1991), learning how to talk to and listen to young children (Lieberman, 1993), emphasizing strengths (McDonough, Chapter 31, this volume), and using "teachable moments" (Zuckerman, Kaplan-Sanoff, Parker, & Young, 1997) all are potentially useful in a range of settings. Teaching specific assessment and intervention methods depends on the purposes, goals, and training needed.

Whenever possible, the emphasis should be on the use of methods that are both reliable and valid. Infant mental health is a new but rapidly growing field, and many assessment and intervention methods are being developed. Often, there is no standard nomenclature, and methods may not have established reliability and validi-

ty. Trainees need to be aware of the methodological advances in infant mental health in order to be able to make appropriate selections for their practices.

Prevention

Clearly, one of the goals of infant mental health is the prevention of problems that may evolve or predispose the young child to short- or long-term difficulties. Because the problems of infancy are multiply determined and may have a wide range of effects (e.g., few specific causes and effects have been identified), it often is not clear which preventive effort will result in a positive outcome. Therefore, the infant mental health professional should be acquainted with multiple "generic" preventive approaches, as well as known specific preventive techniques. Simply establishing a good working relationship with the infant's caregiver can be a most effective and powerful preventive intervention tool, as it allows the professional to intervene in more specific areas. For example, the clinician may provide anticipatory guidance more effectively, may be able to elicit a history of domestic violence, or may inquire empathically about a caregiver's depression. General preventive intervention programs, such as nurse home-visitation programs (Olds, Henderson, Kitzman, & Cole, 1995; Olds et al., 1998), as well as discipline-specific techniques, should be covered.

Professional–Family Relationships

Professional–family relationships ought to be considered core components of an infant mental health training program. Establishing a good working relationship, use of the relationship as a "model" for the parent, and setting boundaries of professional–family relationships are some of the topics that should be covered. Work with caregivers and young children often generates strong feelings in the professional, based on that individual's own experiences, beliefs, attitudes, knowledge level, and work-related expectations and goals. It is important that trainees begin to recognize transference and countertransference issues and begin to develop strategies for acknowledging and dealing with their own powerful feelings and reactions. A number of training programs spend a significant amount of time during training on these issues because of their crucial importance. Use of reflective supervision, as well as group processes, in addition to the didactic components, typically are incorporated in training programs (Hornstein, O'Brien, & Stadtler, 1997; Pawl, 1995; Wieder & Greenspan, 1997).

Interdisciplinary Collaboration

Infant mental health practitioners are likely to work regularly with other disciplines, and many training programs include trainees from different disciplines. Learning to "talk" with individuals across disciplines, with disparate goals and understanding of problems, can be a professional challenge. Still, this is an essential skill for those working with caregivers and young children. Developing and using internal and external referral sources and making good referrals may seem too basic, yet the inability to use other sources of support or care can be a major frustration for infant mental health professionals. Trainees also may benefit from an introduction to consultation and supervision methods.

Legal and Ethical Issues

To varying degrees, each of the foregoing components of training involves ethical dilemmas. For example, a vital issue in clinical infant mental health is the maintenance of appropriate boundaries. This is more challenging in working with infants than in other areas of mental health because of the tradition of home visiting and concrete support articulated by Fraiberg (1980) that extends some of the usual roles and activities of the professional outside the clinic. The question of ownership of infants is another vexing problem most often manifest in legal custody disputes, involving divorcing parents, foster/adoptive and biological parents, or infants who are orphaned. In addition, rights of infants versus rights of parents create challenging dilemmas for clinicians who must resist pressures to overidentify with infants or with parents.

Finally, questions of child maltreatment are not uncommon in infancy, and clinicians must be familiar with reporting laws as well as the legal process involved in permanency planning.

TRAINING DILEMMAS

A number of issues and dilemmas are being identified as training programs develop. As noted previously, infant mental health is not just for patients and clients; the information, methods, and emphases often have personal relevance, as individuals' own childhood and parenting experience, as well as personal values, attitudes, and experiences as parents themselves, are naturally revisited during training. In our experience of providing training to disciplines beyond traditional mental health disciplines, curbside consults regarding personal dilemmas of trainees are almost always a part of the training. One result of this is that we have found it useful to spend considerable time and energy on issues of transference and countertransference in clinical infant mental health. Good supervision is essential, even in non–mental-health training programs.

Another issue for training programs is having relatively few individuals with expertise in infant mental health. Even with a critical mass of experts, the training tends to be rather intensive, so that the number of trainees who can participate in a given program may be limited. Cost-effectiveness of training may be an issue in developing programs, especially at the outset, when expert personnel may be limited.

The relatively small number of professionals from any discipline with whom a common language and knowledge base are shared is another manifestation of this problem. Of course, the lack of widespread knowledge and skill in this area provides both a challenge and an opportunity. There are few with whom to network, especially within circumscribed geographic locations. The scarcity of infant mental health professionals creates a high demand for those with expertise, so the issue of precious resources is a real one. There also is a real ethical dilemma of uncovering problems without being able to follow through with interventions.

Individuals who are trained to identify problems more skillfully and to provide brief interventions for infants and families may be frustrated if clinical demands of time, lack of resources, or administrative procedures interfere with or prevent them from doing their work. Professional burnout is not uncommon in this field for several reasons. First, the acuity and complexity of many of the cases are high. Second, reimbursement is often limited and tailored to succinct office visits when the case may demand many visits in a week, often at homes or day-care centers. Third, professional isolation is not uncommon for infant mental health clinicians not working in major centers. All these issues need to be anticipated in both training and work settings.

On the positive side, better understanding of the impact of early development and experiences on later development often serves as a powerful catalyst for systems change. Nevertheless, because of the multiple issues that affect infant development, system change often must occur at multiple levels and across disparate agencies. Thus, at a macrolevel, the systems change can serve as a model of what must happen for infants and their caregivers.

To date, there is no formal credentialing process in infant mental health. The issues of how and when to credential someone as an expert in infant mental health are just beginning to be articulated. What information is generic to all parent–infant professionals; what does it take to be an expert? Who determines this? Does the infant mental health practitioner need a basic discipline (e.g., nursing, psychiatry, psychology, or social work)? What does the expert do? Is reimbursement possible? There are no clear and simple answers for these questions, but it is likely that they will become more pressing as the field matures.

ILLUSTRATIVE PROGRAMS

Given the many disciplines involved in infant mental health, it would be impossible to list comprehensively all those programs that provide infant mental health training. We have selected a number of programs to describe briefly to illustrate the breadth of training programs in the United States that we believe are centrally involved in infant mental health training.

Harris Professional Development Network

The Harris Foundation in Chicago provides funding to eight sites across the United States, and several others in Israel, that offer training programs in infant mental health (Stott & Gilkerson, 1998). The network consists of a range of disciplines which influence infant functioning and thus benefit from specialized training in infant mental health. The sites include community-based child-care centers, early intervention programs, child welfare and prevention programs, hospitals, and mental health settings. Drawn from Stott and Gilkerson's (1998) overview, we describe briefly specific sites in the United States to convey the range of different training programs involved.

Boston Institute for Early Child Development

Located at Boston University Medical Center, this program is staffed primarily by pediatricians. It trains health care professionals who work with young children, particularly child development fellows and pediatric residents and practitioners. There are education and mentoring programs for child-care teachers, as well. Written and videotaped training materials are provided to professionals throughout the New England region. Community seminars, conferences, and workshops interweave theory and service in early child development.

The Irving B. Harris Training Program in Child Development and Infant Mental Health

This program is staffed by faculty in psychiatry at the University of Colorado Health Sciences Center and offers an advanced fellowship program for mental health and early childhood professionals. Didactics are provided in normal development and developmental psychopathology. Clinical experiences include work in the newborn intensive care nursery and consultation to the state department of education. There also is a training and consultation network for infant mental health professionals throughout Colorado.

The Irving B. Harris Infant Studies Program at The Erikson Institute

The Erikson Institute at Loyola University in Chicago trains infant specialists and early interventionists in outreach, prevention, support, child care, child life, and treatment. Courses in early development, family systems, assessment, and intervention are held, as well as a supervised internship. Postbaccalaureate and master's-level training can lead to certification. A director/supervisor training seminar also is offered. This program makes a thoughtful effort to integrate infant mental health principles into the training of individuals whose frame of reference is more likely to be education.

The Early Childhood Group Therapy Training Program

The Jewish Board of Family and Children's Services in New York City educates an interdisciplinary group of professionals to provide mental health consultation services to preschool and elementary school children, their teachers, and their parents. It provides identification of mental health problems and a variety of treatment modalities to the children and families in a school-based program of outreach. The Jewish Board of Family and Children's Services also has an Institute for Clinical Studies of Infants, Toddlers, and Parents within the organization which trains mental health professionals and directors of extant infant programs in the metropolitan New York area. The faculty and midcareer trainees represent a range of disciplines; the clinical settings are both private and community based. Clinical supervision and education in administration and leadership form the basis of the institute's program curriculum.

Harris Program in Infant Mental Health

The Louisiana State University Medical Center Department of Psychiatry trains mental health professionals who wish to gain expertise in infant mental health. This program is building a large support network of infant mental health specialists. Networking also occurs with systems that have an impact on infant functioning, including the judicial system, law enforcement, child care, early intervention, schools, and child welfare. It offers an extensive didactic series, observations of parents of low-risk, normally developing infants, and clinical training from a variety of sites. The clinical practica include a community college-based child-care center, a community program for mothers and infants at risk for problematic development, and multidisciplinary permanency planning teams for maltreated infants and toddlers.

The Irving B. Harris Training Center for Infant and Toddler Development

The Institute for Child Development at the University of Minnesota is an academic center which provides training and continuing education to professionals who work in infant and toddler development. The Institute for Child Development has had faculty producing some of the most important research in the past 20 years in developmental psychology and developmental psychopathology. The Harris Program has allowed university faculty and students to form a partnership with the community in order to convey important research findings to community practitioners. They provide resource material and education to community members through a variety of seminars and visiting scholar programs.

Yale Child Study Center

At Yale University School of Medicine, faculty in the Child Study Center conduct service-based research with infants and young children. Research projects investigate a variety of serious medical and mental health problems. There is an education module for early childhood and early intervention specialists in the community as well as a community consultation program.

Infant–Parent Program

The Infant–Parent Program at San Francisco General Hospital was founded by Selma Fraiberg 20 years ago. Drawn from the psychoanalytical tradition of discovering infant–parent relationship patterns in the present that are based on parents' previous relationship experiences, this program pioneered home-based treatment of parents and infants (Fraiberg, 1980). Trainees from a variety of mental health disciplines have been trained in intensive psychotherapeutic treatment of disadvantaged families. The emphasis of the training includes a focus on changing maladaptive infant–parent relationship patterns, understanding transference and countertransference in the therapist–parent relationships, and a focus on emotional communications between parents and infants.

Merrill–Palmer Institute/Wayne State University

Another program different from those sponsored by the Harris Foundation offers a graduate certificate in infant mental health for clinicians with master's degrees. The program reflects the principles and practices of Fraiberg's (1980) model of infant mental health, involving understanding the baby in the context of the infant–parent relationship. In addition to course work taken in the departments of psychology, sociology, education, nursing and social work at Wayne State University, trainees also participate in a year-long clinical practicum which provides hands-on experience with referred infants and families. Supervision of this work focuses on integration of theory and practice of infant mental health.

The Infant–Parent Institute

The Infant–Parent Institute in Champaign, Illinois offers a 4-day clinical course for mental health and allied professionals who wish to learn about infant mental health. This course covers attachment, assessment, and treatment of infant–parent dyads. The training is transdisciplinary, involves clinical service delivery, and draws from the literature and guiding principles of several fields. For more extensive training, clinical traineeships include intensive individual supervision, practicum experiences, and training seminars. The clinical practicum experience includes family observation, assessments, and treatment. Working with other systems, including other court consultation, social service agencies, and the public, throughout the practicum is included.

Infant Mental Health at Tulane University School of Medicine

This program is staffed by faculty members in the section of child and adolescent psychiatry and has been involved in the clinical training of a number of mental health professionals, anchored in a community-based intervention program for maltreated infants and toddlers (Larrieu & Zeanah, 1998). In addition, program faculty have provided training for and ongoing consultation with child protective services workers and community clinicians. More intensive training has been provided to public health nurses and to mental health professionals as a part of a state wide preventive/intervention initiative.

From its inception, this program has emphasized a relationship-based approach to understanding infant development (Zeanah, Boris, & Larrieu, 1997), psychopathology (Lyons-Ruth, Zeanah, & Benoit, 1996; Zeanah, Boris, & Scheeringa, 1997), assessment (Zeanah, Boris, & Heller, 1997), and treatment (Larrieu & Zeanah, 1998). The overall goal of this program is to increase the critical mass of mental health and other professionals in Louisiana and elsewhere who are competent in practicing infant mental health. A secondary goal is to increase knowledge about infant mental health among non–mental health professionals who work with infants and caregivers in need.

SUMMARY

In this chapter, we began by stressing the unique features of infant mental health that pose challenges for training programs, including its multidisciplinary nature, developmental orientation, multigenerational focus, and emphasis on prevention. Next, we indicated a number of the disciplines concerned with infant mental health, and we suggested how each may have somewhat different interests in specific topics. We have also indicated general topics that we believe ought to be included in most training programs. Finally, we reviewed a number of emerging issues in infant mental health training.

Perhaps of note, most of the training programs summarized in this chapter either did not exist or have increased in size and scope substantially since the first edition of this volume was published (Zeanah, 1993). Infant mental health training is growing and evolving as rapidly as its young subjects. Grounded in a belief in the importance of understanding infant development in context, these programs and others like them around the world ensure that infant mental health will be well served by future generations of practitioners.

REFERENCES

Benoit, D., & Parker, K. (1994). Stability and transmission of attachment across three generations. *Child Development, 65,* 1444–1456.

Brazelton, T. B., & Cramer, B. (1991). *The earliest relationship.* Reading, MA: Addison-Wesley.

Burnst, B. J., & Burke, J. D. (1985). Improving mental health practices in primary care: Findings from recent research. *Public Health Reports, 100,* 294–300.

Carter, S., Osofsky, J., & Hann, D. (1991). Speaking for the baby: A therapeutic intervention with adolescent mothers and their babies. *Infant Mental Health Journal, 12,* 291–301.

Costello, E. J. (1986). Primary care pediatrics and child psychopathology: A review of diagnostic, treatment, and referral practices. *Pediatrics, 78,* 1044–1051.

Emde, R. N., Bingham, R. D., & Harmon, R. J. (1993). Classification and the diagnostic process in infancy. In C. H. Zeanah, Jr. (Ed.), *Handbook of infant mental health* (pp. 225–235), New York: Guilford Press.

Fenichel, E. (Ed.). (1995). *Zero to Three, 16,* 1–35.

Fenichel, E. (Ed.). (1997). Pediatric primary care. *Zero to Three, 17,* 1–55.

Fraiberg, S. (Ed.). (1980). *Clinical studies in infant mental health*. New York: Basic Books.

Green, M. (Ed.). (1994). *Bright futures: Guidelines for health supervision of infants, children, and adolescents*. Arlington, VA: National Center for Education in Maternal and Child Health.

Haggerty, R. J., Roghmann, K. J., & Pless, I. B. (1975). *Child health and the community*. New York: Wiley.

Hornstein, J., O'Brien, M. A., & Stadtler, A. C. (1997). Touchpoints practice: Lessons learned from training and implementation. *Zero to Three, 17*, 26–33.

Larrieu, J., & Zeanah, C. H. (1998). An intensive intervention for infants and toddlers in foster care. *Child and Adolescent Psychiatric Clinics of North America, 7*, 357–371.

Lieberman, A. F. (1993). *The emotional life of the toddler*. New York: The Free Press.

Lyons-Ruth, K., Zeanah, C. H., & Benoit, D. (1996). Disorder and risk for disorder during infancy and toddlerhood. In E. J. Mash & R. A. Barkley, (Eds.), *Child psychopathology* (pp. 457–491), New York: Guilford Press.

Olds, D. L., Henderson, C. R., Cole, R., Eckenrode, J., Kitzman, H., Luckey, D., Pettit, L., Sidora, K., Morris, P., & Powers, J. (1998). Long-term effects of nurse home visitation on children's criminal and antisocial behavior. *Journal of the American Medical Association, 280*, 1238–1244.

Olds, D. L., Henderson, C. R., Kitzman, H., & Cole, R. (1995). Effects of prenatal and infancy nurse home visitation on surveillance of child maltreatment. *Pediatrics, 95*, 365–372.

Pawl, J. (1995). On supervision. *Zero to Three, 15*, 21–29.

Pruitt, D. (Ed.). (1998). *Your child*. Washington, DC: American Academy of Child and Adolescent Psychiatry.

Spock, B. (1946). *The common sense book of baby and child care*. New York: Duell, Sloan and Pearce.

Stott, F., & Gilkerson, L. (1998). Taking the long view: Supporting higher education on behalf of young children. *Zero to Three, 19*, 27–33.

U.S. Department of Health and Human Services. (1997). *Developing objectives for Healthy People 2010*. Washington, DC: Office of Disease Prevention and Health Promotion.

Weatherston, D. (in press). Infant mental health assessment through careful observation and listening: Unique training opportunities. In H. Fitzgerald & J. Osofsky (Eds.), *WAIMH handbook of infant mental health*. New York: Wiley.

Wieder, S., & Greenspan, S. (1997). Training and supervising developmental specialists in pediatric practice. *Zero to Three, 17,* 16–19.

Zeanah, C. H., Boris, N. W., Heller, S. S., Hinshaw-Fuselier, S., Larrieu, J., Lewis, M., Palomino, R., Rovaris, M., & Valliere, J. (1997). Relationship assessment in infant mental health. *Infant Mental Health Journal, 18*, 182–197.

Zeanah, C. H., Boris, N., & Larrieu, J. (1997). Infant development and developmental risk: A review of the past 10 years. *Journal of the American Academy of Child and Adolescent Psychiatry, 36*, 165–178.

Zeanah, C. H., Boris, N., & Scheeringa, M. (1997). Psychopathology in infancy. *Journal of Child Psychology, Psychiatry and Allied Disciplines, 38*, 81–99.

Zuckerman, B., Kaplan-Sanoff, M., Parker, S., & Young, K. T. (1997). The Healthy Steps for Young Children program. *Zero to Three, 17,* 20–25.

Author Index

❖

Subject Index

❖